FIRST AID FOR THE® Emergency Medicine Boards

Third Edition

BARBARA K. BLOK, MD
Associate Program Director
Denver Health Residency in Emergency Medicine
Associate Professor
Department of Emergency Medicine
University of Colorado School of Medicine
Aurora, Colorado

DICKSON S. CHEUNG, MD, MBA, MPH
Department of Emergency Medicine
Sky Ridge Medical Center
CarePoint, PC
Denver, Colorado

TIMOTHY F. PLATTS-MILLS, MD
Department of Emergency Medicine
University of North Carolina at Chapel Hill
Chapel Hill, North Carolina

Mc Graw Hill Education

New York Chicago San Francisco Athens London Madrid Mexico City
Milan New Delhi Singapore Sydney Toronto

First Aid for the® Emergency Medicine Boards, Third Edition

2 3 4 5 6 7 8 9 0 DSS/DSS 20 19 18 17

ISBN 978-0-07-184913-5
MHID 0-07-184913-0

NOTICE

Medicine is an ever-changing science. As new research and clinical experience broaden our knowledge, changes in treatment and drug therapy are required. The authors and the publisher of this work have checked with sources believed to be reliable in their efforts to provide information that is complete and generally in accord with the standards accepted at the time of publication. However, in view of the possibility of human error or changes in medical sciences, neither the authors nor the publisher nor any other party who has been involved in the preparation or publication of this work warrants that the information contained herein is in every respect accurate or complete, and they disclaim all responsibility for any errors or omissions or for the results obtained from use of the information contained in this work. Readers are encouraged to confirm the information contained herein with other sources. For example and in particular, readers are advised to check the product information sheet included in the package of each drug they plan to administer to be certain that the information contained in this work is accurate and that changes have not been made in the recommended dose or in the contraindications for administration. This recommendation is of particular importance in connection with new or infrequently used drugs.

This book was set in Electra LH Std by Cenveo® Publisher Services.
The editors were Catherine A. Johnson and Cindy Yoo.
The production supervisor was Richard Ruzycka.
Project management was provided by Raghavi Khullar, Cenveo Publisher Services.
The cover designer was Dreamit, Inc.
RR Donnelley/China was printer and binder.

This book is printed on acid-free paper.

Library of Congress Cataloging-in-Publication Data

Blok, Barbara K., author.
First aid for the emergency medicine boards / Barbara K. Blok, Dickson S. Cheung, Timothy Fortescue Platts-Mills.—Third edition.
p. ; cm.
Includes index.
ISBN 978-0-07-184913-5 (pbk. : alk. paper)—ISBN 0-07-184913-0 (pbk. : alk. paper)
I. Cheung, Dickson S., author. II. Platts-Mills, Timothy Fortescue, author. III. Title.
[DNLM: 1. Emergency Treatment—methods—Outlines. 2. Emergency Medicine—methods—Outlines. WB 18.2]
RC86.9
616.02'52—dc23

015032675

DEDICATION

To our families, friends, and loved ones, who endured
and assisted in the task of assembling this guide,

and

To the contributors to this, past, and future editions, who took time to share
their knowledge, insight, and humor for the benefit of residents and clinicians.

Contents

Contributing Authors

Lauren M. Abbate, MD, PHD
Department of Emergency Medicine
University of Colorado School of Medicine
Aurora, Colorado
Chapter 7. Endocrine, Metabolic, Fluid, and Electrolyte Disorders

Sabrina A. Adams, MD
Department of Emergency Medicine
Denver Health Medical Center
Denver, Colorado
Chapter 12. Obstetrics and Gynecology

James Dazhe Cao, MD
Assistant Professor, Department of Emergency Medicine
University of Southwestern Medical Center
Dallas, Texas
Chapter 6. Toxicology

Jenny L. Chua-Tuan, MD, MBA
Chief Resident of Emergency Medicine
Denver Health Medical Center
Denver, Colorado
Chapter 3. Trauma

Andrew P. Coleman, MD, MHS
Department of Emergency Medicine
Denver Health Residency in Emergency Medicine
Aurora, Colorado
Chapter 2. Cardiovascular Emergencies

Stephanie A. Crapo, MD
Assistant Professor, Department of Emergency Medicine
University of North Carolina at Chapel Hill
Chapel Hill, North Carolina
Chapter 10. Thoracic and Respiratory Disorders

Christopher Davis, MD, DTMH
Assistant Professor, Department of Emergency Medicine
University of Colorado School of Medicine
Aurora, Colorado
Chapter 8. Infectious Disease

Jasmeet Dhaliwal, MD
Chief Resident of Emergency Medicine
Denver Health Medical Center
Denver, Colorado
Chapter 2. Cardiovascular Emergencies

C. Scott Forsythe, MD, MPH
Department of Emergency Medicine
University of North Carolina School of Medicine at Chapel Hill
Chapel Hill, North Carolina
Chapter 11. Abdominal and Gastrointestinal Emergencies

Elena D. Garcia, MD
Clinical Instructor
Emergency Medicine
Denver Health Medical Center
Denver, Colorado
Chapter 20. EMS and Disaster Medicine

Graydon Goodman, MD
Attending Physician at Alamance Regional Medical Center
Burlington, North Carolina
Chapter 21. Ethical/Legal Issues

Joseph Hemerka, MD
Resident of Emergency Medicine
Denver Health Medical Center
Denver, Colorado
Chapter 8. Infectious Disease

Cameron G. Isaacs, MD, HO-1
Department of Emergency Medicine
Wake Forest University
Baptist Medical Center
Winston-Salem, North Carolina
Chapter 16. Psychobehavioral Disorders

Janetta L. Iwanicki, MD
Associate Medical Director
Rocky Mountain Poison and Drug Center
Attending Physician
Department of Emergency Medicine
Denver Health and Hospital Authority
Denver, Colorado
Chapter 6. Toxicology

Leah Jacoby, MD
Department of Emergency Medicine
George Washington University School of Medicine
Washington, District of Columbia
Chapter 13. Environmental Emergencies

Brian M. Jekich, MD
Department of Emergency Medicine
Denver Health Medical Center
Denver, Colorado
Chapter 1. Resuscitation

Howard Kim, MD
Resident of Emergency Medicine Denver Health Medical Center
Denver, Colorado
Chapter 6. Toxicology

Sara M. Krzyzaniak, MD
Clinical Assistant Professor of Emergency Medicine
Department of Emergency Medicine
University of Illinois College of Medicine at Peoria
OSF Saint Francis Medical Center
Peoria, Illinois
Chapter 19. Procedures and Skills

Sarah Leeper, MD
Fellow, Global Health and Leadership Program
Department of Emergency Medicine
University of North Carolina at Chapel Hill
Chapel Hill, North Carolina
Chapter 4. Orthopedics

Jesse W. Loar, MD
Emergency Medicine Physician
Emergency Physicians of Porter Hospitals
Littleton, Colorado
Chapter 9. Hematology, Oncology, Allergy, and Immunology

Justin McLean, MD
Denver Health Residency in Emergency Medicine
Denver Health Hospital
Denver, Colorado
Chapter 20. EMS and Disaster Medicine

Abhi Mehrotra, MD, MBA, FACEP
Vice Chair, Strategic Initiatives and Operations
Department of Emergency Medicine
University of North Carolina at Chapel Hill
Chapel Hill, North Carolina
Chapter 21. Ethical/Legal Issues

Marc Quinlan, MD
PGY-IV
Denver Health Residency in Emergency Medicine
Denver, Colorado
Chapter 1. Resuscitation

Elaine M. Reno, MD
Assistant Professor of Department of Emergency Medicine
University of Colorado School of Medicine
Denver, Colorado
Chapter 3. Trauma

Jordan Ryan, MD
Associate Physician
Emergency Physicians at Porter Hospitals
Denver, Colorado
Chapter 18. Renal and Genitourinary Emergencies

Christina L. Shenvi, MD, PhD
Assistant Professor
Assistant Residency Director
University of North Carolina at Chapel Hill
Chapel Hill, North Carolina
Chapter 5. Pediatrics

Jessica J. Slim, MD, MPH
Resident of Emergency Medicine
Denver Health Medical Center
Denver, Colorado
Chapter 15. Neurology

W. Gannon Sungar, DO
Department of Emergency Medicine
Denver Health Medical Center
Denver, Colorado
Chapter 14. Head, Eyes, Ear, Nose, and Throat, and Dental Emergencies

Michael D. Susalla, MD
Resident, Department of Emergency Medicine
Denver Health Medical Center
Denver, Colorado
Chapter 19. Procedures and Skills

Java Tunson, MD
Resident of Emergency Medicine
Denver Health Medical Center
Denver, Colorado
Chapter 6. Toxicology

Jeremy Voros, MD
Denver Health Residency in Emergency Medicine
Denver, Colorado
Chapter 17. Dermatology

Senior Reviewers

Peter Bakes, MD
Swedish Medical Center
Engelwood, Colorado
Chapter 9. Hematology, Oncology, Allergy, and Immunology

David J. Berkoff, MD, FAAEM, CAQSM
Associate Professor
Department of Orthopaedics and Emergency Medicine
University of North Carolina at Chapel Hill
Chapel Hill, North Carolina
Chapter 4. Orthopedics

Michael Breyer, MD
Assistant Professor
Department of Emergency Medicine
University of Colorado School of Medicine
Aurora, Colorado;
Staff Physician Emergency Medicine
Denver Health Medical Center
Denver, Colorado
Chapter 3. Trauma

Jane H. Brice, MD, MPH
Professor and Chair
Department of Emergency Medicine
University of North Carolina at Chapel Hill
Chapel Hill, North Carolina
Chapter 10. Thoracic and Respiratory Disorders and Chapter11. Abdominal and Gastrointestinal Emergencies

Jennie A. Buchanan, MD
Associate Program Director
Denver Health Residency in Emergency Medicine;
Assistant Professor
Department of Emergency Medicine
University of Colorado School of Medicine
Aurora, Colorado;
Staff Physician Emergency Medicine
Denver Health Medical Center
Denver, Colorado;
Attending, Medical Toxicology Rocky Mountain Poison and Drug Center
Denver, Colorado
Chapter 12. Obstetrics and Gynecology

Richard L. Byyny, MD
Associate Professor
Department of Emergency Medicine
University of Colorado School of Medicine
Aurora, Colorado;
Staff Physician
Emergency Medicine
Denver Health Medical Center Denver, Colorado
Chapter 19. Procedures and Skills

Ira Chang, MD
Blue Sky Neurology
Carepoint PC
Swedish Medical Center
Englewood, Colorado
Chapter 15. Neurology

Erica Douglas, MD, FACEP
Associate Medical Director
AirLife Denver
Denver, Colorado
Chapter 20. EMS and Disaster Medicine

Jeffrey Druck, MD
Associate Professor of Department of Emergency Medicine
University of Colorado School of Medicine
Aurora, Colorado
Chapter 17. Dermatology

Casey Glass, MD
Assistant Professor
Department of Emergency Medicine
Wake Forest School of Medicine
Winston Salem, North Carolina
Chapter 16. Psychobehavioral Disorders

Kennon Heard, MD, PhD
University of Colorado
Aurora, Colorado
Chapter 6. Toxicology

Benjamin Honigman, MD
Professor Department of Emergency Medicine
Associate Dean, Clinical Outreach
University of Colorado School of Medicine
Aurora, Colorado
Chapter 8. Infectious Disease

Frank Lansville, DO
CarePoint PC
President, Medical Staff and Medical Director, Emergency Department
The Medical Center of Aurora
Centennial Medical Plaza ED and Saddle Rock ED
Aurora, Colorado
Chapter 18. Renal and Genitourinary Emergencies

Dylan Luyten, MD, FACEP
Associate EMS Medical Director
St. Anthony Hospitals
Lakewood, Colorado
Chapter 1. Resuscitation

Courtney H. Mann, MD
University of North Carolina at Chapel Hill
Chapel Hill, North Carolina
Chapter 5. Pediatrics

Maria Moreira, MD
Program Director
Denver Health Residency in Emergency Medicine;
Associate Professor
Department of Emergency Medicine
University of Colorado School of Medicine
Aurora, Colorado;
Staff Physician Emergency Medicine
Denver Health Medical Center
Denver, Colorado
Chapter 14. Head, Eyes, Ear, Nose, and Throat, and Dental Emergencies

Kristen E. Nordenholz, MD
Associate Professor
Department of Emergency Medicine
University of Colorado School of Medicine
Aurora, Colorado
Chapter 7. Endocrine, Metabolic, Fluid, and Electrolyte Disorders

Neal O'Connor, MD, FACEP
Chief Medical Officer Care Point PC
Greenwood Village, Colorado
Chapter 2. Cardiovascular Emergencies

Timothy F. Platts-Mills, MD
Department of Emergency Medicine
University of North Carolina at Chapel Hill
Chapel Hill, North Carolina
Chapter 21. Ethical/Legal Issues

Gregory Stiller, MD, FACEP, FAWM
Assistant Clinical Professor
University of Texas Health Sciences Center at San Antonio
San Antonio, Texas
Chapter 13. Environmental Emergencies

Introduction

Passing the emergency medicine written certification examination is an important milestone in the process of becoming a board-certified emergency physician. The written exam, formerly called the Written Certification Examination and now referred to by the American Board of Emergency Medicine (ABEM) as the "Qualifying Examination," is used to identify candidates who are ready to take the oral exam, the final step in becoming board certified. The Qualifying Examination measures core knowledge, and, to many who must take it, it is an intimidating hurdle. Every year approximately 10% of examinees fail the test and must retake it the following year. Given that many test takers are completing their residency and may be moving to start a new job in the months leading up to the test, it is clear that there is a need for a focused, easy-to-use review book to help them prepare.

First Aid for the® Emergency Medicine Boards is such a book. The First Aid series is based on the idea that people who have recently prepared for and taken the test know best how to teach others to study for it. We have drawn on the experience of 26 individual chapter`authors and nearly as many senior reviewers, integrating clinical experience, information from existing review books, and the ABEM practice questions to create a book designed to improve your score on the Qualifying Examination. *First Aid for the® Emergency Medicine Boards* contains dozens of challenging cases ("minicases") and reinforces important information in highlighted "key facts" and "mnemonics." Filled with tables and figures, it presents key findings and must-know information in a clear, concise, and highly accessible format that makes it easy to recall both on test day and in the emergency department.

ABOUT THE QUALIFYING EXAMINATION

The Qualifying Examination consists of approximately 305 questions. Candidates are given six-and-a-half hours of time to complete the test. All questions are the multiple choice, **single-best-answer** type. You will be presented with a case scenario and a question, followed by five answer options. Approximately 10% of the questions include a figure (radiograph, photograph, ECG, rhythm strip, or ultrasound image). There are no penalties for wrong answers, so if you find a question unanswerable, make your best guess and move on. Candidates who achieve a score of 75% or higher pass.

The exam is given in the fall of each year at one of 200 PearsonVUE professional computer-based testing centers. Test locations can be found by selecting "Locate a Test Center" on www.pearsonvue.com. Information on registration, fees, and test composition can be obtained from the ABEM website, www.abem.org.

Exam content is defined by ABEM's Model of the Clinical Practice of Emergency Medicine (EM Model). The table lists the relative weight given to different elements of the exam. A minimum of 8% of the questions involve pediatrics cases, and a minimum of 4% of the questions involve geriatrics cases.

HOW TO USE THIS BOOK

As we have done with other books in the First Aid series, we encourage you to read this book early on and throughout your residency, and to supplement it with margin notes. As with general medicine, mastering emergency medicine does not result from a single reading of a textbook but from many readings and multiple experiences treating patients. For common conditions, such as blunt trauma, CHF, and pneumonia, we focus on the kinds of complicated scenarios that you will find on the test. At this point in your career, you will not be tested on your knowledge of basic information. You will not be asked *What is the most common cause of community-acquired pneumonia*? for example. Instead, you are tested on your ability to apply that basic knowledge in the far more challenging situations you are likely to encounter in the ED, where the question is more likely to be *What is the cause of pneumonia in this patient who has just returned from a rat-infested cabin in New Mexico*? For rare conditions, such as an organophosphate overdose, ciguatera toxicity, or high-altitude pulmonary edema, our goal has been to provide simple, clear, memorable explanations. By the time you have read this book two or three times, you should be well prepared to make the right decisions on the exam and in real life.

Some young physicians say that practicing medicine is intuitive and experience based, that once you have done a residency, studying and memorizing are things of the past. For most of us, this is not true. When a patient comes

Relative Weight of EM Model Elements

Condition/Component	Relative Weight (%)
Signs, Symptoms, and Presentations	9
Abdominal and Gastrointestinal Disorders	9
Cardiovascular Disorders	10
Cutaneous Disorders	2
Endocrine, Metabolic, and Nutritional Disorders	3
Environmental Disorders	3
Head, Ear, Eye, Nose, and Throat Disorders	5
Hematologic Disorders	2
Immune System Disorders	2
Systemic Infectious Disorders	5
Musculoskeletal Disorders (Nontraumatic)	3
Nervous System Disorders	5
Obstetrics and Gynecology	4
Psychobehavioral Disorders	3
Renal and Urogenital Disorders	3
Thoracic-Respiratory Disorders	8
Toxicologic Disorders	4
Traumatic Disorders	11
Procedures and Skills	6
Other Components (EMS, Administration, Legal)	3

into the emergency department 15 minutes after eating dark-meat fish with flushing and palpitations, you might know that you need to initiate treatment with diphenhydramine for scombroid poisoning. But this knowledge is hardly intuitive. And, unless you had trained in Florida, you would probably never have seen this disease. For most examinees, study and memorization are a necessary part of test preparation.

In preparing for the exam, take an expansive and a reductionist approach. Be expansive by studying with your reference books and internet resources readily at hand. Supplementing your clinical knowledge with pictures and detailed descriptions of illnesses will help you remember how to identify and manage complex and rare diseases. Be reductionist by preparing notes on the subjects you have difficulty remembering. Linking key words together on paper, "dendritic ulcer → herpes keratitis," for example, and reviewing them regularly is often enough to help you "capture" an important piece of knowledge—and ensure the right answer—on test day.

Most cases you see in an emergency department will require more complex thinking than can be presented in a multiple choice question. We encourage you to accept that the test simplifies complexities in order to provide an objective measure of your knowledge. For evolving and complex situations, such as evaluating the source of chest pain, we describe the current, generally accepted approaches. Please be aware that medicine continually changes, and there are many situations for which we still do not know the best approach.

TEST-PREPARATION STRATEGIES

When you work in the emergency department, knowledge and experience are your friends. The greater your experience with and understanding of a given complaint, the faster you will be able to help your patient. And while it may seem that the amount of information that could be included on an emergency medicine certification exam is unlimited, it is not. Like most of the exams you have taken in the past, this one tests a finite body of knowledge. The material on the exam is readily identifiable and studying can greatly improve your competency with it. In short, you *can* master the content of this exam. What's more, preparing for the exam should make you a more confident and capable emergency physician. You are no longer simply studying for an organic chemistry test; you are preparing for a career as an emergency physician.

How much time you allow for test preparation will depend on your interest in the formal study of the material and how likely you are to pass the exam with minimal preparation. If you consistently score above 85% on in-service or practice examinations and are currently practicing emergency medicine and reading regularly, you probably won't need to study too much. Most people, however, need two to three months to study for the exam. Giving yourself adequate time makes the experience richer and more enjoyable, and enables you to integrate your clinical experience with what you are studying. We recommend that you read this book in its entirety at least two months before the exam date. Use this initial read to identify the gaps in your knowledge and facts that you want to memorize. Use practice test questions, such as those found in PEER VIII, to improve your test-taking skills, to further identify knowledge gaps, and to add to your list of facts to memorize. Two weeks before the test, review the book again, focusing on areas of weakness. Avoid trying to cover new ground, and instead spend your time reviewing core knowledge and memorizing your list of facts.

TEST-TAKING STRATEGIES

Knowing the right answers is the most obvious way to pass the test, but studying is not the only way to prepare. Knowing how to take a multiple choice test can also help. There are five key components.

First, anticipate the answer as you read the question. With most questions, you should already have an answer in mind before you look at the choices. For example, a question might describe a young lady who presents with odd neurologic complaints. She is not obviously sick, and she reports that she had a different neurologic problem two months ago. Just as when you listen to real patients describe their symptoms, a differential should form in your mind. At the top of the list for the test patient should be multiple sclerosis. If you are confident in your answer, you can avoid wasting the time it takes to carefully consider the merits of each answer choice. Instead, you can scan for the one you know is right, check the alternatives to make sure they don't compete with your anticipated answer, and move on.

Second, when you cannot anticipate the answer, use the following guidelines to help you make your choice:

1. **Opposites attract.** If two of the answers are the opposites of each other, one of them is usually the right answer.
2. **Similars attract.** If two answers are similar, one of them is usually the right answer. Test writers don't usually create two similar wrong answers.
3. **Grammar is a guide.** Sometimes wrong answers can be identified through minor grammatical inconsistencies between the question and the answer choice. The right answer should link to the question without grammatical errors, as if it is part of a sentence that was cut neatly in half.
4. **Avoid "always" and "never."** Answers that include *always* and never are almost never correct. This fact has become so well known that you will probably not see these words on the test. If you do, be wary.
5. **Worst-case answers are often right.** One of the goals of emergency medicine training is to teach you to consider life-threatening illnesses first. Be always on the look out for the pulmonary embolus or the ectopic pregnancy, and anticipate the need for immediate surgical consultation and early intubation. The diagnoses of GERD, gastroenteritis, or musculoskeletal low-back pain should be made only after you have ruled out more serious diseases with similar presentations.

Third, don't be flustered if you have difficulty interpreting a figure on the test. Like diagnostic tests in the emergency department, images on the written exam should be used to confirm or refute a clinical suspicion. The question will often guide you to the answer without the image. Use the picture to strengthen your confidence in your answer choice. For example, a 72-year-old man presents with hip pain and difficulty walking after a ground-level fall at home. What is his diagnosis? If you were seeing this patient in the emergency department, you would put hip fracture at the top of the differential. The purpose of the radiograph would be to exclude a hip dislocation (although your exam will usually do this) and to identify the location of the fracture. If the radiograph is negative and the patient really cannot walk without a lot of pain, you will probably proceed to a CT or an MRI to find the fracture that you cannot see on radiograph. Take the same approach to this patient on the test as you would in the emergency department. Determine the answer from the story, and look to the image to confirm your diagnosis. If you can't interpret the image, answer the question without it.

Fourth, read the question carefully. As in the emergency department, there is a danger in being overly confident in a diagnosis. It is good to anticipate an answer as you read, but be sure to read the entire question. Don't be so certain about your diagnosis of glaucoma that you miss the sulfa allergy, the history of sickle cell disease, or COPD. Paying attention to such details can mean the difference between choosing the right answer and a wrong one.

Fifth, be aware that test writers like to mislead test takers. It has been said that writing good test questions is easy—it is writing good test answers that is difficult. A good test answer choice captures the imagination of unprepared test takers, and lures them down the wrong path. Here, again, knowledge is your friend. In this book, we include information about unusual problems to help you hone in on the correct diagnosis and alert you when you are being led astray. For example, strychnine causes muscle convulsions leading to asphyxia two hours after ingestion and is therefore unlikely to be the right answer to any question, but if you don't know that, you might end up choosing it. Of course, good foils sometimes are right answers; knowing the key information covered by each question should help you tell the difference.

Finally, good luck and enjoy your time studying. There are few careers that offer as much opportunity to positively impact the lives of others as that of the emergency physician. The investment you make in yourself by studying will make you a stronger test taker and a more competent emergency physician.

OTHER RESOURCES

There are a number of excellent books that will help you prepare for the written exam. They are listed below, along with sources of practice questions and review courses you can take.

Books for Review

Harwood-Nuss A, Wolfson AB, Linden CH, et al (Eds). *Harwood-Nuss' Clinical Practice of Emergency Medicine*, 4th ed. New York: Lippincott Williams & Wilkins; 2005.

Marx JA, Hockberger RS, Walls RM (Eds). *Rosen's Emergency Medicine Concepts and Clinical Practice*, 6th ed. St Louis, MO: Mosby; 2006.

Rivers C (Ed). *Preparing for the Written Board Exam in Emergency Medicine*, 5th ed. Milford, OH: EMEE, Inc.; 2006.

Tintinalli JE, Galen DK, Stapcyzinski JS. *Emergency Medicine: A Comprehensive Study Guide*, 6th ed. New York: McGraw-Hill; 2004.

Practice Questions

PEER VIII: Physician's Evaluation and Educational Review in Emergency Medicine, 8th ed. Dallas, TX: American College of Emergency Physicians; 2006.

Pennsylvania Chapter, American College of Emergency Physicians Written Board Practice Examination. www.paacep.org.

Promes S. *Emergency Medicine Examination and Board Review*, 3rd ed. New York: McGraw-Hill; 2005.

Written Exam Review Courses

American Physician Institute
Emergency Medicine Qualifying Exam Course
www.thepassmachine.com
1-877-225-8384

Emergency Medicine Review: The Comprehensive CORE CONTENT Board Review Course. Education Medical Services, Inc.
P.O. Box 510222
St. Louis, MO 63151
1-800-MED-TEST

Illinois College of Emergency Physicians, Written Board Review Course
1 S 280 Summit Avenue, Court B-2
Oakbrook Terrace, IL 60181
1-630-495-6400
www.icep.org

LSU Emergency Medicine Written Board Review Course and Clinical Update
Department of Medicine, Section of Emergency Medicine
Louisiana State University School of Medicine
LSUHSC Institute of Professional Education
1600 Canal Street, Suite 1034
New Orleans, LA 70112
1-504-568-5272

Medical University of South Carolina Intensive Review in Emergency Medicine
Office of Continuing Medical Education
261 Calhoun St., Ste. 301
P.O. Box 250189
Charleston, SC 29425
(843) 876-1925

National Emergency Medicine Board Review
4535 Dressler Road NW
Canton, OH 44718
1-800-651-CEME
www.emboards.com

Ohio Chapter American College of Emergency Physicians, Emergency Medicine Review Course
3510 Snouffer Road, Suite 100
Columbus, OH 43235
1-888-OHA-CEP4
www.ohacep.org
Pennsylvania Chapter American College of Emergency Physicians, PaACEPs Emergency Medicine Written Board Review Course

777 East Park Drive, P.O. Box 8820
Harrisburg, PA 17105-8820
1-888-633-5784
www.paacep.org

Preparing for the Written Board Exam in Emergency Medicine
Emergency Medicine Educational Enterprises
200 TechneCenter Drive, #103
Milford, OH 45150
1-800-878-5667
www.emeeinc.com

Acknowledgments

For Chapter 6:

We would like to thank Kennon Heard, MD, Carrie D. Mendoza, MD, Sean H. Rhyee, MD, MPH, and Jason Hoppe, DO, each of who contributed substantially to the first edition of this chapter.

For Chapter 12:

Special thanks to Danielle D. Campagne, MD, author of this chapter in the first edition.

CHAPTER 1

Resuscitation

Marc Quinlan, MD and Brian M. Jekich, MD

Airway Management

DECISION TO INTUBATE

- Failure to maintain a patent airway
  - Impending upper airway obstruction (eg, facial burns, severe angio-edema, penetrating neck trauma, expanding hematoma, foreign body, epiglottitis)
  - Severe maxillofacial trauma
- Loss of protective reflexes
  - Lack of spontaneous swallowing, inability to handle secretions, or loss of gag reflex.
  - Approximately 12%-25% of adults do not have a gag reflex; therefore, **inability** to swallow is a more sensitive indicator for intubation than lack of gag reflex.
  - Decreased level of consciousness (Glasgow Coma Scale [GCS] < 8) not due to a rapidly reversible cause (eg, hypoglycemia, opioid overdose).
- Failure to adequately oxygenate or ventilate
  - Hypoxemia, unresponsive to supplemental oxygen, as measured by pulse oximetry with good waveform
  - Hypercapnia, as measured by arterial blood gas (ABG) or end-tidal CO_2 ($ETco_2$). May be due to diminished central respiratory drive (eg, central nervous system [CNS] injury, sedatives, alcohol) or a peripheral process (eg, Guillain Barré, myasthenia gravis, muscular dystrophy)
- Anticipated clinical deterioration
  - Status epilepticus, poly-trauma (± head injury), certain overdoses (tricyclic antidepressants [TCAs], tiring asthmatic, etc)

KEY FACT

Approximately 12%-25% of adults do not have a gag reflex, thus lack of spontaneous swallowing/pooling of secretions is a more sensitive indicator for intubation.

KEY FACT

Be sure to correlate ABG findings with the patient's clinical status.

KEY FACT

Expectation/knowledge of a patient's clinical course is paramount when considering intubation, especially if the patient is to leave for imaging or trans-facility outreach.

BASIC AIRWAY MANEUVERS

Basic airway maneuvers may prevent further need for intervention.

Airway Positioning

Head tilt with chin lift to extend head on neck, or jaw thrust to elevate mandible if possible C-spine injury.

PATHOPHYSIOLOGY

Posterior displacement of the **tongue and intrinsic muscle relaxation, causing the epiglottis to obstruct the laryngeal inlet,** are the most common causes of upper airway obstruction in the supine unconscious or semiconscious patient.

AIRWAY ADJUNCTS

Oropharyngeal and Nasopharyngeal Airway Placement

INDICATIONS

- Relieve upper airway obstruction from the tongue in the unconscious or semiconscious patient
- Adjunct to **bag-valve-mask (BVM)** ventilation

KEY FACT

Airway adjuncts are temporary and should be replaced by a definitive airway if the causative etiology of the condition is not quickly reversed.

PROCEDURE

- Oropharyngeal airway (OPA)
  - OPAs come in multiple sizes. To determine the appropriate size, the flange of the OPA should be placed at the mouth and the tip should reach the angle of the mandible.

- Insert the device while inverted → rotate 180° once well into the mouth (in order to avoid pushing the tongue posteriorly) → advance distal end into the hypopharynx.
- **Alternatively,** compress the tongue with a tongue depressor and advance the device without inversion. This technique is recommended for pediatric patients, because their smaller mouth may not allow for OPA rotation and can cause soft-tissue injury.
- Should only be used in a deeply **unresponsive** patient who is unable to maintain his or her airway. More responsive patients will gag, possibly leading to vomiting and aspiration.

- Nasopharyngeal airway (NPA)
  - Also known as a nasal trumpet. Patients typically tolerate NPAs more so than OPAs and therefore can be used in the **semiconscious** patient. NPAs also come in various sizes and approximate size can be assessed in a similar fashion; the flange should be placed at the nares and the tip should reach the angle of the mandible.
  - Gently advance into the nostril, preferably with lubrication, until the flared end is resting against the nares.

CONTRAINDICATIONS

- The NPA should **not** be used in patients with mid-face or basilar skull fracture.
- The OPA should **not** be used on the patient with an **intact gag reflex** as can lead to vomiting and subsequently aspiration.

COMPLICATIONS

Epistaxis (NPA), vomiting/aspiration, and worsened obstruction from improper placement (OPA)

Bag-Valve-Mask Ventilation

A bag valve mask (BVM) with reservoir bag (to increase O_2 delivery) is essential for airway management and almost always the initial choice for assisted ventilation.

PEDIATRICS

- Bags should have a minimum volume of 450 mL.
- Pop-off valves should be **avoided** (pressures required to ventilate are often higher than the pop-off threshold). Make sure the pop-off valve is toggled off.

INDICATION

Inadequate oxygenation or ventilation; bridge to intubation

PROCEDURE

- Open airway via jaw thrust and place NPA or OPA adjunct. Then position the mask to cover the mouth and nose.
- If using the **single-handed hold technique,** the thumb and index fingers should be placed on the mask, with the remaining fingers wrapped around mandible in a "C-grip." This is a difficult technique, but may be necessary for a single rescuer.
- The **two-handed technique is markedly preferred.** The thumb and index fingers should be placed on both sides of the mask with remaining fingers wrapped around mandible, creating a double "C-grip." The mandible is then lifted into the mask to form a seal. Next, verify that the oxygen flow rate is at 15 L/min and administer **enough volume in order to achieve chest rise.**

Q

A 23-year-old man arrives to the emergency department (ED) via ambulance after being found down. On examination, he is lying supine on the stretcher and has sonorous respirations with loud upper airway noises during inspiration. Upon inspection of his backpack, multiple bottles of oxycodone are found. What is the first step in managing this patient's airway?

KEY FACT

A patient who easily tolerates an oral airway **needs** intubation.

KEY FACT

What is the appropriate volume to administer with BVM? One that achieves chest rise.

KEY FACT

Avoid pop-off valves as airway pressure in emergency conditions often exceeds the valve pressure.

KEY FACT

Two-handed mask hold obtains better seal!

A

This patient likely has an upper airway obstruction from his tongue falling back against his posterior pharynx. The first step is to perform a chin-lift and jaw-thrust maneuver, which will relieve the obstruction. Subsequently, naloxone should be given and the patient should be monitored on end-tidal CO_2 monitoring to evaluate for recurrence of his opioid toxicity, because it is likely that naloxone's effect will wear off prior to the ingested narcotics.

KEY FACT

If you can't bag a patient, add naso- or oropharyngeal airways, reposition head, and try again.

KEY FACT

Important to keep pediatric cuff pressure < 20 cm H_2O so as to avoid decreased tracheal mucosa blood flow.

KEY FACT

The MacIntosh blade indirectly lifts the epiglottis via the hyoepiglottic ligament.

KEY FACT

Yellow = Yes

COMPLICATIONS

- Inadequate mask seal → Inadequate ventilation
- Gastric distention → emesis and aspiration
- Insufflation of vomitus/blood/debris into trachea → pneumonia/pneumonitis
- Air trapping or pneumothorax
  - Overaggressive ventilation or too large a bag (eg, pediatrics) → volutrauma → pneumothorax.
  - If you suspect air trapping (eg, history of asthma or chronic obstructive pulmonary disease [COPD]), stop bagging and squeeze the chest to help the patient exhale, then bag at a slower rate to increase exhalation time.
- Trouble-shooting BVM problems
  - If you cannot form an appropriate seal: (1) consider two-handed technique; (2) make sure an OPA or NPA is in place; (3) make sure proper mask size is being used; (4) if patient has dentures that have been removed consider replacing dentures; (5) if patient has a beard, considering lubricating with KY jelly.

INTUBATION EQUIPMENT

Endotracheal Tube

- Adult male: 7.5- to 9.0-mm tube.
- Adult female: 7.0- to 8.0-mm tube.
- Nasal intubation: Use slightly smaller tube (by 0.5-1.0 mm).
- **Pediatrics: (age/4) +4 for uncuffed; (age/4) +3.5 for cuffed, or estimated from Broselow tape.**
  - New evidence supports the use of cuffed endotracheal (ET) tube in infants and children and in some instances (eg, high airway resistance, poor compliance, substantial air leak) may be advantageous. In order to avoid tracheal mucosa necrosis, it is crucial to keep cuff pressure < 20 cm H_2O in the pediatric population.

Laryngoscope Blades

- **MacIntosh**
  - Curved, fits into the vallecula
  - Indirectly lifts the epiglottis via the **hyoepiglottic ligament**
  - However, can also be used to pick up the epiglottitis similar to the Miller blade
- **Miller**
  - Straight, inserted under epiglottis to lift it directly
  - Preferred in pediatric patients (especially < 3 years old) or if larynx is fixed by scar tissue
- **Sizing**
  - Premature infants: Size 0
  - Normal infants: Size 1
  - Older children: Size 2
  - Adults: Sizes 3-4

End-Tidal CO_2 Detector

Detecting end-tidal CO_2 ($ETco_2$) (yellow color change or 5% CO_2) after **6 manual breaths** is the best single means of confirming ET tube placement. But, all available information including visualization during placement, auscultation, chest rise, condensation in tube, and closely monitoring vital signs should be applied as well.

- False-positive $ETco_2$
  - May occur if tube is in the supraglottic region, with gastric distention or immediately following sodium bicarbonate administration
  - Indicates that the ET tube is in the airway, **not** the trachea (eg, can have color change with main-stem intubation)
- False-negative or indeterminate result
  - May occur in patients with poor pulmonary perfusion (cardiac arrest, massive pulmonary embolism [PE])
  - CO_2 level > 2% (tan or yellow) = correct placement in cardiac arrest
  - No $ETco_2$ → tube could be anywhere! Provider MUST confirm tube placement

Gum Elastic Bougie

- Helpful when only arytenoids or epiglottis is seen or cord opening is narrow
- Entry into trachea is suggested when the intubator feels ridges of the tracheal rings and resistance at approximately 27-30 cm as the bougie contacts carina
- Secures a path into the trachea over which an ET tube can be guided

DEFINITIVE AIRWAY MANAGEMENT

Orotracheal Intubation (Direct Laryngoscopy)

INDICATIONS

- Failure to maintain or protect the airway
- Failure of oxygenation or ventilation
- Anticipated deterioration

CONTRAINDICATION

There are no absolute contraindications.

PROCEDURE

- Prior to intubation, position the patient at mid chest of the intubating provider and check the blade light, balloon cuff and suction are functioning appropriately. Adjust patient position into the "sniffing position" (slightly flex lower neck and extend at atlanto-occipital joint). Next, open the patient's mouth, insert the blade, and sweep patient's tongue to the left. Advance the **curved blade** into vallecula or **straight blade** under epiglottis, then elevate the epiglottis by lifting blade upward and forward at 45° angle along direction of handle.
- **Tracheal manipulation.**
  - **BURP:** **B**ackward, **U**pward, **R**ightward **P**ressure on thyroid and cricoid cartilage.
  - **Bimanual laryngoscopy: Intubating provider moves trachea into view with right hand.** Assistant holds trachea in preferred position designated by intubating provider. Probably better than BURP but either may be helpful and in many cases the actual movement may be the same.
  - Moves larynx posteriorly and superiorly for better visualization of cords.
  - Insert ET tube through cords and inflate balloon.
- Depth at teeth:
  - 23 cm for adult males
  - 21 cm for adult females
  - Children = 3 × the ET tube size

Q

A 35-year-old unhelmeted motorcyclist presents after high-mechanism accident with a heart rate of 130 bpm and a blood pressure of 130/70 mm Hg. He has a GCS of 3 on arrival and is intubated. Immediately following intubation his blood pressure decreases rapidly to 70/40 mm Hg and becomes more difficult to ventilate. What should you consider first?

KEY FACT

$ETco_2$ is most sensitive after **6** manual breathes.

KEY FACT

$ETco_2$ confirms placement, NOT position and cannot rule out main-stem intubation.

KEY FACT

False-negative $ETco_2$ may occur with low pulmonary perfusion states (massive PE, cardiac arrest, or severe pulmonary edema).

MNEMONIC

Tracheal manipulation of the thyroid and cricoid cartilages:

BURP

Backward
Upward
Rightward
Pressure

KEY FACT

BURP can improve laryngoscopic visualization by 1 full visual grade, on average.

- Confirm tube placement.
  - **$ETco_2$ = best and most readily available method**
  - Gold standard = fiberoptic visualization of tracheal rings through ET tube
  - Esophageal detector device:
    - Syringe-like aspiration device that is inserted into the end of ET tube
    - **No resistance** to pulling plunger = tracheal intubation
    - **Resistance** = esophageal intubation
  - Other methods: Direct visualization, physical examination, pulse oximetry, chest x-ray (CXR)

COMPLICATIONS

- Broken teeth.
- Soft-tissue trauma: Lacerations to pharynx, arytenoid cartilage dislocation, vocal cord damage, etc.
- Laryngospasm.
- Main-stem intubation.
- Postintubation hypotension may be due to pneumothorax, decreased venous return from positive pressure ventilation, or drop in peripheral resistance from induction and paralysis.

Rapid Sequence Intubation

PREPARATION

- Assess for difficult airway and develop backup plan for possible failed airway.
- Monitors, intravenous (IV), equipment.
- Position patient. The patient's head should be elevated such that the patient's ear (external auditory meatus) is level with the sternal notch. This can be easily accomplished by either raising the gurney or placing a support such as bed linens to create a ramp under the patient's head.

PREOXYGENATION

- **3 minutes** on 100% O_2 nonrebreather mask **or 6 vital capacity breaths.**
- Recent studies show that, during the apneic period, concomitant oxygen delivery with a nasal canula at a flow rate of 5 L/min extends the period of adequate oxygen saturation.

PRETREATMENT

- Pretreatment medications can be considered to blunt the adverse effects of laryngoscopy, but evidence is insufficient to support routine use.
  - Pretreatment medications include lidocaine, fentanyl, and atropine.
- Despite lack of evidence showing consistent benefit, conditions where pretreatment medications can be considered include:
  - Reactive airway disease: Lidocaine can be given to mitigate bronchospasm. Physicians should also consider nebulized β-agonist.
  - Myocardial infarction (MI)/dissection/coronary artery disease (CAD): Fentanyl can be used to mitigate tachycardic response to intubation.
  - Elevated intracranial pressure (ICP): Lidocaine can be given to mitigate ↑ in ICP secondary to airway manipulation/agitation.
  - Pediatric: Atropine can be considered for symptomatic bradycardia, but does not consistently prevent reflex bradycardia in the pediatric age group.
- Premedication medications should be given approximately 3 minutes before induction medications (Table 1.1).

A

Physical examination should reveal the etiology: unilateral breath sounds, distended neck veins, and hyperresonant percussive sounds are diagnostic for tension pneumothorax. Do not wait for the CXR because tension pneumothorax is a clinical diagnosis. Vent chest with 10- to 14-gauge angiocatheter (eg, midclavicular line between the second and third ribs or anterior axillary line at the fifth intercostal space in obese patients) and subsequently place chest tube.

KEY FACT

$ETco_2$ is the best single method of confirming ET tube placement.

MNEMONIC

6 Ps of rapid sequence intubation (RSI):

Preparation
Preoxygenation
Pretreatment
Paralysis with induction
Placement of tube
Postintubation management

MNEMONIC

When to consider RSI pretreatment:

PREMED

Pediatric
Reactive airway disease (asthma)
Elevated intracranial pressure (ICP)
Myocardial infarction (MI)
Elevated blood pressure (BP)
Dissection

TABLE 1.1. Pretreatment Medications for Rapid Sequence Intubation

Drug	Mechanism	Indication	Dose (IV)
Lidocaine	↓ ICP ↓ Bronchospastic response to intubation	↓ ICP ↑ IOP Reactive airway disease	1.5 mg/kg
Fentanyl	↓ Sympathetic response to intubation	↓ ICP Intracranial bleed or aneurysm Heart disease Aortic dissection	3 μg/kg
Atropine	May ↓ symptomatic bradycardia due to enhanced vagal tone from laryngoscopy ↓ Bronchorrhea due to ketamine	< 10 y old	0.02 mg/kg

ICP, intracranial pressure; IOP, intraocular pressure; IV, intravenous.

Q

A patient is brought to the ED after being found in a building that collapsed 5 days ago. He has diffuse bruising and an apparent forearm fracture. On arrival, he rapidly decompensates and develops respiratory failure. **What paralytic would you use for intubation?**

PARALYSIS WITH INDUCTION

- Administer induction medication (Table 1.2), immediately followed by paralytic medication (Table 1.3).
- Ketamine should be used with caution in patients with known CAD because it causes tachycardia → demand ischemia.
- For reversal of nondepolarizing neuromuscular blockade, edrophonium (0.5-1 mg/kg IV) can be given after administration of atropine (0.01 mg/kg IV) once partial motor activity has been regained, although is rarely used in emergency department (ED).

TABLE 1.2. Induction Medications for Rapid Sequence Intubation

Drug	Class	Benefit	Side Effect	Dose (IV)
Etomidate	Imidazole derivative	↓ ICP Hemodynamically neutral	Brief myoclonus ↓ Cortisol	0.3 mg/kg
Ketamine	PCP derivative	Bronchodilator Dissociative amnesia Short acting Preserves respiratory drive (awake intubation) Safe in head injury	↑ Secretions ↑ HR Emergence phenomenon	1-2 mg/kg
Midazolam	Benzodiazepine	↓ ICP Anticonvulsant effects	Negative inotropy → ↓ BP	0.1-0.2 mg/kg
Propofol	GABA agonist	↓ ICP ↓ Airway resistance Short onset and duration of action	Negative inotropy, vasodilation → ↓ BP Apnea	1.5-3 mg/kg

BP, blood pressure; GABA, γ-aminobutyric acid; HR, heart rate; ICP, intracranial pressure; IV, intravenous; PCP, primary care provider.

A

A **nondepolarizing agent** (eg, vecuronium, rocuronium) should be used. Upregulation of acetylcholine receptors in the setting of recent (> 3 days) crush injury may lead to exaggerated K^+ release with the use of **succinylcholine**, which can lead to catastrophic effects on cardiac conduction.

TABLE 1.3. Paralytic Agents for Rapid Sequence Intubation

Drug	Onset	Duration	Complication	Dose (IV)
		Depolarizing Agent		
Succinylcholine	45-60 s	5-9 min	Hyperkalemia Fasciculations Trismus/masseter spasm Increased ICP/IOP Malignant hyperthermia Prolonged action if ↓ pseudocholinesterase activity	1.5 mg/kg
		Nondepolarizing Agents		
Vecuronium	2-4 min	40-60 min	Prolonged action in obese/elderly/ hepatorenal dysfunction	0.1 mg/kg
Rocuronium	1-3 min	30-45 min	Tachycardia	1 mg/kg

ICP, intracranial pressure; IOP, intraocular pressure; IV, intravenous.

- Avoid succinylcholine in patients who you suspect are hyperkalemic or are at increased risk for succinylcholine-induced hyperkalemia, such as:
  - Neuromuscular diseases (eg, amyotrophic lateral sclerosis [ALS], multiple sclerosis [MS], muscular dystrophy, myasthenia gravis).
  - Skeletal muscle denervation (stroke, spinal cord injury), major burns, or prolonged abdominal sepsis > 5 days.
  - Malignant hyperthermia history.
  - Not contraindicated in patients with end-stage renal disease, but extra caution is warranted.

KEY FACT

Risk of hyperkalemia with succinylcholine if:
- Neuromuscular disease
- Denervation injury
- Crush injury
- Major burn
- Prolonged abdominal sepsis

Placement of Tube (Intubation)

Postintubation Management

- Confirm tube placement with $ETco_2$ and auscultation.
- **Sedate** with benzodiazepines or propofol to minimize agitation **and** provide analgesia with opioid.
  - Opiates not only control pain, but also blunt sympathetic response to intubation.
- Paralyze **only if necessary** for ventilator synchrony or patient control during imaging or invasive procedures. Recent studies show that prolonged paralyzation leads to increased morbidity and mortality.

MNEMONIC

Difficult bag valve mask (BVM):

BAG'EM

Body mass index (obese)
Airtight seal
Geriatric
Edentulous (without teeth)
Mobility (decreased neck mobility or pulmonary compliance)

PEDIATRIC AIRWAY MANAGEMENT

Pediatric versus Adult Airway Management

Besides the obvious smaller size of the pediatric airway, there are other important anatomic differences compared to the adult airway (Table 1.4). These differences gradually decrease with age. Adult proportions are seen at age 8-10 years.

Recognizing the Difficult Airway

Routinely evaluating patients for markers of difficult intubation, BVM ventilation, and cricothyrotomy allows the emergency physician to thoughtfully plan alternative approaches.

TABLE 1.4. Anatomic and Physiologic Differences in Pediatric Versus Adult Airway Management

Variable	Effect	Technique to Overcome/Address
Large Occiput	When supine, ↑ angle of flexion → obstruction	Place towel under thorax to decrease angle
Smallest airway diameter at cricoid ring	ET tube may pass through cords, but then stops	May need to decrease ET tube size as needed
Anterior/superior larynx	↑ difficulty with direct laryngoscopy	Consider Miller blade or video laryngoscopy
Large/floppy epiglottis	↑ difficulty with direct laryngoscopy	Consider Miller blade or video laryngoscopy
Large tongue	↑ Risk of obstruction	Consider Miller blade or video laryngoscopy
Variable length of trachea	Infant = 5 cm; 18 mo = 7 cm (vs adult = 12 cm)	Depth at teeth = 3 × the ET tube size
↑ O_2 consumption	More rapid desaturation with apnea	High-quality bag valve ventilation

ET, endotracheal.

Q

Emergency medical service (EMS) presents with an obese 75-year-old man with oral cancer status postradiation who is unconscious after a fall. On examination, he is unresponsive, GCS 3, with shallow, sonorous respirations. He has obvious facial trauma, and an old surgical scar on his short neck, and a large beard. How do you prepare for his intubation?

- Difficult BVM
- Difficult mask placement
  - Facial trauma, bearded, no teeth, abnormal facies
- Difficult mask ventilation
  - Obese, airway obstruction, stiff lungs, advanced pregnancy, advanced age (loss of pharyngeal muscle tone), significant ascites
- Difficult laryngoscopy and intubation
  - **General appearance**
    - Predictors of a difficult intubation are often evident at first glance, such as facial disruption or oral bleeding.
  - **Upper airway obstruction**
    - Epiglottitis, angioedema, neck hematoma/masses
  - **Poor oropharyngeal access**
    - Limited mouth opening with < 3 patient fingerbreadths between the upper and lower teeth.
    - Large tongue.
    - Mallampati score (Table 1.5) is assessed by asking patient to open mouth.

TABLE 1.5. Mallampati Score for Oral Access

Class	Visible on Mouth Opening	Difficulty with Oral Access
I	Soft palate, uvula, fauces, tonsillar pillars	None
II	Soft palate, uvula, fauces	None
III	Soft palate, base of uvula	Moderate
IV	Hard palate only	Severe

A

This patient has several markers of a difficult airway, including obesity, facial trauma, facial hair, short neck, and history of surgery/radiation. This is a patient for whom you want to have backup plans in case endotracheal intubation attempts fail. Initially, his beard should be lubricated and a nasopharyngeal airway (NPA) or oropharyngeal airway (OPA) should be placed to better facilitate bag-valve-mask preoxygenation. Subsequently, the provider should be prepared for a difficult airway. Carefully consider the best approach and have a backup plan formulated in advance (eg, video laryngoscopy, adjuncts such as a bougie readily available, rescue device for ventilation such as a supraglottic airway, and a surgical airway option such as a cricothyrotomy kit).

MNEMONIC

Difficult laryngoscopy and intubation:

GOOSE

General appearance
Obstruction
Oral opening
Superior larynx
Extension (head)

MNEMONIC

Difficult cricothyrotomy:

SLICE

Surgery/radiation
Large neck
Infection
Cancer
Expanding hematoma

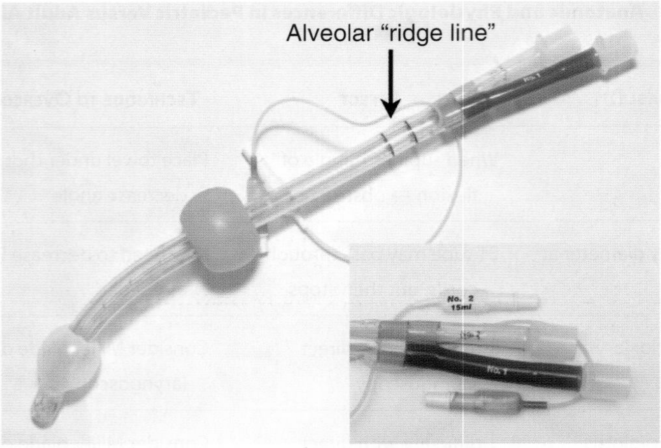

FIGURE 1.1. Combitube. The 37 F Combitube for patients up to 6 ft 6 in in height. (Reproduced, with permission, from Knoop KJ, Stack LB, Storrow AB, et al. *The Atlas of Emergency Medicine*. 3rd ed. New York, NY: McGraw-Hill Education; 2010. Figure 22.59. Photographer: Lawrence B. Stack, MD.)

    - Prominent incisors.
    - Receding mandible: < 3 patient fingerbreadths from the mentum to the hyoid bone.
  - **Superior or high larynx**
    - Distance from the undersurface of the mandible to the laryngeal prominence < 2 patient fingerbreadths
  - **Limited head extension or neck flexion**
    - Cervical spine immobilization, surgical fusion, ankylosing spondylitis, arthritis
- *Difficult cricothyrotomy*
  - Predictors include: Short/obese neck, prior surgery or radiation, presence of mass or hematoma.

Advanced Airway Procedures

Used in the management of the difficult or failed airway

DIFFICULT AIRWAY

- Difficult mask ventilation or endotracheal intubation
- If anticipated by preintubation assessment → perform awake (sedation with **no paralysis**) intubation

FAILED AIRWAY

- Failed intubation ("can't intubate") and failed BVM ventilation ("can't ventilate")
- Advanced airway procedures include:
  - Awake intubation (oral or nasotracheal)
  - Supraglottic airway (eg, laryngeal mask airway)
  - Fiberoptic intubation
  - Video laryngoscopy
  - Translaryngeal jet ventilation
  - Cricothyrotomy
  - Tracheostomy
  - Lighted stylet
  - Retrograde tracheal intubation

Awake Intubation

Indication

Spontaneously breathing patients with an anticipated difficult airway

Procedure

- Administer local airway anesthetic. Options include nebulized or atomized 4% lidocaine and topical benzocaine gel to base of tongue.
- Sedate to blunt airway reflexes.
- Ketamine (10-20 mg/dose): Muscle tone is maintained.
- Perform direct laryngoscopy and intubation once sedated. Wait for vocal cords to open during inspiration to advance tube through cords.
- Confirm placement.

Fiberoptic Awake Intubation

Indications

- Spontaneously breathing patient with an anticipated difficult airway (eg, angioedema with tongue swelling or upper airway infection)
- Suspected laryngeal abnormalities
- Poor mouth opening

Contraindications

- Copious blood or secretions
- Inadequate oxygenation or ventilation (because of time required for procedure)

Procedure

- Anesthetize nasal and/or oral mucosa with topical, nebulized, or atomized vasoconstrictor such as neosynephrine or oxymetazoline.
- Nasopharyngeal approach is preferred due to easier angle of insertion.
- Insert scope "loaded" with ET tube and advance through cords under direct visualization.
- Advance ET tube.
- Confirm placement.
- Following awake intubation, give additional sedation.

> **KEY FACT**
>
> The nasal approach is better tolerated than the oral approach in fiberoptic awake intubation.

Blind Nasotracheal Intubation

Indication

Spontaneously breathing patient with an anticipated difficult airway

Contraindications

- Pediatric patient < 10 years old
- Midface trauma or basilar skull fracture
- ↑ ICP
- Anticoagulation or anticipated need for thrombolysis
- Combative patient
- Apnea

> **KEY FACT**
>
> Blind nasotracheal intubation **cannot** be performed on the apneic patient.

Procedure

- Administer nasal anesthetic, vasoconstrictor, and lubricant.
- Insert the ET tube (usually 1-2 sizes smaller than a corresponding oral tracheal intubation) with the **bevel facing the septum** and gently advance until breath sounds are heard best through tube.
- Advance the tube during inspiration.

- If the procedure is successful, associated coughing and cessation of vocalization occurs. Insert tube to a depth of 28 cm in males and 26 cm in females as measured from the nares.
- Inflate cuff and confirm placement.

Complications

- Ability to vocalize indicates failure of tracheal intubation
- Epistaxis
- Esophageal intubation
- Sinusitis, turbinate damage, retropharyngeal laceration

Video Laryngoscopy

Video laryngoscopy allows direct visualization of the placement of the tube using an external video screen. Because a direct line of sight is not required, it generally allows for tube placement with less manipulation of the head and cervical spine than does direct laryngoscopy. Two such available products are the GlideScope and C-MAC video laryngoscopes. Recent studies show that video-assisted laryngoscopy reduces the rate of difficult intubations and increases the rate of first-attempt intubation success.

Indication

Limited mouth opening or cervical spine mobility

Procedure

- Insert blade in **midline**, without tongue sweep, and slowly advance until epiglottis is visualized. The tip of the blade should be placed into the vallecula as if the provider was using a MacIntosh blade. Unlike direct laryngoscopy, only gentle traction is required to obtain visualization. Pass ET tube through cords and confirm placement.
- It may be necessary to slide the blade back cephalad such that the view of the glottis is in the top half of the video screen to facilitate a favorable angle to pass the ET tube.
- Partially withdraw the stylet to allow the ET tube to advance to the trachea.

Complication

Lens fogging, secretions, or blood may obstruct view.

Laryngeal Mask Airway

The laryngeal mask airway (LMA) is available in the following sizes:

- 1-3: Newborn to 30- to 50-kg child, in 0.5 increments
- 4: 50- to 70-kg adult
- 5: Larger adults

Indication

Rescue device for “can’t intubate” situations

Contraindications

- Complete upper airway obstruction
- Oropharyngeal pathology, trauma, or bleeding
- Increased risk of aspiration (eg, gastrointestinal [GI] bleed)
- Limited utility in patients who require high pressures to ventilate (eg, obese, severe asthma)

Procedure

Open airway via head tilt. Next, insert LMA with opening facing the tongue and advance along the hard palate until tip is well into hypopharynx. Once in position, inflate cuff with 20- to 40-mL air (amount listed on device), which will form the seal around the glottic opening

Intubating Laryngeal Mask Airway

- With an intubating laryngeal mask airway (ILMA), a specialized ET tube can be advanced through the lumen of the LMA allowing for blind tracheal intubation.
- The intubating LMA is subsequently removed using the disposable tube stabilizer to hold the ET tube in place.
- Limitation:
  - ILMA are available in sizes 3, 4, and 5 and are thus limited to patients > 30 kg.

Retrograde Tracheal Intubation

Indication

Rescue device for "can't intubate" situations

Procedure

- First, place needle in cricothyroid membrane. Next, pass a wire through the needle until it emerges from the mouth. Remove the needle and secure the percutaneous part of the wire with a hemostat. Advance an ET tube over wire into trachea.
- Should **not be used** in "can't intubate, can't ventilate" scenario because procedure takes too long to replace cricothyrotomy.

Complications

- Hemorrhage (if cricothyroid artery lacerated)
- Soft-tissue infection

Esophageal Tracheal Combitube (Figures 1.1 and 1.2)

An esophageal tracheal Combitube consists of a twin-lumen tube with a proximal low-pressure cuff that seals the pharyngeal area, a distal cuff that seals the esophagus (or the trachea), and ports for ventilation between the lumens (Figures 1.2 and 1.3).

The KING LT supraglottic airway has similar function, containing a distal cuff to seal the esophagus and a proximal cuff to seal the pharynx. Ventilation occurs through the multiple holes between the 2 cuffs.

Two sizes available:

- 37 F: Small adult/large child
- 41 F: Larger adults

Indications

- Apneic and unconscious adult with:
  - Failed intubation
  - Limited mouth opening

Contraindications

- Intact airway reflexes
- Esophageal disease or caustic ingestion

Q

A 50-year-old man is brought to ED by EMS after being found with agonal respirations in a closed garage with the car running. On arrival, the patient is being ventilated via a King LT, but waking up and regaining spontaneous respiratory effort. How do you want to manage his airway now?

KEY FACT

Ease of use and potential to transition to a definitive airway make the LMA useful in the difficult airway but it doesn't protect against aspiration.

KEY FACT

ILMA are available in sizes 3, 4, and 5 and are thusly limited to patients > 30 kg.

KEY FACT

The Combitube can be used in the setting of upper GI bleed, but not if there is expected esophageal pathology.

A

If you want to keep the patient intubated, an intubating introducer (or gum elastic bougie) can be inserted through the anterior port of the King LT followed by removal of the King LT over the intubating stylet and placement of an ET tube over the stylet into the trachea. If you want to allow the patient to wake up, the King LT can be removed after deflation of the pharyngeal and esophageal cuffs.

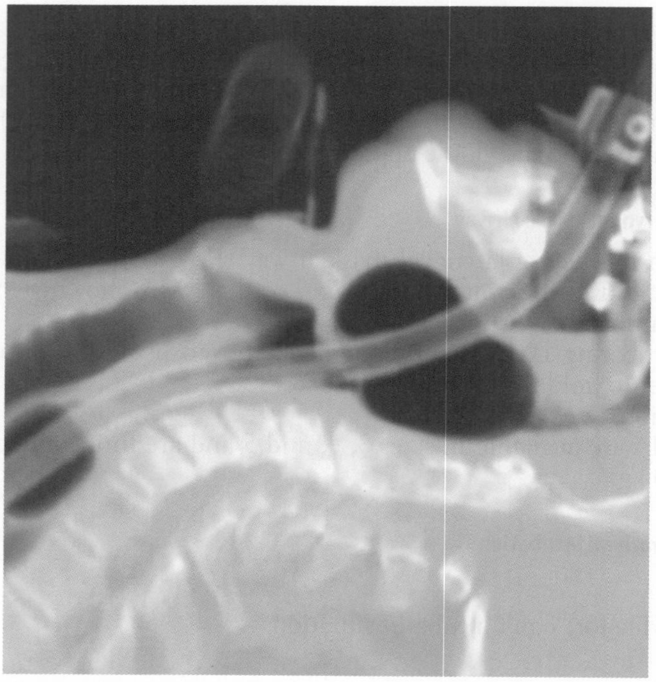

FIGURE 1.2. Esophageal Combitube placement. CT scout film demonstrating esophageal placement of the Combitube. (Reproduced, with permission, from Knoop KJ, Stack LB, Storrow AB, et al. *The Atlas of Emergency Medicine*. 3rd ed. New York, NY: McGraw-Hill Education; 2010. Figure 22.60. Photographer: Steven J. White, MD.)

- Upper airway obstruction
- Children ≤ 4 ft tall because no child/infant sizes available

PROCEDURE

With the provider's nondominant hand, grab and elevate the patient's tongue and jaw. If possible, flex the patient's neck. Next, pass the tube blindly into the pharynx until the marker on the tube is between the patient's teeth. Inflate the pharyngeal balloon with 100 mL of air and the distal white balloon with 5-15 mL of air. Initially, begin ventilation

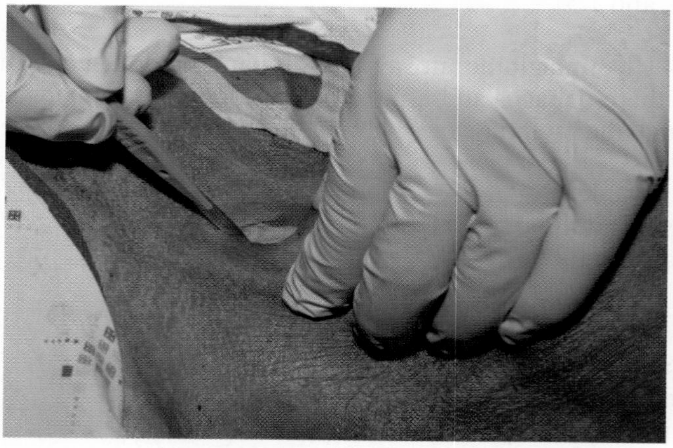

FIGURE 1.3. Incision over cricothyroid membrane. Stabilize the proximal trachea; make a vertical incision over the cricothyroid membrane. (Reproduced, with permission, from Knoop KJ, Stack LB, Storrow AB, et al. *The Atlas of Emergency Medicine*. 3rd ed. New York, NY: McGraw-Hill Education; 2010. Figure 22.88. Photographer: Lawrence B. Stack, MD.)

through the longer (blue) connector. Air entry into the lungs is achieved via holes on the side (this confirms that Combitube is in the esophagus). If air entry occurs into the stomach, this represents a rare tracheal placement, in which case the BVM should be attached to the shorter (clear) tube, facilitating ventilation.

Lighted Stylet

INDICATIONS

- Difficult airway
- Limited mouth opening
- Limited cervical spine mobility

CONTRAINDICATIONS

- Failed airway: Because of time required
- Laryngeal pathology

PROCEDURE

With the nondominant hand, grab the patient's tongue and jaw. Next, insert a lighted stylet "loaded" with ET tube into the oropharynx, with curved tip midline and pointing inferiorly, until it sits in the posterior pharynx. Follow the well-defined glow anteriorly and midline. Once it is below the larynx, it indicates tracheal placement. Advance ET tube and confirm placement.

Needle Cricothyrotomy

Surgical airway of choice in children < 10-12 years old
Provides a temporary airway to oxygenate and ventilate a patient in a failed airway event

INDICATION

Rescue device for **oxygenation** in failed airway

CONTRAINDICATIONS

- Tracheal transection with retraction of the distal end
- Cricoid or laryngeal damage

PROCEDURE

Attach a 12- or 14-gauge needle catheter to a 3-mL syringe and clean anterior neck with a sterilizing solution (eg, iodine). With nondominant hand, locate and stabilize the cricoid membrane. Unfortunately, the laryngeal prominence does not develop until adolescence and therefore, can be difficult to find in infants and younger children. Rather, trace tracheal rings superiorly until cricoid membrane is palpated, or if unable to locate, needle can be placed midline through the tracheal rings. Next, direct the needle catheter inferiorly and insert it (aspirating continuously) through the cricoid membrane into the trachea. Once in the trachea, advance the catheter over the needle. Lastly, attach catheter to jet-ventilation system and oxygenate set to deliver 100% O_2 for 1 second, then release for 4 seconds to allow for expiration.

COMPLICATIONS

- Common: Subcutaneous emphysema, catheter kinking/obstruction, coughing if patient is conscious, CO_2 retention
- Uncommon but serious: Barotrauma, pneumothorax, pneumomediastinum

Q

A 6-year-old boy is in respiratory arrest after being ejected from a car during a rollover accident. He has obvious head and face trauma. You are unable to intubate using direct laryngoscopy or BVM ventilate. What should you do next?

KEY FACT

"A blue patient is bad." Begin ventilation through the Combitube's blue connector.

KEY FACT

A lateral or poorly defined glow indicates improper lighted stylet placement.

KEY FACT

Needle cricothyrotomy can usually support oxygenation requirements, but ventilation may be poor.

KEY FACT

Advantages of needle cricothyrotomy over surgical cricothyrotomy: Simpler, faster, less bleeding, fewer long-term complications, and can be done in patients of all ages.

A

This child has a failed airway ("can't intubate, can't ventilate"). You should immediately perform a needle cricothyrotomy to provide oxygenation. Needle cricothyrotomy is a temporizing measure due to the limited ventilation it provides. While providing temporary transtracheal jet ventilation, preparation should be made for definitive airway management.

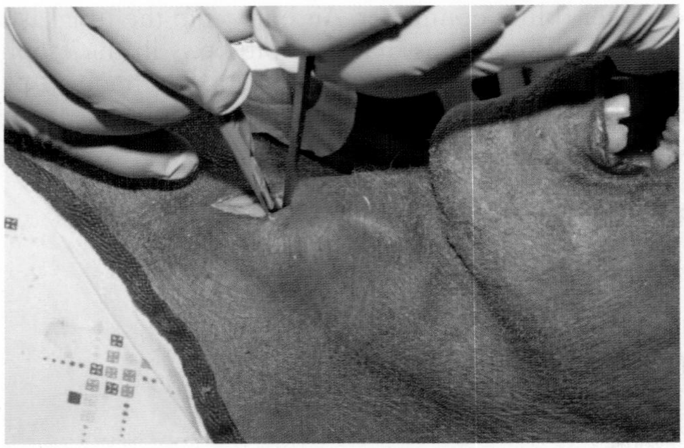

FIGURE 1.4. Horizontal incision through cricothyroid membrane. Insert a tracheal hook through the incision to gain proximal control of the trachea. (Reproduced, with permission, from Knoop KJ, Stack LB, Storrow AB, et al. *The Atlas of Emergency Medicine*. 3rd ed. New York, NY: McGraw-Hill Education; 2010. Figure 22.89. Photographer: Lawrence B. Stack, MD.)

KEY FACT

Surgical cricothyrotomy is contraindicated in patients < 10-12 years old. Needle cricothyrotomy is a better choice in this age group.

Cricothyrotomy

Equipment needed at a minimum: Scalpel, tracheal hook, or tissue-spreading device, 5.5 or 6.0 cuffed ET tube.

Indication

Failed airway

Contraindication

Age: Substitute needle cricothyrotomy for patients < 10-12 years old

Procedure

First, apply sterilizing solution to neck. Next, with nondominant hand, locate cricothyroid membrane. Make a midline vertical skin incision at the level of the cricothyroid membrane (Figure 1.4), while stabilizing the larynx with thumb and middle finger of nondominant hand, make a horizontal incision in the cricothyroid membrane (Figure 1.5). Use a tracheal hook to maintain control of trachea and then bluntly widen the cricothyroid membrane orifice

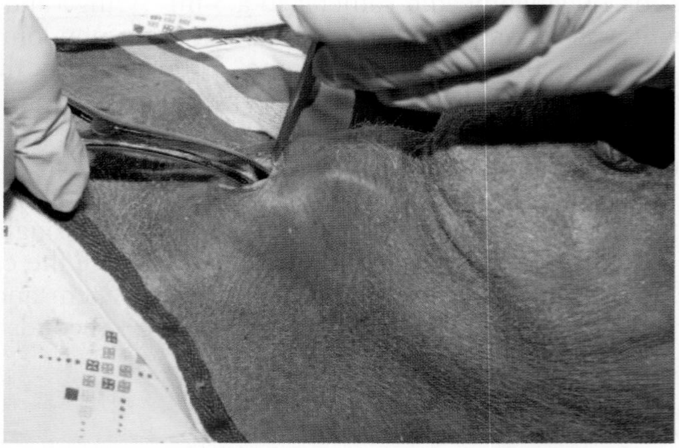

FIGURE 1.5. Insert tracheal dilator. Then rotate dilator cephalad. (Reproduced, with permission, from Knoop KJ, Stack LB, Storrow AB, et al. *The Atlas of Emergency Medicine*. 3rd ed. New York, NY: McGraw-Hill Education; 2010. Figure 22.90. Photographer: Lawrence B. Stack, MD.)

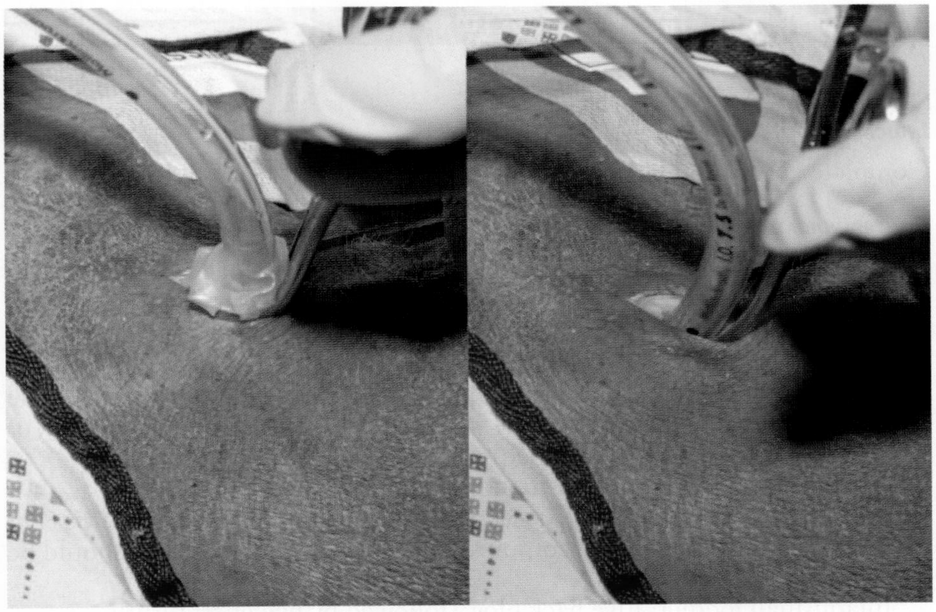

FIGURE 1.6. Insert endotracheal (ET) or tracheostomy tube. Insert a cuffed ET tube or tracheostomy tube and remove dilator. (Reproduced, with permission, from Knoop KJ, Stack LB, Storrow AB, et al. *The Atlas of Emergency Medicine*. 3rd ed. New York, NY: McGraw-Hill Education; 2010. Figure 22.91. Photographer: Lawrence B. Stack, MD.)

with finger or blunt end of scalpel/hemostat (Figure 1.6). Next, you can either place a bougie and subsequently slide ET tube over bougie, or insert the ET tube directly into the tracheostomy (Figure 1.7). Last, confirm placement with $ETco_2$.

Complications

- Bleeding from perithyroid vasculature
- Trachea, esophagus, or recurrent laryngeal nerve injury
- Misplacement of the tube anterior to the trachea into the mediastinum → pneumothorax or pneumomediastinum

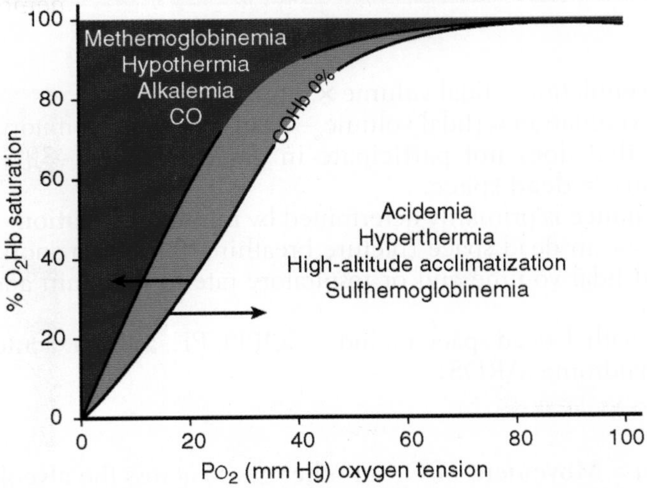

FIGURE 1.7. Oxyhemoglobin dissociation curve at 98.6°F (37°C) and pH 7.40. Hematocrit does not alter this relationship. (Reproduced, with permission, from Hoffman RS, Howland MA, Lewin NA, et al: *Goldfrank's Toxicologic Emergencies*, 10th ed. New York, NY: McGraw-Hill Education; 2015. Figure 29.2.)

MANAGEMENT OF AIRWAY OBSTRUCTION

Abdominal Thrusts

INDICATION

Complete airway obstruction due to tracheal foreign body

CONTRAINDICATION

Breathing/coughing/speaking patient with adequate oxygenation

PROCEDURE

- Child/adult
  - Subdiaphragmatic thrusts are performed while standing behind the patient and grabbing a closed fist located above the patient's umbilicus and well below xiphoid process.
  - Arms wrapped around victim if conscious.
  - Exceptions: Morbidly obese, pregnant and unconscious patients. For these individuals, chest compressions, not abdominal thrusts, should be attempted.
- Infant/small toddler: Five back blows followed by five chest thrusts
  - Direct laryngoscopy with foreign body removal via Magill forceps when available.
  - Perform finger sweep only if foreign body is directly visualized.
- If abdominal thrusts/chest compressions fail, consider using an ET tube to push the foreign body into the right main-stem bronchus, then withdrawing the tube several centimeters to allow ventilation of the left lung.

KEY FACT

Encourage a patient who is speaking or audibly coughing to continue coughing.

KEY FACT

Never perform a blind finger sweep.

Blood Gases

When evaluating the patient in respiratory failure, blood gases can aid in diagnoses, prognosis, and effectiveness of intervention. Acid-base disorders and the use of blood gases to address such disorders are covered separately in Chapter 7, Endocrine, Metabolic, Fluid, and Electrolyte Disorders.

BASIC PRINCIPLES OF PULMONARY PHYSIOLOGY

Ventilation

- Minute ventilation = tidal volume × respiratory rate.
- Alveolar ventilation = (tidal volume – dead space) × respiratory rate.
- The air that does not participate in gas exchange (~30% in normal conditions) = **dead space.**
- **CO_2** clearance is primarily determined by minute **ventilation**.
- An increase in dead space (picture breathing through a snorkel) requires increased tidal volume and or respiratory rate to maintain adequate CO_2 clearance.
- Diseases with ↑ dead space include: COPD, PE, asthma, acute respiratory distress syndrome (ARDS).

KEY FACT

Decreased ventilation or an increase in dead space → increased CO_2 on blood gas.

KEY FACT

An increase in dead space requires increased ventilation rate to maintain CO_2 clearance.

Diffusion

- Diffusion = **Movement of O_2** (or other gases) across the **alveolar-capillary membrane.**
- Factors that determine diffusion: (1) membrane thickness, (2) surface area, (3) the diffusion coefficient, and (4) the partial pressure difference of the gas between the 2 sides of the membrane.

- O_2 is much less soluble than CO_2, therefore more easily affected by diseases of the alveolar-capillary membrane.
- If alveoli fill with fluid (pulmonary edema), the thickness of the respiratory membrane ↑ and diffusion ↓.
- If you ↓ alveolar surface area, as occurs in emphysema, then diffusion ↓.
- In the normal lung, the only way to change diffusion is to change the partial pressure concentration (**therefore supplemental oxygen improves the A-a gradient**).
- Diseases affecting the alveolar-capillary membrane include: Pulmonary edema, interstitial fibrosis, asbestosis, sarcoidosis, and scleroderma.

Q

A 72-year-old man with a past medical history notable for COPD requiring multiple ICU hospitalizations, presents in respiratory distress. He is immediately placed on BiPAP and gradually improves. How do you change BiPAP settings to improve oxygenation and also hypercarbia?

Shunt

- Right-to-left shunt → low Pao_2 and an increased A-a gradient on blood gas
- Physiologic right-to-left shunt = blood flow to alveoli that cannot participate in gas exchange (perfusion without ventilation)
  - Occurs in setting of nonfunctioning alveoli, such as *ARDS*, pneumonia, and atelectasis
- Anatomic right-to-left shunt = blood flow that bypasses the lungs altogether
  - Seen in ventricular septal defect (VSD) or atrial septal defect (ASD) with pulmonary hypertension. Does not improve with supplemental O_2

KEY FACT

Oxygenation is adversely affected by diseases of the alveolar-capillary membrane that decrease diffusion (eg, interstitial fibrosis).

Ventilation-Perfusion Inequality

- Ventilation and blood flow are mismatched in regions of the lung.
- Ventilation-perfusion (V/Q) mismatch can adversely affect CO_2 elimination in addition to oxygenation.
- An area with no ventilation (V/Q = 0) is called a "shunt."
- An area with no perfusion (V/Q = infinity) is called "dead space."
- A low V/Q ratio ↓ gas exchange and is a cause of low Pao_2. Commonly seen in COPD, asthma, hepato-pulmonary syndrome, and pulmonary edema.
- A high V/Q ratio ↓ $Paco_2$ and ↑ Pao_2. Commonly seen in pulmonary embolus because ventilation fails to oxygenate blood.

KEY FACT

Hypoxemia due to an anatomic shunt does not correct with 100% O_2.

O_2 Delivery to Tissues

- 3 principal components determine O_2 delivery to tissues:
  - O_2 content: Amount of O_2 dissolved in blood and carried on hemoglobin
  - Cardiac output = ***Heart rate (HR) × stroke volume***
  - Oxyhemoglobin saturation at a given Pao_2
- The oxyhemoglobin dissociation curve describes the strength with which hemoglobin binds **O_2**.
  - **Right shift of curve = O_2 more readily given up to tissue** (Figure 1.8)
  - Causes of right shift: Acidosis, hyperthermia, increased 2,3-diglycerophosphate (**2,3-DPG**), increased $Paco_2$
  - Causes of left shift: Alkalosis, hypothermia, abnormal hemoglobin, decreased 2,3-DPG, decreased $Paco_2$

KEY FACT

Carbon monoxide replaces O_2 by binding to hemoglobin and shifts the oxyhemoglobin dissociation curve to the left, decreasing the availability of O_2 to tissues.

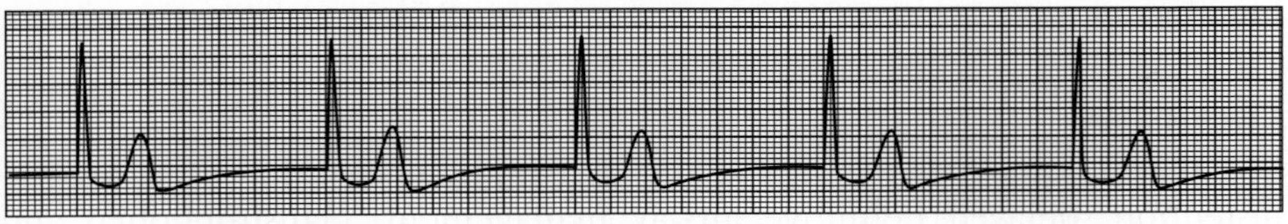

FIGURE 1.8. Sinus arrest with junctional escape rhythm.

To improve oxygenation: Increase Fio_2 and expiratory positive airway pressure (EPAP)
To improve hypercarbia: Increase inspiratory positive airway pressure (IPAP).

Ventilation Techniques

NONINVASIVE VENTILATION

- Contraindications: If patient is apneic, unable to protect his or her airway (eg, upper airway obstruction, inability to swallow or presence of copious secretions), has had recent esophageal or maxillofacial surgery or has an untreated pneumothorax, noninvasive ventilation is contraindicated.
- Patients most likely to succeed solely with noninvasive positive pressure ventilation (NIPPV) are those with more easily reversible causes of respiratory distress, such as COPD exacerbation, pulmonary edema, and asthma.
- Reduces work of breathing, ↑ oxygenation and CO_2 clearance.
- Allows for alveolar recruitment and increased lung volumes.
- Redistributes alveolar fluid.
- Increases cardiac output by not only decreasing preload (eg, ↓ right ventricle [RV] preload → ↑ compliance), but also decreasing afterload (eg, ↑ intrathoracic pressure that ↓ left ventricular [LV] ejection pressure).
- Can assist in chest wall stabilization in patient with chest trauma or following surgery.

Continuous Positive Airway Pressure

- By utilizing constant flow to generate pressure, continuous positive airway pressure (CPAP) provides fixed positive pressure throughout respiratory cycle without pause.
- Recent studies show that CPAP is more effective in reducing the need for ET intubation in patients with acute cardiogenic pulmonary edema.

Bilevel Positive Airway Pressure

- Delivers different levels of pressure during inspiration and expiration.
- Each cycle is triggered by patient initiation of inhalation.
- Inspiratory positive pressure (5-15 cm H_2O) exceeds that of expiratory positive pressure (3-5 cm H_2O) provided.
- **Provides extrinsic** positive end-expiratory pressure **(PEEP) to prevent alveolar collapse.**
- Gastric distention unlikely with peak inspiratory pressure < 25 cm H_2O.
- Recent studies show that bilevel positive airway pressure (BiPAP) is more effective in reducing the need for ET intubation in patients with COPD exacerbation.

KEY FACT

BiPAP is a combination of CPAP with additional inspiratory assist.

Procedure

Make sure that NIPPV mask fits appropriately to limit leaks. Patient reassurance is critical, because placement of the mask can cause a sense of claustrophobia and increased anxiety. Next, start at lower pressure settings (eg, BiPAP: 10/5 cm H_2O or CPAP 5 cm H_2O) and increase pressures gradually until patient responds. Monitor patient closely and consider checking blood gases.

Complication

Volutrauma, pressure necrosis of the skin from an ill-fitting mask, gastric distention, delayed definitive airway management, claustrophobia, and anxiety.

MECHANICAL VENTILATION

Ventilators are either pressure or volume cycled. The ventilator mode should be selected according to the inherent advantages/disadvantages based on the underlying disease process (Tables 1.6 and 1.7).

Initial ventilator setting should be based on review of the underlying pulmonary process (see Table 1.7).

Complications

- **Volutrauma**
  - Over distention of alveoli
  - Prevented by using smaller tidal volumes
- **Barotrauma**
  - Caused by excessive peak inspiratory and mean airway pressures
  - Diagnosed by sudden increase in peak inspiratory pressure
  - Risk increased with severe lung pathology or presence of necrosis
  - **Prevention by lowering plateau pressures** ($\leq$ 30 cm H_2O) appears more important than peak airway pressure
- Loss of upper airway mechanisms **to prevent aspiration**
- **Ventilator-associated pneumonia (VAP)**
  - Risk increases exponentially in relationship to duration of intubation
  - Decrease risk by sitting patients up in bed by at least 30°, if not contraindicated
  - **Early pneumonia** (< 48 hours postintubation): Community-acquired pathogens
  - **Late pneumonia** (> 48 hours postintubation): Nosocomial pathogens, more resistant strains

TABLE 1.6. Common Emergency Department Modes of Ventilation

Mode	Support	Advantages	Disadvantages
Assist volume control	Breaths initiated by patient or ventilator Every breath fully ventilator supported	Set tidal volume delivered unless peak pressure exceeded	May cause high peak inspiratory pressures, hypotension, or hyperventilation
Assist pressure control	Breaths initiated by patient or ventilator Every breath fully ventilator supported	Allows regulation of peak inspiratory pressures (eg, ARDS)	Change in compliance may cause hyper-/hypoventilation, hypotension
SIMV	Spontaneous breaths allowed above mandatory preset number of ventilator-supported breaths	Hemodynamically stable	Greater work of breathing than assist control Discomfort with 2 different ventilated breaths
PSV	Patient triggers each breath	Enables weaning	Requires intact respiratory drive

ARDS, acute respiratory distress syndrome; PSV, pressure support ventilation; SIMV, synchronized intermittent mandatory ventilation.

Q

A 60-year-old smoker with a COPD exacerbation is intubated after failing aggressive noninvasive therapy. What should his initial ventilator settings be?

KEY FACT

VAP
Most common pathogens = Gram negatives (*Pseudomonas, Acinetobacter, Enterobacter*)

A

In a patient with COPD, the initial selected tidal volume and rate should be slightly reduced to avoid hyperinflation and hyperventilation. Begin with 6-8 mL/kg of patient's ideal body weight at 10 breaths/min and 100% FIO_2 and wean as tolerated. If peak pressures are high, decrease tidal volume to allow permissive hypercapnia. Inspiratory flow rate and expiratory time can be increased to avoid hyperinflation from auto-PEEP.

TABLE 1.7. Initial Ventilator Settings

Pulmonary Process	Ventilator Settings
Pulmonary contusion, pneumonia, pulmonary edema	Low tidal volume (Vt) (6 cc/kg) to prevent barotrauma PEEP 5-15 cm H_2O to prevent alveoli collapse Goal plateau pressure < 30 cm H_2O
Asthma/COPD	Slow respiratory rate (10 bpm) Prolonged exhalation phase (I:E 1:3-5) to ↓ intrinsic PEEP Vt < 8 cc/kg Permissive hypercapnia for high peak pressures
ARDS	Low tidal volume (6 mL/kg) to prevent volutrauma Low respiratory rate (10-12 bpm) to maximize recruitment PEEP Inverse I:E ratio (inspiratory time > expiratory time) to improve oxygenation Permissive hypercapnia
Neonates	Best setting = pressure-controlled ventilation
Acidosis without lung injury	Match intrinsic minute ventilation by ↑ rate or tidal volume
Head injury	Avoid hypercapnia, which causes cerebral vasodilation and ↑ ICP Goal $PaCO_2$ = 35

ARDS, acute respiratory distress syndrome; COPD, chronic obstructive pulmonary disorder; ICP, intracranial pressure; PEEP, positive end-expiratory pressure.

- **Hemodynamic instability**
  - High respiratory rate, high mean airway pressure, high PEEP, or inverse ratio ventilation (IRV) may increase intrathoracic pressure, decreasing venous return → decreased cardiac output → hypotension.
  - IRV refers to inspiratory time that exceeds expiratory time. IRV improves oxygenation by increasing mean airway pressure, but may cause auto-PEEP (ie, "breath stacking").
  - May also increase cerebral venous pressure → cerebral ischemia.

Cardiac Conduction and Rhythm Assessment

GENERAL APPROACH

Arrhythmias have a wide range of possible presentations. Some patients may be asymptomatic, while others present with palpitations, dizziness, syncope, or sudden death. A systematic approach to assessing rhythms is essential to accurate diagnosis and management. For additional information, please reference the section "Management of Cardiac Arrest."

Is the patient in cardiac arrest?

- Rhythms that can produce cardiac arrest: **Ventricular fibrillation (VFib), ventricular tachycardia (VT), pulseless electrical activity (PEA), bradycardia, and asystole**

- Understanding the causes of cardiac arrest helps direct not only diagnostic therapy, but also therapeutic therapies

Is the patient stable or unstable?
The definition of stability relates to the ability of the heart to provide sufficient cardiac output.

Signs of instability:
- Cardiac ischemia manifested by chest pain or pulmonary edema
- Circulatory compromise (hypotension, diaphoresis, weak pulses)
- Altered mental status caused by decreased cerebral blood flow

Is the rhythm tachycardic (> 100 bpm [beats/min]) or bradycardic (< 60 bpm)?
Is the rhythm regular or irregular?
Is the rhythm wide or narrow complex?
Rhythm complex width is defined as the width of the QRS. **QRS ≥ 0.12** second is considered wide complex.
- Narrow complex rhythms are conducted through normal pathways and almost always begin above or within the atrioventricular (AV) node.
- Wide complex rhythms result from supraventricular arrhythmia with preexisting or rate-related bundle branch block (BBB), accessory pathway conduction or preexcitation, ventricular arrhythmia, a pacemaker, or the presence of a metabolic abnormality (eg, hyperkalemia) or toxin (eg, TCA overdose).

Are P waves present? If so, are they associated with QRS complexes?
The presence or absence of P waves as well as their relationship with the QRS complexes is important to understanding the origin of the rhythm.

SINUS RHYTHM

- A regular rate between 60 and 100 bpm
- P wave present before every QRS complex with a 1:1 ratio
- Normal intervals: PR interval between 0.12 and 0.2 seconds and a QRS interval < 0.12 second

SINUS DYSRHYTHMIAS

Sinus Bradycardia

- Ventricle rate < 60 bpm
- Can be associated with vasovagal response, hypothermia, medication side effect (eg, β-blockers, calcium channel blockers, digoxin), as well as in healthy adults, especially athletes
- If asymptomatic, typically requires no intervention

Sick Sinus Syndrome

- Occurs because of disease in the sinoatrial (SA) node
- May cause tachycardia-bradycardia syndrome in which heart rate varies significantly
- More common in elderly because SA nodes become increasingly fibrotic with age
- Often manifests as syncope, presyncope, palpitations, or dyspnea

ECG Findings

- Irregular rhythm with pauses in sinus activity
- May miss intermittent dysrhythmia, so ambulatory electrocardiogram (ECG) monitoring may be necessary

Q

A 55-year-old man presents to the ED with acute onset of chest pain, shortness of breath, and diaphoresis. His initial ECG shows acute ST elevation in the anterior leads. You initiate acute coronary syndrome (ACS) protocols and activate the cardiac cath laboratory. Shortly thereafter he complains of lightheadedness. The monitor now shows third-degree AV block with a ventricular escape rhythm at 35 bpm. What should you do first?

KEY FACT

Rhythms that can produce cardiac arrest:
VFib
Pulseless VT
PEA
Asystole
Bradycardia

KEY FACT

Unstable rhythm = Rhythm with associated signs or symptoms of inadequate cardiac output.

KEY FACT

Unstable cardiac rhythms require immediate intervention. Stable rhythms may be further delineated via more investigation.

A

Anterior MI is associated with infranodal conduction damage that is often permanent. Transcutaneous pacing should be initiated and the patient prepped for transvenous pacer placement. Atropine may actually *worsen* the conduction ratio, and therefore should not be used in this setting.

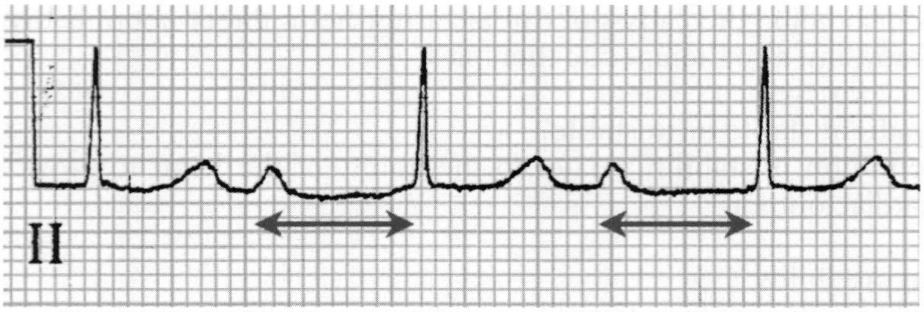

FIGURE 1.9. The PR interval is fixed (double arrows) and is longer than 0.2 second, or 5 small blocks. (Reproduced, with permission, from Knoop KJ, Stack LB, Storrow AB, et al. *The Atlas of Emergency Medicine*. 3rd ed. New York, NY: McGraw-Hill Education; 2010. Figure 23.14B.)

TREATMENT

- Depends on presentation
- Too slow: Rate stimulation with atropine or pacing
- Too fast: Rate control with calcium channel or β-blockers, but risk worsening AV block or sinus arrest
- Definitive therapy: Typically a combination of permanent pacemaker as well as rate control medications

Sinus Arrest (Sinus Block)

Left untreated, sick sinus syndrome (SSS) leads to complete cessation of SA activity

KEY FACT

Sinus arrest or sinus block is often the result of untreated sick sinus syndrome.

ECG FINDINGS (FIGURE 1.9)

- No P waves
- Escape pacemaker activity
- Usually from the AV node or bundle of His (40-60 bpm) but may be ventricular escape (< 40 bpm)

TREATMENT

- Acute care: Often requires emergent temporary transcutaneous or transvenous pacing ± atropine
- Definitive care: Permanent pacemaker

ATRIOVENTRICULAR BLOCKS

- Involve the atrioventricular (AV) node and/or proximal His bundle ("infranodal" AV block)
- See Table 1.8 for differentiating characteristics:
  - First-degree AV block (**Regular**)
  - Second-degree AV block type I (Wenckebach, Mobitz I) (**Irregular**)
  - Second-degree AV block type II (Mobitz II) (**Irregular**)
  - Third-degree AV block (complete heart block) (**Regular**)

First-Degree AV Block

First-degree AV block is common and is often a normal variant in a healthy heart. It results from prolonged conduction of the atrial impulse, typically at the AV node, without the loss of conduction of a single impulse.

CAUSES

- Normal variant in a healthy heart
- Acute coronary syndrome (ACS) (usually **inferior MI**)

TABLE 1.8. Distinguishing Characteristics of AV Blocks

Type of AV Block	ECG	Rhythm	QRS Duration
First degree	PR > 0.20 s All P waves conduct	Regular	Narrow[a]
Second-degree Type I (Wenckebach, Mobitz)	Progressive prolongation of PR interval until QRS dropped Block typically at AV node	Irregular (unless fixed conduction)	Narrow[a]
Second-degree Type II (Mobitz II)	Constant PR interval Block typically infranodal	Irregular (unless fixed conduction)	Usually wide
Third degree	Complete disruption of AV conduction	Regular	Varies by origin of escape rhythm

AV, atrioventricular; ECG, electrocardiogram.

[a]In the absence of other conduction abnormalities.

- Infectious disease (eg, Lyme disease, myocarditis)
- Infiltrative myocardial disease (eg, sarcoidosis)
- Structural heart disease (congenital or surgical)
- Medications (digoxin toxicity, β-blockers)

ECG Findings (Figure 1.10)

- Regular rhythm
- All P waves conducted (eg, there is a QRS for every P wave)
- PR interval > 0.2 second
- PR interval constant

Treatment

Usually no treatment required

Second-Degree AV Block Type I (Wenckebach, Mobitz I)

Characterized by progressive prolongation of the PR interval, secondary to prolongation of the AV-nodal refractory period, eventually culminating in a nonconducted P wave

Causes

- Medication side effect (eg, digitalis, β-blockers, calcium channel blockers)
- Normal variant (eg, increased vagal tone)
- Can occur in ACS and should increase physician's concern for an **inferior MI**
- Infection (eg, myocarditis, rheumatic fever)

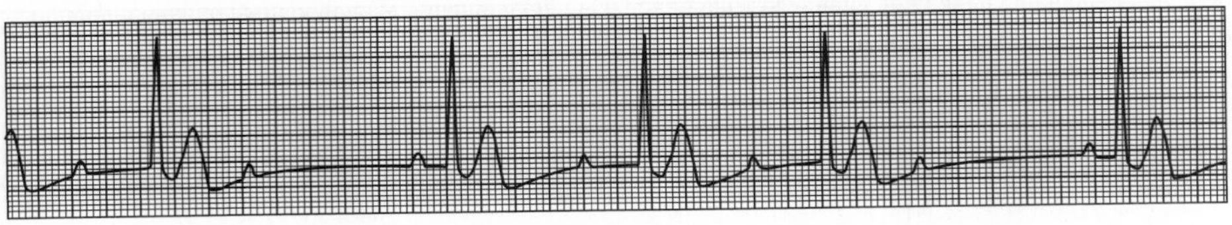

FIGURE 1.10. Second-degree AV block type I.

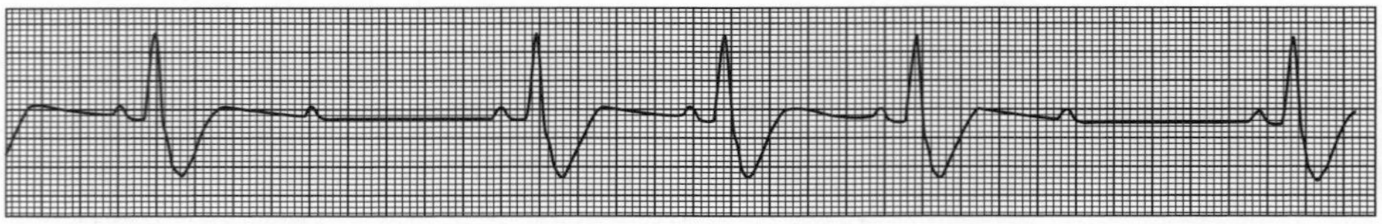

FIGURE 1.11. **Second-degree AV block type II.**

ECG Findings (Figure 1.11)

- Irregular rhythm; QRS complexes appear "grouped."
- PR **progressively elongates** until 1 QRS complex is dropped (eg, some, **NOT all,** dropped).
- P waves regular.
- Not all P waves conducted past AV node.
- PR interval generally > 0.2 second and QRS interval generally < 0.12 second.

KEY FACT

First-degree heart block, Wenckebach, and right bundle branch block (RBBB) can all occur in a healthy heart.

Treatment

- Unlikely to cause serious signs or symptoms.
- If evidence of hypoperfusion, give atropine 0.5 mg IV every 5 minutes (max dose 2 mg).
- Permanent pacemaker rarely required.

KEY FACT

Second-degree AV block type II (Mobitz II) = damage to the infranodal conducting system.

Second-Degree AV Block Type II (Mobitz II)

A significant rhythm associated with damage to the conducting system below the AV node (eg, **infranodal**). Progression without warning to complete heart block can occur, making this rhythm more concerning that Mobitz I.

Causes

Mobitz II, unlike the previously described AV blocks, does **not** occur in healthy hearts. Causes include:

- ACS (commonly **anteroseptal MI)**
- Hyperkalemia
- Fibrosing disease (eg, Lenegre disease)
- Infiltrative myocardial disease (eg, sarcoidosis, amyloidosis)
- Structural heart disease (congenital or surgical)
- Autoimmune disease (eg, lupus)

ECG Findings (Figure 1.12)

- PR interval constant
- P waves regular
- QRS complex regularly or randomly dropped
- QRS duration typically prolonged secondary to infranodal block

KEY FACT

Inferior MI → reversible AV block. Anteroseptal MI → permanent infranodal conduction system damage.

Treatment

- Symptomatic bradycardia → transcutaneous pacing and transvenous pacemaker placement.
- Atropine is **not** helpful and may actually **worsen** conduction ratio.
- Admission (unless chronic or asymptomatic).

KEY FACT

Atropine may actually worsen the conduction ratio with infranodal AV block (Mobitz II or infranodal third degree).

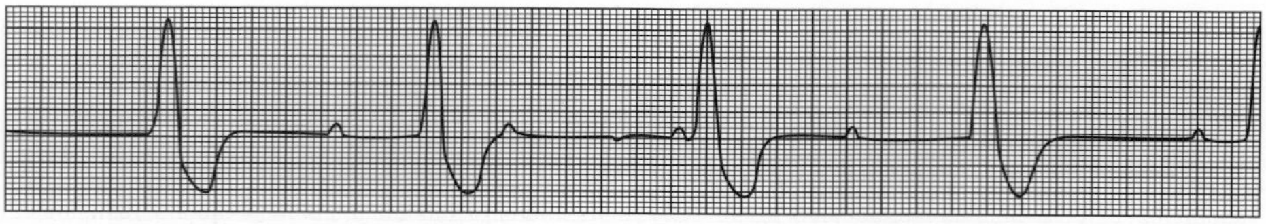

FIGURE 1.12. **Third-degree AV block.**

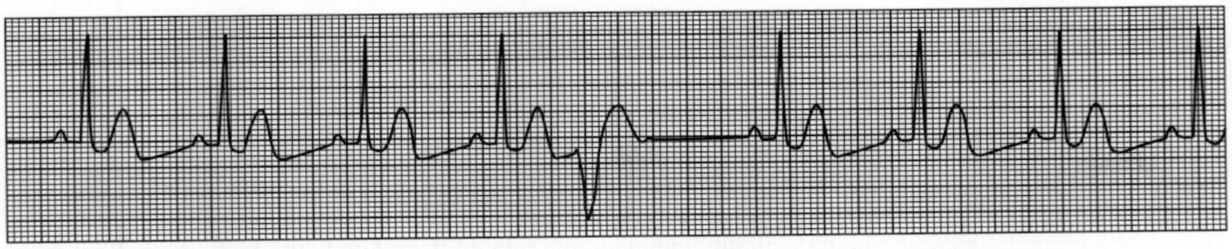

FIGURE 1.13. Premature ventricular contraction.

Third-Degree AV Block

Characterized by complete loss of AV conduction leading to a generally unstable rhythm notable for junctional and ventricular escape rhythms. Side effects include syncope, hypotension, and even death. Third-degree AV block can be due to damage to the AV node or the infranodal conducting system.

Causes

Causes are similar to second-degree AV block: congenital, medications (eg, β-blockers, calcium channel blockers, digoxin, etc), acute ischemia.

In the setting of ACS, third-degree AV block may be either nodal or infranodal.

- **Nodal** third-degree AV block is seen primarily with inferior MI and is typically transient.
- **Infranodal** third-degree AV block is seen in large anteroseptal MI from damage to the infranodal conducting system and is often permanent.

ECG Findings (Figure 1.13)

- No P waves conducted
- Nodal block → junctional escape rhythm (40-60 bpm), narrow complexes
- Infranodal block → ventricular escape rhythm (< 40 bpm), wide complexes
- Therefore, QRS duration depends on location of escape rhythm

Treatment

- Nodal
  - Atropine and transcutaneous pacing if symptomatic
  - Temporary transvenous pacemaker often required
- Infranodal
  - **Avoid: Atropine** (may worsen the conduction rate)
  - Isoproterenol (to increase ventricular rate) and transcutaneous pacing if symptomatic, until transvenous pacemaker placement
  - If congenital and asymptomatic, may not require immediate therapy

> **KEY FACT**
>
> Inferior MI → third-degree AV block with junctional escape (40-60 bpm) and narrow complexes. Anterior MI → third-degree AV block with ventricular escape (< 40 bpm) and wide complexes.

EXTRASYSTOLES

- Extrasystoles are ectopic impulses occurring **in addition to** regular sinus beats.
- Most extrasystoles are the result of enhanced automaticity, with resultant pattern based on location of ectopic foci.

Premature Atrial Contraction

Causes

Typically a normal variant; less likely because of ischemia, lung disease, hyperthyroidism, caffeine, nicotine

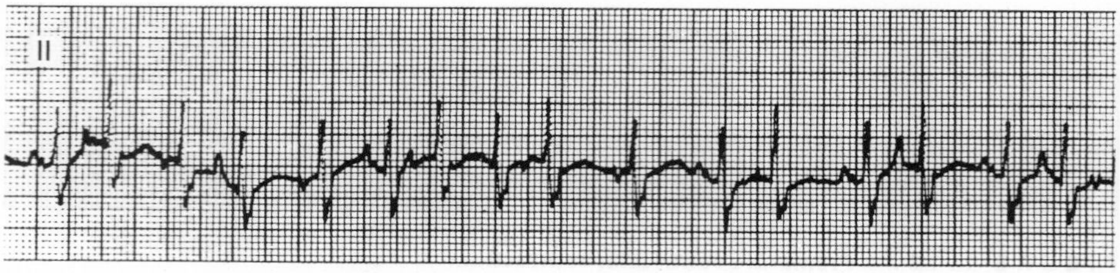

FIGURE 1.14. Multifocal atrial tachycardia. (Reproduced, with permission, from Tintinalli JE, Kelen GD, Stapczynski JS. *Emergency Medicine: A Comprehensive Study Guide.* 6th ed. New York, NY: McGraw-Hill; 2004:184.)

ECG Findings

- Premature beat with preceding P wave
- Narrow or wide QRS complex depending on timing
- Premature atrial contraction (PAC) P wave is **different** from a normal sinus P wave
- **Noncompensatory pause** (sinus node is depolarized early by the premature beat → next cycle of automated depolarization starts early → next normal beat is earlier than expected)

Complication

Precipitation of atrial tachycardia (AT), atrial flutter, atrial fibrillation (AFib)

Premature Ventricular Contraction

Causes

- Occasional premature ventricular contractions (PVCs) occur in healthy adults.
- Other etiologies: Stimulants (eg, caffeine, nicotine, cocaine), catecholamine surge (eg, pain), ischemia, electrolyte *abnormalities* (eg, hypokalemia), and medication toxicity.

ECG Findings (Figure 1.14)

- Premature wide QRS without preceding P wave
- Appropriate discordance present (ST segment, T wave opposite major QRS deflection)
- Interpolated between normal beats
- **Fully compensatory pause** (typically seen on a nonconducted P wave within the PVC; the PVC itself does not "reset" the sinus node and P waves continue at regular intervals after the PVC)
- ≥ 3 PVCs = nonsustained VT

DYSRHYTHMIAS

> **KEY FACT**
>
> **Three mechanisms of tachydysrhythmias:**
> Increased automaticity
> Reentry
> Triggered rhythm

Dysrhythmias can be grouped based on whether the resulting ventricular rate is too slow or too fast.

Rates that are slow (bradydysrhythmias) can result from the following:

- Disordered impulse generation
- Abnormal impulse conduction

Rates that are too fast (tachydysrhythmias) may result from 3 mechanisms:

- **Increased automaticity** of a sinus or ectopic focus
- **Reentry** via AV node or accessory pathway
- **Triggered arrhythmia** (eg, R on T)

TABLE 1.9. Tachycardia Differential Diagnosis

	Regular	Irregular
Narrow	Sinus tachycardia Atrial tachycardia Atrial flutter with fixed block AVNRT	Sinus tachycardia with PACs Atrial fibrillation MAT Atrial flutter with variable block
Wide	Regular SVT with BBB Regular SVT with preexcitation Ventricular tachycardia V paced	Irregular SVT with BBB Irregular SVT with preexcitation Ventricular fibrillation Torsade de pointes

AVNRT, AV-nodal reentrant tachycardia; BBB, bundle branch block; MAT, multifocal atrial tachycardia; PAC, premature atrial contraction; SVT, supraventricular tachycardia.

Q

A 52-year-old man is brought to the ED by ambulance complaining of palpitations, shortness of breath, and chest pain. He is diaphoretic and pale, speaking in 3-word sentences and clutching his chest. After being transferred to a gurney, cardiac monitor demonstrates a wide complex rhythm at 175 bpm. His BP is 85/60 mm Hg and his respiratory rate (RR) is 30 breaths/min. How should you proceed?

Tachydysrhythmias

The differential diagnosis for tachydysrhythmias can be narrowed by assessing whether the rhythm is regular or irregular, wide or narrow, and whether p waves are present (Table 1.9).

NARROW COMPLEX TACHYCARDIAS

Sinus Tachycardia

Diagnosis and Causes

There are many causes of sinus tachycardia, including:

- HR increases to maintain cardiac output (eg, in setting of exercise)
  - Decreased effective circulating volume (eg, hypovolemia, anemia, abnormal hemoglobin function)
  - Impaired cardiac function (MI, ACS, valvular disease, tamponade)
  - PE
  - Hypoxia
- **Metabolic/endocrine derangements**
  - Diabetic ketoacidosis (DKA)
  - Hyperthyroidism
  - Adrenal insufficiency
  - Fever/sepsis/systemic inflammatory response syndrome (SIRS)
  - Drug ingestions (sympathomimetics)
  - Drug/alcohol withdrawal
  - Anxiety or pain

ECG Findings

- Regular rhythm
- P waves precede all QRS complexes
- Atrial rate typically 100-160 bpm

Treatment

Treat the underlying condition.

Atrial Tachycardia

Atrial tachycardia (AT) results when an ectopic atrial focus becomes the dominant pacemaker within the right or left atrium.

A

This patient has a wide complex tachycardia and is symptomatic with chest pain, shortness of breath, and hypotension. You are not given any further information to differentiate this rhythm from supraventricular tachycardia (SVT) with aberrancy, so treat the rhythm as unstable VT. Start with immediate **synchronized** cardioversion at 100 J.

KEY FACT

Atrial tachycardia with AV block (typically 2:1) is classic for digoxin toxicity!

KEY FACT

Atrial tachycardia is typically due to an underlying medical (not a cardiac) condition.

KEY FACT

Vagal maneuvers and adenosine are typically unsuccessful in AT and MAT.

CAUSES

- Can be triggered by a PAC (especially in individuals with structural heart disease)
- Electrolyte abnormalities
- Drugs (think **digoxin**, especially if 2:1 or higher grade AV block noted!)
- Fever
- Hypoxia

ECG FINDINGS

- Regular narrow complex tachycardia
- P wave before each QRS
- P waves with abnormal morphologies (eg, inverted in inferior leads)
- Atrial rate typically 130-250 bpm

TREATMENT

- Usually self-limited, does not require therapy.
- If not, treat the underlying condition.
- For hemodynamically stable patient with symptomatic AT:
  - Rate control with diltiazem, β-blockers
- For hemodynamically unstable patient:
  - Electrical cardioversion (likely to be unsuccessful if secondary to enhanced automaticity) or amiodarone

Multifocal Atrial Tachycardia

A subset of AT, multifocal atrial tachycardia (MAT) occurs when multiple ectopic foci stimulate the atria.

CAUSES

Often associated with **COPD**, and less frequently with hypoxia and electrolyte disturbances (eg, hypokalemia, hypomagnesemia)

ECG FINDINGS (FIGURE 1.15)

- Irregular narrow complex tachycardia.
- ≥ 3 P wave morphologies present.
- Atrial rate > 100 bpm (defined as wandering atrial pacemaker if 60-100 bpm).
- P wave before each QRS.
- PP, PR, and RR intervals **vary**.

TREATMENT

- Usually a stable rhythm not requiring antiarrhythmic therapy (treat the underlying condition).
- If unstable, rate control with verapamil, β-blockers.
- Direct current (DC) cardioversion is frequently ineffective in converting MAT to sinus rhythm and an aberrant rhythm will likely recur.

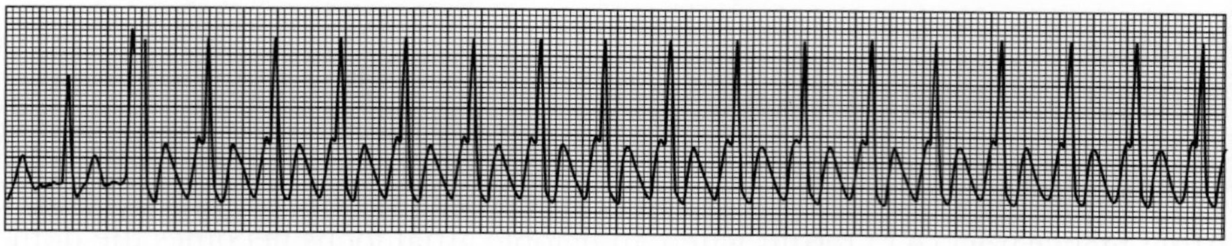

FIGURE 1.15. Atrial flutter.

Supraventricular Tachycardia

Supraventricular tachycardia (SVT) is a broad category that includes macro-reentrant circuits (AVRT), micro-reentrant circuits (AVNRT), atrial reentrant circuits (atrial flutter), AFib, and enhanced automaticity (sinus tachycardia, MAT, AT).

Atrial Flutter

Atrial flutter is a type of SVT caused by a reentry circuit in the right atrium. Because of the length of the circuit, the atrial depolarization rate is typically predictable (~300 bpm) and no coordinated atrial contraction activity is present.

Causes

- Idiopathic
- Valvular heart disease
- Cardiomyopathies
- Post-CABG (coronary artery bypass grafting)
- Electrolyte, metabolic, or hormonal (eg, hyperthyroidism) abnormalities
- PE
- Chronic lung disease

ECG Findings (Figure 1.16)

- Hallmark: ECG with characteristic "saw tooth pattern."
- Regular atrial rate ranges from 250 to 350 bpm.
- In the absence of a atopic conduction tract, AV node refractory period typically conducts every 2 to 3 atrial impulses, thus, classically, the ventricular rate is 150 bpm secondary to 2:1 conduction.

KEY FACT

The ventricular rate in untreated atrial flutter is typically 150 bpm due to 2:1 conduction of atrial impulses.

Diagnosis

If unable to determine via ECG, **adenosine** can be used to block the AV node and "uncover" the underlying atrial tachycardic rhythm.

Treatment

- If patient **unstable** → synchronized cardioversion.
  - Unlike AFib, atrial flutter is **very sensitive** to conversion and often successful with minimal energy (eg, 25-50 J)
- If patient stable → rate control with AV-node blocking agents (eg, diltiazem or β-blockers).
- Chemical conversion can be attempted, but unlike AFib, atrial flutter is more resistant to chemical conversion. Medications that can be considered include amiodarone, ibutilide (class III), procainamide.

KEY FACT

If antidromic conduction of an accessory pathway is **suspected (eg, delta wave or wide complex tachycardia),** AVOID AV-nodal blocking drugs!

Atrial Fibrillation

Atrial fibrillation (AFib) is **disorganized** chaos. Multiple reentry atrial circuits generate 300-600 atrial impulses per minute with **no** associated organized atrial contraction. As with atrial flutter, the ventricular rate is limited by the AV node or accessory pathway refractory period.

KEY FACT

Alcohol use is commonly associated with AFib.

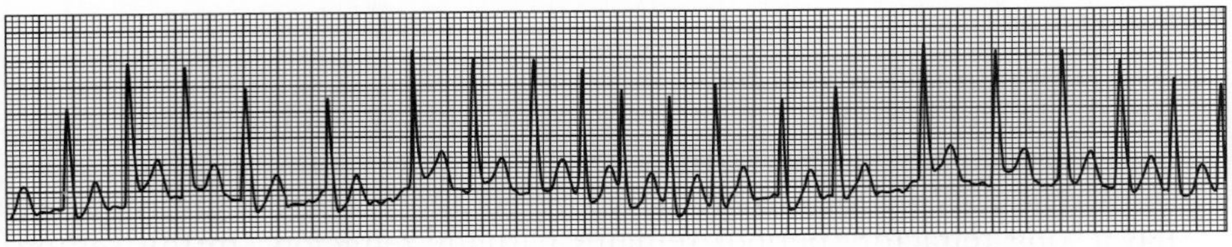

FIGURE 1.16. Atrial fibrillation.

CAUSES

Causes are similar to atrial flutter (valvular heart disease, cardiomyopathy, pericarditis, hyperthyroidism, PE, postcardiac surgery), but one should also consider hypertensive heart disease, congestive heart failure (CHF), acute alcohol intoxication (eg, "holiday heart"), as well as idiopathic causes (eg, lone AFib)

KEY FACT

QRS complexes are narrow in AFib unless there is a preexisting conduction block or an accessory pathway.

ECG FINDINGS (FIGURE 1.16)

- Hallmark: Irregularly irregular QRS pattern (often most notable in inferior leads or V_1). QRS complex is typically narrow unless accessory pathway conduction present (eg, Wolff-Parkinson-White [WPW] syndrome)
- P waves ABSENT
- Ventricular rates limited by AV node refraction (typically < 175 bpm)
- Ventricular rates > 200 bpm **strongly suggest presence** of an accessory pathway

TREATMENT

- If **unstable** → synchronized direct current cardioversion
  - Recent studies suggest that for AFib present for > 24-48 hours, increased levels of energy should be considered (eg, consider starting at 200 J or 360 J, instead of the previously considered 50-100 J). Consider sedation, if time allows.
- If stable → treatment depends on time of onset and etiology
  - New-onset/newly recurrent AFib (eg, < 48 hours duration), cardioversion can be considered an option. Outside that window, a transesophageal echocardiogram can assess for intracardiac thrombus and, if not present, cardioversion can be considered.
  - Conversion can also be accomplished via pharmacologic conversion. Most common agents include amiodarone, ibutilide (class III), dofetilide (class III), procainamide (class IA)
  - Patient with more chronic symptoms, or if the time frame of symptom onset is uncertain, pharmacologic rate control should be considered first-line treatment because it is more important than actual rhythm. Rate control with AV-node blocking agents (eg, diltiazem or β-blockers), with goal heart rate < 120 bpm. Anticoagulation must also be considered. The physician can reference the **$CHADS_2$** score (Table 1.10) for treatment guidelines.

KEY FACT

AV-nodal blocking drugs should be avoided in AFib or AFlutter if an accessory pathway is suspected.

COMPLICATIONS

- If an accessory pathway is suspected, AVOID AV-nodal blocking drugs, because these agents can augment conduction down the bypass tract, paradoxically increasing the ventricular rate and risking degeneration to VFib.
- If an accessory pathway is suspected, and the patient is stable, procainamide should be considered because it has no effect on AV conduction.
- Stroke secondary to increased embolic/thrombolic risk.

AV-Nodal Reentrant Tachycardia

PATHOPHYSIOLOGY

- Also known as paroxysmal SVT.
- Results from the formation of a reentrant pathway within the AV node. More specifically, a PAC arrives when the slow pathway (which has a short refractory period) has fully recovered and the fast pathway (which has a long refractory period) remains partially refractory. In this setting, the impulse travels down the slow pathway **only**, because the fast pathway

TABLE 1.10. CHADS$_2$ Score to Predict Risk of Stroke in Patients with Chronic Atrial Fibrillation

	Variable	Points
C	CHF	1
H	Hypertension	1
A	Age > 75 y	1
D	Diabetes	1
S	Prior TIA or stroke	2

Score and Treatment Guidelines:

0: nothing or full-dose aspirin

1: full-dose aspirin

> 1: warfarin with INR goal between 2 and 3

CHF, congestive heart failure; INR, international normalized ratio; TIA; transient ischemic attack.

remains refractory. But, by the time it arrives at the distal AV node, the fast pathway is no longer refractory, allowing it to travel retrograde up the fast pathway establishing the reentry circuit, while activating the Bundle of His in a typical anterograde fashion.

- AV-nodal reentrant tachycardia (AVNRT), in the absence of cardiopulmonary disease, is usually a clinically stable dysrhythmia.

Causes

Typically abrupt onset with/without inciting event. Can occur in setting of emotional stress, exercise, or stimulant use (eg, nicotine, caffeine, amphetamines).

ECG Findings (Figure 1.17)

- Hallmark: Narrow QRS, rate between 140 and 280 bpm, with **no** visible P waves.
- Inverted P waves (representing retrograde conduction) are buried in the QRS complex and thus typically not present (if visible, typically seen in leads II, III, and aVF).

Treatment

- If patient unstable → synchronized DC cardioversion (100-200 J), unless adenosine immediately available.
- If patient stable → first attempt vagal maneuvers and if that fails consider adenosine 6-mg IV bolus followed by 12-mg IV bolus if ineffective after 2 minutes. If rhythm remains refractory, consider diltiazem, verapamil, or β-blockers.

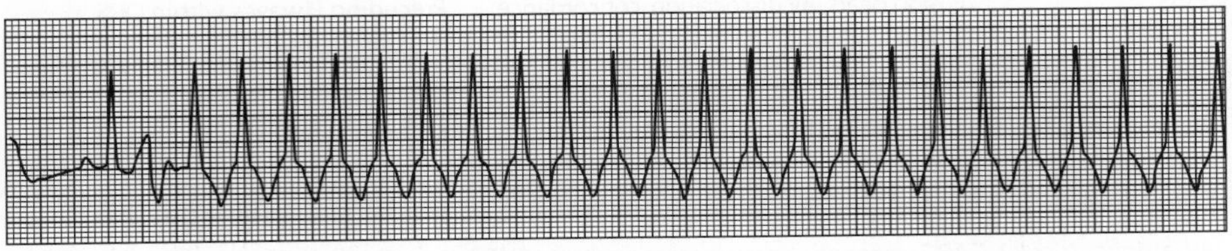

FIGURE 1.17. AV-nodal reentrant tachycardia.

KEY FACT

Vagal maneuvers and adenosine will be effective in the vast majority of patients with AVNRT.

- Vagal maneuvers:
  - Valsalva (at least 10-second strain phase).
  - Carotid sinus massage (ensure no carotid bruit present prior to attempting and even if absent, be wary in elderly population as increased risk of embolic event). Steady pressure or circular massage along the carotid pulse for 5-10 seconds.
  - Diving reflex: Immerse face in cold water for 10-20 seconds (more effective in infants).
- Ablation may be considered in recurrent episodes poorly controlled by medical management.

WIDE COMPLEX TACHYCARDIAS

Pathophysiology

- QRS duration > 0.12 second
- Can originate from:
  - Ventricles (eg, Vtach)
  - Supraventricular with aberrant AV conduction (eg, accessory pathway)

KEY FACT

When in doubt, treat any wide complex tachycardia as VT!

Ventricular Tachycardia

Initially, it can be difficult to distinguish whether a wide complex tachycardia is ventricular tachycardia (VT) or SVT with an accessory pathway. That said, the consequences of VT are typically more grave than those associated with SVT; therefore, all new wide complex tachycardias should be initially presumed VT. In short, SVT with aberrancy should be a diagnosis of **exclusion**. An approach using a combination of historical clues and general ECG characteristics (Table 1.11) can assist the provider in delineating between VT and SVT.

- **Monomorphic VT**
  - Most common form of VT
- Ectopic beats are morphologically the same (eg, QRS is morphologically consistent), with regular pattern, and rate of 150-200 bpm.
- **Polymorphic VT**
  - QRS morphology continuously varies (usually requires > 1 ECG lead to see variation)
  - Usually hemodynamically unstable requiring urgent defibrillation
  - Most often due to cardiac ischemia in absence of QT prolongation

TABLE 1.11. Differentiating VT from SVT with Aberrancy

Feature	VT	SVT
Age (in years)	> 50	< 40
Medical history	MI, CHF, CABG, previous VT	Previous SVT
ECG	Fusion beats, AV dissociation, concordance, QRS > 0.12, extreme left axis	Preceding P waves within QRS complex, QRS < 0.12, normal axis
Vagal maneuvers	No response to vagal maneuvers	Slows or terminates with vagal maneuvers

AV, atrioventricular; CABG, coronary artery bypass grafting; CHF, congestive heart failure; MI, myocardial infarction; VT, ventricular tachycardia; SVT, supraventricular tachycardia.

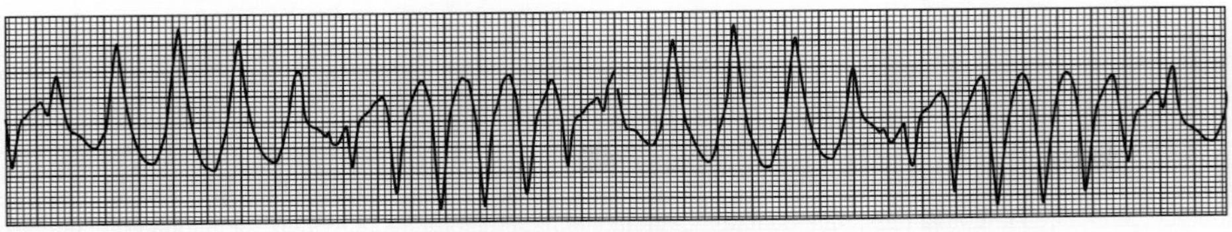

FIGURE 1.18. Torsades de pointes (atypical ventricular tachycardia).

Common variants of VT include:

- **Torsade de pointes (eg, "twisting of the points")**
  - Paroxysmal form of polymorphic VT.
  - Occurs secondary to a prolonged QT interval (that can be acquired, more common, or congenital, more rare).
  - Acquired QT prolongation is commonly associated with medications such as haloperidol, TCAs, antibiotics (eg, macrolides, erythromycin), methadone, antihistamines, antiemetics, anticonvulsants, and electrolyte abnormalities (eg, hypokalemia, hypomagnesemia, and hypocalcemia).
  - Typically presents with polymorphic VT (often described as sinusoidal), with a shifting QRS axis, and rates > 200 bpm (Figure 1.18).
  - Treatment: Unstable patients are treated with DC conversion (although synchronization is impossible) as well as IV magnesium sulfate (1-2 g over 1 minute, then 1-2 g/h infusion), even if patient has normal Mg+ levels. If refractory, consider overdrive pacing (external or transvenous) and avoid drugs that can prolong repolarization (eg, procainamide).
- **Bidirectional VT**
  - Unique form of VT where QRS axis changes (eg, 180° from left to right with each alternate beat) and is typically associated with **severe digitalis toxicity**.
  - Treatment: DC cardioversion typically unsuccessful in setting of severe digitalis toxicity. Consider continuous cardiopulmonary resuscitation (CPR) coupled with high-dose Digoxin Immune Fab.
- **Brugada syndrome**
  - Hereditary syndrome characterized by structurally **normal** heart, associated with ventricular dysrhythmias → syncope and sudden cardiac death (Figure 1.19).

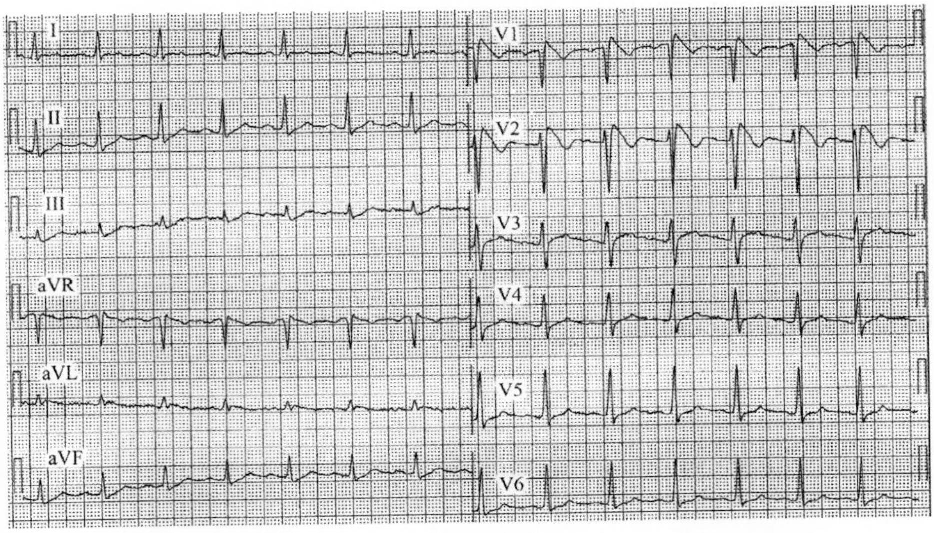

FIGURE 1.19. Typical ECG for Brugada syndrome. (Reproduced, with permission, from Fuster V, Walsh RA, O'Rourke RA, Poole-Wilson P. *Hurst's The Heart*. Vol 2. 12th ed. New York, NY: McGraw-Hill; 2008:1661.)

Q

A 45-year-old man presents to the ED complaining of palpitations. He has a history of alcohol abuse and chronic pain, for which he takes a TCA. He is awake and alert with a BP of 120/60 mm Hg and an initial pulse of 90 bpm. The monitor shows intermittent runs of torsade de pointes. What is your initial treatment for this patient?

KEY FACT

Torsade is due to prolongation of repolarization (QT interval).

A

Torsade is a type of polymorphic VT that occurs in the setting of prolonged repolarization, which in this patient is likely due to hypokalemia, hypomagnesemia, and/or TCA use. Because he is stable, begin treatment with a magnesium sulfate infusion. If this is unsuccessful, try shortening repolarization by increasing the ventricular rate via isoproterenol infusion or overdrive pacing.

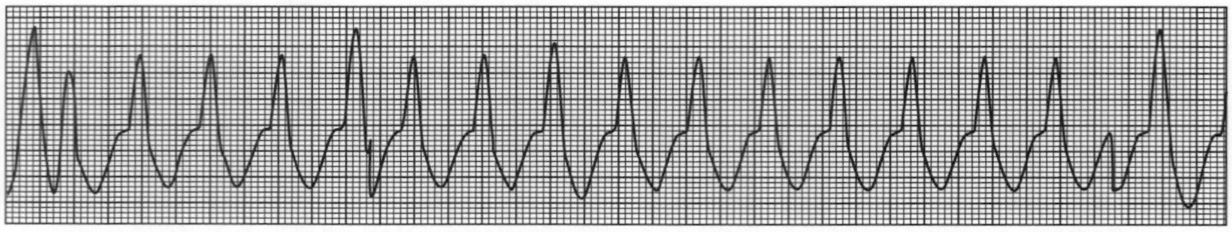

FIGURE 1.20. Ventricular tachycardia.

- Results from an inherited sodium channelopathy and most commonly seen in younger men of Asian descent.
- Hallmark: Coved/downward humped ST segment in V_1-V_3 (Figure 1.20), that can simulate a right bundle branch block (RBBB), **and** history of symptoms (eg, syncope).
- ECG findings **often** transient.
- Treatment: Patients with syncope and Brugada-pattern on ECG **require** implanted defibrillator. Patients with no symptoms, but Brugada-pattern on ECG, should be referred to cardiology.

Causes

Causes of VT include:
- Structural heart disease (CAD, cardiomyopathy most common)
- Trauma
- Hypothermia
- Hypoxia
- Severe electrolyte abnormalities
- Familial disorders (eg, Brugada syndrome, congenital long QT syndrome)
- Medications that prolong QT

KEY FACT

In the patient with prior MI, wide complex tachycardia is nearly always VT.

ECG Findings Associated with VT (Figure 1.21)

- VT originates within or below the bundle of His and therefore presents with a regular **wide** complex tachycardia (eg, QRS > 0.12 second)
- Inappropriately concordant QRS complexes (monophasic with same polarity) across the precordial leads
- AV dissociation (**especially** atrial rate slower than ventricular rate)
- Fusion complexes (ventricle **simultaneously** activated by supraventricular and ventricular impulse)
- Capture beats (QRS with sinus morphology reflecting normal conduction for single beat)

Brugada ECG Criteria for VT

- Absence of RS complexes in all precordial leads
- If RS complex present → RS duration > 0.1 second
- Presence of AV dissociation
- Presence of specific VT morphology

If **any** of the above the criteria are met, the diagnosis = VT. Only if **none** of the criteria are met can the diagnosis of SVT be considered.

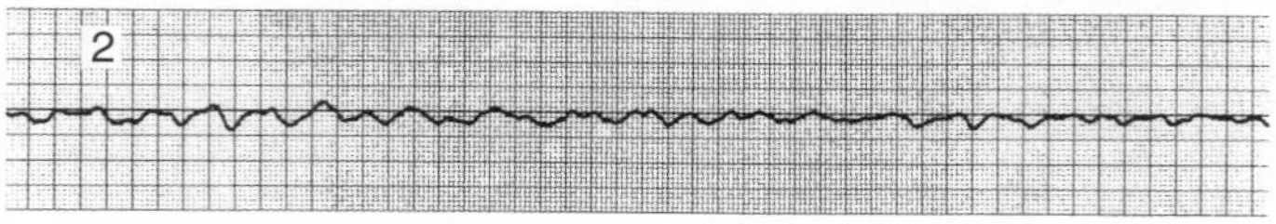

FIGURE 1.21. Ventricular fibrillation. (Reproduced, with permission, from Tintinalli JE, Kelen GD, Stapczynski JS. *Emergency Medicine: A Comprehensive Study Guide.* 6th ed. New York, NY: McGraw-Hill; 2004:191.)

TREATMENT

- **Pulseless** → immediate cardioversion (see the section "Management of Cardiac Arrest")
- **Unstable** → synchronized cardioversion starting at 100 J (sedate if possible)
- **Stable**
  - First-line pharmacotherapy: Amiodarone 150 mg IV over 10 minutes (repeat if necessary) followed by continuous infusion of 1 mg/min for 6 hours and 0.5 mg/min for another 18 hours, or procainamide 20-50 mg/min until arrhythmia terminates, hypotension, or QRS is prolonged by > 50%, or a total of 17 mg/kg.
  - Second-line pharmacotherapy: Lidocaine 1.0-1.5 mg/kg IV every 5 minutes up to 3 mg/kg/h.
  - **Or** synchronized cardioversion.
- Refractory stable VT → synchronized cardioversion as previously

Ventricular Fibrillation

Ventricular fibrillation (Vfib) is total disorganized ventricular depolarization. With ventricle impulse rates ranging up to 500 bpm, total loss of synchronized ventricular contraction occurs, leading to complete loss of cardiac output.

ECG FINDINGS (FIGURE 1.22)

- Chaotic irregular zigzag pattern of varying amplitude
- No identifiable p waves or QRS complexes
- Rate varying between 150 and 500 bpm
- As time passes, amplitude typically decreases (eg, initially coarse → fine)

CAUSES

MI, cardiomyopathy, degradation of VT (especially Brugada and torsade de pointes), PE, hypothermia, drowning, electrical injuries

TREATMENT

Defibrillation (for more information, reference the section "Management of Cardiac Arrest")

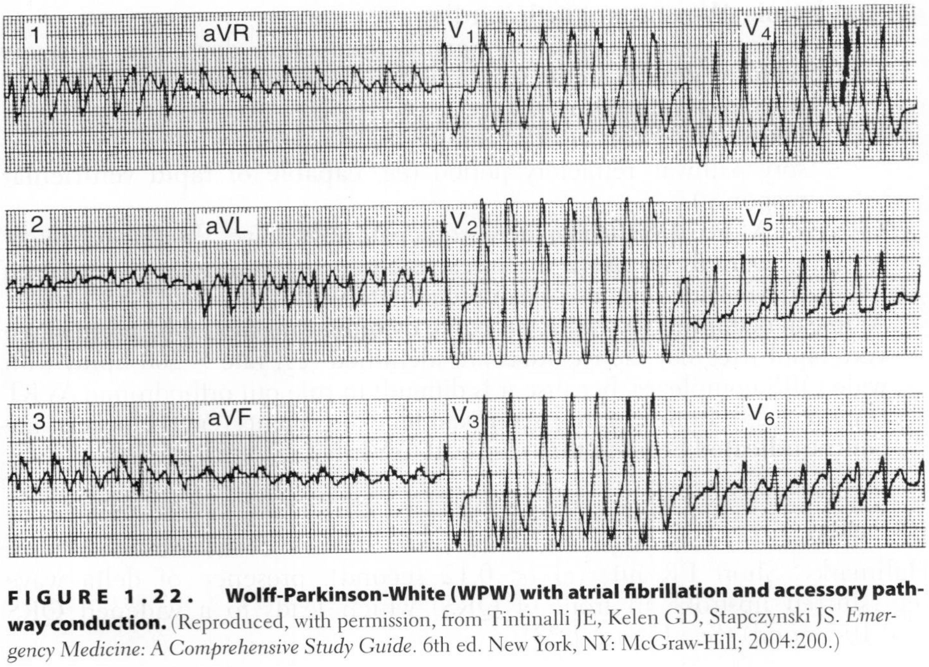

FIGURE 1.22. Wolff-Parkinson-White (WPW) with atrial fibrillation and accessory pathway conduction. (Reproduced, with permission, from Tintinalli JE, Kelen GD, Stapczynski JS. *Emergency Medicine: A Comprehensive Study Guide*. 6th ed. New York, NY: McGraw-Hill; 2004:200.)

PREEXCITATION AND ACCESSORY PATHWAY SYNDROMES

KEY FACT

The bundle of Kent bypasses the AV node and His/Purkinje system in WPW connecting the atrium directly to the ventricle.

KEY FACT

A bypass tract may be completely hidden on the resting ECG.

KEY FACT

Conduction in orthodromic AVRT is limited by the refractory period of the AV node, whereas antidromic AVRT can conduct at very rapid ventricular rates due to the shorter refractory period of the accessory pathway.

Preexcitation refers to an accessory pathway that allows for ventricular depolarization that **bypasses** the AV node. This unique syndrome allows for the formation of AV reentrant circuits that can lead to sustained tachycardias at very high heart rates that lead to a nonperfusing rhythm.

Wolff-Parkinson-White Syndrome

- Wolff-Parkinson-White (WPW) syndrome is the most common type of atrioventricular reentrant tachycardia (AVRT) or accessory pathway syndrome.
- The accessory pathway in WPW = Bundle of Kent. The bundle of Kent bypasses the AV node, connecting the atrium directly to the ventricle.

Pathophysiology

- **Conduction in sinus rhythm:**
  - Impulses travel down both the accessory pathway **and** the AV node to the ventricle → **shortened PR** (secondary to shorter refractory period) and slurred upstroke of QRS complex (**delta wave**) on resting ECG.
  - It is possible that the bypass tract is **completely hidden** during normal conduction.
- **Tachyarrhythmias**
  - Coupling the impulses from the AV node with an accessory pathway, a reentry circuit can be formed → sustained tachycardias (eg, orthodromic/antidromic AVRT, AFib, atrial flutter). There are 2 types of reentry circuits:
  - **Orthodromic AV-reentrant tachycardia**
    - Reentry circuit with anterograde conduction down the AV node to the ventricular myocardium and retrograde conduction up the accessory pathway
    - **Hallmark**: Narrow QRS complex and rate controlled by AV node refractory period (eg, constrained rate)
    - Fortunately, more common (90%) than antidromic AVRT
- **Antidromic AV-reentrant tachycardia**
    - Reentry circuit with anterograde conduction down the accessory pathway directly to the ventricular myocardium and retrograde conduction via the AV node.
    - **Hallmark:** Wide QRS complex and rate-controlled by accessory pathway refractory period (eg, **capable of rapid ventricular response).**
      - More specifically, accessory pathways have shorter refractory periods → **more** impulses reaching the ventricle → very high ventricular rates → can precipitate VFib
- AFib can occur in this setting, therefore **extreme** care should be taken when very rapid irregular tachycardias are identified (eg, rate > 200 bpm) with wide QRS complexes, because it is difficult to rule out orthodromic AVRT (Figure 1.23). In this setting, AV nodal blocking agents (eg, β-blockers) are **contraindicated** because they can lead to VFib.

ECG Findings

Hallmarks: Short PR interval (< 0.12 second); presence of delta wave (eg, slurred upstroke in front of QRS) which leads to a widened QRS (> 0.10 second) (See Figure 1.23).

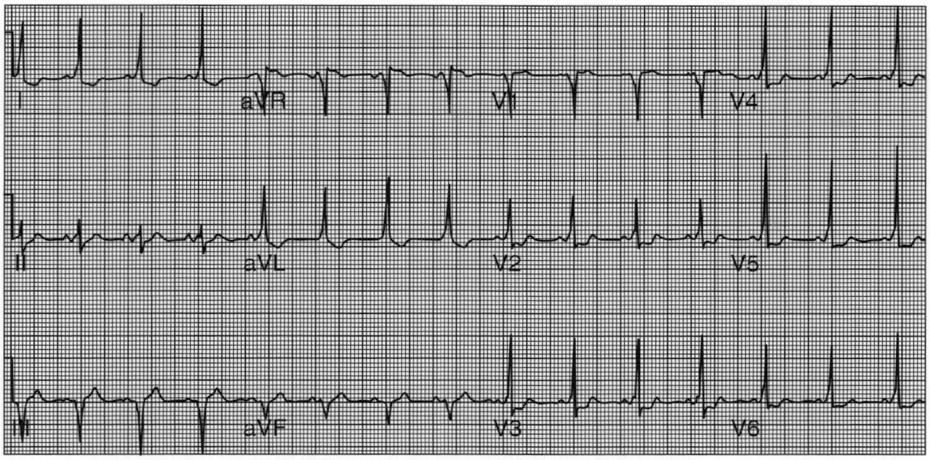

FIGURE 1.23. Delta wave on resting ECG.

Q

During resuscitation of a witnessed arrest, you ensured that CPR was minimally interrupted and proper technique was employed. However, the patient still suffered hypoxic cerebral and cardiac injury. Why?

Treatment

- Narrow complex tachycardia (orthodromic)
  - Implies conduction through the AV node → can treat similar to AVNRT (earlier)
- Wide complex tachycardia (antidromic)
  - Implies AV conduction **through the accessory pathway**.
  - **Avoid all AV blocking agents** (may precipitate VFib).
  - **Stable patient**: Medical therapy with IV procainamide or ibutilide.
    - Prolongs accessory pathway refractory period
    - Shortens AV node refractoriness and increases transmission through AV node
  - **Unstable patient**: Perform synchronized electrical cardioversion (50-100 J).

KEY FACT

WPW with narrow complex tachycardia → treatment is similar to AVNRT (AV blocking drugs **are** OK).

KEY FACT

Therapeutic options for patients with WPW who present with rapid AFib are procainamide, ibutilide, or electrical cardioversion.

Lown-Ganong-Levine Syndrome

- Accessory pathway = James fibers.
- Pathway connects the atria directly to the His bundle.
- ECG shows a **very short** PR interval with **normal** P waves and QRS complexes (eg, no delta waves).

Management of Cardiac Arrest

KEY FACT

Pediatric cardiac arrest is most commonly due to hypoxia or shock.

The 4 causes of sudden cardiac arrest (SCA) include VFib, pulseless VT, PEA, and asystole.

In comparison to the adult population, a primary cardiac event is uncommon in children. Pediatric arrest is most commonly **secondary** to hypoxia or shock.

BASIC CARDIOPULMONARY RESUSCITATION

The basic tenet of cardiopulmonary resuscitation (CPR) is to generate enough blood flow to provide oxygen to the brain and heart. Immediate CPR is vital to preventing anoxic brain injury and maximizing the likelihood of restoring spontaneous circulation.

A

Even properly performed closed chest CPR only provides 25% of prearrest cardiac output. Coronary and cerebral blood flow also falls to 5% and 10%, respectively. Early CPR and defibrillation for witnessed cardiac arrest are critical to improving chances of survival.

TABLE 1.12. CPR in the Emergency Department

	Pediatric	Adult
	Ventilation	
Rate (breaths/min)	BVM: 8-10	BVM: 8-10
	Compression	
Position	Lower half of sternum Infant: 2 thumb-encircling hands Child: Heel of hand or as for adults	Lower half of sternum Heel of one hand, other hand on top
Depth	1/3-1/2 depth of chest	~2 in
Rate	100/min	100/min
Ratio to ventilation	BVM: 15:2 (pause for 2 breaths every 15 compressions) ET tube: No pauses for ventilation	BVM: 30:2 ET tube: No pauses for ventilation
Defibrillation	Use pediatric pads when possible No recommendations for infants	Use adult pads

BVM, bag valve mask; CPR, cardiopulmonary resuscitation; ET, endotracheal.

Initial step for health care providers:

- For sudden collapse (all ages) → phone or call for automated external defibrillator (AED) prior to initiating CPR
- For arrest likely due to asphyxia → immediate CPR prior to calling for help

The technique for adult and pediatric CPR in the ED assumes that multiple providers are present (Table 1.12).

Chest Compressions

The 2010 advanced cardiac life support (ACLS) guidelines recommend beginning CPR in adults with 30 chest compressions, before giving rescue breaths. Chest compressions may either push the blood out by direct compression of the heart (**cardiac pump theory**) or create flow via a pressure gradient between the intrathoracic arteries of the chest and the extrathoracic arteries of the body (**thoracic pump theory**). The goal is to maximize coronary perfusion pressure (CPP) = aortic diastolic pressure – left ventricular end diastolic pressure. CPP of at least 15 mm Hg is needed to achieve return of spontaneous circulation (ROSC).

KEY FACT

CPP = aortic diastolic pressure – left ventricular end diastolic pressure. CPP of at least 15 mm Hg is needed to achieve ROSC.

Airway and Breathing

Assess airway patency by opening the airway with a head tilt and chin lift (jaw thrust alone if suspected cervical spine trauma) and administer 2 rescue breaths. Perform early endotracheal intubation, or place a supraglottic airway device with end-tidal CO_2 monitoring. Do not delay CPR for basic or advanced airway maneuvers. Airway should be addressed early if the cause of SCA is a hypoxic respiratory arrest.

Principles of high-quality CPR (goal is to maintain CPP)

- Compression rate at least 100/min with adequate compression depth and complete recoil between each compression ("push hard, push fast").
- Minimize interruptions in chest compressions.
- Avoid excessive ventilation, which decreases venous return and CPP.
- If end-tidal CO_2 < 10 mm Hg, attempt to improve CPR quality.

NEONATAL RESUSCITATION

Newborn resuscitation differs from adult and pediatric resuscitation in that the initial approach focuses almost entirely on management of the airway and breathing. A primary cardiac etiology is uncommon.

Immediately after delivery, the infant airway should be suctioned with a bulb syringe (mouth, then nares) only if obvious airway obstruction is present or if the infant is nonvigorous with meconium-stained amniotic fluid. The infant should be placed under a warmer, dried, and positioned to open airway (head tilt); stimulated; and assessed for respiratory effort and HR.

Indications for further neonatal resuscitation:

- Apnea
- HR < 100 bpm

TREATMENT

- Place infant in radiant warmer.
- **Airway:**
  - **If meconium present** and unresponsive → immediate intubation and perform endotracheal suctioning.
  - Otherwise, warm infant and provide tactile stimulation.
- **Reassess RR and HR** after 30 seconds.
  - **If still bradycardic or apneic, initiate positive pressure ventilation** via BVM with room air at 40-60 breaths/min. If persistently hypoxemic, provide supplemental oxygen.
- Reassess RR and HR after 30 seconds.
  - If apneic or HR < 100 bpm (by umbilical pulse or auscultation of precordium) after BVM → **intubate and ventilate**.
- **Reassess HR** after 30 seconds.
  - If HR < 60 bpm → begin **chest compressions**.
    - Thumbs just below nipple line with hands encircling the chest or two-finger technique
    - Depth = 1/3 depth of chest
    - Compression rate = 90/min: Ventilation rate = 30/min
      - Compression: ventilation ratio **3:1** (with pauses for ventilation)
- **Reassess HR** after 30 seconds.
  - If HR < 60 bpm → begin **drug therapy**
    - Epinephrine 0.1-0.3 mL/kg IV using 0.1-mg/mL epinephrine (also labeled 1:10,000) (0.01-0.03 mg/kg).
    - Narcan 0.1 mg/kg IV/IO (intraosseous): Use is controversial and no longer recommended in American Heart Association (AHA) guidelines. For persistent respiratory depression suspected due to maternal narcotic use, support respiratory status with intubation and ventilation.
    - Glucose 5 mL/kg of D_{10W}.
    - Normal saline (NS) bolus: 10 mL/kg infused over 5-10 minutes.

Q

You are called to assess a newborn that was just delivered in your ambulance bay. He has been placed under a warmer and is being dried. On examination, he has spontaneous respirations, poor tone, and a HR of 90 bpm. There was no meconium present on delivery. What is your first step in the management of this neonate?

KEY FACT

Factors that worsen CPP:

Interrupting chest compressions
Overventilation
Improper technique

KEY FACT

Indications for neonatal resuscitation:

Apnea
HR < 100 bpm

A

This neonate needs further resuscitation because his HR is < 100 bpm. The focus should initially be on airway and breathing, beginning with (if no meconium is present) positive pressure ventilation via BVM at a rate of 40-60 breaths/min. Room air should be used initially, with supplemental O_2 administration as guided by pulse oximetry. If the HR is not improved after 30 seconds, intubate and provide further positive pressure ventilation. A HR < 100 bpm after an additional 30 seconds is indication for chest compressions followed by cardiac drugs, fluid bolus, and supplemental glucose.

KEY FACT

Drug therapy in neonatal resuscitation:

Epinephrine
Glucose
NS fluid bolus

KEY FACT

Shorter time from onset of SCA to defibrillation = single best determinant of ROSC and neurologically intact survival in cardiac arrest.

MNEMONIC

The treatable causes of cardiac arrest, 6 Hs and 5 Ts:

Hypoxia
Hydrogen ion overload (acidosis)
Hyperkalemia/hypokalemia
Hypoglycemia
Hypothermia
Hypovolemia
Toxins
Tamponade (cardiac)
Tension pneumothorax
Thromboembolism (PE)
Thrombosis (coronary)

PULSELESS VENTRICULAR TACHYCARDIA AND VENTRICULAR FIBRILLATION

The 2010 ACLS cardiac arrest algorithms emphasize the importance of high-quality, uninterrupted CPR with early defibrillation. For patients with a shockable rhythm (VFib or pulseless VT), the goal for defibrillation is within 3 minutes of witnessed SCA. Early defibrillation has been associated with increased likelihood of ROSC and survival to hospital discharge.

Treatment

- See Figure 1.24 for ACLS algorithm.
- Provide O_2 via BVM when available, but do not delay CPR.
- **Immediate CPR and rapid defibrillation.**
  - 360-J monophasic or 200-J biphasic asynchronous.
  - Administer **single** shock.
- **Immediately resume CPR** after defibrillation (don't pause to check rhythm).
- **CPR 2 minutes → check rhythm** → defibrillate, if indicated → immediately resume CPR.
- **CPR 2 minutes → check rhythm** → defibrillate, if indicated; repeat until ROSC achieved or alternative rhythm is detected.
- Epinephrine 1 mg IV/IO every 3-5 minutes or vasopressin 40 units IV/IO can replace first or second dose of epinephrine.
- Secure an advanced airway (supraglottic device or endotracheal intubation) and monitor end-tidal CO_2. Give 8 breaths/minute with an approximate tidal volume of 600 mL.
- **Amiodarone**: First dose: 300 mg IV bolus. Second dose: 150 mg IV.
  - Lidocaine 1 mg/kg IV may be given if amiodarone is unavailable.
  - Magnesium sulfate 2 g IV should be given for polymorphic VT due to torsade de pointes.
- Treat reversible causes (Hs and Ts).
- Continue to evaluate for shockable rhythm every 2 minutes. If present, administer shock.
- ROSC is indicated by sustained pulse and blood pressure ± abrupt sustained increase in end-tidal CO_2 > 40 mm Hg. If ROSC detected → postresuscitation therapy.
- Change of rhythm to PEA or asystole should initiate those algorithms (see the next section).

PULSELESS ELECTRICAL ACTIVITY

Pulseless electrical activity (PEA) patients may be differentiated into 2 groups:

- Those with electrical activity and echocardiographic evidence of cardiac motion
- Those with electrical activity in the absence of any cardiac motion
  - Patients in this group have a worse outcome than those with cardiac motion.

PEA often results from reversible causes but can be a terminal rhythm after prolonged VFib/VT. These must be aggressively pursued and managed if present. PEA is generally the result of one or more of the Hs and Ts.

ECG Findings

- Will vary with underlying cause and duration of systemic abnormality
- Hyperkalemia → wide QRS → sinusoidal rhythm
- Hypovolemia or tamponade → marked sinus tachycardia

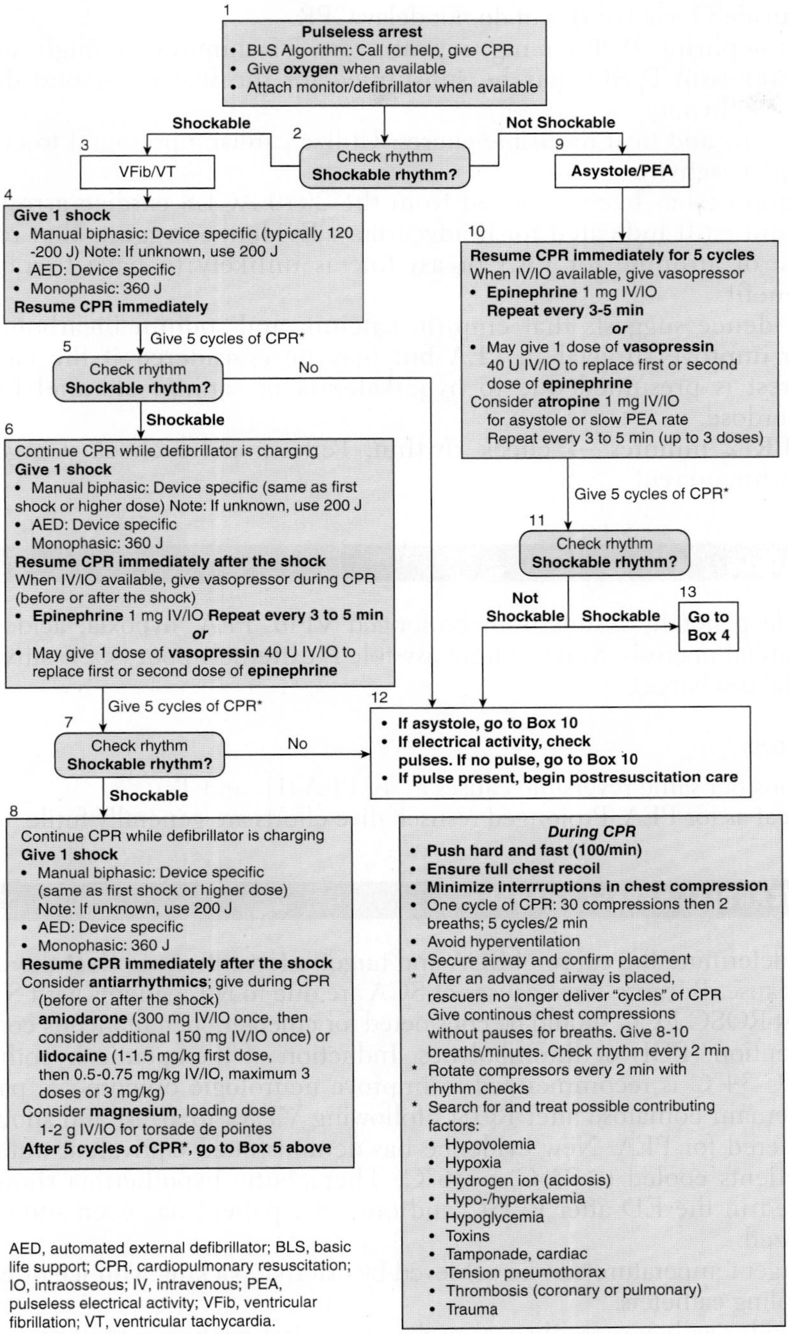

FIGURE 1.24. ACLS algorithm. (Reproduced with permission from McKean SC. Ross JJ, Dressler DD, et al: *Principles and Practice of Hospital Medicine*. New York, NY: McGraw-Hill Education; 2012.)

- Severe acidosis or hypoxia → bradysystolic rhythm
- ACS → ischemia/ST-elevation myocardial infarction (STEMI)

TREATMENT

- See Figure 1.24.
- Administer immediate high-quality CPR and **limit interruptions**.

- Provide O_2 via BVM, but do not delay CPR.
- Epinephrine IV/IO 1 mg, repeat every 3-5 minutes. A single dose of vasopressin IV/IO may be substituted for the first or second dose of epinephrine.
- Identify and treat reversible causes: Utilize cardiac ultrasound to evaluate cardiac activity.
- Atropine has been removed from the 2010 ACLS cardiac arrest algorithm (still indicated for bradycardia). Evidence suggests that routine use of atropine for PEA or asystole is unlikely to have therapeutic benefit.
- Evidence suggests that empiric calcium and sodium bicarbonate do no improve survival in PEA but may be considered if the cause of arrest is presumed due to hyperkalemia or sodium channel blocker overdose.
- **CPR 2 minutes → check rhythm.** Perform pulse check if organized rhythm present.

KEY FACT

Empiric use of calcium and sodium bicarbonate is not recommended for PEA unless hyperkalemia or sodium channel blocker overdose is suspected.

ASYSTOLE

Asystole generally results from prolonged VFib, PEA, hypoxia, acidosis, or myocardial necrosis. Survival from asystole is extremely poor (< 2% survival to hospital discharge).

Treatment

- Consider same reversible causes as for PEA (Hs and Ts).
- Treat as for PEA. Prolonged resuscitative efforts are generally futile.

POSTCARDIAC ARREST THERAPY

First, determine the cause of SCA and target interventions to treat the underlying cause. Because most causes of SCA are due to MI, patients with STEMI on post-ROSC ECG should be considered for emergent percutaneous coronary intervention (PCI) or thrombolytics. Induction of therapeutic hypothermia to 32°C-34°C is recommended to improve neurologic outcome in patients who remain comatose after ROSC following VT/VFib arrest and should be considered for PEA. New evidence has demonstrated equivalent outcomes for patients cooled to 33°C or 36°C. Therapeutic hypothermia should be initiated in the ED after ROSC and once the patient has been sufficiently stabilized.

- Target temperature can be achieved by external packing with ice or central cooling catheters.
- Bladder catheter, esophageal probe, or central cooling catheter is used to monitor temperature.
- Sedation (and neuromuscular blockade, if necessary) is used to prevent shivering.
- Rewarming is achieved passively or with central catheter system over 12-24 hours.
- Support hemodynamic status with crystalloids, vasopressors/inotropes, and blood products as indicated by the cause of SCA.

CARDIAC ARREST MEDICATIONS (TABLE 1.13)

Route of administration:

- Time to drug administration is important.
- The **most rapidly available route** should be used.

TABLE 1.13. Medications for Cardiac Arrest

Drug	Dose (IV/IO)	Mechanism
Epinephrine	Adult: 1 mg Pediatric: 0.01 mg/kg	α, β-Adrenergic receptor agonist → ↑ coronary and cerebral perfusion pressures
Vasopressin	Adult: 40 units	Nonadrenergic peripheral, coronary, and renal vasoconstrictor
Atropine	Adult: 1 mg Pediatric: 0.02 mg/kg (minimum 0.1 mg, maximum 0.5-1 mg)	Parasympatholytic No longer recommended for asystole or PEA
Amiodarone	Adult: 300 mg, repeat at 150 mg Pediatric: 5 mg/kg, repeat up to 15 mg/kg (maximum 300 mg)	Class III antidysrhythmic (blocks K^+ channels); α, β-adrenergic-receptor antagonist Increases short-term survival to hospital admission compared to lidocaine
Lidocaine	Adult: 1-1.5 mg/kg, repeat at 0.5-0.75 mg/kg every 5-10 min PRN (maximum 4 mg/kg) Pediatric: 1 mg/kg every 5-10 min PRN (maximum 100 mg)	Class Ib antidysrhythmic (blocks fast Na^+ channels) Consider if amiodarone unavailable
Magnesium	Adult: 1-2 g Pediatric: 25-50 mg/kg (maximum 2 g)	↑ Mg levels → improved QT intervals

IO, intraosseous; IV, intravenous; PEA, pulseless electrical activity; PRN, as needed.

- Establish IO access if peripheral IV access is not available.
- Central venous access.
  - Provides the fastest drug delivery to the central circulation, but **not** preferred if delayed or interrupts CPR.
- Peripherally administered drugs should be followed by 20-mL flush and elevation of extremity.
- Endotracheal administration:
  - If IV/IO access unavailable, lidocaine, epinephrine, and vasopressin can be administered via endotracheal route.
  - Achieves lower serum drug levels compared to IV/IO routes.
  - Use 2-2.5 times the IV dose (10 × the IV dose in pediatrics), dilute in 10-mL NS, administer directly in ET tube followed by 5 breaths.

> **KEY FACT**
>
> Central venous access provides the fastest drug delivery to the central circulation, but should **not** delay CPR. IO access is rapid and safe for administering ACLS drugs.

Epinephrine

First-line medication for cardiac arrest; associated with improved rates of ROSC, but no difference in survival.

> **KEY FACT**
>
> Epinephrine has been shown to increase coronary and cerebral perfusion pressures during CPR but does not improve survival.

Mechanism of Action

- α- and β-Adrenergic-receptor stimulation → increased coronary and cerebral perfusion pressures during CPR
- Negative effects: Increased myocardial work and myocardial oxygen consumption

DOSE

- Adult: 1 mg IV/IO every 3-5 minutes.
  - ET tube dose: 2-2.5 mg every 3-5 minutes
- Pediatric: 0.01 mg/kg IV/IO (maximum single dose: 1 mg) every 3-5 minutes.
  - ET tube dose: 0.1 mg/kg
- Higher doses have **not** been shown to improve survival, but may be indicated for β-blocker or calcium channel blocker overdose.

Vasopressin

No survival benefit or difference in ROSC over epinephrine.

> **KEY FACT**
>
> Vasopressin is a nonadrenergic peripheral vasoconstrictor.

MECHANISM OF ACTION

- Nonadrenergic peripheral vasoconstrictor without inotropic or chronotropic effects
- Coronary and renal vasoconstriction

DOSE

- Adult: 40 units IV/IO to replace either the first or second dose of epinephrine.
- Following the administration of vasopression, continue to give epinephrine every 3-5 minutes as indicated.
- Pediatrics: Not recommended.

Atropine

According to 2010 AHA guidelines, atropine is no longer recommended for routine use in asystole or PEA.

MECHANISM OF ACTION

Competitive antagonism of muscarinic acetylcholine receptors (parasympatholytic) → ↑ HR, ↑ SVR, ↑ BP

DOSE

- Adult: 0.5 mg IV every 3-5 minutes, maximum dose 3 mg
- Pediatric: 0.02 mg/kg every 3-5 minutes, maximum dose 1 mg

Amiodarone

Amiodarone is indicated for pulseless VT and VFib unresponsive to CPR, shock, and vasopressors. It has many indications outside cardiac arrest, including treatment of tachydysrhythmias.

MECHANISM OF ACTION

- A class III antidysrhythmic
- K^+ channel blockade → prolongation of repolarization (phase 3)
- Has multiple other effects (sodium/calcium channel effects, α-, β-blockade)

DOSE

- Adult: 300 mg IV/IO, followed by 150 mg IV/IO in 3-5 minutes for unstable tachydysrhythmias; 150 mg for stable tachydysrhythmias, repeated every 10 minutes as needed
- Pediatric: 5 mg/kg IV/IO, may repeat twice up to maximum of 300 mg

COMPLICATIONS

Hypotension, bradycardia, prolonged QT interval, long-term pulmonary toxicity

Lidocaine

Second-line treatment for VT and VFib

MECHANISM OF ACTION

- Class Ib antidysrhythmic
- Blocks fast sodium channels → stabilization of membranes/suppresses automaticity

DOSE

- Adult: 1-1.5 mg/kg IV/IO, may be repeated at 0.5-0.75 mg/kg every 5-10 minutes if needed to max of 3 mg/kg
- Pediatric: 1 mg/kg IV/IO to maximum dose of 100 mg

COMPLICATIONS

Hypotension, bradycardia with block, seizures

Magnesium

Used in the treatment of VT or VFib associated with torsade de pointes and prolonged QT

MECHANISM OF ACTION

Increases serum magnesium levels → shortened QT intervals, termination of torsade de pointes

DOSE

- Adult: 1-2 g diluted in 10-mL D_5W IV/IO infused over 15 minutes
- Pediatric: 25-50 mg/kg IV/IO (max: 2 g)

COMPLICATIONS

Hypermagnesemia can cause decreased reflexes and at high levels decreased respiratory drive, heart block, and asystole.

> **KEY FACT**
>
> **Magnesium treats:**
> Torsade de pointes
> Preeclampsia
> Severe asthma

Glucose

May be a critical intervention in the pediatric population. Hypoglycemia should be considered in PEA or drug overdoses. Empiric glucose is generally safe in undifferentiated SCA and may help prevent neuroglycopenia during cardiac arrest.

DOSE

- 0.5–1 g/kg IV/IO ($D_{50}W$ 1 mL/kg adults, $D_{25}W$ 2 mL/kg pediatrics, $D_{10}W$ 5 mL/kg neonates)

Dextrose Therapy Rule of 50: Dextrose concentration × volume = 50

Adult: D_{50}, 1 mL/kg (50 × 1)

Pediatric: D_{25}, 2-4 mL/kg (25 × 2)

Neonate: D_{10}, 5-10 mL/kg (10 × 5)

> **KEY FACT**
>
> Empiric lytics for PEA have no survival benefit unless cause of arrest is due to massive PE.

Interventions Not Recommended for Routine Use During Cardiac Arrest

The following interventions are unlikely to have therapeutic benefit and are therefore not recommended in the routine management of cardiac arrest per 2010 AHA guidelines:

- Atropine
- Sodium bicarbonate and calcium (special situations only: hyperkalemia, TCA overdose)
- Magnesium sulfate (unless SCA due to torsade de pointes with prolonged QT interval)
- Fibrinolysis (can be considered when PE is known or presumed cause of cardiac arrest, otherwise no improvement in survival and increases risk of intracranial bleeding)
- Cardiac pacing in the treatment of asystole or PEA

KEY FACT

Cardiac pacing is not recommended in the treatment of asystole or PEA.

Permanent Pacemakers

Indications (Class I) for permanent pacemaker placement include:

- Third-degree and advanced second-degree AV block resulting in:
  - Symptomatic bradycardia, CHF, ventricular arrhythmias, or exercise intolerance

Ventricular escape rate < 40 bpm or asystolic periods > 3 seconds

- Asymptomatic atrial fibrillation with ventricular rate < 40 bpm
- Following AV nodal ablation or heart surgery
- Neuromuscular disease with AV block (myotonic muscular dystrophy)
- Chronic fascicular block with associated type II second- or third-degree AV block
- Symptomatic sustained SVT
- Symptomatic sinus dysfunction

Individual pacer function is determined by a 3- to 5-letter code, employed by the North American Society of Pacing and Electrophysiology (Table 1.14).

MNEMONIC

VVI pacemaker

Ventricular paced
Ventricular sensed
Inhibited (response to sensing)

PACEMAKER MALFUNCTION

CAUSES

Failure to capture

- Lead displacement (most common), fracture (rare), or disconnection.
- Failure of pacemaker to generate signal.
- Battery depletion.

TABLE 1.14. Interpretation of Pacemaker Codes

1ST LETTER	2ND LETTER	3RD LETTER	4TH LETTER	5TH LETTER
CHAMBER PACED	**CHAMBER SENSED**	**RESPONSE TO SENSING**	**PROGRAMMABLE FUNCTIONS**	**ANTITACHYCARDIA FEATURES**
V = ventricle	**V** = ventricle	**T** = triggered	**P** = programmable rate, output, or both	**P** = antitachycardia pacing
A = atrium	**A** = atrium	**I** = inhibited	**M** = multiprogrammability of rate, output, sensitivity, etc	**S** = shock
D = dual	**D** = dual	**D** = dual	**C** = communication function (telemetry)	**D** = dual
O = none	**O** = none	**O** = none	**R** = rate modulation **O** = none	**O** = none

- Exit block: Failure of myocardial depolarization due to fibrosis, metabolic derangement, ischemia, hypoxia, or class III antiarrhythmics.
- If patient is unstable, use external transcutaneous pacing.

Undersensing

- Failure of pacemaker to sense native impulses (eg, native QRS voltage too low → paced beats in addition to native beats)
- May cause pacer to discharge on T wave → arrhythmia
- Causes are similar to "failure to pace" (battery exhaustion, lead displacement, improper programming, poor lead contact with endocardium)

Oversensing

- Inappropriate pacemaker sensing of "false" extracardiac impulses with pacer in inhibit ("I") mode, causes inappropriate inhibition of pacemaker impulse → no paced beat
- False impulses: Pectoralis muscle contraction, electrocautery, digital cell phones, magnetic resonance imaging (MRI)
- Treatment: Magnet placement

Pacemaker-Mediated Tachycardia

- Reentrant dysrhythmia: **Native ventricular depolarization → retrograde atrial depolarization** → pacemaker sensing → ventricular output via pacer wire ("endless loop tachycardia").
- PVC → retrograde atrial depolarization → sensed by atrial lead → paced ventricular impulse → retrograde atrial depolarization, etc.
- Treatment: Interrupt 1 limb of reentrant circuit with Valsalva maneuver/adenosine. Place a cardiac magnet which terminates pacemaker sensing and arrhythmia.

Runaway Pacemaker

- Pulse generator discharges at rate above preset upper limit, making pacemaker entirely responsible for malfunction **independent of myocardium**, unlike pacemaker-mediated tachycardia.
- Rare; caused by electrical malfunction or unintended pacemaker reprogramming.
- Dual chamber pacemaker in synchronous (demand) AV pacing mode.
- **Treatment: Cardiac magnet to convert pulse generator to asynchronous or "fixed rate" mode** (preset regardless of native electrical activity) should be attempted. May be ineffective in cases of true pacemaker malfunction.
- In cases of hemodynamic compromise, definitive therapy requires reprogramming the atrial refractory period or removal of pulse generator.

> **KEY FACT**
>
> **Pacemaker malfunction simplified:**
> Undersensing = "Overpacing"
> Oversensing = "Underpacing"

SYMPTOMS/EXAMINATION

- With the exception of runaway pacemaker, symptoms are similar to those that prompted pacemaker placement.
- Syncope or near syncope.
- Dyspnea, chest pain, or palpitations.

DIAGNOSIS

- Evaluation of rhythm strip and ECG (Table 1.15).
- CXR for wire fracture/displacement.
- Fractures are usually close to generator or within the heart.
- Ultrasound to assess for cardiac tamponade due to ventricular rupture.
- Electrolytes, cardiac enzymes, and drug levels (eg, digoxin, flecainide).
- Pacemaker interrogation/battery assessment via cardiologist.

TREATMENT

- Depends on the underlying malfunction
- Often requires reprogramming by cardiologist
- **Magnet placement** (oversensing and runaway pacemaker)

> **KEY FACT**
>
> Placing a magnet over the pacemaker generator converts the pacemaker to a fixed-rate pacing mode, disables sensing, and turns off the er the pacemaker ge.

TABLE 1.15. ECG Findings in Pacemaker Malfunction

ECG Finding	Pacemaker Malfunction
Absence of pacer spikes when indicated	Failure to output signal
Pacer spikes, but no depolarization	Failure to capture signal
Pacer spikes despite native beats	Undersensing native beats
Absence of pacer spikes with external motion or interference pattern	Oversensing

ECG, electrocardiogram.

- Converts pacer to preset fixed rate and disables sensing function
- Turns off "inhibit" function

KEY FACT

Pacemaker syndrome occurs due to loss of AV synchrony, most commonly with VVI pacemakers.

PACEMAKER SYNDROME

Most commonly seen with VVI pacemakers because of atrial contractions against a closed AV valve, but can occur in DDI if sinus node discharge rate > programmed pacemaker rate.

Pathophysiology

- Atrial contractions against closed AV valve →
  - ↑ Atrial pressures → pulmonary and hepatic congestion
  - ↓ Ventricular filling (loss of "atrial kick") → decreased cardiac output (by 20%-50%)

Symptoms and Examination

- Malaise, fatigue, dyspnea, orthopnea, cough, throat fullness
- Light-headedness, orthostatic dizziness, near-syncope, or syncope
- Sense of pulsations in neck or abdomen
- Heart failure symptoms, chest pain, right upper quadrant (RUQ) pain

Diagnosis/Treatment

- Diagnosis is primarily clinical → difficult to differentiate from true pacemaker malfunction.
- ECG to evaluate for **AV** dissociation or ventriculoatrial (**VA**) conduction.
- Interrogate pacer to rule out malfunction and reprogram setting.
- Often resolves after change to dual chamber pacemaker.

Complications

Increased risk of atrial fibrillation, thromboembolic events, and heart failure

Implantable Cardioverter-Defibrillators

Implantable cardioverter-defibrillators (ICDs) reduce mortality in patients at high risk for sudden cardiac death from VT and VFib. They are programmed to analyze the cardiac rhythm, perform antitachycardia pacing, generate an electrical charge, and deliver an electrical shock. All new-generation ICDs have ventricular pacing abilities.

EVALUATION OF A DELIVERED SHOCK

Patient-reported shocks may be appropriate (underlying VT or VFib), inappropriate, or phantom (patients perceive shock that did not occur). Contemporary ICDs can treat ventricular arrhythmia with antitachycardia pacing, cardioversion, or defibrillation and are better at recognizing SVT. Only interrogation of the device or monitoring during an event can differentiate appropriate from inappropriate shocks.

Appropriate shocks may result from associated:

- Ventricular dysrhythmia
- Electrolyte abnormalities
- Myocardial ischemia
- Medications (proarrhythmic drugs or medication noncompliance)

Inappropriate shocks may be because of:

- Recurrent nonsustained VT
- SVT with rapid ventricular response inappropriately sensed as VT
- Oversensing T waves as QRS complexes
- Artifact oversensing (muscular activity, shivering, or fasciculations from succinylcholine)
- Broken/displaced ventricular lead

Diagnosis

- External cardiac monitoring during ICD event.
- ECG and laboratory test results to evaluate for ischemia or electrolyte abnormalities.
- Postshock ECG may demonstrate transient ST elevation or depression for 5-15 minutes.
- CXR to evaluate leads.
- Device interrogation.
- All patients with repetitive shocks (≥ 2) warrant diagnostic evaluation.
- Stable patient with single isolated shock may warrant less extensive evaluation.

Treatment

- Identify and treat contributing conditions.
- Inappropriate shocks may be prevented with magnet deactivation of the ICD.
- Magnet placement will disable tachyarrhythmia detection/therapy without affecting backup pacing, but return of function after magnet removal is manufacturer dependent.
- Device interrogation for possible reprogramming, as indicated by cardiologist, will prevent inappropriate removal of vital functions.
- IV antiarrhythmic drugs (amiodarone) for persistent ventricular ectopy/VT/VFib.

IMPLANTABLE CARDIOVERTER-DEFIBRILLATOR FAILURE

Causes

- **Component failure**.
  - Lead fracture/displacement.
- Battery depletion.
- Interference with pacemakers.
- **Inadvertent inactivation:** Any strong magnetic force can cause temporary or permanent (depending on device) failure.

Q

A 58-year-old man presents to the ED complaining of recurrent implantable cardioverter-defibrillators (ICDs) firing. On the monitor, you see a narrow complex tachycardia at a rate of 150 bpm, which is temporarily converted to sinus rhythm with ICD firing. The patient is hemodynamically stable during the tachydysrhythmia, but has considerable discomfort with each firing. How do you prevent the inappropriate ICD firing in this patient?

KEY FACT

VT/VFib should be the assumed cause of ICD firing until proven otherwise.

Preventing the underlying tachydysrhythmia and/or ICD reprogramming is the definitive treatment, but placing a ring magnet over the generator site will temporarily inactivate the ICD.

- **Resistant VT or VFib:** Device functioning, but rhythm resistant to internal defibrillation.

Symptoms/Examination

May range from asymptomatic (found on device evaluation) to cardiac arrest

Treatment

- Definitive treatment is device reprogramming or replacement.
- Perform usual ACLS protocols. There is no risk from ICD for CPR providers.
- Perform external defibrillation for VT/VFib not resolved with internal defibrillation.
- Use standard paddles, place them front and back of chest, ≥ 10 cm away from generator.

Volume Assessment

NEONATES

KEY FACT

Neonates may present with respiratory distress as a sign of volume loss.

Newborns have very poor cardiac reserve and as a result progress rapidly to circulatory collapse in the setting of even moderate volume loss. High rates of water loss from kidneys, skin, and lungs.

Symptoms/Examination

- **Tachycardia:** Any increase of HR above the normal range for age.
- **Respiratory distress:** Nasal flaring or grunting. This is a sign of increasing stress and may be seen when volume loss is > 5%.
- **Lethargy:** Seen in moderate-to-severe volume loss (10%-15%).
- **BP drop:** Is the final sign of severe volume loss (> 15%) in a neonate and is often precipitous.
- Subacute volume loss may occur over a period of days and presents with changes in skin turgor ("doughiness" of the skin), decreased frequency of wet diapers, sunken eyes and fontanelle, dry mucous membranes, lack of tears, cap refill > 2 seconds, and cool or mottled extremities.

Treatment

- IV rehydration with isotonic fluids at 10-20 mL/kg. Electrolytes and glucose must also be corrected.

PEDIATRICS

KEY FACT

Pediatric hypotension = systolic blood pressure < 70 mm Hg + (2 × age in years).

Volume assessment in children is made difficult by the normal variation of vital signs seen with increasing age. Thus, some knowledge of normal vital signs is important (Table 1.16). When available, the change in weight from baseline is the most accurate objective measure of the degree of volume loss (eg, 1-kg weight loss = 1-L fluid loss).

After the neonatal stage, cardiac reserve becomes substantially better. As a result, even significant volume loss may be well compensated for by increasing HR. However, when compensation fails, cardiovascular collapse may result.

TABLE 1.16. Normal Vital Signs for Pediatric Patients

Age	HR (bpm)	RR (breaths/min)	Systolic BP (mm Hg)
Neonates, 0-28 days	120-160	30-50	> 60
Infants, 1-12 months	100-120	20-30	70-95
Children, 1-8 y	80-100	20-30	80-110

BP, blood pressure; HR, heart rate; RR, respiratory rate.

Q

A 17-month-old boy is brought in by his parents after 3 days of nonbloody diarrhea. The child has had 6-8 soiled diapers a day, although in the 4 hours prior to presentation the diaper has not required changing. On presentation, the child is noted to be clinging to his mother but not crying. His mucous membranes are dry and his eyes appear sunken. His HR is 140 bpm and his SBP is 80 mm Hg. What is the initial indicator of volume loss in the pediatric patient? What is the most appropriate first treatment?

Symptoms/Examination

- **Mild volume loss (3%-5%)**
  - Normal examination with history of volume loss
  - May report increased thirst or decreased urine output (UOP)
- **Moderate volume loss (6%-9%)**
  - Presents with irritability, restlessness, and history of decreased tears or urine output
  - Tachycardia, orthostatic hypotension, deep respirations, cool extremities with delayed capillary refill, decreased skin turgor, sunken eyes and fontanelle

Treatment

- ORT is recommended for mild-to-moderate volume loss.
- Laboratory testing is not indicated for mild-to-moderate volume loss.
- **Severe volume loss (> 10%).**
  - Presents with lethargy, somnolence, and signs of shock
  - Marked tachycardia, weak pulses, hypotension, delayed capillary refill, cold and mottled extremities, minimal urine output, and sunken eyes and fontanelle

KEY FACT

Evidence shows that delayed capillary refill, decreased skin turgor, and deep respirations predict > 5% volume loss.

Treatment

- Aggressive IV volume repletion with 20-mL/kg isotonic fluid bolus is critical to prevent ischemic tissue injury.
- Laboratory testing may show a metabolic acidosis, hypo/hyperkalemia, and hypo/hypernatremia.

ADULTS

Adults and older children have similar cardiac reserve. However, adults have less vascular tone, causing hypotension with less volume loss. Volume status can be estimated more precisely in adults than in children, because physical findings are more predictable with progressive hypovolemia. The American College of Surgeons Advanced Trauma Life Support (ATLS) guidelines suggests a means of correlating blood loss in adult trauma patients based on appearance and vital signs (Table 1.17). Recent evidence calls into question the validity of the ATLS guidelines, because they may be unreliable or absent in hypovolemic patients and do not always correlate with the severity of illness. Signs and symptoms of hypovolemia are similar regardless of the actual mechanism of volume loss, but should be used in conjunction with historical and laboratory data. Adjuncts for evaluation of volume status include bedside ultrasound, central venous pressure (CVP) monitoring, and arterial waveform monitoring.

A

This child has lost a moderate volume of fluid. Because infants and young children are fairly HR dependent for their cardiac output, tachycardia is the initial indicator of moderate volume loss. The initial treatment should be a trial of oral rehydration therapy (ORT).

TABLE 1.17. Guidelines for Correlating Volume Loss in Adults

Hemorrhage Class	Volume Loss	HR	BP	CNS
I	< 15% (< 750 mL)	< 100	Normal	Normal
II	15%-30% (750-1500 mL)	> 100	Orthostatic	Anxious
III	30%-40% (1500-2000 mL)	> 120	Hypotension	Confusion, agitation
IV	> 40% (> 2000 mL)	> 140	Severe hypotension	Obtunded

BP, blood pressure; CNS, central nervous system; HR, heart rate.

Symptoms/Examination

- Cardiovascular: Tachycardia, hypotension, narrow pulse pressure (diastolic BP may rise in early shock due to vasoconstriction, but later falls after compensation fails), decreased jugular venous pressure.
- Respiratory: Tachypnea, depressed respiratory drive may indicate impending respiratory arrest.
  - Neurologic: Mental status changes including anxiety, agitation, and confusion progressing to obtundation, seizures, and coma.
  - Skin: Cool and clammy skin with poor capillary refill, dry mucous membranes.
  - Renal: Decreased UOP (< 0.5-1 mL/kg/h).

Shock

KEY FACT

A "normal" blood pressure does not exclude the diagnosis of shock, and hypotension may occur in the absence of shock.

Shock is characterized by a reduction in systemic perfusion causing inadequate tissue O_2 delivery to meet demand, resulting in anaerobic metabolism and the formation of lactic acid. Oxygen deprivation is initially reversible, but will progress to cellular death, end-organ damage, multiorgan dysfunction, and death, if not corrected. Shock can be divided into 4 categories: **hypovolemic, cardiogenic, obstructive, and distributive**.

Symptoms/Examination

- See Figure 1.25 for algorithmic approach to evaluating undifferentiated shock.
- Vary with etiology of shock (see individual shock sections).
- Common features: Tachycardia, hypotension, altered mental status, oliguria, negative base deficit, lactic acidosis.

KEY FACT

Laboratory evidence for inadequate tissue oxygenation:

Base deficit more negative than −2 mEq/L
Serum lactate > 4 mmol/L
Multiorgan dysfunction

Diagnosis

- Suspected from clinical findings defined by each type of shock (Table 1.18)
- Evidence of inadequate tissue oxygenation by laboratory studies
- **Base deficit**
  - Estimate of O_2 debt: Amount of strong base needed to normalize pH of 1 L of blood
  - If more negative than −2 mEq/L may represent early shock before HR or BP
- **Lactic acidosis:** Defined as serum lactate > 4 mmol/L
  - Correlates with O_2 debt (released primarily from muscle and intestine)

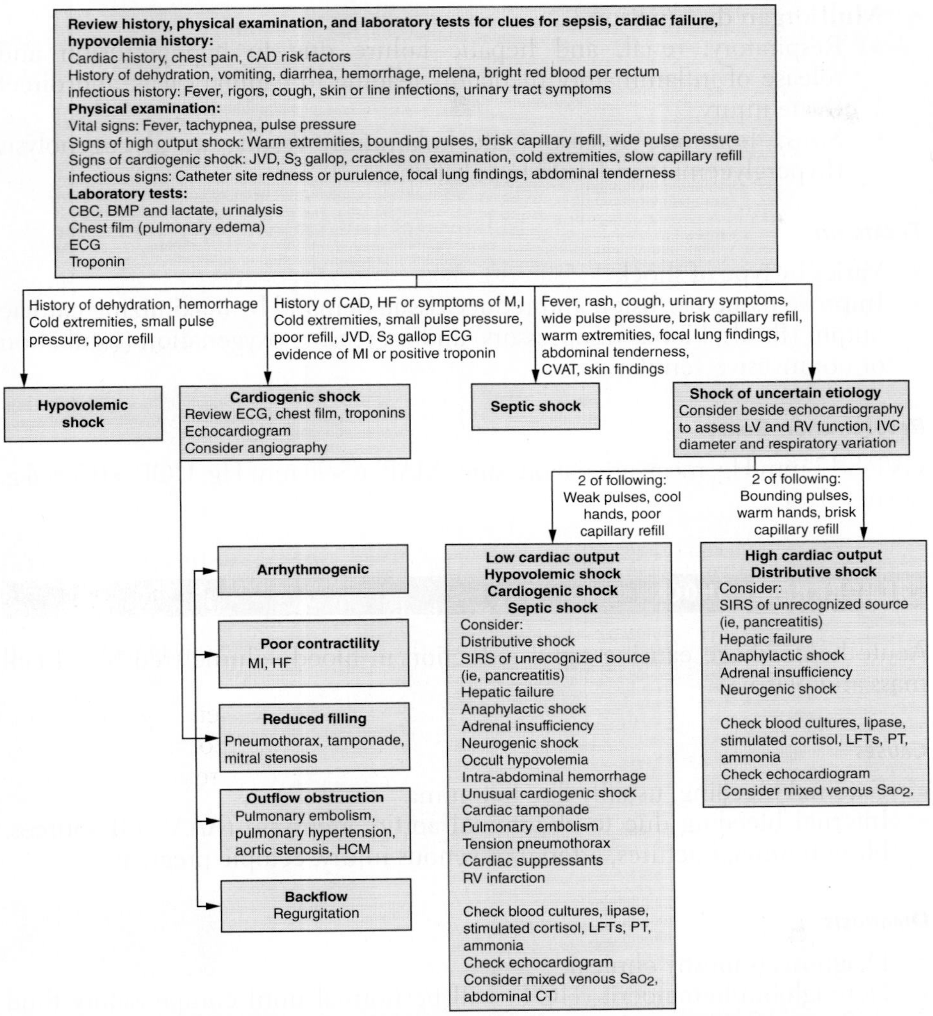
Review history, physical examination, and laboratory tests for clues for sepsis, cardiac failure, hypovolemia history:
Cardiac history, chest pain, CAD risk factors
History of dehydration, vomiting, diarrhea, hemorrhage, melena, bright red blood per rectum
infectious history: Fever, rigors, cough, skin or line infections, urinary tract symptoms
Physical examination:
Vital signs: Fever, tachypnea, pulse pressure
Signs of high output shock: Warm extremities, bounding pulses, brisk capillary refill, wide pulse pressure
Signs of cardiogenic shock: JVD, S3 gallop, crackles on examination, cold extremities, slow capillary refill
infectious signs: Catheter site redness or purulence, focal lung findings, abdominal tenderness
Laboratory tests:
CBC, BMP and lactate, urinalysis
Chest film (pulmonary edema)
ECG
Troponin
History of dehydration, hemorrhage Cold extremities, small pulse pressure, poor refill
History of CAD, HF or symptoms of M,I Cold extremities, small pulse pressure, poor refill, JVD, S3 gallop ECG evidence of MI or positive troponin
Fever, rash, cough, urinary symptoms, wide pulse pressure, brisk capillary refill, warm extremities, focal lung findings, abdominal tenderness, CVAT, skin findings
Hypovolemic shock
Cardiogenic shock
Review ECG, chest film, troponins
Echocardiogram
Consider angiography
Septic shock
Shock of uncertain etiology
Consider beside echocardiography to assess LV and RV function, IVC diameter and respiratory variation
2 of following: Weak pulses, cool hands, poor capillary refill
2 of following: Bounding pulses, warm hands, brisk capillary refill
Arrhythmogenic
Poor contractility
MI, HF
Reduced filling
Pneumothorax, tamponade, mitral stenosis
Outflow obstruction
Pulmonary embolism, pulmonary hypertension, aortic stenosis, HCM
Backflow
Regurgitation
Low cardiac output
Hypovolemic shock
Cardiogenic shock
Septic shock
Consider:
Distributive shock
SIRS of unrecognized source (ie, pancreatitis)
Hepatic failure
Anaphylactic shock
Adrenal insufficiency
Neurogenic shock
Occult hypovolemia
Intra-abdominal hemorrhage
Unusual cardiogenic shock
Cardiac tamponade
Pulmonary embolism
Tension pneumothorax
Cardiac suppressants
RV infarction
Check blood cultures, lipase, stimulated cortisol, LFTs, PT, ammonia
Check echocardiogram
Consider mixed venous SaO2, abdominal CT
High cardiac output
Distributive shock
Consider:
SIRS of unrecognized source (ie, pancreatitis)
Hepatic failure
Anaphylactic shock
Adrenal insufficiency
Neurogenic shock
Check blood cultures, lipase, stimulated cortisol, LFTs, PT, ammonia
Check echocardiogram
Consider mixed venous SaO2,

BMP, basic metabolic profile; CAD, coronary artery disease; CBC, complete blood count; CVAT, costovertebral angle tenderness; ECG, electrocardiogram; HCM, hypertrophic cardiomyopathy; HF, heart failure; IVC, inferior vena cava; JVD, jugular venous distention; LFTs, liver function tests; LV left ventricle; MI, myocardial infarction; PT, prothrombin time; RV; right ventricle; SIRS, systemic inflammatory response syndrome.

FIGURE 1.25. Approach to undifferentiated shock. (Reproduced with permission from Stern SC, Cifu AS, Altkorn D, eds. *Symptom to Diagnosis: An Evidence-Based Guide*. 3rd ed. New York, NY: McGraw-Hill Education; 2015.)

TABLE 1.18. Differentiating Types of Shock

Type of Shock	Extremities	Pulse Pressure	CVP	Tissue Perfusion/$Scvo_2$
Cardiogenic	Cool	Narrow	High	Low
Obstructive	Cool or warm	Narrow	High	Low
Hypovolemic	Cool	Narrow	Low	Low
Distributive	Warm	Wide	Low or nil	High or low

CVP, central venous pressure.

Q

A 45-year-old man is brought to the ED by ambulance after a 2-day history of abdominal pain and bloody diarrhea. On presentation, he is lethargic and has a HR of 140 bpm and a BP of 90/60 mm Hg. What are the indicators of shock in this patient?

A

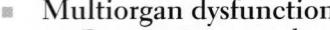

Diminished end-organ perfusion is a good indicator of shock in addition to abnormal vital signs. Bedside clinical markers include tachycardia, hypotension, mental status changes, and decreased urine output. Blood gas may demonstrate increased base deficit or lactate production.

- **Multiorgan dysfunction**
  - Respiratory, renal, and hepatic failure due to hypoperfusion and release of inflammatory mediators leading to capillary leak and direct tissue injury.
  - Stress hormone release (catecholamines) results in glycogenolysis (hyperglycemia) and mild hypokalemia.

Treatment

- Varies by type of shock
- Improve tissue perfusion and reduce tissue demand by maximizing cardiac output (fluids, blood, vasopressors) and increasing oxygenation (intubation or noninvasive ventilation)

Resuscitation Goals

CVP 8-12 mm Hg, mean arterial pressure (MAP) 65-90 mm Hg, UOP > 0.5 cc/kg, $Scvo_2$ > 70%

KEY FACT

In acute hemorrhagic shock, the initial hemoglobin may be deceptively normal.

HEMORRHAGIC SHOCK

Acute hemorrhage causing rapid reduction in blood volume (red blood cell mass and plasma)

Causes

- External bleeding, usually due to trauma
- Internal bleeding due to abdominal aortic aneurysm (AAA), GI sources, blunt trauma, fractures, arterial or venous injury, ectopic pregnancy

Diagnosis

- Diagnosis is mostly clinical.
- Hemoglobin/hematocrit (HCT) will be normal until compensatory fluid shifting or fluid resuscitation has occurred.
- Focused Assessment with Sonography for Trauma (FAST) scan, chest and pelvis x-rays, and other indicated imaging for trauma patients.

Treatment

- Ensure adequate oxygenation and ventilation.
- **Volume resuscitation**.
  - **Isotonic crystalloid** (NS or lactated Ringer [LR]) boluses through large-bore peripheral IV lines, central line, or IO lines
  - 2 L in adults and 20 cc/kg in neonates, infants, and young children
- **Blood transfusion**, if no response to fluid boluses (max 50 mL/kg), ongoing hemorrhage, or if impending cardiovascular collapse.
  - When time is critical, the use of O-negative blood is standard (O positive in men is also acceptable).
  - 2 units packed red blood cells (PRBCs) in adults initially. Then transfuse PRBCs, fresh frozen plasma (FFP), and platelets in a 1:1:1 ratio for ongoing severe hemorrhage or shock.
  - 10-15 mL/kg PRBC in neonates, infants, and young children.
- **Hemorrhage control**.
  - Identify and control source of bleeding.
- Fix hereditary or acquired bleeding diatheses:
  - Platelets when platelet count is < 50,000/μL for active bleeding.
  - FFP for patients on warfarin with an elevated INR and significant bleeding, liver failure, or requiring massive transfusion.

KEY FACT

Indications for PRBC transfusion in hemorrhagic shock:

- No response to 2 fluid boluses
- Ongoing hemorrhage
- Impending cardiovascular collapse

- Prothrombin complex concentrate (PCC) or recombinant factor VIIa can be considered for coagulopathy from warfarin or liver failure.
- For hemophiliacs, factor replacement is preferred, but FFP and/or cryoprecipitate may be considered if limited by cost or availability.

NONHEMORRHAGIC HYPOVOLEMIC SHOCK

Nonhemorrhagic hypovolemic shock arises when volume intake is insufficient to make up for volume losses. Extracellular fluid (ECF) volume contraction causes loss of plasma volume and may result in hypotension due to decreased venous return and cardiac output.

CAUSES

- Inadequate intake/fluid restriction
- Excessive output: Renal diuresis, GI losses, insensible losses (skin, respiratory), third space (burns, pancreatitis, peritonitis)
- Metabolic derangements (hyperglycemia, inborn error of metabolism)

DIAGNOSIS

- Hematocrit and hemoglobin levels are high due to hemoconcentration.
- Blood urea nitrogen (BUN):creatinine (Cr) ratio > 20:1 (prerenal azotemia).
- Sodium is usually elevated secondary to free water loss.
- In DKA and hyperosmolar states, sodium may be factitiously low.

TREATMENT

- Ensure adequate ventilation and oxygenation.
- **Immediate isotonic crystalloid intravascular volume resuscitation.**
  - NS or LR bolus 30 mL/kg initially in adults, then reassess
  - NS or LR bolus 20 mL/kg in neonates and pediatrics
- **Restore total body water and sodium.**
  - Adults: 1/2 NS with or without 5% dextrose at a rate of 100-200 cc/h
- **Pediatrics.**
  - **Deficit fluids:** Percent fluid loss × weight (kg) = L deficit (ie, 10% loss in 20-kg child = 2-L fluid deficit). Replace one-half the deficit over first 8 hours and remainder over next 16 hours.
  - **Maintenance fluids:** Calculate maintenance fluids (Table 1.19) and add to deficit replacement.
  - **Solution:** Use $D_5$1/4 NS for infants and $D_5$1/2 NS in children.
  - Treatment of the underlying cause should occur simultaneously.

TABLE 1.19. Calculating Maintenance Fluids

PATIENT WEIGHT	DAILY MAINTENANCE FLUIDS[a]
For the first 0-10 kg	100 mL/kg/d
For the next 10-20 kg	50 mL/kg/d
From 20-70 kg	20 mL/kg/d

[a]Add up total mL and divide by 24 to obtain hourly rate.

Q

A 67-year-old man with a history of diabetes and hypertension presents to the ED complaining of 2 days of chest pain and shortness of breath. On examination, he appears ill with BP 80/50 mm Hg, HR 140 bpm, RR 30 breaths/min, and temperature 37°C. He has evidence of poor perfusion including cool extremities, bilateral rales, and jugular venous distention (JVD). ECG shows sinus tachycardia with anterior ST-segment elevation. Chest x-ray shows pulmonary edema and bedside cardiac ultrasound shows reduced left ventricular ejection fraction. What is the best initial management of this patient?

KEY FACT

Deficit fluids (in liters) = % fluid loss resuscitation

KEY FACT

Replace one-half the deficit over first 8 hours, the rest over the next 16 hours.

A

This patient is in cardiogenic shock from acute ST-elevation MI. The goal of treatment is to support oxygenation and ventilation with NIPPV, administration of aspirin and heparin, and improvement in myocardial contractility and pump function by initiating inotropes (dobutamine, dopamine or norepinephrine). Emergent PCI for early revascularization should be considered in consultation with a cardiologist.

KEY FACT

Acute MI is the most common cause of cardiogenic shock.

KEY FACT

Cardiogenic shock will occur if 40% of the left ventricle loses contractile function.

CARDIOGENIC SHOCK

Characterized by reduced cardiac output resulting in decreased oxygen delivery to the tissues with signs of end-organ hypoperfusion.

Cardiac output (CO) is the product of HR and stroke volume (SV).

$$\text{CO (L/min)} = \text{HR (bpm)} \times \text{SV (L)}$$

Stroke volume is the interrelation of preload, afterload, and contractility. Problems in any of the determinants of cardiac output may cause cardiogenic shock.

Etiology

Most commonly (80% of cases) due to acute MI due to ischemia. Other causes include myocardial dysfunction (myocarditis, cardiomyopathy), valvular heart disease (papillary muscle rupture, critical aortic stenosis), brady/tachydysrhythmias, aortic dissection, medication overdose (β-blockers or calcium channel blockers), ventricular septal rupture, cardiac tamponade, and traumatic contusion (rare).

Symptoms/Examination

- Chest pain, dyspnea, syncope, oliguria, altered mental status
- Hypotension, tachycardia, tachypnea, rales, jugular venous distention (JVD), abdominal jugular reflex, narrow pulse pressure, gallop rhythm, new murmur, peripheral edema, diaphoresis, cool/clammy extremities

Diagnosis

- **ECG**: Ischemic causes or arrhythmia
- **CXR**: Pulmonary congestion
- **Echocardiography**: Reduced ejection fraction (CO < 2 L/min/m^2) and valvular rupture or stenosis
- **Laboratory test results**: Elevated troponin, lactate, Cr, and low serum bicarbonate

Treatment

- Identify the underlying cause, because most cases are due to acute MI early revascularization with PCI, coronary bypass surgery, or thrombolytics.
- Ensure adequate ventilation and oxygenation using NIPPV or mechanical ventilation for hypoxia or respiratory failure due to pulmonary congestion.
- Improve myocardial contractility and pump function (consider early PCI) in addition to:
  - Small fluid bolus for hypotension without signs of pulmonary congestion (eg, RV infarct).
  - Inotropes for reduced cardiac output and RV/LV dysfunction:
  - Dobutamine: β_1-Adrenergic agonist → improves myocardial contractility and augments diastolic coronary blood flow. Secondary m2-adrenergic agonism causes peripheral vasodilation, limiting use in severely hypotensive patient and may require the addition of a second agent such as norepinephrine.
  - Norepinephrine: α- > β_1-Adrenergic leading to increased SVR with smaller increases in inotropy/chronotropy. Recommended for undifferentiated or mixed shock but may be deleterious in pure cardiogenic shock.
  - Dopamine: At high doses (15 μg/kg/min) has α- and β_1-adrenergic effects offering increased inotropy and SVR. Also associated with higher rates of tachydysrhythmias, so it is no longer recommended as first line.

- Milrinone: Phosphodiesterase inhibitor → positive inotrope and vasodilator (hypotension limits use); may be useful for cardiogenic shock due to pulmonary hypertension.
- Intra-aortic balloon pump decreases afterload and increases diastolic BP (improves CPP) as bridge to revascularization or valvular repair.
- For patients with acute MI: Aspirin, heparin, and GpIIb/IIIa inhibitors.
- Amiodarone is first line for dysrhythmias complicating cardiogenic shock; avoid β-/calcium channel blockers and other negative inotropes (procainamide, lidocaine).

OBSTRUCTIVE SHOCK

Obstructive shock occurs when extracardiac obstruction impedes cardiac filling (reduces preload) or impairs cardiac output (increased afterload).

ETIOLOGIES

Etiologies include:

- Cardiac tamponade, constrictive pericarditis (impaired RV diastolic filling)
- Tension pneumothorax (impaired RV filling due to obstructed venous return)
- PE (increased RV afterload, reduced LV preload)
- Aortic dissection (increased left ventricular afterload, reduced preload if tamponade present)

SYMPTOMS/EXAMINATION

- Chest pain, SOB, altered mental status
- Hypotension, tachycardia, tachypnea, JVD, muffled heart sounds, pulsus paradoxus, cool extremities, friction rub, new murmur, signs of deep vein thrombosis (DVT), chest trauma

TREATMENT

- Determined by cause; goal is to relieve obstruction to flow.
- Pericardiocentesis (tamponade), finger followed by tube thoracostomy (tension pneumothorax), thrombolysis (massive PE), afterload reduction (aortic dissection).

DISTRIBUTIVE SHOCK

Distributive shock is characterized by impaired tissue oxygenation due to peripheral vasodilation with low SVR with normal or reduced cardiac output. There are 5 major causes of distributive shock: **sepsis/SIRS, anaphylaxis, neurogenic shock, rewarming in severe hypothermia, and endocrinologic (adrenal crisis, thyroid storm). Toxic shock syndrome (TSS)** is a variant of septic shock and is discussed briefly in the section "Toxic Shock Syndrome."

Septic Shock

Sepsis is a clinical syndrome due to systemic inflammation in the presence of infection. The SIRS is because of a complicated cascade of cytokines and other immune and inflammatory modulators producing peripheral vasodilation, capillary leak, and myocardial dysfunction.

DEFINITION

- Sepsis: Presence of SIRS plus infection.
  - Gram-positive organisms more common cause than gram-negative organisms

Q

A 75-year-old woman is brought in from a nursing home for altered mental status. On examination, she has decreased mentation, bounding heart sounds, rhonchorous breath sounds, and extremities are warm to the touch. Her vital signs are temperature 39.2°C, HR 120 bpm, BP 66/30 mm Hg, and RR 32 breaths/min. A chest x-ray shows bilateral infiltrates consistent with pneumonia. Laboratory test results return with a lactate of 5 mmol/L. After an initial fluid bolus with NS 30 mL/kg, the patient's BP is 78/60 mm Hg. What is the next step in management?

KEY FACT

Five causes of distributive shock:

Sepsis/SIRS
Anaphylaxis
Rewarming (after severe hypothermia)
Endocrinologic (adrenal crisis, thyroid storm)
Neurogenic shock

A

This patient is in septic shock from pneumonia. She has evidence of end-organ hypoperfusion and lactic acidosis, and persistent hypotension after an appropriate fluid bolus. A central venous catheter should be placed and the patient should be started on norepinephrine for a goal MAP > 65 mm Hg. Her respiratory status should be supported with mechanical ventilation, particularly if she remains altered. Broad-spectrum antibiotics should be initiated within 1 hour of the patient's arrival.

KEY FACT

Resuscitation goals in septic shock: Give antibiotics within 1 hour. Early intubation to improve oxygenation. Administer > 30-mL/kg fluid bolus. Begin norepinephrine if MAP remains < 65 mm Hg, or lactate > 4 mmol/L. Transfuse PRBCs if hemoglobin < 7g/dL. Begin dobutamine if $Scvo_2$ remains < 70%.

- Noninfectious causes of SIRS include trauma, pancreatitis, ingestions, burns, myocardial ischemia, pulmonary embolism, GI bleed, and drug reactions.

SYMPTOMS/EXAMINATION

- Cough, dysuria, headache, abdominal pain, arthralgias, vomiting, diarrhea, chills
- Hypo-/hyperthermia, tachycardia, tachypnea, wide pulse pressure, warm extremities, altered mental status, oliguria, skin rash

DIAGNOSIS

- Based on clinical criteria (Table 1.20)

TREATMENT

- Early intubation and mechanical ventilation to decrease work of breathing (lung-protective ventilation goals: tidal volume 6 cc/kg, plateau pressures < 30 cm H_2O, apply PEEP).
- **Targeted resuscitation goals within the first 6 hours of presentation:**
  - MAP > 65 mm Hg, CVP 8-12 mm Hg, UOP > 0.5 mL/kg/h, central venous oxygen saturation ($Scvo_2$) > 70%.
  - Administer broad-spectrum antibiotics within 1 hour of identification of septic shock.
    - Empiric (source unknown) coverage for non-neutropenic patient:
    - Neonates: Ampicillin + cefotaxime.
    - Child: Vancomycin + cefotaxime.
    - Adult: Vancomycin + third- or fourth-generation cephalosporin, piperacillin-tazobactam, or carbapenems.

TABLE 1.20. Clinical Criteria for Diagnosis of SIRS and Sepsis

SIRS
Two or more of the following:
HR > 90 bpm
Temperature < 36°C or > 38°C
RR > 20 breaths/min or $Paco_2$ < 32 mm Hg
WBC < 4000 cells/mm³ or > 12,000 cells/mm³ or > 10% immature neutrophils
SEPSIS
SIRS + infection
SEVERE SEPSIS
Sepsis + organ dysfunction, hypoperfusion, or hypotension
SEPTIC SHOCK
Sepsis + impaired perfusion or hypotension (SBP < 90 mm Hg or reduction > 40 mm Hg from baseline) despite adequate fluid resuscitation

HR, heart rate; RR, respiratory rate; SBP, systolic blood pressure; SIRS, systemic inflammatory response syndrome; WBC, white blood cell.

- Obtain aerobic and anaerobic blood cultures before administration of antibiotics.
- Maximize blood pressure through use of fluids and/or pressor agents:
  - Crystalloid fluid bolus 30 mL/kg; avoid albumin or hydroxyethyl starches.
  - Insert central line and initiate vasopressors for MAP < 65 mm Hg or CVP < 8 cm H_2O after initial fluid bolus.
  - Vasopressors: Norepinephrine is first line; add epinephrine or vasopressin for persistent hypotension. If $Scvo_2$ < 70% or evidence of diminished cardiac output after fluids and pressors, consider adding dobutamine (β_2-agonist).
  - If hemoglobin < 7 g/dL or there is active bleeding → transfuse PRBCs.
  - Consider corticosteroids (hydrocortisone 200-300 mg/d in divided doses 3-4 times per day) to treat relative adrenal suppression if refractory hypotension after appropriate fluids and vasopressors.

COMPLICATIONS

- Multisystem organ dysfunction
- Respiratory failure and adult respiratory distress syndrome (ARDS)
- Disseminated intravascular coagulation (**DIC**) (activation of both hemostatic and fibrinolytic systems)

Toxic Shock Syndrome

CAUSES

Inflammatory cascade similar to that seen in sepsis, caused by preformed exotoxin release from *Staphylococcus* or *Streptococcus* species

TWO DISTINCT SYNDROMES

Staphylococcal toxic shock syndrome (StTSS)

- Because of **colonization with exotoxin-producing strain of S *aureus***
- Historically associated with tampon use (commonly due to TSS toxin-1), but also can result from surgical wounds, nasal packing, burns (commonly due to enterotoxins A, B, C)

Streptococcal toxic shock syndrome (STSS)

- Typically due to **skin and soft tissue infections** with exotoxin-producing strain of group A *Streptococcus* (GAS). Exotoxins act as superantigens bypassing the antigen-mediated immune response causing overwhelming cytokine release which produces the clinical syndrome.

> **KEY FACT**
>
> Staphylococcal toxic shock syndrome (StTSS) results from **colonization** with exotoxin-producing *Staphylococcus aureus*. Streptococcal toxic shock syndrome (STSS) results from **infection** with exotoxin-producing group A *Streptococcus* (GAS).

SYMPTOMS/EXAMINATION

- Vomiting, diarrhea, chills, sore throat, headache, myalgias
- Profound hypotension, tachycardia, tachypnea, mucus membrane hyperemia, rash (diffuse erythroderma), altered mental status, oliguria

DIAGNOSIS

Based on established clinical criteria (Table 1.21)

TREATMENT

- Treatment strategy is the same as for patients with septic shock. Aggressive fluid resuscitation often requiring 4-20 L and early use of vasopressors as hypotension and capillary leak from massive cytokine release is profound.
- Antibiotic regimen should cover methicillin-resistant *Staphylococcus aureus* (MRSA) as well as GAS. Recommended regimens include β-lactam plus clindamycin (inhibits protein synthesis/toxin production) and vancomycin.

TABLE 1.21. CDC Criteria for the Diagnosis of StTSS and STSS

CDC Criteria for TSS
Fever > 38.9°C (102°F)
Rash
(Diffuse, blanching, erythroderma ["sunburn"] with desquamation approximately 1-2 wk later)
Hypotension with SBP < 90 mm Hg
Evidence of involvement of ≥ 3 organ systems (GI, muscular, mucus membranes, renal, hepatic, CNS, hematologic) If obtained, negative serologic evidence of: Rocky Mountain spotted fever Leptospirosis Measles Hepatitis B Antinuclear antibody VDRL Monospot
CDC Criteria for STSS
Isolation of group A *Streptococcus* (CSF, surgical wound, throat, blood)
Hypotension with SBP < 90 mm Hg
Involvement of ≥ 2 organ systems

CDC, Centers for Disease Control and Prevention; CNS, central nervous system; CSF, cerebrospinal fluid; GI, gastrointestinal; SBP, systolic blood pressure; STSS, streptococcal toxic shock syndrome; StTSS, staphylococcal toxic shock syndrome; TSS, toxic shock syndrome; VDRL, venereal disease research laboratory.

- Adjunctive therapies include intravenous immunoglobulin (IVIG) (pooled immunoglobulin to toxic shock toxin) and hyperbaric oxygen.

Anaphylaxis and Anaphylactic Shock

See Chapter 9, Hematology, Oncology, Allergy, and Immunology.

Neurogenic Shock

Neurogenic shock occurs when an acute spinal cord injury above the level of T5 causes loss of vasomotor tone below the level of the lesion, leading to loss of systemic vascular resistance and hypotension. Neurogenic shock differs from spinal shock which is a temporary loss of spinal reflexes below the level of a complete or incomplete spinal cord injury characterized by flaccid paralysis with hypotension and bradycardia. In the trauma patient, hemorrhagic shock is a more likely cause of hypotension and may accompany the presence of neurogenic shock. Other causes of neurogenic shock include spinal cord compression by neoplasms or epidural hematoma.

Symptoms/Examination

- Hypotension, bradycardia, vasodilation producing warm extremities.

- Neurologic deficits correlate to a spinal cord level T5 and above, but typically include flaccid paralysis, loss of sensation and deep tendon reflexes, intestinal ileus, and priapism (males).
- Hemorrhage should be excluded as a concomitant cause of shock in trauma patients.

> **KEY FACT**
>
> Shock in a trauma patient should **always** be presumed to be secondary to hemorrhage.

Diagnosis

- Physical examination showing motor and sensory deficits consistent with a spinal level.
- Radiographic evidence of vertebral fracture or cord compression (CT, MRI).

Treatment

- Resuscitation with crystalloid bolus and blood products for concomitant hemorrhage.
- Atropine for hemodynamically unstable bradycardia.
- Avoid over aggressive fluid resuscitation as this may worsen spinal cord edema. After initial fluid bolus, start vasopressors to improve cord perfusion and maintain MAP 85-90 mm Hg. Dopamine is first line and phenylephrine can be added if no response to dopamine.
- Monitor UOP as a measure of adequate perfusion.
- No role for high-dose corticosteroids in acute spinal cord injury.

> **KEY FACT**
>
> Neurogenic shock is characterized by hypotension, bradycardia, and flaccid paralysis and is seen with spinal cord injury above T5.

Fluid Resuscitation

There are numerous options for fluid resuscitation available to the emergency physician, including crystalloids, colloids, and blood products. No mortality difference has been identified for resuscitation with crystalloid versus colloid, but crystalloid is generally preferable.

CRYSTALLOIDS

Isotonic Fluids

Isotonic electrolyte solutions, include NS (0.9% NaCl) and Ringer lactate (NaCl, $CaCl_2$, KCl, Na-lactate)

> **KEY FACT**
>
> One-third of the volume of infused crystalloid remains intravascular after 20 minutes.

Characteristics

- Do not aid in O_2 transport
- Hypo-oncotic → one-third of the volume infused remains in the intravascular space after 20 minutes

Clinical Indications

- Clinically significant hypovolemia/shock.
- Regardless of the cause of hypovolemia, crystalloids should be administered first.

Hypertonic Saline

- Hypertonic (7.5%) saline has been suggested as an alternative to isotonic saline in trauma to promote fluid shift from the extravascular to intravascular space.
- While hypertonic saline may effectively decrease intracranial pressure in head injury, no mortality benefit has been demonstrated for volume resuscitation compared to isotonic saline.

KEY FACT

There is no proven benefit of colloids over crystalloids in volume resuscitation.

KEY FACT

Albumin has the potential for infectious or allergic complications.

COLLOIDS

Colloid solutions contain large-molecular-weight particles of high osmolarity that enable fluid to remain in the intravascular space and draw fluid from the interstitial space. Colloids do not augment O_2-carrying capacity.

Available Products

Albumin, bovine, or human protein

- 5% albumin solution at 0.5-1 g/kg/dose, repeat as needed
- 100 mL approximately equivalent to 1 L of crystalloid
- Potential for infectious complications or allergic reactions

Dextrans

- Highly branched polysaccharides
- May interfere with hemostasis
- Maximum dosage 20 mL/kg

Gelatins

- Modified derivatives of bovine collagen
- Dilutional coagulopathy seen with high-volume infusions

Polystarches

- Pentastarch and hetastarch most commonly used.
- Limited usefulness secondary to dilutional coagulopathy and platelet inhibition. Large volume resuscitation with polystarches is associated with higher rates of kidney injury and mortality.

Clinical Indications

- Colloid solutions are never indicated as primary therapy for volume resuscitation.
- Associated with increased mortality in sepsis and trauma patients compared to crystalloids.
- Albumin 25%: Indicated for the treatment of spontaneous bacterial peritonitis and for patients receiving large-volume paracentesis.
- Hyper-oncotic starches are inferior to crystalloids for volume resuscitation in hypovolemic shock and should generally be avoided.

REVIEW QUESTIONS

QUESTIONS

1. A 35-year-old previously healthy man presents to the emergency department (ED) with 3 days of profuse vomiting and watery diarrhea. Vital signs are HR 130 bpm and BP 90/60 mm Hg. Examination shows a pale dehydrated appearing man with no focal abdominal tenderness. The preferred resuscitation includes:
   A. 1-mL/kg 5% albumin bolus followed by normal saline (NS) infusion at 100 mL/h
   B. 30-mL/kg NS bolus followed by maintenance infusion of NS
   C. 1-L NS bolus and administration of 2 units packed red blood cells (PRBCs)
   D. Pentastarch 10% 500-mL bolus followed by 2-L NS

2. A 64-year-old woman with unknown medical history is brought to the ED with 10 minutes of cardiopulmonary resuscitation (CPR) in progress after she was found pulseless and apneic. On ED arrival the patient's cardiac rhythm shows pulseless electrical activity (PEA). Which of the following is the best initial management?
   A. Continue CPR, place a supraglottic airway, monitor end-tidal CO_2, and administer epinephrine 1 mg every 3-5 minutes.
   B. Administer amiodarone 300 mg intravenous (IV) followed by epinephrine 1 mg IV every 3-5 minutes.
   C. After 2 minutes of CPR pause, perform endotracheal intubation and then immediately resume CPR.
   D. Initiate transcutaneous pacing and start an epinephrine drip.
   E. Administer IV thrombolytics for presumed massive pulmonary embolism.

3. For patients presenting with cardiogenic shock due to acute myocardial infarction (MI), which of the following describes the best approach to management?
   A. Dopamine is a first-line vasopressor.
   B. Revascularization with lytics is preferred to percutaneous coronary intervention (PCI).
   C. Cardiogenic pulmonary edema due to papillary muscle rupture should be managed with nitrates, diuretics, and heparin.
   D. Supportive care with inotropes, noninvasive positive pressure ventilation (NIPPV), and anticoagulation is bridge to PCI or lytics.
   E. β-Blockers are indicated to reduce myocardial oxygen demand.

4. A 77-year-old man presents with 1 week of cough and lethargy. He is found to be febrile with HR 110 bpm, BP 76/38 mm Hg, and oxygen saturation 77% on room air. He is placed on supplemental oxygen and given NS 30-mL/kg IV bolus. Which of the following best describes resuscitation of this patient?
   A. Transfuse PRBCs for Hgb < 9.
   B. Colloid infusion with albumin is equally effective to crystalloid and should be considered.
   C. Place a central venous catheter and initiate norepinephrine infusion if after initial NS bolus the mean arterial pressure (MAP) < 65 mm Hg.
   D. Avoid endotracheal intubation because it may worsen venous return and precipitate cardiovascular collapse.
   E. Administration of broad-spectrum antibiotics within 6 hours is ideal.

5. A 23-year-old man is brought to the ED after a motor vehicle collision. The patient's vital signs are HR 66 bpm and BP 82/68 mm Hg. Which of the following statements is correct?
   A. Spinal shock is the most likely cause of hypotension in this patient.
   B. Initial hematocrit is a reliable predictor of blood loss in this patient.
   C. If the patient requires blood products, the ideal ratio of red blood cells to plasma to platelets after an initial fluid bolus and infusion of 2 units of PRBCs is 4:1:1.
   D. Once hemorrhagic shock has been excluded, the patient should be started on dopamine infusion to keep MAP > 85 mm Hg.
   E. If a spinal cord injury is suspected, early administration of high-dose corticosteroids decreases long-term morbidity.

6. What is the most sensitive physical examination procedure to assess for a patient's ability to protect their airway?
   A. Gag reflex present
   B. Ability to swallow spontaneously
   C. No evidence of pooling of secretions in the posterior pharynx
   D. Ability to speak

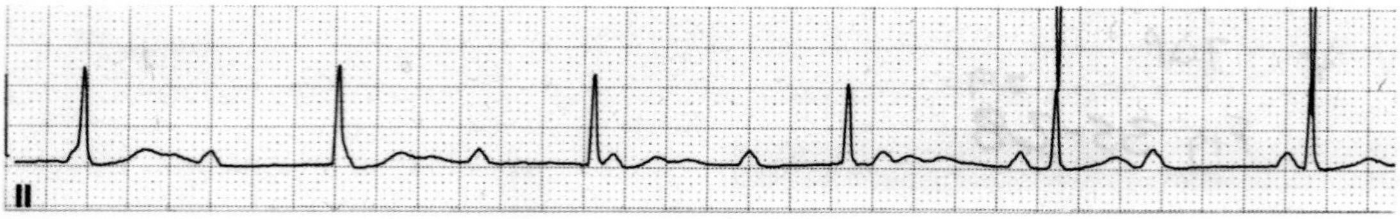

FIGURE 1.26. (Reproduced, with permission, from Stone CK. Humphries RL. *Current Diagnosis & Treatment: Emergency Medicine*. 7th ed. New York, NY: McGraw-Hill Education; 2011. Figure 35-29.)

7. A 5-year-old boy presents with severe respiratory distress after eating a peanut. The patient has a known nut allergy. The patient has notable angioedema, bilateral wheezing, and stridor. Despite pharmaceutical treatment with epinephrine, methylprednisolone, and diphenhydramine, the patient continues to rapidly decompensate. The decision is made to intubate. Following rapid sequence intubation (RSI), the emergency medicine physician is unable to visualize the cords with direct laryngoscopy and bag-valve-mask ventilation is attempted. Despite appropriate bagging with an oropharyngeal airway in place, the patient's oxygen saturation continues to fall and he becomes bradycardic. What is the next appropriate step?
   A. Video laryngoscopy
   B. Cricothyrotomy
   C. Needle cricothyrotomy
   D. Attempt nasal intubation

8. A 55-year-old man presents to the ED 2 days after accessory pathway ablation. He states that he was started on new medications, but cannot remember their names. He denies chest pain, but is noting fatigue, light-headedness, and shortness of breath. His electrocardiogram (ECG) is shown below. Patient becomes less responsive and repeat vitals show a heart rate of 25 bpm and blood pressure of 70/40 mm Hg. What is the next step?
   A. Transcutaneous pacing.
   B. Synchronized cardioversion.
   C. Emergent pericardiocentesis.
   D. Activate ST-elevation myocardial infarction (STEMI) protocol and prepare patient for cath laboratory.

9. An 18-year-old girl has a known history of Wolff-Parkinson-White (WPW). She presents to the ED complaining of palpitations. Her ECG shows a wide complex tachycardia at a rate of 250 bpm. The rest of her vitals are reassuring, and she is denying chest pain or shortness of breath. What is the first-line treatment for her condition?
   A. Cardioversion
   B. Adenosine
   C. Esmolol
   D. Procainamide

ANSWERS

1. **B.** This patient is presenting with nonhemorrhagic hypovolemic shock, presumably due to gastrointestinal (GI) losses. He should be aggressively resuscitated with isotonic crystalloids, either NS or lactated Ringer (LR) is appropriate. Colloids are equivalent to crystalloids in hypovolemic shock, but this patient requires large volume replacement making crystalloid preferable. Hyperoncotic starches are associated with worse outcome in patients with shock and should be avoided.

2. **A.** Management of PEA emphasizes high-quality CPR with end-tidal carbon dioxide monitoring, epinephrine, and a focus on treating the underlying cause. Consider the 6Hs and 5Ts for potentially treatable causes of PEA. CPR should never be interrupted for intubation. Amiodarone and other antiarrhythmic drugs have not been shown to be effective for PEA.

3. **D.** This patient has cardiogenic shock due to acute MI. Management of cardiogenic shock emphasizes inotropic support with preferably dobutamine or dopamine (second line). Most causes of cardiogenic shock are due to acute myocardial ischemia and require revascularization therapy. PCI is preferred to lytics when available. In general, preload reduction with nitrates and diuretics should be avoided. Negative inotropes and chronotropes like β-blockers will worsen cardiogenic shock and are contraindicated.

4. **C.** The patient is presenting with septic shock due to pneumonia. He should be resuscitated with 30-mL/kg crystalloids, not colloids. Colloids are associated with increased mortality in patients with septic shock. If the patient remains hypotensive after fluid bolus, a central venous catheter should be placed and he should be started on norepinephrine. Respiratory support should be provided in the form of endotracheal intubation. Prior studies suggested transfusing to hemoglobin > 10 g/dL, but current Surviving Sepsis Guidelines recommend transfusing for hemoglobin value < 7.

5. **D.** This patient has signs of neurogenic shock due to spinal cord injury, including bradycardia and hypotension. In trauma patients with neurogenic shock, hemorrhagic shock is the most likely cause of hypotension and should be excluded before assuming neurogenic shock. Management of neurogenic shock requires consultation with a spine surgeon and initiation of dopamine or phenylephrine to maintain spinal perfusion pressure > 85 mm Hg. There is currently no role for high-dose steroids in spinal cord injury. The initial hematocrit value is an unreliable indicator or degree of blood loss in trauma patients.

6. **D.** When assessing the airway all the options listed are reassuring findings, but the patient's ability to speak is the most sensitive examination finding when assessing the patency of an airway.

7. **C.** This is a can't intubate/can't ventilate situation and in turns represents a failed airway. In an older individual, a cricothyrotomy would be the appropriate next step, but due to his age, needle cricothyrotomy would be the appropriate next step.

8. **A.** The patient has complete heart block and is rapidly decompensating. Pads should be placed and he should be transcutaneously paced and prepared for transvenous pacing and permanent pacemaker placement.

9. **D.** The patient has known WPW and her wide QRS complex with rapid rate likely represents antidromic tachydysrhythmia. As such, all AV blocking agents should be avoided. She does not warrant emergent cardioversion because she is otherwise stable. Procainamide is the most appropriate option because it should slow conduction via the accessory pathway and hopefully end the antidromic reentry cycle.

CHAPTER 2

Cardiovascular Emergencies

Andrew P. Coleman, MD, MHS and Jasmeet Dhaliwal, MD

Disorders of Arterial Circulation

PERIPHERAL ARTERIAL DISEASE

The vast majority of peripheral arterial disease (PAD) in the United States and Western Europe is due to atherosclerotic arterial disease. Factors contributing to the development of atherosclerosis include cigarette smoking, hyperlipidemia, hypertension (HTN), and diabetes mellitus.

Thromboangiitis obliterans (**Buerger disease**) is an idiopathic cause of PAD more commonly seen in the Middle and Far East. It occurs almost exclusively in smokers, and is most common in young males.

Pathophysiology

- Atherosclerotic PAD: Peripheral vascular atherosclerotic lesions reduce arterial luminal diameter and blood flow → tissues ischemia when blood flow does not meet O_2 demand
- **Buerger disease:** Inflammation of small and medium-size vessels → thrombus formation and subsequent fibrosis → tissue ischemia

Symptoms

- Claudication: Fatigue, pain, or weakness in involved extremity or digit.
- Exertional symptoms become rest symptoms as disease progresses.
- Painful ulcerations.
- **Leriche syndrome:** Triad of bilateral hip claudication, erectile dysfunction, absent femoral pulses = aortoiliac occlusive disease.
- Buerger disease can present with claudication of distal extremities, isolated joint pain, or superficial thrombophlebitis.

KEY FACT

Claudication of distal extremities in a young smoker = Buerger disease

Examination

Patients with PAD will exhibit muscular atrophy, shiny or scaly skin, evidence of poor wound healing, digital ulcerations, loss of hair follicles, diminished pulses, and slowed capillary refill.

KEY FACT

The ankle brachial index (ABI) is a ratio of ankle-to-arm BP. A BP cuff is slowly deflated until distal pulses become audible on Doppler. ABI < 0.9 is diagnostic of PAD. Claudication occurs at ABI < 0.6. Resting angina typically occurs at < 0.26.

Differential

- Spinal stenosis or nerve root compression is another cause of intermittent claudication.
- Ethyl alcohol (EtOH) abuse, diabetes, and chemotherapy may cause neuropathic pain.

Diagnosis

- Suspect based on history and examination.
- Ankle brachial index (ABI) ≤ 0.9 is highly sensitive and specific for the diagnosis.
- **Duplex ultrasound**, comprised of Doppler waveform analysis and color-coded ultrasound imaging, is a noninvasive and accurate diagnostic modality for both PAD and venous disease.
- **Arteriography** has long been the definitive test for peripheral arterial anatomy but is invasive and associated with contrast-related and catheter-related complications.
- Shows diffuse atherosclerosis, irregular cutoff of contrast flow, increased collaterals.

TREATMENT

- Risk-factor modification: Smoking cessation, antihypertensive therapy, lipid-lowering therapy, glycemic control
- Antithrombotic therapy (aspirin, clopidogrel, warfarin)
- Immediate surgical intervention if limb-threatening ischemia:
  - Stents or arterial bypass surgery
- Wound care for ulcerations
- **Smoking cessation** = Only effective therapy for Buerger disease

> **KEY FACT**
>
> Diabetic patients may have a paradoxically normal ABI due to calcification and noncompressibility in the dorsalis pedis and posterior tibial arteries.

ARTERIAL ANEURYSM

Aneurysms can occur anywhere in the arterial system but are most common in the abdominal aorta. Of those occurring in the peripheral arteries, popliteal artery aneurysm is the most common (bilateral in > 50%).

Arteries are composed of 3 layers: tunica intima (inner layer), tunica media, and tunica adventitia (outer layer).

PATHOPHYSIOLOGY

Inciting causes of arterial wall injury include, most commonly, atherosclerosis and loss of elastin and collagen, and less commonly, infection, trauma, connective tissue diseases, and arteritis. Constant shear stress at the vessel wall contributes to weakening of the media and, eventually, dilation or "ballooning" of all 3 vessel wall layers, or a **true aneurysm**.

Trauma to the vessel wall may also result in injury to and eventual disruption of the intima and media such that blood can communicate between the arterial lumen and **pseudoaneurysm**, which is merely a thin layer of adventitia or surrounding soft tissue.

Aneurysms naturally enlarge over time. **Complications** are caused by rupture (unlikely with peripheral artery aneurysms), impingement of adjacent structures, thrombosis, or embolism.

ABDOMINAL AORTIC ANEURYSM

Abdominal aortic aneurysms (AAAs) are usually true aneurysms and most commonly involve the abdominal aorta below the renal arteries and inferior mesenteric artery. The normal adult infrarenal aorta has a diameter of 2 cm and a diameter > 3 cm defines AAA.

The **primary risk factors** for AAA include having a first-degree relative with AAA, comorbid coronary artery disease (CAD) or occlusive peripheral vascular disease, older age (mean age at diagnosis is 65-70 years), and smoking history.

> **KEY FACT**
>
> An AAA of any size can rupture, but those > 5 cm are more likely to rupture.

An AAA of any size **can** rupture, but the likelihood ↑ with increasing size. The most common location of rupture in patients who survive to hospital presentation is in the retroperitoneum. Rupture is associated with 80%-90% overall mortality (many patients do not even reach the hospital).

SYMPTOMS

Unruptured aneurysms are usually asymptomatic. Occasionally they may manifest as an abdominal mass or fullness, or a sensation of abdominal pulsations. Rarely, expansion can cause duodenum compression/obstruction or ureteral obstruction/colic.

In contrast, a **rapidly expanding or ruptured AAA** may be associated with abdominal, back, and/or flank pain and nausea/vomiting. In cases of the latter, syncope may occur. Rupture may occur directly into the gastrointestinal (GI) tract or the inferior vena cava (IVC). The former manifests as a GI bleed, normally a rare complication but the leading diagnosis in a patient with a history of aortic graft placement who presents with GI bleeding. The latter results in the formation of an arteriovenous (AV) fistula, leading to high-output congestive heart failure (CHF). Classically, this may lead to the painless hematuria associated with AAA.

KEY FACT

The most common location of AAA rupture in emergency department (ED) patients = retroperitoneum.

Examination

Abdominal tenderness, distension, and/or pulsatile abdominal mass may be present in the setting of a ruptured AAA. Vital signs may be normal if rupture occurs into the retroperitoneum with subsequent tamponade. In this case, periumbilical and flank ecchymoses may be present (**Cullen** and **Grey-Turner sign**, respectively). Melena and hematemesis may occur in cases of aortoenteric rupture, and signs of heart failure will accompany AV rupture.

Diagnosis

KEY FACT

Triad of abdominal pain, hypotension, pulsatile abdominal mass = AAA until proven otherwise.

The diagnosis should be considered in any patient > 50 years old presenting with pain in the abdomen, flank, or back (especially when associated with hematuria), or with unexplained hypotension or syncope.

Bedside ultrasound can be used to obtain rapid and reliable aortic diameter measurements and evaluate for free fluid in patients with possible AAA, making it the modality of choice in the unstable patient (Figure 2.1).

In cases in which ultrasound is unavailable and the patient is stable enough to travel to the radiology suite, computed tomography (CT), ideally with intravenous (IV) contrast, is appropriate and may show the location of rupture if present or provide alternative diagnoses for a patient's symptoms (Figure 2.2).

Magnetic resonance imaging (MRI) and aortography have no place in the emergent evaluation of a possible ruptured AAA.

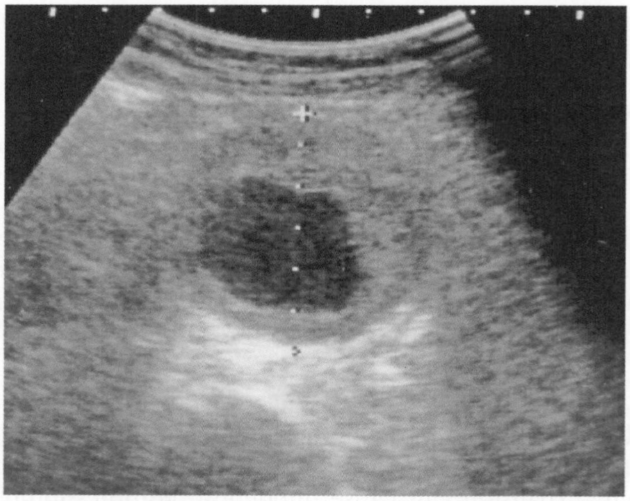

FIGURE 2.1. Transabdominal ultrasound showing 6-cm abdominal aortic aneurysm (AAA).

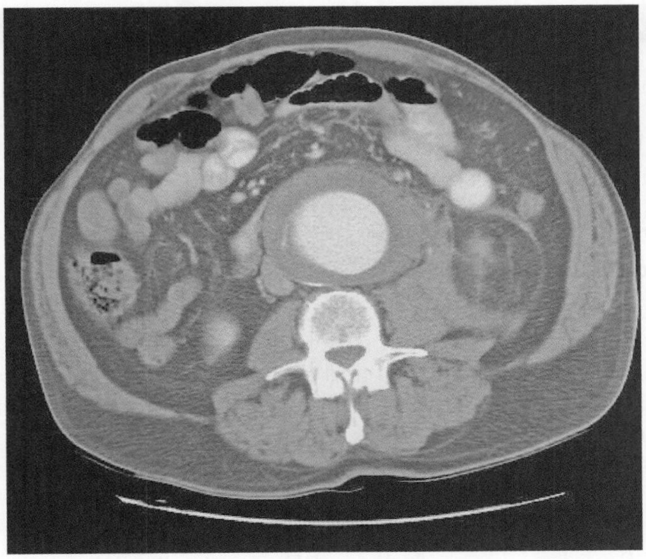

FIGURE 2.2. Contrast-enhanced abdominal CT showing large AAA with rupture. (Used with permission from Matthew J Fleishman, MD, Radiology Imaging Associates. Englewood, Colorado.)

Differential

The rapidly expanding or ruptured AAA may present clinically like renal colic, muscular back pain, pancreatitis, intestinal ischemia, diverticulitis, biliary disease, and, uncommonly, bowel obstruction, upper GI bleed, and heart failure. Because it may cause coronary hypoperfusion, chest pain, and electrocardiogram (ECG) changes in patients with CAD, ruptured AAA can also present like acute coronary syndrome (ACS).

Treatment

Ruptured aneurysms require immediate surgical intervention with operative or endovascular repair. It is reasonable to resuscitate a hypotensive patient with a ruptured AAA with fluids and blood to a systolic blood pressure (SBP) of 80-100 mm Hg ("permissive hypotension") if it can be done quickly and/or there is a delay in operating room (OR) readiness, but in general transfer of hypotensive patients to the OR should not be delayed by prolonged attempts at resuscitation in the emergency department (ED) or trips to the radiology suite for imaging.

In cases of cardiac arrest, ED thoracotomy and aortic cross-clamping may be considered.

Complications

In addition to rupture, atherosclerotic aneurysms can cause **atheroembolism**, in which microemboli travel to and obstruct distal small vessels, leading to **blue toe syndrome**.

Acute (iatrogenic) complications of AAA endovascular grafting includes vascular injury to the renal, mesenteric, or Adamkiewicz artery (the latter causes an anterior cord syndrome). Chronic complications include infection, thrombosis, migration, kinking, aortoenteric fistula formation, pseudoaneurysm at anastomosis site, and **endoleak**, in which blood leaks between the graft and the aneurysm, leading to continued growth and/or aneurysmal rupture.

THORACIC AORTIC ANEURYSM

Thoracic aortic aneurysm (TAA) is most often an incidental finding on chest x-ray (CXR) and is defined by a **thoracic aorta diameter of > 4.5 cm**. Risk factors are similar to those for AAA. Risk of rupture is high when diameter ≥ 6 cm. It may be saccular (involving only a portion of the total vessel circumference) or fusiform (symmetrical expansion of the entire circumference).

Symptoms and Examination

As in the case of AAA, TAA is asymptomatic unless it is rapidly expanding, ruptured, or compressing adjacent structure. When ruptured, it will present as chest or back pain in an acutely ill and likely hypotensive patient. When associated with a bicuspid aortic valve, the clinical picture will be similar to that of acute aortic insufficiency. Hoarseness, cough, and wheezing may occur due to compression of the recurrent laryngeal nerve and trachea.

Differential

Includes ACS, pulmonary embolism (PE), aortic dissection, pneumothorax, and esophageal rupture

Diagnosis

CXR is normal in 40% of cases, but may show a wide mediastinum or large aortic knob.

CT is confirmative and is most appropriate in stable patients in whom the diagnosis is unknown.

Transesophageal echocardiography (TEE) is most appropriate in the unstable patient.

Treatment

The unstable patient with TAA is treated similarly to the patient with aortic dissection, in which resuscitation, aggressive BP and heart rate (HR) control, and immediate surgical consult are the priorities. As is the case with incidentally diagnosed AAA, patients with asymptomatic TAA are appropriate for outpatient follow-up.

AORTIC DISSECTION

Aortic dissections are classified by their location (Figure 2.3). Location has important implications for management and prognosis: dissection of the ascending aorta, comprising 62% of dissections, is highly lethal and is managed surgically, whereas descending dissections (38% of dissections) have a better prognosis and are typically managed medically.

The most common predisposing risk factor (Table 2.1) for aortic dissection = uncontrolled HTN.

Pathophysiology

- Disruption of intima of aortic wall → blood travels (dissects) into media, creating false lumen.
- Dissection can propagate down/up the aorta through the false lumen:
  - Proximally into aortic root → right coronary artery involvement and myocardial infarction (MI), tamponade, aortic regurgitation (AR)
  - Into carotid artery → stroke symptoms

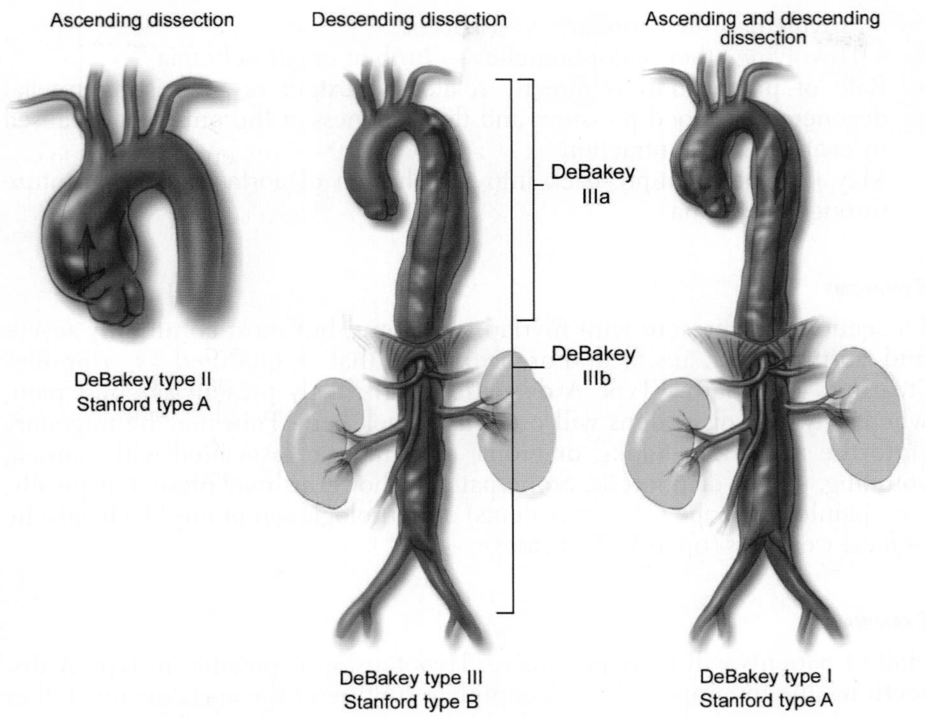

FIGURE 2.3. Illustration of the classification schemes for aortic dissection based on which portions of the aorta are involved. Dissection can be confined to the ascending aorta (left) or descending aorta (middle), or it can involve the entire aorta (right). (Reproduced, with permission, from Creager MA, Dzau VS, Loscalzo J, eds. *Vascular Medicine*. Philadelphia, PA: WB Saunders; 2006. Figure 35.2).

Q

A 55-year-old man with a history of poorly controlled HTN presents after a syncopal event while lifting weights at the gym. He complains of severe, sharp, left-chest pain radiating to his back, and he is diaphoretic and anxious appearing. Initial BP is 88/55 mm Hg and HR is 122 bpm. Examination reveals equal breath sounds, prominent jugular venous distention (JVD), distant heart tones, and weak radial pulses. His ECG is nondiagnostic. What is the most likely diagnosis and what is the confirmatory study of choice?

TABLE 2.1. Risk Factors for Aortic Dissection

Uncontrolled hypertension
Advancing age
Connective tissue disease (eg, Marfan syndrome and Ehlers-Danlos syndrome)
Congenital heart disease (eg, bicuspid aortic valve)
Giant cell arteritis
Annuloaortic ectasia
Family history
Stimulant abuse
Latrogenic (catheterization or surgery)

A

This patient has a proximal aortic dissection with associated tamponade. Bedside transthoracic ECG will demonstrate an effusion. Either transesophageal ECG or chest CT angiography (CTA) can be used to confirm the presence of a proximal dissection. Study choice depends on the availability of these modalities in a particular medical center.

KEY FACT

Patient with chest pain and neurologic symptoms? Consider aortic dissection!

KEY FACT

A new AR murmur in a patient with acute chest pain is highly suggestive of proximal aortic dissection.

    - Involving spinal cord artery → paresis
    - Involving other major branches → limb or organ ischemia
- Rate of propagation is directly related to extent of preexisting medial degeneration, blood pressure, and the steepness of the pulse wave caused by each cardiac contraction.
- May ultimately empty back into true lumen of aorta (rare), or rupture through adventitia.

Symptoms

Dissection may present with myriad symptoms, but most commonly severe and abrupt chest, neck, and/or back pain that is qualified as "ripping," "tearing," or "sharp." Type A dissections will likely present as chest pain, whereas type B dissections will present as back pain. Pain may be migratory (into the abdomen, flanks, or groin) and may be associated with nausea, vomiting, and/or diaphoresis. Some patients, however, may present atypically, with painless syncope (~9% of patients) or neurologic symptoms like headache or focal weakness (up to 17% of cases).

Examination

Half of patients will be hypertensive. Hypotension is possible in **type A dissections** due to tamponade or if complete rupture of the aorta occurs. Other signs of proximal dissection include AR, upper extremity blood pressure asymmetry, or low/absent blood pressure ("pseudohypotension") due to subclavian artery involvement, altered mental status (AMS), or stroke symptoms due to carotid or vertebral artery involvement.

Type B dissections may result in asymmetric blood pressure or pseudohypotension in the lower extremities, mesenteric ischemia, refractory HTN due to renin secretion in cases of renal artery involvement, or paraparesis or peripheral neuropathy due to anterior spinal artery involvement.

Differential

Includes ACS, PE, pneumothorax, ruptured aneurysm, esophageal perforation, stroke

Diagnosis

- The **mortality rate** of aortic dissection is > 1% per hour, and thus diagnosis is highly time sensitive.
- **D-dimer** has a sensitivity of about 90% (but poor specificity) which may be helpful ruling out a dissection.
- **ECG** will in 15% of cases show inferior/posterior ischemia indicating right coronary artery (RCA) involvement. More commonly it will show evidence of left ventricular hypertrophy (LVH) (26%) suggestive of chronic HTN.
- **CXR** will be abnormal in > 85% of patients (Figure 2.4). Abnormal findings include widened mediastinum (62%); loss of aortic know (50%); pleural capping; and the "calcium sign," or aortic shadow extension > 5 mm from an aortic calcification (14%).
- **Bedside transthoracic echocardiography (TTE)** is a useful bedside screening test to evaluate for enlarged aortic root and tamponade, but has a poor sensitivity. If available, **TEE** has sufficient sensitivity (98%) to rule out type A and all but the most distal type B dissections.
- **CT angiogram** is the diagnostic test of choice at most institutions (Figure 2.5) and has largely supplanted **aortography**.

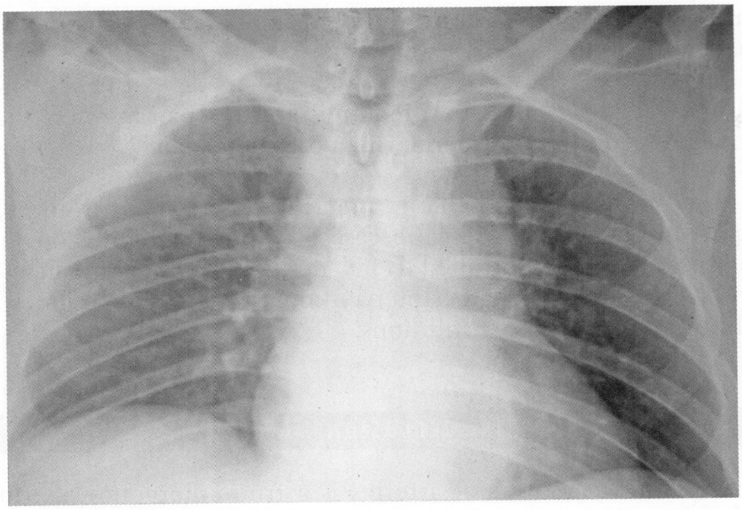

FIGURE 2.4. Anteroposterior (AP) chest radiograph showing widened mediastinum and loss of aortic knob in patient with aortic dissection. (Used with permission from Matthew J Fleishman, MD, Radiology Imaging Associates. Englewood, Colorado.)

Treatment

The rate of dissection extension is directly related to blood pressure and steepness of the pulse wave caused by each cardiac contraction. Therefore, treatment is aimed at reducing sympathetic tone via adequate pain control, SBP to **100-120 mm Hg**, and heart rate to **< 60 bpm**. Blood pressure and heart rate reduction is accomplished with IV β-blockers such as esmolol or labetalol (or selective β-blockers such as metoprolol or atenolol in cases of severe asthma/chronic obstructive pulmonary disease [COPD]). Nitroprusside may be added if monotherapy with a β-blocker does not achieve the blood pressure goal.

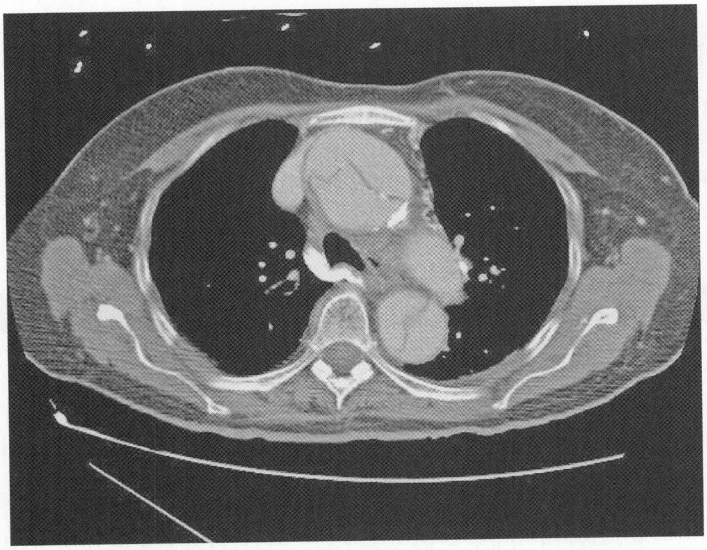

FIGURE 2.5. Contrast-enhanced chest CT showing type A aortic dissection. (Used with permission from Matthew J Fleishman, MD, Radiology Imaging Associates. Englewood, Colorado.)

Hypotensive patients will require fluids, pressors, and pericardiocentesis if tamponade is present.

KEY FACT

Initial drug of choice in aortic dissection is IV esmolol (or labetalol) → decrease shearing forces.

Type A dissections will ultimately require surgical repair to resect the area of dissection and reconstruct the aorta with a prosthetic graft.

Type B dissections are amenable to medical management in the ICU, but also require surgical consult in the case of rupture, progression, impaired distal perfusion, or uncontrolled HTN despite maximal medical therapy (indications for surgical repair). Interventional vascular techniques are also currently available in some institutions.

ACUTE PERIPHERAL ARTERIAL OCCLUSION

Acute occlusion of peripheral arteries is a true emergency, as infarction of distal extremity tissue will occur in 4-6 hours without revascularization, resulting in amputation and even death. Acute arterial occlusion is most commonly caused by **acute arterial thromboembolism**, but may also be caused by **acute thrombotic occlusion** (aka, thrombosis in situ). Because each disease is managed differently, it is vital to differentiate them clinically.

ACUTE ARTERIAL THROMBOEMBOLISM

KEY FACT

The most common site of acute arterial embolism = bifurcation of common femoral artery.

Pathophysiology

Step 1: Thrombus formation occurs in places where there is turbulent or static blood flow, most commonly the left ventricle of patients with a history of MI (60%-70%). Additional sources of thrombi include the **left atrium** in patients with mitral valve disease or atrial fibrillation or within a large arterial aneurysm.

Step 2: Embolization occurs when thrombus is launched out into systemic circulation, most commonly landing at the bifurcation of the common femoral artery (35%-50% of cases), within the large arteries of the upper extremity, or the popliteal artery.

Result: Because most patients with thromboembolism are not affected by atherosclerosis, they will not have collateral circulation. Without collateral circulation, thromboembolism results in acute occlusion, leading to limb-threatening ischemia.

ACUTE THROMBOTIC OCCLUSION (THROMBOSIS IN SITU)

Pathophysiology

Step 1: Atherosclerosis develops over years, secondary to smoking, HTN, high cholesterol, diabetes, etc. Trauma and vasculitis are much less common inciting factors.

Step 2: Either through plaque rupture or the development of turbulent/sluggish flow, thrombus forms.

Result: Distal ischemia results, but because collateral circulation has had time to develop, limb-threatening ischemia is less likely.

SYMPTOMS AND EXAMINATION

Patients with acute arterial occlusion present with signs of **limb-threatening ischemia**. These signs comprise the 6 Ps of acute occlusion:

THE 6 PS OF ACUTE ARTERIAL OCCLUSION		
Pain	Pallor	Paresthesias
Pulselessness	Paralysis	Poikilothermia

> **KEY FACT**
>
> In acute arterial occlusion, surgical embolectomy must occur within 4-6 hours to preserve limb function.

DIFFERENTIAL

Because they require different treatments, acute arterial thromboembolism and acute thrombotic occlusion must be differentiated from one another (Table 2.2). Other differential diagnoses include:

- **Atheroembolism**, caused by atherosclerotic plaque particles called **microemboli**, which, as the name suggests, are much smaller and therefore only obstruct the most distal small vessels, causing blue toe syndrome but leaving pulses intact.
- Infectious emboli from bacterial endocarditis (discussed later).
- Malignant emboli from melanoma or lung cancer.
- Foreign body emboli (eg, bullet fragment embolism).
- Raynaud disease.
- Vasculitis.

> **KEY FACT**
>
> Raynaud disease is characterized by a triphasic response to cold or emotion (fingers become white, then blue, then red) followed by spontaneous resolution.

DIAGNOSIS

Limb-threatening ischemia is a clinical diagnosis that is made in a patient presenting with acute pain in a pulseless extremity. An attempt should be made to distinguish between thromboembolism and thrombosis based on the patient's past medical history and physical examination.

If the etiology of acute arterial occlusion is unclear, angiography can be used prior to embolectomy to differentiate between thromboembolism and thrombosis in situ.

In cases of incomplete occlusion, pulses may be decreased or grossly symmetrical, depending on the degree of arterial occlusion.

- **Ankle-brachial blood pressure comparisons** performed at the bedside will be < 0.9.
- **Doppler ultrasonography** will reveal biphasic or uniphasic signal (normal arterial signal is **triphasic**).
- **Duplex ultrasound** combines Doppler signal analysis of blood flow with B-mode ultrasound imaging of the vascular structure and occlusion.
- **Arteriography** is used to differentiate thromboembolism and thrombosis in situ when the clinical picture is unclear, and to determine the feasibility of bypass grafting in the latter.

> **KEY FACT**
>
> Limb-threatening ischemia due to thromboembolism or thrombosis mandates immediate heparinization and surgical consult for embolectomy. Intra-arterial thrombolysis takes 6-72 hours, outside the time window for irreversible limb ischemia.

TREATMENT

- Acute thromboembolism: heparin + **Fogarty catheter embolectomy**
- Thrombosis in situ with limb-threatening ischemia: Heparin + embolectomy + bypass grafting
- Arterial thrombosis without limb-threatening ischemia: heparinization ± thrombolysis

TABLE 2.2. Characteristics and Management of Acute Arterial Embolism and Arterial Thrombosis

	Acute Arterial Embolism	Acute Thrombotic Occlusion (Thrombosis in situ)
Pathophysiology	Step 1: Distant thrombus formation, usually the left ventricle or atrium Step 2: Embolization to mid-sized artery, usually at point of bifurcation	Atherosclerotic plaque alters normal blood flow and causes endothelial injury, allowing formation of a blood clot (thrombosis) at the site of injury (in situ)
Patient characteristics	May have history of recent MI, cardiac valve disease, and/or atrial fibrillation. History of peripheral atherosclerosis is **uncommon**, so well-developed collateral circulation is **absent**	History of atherosclerosis, stroke, MI, cardiac dysrhythmias, renal disease, claudication, and/or neuropathy. Because peripheral atherosclerosis is **common**, collateral circulation is often **present**
Presentation symptoms	In the absence of collateral circulation, embolism results in limb-threatening ischemia, causing severe, sudden-onset, "shocking" pain	Because of collateral circulation, thrombosis usually presents subacutely as non–limb-threatening ischemia. Patient may endorse claudication
Physical examination signs		
Limb-threatening ischemia	Common (see 6 Ps of acute arterial occlusion)	Uncommon, though possible
Peripheral vascular disease	Uncommon	Muscular atrophy, hair loss, shiny/scaly skin, ulcers
Proximal/contralateral pulses	Strong	Faint/absent
Line of demarcation	Sharp	Diffuse or absent
Testing	Not needed if signs of limb-threatening ischemia Bedside ABI Color-coded Doppler or Duplex ultrasonography Invasive contrast arteriography CT angiography	Not needed if signs of limb-threatening ischemia Bedside ABI Color-coded Doppler or Duplex ultrasonography Invasive contrast arteriography CT angiography
Treatment of limb-threatening ischemia	Fogarty catheter embolectomy Amputation if irreversible ischemia	Fogarty embolectomy **plus** vascular bypass grafting Amputation if irreversible ischemia or lesion cannot be bypassed
Treatment of non–limb-threatening ischemia	Fogarty catheter embolectomy	Immediate heparinization Consider intra-arterial thrombolytic therapy

ABI, ankle brachial index; CT, computed tomography; MI, myocardial infarction.

Disorders of Venous Circulation

DEEP VENOUS THROMBOSIS

Deep venous thrombosis (DVT) can occur anywhere in the deep venous system, but is most common in the deep veins of the legs. The "deep" venous system constitutes a network of veins that extend from the calf veins to the femoral (which is, in fact, a deep vein, although it is often called the "superficial femoral vein") and iliac veins. The superficial veins in the legs include the greater and short saphenous veins and the perforator veins.

TABLE 2.3. Clinical Risk Factors for Deep Venous Thrombosis

T	Trauma, travel
H	Hypercoagulable, hormone replacement
R	Relatives, recreational drugs (intravenous drugs)
O	Old (age > 60 y)
M	Malignancy
B	Birth control pill, blood group A
O	Obesity, obstetrics
S	Surgery, smoking
I	Immobilization
S	Sickness

(Reproduced, with permission, from Tintinalli JE, Kelen GD, Stapczynski JS. *Emergency Medicine: A Comprehensive Study Guide*. 6th ed. New York, NY: McGraw-Hill; 2004:409.)

There are many clinical factors that increase the susceptibility to DVT formation (Table 2.3).

PATHOPHYSIOLOGY

- Damage to the vessel wall, venostasis, or hypercoagulable state (Virchow triad) → thrombus formation.
- Once formed, thrombus can propagate or embolize distally.
- Massive thrombus can cause vasospasm of adjacent artery.

> **KEY FACT**
>
> Virchow triad: venous injury, venostasis, hypercoagulable state

SYMPTOMS/EXAMINATION

The signs and symptoms in a patient with DVT are often nonspecific and may be completely absent. They include unilateral limb swelling and/or pain, a tender palpable cord, erythema and warmth, distended collateral veins, and/or **Homans sign** (pain in calf or posterior knee with passive dorsiflexion of foot).

Severe manifestations of DVT include the following:

- **Phlegmasia cerulean dolens (painful blue leg)** = massive iliofemoral thrombosis causing acute, massive edema due to **venous** insufficiency, severe pain, and cyanosis
- **Phlegmasia alba dolens (painful white leg)** = massive iliofemoral thrombosis causing **arterial** spasm and a swollen, pale leg

> **KEY FACT**
>
> Phlegmasia cerulean dolens (painful blue leg) = massive thrombosis with venous insufficiency.
>
> Phlegmasia alba dolens (painful white leg) = massive thrombosis with arterial spasm.

DIFFERENTIAL

- **Superficial thrombophlebitis**
- Cellulitis
- Lymphedema
- Musculoskeletal injury
- Baker cyst

DIAGNOSIS

- **Wells criteria for DVT** (Table 2.4).
  - Initial step in establishing diagnosis.
  - Estimates the pretest likelihood of DVT.
  - Score ≤ 2 indicates a **low or moderate pretest risk** for DVT.
  - Score > 2 indicates a **high pretest risk** for DVT.

TABLE 2.4. Wells Pretest Probability for Predicting DVT

CRITERIA	SCORE
Active cancer	1
Paralysis/immobilization	1
Bedridden 3 d/surgery in last 4 wk	1
Tender along deep vein (localized)	1
Entire leg swollen	1
Unilateral calf swelling (> 3 cm)	1
Pitting edema, 1 leg	1
Collateral superficial nonvaricose vein	1
Previous documented DVT	1
Alternative diagnosis likely	–2

Score ≤ 2 = low or moderate risk for DVT
Score > 2 = high risk for DVT
DVT, deep venous thrombosis.

- **D-dimer.**
  - Fibrin breakdown product.
  - Indicates presence of a clot (somewhere) within **past 72 hours**, increases in relation to size of new clot burden, and declines in the presence of chronic clot (half-life is 8 hours).
  - Elevated levels may be seen in sepsis, pregnancy, trauma, MI, liver disease, cancer.
  - Enzyme-linked immunosorbent assay (ELISA) (quantitative) is more accurate than latex agglutination (qualitative).
- **Duplex ultrasound** = study of choice.
  - Ultrasound with color Doppler flow evaluation
  - 95% sensitivity/specificity for proximal DVT of leg
  - May not identify calf vein or iliac vein thrombosis
- **Venography:** Gold standard, but rarely used (invasive, radiation, cost).
- **MRI.**
  - Highly sensitive for DVT
  - Useful for DVT in iliac vein or vena cava where ultrasound cannot be used
- A clinical diagnosis is established using a combination of the previously listed modalities (Table 2.5).

KEY FACT

D-dimer measured by ELISA is more accurate than the latex agglutination method.

TREATMENT

- **Immediate anticoagulation** with unfractionated heparin or low-molecular-weight (LMW) heparin.
  - LMW heparin requires dose adjustment in renal failure.
  - Does not prevent investigation for hypercoagulable state.

TABLE 2.5. Clinical Evaluation for DVT

Low or moderate pretest risk
If D-dimer normal → no DVT present
If D-dimer elevated → obtain extremity ultrasound to exclude DVT
High pretest risk
Obtain extremity ultrasound to exclude DVT
If ultrasound negative but D-dimer elevated → plan repeat ultrasound in 5-7 d
If ultrasound and D-dimer both negative → no DVT present
Suspected pelvic vein or vena caval thrombosis
Obtain CT with contrast or MR venography

CT, computed tomography; DVT, deep venous thrombosis; MR, magnetic resonance.

- If heparin contraindicated (eg, heparin-induced thrombocytopenia), use thrombin inhibitor, such as lepirudin or danaparoid.
- **Long-term anticoagulation:** 3 months of warfarin, started in the ED.
- **Thrombolysis** is **not** more effective than heparin for preventing PE.
  - May accelerate clot lysis and **reduce complications of venous insufficiency** in massive thrombosis
  - Contraindications: As with MI
- **IVC filter** indications include:
  - Contraindication to or complication of anticoagulation (bleeding, heparin-induced thrombocytopenia)
  - Propagation of DVT despite adequate anticoagulation with warfarin and heparin
  - Presence of free-floating nonadherent iliofemoral thrombus > 5 cm
  - Massive clot burden
  - Permanent IVC filter placement **increases** long-term DVT risk
- Many possible clinical scenarios exist in the treatment of DVT (Table 2.6).

Complications

- PE
- Chronic venous insufficiency
- SVC syndrome (upper extremity clot)
- Heparin-induced thrombocytopenia, warfarin skin necrosis, bleeding (from therapy)
- Postphlebitic syndrome

PULMONARY EMBOLISM

By far, the most common source of pulmonary embolism (PE) is thrombus in the lower extremity deep venous system. Risk factors are therefore identical to DVT (see Table 2.3). Other possible emboli include venous thrombi from other parts of the body, fat, amniotic fluid, foreign bodies, and tumor.

Pathophysiology

- Thrombus formed in venous system → embolizes to lung → acute obstruction of the pulmonary arterial system and pulmonary ischemia/infarction

Q

A 40-year-old woman 1 week status-post mastectomy presents with mild right-sided pleuritic chest pain and dyspnea. Her initial BP is 124/72 mm Hg, HR is 122 bpm, O_2 saturation is 90% on room air, and temperature is 100.4°F = (38°C). Examination reveals equal breath sounds with no rales or rhonchi. There is no redness or swelling over the chest wall. There is no swelling in the legs. What is the study of choice in this patient?

KEY FACT

Thrombolysis is **not** more effective than heparin for preventing PE in DVT.

A

CT angiogram of chest to evaluate for PE. Because this patient has a high pretest probability for PE, a D-dimer is not indicated. CT can also detect abscess or pneumonia in this patient.

TABLE 2.6. Clinical Considerations in the Treatment of DVT

Proximal DVT Immediate anticoagulation with heparin and warfarin until INR therapeutic
Massive DVT Vascular surgery consult for thrombectomy Consider thrombolysis Consider IVC filter placement
Isolated calf vein thrombosis These veins have a low risk for embolization **but**: At least 25% will propagate proximally, where they **may** embolize Options include anticoagulation (for high-risk patients) or ASA and follow-up ultrasound in 3-7 d
Proximal greater saphenous vein clot Too close to the deep system for comfort! Anticoagulate
Recurrent DVT on adequate warfarin Add heparin Indication for IVC filter placement
Propagation of DVT on adequate warfarin and heparin Indication for IVC filter placement
Upper extremity venous thrombosis 50% associated with indwelling catheters. Thrombosis above the elbow requires definitive treatment. If no contraindications, anticoagulate for 3 mo.

DVT, deep venous thrombosis; INR, international normalized ratio; IVC, inferior vena cava; ASA, acetylsalicylic acid.

KEY FACT

Symptoms in PE are sudden in **onset only in half of patient presentations**!

- Large emboli → obstruction of right ventricular outflow and circulatory collapse

Risk Factors for ED Patients

- Strongest risk factors are surgery within 4 weeks requiring general anesthesia and trauma within 4 weeks requiring hospitalization.
- Other strong risk factors include limb/generalized immobility, estrogen use, and hypercoagulability.
- Moderate risk factors include history of PE/DVT and carcinoma.

Symptoms

- Strongest association with PE: Hemoptysis
- Most common complaint: Dyspnea
- Chest pain: Classically pleuritic (but not always), but commonly absent
- Classic misconception: PE presents with sudden-onset chest pain (CP) or SOB (< 50% of cases present with sudden-onset symptoms)

EXAMINATION

- Tachypnea: Most common finding
- Tachycardia
- Clear lungs (but may hear rales/wheezes)
- Hypoxia
- Unilateral leg swelling if concomitant DVT
- Evidence of acute right heart failure, hypotension if massive

DIAGNOSIS

Diagnosis should be suspected in any patient presenting with dyspnea, unexplained hypoxia, or chest pain, especially in the presence of risk factors.

Multiple tools are available to risk stratify patients for PE; diagnostic evaluation should be based on individual risk assessment. The Wells clinical prediction rule is a useful risk stratification tool (Table 2.7).

- **ECG:** Abnormal in most, but not diagnostic.
  - Tachycardia and nonspecific ST-T changes most common.
  - **Any** evidence of right heart strain: Classic is S wave in lead I, Q wave in lead III, and T-wave inversion in lead III ($S_1Q_3T_3$ pattern).
  - Also new right bundle branch block (RBBB) or incomplete RBBB.
  - T-wave inversion in the anterior precordial leads and/or inferior leads, especially if new, is a PE until proven otherwise.
- **Arterial blood gas (ABG):** May demonstrate respiratory alkalosis, hypoxemia, and a widened A-a gradient; a normal ABG does not exclude PE.
- **CXR:** Useful to rule out other causes of SOB/CP, may show clues suggestive of PE:
  - **Hampton hump** = Pleural-based, wedge-shaped density indicating infarcted lung.
  - **Westermark sign** = ↓ vessel markings distal to embolus (oligemia) (**rarely** seen).

KEY FACT

Most common ECG in PE = tachycardia and nonspecific ST-T changes.

Classic ECG finding = $S_1Q_3T_3$

KEY FACT

A-a gradient at sea level: 150 – (Po_2 + Pco_2/0.8)

KEY FACT

Normal A-a gradient = Age/4 + 4

TABLE 2.7. Wells Clinical Prediction Rule for PE

CLINICAL FEATURE	POINTS
Clinical symptoms of DVT	3
Other diagnosis less likely than PE	3
Heart rate > 100 bpm	1.5
Immobilization or surgery within past 4 wk	1.5
Previous DVT or PE	1.5
Hemoptysis	1
Malignancy	1
High risk for PE: > 6 points **Moderate risk for PE: 2-6 points** **Low risk for PE: < 2 points**	

DVT, deep venous thrombosis; PE, pulmonary embolism.

Note: Newer studies are dichotomizing patients into a modified Wells score: low (≤ 4 points) or high (> 4 points) risk.

TABLE 2.8. PERC Rule

Low pretest probability for PE by the treating clinician's estimate, plus:	
Age < 50 y	Pulse < 100 bpm
Oxygen saturation > 94%	No hemoptysis
No unilateral leg swelling	No recent major surgery or trauma
No prior PE or DVT	No hormone use

DVT, deep venous thrombosis; PE, pulmonary embolism; PERC, pulmonary embolism rule-out criteria.

Note: If a low pretest probability patient satisfies all these criteria, their risk of having a PE is < 2%, or equivalent to the same patient having a negative D-dimer assay.

KEY FACT

A negative D-dimer **or** meeting all PERC virtually excludes PE in a low clinical suspicion patient.

- **D-dimer:** Described in the section "Deep Venous Thrombosis."
  - Test virtually excludes PE in a low-risk patient, and some evidence supports its use in intermediate-probability patients as well.
- **Pulmonary embolism rule-out criteria (PERC):** If all these criteria apply, the patient's risk of having a PE is < 2%, which is equivalent to the same patient with a negative D-dimer (Table 2.8).
- **CT angiography** (Figure 2.6): Study of choice in many centers.
  - High sensitivity and specificity.
  - Preferred over ventilation-perfusion (V/Q) scan in early pregnancy due to **lower** fetal radiation exposure.
  - A high-risk patient with a negative CT angiogram requires further testing to rule out PE, such as V/Q scan (described below), D-dimer testing, DVT ultrasound, or pulmonary arteriography.

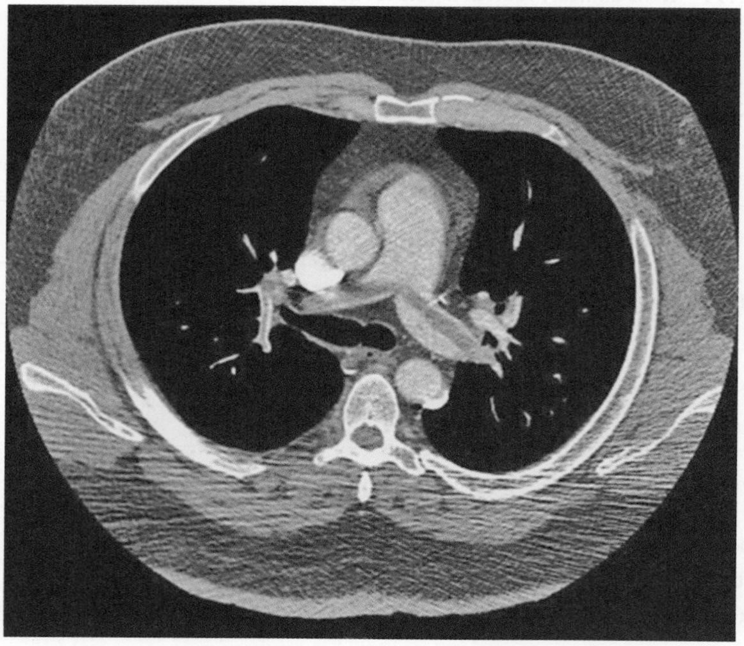

FIGURE 2.6. Contrast-enhanced helical chest CT, showing large filling defect in both pulmonary arteries from a saddle pulmonary embolus. (Used with permission from Matthew J Fleishman, MD, Radiology Imaging Associates. Englewood, Colorado.)

- **V/Q scan:** Matches inhaled radionuclide distribution (ventilation) to pulmonary vasculature radionuclide (perfusion).
  - **Normal** perfusion = No PE
  - High probability = Definite PE
  - Low probability with low clinical suspicion = No PE
  - Indeterminate test results are common, mandating further testing
  - Indications include renal failure, contrast allergy
  - Less useful if underlying lung disease or abnormal CXR
- **Pulmonary arteriography:** Classic gold standard, but mostly supplanted by chest CT.
- **Duplex ultrasound.**
  - Presumptive PE if positive for DVT in correct clinical setting (negative test **not** helpful in excluding PE)

Treatment

- **Immediate anticoagulation** with unfractionated heparin infusion or LMW heparin.
  - If heparin is contraindicated use the factor Xa inhibitor, fondaparinux.
  - If pretest probability of PE is > 30%, anticoagulate prior to obtaining the CT angiogram.
- **Thrombolysis** should be used if there is clinical evidence of massive PE (SBP < 90 mm Hg for > 15 minutes or baseline SBP reduction > 60 mm Hg, severe hypoxemia, cardiac arrest, evidence of right heart strain).
  - tPA is preferred agent (100 mg over 2 hours).
  - Contraindications similar to thrombolytics in MI (see Table 2.7).
  - No evidence that mortality is lowered, but will improve right heart function.
- **Embolectomy.**
  - May be used independently of or in conjunction with thrombolysis
  - Can be beneficial in cases of large embolism that does not resolve alone with thrombolytics or in patients with contraindications to thrombolytics (eg, recent stroke or brain metastases)
- **IVC filter:** Used in patients with contraindications to anticoagulation or with recurrent PE on anticoagulation.

> **KEY FACT**
>
> Indications for thrombolysis in PE = hypotension, severe hypoxemia, cardiac arrest, evidence of right heart strain on echocardiogram.

Complications

- Cardiac arrest and death
- Development of pulmonary HTN

VENOUS INSUFFICIENCY

Chronic elevation of venous pressure can compromise the integrity of valves in the deep and perforating veins in the leg. This results in edema, varicose veins, and chronic changes in the skin and soft tissues.

Causes

- DVT: Most common
- Trauma
- Others: Varicose veins, pelvic vein obstruction, AV fistula

Examination

Edema (early), stasis dermatitis/varicose veins/ulceration (late)

Differential

- CHF
- Renal disease

- Lymphedema
- Arterial insufficiency

TREATMENT

- Treat the underlying condition.
- Elevation, avoidance of prolonged dependency, compression.
- Wound care for skin breakdown/ulceration.
- Antibiotics, if infection is present.

Disturbances of Cardiac Rhythm

BUNDLE BRANCH BLOCKS

Right Bundle Branch Block

Right bundle branch block (RBBB) results from failure of conduction of the right bundle. Right ventricular activation occurs via conduction through the left ventricle and is therefore delayed and slowed.

KEY FACT

RBBB can occur in a healthy heart.

CAUSES

RBBB may occur in a healthy heart but is typically caused by either acute or chronic right-sided heart strain (pulmonary HTN, COPD, PE, cardiomyopathy).

KEY FACT

Law of Appropriate Discordance: The T waves should be deflected in the direction opposite to the terminal deflection of the rR′ or rSR′ complexes.

ECG FINDINGS (FIGURE 2.7)

- QRS duration ≥ 0.12 second
- Terminal R in V_1 (rR′, rSR′), with appropriately discordant T waves (Ts deflected opposite the rR′ or rSR′ waves)
- Large, "slurred" S wave in V_6

TREATMENT

Treat the underlying condition.

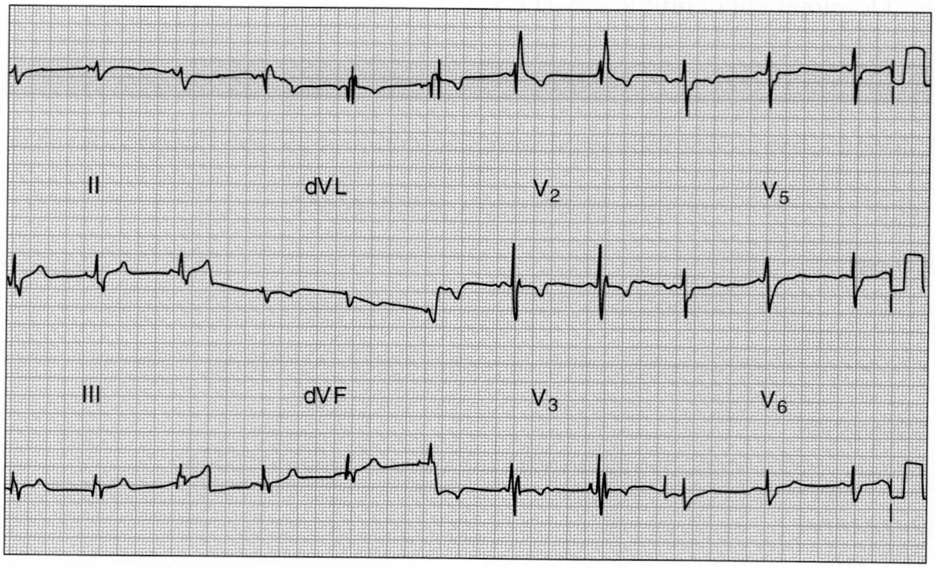

FIGURE 2.7. Right bundle branch block.

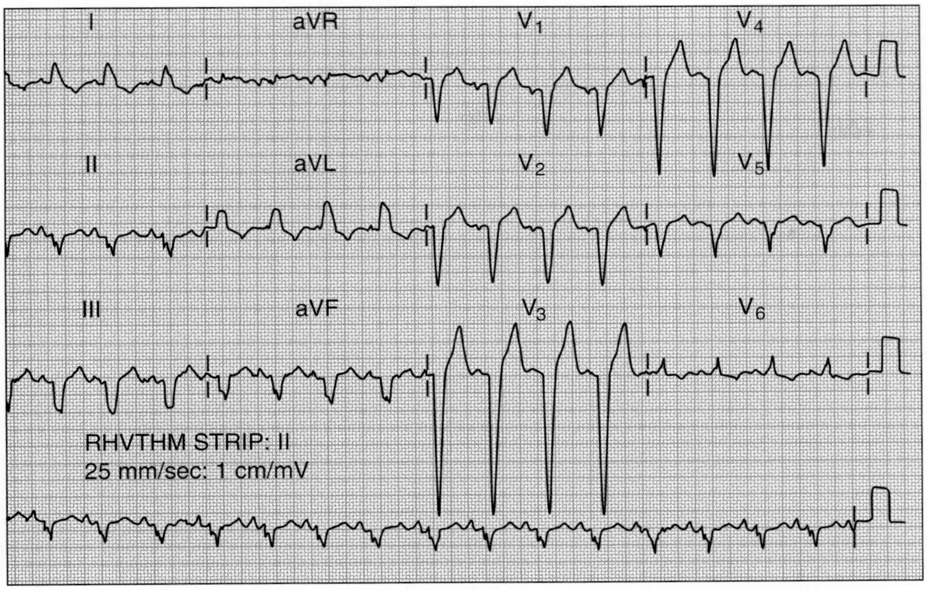

FIGURE 2.8. Left bundle branch block.

Left Bundle Branch Block

In left bundle branch block (LBBB), both the left anterior and posterior fascicles are blocked and electrical conduction to the L ventricle is delayed (after R ventricular conduction) and slowed.

Causes

LBBB does **not** occur in a healthy heart. Causes include chronic HTN, valvular disease, ischemia, cardiomyopathy, myocarditis, congenital heart disease (CHD), and following cardiac surgery.

ECG Findings (Figure 2.8)

- Symmetric slurring through entire QRS complex, with QRS duration ≥ 0.12 second
- QS or rS in V_1
- Monophasic R in V_6
- Appropriately discordant ST segments

Left Anterior Fascicular Block

Left anterior fascicular block (LAFB) results from failure of conduction of the left anterior fascicle of the left bundle.

Causes

Causes are similar to LBBB.

ECG Findings (Figure 2.9)

- QRS duration < 120 milliseconds
- Leftward QRS axis of > –30° (usually –45° to –60°)
- **LAFB = LAD** (left axis deviation)
- rS in inferior leads (II, III, aVF) and qR in lateral leads (I and aVL)

Treatment

Treat the underlying condition.

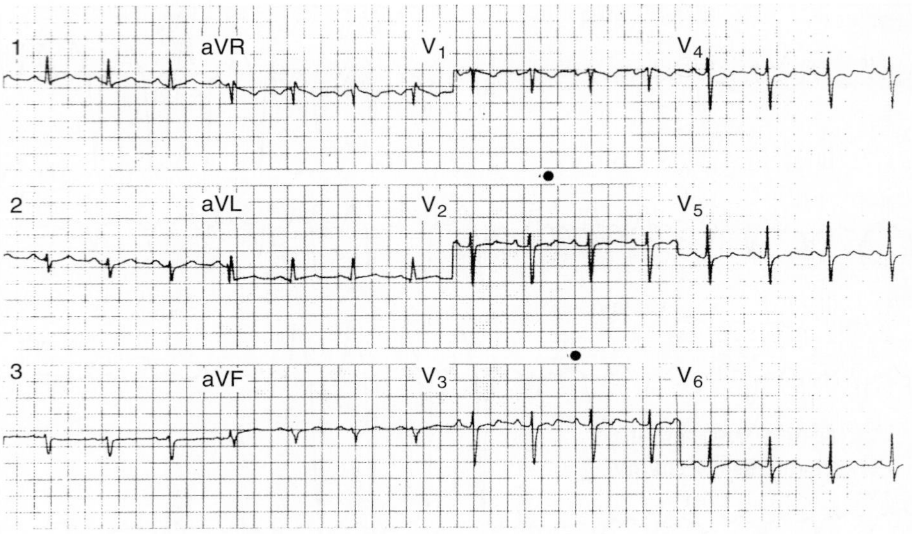

FIGURE 2.9. Left anterior fascicular block. (Reproduced, with permission, from Tintinalli JE, Kelen GD, Stapczynski JS. *Emergency Medicine: A Comprehensive Study Guide*. 6th ed. New York, NY: McGraw-Hill; 2004:195.)

Left Posterior Fascicular Block

Left posterior fascicular block (LPFB) results from damage to the L posterior fascicle of the L bundle.

Causes

Causes are similar to LBBB.

KEY FACT

LAFB = Q1S3
LPFB = S1Q3

ECG Findings (Figure 2.10)

- QRS duration < 120 milliseconds
- Rightward QRS axis of > +90°
- qR in inferior leads (II, III, aVF) and rS in lateral leads (I and aVL)
- Similar ECG pattern seen in right ventricular hypertrophy (RVH)

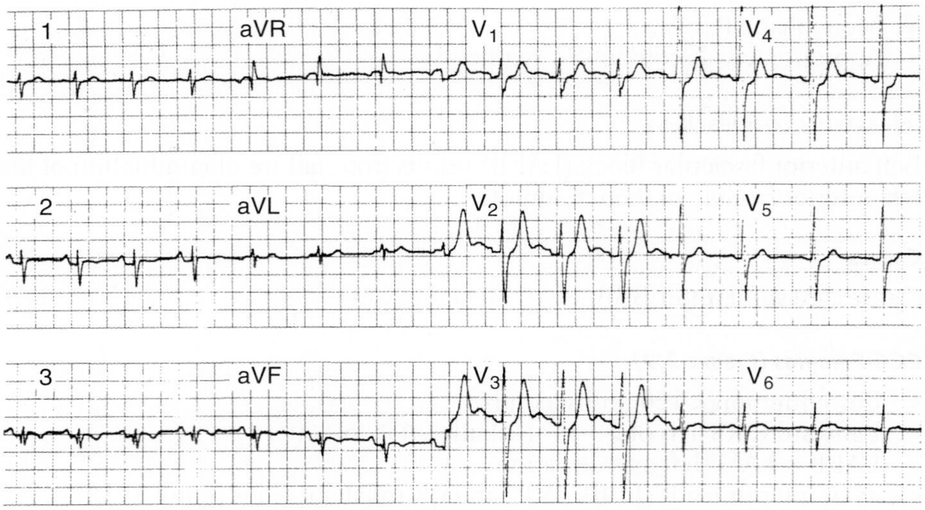

FIGURE 2.10. Left posterior fascicular block. (Reproduced, with permission, from Tintinalli JE, Kelen GD, Stapczynski JS. *Emergency Medicine: A Comprehensive Study Guide*. 6th ed. New York, NY: McGraw-Hill; 2004:195.)

TREATMENT

Treat the underlying condition.

Bifascicular Block

Bifascicular block occurs when any 2 of the 3 major infranodal pathways (right bundle branch, left anterior fascicle, left posterior fascicle) are blocked.

ECG FINDINGS

- LBBB **or**
- RBBB + LAFB **or**
- RBBB + LPFB

TREATMENT

- Transvenous pacing for symptomatic bradycardia
- May require permanent pacing if associated with high-degree AV block

> **KEY FACT**
>
> **Bifascicular blocks:**
> - LBBB
> - RBBB + LAFB
> - RBBB + LPFB

Trifascicular Block

Trifascicular block occurs when any combination of 3 fascicular blocks are found concomitantly.

ECG FINDINGS

- Bifascicular block + first-degree AV block (AVB) **or**
- Alternating RBBB and LBBB

TREATMENT

- Transvenous pacing for symptomatic bradycardia
- May require permanent pacing if associated with high-degree AV block

> **KEY FACT**
>
> **Trifascicular blocks:**
> - Bifascicular block + first-degree AV block
> - Alternating RBBB and LBBB

VENTRICULAR HYPERTROPHY

Right Ventricular Hypertrophy

Increased right ventricular mass results from chronic exposure to elevated right-sided pressures.

CAUSES

Causes include mitral or pulmonic stenosis, pulmonary HTN, chronic PE, and left-to-right shunts.

ECG FINDINGS (FIGURE 2.11)

- Right-axis deviation
- R wave > S wave in V_1 (rule out posterior MI)
- Deep S wave in V_6
- Inverted T waves in right precordial leads (right ventricular strain)

Left Ventricular Hypertrophy

Increased left ventricular (LV) mass results in prominent L-sided depolarization forces.

CAUSES

Includes chronic HTN (most common etiology), chronic CAD and ischemia, aortic stenosis, aortic or mitral regurgitation (MR), CHD, and hypertrophic cardiomyopathy (HCM)

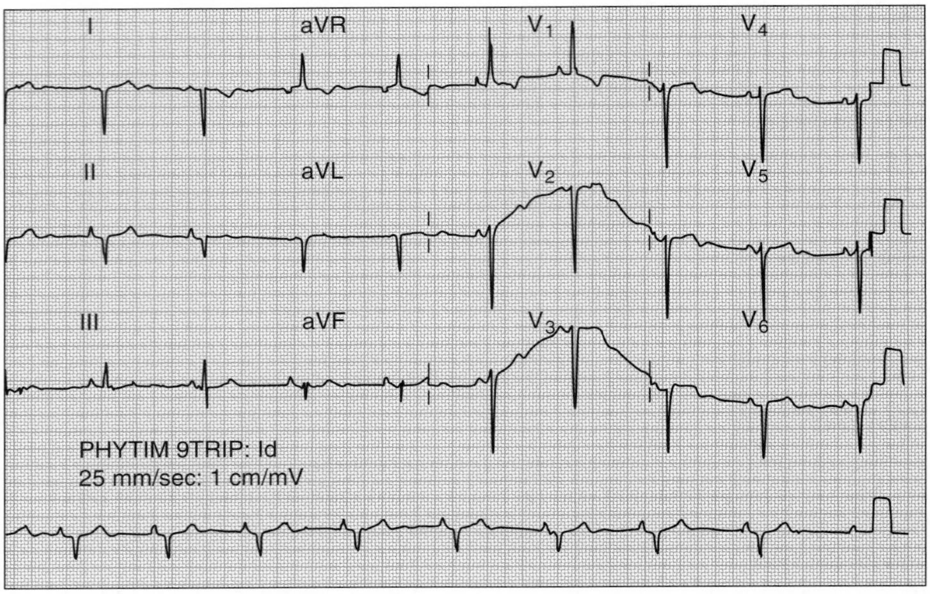

FIGURE 2.11. Right ventricular hypertrophy.

ECG Findings (Sokolow–Lyon Criteria) (Figure 2.12)

- S in V_1 + R in V_5 (or V_6) ≥ 35 mm or R in aVL ≥ 11 mm.
- May see T-wave strain pattern.
- ECG criteria have poor sensitivity and good specificity.
- False positives may occur in very thin patients.

ELECTROLYTE DISTURBANCES

Hyperkalemia

Hyperkalemia alters cardiac membrane polarization. The degree of ECG changes depends somewhat on the rapidity of onset (slowly developing hyperkalemia → ECG findings at higher K^+ concentrations).

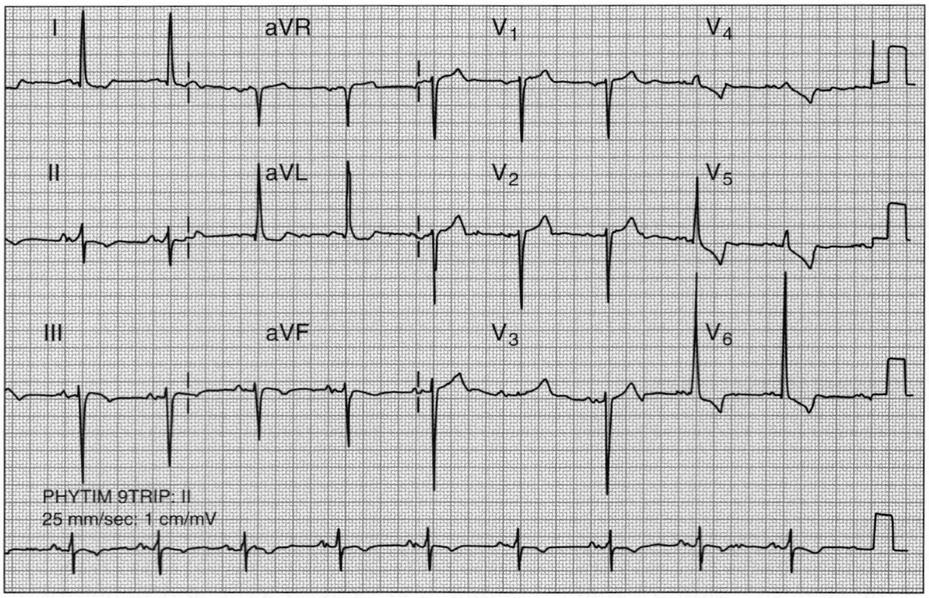

FIGURE 2.12. Left ventricular hypertrophy.

ECG Findings (Figure 2.13)

- $K^+ = 6.5$-7.5 ng/dL: Tall peaked T waves (earliest), PR prolongation.
- K^+ 7.5-8.0 ng/dL: P wave flattens, QRS widens.
- $K^+ > 9.0$ ng/dL: Sine wave pattern on ECG, anticipate cardiac arrest.
- Serum potassium levels and ECG findings are loosely related and depend on other factors including pH. A K^+ of 7.5 will cause sine waves in some patients.
- May also present with bradyarrhythmias with or without the classic ECG findings previously listed.

KEY FACT

Tall, peaked T waves are the earliest ECG finding in hyperkalemia.

Hypokalemia

Hypokalemia alters membrane polarization.

ECG Findings (Figure 2.14)

- Flattening of the T wave (earliest sign)
- Prominent U waves following T waves
- ST depression at low levels

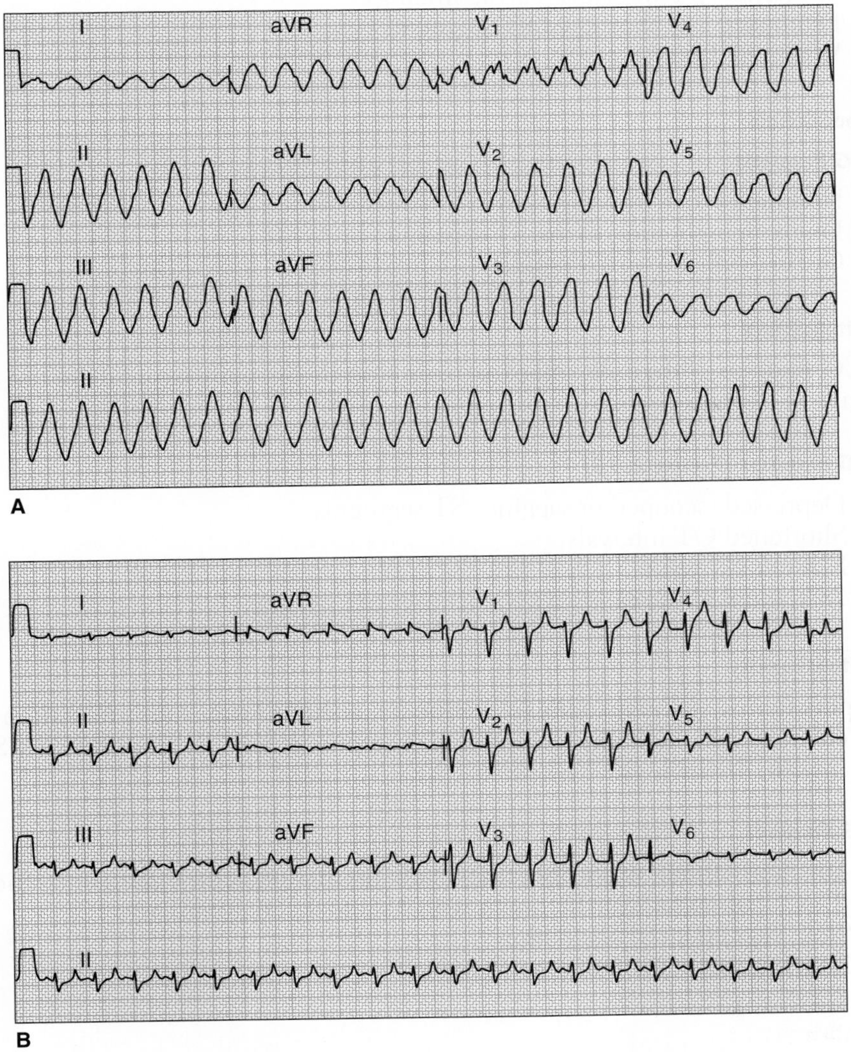

FIGURE 2.13. Hyperkalemia. (**A**) ECG showing sine wave complexes in severe hyperkalemia ($[K^+] = 9.2$ ng/dL). (**B**) ECG after treatment. Note peaked T waves and flattened P waves.

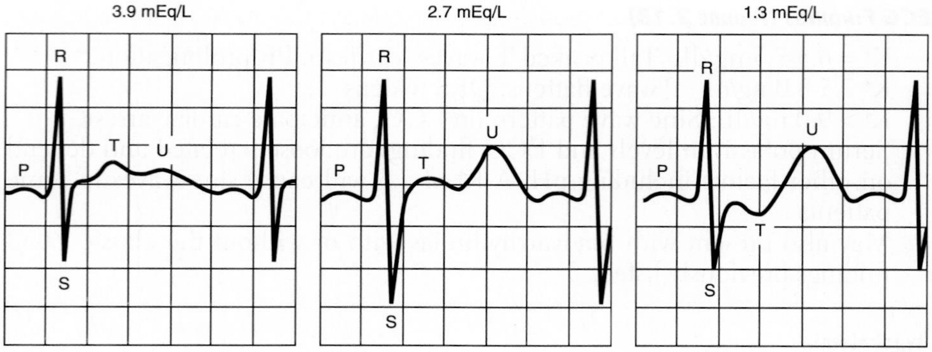

FIGURE 2.14. Hypokalemia. ECG changes with hypokalemia. Note progressive flattening of T waves and development of prominent U waves and ST-segment depression. (Reproduced, with permission, from Morgan GE, Mikhail MS, Murray MJ. *Clinical Anesthesiology*. 4th ed. New York, NY: McGraw-Hill; 2006:679.)

Hypercalcemia

ECG Findings

- Shortened QT intervals (classic finding)
- Depressed and shortened ST segments
- Widened T waves

Hypocalcemia

ECG Findings

- Hallmark = QT prolongation
- Due to lengthening of the ST segment
- Occurs with $Ca^+ < 6.0$ mg/dL

Digitalis Effect

ECG findings of **digitalis effect** are common in digoxin users and are not evidence of digitalis toxicity.

ECG Findings (Figure 2.15)

- Depressed (scooped or sagging) ST segments
- Shortened QT intervals
- Flattened T waves
- Prominent U waves

Digitalis Toxicity

Hyperkalemia → give digoxin antibody; avoid routine administration of IV calcium although this is not as dangerous previously considered. (See Chapter 6, Toxicology.)

ECG Findings

- Any dysrhythmia is possible (especially premature ventricular contractions [PVCs], atrial tachyarrhythmias with AV block, bradycardia).
- Slow, regular atrial fibrillation.
- Bidirectional ventricular tachycardia.

Hypothermia

Core temperature < 35°C (95°F). The risk of arrhythmia increases as core temperature drops, especially < 30°C (86°F).

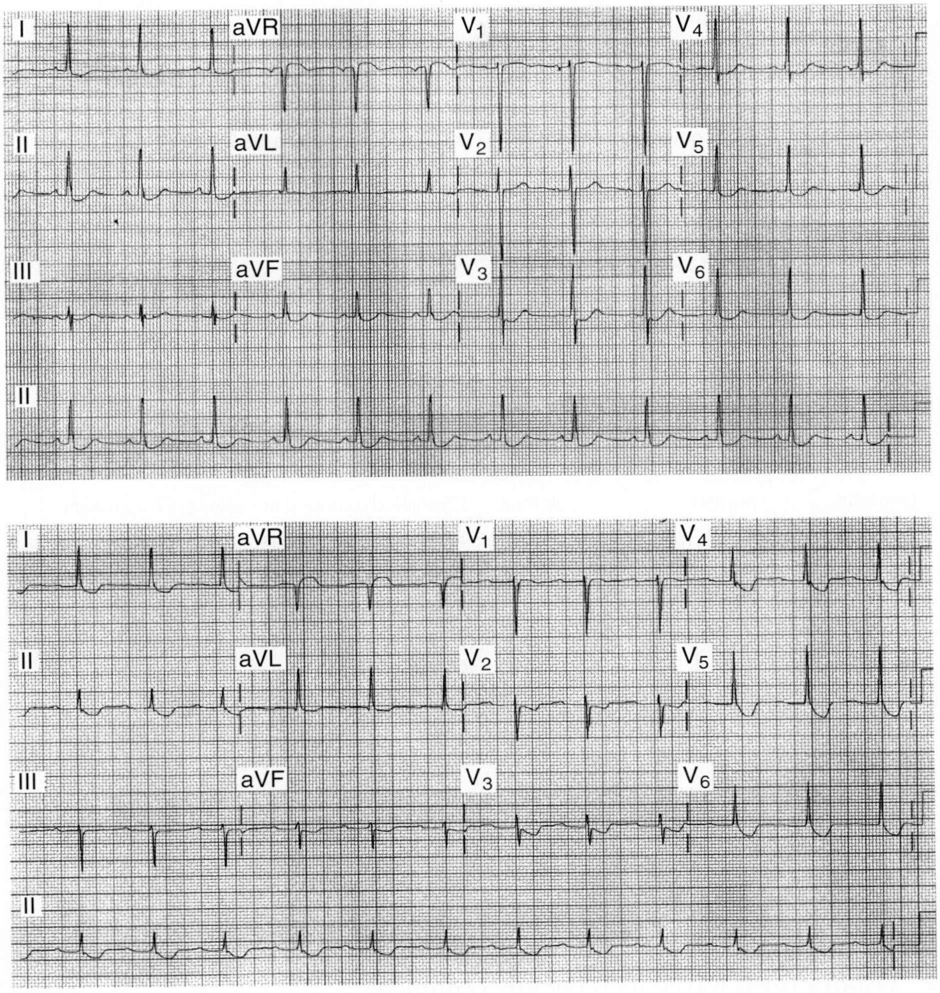

FIGURE 2.15. ECG findings of digitalis effect. Note scooped ST segments and flattened T waves. (Reproduced, with permission, from Tintinalli JE, Stapczynski JS, Ma OJ, et al. *Tintinalli's Emergency Medicine*. 7th ed. New York, NY: McGraw-Hill; 2011:1262.)

ECG Findings (Figure 2.16)

- Cardiac conduction abnormalities result in prolongation of all cardiac intervals.

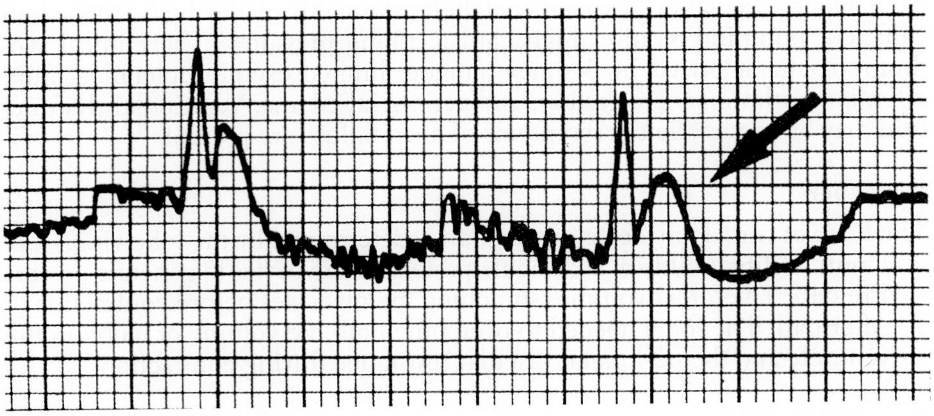

FIGURE 2.16. Osborn wave or J wave, indicating hypothermia. (Reproduced, with permission, from Tintinalli JE, Kelen GD, Stapczynski JS. *Emergency Medicine: A Comprehensive Study Guide*. 6th ed. New York, NY: McGraw-Hill; 2004:1180.)

TABLE 2.9. Summary of ECG Essentials

	Axis	QRS	Characteristic ECG Findings
RBBB	Right or vertical	Wide	rR′ or rSR′ in V_1 **and** large S wave in V_6
LBBB	Left	Wide	QS or rS in V_1 **and** monophasic R or RSR′ in V_6
LAFB	Left (> −30°)	Normal	Q in I, S in III (Q_1S_3)
LPFB	Right	Normal	S in I, Q in III (S_1Q_3)
RVH	Right	Normal	R wave > S wave in V_1 **and** deep S wave in V_6
LVH	Left or horizontal	Normal	S in V_1 + R in V_5 (or V_6) ≥ 35 mm **or** R in aVL ≥ 11 mm
Digitalis effect	Normal	Normal	Depressed (scooped or sagging) ST segments Shortened QT intervals Flattened T waves Prominent U waves
Hypothermia	Normal	Normal or wide	Osborn J waves

ECG, electrocardiogram; LAFB, left anterior fascicular block; LBBB, left bundle branch block; LPFB, left posterior fascicular block; LVH, left ventricular hypertrophy; RBBB, right bundle branch block; RVH, right ventricular hypertrophy.

- Typical progression from sinus bradycardia to atrial fibrillation to ventricular fibrillation.
- **Osborn (or J) waves** at end of QRS complex.
  - Characteristic but **can** be seen in other heart conditions

See Table 2.9 for summary of ECG essentials.

Diseases of the Myocardium

Heart failure exists when impaired pumping ability of heart leads to insufficient blood circulation to meet metabolic demands of the body, OR when sufficient pumping requires high cardiac filling pressures. The clinical syndrome is characterized by dyspnea, fatigue, limited exercise tolerance, fluid retention, pulmonary congestion, and peripheral edema. Ventricular **dysfunction** may be present before symptoms of heart failure are present.

Physiology

The force of cardiac myocyte contraction is determined by the following:

- **Contractility:** Ability of contractile proteins in myocytes to generate **power**
- **Preload:** The force (volume) stretching the myocytes **before** contraction
- **Afterload:** The force needed to overcome both the volume of blood in the ventricle and the peripheral vascular resistance **during** contraction

Pathophysiology

Initial insult to myocytes leads to compensatory neurohormonal response that eventually causes more damage.

TABLE 2.10. Common Causes of Heart Failure

Ischemic heart disease[a] (most common)
Cardiomyopathy
Congenital heart disease
Valvular disease
Hypertension
Myocarditis
Constrictive pericarditis
Tamponade/pericardial effusion
Pulmonary disease (from pulmonary HTN)
High-output states (thyrotoxicosis, anemia, beriberi, Paget disease, arteriovenous fistula, pregnancy)

HTN, hypertension.

Underlying disease process leads to → initial insult → myocyte death and hypertrophy

- Myocyte death → ↓ contractility and ↓ ejection fraction (EF) → neurohormonal response → ↑ aldosterone, renin and circulating catecholamines → pathologic fluid retention and ↑ afterload
- Myocyte hypertrophy → ↓ compliance → poor ventricular filling with preserved EF

Common causes of initial myocyte dysfunction leading to **heart failure** (Table 2.10):

SYSTOLIC VERSUS DIASTOLIC DYSFUNCTION

Systolic Dysfunction

- Most common cause is ischemic heart disease.
- Impaired contractility and eventual pathologic increase afterload and preload.
- EF < 40%.

Diastolic Dysfunction

- Most common cause is HTN. Also caused by HCM.
- **Impaired relaxation and ventricular filling.**
- Preserved ejection fraction.
- Small changes in ventricular filling can have significant effects on cardiac output.

Other terms used to classify heart failure are based on clinical presentation:

- Left-sided vs right-sided
- High-output vs low-output
- Acute vs chronic

KEY FACT

Relaxation of myocytes is an active process requiring calcium and energy.

Systolic and diastolic dysfunctions typically occur in combination. The predominant type dictates the treatment strategy.

In diastolic dysfunction, cardiac output is dependent on preload.

Diastolic dysfunction is also referred to as HFpEF—"Heart Failure with preserved Ejection Fraction"

In systolic dysfunction, cardiac output is dependent on afterload and contractility.

CAUSES (TABLE 2.11)

Decompensation from baseline may be acute or gradual in onset, depending on prior history of heart failure and underlying etiology. Cardiogenic pulmonary

TABLE 2.11. Precipitants of Acute/Decompensated Heart Failure

Precipitant	Key Points and Examples
Myocardial infarction or ischemia	Always consider occult ACS in elderly with heart failure
Acute hypertension	aka "Hypertensive emergency"
Acute valvular dysfunction	Mitral insufficiency from MI; aortic insufficiency from dissection; AS
Volume overload (sodium excess)	Diet or medication noncompliance; IV fluids or transfusions
Acute hypoxia	COPD exacerbation, PNA; leads to myocardial strain
Myocarditis	Recent viral illness
Systemic infection	Sepsis cytokines cause myocyte dysfunction
Dysrhythmia	Atrial fibrillation in diastolic dysfunction
Anemia	Acute—think GI bleed; chronic anemia is common
Thyroid dysfunction	Hypothyroid causes poor contractility; hyperthyroid causes prolonged tachycardia and associated high-output failure
Pregnancy	High-output failure

ACS, acute coronary syndrome; AS, aortic stenosis; COPD, chronic obstructive pulmonary disease; GI, gastrointestinal; IV, intravenous; MI, myocardial infarction; PNA, peptide nucleic acid.

edema is classic finding in left-sided heart failure. It occurs when rise in LV end-diastolic pressures leads to rapid elevation of pulmonary capillary hydrostatic pressure, which forces fluid from the intravascular space into the alveolar space.

KEY FACT

Paroxysmal nocturnal dyspnea is highly predictive of CHF.

Symptoms

- Presents with new or worsening dyspnea at rest, dyspnea with exertion, paroxysmal nocturnal dyspnea, orthopnea, fatigue, weakness, lower extremity edema, and/or abdominal distention.
- Symptoms of ACS, dysrhythmia, infection, and thyroid dysfunction may identify etiology.

KEY FACT

Previously healthy patients with acute left-sided heart failure may not have JVD, peripheral edema, or cardiomegaly.

Examination

- Typically hypertensive (normotensive or hypotensive patients have worse prognosis).
- Jugular venous distention (JVD), peripheral edema, hepatojugular reflex, and S_3 gallop.
- Tachypnea, rales, and/or "cardiac" wheezes.
- Severe cardiac dysfunction → intense sympathetic activation → cool, clammy, slow cap refill.
- Right-ventricular failure may present without evidence of pulmonary edema.
- Look for evidence of underlying cause/event: Infection, DVT/PE, valvular disease.

Differential

- Causes of noncardiogenic alveolar filling → PNA, ARDS, altitude, inhalational injuries, diffuse alveolar hemorrhage
- Asthma, COPD, PE, tamponade, anaphylaxis

Diagnosis

- **ECG**
  - Look for LVH, ischemia, dysrhythmias.
- **Upright CXR**
  - Enlarged cardiac silhouette (70% of cases).
  - **Progression of lung field changes on CXR.**
    - Vascular congestion (cephalization of vessels) → interstitial edema (Kerley B lines, haziness) → alveolar infiltrates (butterfly pattern, effusions)
  - Normal heart size? Suspect noncardiogenic pulmonary edema (Figure 2.17), acute valve failure, or diastolic dysfunction.
  - CXR findings may lag behind clinical findings.
- **Laboratory tests**
  - Complete blood count (CBC), BMP, and troponin to identify cause for decompensation → anemia, renal dysfunction, electrolyte derangement, MI, or myocardial injury.
- **B-type natriuretic peptide (BNP) or N-terminal-pro BNP (NT-pro-BNP)**
  – Order if diagnosis is unclear or for prognosis in patient with history of heart failure.
  – Released in response to ventricular myocyte stretch.
  – < 100 pg/dL makes heart failure unlikely, whereas > 500 pg/dL makes heart failure highly probable.
  – Should be compared to patient's baseline values.
  – Correlates to ventricular function, NYHA Class and prognosis.
  – Also elevated in the elderly, renal failure, PE, or cor pulmonale.

> **KEY FACT**
>
> Lack of cardiomegaly plus normal ECG have high negative predictive value against heart failure.

> **KEY FACT**
>
> BNP < 100 pg/mL makes heart failure unlikely.

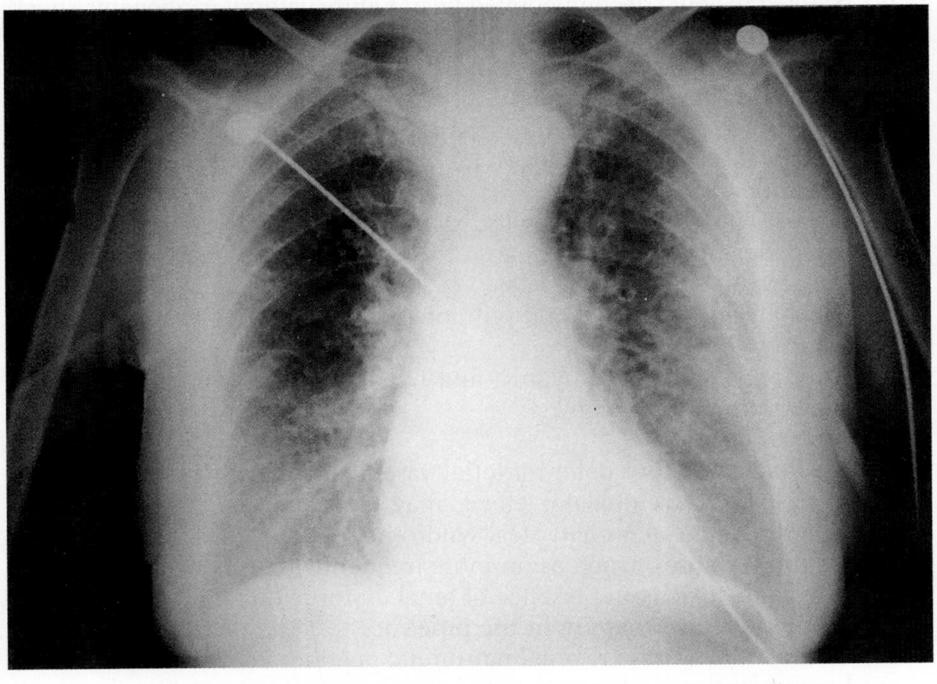

FIGURE 2.17. Mild-to-moderate pulmonary edema with cephalization of pulmonary vasculature. (Reproduced, with permission, from Stone CK, Humphries RL. *Current Diagnosis & Treatment Emergency Medicine*. 7th ed. New York, NY: McGraw-Hill Education; 2011. Figure 13.5.)

- **Bedside ultrasound and echocardiogram**
  - Used to assess wall motion abnormalities, ejection fraction, valvular function, and structural heart disease. Can also exclude tamponade

Treatment

Intensity of treatment depends on severity of presentation. Generally, these patients present with pulmonary edema. Basic tenets of treatment are to (1) improve gas exchange and arterial O_2 saturation, (2) reduce cardiac workload by decreasing preload and afterload, (3) address excess sodium and water, and (4) improve contractility.

Treatment of Acute Heart Failure with Adequate Perfusion

- Position patient upright.
- Supplemental O_2 to maintain arterial saturation >90%.
- **Noninvasive positive pressure ventilation.**
  - **Bilevel positive airway pressure** (BiPAP) or **continuous positive airway pressure** (CPAP)
  - Mechanism: ↑ Oxygenation, ↓ work of breathing, ↓ preload and afterload
  - No change in mortality
- **Nitroglycerin (NTG).**
  - Mainstay of therapy for flash pulmonary edema.
  - Sublingual, then IV if needed.
  - Mechanism: ↓ Preload by venodilation, ↓ afterload (at high doses) via arterial vasodilation, direct coronary vasodilator (good in ischemia).
  - Caution: Avoid in hypotension, concomitant PDE5 inhibitor use (sildenafil, tadalafil), severe aortic stenosis, and RV infarction.
- **Morphine sulfate.**
  - Mechanism: ↓ Myocardial **O_2** consumption by ↓ catecholamines, ↓ preload from mild vasodilator effect, ↓ pain and anxiety
  - Caution: May ↑ mortality
- **Nesiritide.**
  - Studied in acute decompensated heart failure without cardiogenic shock.
  - Mechanism: Recombinant BNP; antagonizes renin-aldosterone system and sympathetic nervous system → diuresis, ↓ preload via venodilation, ↓ afterload via vasodilation.
  - Caution: No benefit to routine use in place of or in addition to NTG therapy. Meta-analyses suggest increased mortality with its use.
- **Furosemide.**
  - For patients with evidence of subacute volume overload; **not for use in rapid decompensation** because these patients are often volume neutral or even dehydrated.
  - Mechanism: ↓ Preload and pulmonary congestion by reducing plasma volume.
  - Caution: Can lead to hypoK^+ and hypoMg^+; furosemide drip is NOT superior to bolus therapy.
- **Nitroprusside.**
  - Mechanism: More potent arterial vasodilator than NTG, ↓ afterload, ↓ preload via venodilator effect, may dilate normal coronaries more than diseased → coronary steal syndrome
  - Caution: Causes hypotension more frequently than NTG and can lead to cyanide toxicity in presence of renal dysfunction
- **Other medications that are in the pipeline.**
  - Urodilantin: Synthetic renal natriuretic peptide
  - Levosimendan: Calcium-sensitizing inotropic agent
  - Relaxin: Vasodilatory hormone

Table 2.12 summarizes the medications for acute heart failure with adequate perfusion.

MNEMONIC

Pneumonic for heart failure treatment:

LMNOP

Lasix
Morphine
Nitrates
Oxygen
Positioning

KEY FACT

Nitroprusside may dilate normal coronaries more than diseased coronaries, causing a coronary steal syndrome.

TABLE 2.12. Medications for Acute Heart Failure with Adequate Perfusion

Medication	Beneficial Effects	Deleterious Effects
Nitroglycerin	↓ Preload ↓ Afterload (high doses) Coronary vasodilation	Severe hypotension with: Viagra use Aortic stenosis Hypertrophic cardiomyopathy RV infarct
Morphine	↓ Catecholamines ↓ Preload (mild) ↓ Anxiety, pain	CNS and respiratory depression Associated with ↑ mortality
Furosemide	Possible venodilator effect (↓ preload) Delayed diuresis	Hypotension from hypovolemia Hypokalemia
Nitroprusside	↓ Afterload ↓ Preload Coronary vasodilation	Coronary steal Hypotension
ACE inhibitors	↓ Afterload	Hyperkalemia Renal failure

ACE, angiotensin-converting enzyme; CNS, central nervous system; RV, right ventricular.

Treatment of Acute Heart Failure with Hypotension

- Pulmonary edema + poor perfusion (cool extremities) = cardiogenic shock.
- Hypovolemia often present, so correct any underlying hypovolemia **first** with judicious fluid challenge to maximize preload. If still hypotensive despite adequate preload, proceed to vasopressors/inotropes and intra-aortic balloon pump.
- If ACS is present, definitive therapy is coronary revascularization.
- If tachyarrhythmia or bradyarrhythmia is present, normalize rate.
- **Norepinephrine.**
  - First-line therapy. Temporizing measure pending rescue strategy
  - Mechanism: ↑ Systemic vascular resistance, ↑ BP and coronary perfusion pressure, will ↑ HR and myocardial O_2 demand
- **Dopamine.**
  - Mechanism: Catecholamine and norepinephrine precursor; ↑ cardiac output and ↑ systemic vascular resistance; does NOT have clinically significant renal-sparing effect at any dose
- **Epinephrine.**
  - Mechanism: α- and β-Receptor agonist; ↑ cardiac output and ↑ systemic vascular resistance
- **Dobutamine.**
  - Mechanism: Primarily a β-1 agonist. ↑ cardiac output and ↓ systemic vascular resistance.
  - Caution: May exacerbate hypotension (vasodilator effect).
- **Amrinone and milrinone.**
  - Mechanism: PDE3 inhibitor; ↑ cardiac output and ↓ systemic vascular resistance without changing HR or BP

KEY FACT

Norepinephrine will ↑ HR and myocardial O_2 demand.

- **Intra-aortic balloon pump.**
  - Bridge to revascularization, valve repair, or LVAD/transplant
  - Mechanism: Inflates during diastole and deflates during systole; ↑ cardiac output primarily by ↓ systemic vascular resistance
  - Caution: Contraindicated in acute AR

Complications

- Dysrhythmias and sudden death
- Intracardiac thrombus and embolism
- Progression of disease

STABLE CHRONIC HEART FAILURE

Symptoms

- Dyspnea on exertion, orthopnea, paroxysmal nocturnal dyspnea, fatigue.
- The New York Heart Association (NYHA) classifies heart failure based on severity of symptoms (Table 2.13). These classifications have prognostic and treatment implications.
- More recent guidelines from the AHA/ACC recommend use of stages to guide therapy (Table 2.14).

Treatment

- Lifestyle modification.
- Treat the underlying etiology when possible.
- Treatment for diastolic failure focuses on diuresis, BP control, and prevention of tachycardia.
- **Angiotensin-converting-enzyme (ACE) inhibitors (ACEIs).**
  - Mortality and hospitalizations, beneficial effects on LV remodeling
  - Caution: Can cause renal failure, hyperkalemia, cough, angioedema. No mortality benefit in diastolic failure
- **Angiotensin receptor blockers (ARBs).**
  - If ACEI not tolerated
- **Hydralazine with nitrates.**
  - ↓ Mortality in black patients; may also use in ACEI/ARB intolerance
- **β-Blockers.**
  - ↓ Mortality and improved symptoms with chronic use
  - Caution: Contraindicated in decompensated heart failure
- **Loop and thiazide diuretics.**
  - Improves symptoms but no mortality benefit
- **Digoxin.**
  - Reduces hospitalizations but no mortality benefit

TABLE 2.13. NYHA Functional Classification for Chronic Heart Failure

Class	Functional Ability
Class I	(Mild) No limitation of ordinary physical activity
Class II	(Mild) Mild dyspnea, fatigue, or palpitations with ordinary physical activity
Class III	(Moderate) Symptoms with less than ordinary physical activity
Class IV	(Severe) Symptoms present at rest

NYHA, New York Heart Association.

TABLE 2.14. AHA/ACC Stages of Heart Failure

STAGE	DESCRIPTION	RECOMMENDED THERAPIES
Stage A	No symptoms of HF + risk factors (DM, HTN, CAD, etc)	Risk factor modification. Treat DM, HTN, CAD, lipids.
Stage B	No symptoms of HF + Evidence of structural heart disease	Add ACEI/ARB. Add β-blocker if has CAD.
Stage C	+ Symptoms of HF (now or in past) + Evidence of structural heart disease	Add diuretics, Na restriction. Consider digoxin and nitrates. Consider aldosterone antagonists, ICD, CRT.
Stage D	Refractory symptoms of HF despite maximal medical therapy	IV inotropes, ventricular assist device, transplant

ACC, AHA, American Heart Association; CAD, coronary artery disease; CRT, cathode ray tube; DM, diabetes mellitus; HF, hydrogen fluoride; HTN, hypertension; ICD, implantable cardioverter-defibrillators; IV, intravenous.

- **Aldosterone antagonists.**
  - Improve mortality in NYHA II-IV and left ventricular ejection fraction (LVEF) <35%
  - Caution: Cause hyperK^+
- **Cardiac resynchronization therapy (CRT).**
  - Improves mortality if LVEF < 35% and wide QRS (>120 milliseconds)
- **Implantable cardiac defibrillator (ICD).**
  - Mortality benefit in primary prevention of sudden cardiac death if LVEF < 30%
- **Salvage therapies in NYHA Class IV and AHA heart failure Stage D:**
  - Mechanical assist device
  - Heart transplant
  - Inotrope infusion

Q

A 32-year-old woman presents to the ED with 2 days of progressive shortness of breath. She is 3 weeks postpartum after an uneventful pregnancy and vaginal delivery. On examination, the patient is in mild respiratory distress, has bilateral rales and JVD, and is tachycardic to a rate of 120 bpm. Bedside echocardiogram shows dilated chambers and poor systolic function. How should she be treated and what is her prognosis?

Cardiomyopathy

Cardiomyopathies encompass a group of diseases that alter the physical and electrical composition of the myocardium. These diseases can lead to impaired cardiac pump function and symptomatic heart failure. They can also lead to electrical dysfunction and arrhythmia. The definition and classification of cardiomyopathy vary across professional societies. Based on the World Health Organization classification, there are 5 types of cardiomyopathy:

- Dilated
- Restrictive
- Hypertrophic
- Arrhythmogenic right ventricular dysplasia
- Unclassified

Extrinsic causes of cardiomyopathy include HTN, valvular disease, ischemia, systemic disease, and inflammation.

KEY FACT

Cardiomyopathy
Five types of cardiomyopathy:
1. Dilated
2. Restrictive
3. Hypertrophic
4. Arrhythmogenic right ventricular dysplasia
5. Unclassified

DILATED CARDIOMYOPATHY

Dilated cardiomyopathy is a spectrum of disorders resulting in depressed myocardial systolic function and pump failure.

A

The patient has peripartum dilated cardiomyopathy. Treatment mirrors that of CHF, including ACEIs (or hydralazine + nitrates if still pregnant), β-blockers, and diuretics. Refractory cases may require cardiac transplant. Peripartum cardiomyopathy has a better prognosis than most dilated cardiomyopathies: 50% of these patients will recover completely. Even if her cardiac function normalizes, this patient is at high risk of recurrence with any future pregnancy.

Causes

Both primary and secondary causes exist:

- 30%-40% are genetic—35 genes for myocyte cytoskeleton and sarcomere proteins found.
- Risk factors include alcohol and tobacco use, pregnancy, HTN, and myocarditis.
- Peripartum cardiomyopathy:
  - Most common in older multiparous women, twin gestation, and in first 2 months postpartum (but can occur from last month of pregnancy to 5 months postpartum).
  - Increased risk with tocolytics and preeclampsia.
  - 50% will have complete resolution.
  - Elevated risk of relapse with future pregnancies.

Pathophysiology

Myocardial cell death and fibrosis → cardiac chamber dilation and systolic dysfunction

Symptoms

Same as those with L heart failure: Dyspnea, orthopnea, chest pain, lower extremity edema

KEY FACT

Amyloidosis can cause a dilated or a restrictive cardiomyopathy.

Examination

Rales, laterally displaced point of maximal impulse (PMI), JVD, lower extremity edema

Diagnosis

- ECG is nonspecific, but may include poor R wave progression, interventricular conduction delay, LBBB, frequent premature atrial complexes, and ventricular tachycardia.
- CXR indicates cardiomegaly.
- Echocardiogram demonstrates LV dilation, LVEF <45%, variable wall motion abnormalities.
- Endomyocardial biopsy findings usually nonspecific.

Treatment

- Similar to treatment for CHF.
- Mortality benefit found for ACEIs/ARBs, β-blockers, nitrates + hydralazine, spironolactone, ICDs.
- ACEIs contraindicated in pregnancy → hydralazine and nitrates are alternatives.
- Diuretics and digitalis: Improve symptoms, but not survival.
- Severe cases require transplantation.

KEY FACT

Diuresis and digoxin improve symptoms in dilated cardiomyopathy, but do not improve survival.

Complications

- Sequelae of progressive heart failure—dysrhythmias, sudden death, mural thrombi, and systemic emboli
- 75% mortality within 5 years → #1 cause for cardiac transplant in kids and adults

RESTRICTIVE CARDIOMYOPATHY

Restrictive cardiomyopathy is characterized by myocardial infiltration that results in restricted ventricular filling and diastolic dysfunction but preserved systolic function. Least common cardiomyopathy.

Causes

Systemic disorders associated with restrictive cardiomyopathy include amyloidosis (most common in the United States), sarcoidosis, hemochromatosis, scleroderma, glycogen storage diseases, and tropical endomyocardial fibrosis (most common cause worldwide).

Pathophysiology

Fibrotic process reduces the size and compliance of the left ventricle → reduced filling of L ventricle → ↑ diastolic pressures and ↓ diastolic volumes.

Symptoms

Symptoms include exercise intolerance in adults and failure-to-thrive in children. Right-sided heart failure symptoms (dyspnea and edema) may predominate in tropical endomyocardial fibrosis.

Examination

Findings include **Kussmaul sign** (increase in jugular venous pressure during inspiration), rales, S_3 or S_4 gallop, JVD, hepatojugular reflex, and peripheral edema.

Differential

Important to exclude **constrictive pericarditis**. May be misdiagnosed as HTN-related diastolic dysfunction

Diagnosis

- ECG: Nonspecific, decreased voltages, conduction abnormalities.
- CXR: Mild (if any) cardiomegaly.
- Echocardiogram: Normal LV size and systolic function, dilated atria.
- Characteristic **"dip and plateau"** (also seen with constrictive pericarditis) of LV pressures on catheterization.
- Biopsy is definitive.

Treatment

- Limited treatment modalities because most underlying causes are untreatable
- Diuretics, ACEIs/ARBs, nitrates + hydralazine, rhythm control
- Transplant necessary in some patients

Complications

- Progressive heart failure → 90% die within 10 years

HYPERTROPHIC CARDIOMYOPATHY

Hypertrophic cardiomyopathy (HCM) was previously referred to as idiopathic hypertrophic subaortic stenosis (IHSS). This is often an autosomal dominant disorder, so always ask about sudden death or early cardiac disorders in family members. It is characterized by asymmetric thickening of the LV septal wall.

Pathophysiology

- Autosomal dominant defect in a sarcomere protein that has variable phenotype depending on environmental factors.
- Compensatory hypertrophy of LV is asymmetric and leads to LV outflow tract obstruction and diastolic dysfunction.

Q

A 17-year-old adolescent boy presents to the ED after passing out during basketball practice. He has no symptoms now, but his mother insisted he come in because his cousin died while playing basketball 2 years ago. On examination, there is a systolic murmur that worsens with standing. What is the most likely diagnosis?

KEY FACT

Restrictive cardiomyopathy leads to diastolic dysfunction.

KEY FACT

Consider restrictive cardiomyopathy in the patient presenting with CHF without cardiomegaly or systolic dysfunction.

A

Hypertrophic cardiomyopathy. Syncope is an independent predictor of sudden cardiac death in patients with HCM. This patient requires hospitalization for further monitoring and evaluation.

KEY FACT

Murmur of HCM ↓ LV filling (standing, Valsalva) = ↑ murmur. ↑ LV filling (squatting, leg elevation) = ↓ murmur. This is the opposite of aortic stenosis!

KEY FACT

β-Blockers and/or calcium channel blockers are the mainstay of therapy for HCM.

Symptoms

- Average age at diagnosis is 30-40 years old.
- Symptoms include dyspnea, **exertional syncope** or sudden cardiac death, chest pain, decreased exercise tolerance, and palpitations.

Examination

- S_4 gallop and loud crescendo–decrescendo systolic murmur heard best at the left lower sternal border.
- Murmur increases with ↓ LV filling (standing, Valsalva) by increasing obstruction of LV outflow tract. Murmur decreases with ↑ LV filling (squatting, leg elevation, or Trendelenburg) by lessening obstruction.
- Paradoxically split S_2 and bifid arterial pulse sometimes present.

Differential

- Aortic stenosis, pulmonary stenosis, ventricular septal defect (VSD), MR, ACS

Diagnosis

- Suspect in any young person with exertional syncope, family history of sudden death or characteristic murmur. **Echocardiography is the most important study**.
- ECG: 90% have abnormal ECG. Abnormalities include left atrial enlargement and LVH, **septal Q waves**, absent R waves in lateral leads.
- CXR: Mild cardiomegaly or normal size.
- Echocardiogram: Asymmetric LV hypertrophy, LV outflow tract narrowing, reduced septal motion, and small LV cavity.

Treatment

- β-Blockers and calcium channel blockers to decrease outflow obstruction, prolong diastolic filling time, and reduce myocardial O_2 demand.
- **Avoid** inotropes and nitrates, which will worsen obstruction.
- Counsel avoidance of intense exertion until cardiology evaluation.
- Family members should undergo screening and genetic counseling.
- Endocarditis prophylaxis no longer routinely recommended.
- Treat atrial fibrillation → may cause precipitous decline in cardiac output.
- Admit for monitoring if syncope, near-syncope, or presence of dysrhythmia.
- Nonpharmacologic interventions include septal myomectomy, ethanol septal ablation, dual chamber pacing, and implantable defibrillator, as necessary.

Complications

Complications include heart failure, dysrhythmias (atrial fibrillation, PVCs most common), exertional syncope, and sudden cardiac death.

ARRHYTHMOGENIC RIGHT VENTRICULAR DYSPLASIA

As the name implies, this cardiomyopathy is characterized by right ventricular dysplasia and ventricular dysrhythmias. It is an autosomal dominant disorder common in regions of Italy.

Pathophysiology

- Replacement of right ventricle myocardium with fibrofatty tissue.
- Overall cardiac function is normal.

SYMPTOMS/EXAMINATION

- Sudden cardiac death or ventricular dysrhythmias
- Normal examination

DIAGNOSIS

- ECG: May see **RBBB pattern**.
- CXR: Normal.
- Echocardiogram: Right ventricular enlargement and dysfunction.
- Biopsy is confirmatory.

TREATMENT

- Antidysrhythmics and/or AICD to prevent sudden death

UNCLASSIFIED CARDIOMYOPATHIES

Takotsubo Cardiomyopathy (aka "Broken Heart" Syndrome and Stress Cardiomyopathy)

Also known as "broken heart" syndrome and stress cardiomyopathy. The syndrome was named after the characteristic apical-ballooning pattern of the LV seen on ventriculography in these patients. The shape of the LV resembles a **takotsuboz**, which means octopus trap in Japanese.

PATHOPHYSIOLOGY

Regional LV dysfunction (most commonly seen in the apex) thought to be caused by stress hormones or microvascular spasm. Originally reported in postmenopausal Japanese women undergoing significant social stressors, but now widely reported with a broad range of precipitating events.

SYMPTOMS/EXAMINATION

- Presents with chest pain and dyspnea on exertion. Mimics ACS.
- Examination can be normal or show evidence of heart failure.

DIAGNOSIS

- Mimics ST-elevation myocardial infarction (STEMI) but is characterized by a normal left heart catheterization.
- ECG: ST elevations in V_1 through V_3 (mimics anterior STEMI). Later findings include T-wave inversions and prolonged QTc.
- Troponin elevated.
- CXR: Normal or enlarged cardiac size.
- Echocardiogram: Classic finding is apical akinesis and ballooning but wall motion abnormalities in LV base also seen. Generally do not follow pattern expected for coronary artery distribution.
- Left heart catheterization is normal.

TREATMENT

Diagnosis not made until after catheterization so treat just like ACS. Thereafter, β-blockers and ACEIs are the mainstay of treatment. Nearly all patients recover completely.

MYOCARDITIS

Myocarditis is characterized by inflammation of the myocardium. Infectious agents, inflammatory disorders, and toxic exposures can all cause myocarditis. A number of **infectious agents** have been implicated (Table 2.15).

- Viral agents are the most common etiology in the United States.
- Chagas disease is the most common etiology worldwide.

Q

A 25-year-old man presents with flu-like symptoms, chest pain, and worsening shortness of breath. He has no past medical history, but recently returned from a 2-week camping trip to Central America. On examination, the patient has bilateral rales, S_3, and JVD. His ECG shows tachycardia and nonspecific T-wave changes. Echocardiogram shows diffuse hypokinesis. What is the most likely etiologic agent in this patient?

KEY FACT

Takotsubo cardiomyopathy usually presents in a manner indistinguishable from STEMI.

KEY FACT

LLSA Article: Myocarditis. *N Engl J Med*. April 2009;360(15):1526-1538.

A

This patient likely has myocarditis from the parasite *Trypanosoma cruzi*. Chagas disease, which results from infection with *Trypanosoma cruzi*, is the most common etiology of myocarditis worldwide. It is especially common in Latin America.

TABLE 2.15. Infectious Agents Implicated in Myocarditis

Viral	Bacterial	Parasitic
Coxsackie B virus	β-Hemolytic *Streptococcus* (rheumatic fever)	*Trypanosoma cruzi* (Chagas disease)
Adenovirus	*Mycoplasma pneumoniae*	*Trichinella spiralis* (Trichonosis)
Hepatitis B and C	*Corynebacterium diphtheriae* (Diphtheria)	
HIV	*Borrelia burgdorferi* (Lyme disease)	
Echovirus	*Mycobacterium tuberculosis*	

HIV, human immunodeficiency virus.

Myocarditis may also result from **autoimmune diseases, chemical exposure, or drugs**. These include Kawasaki disease, sarcoidosis, systemic lupus erythematosus (SLE), penicillins, sulfonamides, and cocaine.

PATHOPHYSIOLOGY

- Direct invasion, damage from the host inflammatory/autoimmune response, and direct toxicity of circulating chemicals → myocardial damage
- Often associated with pericarditis

KEY FACT

Flu-like symptoms and new CHF? Suspect myocarditis.

SYMPTOMS

- Flu-like symptoms are common: Fever, fatigue, myalgias, vomiting, diarrhea.
- Other symptoms include retrosternal chest pain, dyspnea, palpitations, syncope, or near syncope.

EXAMINATION

- Fever, sinus tachycardia beyond what would be expected from fever
- Signs of heart failure including rales, peripheral edema, and JVD

DIAGNOSIS

- Suspect in any patient presenting with flu-like symptoms and CHF.
- White blood count (WBC) and erythrocyte sedimentation rate (ESR) are only sometimes elevated and so do not have diagnostic utility.
- Elevated troponin.
- ECG: Sinus tachycardia, wide QRS, low QRS voltage, prolonged QTc, ST elevations, nonspecific ST-T changes.
- CXR: Usually normal, but may show cardiomegaly or pulmonary edema.
- TTE: Dilated chambers and hypokinesis (can be global or focal).
- Biopsy: Poor sensitivity and specificity depending on tissue sampled. High false negative.
- Contrast-enhanced MRI may be gold standard in future.

TREATMENT

- Address infectious etiology, if identified.
- Treat heart failure as with other causes (ACEI, β-blockers, diuresis).
- Steroids and intravenous immunoglobulin (IVIG) have not consistently shown benefit in studies (except in Kawasaki).
- IV inotropes, balloon pump, extracorporeal membrane oxygenation (ECMO), or ventricular assist device for fulminant heart failure. Transplant may be needed.

COMPLICATIONS

Complications include sudden death, dysrhythmia, dilated cardiomyopathy, heart failure, and mural thrombus with systemic emboli.

ISCHEMIC HEART DISEASE

Ischemic heart disease consists of a spectrum of illness from asymptomatic coronary CAD to stable angina pectoris to unstable angina (UA) to non–ST-elevation myocardial infarction (*NSTEMI*) to STEMI. Acute coronary syndrome (ACS) refers to the constellation of diseases caused by acute ischemia, and thus includes UA, NSTEMI, and STEMI.

Stable Angina

Stable angina pectoris results when a fixed coronary plaque prevents sufficient blood supply through a coronary artery at times of increased O_2 demand. This results in predictable chest discomfort during periods of physical or emotional stress. Stable angina is resolved by alleviating the increased O_2 demand with rest or by increasing myocardial oxygen supply with supplemental oxygen, blood transfusion for severe anemia, or vasodilators such as nitroglycerin. Symptoms usually last only a **few minutes** after cessation of activity or use of nitroglycerin.

It is divided into 4 classes by the Canadian Cardiovascular Society:

- **Class I:** Angina with strenuous physical activity
- **Class II:** Slight limitation of normal physical activity
- **Class III:** Severe limitation of normal physical activity
- **Class IV:** Inability to perform any physical activity without symptoms

ACUTE CORONARY SYNDROMES

Unstable Angina

Unstable angina (UA) is angina occurring with minimal exertion or at rest, new-onset angina (within last 2 months), or an increasing frequency or duration of previously stable angina.

UA is part of the continuum of ACS and overlaps with NSTEMI. A patient experiencing severe UA has a prognosis and risk profile similar to that of a patient with a mild NSTEMI. Some differentiate UA from NSTEMI in that the latter can be detected by an elevation in cardiac markers.

Short-term, high-risk factors for death or nonfatal AMI in patients with UA include:

- Rest pain > 20 minutes
- CHF or pulmonary edema
- Rest pain with dynamic ECG changes
- Chest pain with new or worsening MR murmur
- Chest pain with hypotension

Acute Myocardial Infarction

Acute myocardial infarction (AMI) can be categorized by the type of infarction (Table 2.16) and the ECG findings present at diagnosis (NSTEMI or STEMI). The "**Universal Definition**" of AMI is myocardial cell death and necrosis as diagnosed by a rise and fall of cardiac enzymes in combination with 1 of the following clinical findings: (1) appropriate clinical presentation

Q

A 65-year-old man presents via emergency medical service (EMS) with substernal chest pressure, diaphoresis, and shortness of breath. His initial ECG demonstrated ST elevation in leads II, III, and aVF. Following a sublingual nitroglycerin, his BP dropped from 130/75 to 85/50 mm Hg and his chest pain worsened. What caused his drop in blood pressure? How could this have been avoided, and what is the most appropriate initial therapy for his hypotension?

KEY FACT

Coronary heart disease is the number 1 cause of death in the United States, with > 500,000 deaths annually.

KEY FACT

UA = new-onset angina, angina with ↑ frequency or duration, angina with minimal exertion/rest

A

Patients suffering from a MI involving the RV are often very preload dependent, so nitroglycerin can cause a precipitous drop in BP. A right-sided ECG should be performed on all patients with inferior (II, III, aVF) ST elevation. ST elevation in lead V_4R indicates RV infarction; nitroglycerin is generally contraindicated. This patient should be given boluses of a crystalloid until his vital signs stabilize. Administration of inotropes or vasopressors may also be required.

TABLE 2.16. Universal Classification of Myocardial Infarction

Type	Type of Ischemia	Description
Type 1	Spontaneous myocardial infarction	Intraluminal thrombus in coronary artery leading to decreased myocardial blood flow or distal platelet emboli with ensuing myocyte necrosis.
Type 2	Myocardial infarction secondary to an ischemic imbalance	Condition other than CAD contributes to imbalance between myocardial oxygen supply and/or demand.
Type 3	Myocardial infarction resulting in death when biomarker values are unavailable	Cardiac death with symptoms suggestive of myocardial ischemia and presumed new ischemic ECG changes or new LBBB, but death occurring before cardiac markers drawn.
Type 4	Myocardial infarction related to PCI	Myocardial infarction associated with PCI.
Type 5	Myocardial infarction related to CABG	Myocardial infarction associated with CABG.

CABG, coronary artery bypass grafting; CAD, coronary artery disease; ECG, electrocardiogram; LBBB, left bundle branch block; PCI, percutaneous coronary intervention.

(chest pain or "anginal equivalent"), (2) ECG changes indicative of ischemia, (3) pathologic Q waves on ECG, or (4) identification of coronary artery abnormality noted by new finding on cardiac imaging or culprit lesion on catheterization.

- NSTEMI is an AMI occurring without ST elevations on the ECG.
- STEMI is an AMI occurring with 1 of following ECG findings: (1) ≥ 1 mm ST elevation in ≥ 2 contiguous standard limb leads, (2) ≥ 2 mm ST elevation in ≥ 2 contiguous precordial leads, OR (c) new LBBB.

Pathophysiology

ACS results from insufficient O_2 supply to meet cardiac muscle demands:

- Progressive growth of atherosclerotic lesions within the coronary arteries → ↓ luminal diameter and ↓ coronary blood flow
- Acute coronary artery plaque disruption → exposed thrombogenic endothelium → platelet aggregation and thrombus formation
- Coronary artery vasospasm (eg, Prinzmetal angina)
- Other causes: Dissection of the coronary arteries, embolic disease, excess demand states, vasculitis, severely compromised oxygen carrying capacity

Symptoms

- Classic symptoms include chest pain or pressure (may radiate to the back, chest, jaw, or either arm), shortness of breath, sweating, nausea, and impending sense of doom.
- Exertional chest pain (LR6 + 2.4), radiation of pain to right arm (LR 4.7), associated dyspnea or diaphoresis (LR 2.4), and nausea/vomiting (LR 1.9) can help identify ACS. Pleuritic, positional, or reproducible pain with palpation points away from ACS (LR < 0.31). However, no symptom has sufficient sensitivity or specificity to rule-in or rule out ACS.

- Nearly one-third of patients with acute MI will have atypical or silent presentations. Be especially suspicious in diabetics, the elderly, and women. These atypical symptoms include fatigue or generalized weakness, shortness of breath without chest pain, epigastric abdominal pain or "indigestion," and mental status change.
- Resolution of symptoms with antacids, GERD (gastroesophageal reflux disease)-related medications, or nitroglycerin does not exclude cardiac etiology for symptoms.

Risk factors for CAD are more common in patients with ACS but do not predict presence or absence of ACS. They include:

- Smoking, HTN, diabetes, hyperlipidemia, family history, advanced age, male gender, cocaine use, **SLE**, rheumatoid arthritis, human immunodeficiency virus (HIV), obesity, postmenopausal state

KEY FACT

ACS in diabetic, elderly patients, and women commonly presents with atypical symptoms.

Examination

- Often nonspecific and may include pallor, diaphoresis, and tachypnea.
- Listen for new heart murmur (MR or septal rupture).
- Reproducible chest pain is present in 15% of patients with proven MI.

KEY FACT

A normal initial ECG does not rule out MI, even if performed while the patient is experiencing pain!

Differential

PE, aortic dissection, cardiac tamponade, myocarditis, pericarditis, pneumothorax, pneumonia, musculoskeletal pain, gastroesophageal reflux (a diagnosis of exclusion, rarely the correct answer on boards), esophageal rupture, Mallory-Weiss syndrome, biliary disease, pancreatitis

KEY FACT

Always get a RIGHT-sided ECG to look for RV infarct in inferior wall MI. Patients with RV infarct are preload dependent. NTG is contraindicated!

Diagnosis

Diagnosis of ACS made with combination of symptoms, ECG findings and biomarkers. See "Universal Definition" given earlier.

ECG Findings Suggestive of AMI

- **Hyperacute T waves**
  - Tall, symmetric T waves, especially in the anterior precordial leads
  - Earliest ECG finding in acute MI but transient
  - Differential includes hyperkalemia, LVH, pericarditis
- **ST-segment elevation**
  - Domed, **"tombstone morphology"**
  - Occurring in a regional distribution (Table 2.17)
  - Dynamic—waxing and waning with time
  - May be associated with evolving Q waves (infarct)
  - May only appear on ECG with posterior leads for posterior MI (or ST depressions in V_1 and V_2) or right-sided leads for RV infarction (Figure 2.18)
- **Reciprocal ST-segment depression**
  - Changes in region electrically opposite to that of injury
  - Indicates a larger area of injury, lower ejection fraction, and ↑ mortality
- **T-wave inversions in regional distribution**
  - May occur before or after ST elevation.
  - **Wellens T waves**—deep symmetric or biphasic T wave inversions in the anterior precordial leads suggest LAD lesion (Figure 2.19).
  - Differential includes LVH, BBB, pacer, myocarditis, and pericarditis.
- **New LBBB**
  - **Prexisting LBBB or ventricular-paced rhythm:**
    - LBBB follows **Law of Appropriate Discordance:** It is **appropriate** for the ST-segment elevation/depression to be **discordant** with the direction of the primary QRS vector.
  - Sgarbossa criteria score ≥ 3 is strongly predictive of acute MI (Table 2.18).

KEY FACT

ST depression and prominent R waves in V_1, V_2 = posterior STEMI. Obtain leads V_7 through V_9.

KEY FACT

ECG findings suggestive of MI:

- Hyperacute T waves
- ST-segment elevation
- Reciprocal ST-segment depression
- T-wave inversions in regional distribution
- New LBBB

KEY FACT

Hyperacute T waves are the earliest ECG finding of STEMI.

TABLE 2.17. Regional ECG Findings in the Setting of MI

Region of ST Elevation	Region of Infarct	Affected Vessel	Special Considerations
II, III, aVF (Reciprocal changes in aVL)	Inferior	Right coronary artery—posterior descending branch	Anticipate RV or posterior infarct.
V_3, V_4 (Reciprocal changes in II, III, aVF)	Anterior	Left anterior descending—diagonal branch	Anticipate BBB, LV dysfunction, complete heart block.
V_1, V_2	Septal	Left anterior descending—septal branch	Anticipate BBB.
V_5, V_6, and I, aVL	Lateral	Left circumflex—circumflex or diagonal branch	Anticipate LV dysfunction with CHF.
On R-sided ECG: V_4R (see Figure 2.11.)	Right ventricle	Right coronary artery—proximal branches	Anticipate hypotension with clear lungs. Preload dependent.
Posterior ECG: V_7 to V_9 *Note:* ST **depression** in V_1, V_2 with prominent R waves suggests posterior STEMI; tall, upright T wave in V_1 instead of normally inverted T wave also suggestive	Posterior	Left circumflex—posterior circumflex **or** right coronary artery—posterior descending	Rarely occurs in isolation, usually with inferior or lateral MI. Anticipate LV dysfunction.

BBB, bundle branch clock; CHF, congestive heart failure; ECG, electrocardiogram; LV, left ventricular; MI, myocardial infarction; RV, right ventricular; STEMI, ST-elevation myocardial infarction.

KEY FACT

A normal ECG does **not** rule out ACS. The initial ECG is nondiagnostic in many patients with MI.

Differential Diagnosis of ST Elevation on ECG

- LV aneurysm
  - History of prior MI
  - ECG with anterior (usually) Q waves and ST elevation
  - ST without dynamic or reciprocal changes
  - Can be visualized on echocardiography
- Benign early repolarization (Figure 2.20)
  - Characterized by 1-4 mm of J-point elevation in precordial leads with upwardly concave morphology
  - Frequently associated with notching at J point (junction of QRS complex and ST segment)
  - Rarely seen in leads V_1 and V_2

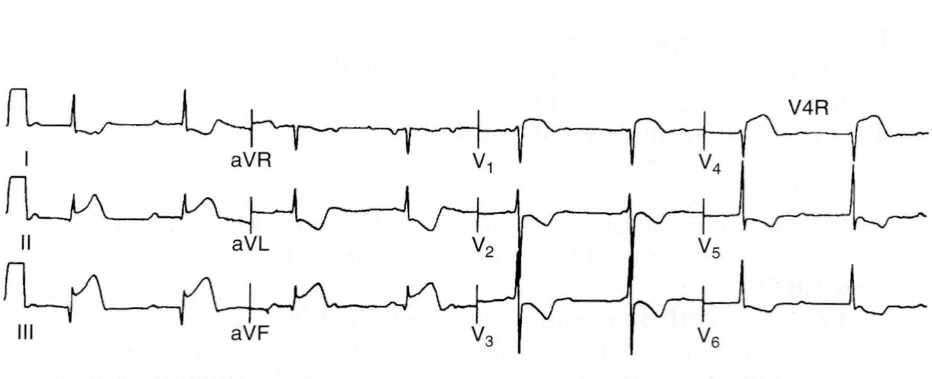

FIGURE 2.18. Right-sided ECG in patient with inferior myocardial infarction (MI). (Reproduced, with permission, from Fuster V, Alexander RW, O'Rourke RA. *Hurst's The Heart*. 12th ed. New York, NY: McGraw-Hill; 2008:300.)

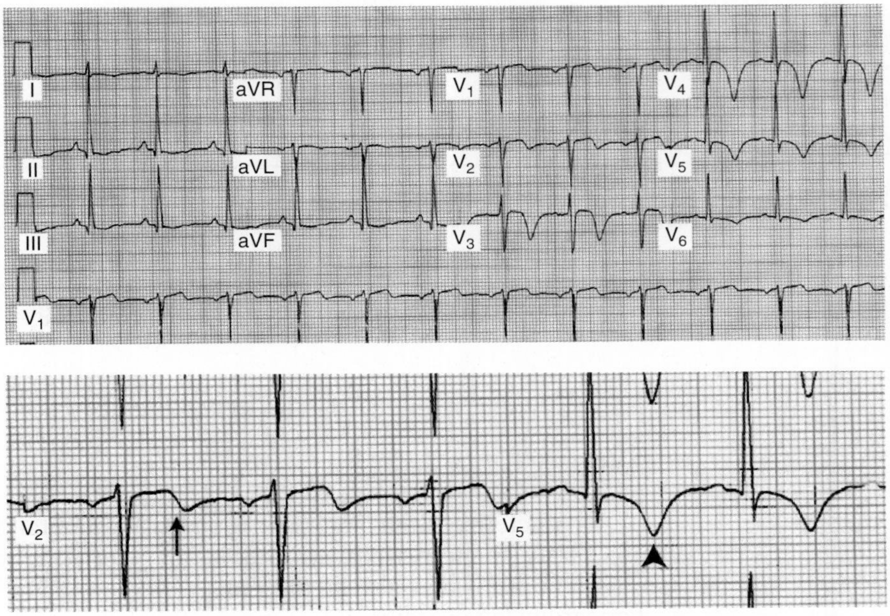

FIGURE 2.19. Wellens waves. Arrow indicates biphasic T wave; arrowhead indicates deeply inverted T wave. Both findings are consistent with a proximal LAD lesion. (Reproduced, with permission, from Koop KJ, Stack LB, Storrow AB, Thurman RJ. *The Atlas of Emergency Medicine*. 3rd ed. New York, NY: McGraw-Hill; 2010.)

TABLE 2.18. Sgarbossa Criteria for the Diagnosis of AMI With Preexisting LBBB

ECG Finding	Point Value
Concordant ST elevation > 1 mm	5
Concordant ST depression > 1 mm in V1, V2, or V3	3
Discordant ST elevation > 5 mm	1

AMI, acute myocardial infarction; ECG, electrocardiogram; LBBB, left bundle branch block.

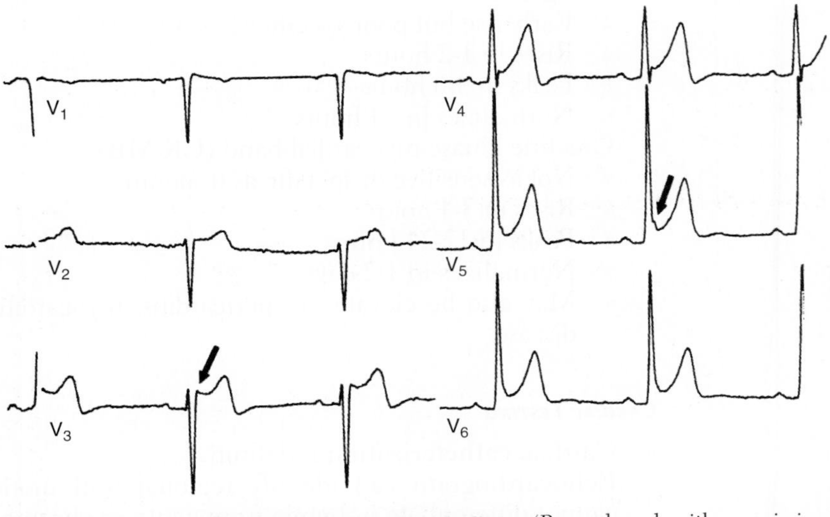

FIGURE 2.20. Early repolarization ECG findings. (Reproduced, with permission, from Fuster V, Alexander RW, O'Rourke RA. *Hurst's The Heart*. 12th ed. New York, NY: McGraw-Hill; 2008:303.)

TABLE 2.19. Timeline for Serum Markers in the Evaluation of ACS

MARKER	RISES	PEAKS	NORMALIZES
Troponin	2-6 h	12-24 h	7-10 d
Myoglobin	1-2 h	4-6 h	24 h
CK-MB	3-4 h	12-24 h	1-2 d

ACS, acute coronary syndrome; CK-MB, creatine kinase-myocardial band.

- LVH (see Figure 2.12)
  - May mimic or obscure ACS.
  - Characterized by a large S wave in V_1, V_2, and tall R wave in V_5, V_6.
  - "Strain" pattern with asymmetrically inverted T waves in inferior and lateral leads may also be present.
- Pericarditis/myocarditis
  - Diffuse ST elevations in multiple regions
  - PR depression
  - Common finding for several minutes following electrical cardioversion
- Also consider PE, hyperkalemia, cerebral hemorrhage, Brugada syndrome, arrhythmogenic right ventricular cardiomyopathy

Serum Markers

- May be normal early despite ongoing ischemia → must check serial measurements
- Become elevated in NSTEMI and STEMI (Table 2.19)
- **Troponin I**
  - Most sensitive and specific but delayed rise
  - Traditional troponin assays rise in 3-6 hours after symptom onset
  - New highly sensitive assays are more likely to rise within 2-3 hours
  - Peaks at 12-24 hours
  - Normalizes in 7-10 days
  - Unlike troponin T, is **not** elevated in skeletal muscle disease
- **Myoglobin**
  - Early rise but poor specificity
  - Rises in 1-2 hours
  - Peaks in 4-6 hours
  - Normalizes in 24 hours
- Creatine kinase-myocardial band (**CK-MB**)
  - Not as sensitive or specific as troponin
  - Rises in 3-4 hours
  - Peaks in 12-24 hours
  - Normalizes in 1-2 days
  - May also be elevated in pericarditis, myocarditis, and skeletal muscle disease

Cardiac Testing

- **Cardiac catheterization** is definitive.
- **Echocardiogram** can identify regional wall motion abnormalities, but cannot differentiate ischemia from acute or chronic infarction and **cannot reliably** detect subendocardial ischemia.

TABLE 2.20. Cardiac Stress Testing Modalities

Method	Advantages	Limitations
Treadmill	Cheap Rapid Wide availability	Contraindicated in high-risk patients Inability to exercise to 85% max HR (arthritis, COPD, deconditioning, etc)
Chemical stress	Side effects rapidly reversible Useful for patients with exercise limitations	False negatives with methylxanthines, including caffeine Risk of induced arrhythmia or heart block
Stress ECG	Cheap Wide availability	Baseline ECG abnormalities Lowest sensitivity
Stress TTE	No radiation Evaluates cardiac function	Operator dependent Misses small or subendocardial lesions
Nuclear	Best sensitivity Less operator dependent Can delay up to 3 h between isotope administration and imaging	Radiation exposure Most expensive Limited by adipose tissue

COPD, chronic obstructive pulmonary disease; ECG, electrocardiogram; HR, heart rate; TTE, transthoracic echocardiogram.

- **Perfusion imaging** during symptoms.
  - IV radionuclide (eg, thallium 201, technetium 99m-sestamibi) is taken up by myocardium.
  - Uptake is proportional to blood flow, so areas with poor perfusion are demonstrated.
- **Electron beam CT (EBCT)** is a new technology that shows calcium plaques in arteries.
- **Exercise stress testing** is safe in low-risk patients but in others it should be performed only after the patient has had 8-12 hours free of active ischemic or heart failure symptoms. False-positive and false-negative results are common. Other stress testing modalities used to evaluate CAD can be seen in Table 2.20.

Treatment (Table 2.21)

STEMI treatment involves immediate fibrinolysis or percutaneous coronary intervention (PCI). UA and NSTEMI have the same treatment pathways which are based on clinical risk assessment.

TABLE 2.21. ED Core Measures for ACS in 2015

ASA on arrival
Time to ECG
If STEMI: • Door-to-balloon time < 90 min **Or** • Door to needle (fibrinolytics) < 30 min

ACS, acute coronary syndrome; ASA, acetylsalicylic acid; ECG, electrocardiogram; ED, emergency department; STEMI, ST-elevation myocardial infarction.

KEY FACT

In patients who present to the ED with chest pain, the ECG should be interpreted by the physician **within 10 minutes** of patient's arrival.

MNEMONIC

In ACS, remember:

MONAB

Morphine
Oxygen
Nitrates
Aspirin
β-Blocker (within 24 hours)

> **KEY FACT**
>
> Morphine has not been shown to ↓ mortality in ACS.

> **KEY FACT**
>
> Always ask the patient about use of sildenafil (Viagra) or other phosphodiesterase inhibitors before administering nitroglycerin.

> **KEY FACT**
>
> Aspirin is the most cost-effective treatment available for patients with ACS. It independently reduces mortality of patients with AMI and is synergistic with fibrinolysis and PCI.
>
> In aspirin allergy, give 300-600 mg loading dose of clopidogrel.

> **KEY FACT**
>
> LLSA Article: ECG Activation of Cath Lab. *Am Heart J.* 2010;160(6):995-1003.

General Medications Used in STEMI and UA/NSTEMI

- **Morphine**
  - Sympatholytic, ↓ myocardial O_2 consumption, mild vasodilator, ↓ preload.
  - Analgesic for intractable chest pain. No proven ↓ in mortality.
  - Contraindicated in patients with SBP < 100 mm Hg.
  - Typical dose is 0.05-0.1 mg/kg IV.
- **O_2**
  - Evidence suggests hyperoxia may lead to ↑ mortality in AMI—aim for O_2 sat > 90%
- **NTG**
  - Dilates coronary arteries and relaxes vascular smooth muscle, resulting in decreased preload/afterload and decreased myocardial O_2 demand.
  - No mortality benefit but reduces symptoms. Commonly causes headache.
  - 0.4 mg sublingual q5min prn × 3, then IV drip if symptoms persist.
  - Symptomatic response does not rule cardiac disease in or out.
  - Contraindications: Hypotension (SBP < 90 mm Hg), RV infarct, concomitant use of PDE inhibitor within 24-48 hours (24 hours for sildenafil, 48 hours for tadalafil).
- **Aspirin**
  - Antiplatelet agent—irreversibly inhibits platelet cyclooxygenase activity, thereby inhibiting the formation of thromboxane A_2. Effect of 1 dose lasts 8-10 days.
  - Onset of action is **minutes**.
  - ↓ Long-term mortality and **synergistic** with fibrinolysis.
  - Administer rectally when patients cannot tolerate medications by mouth.
  - Dose 162-325 mg orally (PO) (chewed, nonenteric coated) or when needed (PR).
  - Aspirin allergy: Use clopidogrel 300 mg PO if < 75 years and 75 mg PO if ≥ 75 years.
- **β-Blockers**
  - Block sympathetic stimulation, reducing heart rate and ↓ myocardial O_2 consumption.
  - ↓ Incidence of ventricular fibrillation and recurrence of AMI but ↑ shock.
  - No mortality benefit when given early (eg, in ED).
  - Give orally **within 24 hours of hospitalization**.
  - Relative contraindications include:
    - SBP < 120 mm Hg
    - HR < 60 or > 110 bpm
    - LV failure with pulmonary edema
    - Second- and third-degree heart block
    - Severe reactive airway disease
  - IV administration should NOT be used unless hypertensive and no contraindications.

Reperfusion Therapy: PCI and Fibrinolysis

Indications for immediate reperfusion therapy are (1) symptom onset < 12 hours or ongoing evidence of ischemia at 12-24 hours AND (2) ≥ 1- to 2-mm ST elevation in regional distribution or new LBBB (Table 2.22).

Primary PCI

- Consists of immediate catheterization, angioplasty, and stent placement across culprit lesion.

TABLE 2.22. ECG Indications for Reperfusion Therapy in STEMI

1-mm ST elevation in 2 contiguous limb leads
2-mm ST elevation in 2 contiguous precordial leads
New LBBB[a]

ECG, electrocardiogram; LBBB, left bundle branch block; STEMI, ST-elevation myocardial infarction.

[a]LBBB must be present in setting of chest pain or "anginal equivalent" to be considered STEMI equivalent.

- Preferred method of reperfusion at PCI-capable centers.
- Goal door-to-balloon is ≤ 90 minutes at PCI-capable center.
- At non-PCI-capable centers, transfer to PCI-capable center preferred if:
  - Door-to-balloon **time** < 120 minutes (including transfer) < 120 minutes AND door-to-balloon time (including transfer) minus door-to-needle time (at non-PCI center) is < 60 minutes. (eg, if you can get patient to PCI center and get lesion stented within 120 minutes AND the delay between giving lytics at non-PCI center and PCI is < 1 hour → transfer patient)
  - **Time** to presentation > 3 hours after onset of symptoms
  - High-**risk** presentation (cardiogenic shock)
  - High **risk** for thrombolytics (≥75 years old, other relative contraindication)
- The American Heart Association recommends that PCI be performed in a center which does > 200 PCIs per year.

Fibrinolysis

- IV thrombolytics → activate plasminogen → degrade fibrin clots → open coronary artery.
  - Fibrin-specific lytics: Tenecteplase (TNK), alteplase (tPa), and reteplase (rPA) (Table 2.23)
  - TNK marginally more effective, minimally safer, and easier to dose

TABLE 2.23. Dosing for fibrinolytic agents in STEMI

Medication	Administration	Dosage
Tenecteplase (TNK)	Single bolus	< 60 kg → 30 mg 60-69 kg → 35mg 70-79 kg → 40 mg 80-89 kg → 45 mg ≥ 90 kg → 50 mg
Alteplase (tPA)	Bolus and infusions with ceiling doses	15 mg IVP; then 0.75 mg/kg × 30 min (max 50 mg); then 0.5 mg/kg × 60 min (max 35 mg) Total dose not to exceed 100 mg
Reteplase (rPA)	Double bolus	10 units IVP q30min × 2 doses

STEMI, ST-elevation myocardial infarction.

TABLE 2.24. Contraindications to Fibrinolytic Therapy in Acute Myocardial Infarction

Absolute Contraindications
Previous hemorrhagic stroke at any time
Bland CVA in past year
Known intracranial neoplasm
Active internal bleeding (excluding menses)
Suspected aortic dissection or pericarditis
Relative Contraindications
Severe uncontrolled blood pressure (> 180/100 mm Hg)
History of chronic severe hypertension
History of prior CVA or known intracranial pathology not covered in contraindications
Current use of anticoagulants with known INR > 2-3
Known bleeding diathesis
Recent trauma (past 2 wk)
Prolonged CPR (> 10 min)
Major surgery (< 3 wk)
Noncompressible vascular punctures (including subclavian and internal jugular central lines)
Recent internal bleeding (2-4 wk)
Prior streptokinase (should not receive streptokinase)
Pregnancy
Active peptic ulcer disease
Other medical conditions likely to increase risk of bleeding

CPR, cardiopulmonary resuscitation; CVA, cardiovascular accident; INR, international normalized ratio.

(Reproduced, with permission, from Tintinalli JE, Kelen GD, Stapczynski JS. *Emergency Medicine: A Comprehensive Study Guide*. 6th ed. New York, NY: McGraw-Hill; 2004:353.)

KEY FACT

PCI is preferred to fibrinolysis in STEMI if symptoms have been present for ≥ 3 hours **or** if expected door-to-balloon time is within 1 hour of door-to-needle time.

- Fibrinolysis should occur if presentation within 3 hours of symptom onset and unable to meet previous criteria for transfer to PCI center.
- Goal door-to-needle time is ≤ 30 minutes.
- Higher risk than PCI if patient ≥ 75 years due to ICH risk.
- Other contraindications to thrombolytics (Table 2.24).

ADJUNCTIVE TREATMENTS: ANTIPLATELET AGENTS, ANTICOAGULANTS, AND OTHERS

Adjuncts to reperfusion should be utilized in coordination with the team of providers involved in caring for the patient with a STEMI. See Table 2.25 for summary of antiplatelet and anticoagulant agents used in the treatment of STEMI. See Table 2.26 for a summary of other medications used in the treatment of STEMI.

Nonprimary PCI for STEMI

- No benefit to pretreatment with lytics prior to PCI ("facilitated PCI").
- No benefit to PCI in delayed fashion (1 week after AMI) of occluded coronary artery.
- If continued ischemia present after fibrinolysis (persistent ST elevations or symptoms), rescue PCI can be of benefit.
- Angiography within 24 hours of successful fibrinolysis appears beneficial.

TABLE 2.25. Antiplatelet and Anticoagulants Used as Adjuncts to Reperfusion in the Treatment of STEMI

Agent	Mechanism of Action	Effect/Benefits in PCI vs Fibrinolysis	Contraindications
P2Y12 Inhibitors **Clopidogrel** **Prasugrel** **Ticagrelor**	Antiplatelet Irreversibly inhibits platelet aggregation via ADP-receptor antagonism Onset of action = 3-6 h	PCI: ↓ Mortality; prasugruel and ticagrelor have fewer CV complications than clopidogrel Lytics: ↓ Mortality Give clopidogrel in aspirin allergy	Planned CABG within 5 d (No prospective criteria exist to determine need for CABG) Prasugrel contraindicated if prior CVA or TIA
GP IIb/IIIa inhibitors **Abciximab** **Eptifibatide** **Tirofiban**	Antiplatelet Blocks final common pathway of platelet aggregation by inhibiting the GP IIb/IIIa receptor on platelet surface	PCI: ↓ Mortality, MI and urgent revascularization Lytics: No indication for use	Active internal bleeding Bleeding < 30 d Platelet count < 150,000 History of intracranial hemorrhage, AVM, aneurysm, or stroke < 30 d Major surgery or trauma < 30 d
Heparin **UFH** **LMWH**	Antithrombin Binds antithrombin III → inactivates thrombin and activated factor X → ↓ clot formation and propagation Synergistic effect with aspirin UFH: target aPTT 1.5-2.5 × control	PCI: No mortality benefit but recommended Lytics: ↑ Vessel patency LMWH superior to UFH for both indications in recent trials	Use bivalirudin if HIT present and PCI planned LMWH requires renal adjustment

ADP, adenosine diphosphate; AVM, arteriovenous malformation; CABG, coronary artery bypass grafting; CV, cardiovascular; CVA, cardiovascular accident; GP, glycoprotein; HIT, heparin-induced thrombocytopenia; LMWH, low-molecular-weight heparin; MI, myocardial function; PCI, percutaneous coronary intervention; STEMI, ST-elevation myocardial infarction; TIA, transient ischemic attack; UFH, unfractionated heparin.

TABLE 2.26. Other Medications Commonly Used in the Treatment of STEMI

Agent	Mechanism of Action	Effect/Benefits in PCI vs Fibrinolysis	Contraindications
Morphine **O**xygen **N**itroglycerin **A**spirin β-Blockers	See above for discussion of "MONAB"		
ACE inhibitors and ARBs	Reduce adverse LV remodeling via inhibition of pathologic RAAS activation after AMI ARBs have same effect as ACE Inhibitors	↓ Incidence of CHF, sudden death, and subsequent MIs ↓ Mortality benefit if EF < 40%, anterior MI or prior MI Generally start within 24 h	Pregnancy History of angioedema SBP < 100 mm Hg Renal failure Hyperkalemia
Statins	HMG coreductase inhibitor	PCI: ↓ Periprocedural myonecrosis (high-dose statin)	No risk or safety data for statins when used in setting of STEMI
Calcium channel blockers	Nondihydropyridine CCB	Rate control if SVT present and patient cannot tolerate β-blocker Useful in coronary vasospasm	Increases mortality outside this narrow indication

ACE, angiotension-converting enzyme; ARBs, angiotensin receptor blockers; AMI, acute myocardial infarction; CCB, calcium channel blocker; CHF, congestive heart failure; EF, ejection fraction; HMG, LV, left ventricular; MI, myocardial function; PCI, percutaneous coronary intervention; RAAS; SBP, systolic blood pressure; STEMI, ST-elevation myocardial infarction; SVT, supraventricular tachycardia.

Conservative and Invasive Strategies

- In UA and NSTEMI, patients are stratified according to their risk of death, MI, and need for urgent revascularization (TIMI Risk Score is used for this purpose). Based on risk, they receive **conservative** or **early invasive** treatment strategies.
- **Conservative strategy**: Medical treatment with coronary angiography only if ischemia recurs or if stress test is strongly positive.
- **Early invasive strategy**: Angiography within 24-72 hours.
- TIMI Risk Score
  - 1 point each for: (1) age ≥ 65, (2) ≥ 3 CAD risk factors, (3) known CAD (≥ 50% stenosis on prior angiography), (4) aspirin use in last 7 days, (5) ST deviation ≥ 0.5mm on ECG, (6) ≥ 2 anginal events ≤ 24 hours, or (7) positive cardiac biomarker (troponin)
  - Score ≥ 3 confers benefit to early invasive strategy → heparin, GP IIb/IIIa inhibitor, and early angiography

Medications Used to Treat UA/NSTEMI

With the exceptions of aspirin, morphine, nitroglycerin, and oxygen, medications should be selected in coordination with the team of providers involved in caring for the patient with UA/NSTEMI. See Table 2.27 for summary of medications used in the treatment of UA/NSTEMI.

COMPLICATIONS

Complications of AMI (Table 2.28):

Divided into early and late complications

Early Complications

- Stroke
  - Embolic stroke from LV thrombus and atrial fibrillation as well as carotid disease predisposes patients with MI
  - Hemorrhagic stroke more common in fibrinolysis (~1%) versus PCI (~0.1%)
- LV failure (systolic and diastolic dysfunctions)
  - Ranges from mild pulmonary congestion to cardiogenic shock
  - Treat with revascularization, diuresis, afterload reduction, inotropes, and mechanical support (eg, balloon pump, LVAD) as needed
- Bradydysrhythmias and AVB
  - AV node can be affected in inferior MI → transient AV block.
  - Infranodal block at bundle of His in anterior MI → poor prognosis.
  - Treat with observation if first-degree AVB or second-degree Mobitz Type I.
  - Treat with atropine (if within first 24 hours).
  - Begin transcutaneous and prepare for transvenous pacing if symptomatic bradycardia, third-degree AVB, second-degree Mobitz Type II with BBB block, or alternating LBBB/RBBB.
- Tachydysrhythmias
  - Accelerated idioventricular rhythm is common after reperfusion; benign and does not require treatment (Figure 2.21).
  - Atrial fibrillation, sinus tachycardia, ventricular tachycardia, and ventricular fibrillation all fairly common after AMI.
  - Treat in accordance with ACLS.
- LV free wall rupture
  - Rapid decline to PEA with pericardial effusion seen on bedside ultrasound.
  - Can occur in first 24 hours or 3-5 days after transmural MI.
  - Treatment is pericardiocentesis as temporizing measure and surgical repair.

TABLE 2.27. Medications Commonly Used in the Treatment of UA/NSTEMI

Agent	Mechanism of Action	Effect/Benefits in PCI vs Fibrinolysis	Contraindications
Morphine **O**xygen **N**itroglycerin **A**spirin **β**-Blockers	See above for discussion of "MONAB"		
ACE inhibitors and ARBs	Reduce adverse LV remodeling via inhibition of pathologic RAAS activation after AMI ARBs have same effect as ACE Inhibitors	↓ Incidence of CHF, sudden death, and subsequent MIs ↓ Mortality benefit if EF < 40%, anterior MI or prior MI Generally start within 24 h	Pregnancy History of angioedema SBP < 100 mm Hg Renal failure Hyperkalemia
P2Y12 inhibitors **Clopidogrel** **Prasugrel** **Ticagrelor**	Antiplatelet Irreversibly inhibits platelet aggregation via ADP-receptor antagonism Onset of action = 3-6 hours	Synergistic with ASA → reduce stroke and MI risk ↑ Benefit if given hours prior to PCI due to delayed onset of action	Planned CABG within 5 d (No prospective criteria exist to determine need for CABG) Prasugrel contraindicated if prior CVA or TIA
GP IIb/IIIa inhibitors **Abciximab** **Eptifibatide** **Tirofiban**	Antiplatelet Blocks final common pathway of platelet aggregation by inhibiting the GP IIb/IIIa receptor on platelet surface	Used in addition to PO antiplatelet agents (ASA + P2Y12 inhibitors) in patients undergoing PCI NO BENEFIT to starting prior to PCI and increased bleeding	No benefit to starting in ED
Heparin **UFH** **LMWH**	Antithrombin Binds antithrombin III → inactivates thrombin and activated factor X → ↓ clot formation and propagation Synergistic effect with aspirin UFH: target aPTT 1.5-2.5 × control	↓ Mortality LMWH ↓ mortality and MI relative to UFH	Use bivalirudin if HIT present and PCI planned LMWH requires renal adjustment

ACE, angiotension-converting enzyme; ADP, adenosine diphosphate; AMI, acute myocardial infarction; ARBs, angiotensin receptor blockers; ASA; acetyl-salicylic acid; CHF, congestive heart failure; CABG, coronary artery bypass grafting; CVA, cardiovascular accident; ED, emergency department; EF, ejection frac-tion; GP, glycoprotein; HIT, heparin-induced thrombocytopenia; LMWH, low-molecular-weight heparin; LV, left ventricular; MI, myocardial function; NSTEMI, non–ST-elevation myocardial infarction; PCI, percutaneous coronary intervention; PO, by mouth; RAAS; TIA, transient ischemic attack; UA, unstable angina; UFH, unfractionated heparin.

- Rupture of intraventricular septum
  - Rapid decline with new harsh, loud holosystolic murmur at left sternal border.
  - Treat with inotropes, mechanical support (eg, balloon pump), and vasopressors as bridge to surgical repair.
- Papillary muscle rupture
  - Pulmonary edema with new holosystolic, MR murmur 3-5 days after inferior MI (papillary muscle usually supplied by posterior descending artery)
  - Treat with diuretics, afterload reduction, intra-aortic balloon pump, and surgical repair.
- Infarct pericarditis
  - New pleuritic, positional chest pain in first week after MI due to transmural infarct.
  - ECG abnormalities often masked by changes from MI.
  - Treat supportively.

TABLE 2.28. Complications of Myocardial Infarction

	Clinical Features	Treatment
Early Complications		
CHF	Ranging from mild congestion (Killip II MI) to pulmonary edema (Killip III MI) (15%-40% mortality)	Standard MI therapy Diuresis Reperfusion
Cardiogenic shock	Pulmonary congestion and peripheral hypoperfusion (Killip IV MI; 80% mortality)	Reperfusion Inotropes Balloon pump
Bradydysrhythmias and AV block	Inferior MI: AV nodal, proximal to His bundle Stable and transient Anterior MI: Infranodal at lower His bundle, poor prognosis Respond poorly to therapy	Observation Transvenous pacing if: Symptomatic bradycardia, second-degree AV block type II, new bifascicular block with first degree AV block, bilateral BBB
Tachydysrhythmias	Occur in majority of patients	ACLS
Left ventricular free wall rupture	Rapid decline to PEA, pericardial effusion on ultrasound	Pericardiocentesis and surgical repair
Rupture of inter-ventricular septum	Rapid decline with new, harsh, systolic murmur	Surgical repair
Papillary muscle rupture	Days 3-5 after inferior MI Acute pulmonary edema with new systolic murmur	Surgical repair
Infarct pericarditis (different from Dressler syndrome)	Transmural infarct ECG abnormalities often masked by evolutionary changes	Supportive care
Late Complications		
LV thrombus	Stroke or emboli	Anticoagulation
Pleuropericarditis (Dressler syndrome)	2-10 wk post-MI fever, leukocytosis, friction rub, pericardial or pleural effusion	NSAIDs and steroids
LV aneurysm	Following large MI (anterior most common) CHF, dysrhythmias, thromboemboli, persistent ST elevation on ECG	Anticoagulation, surgery

ACLS, advanced cardiac life support; AV, atrioventricular; BBB, bundle branch block; CHF, congestive heart failure; ECG, electrocardiogram; LV, left ventricular; MI, myocardial function; NSAID, nonsteroidal anti-inflammatory drug; PEA, pulseless electrical activity.

Late Complications

- LV thrombus
  - Can lead to embolic stroke.
  - Treat with anticoagulation.
- Dressler syndrome
  - Chest pain and fever 2-10 weeks after MI.
  - Treat with high dose aspirin, nonsteroidal anti-inflammatory drugs (NSAIDs).

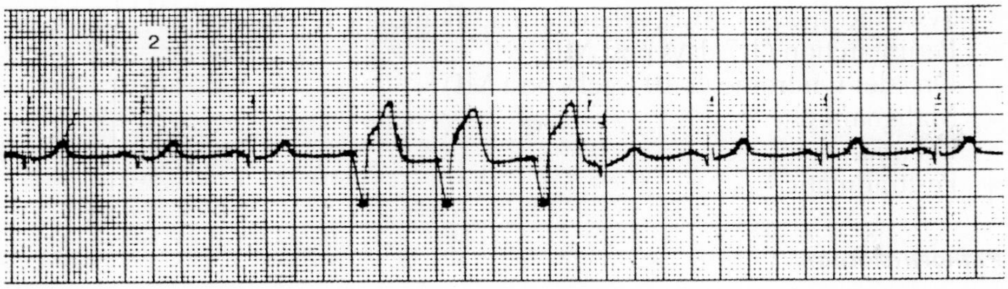

FIGURE 2.21. Accelerated idioventricular rhythms. (Reproduced, with permission, from Tintinalli JE, Kelen GD, Stapczynski JS. *Emergency Medicine: A Comprehensive Study Guide*. 6th ed. New York, NY: McGraw-Hill; 2004:189.)

- LV aneurysm
  - CHF, dysrhythmias, thromboemboli, persistent ST elevation on ECG after large MI (usually anterior).
  - Treat with anticoagulation and surgery.

Special Groups in Acute Coronary Syndrome

Women and the Elderly

- Prolonged atypical prodromal symptoms: Fatigue, shortness of breath, anxiety, indigestion
- Often associated with delay in seeking care

Cocaine-Associated Chest Pain

- Arterial vasoconstriction, sympathetic stimulation, increased platelet aggregation, accelerated atherosclerosis and thrombosis.
- Atypical symptoms: Dyspnea, diaphoresis, nausea.
- Greatest risk within first hour after use.
- ECG changes more atypical.
- 0.7%-6% of patients with cocaine-related chest pain have AMI.
- Only one-third of cocaine-associated MIs have significant CAD on cardiac catheterization.
- Treat with O_2, NTG, ASA, **benzodiazepines**. There is a theoretical risk of precipitating a hypertensive crisis through unopposed α-adrenergic effects if β-blockers (including labetalol) are given to patients with recent cocaine use.
- Complications are extremely rare if they do not present within 12 hours of symptom onset.

Ischemic heart disease is the most common cause of heart failure in the United States.

KEY FACT

LLSA Article: Cocaine-related chest pain: *Circulation*. April 2008;117:1897-1907.

Diseases of the Pericardium

PERICARDITIS

The pericardium may become inflamed for a variety of reasons. The resulting clinical presentation is sometimes confused with acute MI. The **vast majority** of cases are **idiopathic** (80%). Identified causes include:

- Infectious: viral (eg, Coxsackie, adenovirus), bacterial (uncommon), fungal, parasitic (eg, Rickettsia)
- Medications: Procainamide, hydralazine, INH

- Systemic diseases: SLE, scleroderma, rheumatic fever
- Periinfarction (1-7 days post MI)
- Dressler syndrome (2-10 weeks post MI)
- Malignancy
- Uremia
- Posttraumatic

Pathophysiology

Inflammation of pericardium → pericardial thickening and effusion

Symptoms

Classically presents as retrosternal, pleuritic, sharp chest pain **relieved by leaning forward** and exacerbated by lying down and taking deep breaths. May be preceded by fevers and myalgias

Examination

The **pericardial friction rub** is the classic finding. It is best heard over the left sternal border using the diaphragm of the stethoscope while the patient is leaning forward.

Differential

- Myocarditis
- ACS (regional ST elevation with reciprocal T-wave inversions and ST depression, ST elevation in lead III > lead II, and/or new Q waves = acute MI)

Diagnosis

- Suspect in any patient presenting with chest pain and fever (although fever is not a necessary finding)
- ECG (Table 2.29 and Figure 2.22)
  - Stage 1 (first hours to days): PR depression and diffuse ST elevation (may see reciprocal depression in aVR and V1) with concave-up segments
  - Stage 2: ST and PR segments normalize, T waves flatten
  - Stage 3: Diffuse T-wave inversions
  - Stage 4: Returns to normal (occasionally T-wave inversions are permanent)
- CXR: Usually nonspecific, but may show cardiomegaly if a pericardial effusion is present

TABLE 2.29. Progression of ECG Changes in Acute Pericarditis

ECG in Acute Pericarditis	
Stage 1	PR depression and diffuse ST elevation
Stage 2	ST and PR normalize, T waves flatten
Stage 3	Diffuse T-wave inversion
Stage 4	Returns to normal

ECG, electrocardiogram.

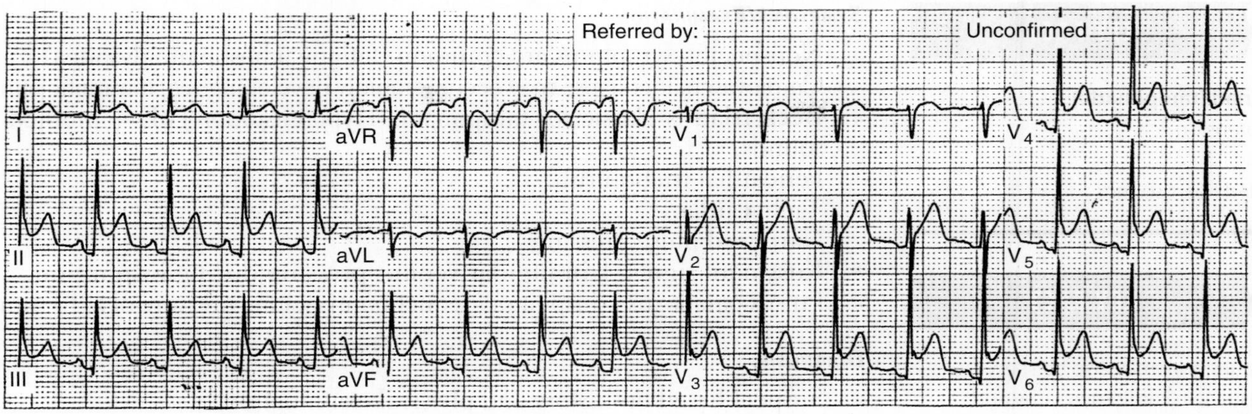

FIGURE 2.22. **Pericarditis with ST elevation in multiple regions.** (Reproduced, with permission, from Fuster V, Alexander RW, O'Rourke RA. *Hurst's The Heart*. 12th ed. New York, NY: McGraw-Hill; 2008:303.)

- Echocardiogram: To evaluate for pericardial effusion and tamponade (see later in the chapter)
- Laboratory studies: Expect leukocytosis, ↑ ESR, ↑ cardiac enzymes, ↑ blood urea nitrogen (BUN)/Cr (if uremic etiology)

KEY FACT

PR depression is specific for pericarditis.

Treatment

- Treat the underlying etiology if known.
- Traditionally, the first-line therapy has been NSAIDs (indomethacin or ibuprofen). Newer recommendations suggest benefit from **combination therapy** using NSAIDs and colchicine.
- Narcotics for intractable pain.
- Steroids in patients with ongoing symptoms or inability to tolerate NSAIDs.
- Mild cases attributed to viral origin can usually be managed as outpatients.

Complication

- Pericardial tamponade
- **Constrictive pericarditis**
  - Fibrotic change reduces diastolic filling.
  - Kussmaul sign: Increase in JVP during inspiration.
  - "Dip and plateau" LV filling (or diastolic) tracing.

PERICARDIAL EFFUSION AND TAMPONADE

While cardiac tamponade results from a pericardial effusion, **not all effusions** cause tamponade. An effusion that develops slowly allows for the pericardium to stretch and the LV volume to increase in response to the fluid, decreasing the likelihood of tamponade.

Etiologies

Most common etiologies of pericardial effusion:

- Malignancy
- Trauma
- Postinfarction
- Radiation
- Postoperative, including CABG (coronary artery bypass grafting) patients
- Pericarditis
- Renal failure

KEY FACT

Cardiac surgery patients can develop effusions despite prior pericardiotomy.

KEY FACT

Beck triad (tamponade):
Hypotension
JVD
Muffled heart sounds

KEY FACT

Kussmaul sign—may also be seen with restrictive cardiomyopathy and constrictive pericarditis.

KEY FACT

Electrical alternans = pericardial effusion

KEY FACT

Echocardiogram confirmation of tamponade = RV collapse during diastole

KEY FACT

HTN = SPB ≥ 140 mm Hg or a DBP ≥ 90 mm Hg

SYMPTOMS/EXAMINATION

- Nonspecific symptoms are common (fatigue, chest pain, dyspnea).
- Cardiovascular collapse may occur if rapidly developing (eg, traumatic effusion).
- **Beck triad** is classic for tamponade: Hypotension + JVD + muffled heart sounds.
- Pericardial friction rub.
- Tachycardia.
- Narrowed pulse pressure.
- **Kussmaul sign = ↑ in jugular venous pressure during inspiration**.
- Pulsus paradoxus = inspiratory reduction in systolic pressure of > 10 mm Hg.

DIAGNOSIS

- Suspect based on history and physical examination
- ECG
  - Low QRS voltage = Nonspecific
  - **Electrical alternans** = Variation of height of the QRS complexes because of the heart swinging within the pericardial effusion
- Echocardiogram—diagnostic study of choice
  - Tamponade physiology represented by **right ventricular collapse during diastole** and IVC dilation with < 50% diameter reduction during inspiration.
  - Magnitude of the effusion can be evaluated.

TREATMENT

Without tamponade: Supplemental O_2, IV fluids to increase LV filling, consult CT surgery and/or cardiology, and prepare for pericardiocentesis

With tamponade: Tachycardia and hypotension suggestive of pericardial tamponade → **immediate pericardiocentesis**

Hypertension

Hypertension (HTN) is defined as a SPB ≥ 140 mm Hg or a diastolic blood pressure (DBP) ≥ 90 mm Hg. HTN is a major risk factor stroke, heart disease, renal failure, vascular disease, and retinal disease. It is the single most common chronic medical condition in the United States.

The Joint National Committee on Prevention, Detection, Evaluation, and Treatment of High Blood Pressure has stratified BP into categories (Table 2.30). These categories are based on the average of at least 2 measurements taken on a seated patient during 2 different outpatient clinic visits.

TABLE 2.30. Classification of Blood Pressure for Adults

CATEGORY	SYSTOLIC (MM HG)		DIASTOLIC (MM HG)
Normal	< 120	and	< 80
Prehypertension	120-139	or	80-89
Stage 1 HTN	140-159	or	90-99
Stage 2 HTN	≥ 160	or	100

HTN, hypertension.

TABLE 2.31. Causes of Secondary Hypertension

Category	Examples
Renovascular	Renal artery stenosis Fibromuscular dysplasia
Renal parenchymal	Glomerulonephritis Chronic pyelonephritis
Hormonal	Estrogens 1° hyperaldosteronism Glucocorticoids
Illicit drug intoxication/withdrawal	Cocaine intoxication Alcohol withdrawal
Circulating catecholamines	Pheochromocytoma Tyramine Clonidine withdrawal
Other: Coarctation, obstructive sleep apnea, hypercalcemia	

Q

A 65-year-old man with a history of HTN treated with lisonopril and atenolol presents with a 6-hour history of headache, vomiting, and progressive confusion. Initial BP is 220/130 mm Hg and remains on repeat measurement. Emergent head CT shows no hemorrhage. What is the goal for managing this patient's blood pressure?

Etiology

- **Essential (primary)** HTN comprises > 90% of all cases of HTN. Although no specific cause has been identified, most cases have a common end pathway of activation of the renin–angiotensin system.
- **Secondary HTN:** Underlying cause has been identified (Table 2.31).
- In the ED, elevated blood pressure can be classified as asymptomatic elevated blood pressure without a history of HTN, uncontrolled HTN, or hypertensive emergency (the term "hypertensive crisis" is no longer used).

ASYMPTOMATIC ELEVATED BLOOD PRESSURE AND UNCONTROLLED HYPERTENSION

Patients with persistent elevations of BP without any evidence for end-organ damage

Symptoms/Examination

- Elevated BP in the ED is moderately predictive of undiagnosed chronic HTN.
- High triage BPs frequently fall with observation only (regression to the mean).
- Use appropriately sized cuff:
  - Too large → falsely low reading
  - Too small → falsely elevated reading
- Evidence of chronic HTN:
  - Retinal: AV nicking, narrowing of arterial diameter
  - Cardiac: S_4 gallop, signs of LVH
- Coarctation: Upper extremity HTN, systolic murmur (best over back), delayed femoral pulses
- Renovascular disease: Flank bruits
- Pheochromocytoma: Palpitations, apprehension, malaise, tachycardia, diaphoresis

KEY FACT

Coarctation → upper extremity HTN, systolic murmur, delayed femoral pulses.

A

Reduce MAP by 10-20% within 30-60 minutes with a titratable agent with a predictable blood pressure response such as nicardipine.

TABLE 2.32. Risk Factors for Complications from HTN

African American
Male
Early age of onset
DBP > 115 mm Hg
Smoking
Diabetes
Hypercholesterolemia
Obesity
Alcoholism
Evidence of chronic end-organ dysfunction

DBP, diastolic blood pressure; HTN, hypertension.

KEY FACT

PCP referral is the most important ED intervention for asymptomatic HTN.

TREATMENT

- Routine ED screening for end-organ damage is unnecessary.
- Identify and correct underlying secondary causes.
- Lifestyle and dietary changes: Mild sodium restriction, weight loss (if needed), decreased cholesterol and fat intake, exercise, smoking cessation.
- Referral to primary care physician (PCP) for recheck if BP > 140/90 mm Hg.
- Consider initiation of antihypertensive therapy if:
  - Stage 2 HTN.
  - ≥ 2 risk factors (Table 2.32) for complications.
  - Prompt primary care follow-up is unavailable.
- Rapidly lowering blood pressure in asymptomatic patients is **not necessary** and may be harmful.
- Treatment can be initiated with thiazide diuretic, dihydropyridine (DHP) calcium channel blocker, or ACEI.

KEY FACT

Hypertensive emergency = HTN with acute end-organ dysfunction

HYPERTENSIVE EMERGENCY

Hypertensive emergency is defined as HTN with evidence for acute end-organ ***dysfunction***. The absolute BP is not as important as the presence of dysfunction. The heart, brain, and kidneys are the organs most frequently affected (Table 2.33).

Stroke syndromes are often considered a form of hypertensive emergency, though the extreme elevations of BP may be a response to the stroke and not an immediate cause.

TABLE 2.33. Types of Hypertensive Emergencies

Myocardial ischemia
Pulmonary edema
Acute aortic dissection
Hypertensive encephalopathy
Intracranial hemorrhage
HELLP syndrome/eclampsia
Acute renal failure
Uncontrolled bleeding

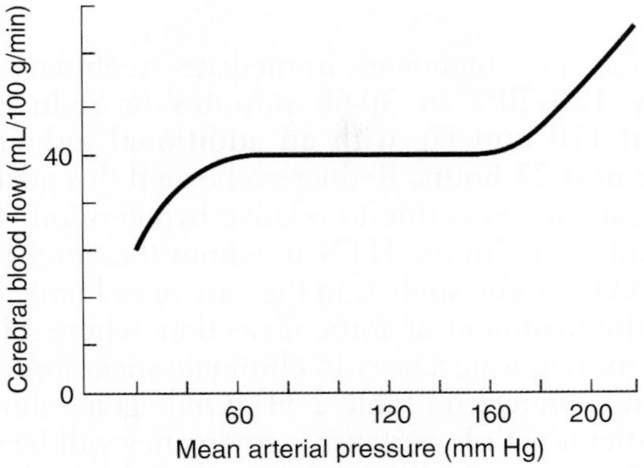

FIGURE 2.23. The normal cerebral autoregulation curve. (Reproduced, with permission, from Morgan GE, Mikhail MS, Murray MJ. *Clinical Anesthesiology*. 4th ed. New York, NY: McGraw-Hill; 2006:616.)

Pathophysiology

- In the heart, an abrupt, severe elevation of BP → acute LV failure or increase myocardial O_2 demand → ischemia and pulmonary edema.
- In the brain, an abrupt rise in BP that exceeds the upper limits of cerebral autoregulation (typically MAP > 160 mm Hg; see Figure 2.23) → hypertensive encephalopathy.
- Cerebral autoregulation = adjusting cerebrovascular resistance to maintain constant cerebral blood flow despite changes in cerebral perfusion pressure.
- Chronic HTN is accommodated by gradual changes in cerebral autoregulation. This makes rapidly lowering BP potentially dangerous, because the brain may come to depend on an elevated BP to maintain constant cerebral blood flow.
- In the kidney a sustained elevation of blood pressure → ↓ renal perfusion, ischemia, and renal impairment.
- Other presentations include uncontrolled bleeding, eclampsia, aortic dissection.

Symptoms

- Most common are dyspnea, chest pain, headache, AMS, or focal neuro deficit
- Chest pain, dyspnea, nausea if myocardial ischemia
- Dyspnea, cough, pink-tinged sputum if pulmonary edema
- Tearing pain in chest or upper back if aortic dissection
- Severe headache, nausea, vomiting, confusion, visual changes if hypertensive encephalopathy

Examination

- Blood pressure is often markedly elevated, exceptions being eclampsia and aortic dissection with tamponade.
- Evidence of end-organ damage may include:
  - S_3, new murmur, unequal pulses
  - Rales, wheezing, hypoxia, respiratory distress
  - Decreased mental status, seizures, focal deficits
  - Papilledema, retinal hemorrhages

Diagnosis

- Clinical examination or studies showing evidence of end-organ damage
- Elevated creatinine, evidence of hemolysis, pulmonary edema, etc

KEY FACT

Cerebral perfusion pressure = MAP – ICP (or MAP – JVP if jugular venous pressure > ICP)

KEY FACT

$MAP = P_{diastolic} + 1/3(P_{systolic} - P_{diastolic})$

KEY FACT

Cerebral autoregulation is effective between a MAP of 60 and 160 mm Hg.

KEY FACT

Nitroprusside can cause cyanide toxicity.

Treatment

Hypertensive emergency mandates immediate treatment, with a goal to **reduce MAP by 10%-20% in 30-60 minutes or reduction of diastolic pressure to about 110 mm Hg with an additional reduction in MAP by 5%-15% over the next 23 hours**. Reduction beyond this goal puts the patient at risk for end-organ ischemia due to relative hypotension. This is especially true for the patient with chronic HTN in whom the cerebral autoregulation curve has shifted to the right, such as in the case of ischemic stroke. An exception to this is in the treatment of aortic dissection, where a lower SBP in the range of 100-120 mmHg is necessary to eliminate shear forces. A short-acting, titratable IV agent is preferred (Table 2.34). Oral agents should **not** be used. Of note, many patients with hypertensive emergency will be volume depleted due to pressure natriuresis. If given antihypertensives prior to volume, may have precipitous drop in blood pressure.

- **Nicardipine**
  - DHP calcium channel blocker.
  - ↓ Peripheral vascular resistance.
  - ↓ Cerebral vasospasm (used for SAH or ICH).
  - Avoid in liver failure and aortic stenosis.
  - Clevidipine is new DHP calcium channel blocker with extremely short half-life that is metabolized by plasma esterases. Will likely be part of future practice in ED.
- **Labetalol**
  - α_1-, β-Adrenergic blocker
  - 7 × more potent β-blockade than α-blockade
  - Effective as single agent
  - As with all β-blockers, caution in asthma/COPD and in acute cocaine intoxication

TABLE 2.34. Antihypertensive Agents for Hypertensive Emergencies

Condition	Agent of Choice
Encephalopathy, ischemic stroke, hemorrhagic stroke	Nicardipine Labetalol
Acute pulmonary edema	Nitroglycerin Nicardipine Lasix
Myocardial ischemia	Nitroglycerin Labetalol
Aortic dissection	Esmolol or Labetalol (first) + nicardipine Sodium nitroprusside + metoprolol
Catecholamine crisis	Nicardipine Benzodiazepines Diltiazem Phentolamine
Eclampsia	Magnesium Labetalol Nicardipine Hydralazine

- **NTG**
  - First-line agent for cardiogenic pulmonary edema
  - Venous >> arteriolar dilation
  - Contraindicated in preload-dependent patients or with recent PDE5 inhibitor use
- **Esmolol**
  - β_1-Adrenergic blocker
  - Very short acting
  - Often used with nicardipine to blunt tachycardia
- **Fenoldopam**
  - Peripheral dopamine-1 receptor agonist
  - Improves renal function acutely
- **Phentolamine**
  - Pure α-blocker
  - Indicated for hypertensive emergency in setting of cocaine/amphetamine intoxication or pheochromocytoma
- **Sodium nitroprusside**
  - Activity is via nitric oxide release, results in arterial and venous dilation.
  - Cerebral vasodilator (careful in stroke syndromes).
  - Dilates normal coronary arteries > diseased → **coronary steal**.
  - Metabolized to **cyanide**, limiting dosing amount and duration.
  - Contraindicated in pregnancy and with PDE5 inhibitor usage.
  - Continuous BP monitoring recommended.
  - Dose response is unpredictable.
- **Hydralazine**
  - Direct arteriolar vasodilator (watch for reflex tachycardia)
  - Relatively unpredictable dose response
  - Safe in pregnancy (as is labetalol)

KEY FACT

In hypertensive emergencies, reduction of MAP > 20% puts the patient at risk for end-organ ischemia due to relative hypotension.

Disorders of the Cardiac Valves

Most common valvular lesion: Mitral valve prolapse.

Most common **congenital** valvular lesion: Bicuspid aortic valve.

Rheumatic heart disease remains a common cause of valvular pathology worldwide, but is rare in developed countries.

Table 2.35 summarizes the causes and examination findings for common valvular lesions.

AORTIC VALVULAR DISORDERS

Aortic Stenosis

The most common causes are calcific valve degeneration (patients > 65 years), congenital bicuspid valve (younger patients), and rheumatic heart disease (less common). Rheumatic aortic stenosis should be suspected if there is concomitant mitral valve disease.

Pathophysiology

- LV outflow tract is obstructed → LVH, ↓ cardiac output, and eventual dilated cardiomyopathy with hypertrophy.
- Usually no signs or symptoms until the aortic outflow tract is reduced by at least 75% (to < 1 cm).
- Survival is 2-5 years from onset of symptoms without valve replacement.

KEY FACT

Classic triad of symptomatic aortic stenosis: Angina, syncope, CHF

TABLE 2.35. Valvular Lesions With Associated Physical Findings

Valvular Lesion	Common Etiologies	Murmur	Physical Findings
Aortic stenosis	Calcific valve degeneration Bicuspid aortic valve (< 65 y)	Crescendo–decrescendo **systolic** Radiating → neck	Paradoxically split S_2 Narrowed pulse pressure Diminished and slow-rising carotid pulse
Aortic regurgitation	**Acute** Endocarditis Aortic dissection **Chronic** Rheumatic heart disease Bicuspid aortic valve	Blowing **diastolic** Heard best at left sternal border	**Acute** Pulmonary edema and CV collapse **Chronic** Widened pulse pressure Rapid ↓ and ↑ of carotid pulse Nail pulsations To-and-fro murmur over femoral artery Soft mid-diastolic rumble
Mitral stenosis	Rheumatic heart disease	**Diastolic** Heard best at apex	Loud S_1
Mitral regurgitation	**Acute** Endocarditis ACS **Chronic** Rheumatic heart disease	Loud **holosystolic** Heard best at apex Radiating → base	**Acute** Pulmonary edema and CV collapse **Chronic** LV heave
Mitral valve prolapse	Unknown, likely congenital	Late **systolic** heard best at left lateral heart border	Early to mid **systolic click**

ACS, acute coronary syndrome; CV, cardiovascular; LV, left ventricular.

Symptoms

- The **classic triad** of symptomatic aortic stenosis is angina, syncope, and symptoms of CHF.
- Sudden death from dysrhythmias or acute onset of failure may occur.

Examination

- Crescendo–decrescendo systolic murmur radiating to the neck
- Narrowed pulse pressure due to drop in SBP
- Low-amplitude (**parvus**) and slow-rising (**tardus**) carotid pulse
- Heaving, prolonged apical impulse
- CHF symptoms

Diagnosis

- **ECG:** LVH with strain, LBBB.
- **CXR:** LVH, pulmonary congestion (if CHF is present).
- **Echocardiography:** Confirms the diagnosis, allows measurement of valve area.
- Exercise stress testing may provoke dysrhythmias and is contraindicated.

Treatment

- Cautious fluid administration if hypotensive; gentle diuresis if CHF is present.

- Rule out ACS in acute presentations.
- Prophylaxis for endocarditis.
- Intra-aortic balloon pump may be bridge to definitive treatment (aortic valve replacement).
- **Avoid:**
  - Preload or afterload reducers (**no nitroglycerin**)
  - Negative inotropes (can cause acute decompensation and severe hypotension)

> **KEY FACT**
>
> Avoid nitrates and negative inotropes in the treatment of aortic stenosis because they may lead to severe hypotension refractory to therapy.

> **KEY FACT**
>
> Aortic stenosis patients with heart failure require emergent valve replacement.

Aortic Regurgitation (Aortic Insufficiency)

Aortic regurgitation (AR) may be acute or chronic. It is important to make this differentiation, because AR regurgitation is a surgical emergency requiring immediate valve replacement.

Etiologies

- Acute AR: Infective endocarditis (IE), aortic dissection with proximal extension, trauma, prosthetic valve dysfunction
- Chronic AR: Rheumatic heart disease, bicuspid aortic valve, dilation of the aortic root (Marfan syndrome, ankylosing spondylitis, rheumatoid arthritis)

> **KEY FACT**
>
> Acute AR? Consider endocarditis, aortic dissection, and trauma.

Pathophysiology

- Acute aortic valve failure → rapid rise in LV diastolic pressure → acute pulmonary edema and cardiogenic shock
- Chronic aortic valve failure → compensatory LVH, gradual LV dilation → gradual onset of heart failure symptoms

> **KEY FACT**
>
> Acute AR is a **surgical** emergency.

Acute Aortic Regurgitation

Symptoms

- Abrupt onset of dyspnea
- If due to endocarditis, patient may endorse IV drug use or recent fevers
- If due to aortic dissection, at-risk patient may complain of chest pain

Examination

- Tachycardia, tachypnea
- Pulmonary edema and cardiovascular collapse
- High-pitched blowing **diastolic** murmur heard best at left sternal border
- **Normal pulse pressure**

Diagnosis

- Suspect based on history and physical examination.
- CXR: Pulmonary edema.
- Echocardiography confirms diagnosis.

Treatment

- Standard treatment for pulmonary edema
- Nitroprusside for afterload reduction
- Dobutamine (in addition to nitroprusside) if hypotensive
- Immediate valve replacement
- Antibiotics: If endocarditis suspected
- **Avoid:** Intra-aortic balloon pump (may worsen regurgitation and is contraindicated in aortic dissection)

> **KEY FACT**
>
> Aggressive afterload reduction is key to stabilizing the patient with acute AR. Intra-aortic balloon pump is contraindicated.

Chronic Aortic Regurgitation

Symptoms

Gradual onset of dyspnea on exertion, orthopnea, nocturnal dyspnea

KEY FACT

Chronic AR is associated with many CV examination findings, including CHF, widened pulse pressure, pulsations of nailbeds, "water hammer" pulse, and a to-and-fro femoral artery murmur.

Examination

- CHF
- High-pitched blowing diastolic murmur heard best at left sternal border
- Widened pulse pressure (opposite of AS)
- **Austin Flint murmur** (soft mid-diastolic rumble)
- **"Water hammer" pulse** (rapid rise and fall of carotid pulse)
- **Quincke sign** (pulsations of nailbeds)
- **Duroziez murmur** (to-and-fro murmur over femoral artery)
- **De Musset sign** (head bobbing with each heartbeat)

Diagnosis

- Suspect diagnosis based on history and physical examination.
- ECG: LVH, left atrial enlargement.
- CXR: CHF.
- Echocardiography confirms diagnosis.

Treatment

- Nifedipine for asymptomatic AR
- Afterload reducers, digoxin, hydralazine, and surgical referral for elective valve replacement for symptomatic AR
- Prophylaxis for endocarditis

MITRAL VALVULAR DISORDERS

Mitral Stenosis

Mitral valve stenosis most commonly results from **rheumatic heart disease**. Other causes include atrial myxoma, congenital abnormalities, and calcific valve degeneration. Atrial fibrillation is the most commonly associated complication.

Pathophysiology

- Mitral valve narrowing → increasing pressures across the mitral valve → left atrial hypertrophy and eventual dilation with left heart failure
- Increased pulmonary venous pressure → pulmonary edema, pulmonary HTN

KEY FACT

Left atrial overload in mitral stenosis → pulmonary edema and atrial fibrillation

Symptoms

- Insidious progression of fatigue and dyspnea on exertion (early), orthopnea and peripheral edema (late)
- Palpitations (from atrial fibrillation)
- Hemoptysis from ruptured bronchial vein (classic, but uncommon)

Examination

- Loud S_1 followed by diastolic opening snap and low-pitched rumbling diastolic murmur heard best at the apex
- Pulmonary edema if severe disease

Diagnosis

- Suspect diagnosis based on symptoms and examination.
- ECG: Left atrial enlargement, possibly atrial fibrillation.

- CXR: Often normal, may see left atrial enlargement, CHF.
- Echocardiogram is confirmatory.

TREATMENT

- Treat atrial fibrillation (consider anticoagulation).
- Prophylaxis for endocarditis.
- Cautious diuretic use.
- Percutaneous mitral balloon valvulotomy or operative valve repair/replacement.

COMPLICATIONS

- Atrial fibrillation (very common)
- Massive **pulmonary hemorrhage**
- Pulmonary HTN and right heart failure
- Systemic emboli from left atrial thrombus

Mitral Regurgitation

Mitral valve regurgitation (MR) may be acute or chronic. As with AR, it is important to make this differentiation, because acute MR is a surgical emergency requiring **immediate** valve replacement.

ETIOLOGIES

- Acute MR: Chordae rupture or papillary muscle dysfunction following MI (typically within 2-7 days), perforation of a valve leaflet from endocarditis or trauma (rare)
- Chronic MR: Most commonly occurs due to ischemic heart disease and cardiomyopathy (in the United States) or rheumatic heart disease (developing world); less commonly occurs due to connective tissue disorders (Ehlers-Danlos and Marfan)

PATHOPHYSIOLOGY

- Acute injury or dysfunction of the valve, papillary muscle, or chordae tendineae → acute valve failure → acute left atrial overload → pulmonary edema
- Chronic valve failure → compensatory dilation of left atrium and gradual onset of CHF

Acute Mitral Regurgitation

SYMPTOMS

- Abrupt onset of dyspnea, tachypnea
- Cardiogenic shock
- Chest pain
- Symptoms of the underlying disease process (endocarditis, MI, trauma)

EXAMINATION

- Loud holosystolic murmur heard best at the apex, with radiation to the base or axilla
- LV heave
- Pulmonary edema

DIAGNOSIS

- ECG: **Absence** of left atrial enlargement and LVH
- CXR: Normal cardiac silhouette, pulmonary edema

TREATMENT

- Standard treatment for pulmonary edema.
- Nitroprusside for afterload reduction.

Q

A 67-year-old man presents to the ED with sudden onset of chest pain and shortness of breath. He is 5 days status-post inferior wall MI. On examination, the patient has pulmonary edema and a loud holosystolic murmur heard best at the left lateral sternal border, with radiation to the base. What is the most appropriate initial management?

KEY FACT

Acute MR is a surgical emergency.

KEY FACT

Acute MR? Treat with nitroprusside, dobutamine (if hypotensive), and intra-aortic balloon pump until definitive treatment.

A

Based on the presentation following recent MI, this patient likely has acute mitral valve regurgitation from papillary muscle rupture. This is a surgical emergency that requires immediate valve replacement. Nitroprusside and dobutamine can be used together to help improve forward flow. Intra-aortic balloon pump may also be used as a bridge to surgery.

- Dobutamine (in addition to nitroprusside) if hypotensive.
- Intra-aortic balloon pump as bridge to surgery.
- **Immediate** valve replacement.
- Treat the underlying disease process.

Complications

Includes acute pulmonary edema and cardiogenic shock

Chronic Mitral Regurgitation

Symptoms

- Often asymptomatic
- Gradual progression of dyspnea on exertion and fatigue
- Palpitations (from atrial fibrillation)

Examination

- Holosystolic murmur heard best at the apex with radiation to the base or axilla
- S_3 heart sound

Diagnosis

- ECG: Left atrial enlargement, LVH, atrial fibrillation (common)
- CXR: CHF in advanced cases

KEY FACT

Atrial fibrillation and systemic emboli are common in chronic MR.

Treatment

- Treat CHF and atrial fibrillation (consider anticoagulation)
- Anticoagulate if systemic embolization occurs
- Endocarditis prophylaxis
- Valve replacement

Complications

Include atrial fibrillation (very common), systemic emboli from left atrial thrombus, and endocarditis. If untreated/unrepaired for long period of time, LV dysfunction occurs.

Mitral Valve Prolapse

This is one of the most common valvular disorders. The prototypical patient is a young, thin female (though more recent data suggests nearly equal prevalence in men and women, < 1%). It is an autosomal dominant condition with variable penetrance. There is a possible association with anxiety disorders and low body weight.

Pathophysiology

Abnormal proliferation of valve leaflet → abnormal stretching of valve leaflets during systole

KEY FACT

In mitral valve prolapse, decreasing the LV volume will accentuate the click and move it closer to S_1.

Symptoms

Though usually asymptomatic, mitral valve prolapse (MVP) may present with atypical chest pain, palpitations, light-headedness, and dyspnea.

Examination

Classically, MVP may be heard as an early/midsystolic click with high-pitched late systolic murmur heard best at the left lateral heart border and increased with Valsalva and standing.

DIAGNOSIS

- ECG: Nonspecific ST-T wave changes, paroxysmal supraventricular tachycardia (PSVT)
- CXR: No specific findings
- Echocardiography: Confirmatory

TREATMENT

- No treatment if asymptomatic.
- Prophylaxis for endocarditis if regurgitation or thickened valve leaflets.
- β-Blockers may help with atypical chest pain.

COMPLICATIONS

While usually a benign condition, MVP is the most common cause of MR in the United States. Stroke and endocarditis may occur. Finally, MVP is associated with tachydysrhythmias (PSVT, Wolff-Parkinson-White [WPW] syndrome, PACs, PVCs, and ventricular tachycardia [VT]) and sudden death.

> **KEY FACT**
>
> Thickened or redundant mitral valve leaflets and evidence of MR are the best predictors of serious complications and sudden death in MVP.

TRICUSPID REGURGITATION

CAUSES

The most common causes are right ventricular dilation (from pulmonary HTN), endocarditis, and rheumatic heart disease.

SYMPTOMS AND EXAMINATION

May include fatigue, dyspnea, and lower extremity swelling. Auscultation reveals a holosystolic murmur best heard at the left lower sternal border, right sternal border, or at the subxiphoid area. There is little radiation of the murmur.

DIAGNOSIS

- ECG: Right atrial and ventricular enlargement, atrial fibrillation (in the majority of cases).
- Echocardiography is confirmatory.

TREATMENT

- Treat atrial fibrillation.
- Endocarditis prophylaxis.

PROSTHETIC VALVULAR DISORDERS

Prosthetic heart valves may be mechanical or bioprosthetic (porcine or bovine). Mechanical valves have a metallic sound on auscultation and uncommonly fail. Both mechanical and bioprosthetic valves require lifelong anticoagulation. Complications include paravalvular leak, valve thrombosis, endocarditis, and systemic embolization.

> **KEY FACT**
>
> Mechanical valve failure → CHF, muted valve sounds **with** presence of regurgitation murmur.
>
> Valve thrombosis → CHF, muted mechanical valve sounds **without** regurgitation murmur.

Valve Failure

Ranges from gradually worsening paravalvular leak to abrupt mechanical valve failure.

SYMPTOMS/EXAMINATION

- Vary with location and rapidity of valve failure
- Findings of severe anemia (due to hemolysis)
- Findings consistent with aortic/MR (acute or chronic)
- Muted mechanical valve sounds, if mechanical valve failure

TREATMENT

- Standard treatment for aortic/MR
- Valve replacement

Valve Thrombosis

Thrombus is more likely to form on a mechanical valve and can cause systemic embolization or valve thrombosis. **Mitral valve prostheses have twice the risk of embolization compared to aortic valve prostheses**, and thus INR goals in the former are higher (3-3.5) than in the latter (2.5-3).

> **KEY FACT**
>
> Mechanical mitral valves are in a chronic low-flow state; risk of thrombosis is increased compared to mechanical aortic valves.

SYMPTOMS/EXAMINATION

- If sudden: Acute onset of hypotension, CHF
- Muted mechanical valve sounds
- May have a more gradual course

TREATMENT

Anticoagulation and valve replacement

INFECTIVE ENDOCARDITIS

Infective endocarditis (IE) is an infection of the endocardium that typically involves the valves and adjacent structure. A wide range of infecting organisms has been identified. Of the organisms, *Staphylococcus aureus* is considered to be the most virulent, with a rapid destruction of affected valves.

Risk factors for endocarditis include any process that is characterized by or can cause injury to the endocardium: CHD, rheumatic heart disease, injection drug use (IDU), prosthetic valves, MR, and cardiac pacemaker placement.

PATHOPHYSIOLOGY

- The presence of a foreign body or the disruption of normal flow through the valves → turbulence → platelet aggregation and fibrinogenesis → thrombus formation.
- Thrombus acts as a nidus for implantation of circulating bacteria/virus/fungi (Table 2.36).
- Staphylococci and streptococci are by far the most common causative organisms.
  - Fungal endocarditis (most commonly *Candida* or *Aspergillus*) may occur in the immunocompromised or in IVD users.
  - HACEK organisms are difficult to isolate and may cause IE in immunocompromised patients (***H**aemophilus* species, ***A**ctinobacillus actinomycetemcomitans*, ***C**ardiobacterium hominis*, ***E**ikenella corrodens*, ***K**ingella* species).

> **KEY FACT**
>
> **R-sided endocarditis**—think IDU, acute/fulminant course, *S aureus*.
>
> **L-sided endocarditis**—think native valve disease, indolent course, streptococci.

> **KEY FACT**
>
> IDU + fever = endocarditis until proven otherwise

SYMPTOMS

Fever and malaise are most common. Other symptoms include constitutional (malaise, weakness) as well as dyspnea, body aches, and back pain.

EXAMINATION

- Regurgitation murmur
- Immunologic phenomena: Osler nodes, Roth spots
- Vascular phenomena: Arterial emboli, septic pulmonary emboli, Janeway lesions

> **KEY FACT**
>
> Osler nodes are tender (Osler = Ouch), Janeway lesions are not.

TABLE 2.36. Etiologies of Endocarditis

Predisposing Factors	Location	Usual Pathogens
Prosthetic valve < 60 d (early)	Replaced valve	*Staphylococcus* sp[a] *Enterobacteriaceae* Diphtheroids Fungi
IDU	Tricuspid valve most often	*Staphylococcus aureus*
Native valve	Mitral > aortic >> tricuspid	Streptococci (viridans or others)[a] Staphylococci Enterococci
Prosthetic valve > 60 d (late)	Replaced valve	Same as native valve
Pacemaker, implantable defibrillator	Infection of pacemaker pocket, leads	*S aureus* *Staphylococcus epidermidis*

IDU, injection drug use.

[a]Most common organism.

Diagnosis

- Presumptive diagnosis based on predisposing condition and presence of fever.
- Obtain 3 cultures from 3 different sites, with at least 1 hour between first and last.
- Obtain echocardiogram (transesophageal sensitivity >> transthoracic sensitivity).
- Apply Duke criteria (Table 2.37).

TABLE 2.37. Duke Criteria for Establishing the Diagnosis of Endocarditis

Major criteria	Positive blood cultures (≥ 2 separated by site and time) Major echocardiogram findings (vegetations, abscess, new regurgitation, dehiscence of prosthetic valve)
Minor criteria	Predisposing conditions Fever Embolic disease Immunologic phenomena Single positive blood culture Nonmajor echocardiogram findings
Diagnosis requires: 2 major criteria, **or** 1 major + 3 minor criteria, **or** 5 minor criteria	

TREATMENT

- Antibiotics: Empiric therapy started while awaiting culture results
  - Native valves: Vancomycin + gentamicin
  - Injection drug use: Vancomycin
  - Prosthetic valves: Vancomycin + gentamicin
- Surgical valve repair or replacement as needed

COMPLICATIONS

- Valvular destruction with resulting CHF
- Septic emboli and sequelae
  - CNS abscesses, mycotic aneurysm, meningitis
  - Septic pulmonary emboli
  - Paraspinal abscesses

PROPHYLAXIS FOR ENDOCARDITIS

The following populations need antibiotics prior to procedures (*high-risk groups):

- *Prosthetic heart valve
- *Prior IE
- *Cyanotic CHD or unrepaired CHD
- Acquired valvular heart disease
- Mitral valve prolapse with murmur

Recommended antibiotics for prophylaxis are listed in Table 2.38. An equivalent IV antibiotic should be chosen for patients unable to take the oral recommendations. No prophylaxis is needed for clean procedures (laceration repairs, Foley catheter placement, intubation).

TABLE 2.38. Antibiotic Recommendation for Endocarditis Prophylaxis

Prophylaxis for Dental, Oral, Respiratory, and Esophageal Procedures	
Standard	Amoxicillin
Penicillin allergy	Clindamycin **or** Cephalexin **or** Azithromycin
Prophylaxis for Genitourinary and Gastrointestinal (Nonesophageal) Procedures	
Moderate-risk patients	Amoxicillin PO
Moderate-risk patients allergic to penicillin	Vancomycin IV
High-risk patients	Ampicillin + gentamicin IV
High-risk patients allergic to penicillin	Vancomycin + gentamicin IV

PO, by mouth; IV, intravenous.

Syncope

Syncope is defined as a transient loss of consciousness and postural tone with subsequent spontaneous recovery to baseline. It results from transient cerebral hypoperfusion from a variety of causes (Table 2.39). It is most commonly benign but can be caused by life-threatening conditions. A postictal period is notably absent, differentiating syncope from seizure.

Symptoms/Examination

- Transient loss of consciousness.
- Complete recovery without intervention.
- Other symptoms and examination findings vary with underlying etiology.
- Table 2.40 lists the classic presentations of syncope.

Differential

- It may be difficult to differentiate syncope from seizure.
  - A history of seizures makes a seizure more likely.
  - In rare instances, true syncope leads to seizure.

TABLE 2.39. Causes of Syncope

Acutely life-threatening vascular catastrophe
Aortic dissection, ruptured AAA, ruptured ectopic, subarachnoid hemorrhage, tamponade, PE, severe hemorrhage (GI, retroperitoneal, etc)
Obstruction to cardiac flow
Aortic stenosis, hypertrophic cardiomyopathy, congenital heart disease, myxoma
Primary dysrhythmia
Tachyarrhythmia, heart block, sinus pause/arrest
Preexcitation/accessory pathway
Prolonged QT
Brugada syndrome
Arrhythmogenic right ventricular dysplasia
Neurocardiogenic or reflex mediated
Abnormal autonomic response to stimulus → vagal hyperactivity and symptoms
Classic vasovagal, carotid sinus syndrome, cough, micturition
Medication induced
Orthostatic
Hypoglycemia
Neurologic
Transient ischemic attack, subclavian steal, migraine
Psychiatric (hyperventilation)

AAA, abdominal aortic aneurysm; GI, gastrointestinal; PE, pulmonary embolism.

TABLE 2.40. Classic Presentations of Syncope

Presentation	Suspected Diagnosis
17-y-old man, syncope during running	Hypertrophic cardiomyopathy
29-y-old woman, syncope and abdominal pain	Ectopic pregnancy
68-y-old man, syncope and abdominal or flank pain	Abdominal aortic aneurysm
34-y-old woman, sudden severe headache and syncope	Subarachnoid hemorrhage
72-y-old man with history of MI and CHF, syncope at home	Dysrhythmia
40-y-old woman, syncope while standing in line, prodrome of nausea, sweating, warmth	Vasovagal
78-y-old woman with cancer, sudden onset of SOB and syncope	PE

CHF, congestive heart failure; MI, myocardial function; PE, pulmonary embolism; SOB.

- Both may be associated with extremity movement and urinary incontinence.
- A classic aura, postictal confusion, and muscle pain suggest seizure.

KEY FACT

LLSA Article: EKG findings in syncope. *Acad Emerg Med.* 2011;18(7):714-718.

Diagnosis

- Complete history and examination are critical to guide the ordering of tests.
- ECG should be done in all cases to screen for underlying cardiovascular disease, dysrhythmias, presence of familial disorder (eg, Brugada syndrome; see Figure 2.24), or electrolyte abnormalities.
- Pregnancy test should be performed on all women of child-bearing age.
- Echocardiography: To screen for underlying cardiovascular disease if diagnosis remains unclear.

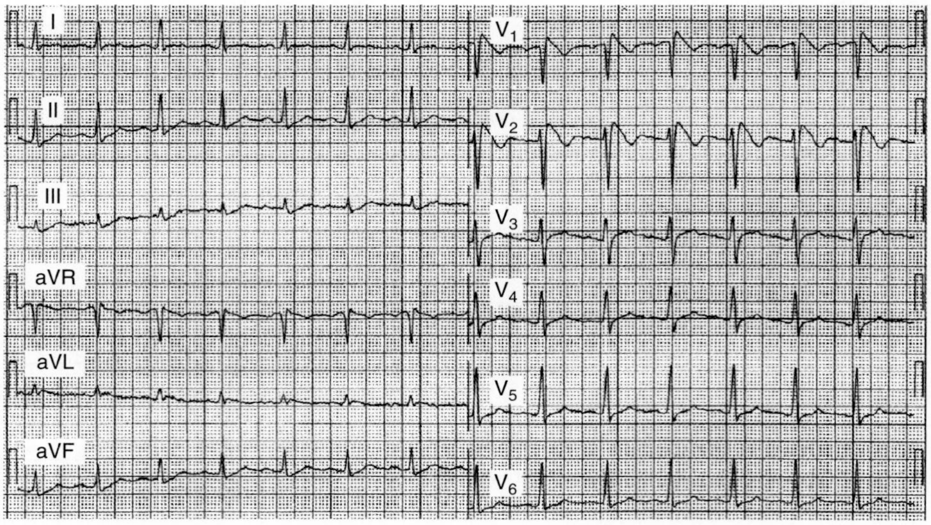

FIGURE 2.24. Typical ECG of Brugada syndrome. (Reproduced, with permission, from Fuster V, Alexander RW, O'Rourke RA. *Hurst's The Heart.* 12th ed. New York, NY: McGraw-Hill; 2008:1837.)

- Patients at high risk for cardiac etiology:
  - Risk increases with increasing age
  - History of ventricular dysrhythmias
  - History of CHF
  - Abnormal ECG
  - Syncope during exertion or supine
  - Syncope associated with chest pain or shortness of breath
  - Persistently low blood pressure (SBP < 90 mmHg)
- Patients at low risk for cardiac etiology:
  - Young patient, normal physical examination, normal ECG
  - Clinical presentation suggestive of vasovagal syncope

Treatment

- Resuscitation, as needed.
- Identifying and treating the underlying etiology is the mainstay of treatment.
- Admit for monitoring and echocardiogram: If no identifiable cause in high-risk patient.
- There is no well-validated clinical decision instrument that identifies high-risk patients with high specificity and sensitivity.

KEY FACT

In patients who present with syncope, the following factors increase the risk of dysrhythmia or sudden death:

1. Increasing age
2. History of ventricular dysrhythmias
3. History of CHF
4. Abnormal ECG

REVIEW QUESTIONS

QUESTIONS

1. A 30-year-old man with past medical history presents with a syncopal episode without prodrome while playing recreational softball. On examination, his vitals are temp 37.6°C (99.7°F), pulse 78 bpm, BP 135/78 mm Hg, RR 16 breaths/min, and 92% on room air. No evidence of trauma is found and the patient is alert and oriented. Auscultation of the heart reveals a 4/6 systolic murmur heard best at the left second rib space adjacent to the sternum. An electrocardiogram (ECG) is performed and shows a normal QTc and QRS interval, but does show voltage criteria for left ventricular hypertrophy (LVH) and deep narrow Q waves in leads I, aVL, and V_5 and V_6. While auscultating the heart, you ask the patient to (1) Valsalva and then (2) squat. How will the intensity of the suspected murmur be affected?
   A. Decrease, decrease
   B. Increase, decrease
   C. Increase, increase
   D. Decrease, increase

2. You work in the emergency department (ED) of a rural hospital with no percutaneous coronary intervention (PCI) capability. The nearest PCI center is 50 minutes away. A 78-year-old man with a history of smoking, diabetes, and hypertension presents with chest pain that has been ongoing for 5 hours. His vital signs are temp 37.5°C, pulse 74 bpm, BP 147/89 mm Hg, RR 15 breaths/min, and 94% on room air. Pulses are equal in all 4 extremities. Auscultation of the lungs and heart is normal. An ECG is performed and shows ST elevations in his lateral leads with reciprocal ST depressions. A chest x-ray is normal. Aspirin and nitroglycerin are administered with resolution of pain but persistence of ECG changes. What is the next step in management?
   A. Give fibrinolytics and admit to your hospital.
   B. Give fibrinolytics and transfer to a PCI center.
   C. Transfer to a PCI center without giving fibrinolytics.
   D. Do not give fibrinolytics but start a heparin drip and admit to your hospital.

3. A 44-year-old man presents to the ED after noting his blood pressure was 180/100 mm Hg at a local pharmacy. He states he was just checking his blood pressure on the blood pressure machine and was advised to seek immediate medical attention. He denies any symptoms. The patient's vitals are 37.1°C, pulse 72 bpm, BP 185/105 mm Hg, RR 18 breaths/min, and 95% on room air. A physical examination, including direct funduscopic examination, is normal. What is the most appropriate next step in management?
   A. Administer intravenous (IV) labetalol.
   B. Administer IV hydralazine.
   C. Administer IV fluids.
   D. Discharge home and refer to primary care physician (PCP) for outpatient BP management.

4. A 66-year-old woman with a history of hypertension presents with 4 hours of sub-sternal chest pain radiating to her right arm and jaw. Her vital signs are 37.2°C, pulse 81 bpm, BP 155/90 mm Hg, RR 18 breaths/min, and 96% on room air. A physical examination is normal. ECG shows ST-segment depressions in leads I, aVL, V_5, and V_6 but no ST-segment elevations. Aspirin and nitroglycerin are administered and the patient is now chest pain-free. A chest x-ray is performed and is unremarkable. Laboratory results are still pending. A few minutes later the patient complains of light-headedness and her blood pressure is noted to be 100/60 mm Hg. Her extremities are cold and auscultation of the chest reveals a loud, harsh murmur at the left sternal border that is softer, but still present during diastole. An ECG is repeated and is unchanged. Of the following options, what is the best next step in management?
   A. Activate the cath laboratory.
   B. Administer alteplase (tPA).
   C. Emergently consult cardiothoracic surgery.
   D. Administer IV phenylephrine.

5. A 64-year-old African American woman with a history of congestive heart failure presents with dyspnea on exertion and orthopnea. Her home medications include lisinopril, metoprolol, furosemide, and a combination pill of isosorbide dinitrate and hydralazine. Which of her medications does NOT provide a mortality benefit in the long-term treatment of congestive heart failure?
   A. Lisinopril
   B. Metoprolol
   C. Furosemide
   D. Isosorbide dinitrate + hydralazine

6. A 68-year-old man with a history of severe chronic obstructive pulmonary disease (COPD) and poorly controlled hypertension presents to the ED complaining of sudden-onset tearing back pain. On examination, his vitals are BP 185/115 mm Hg, HR 105 bpm, RR 20 breaths/min, and O_2 sat 96% on room air. He is diaphoretic and vomits several times during examination. His examination is otherwise normal. Which of the following treatments is the best agent to start first?
   A. Nitroglycerin tablets sublingual
   B. Esmolol IV infusion
   C. Nifedipine IV infusion
   D. Nitroprusside IV infusion

7. A chest x-ray is obtained of the patient mentioned in Question 6 while IV medications are started. The chest x-ray is normal. The diagnostic test of choice at this time is:
   A. D-dimer testing
   B. Transthoracic echocardiogram
   C. Computed tomography (CT) angiography
   D. Aortography

8. You identify a 6-cm abdominal aortic aneurysm (AAA) by bedside ultrasound in a patient presenting with abdominal pain and syncope. Her BP is 85/50 mm Hg and her HR is 135 bpm. After going through a primary survey, your next priority should be:
   A. Infusing 2 L of IV saline followed by O+ blood as needed to stabilize the patient
   B. Starting pressors in combination with fluids to improve end-organ perfusion
   C. Getting a STAT CT scan to localize the site of the bleeding followed by immediate transfer to the OR
   D. Transferring the patient to the OR

9. A 42-year-old woman presents with worsening dyspnea over the past few days. She has had a cough and some viral symptoms. She has no medical or surgical history, has never been hospitalized, and takes no medications. Her vital signs are BP 120/75 mm Hg, HR 85 bpm, RR 16 breaths/min, O_2 sat 96% on room air, and temperature 36.4°C. Her physical examination is normal. Which of the following is the most efficient method of ruling out pulmonary embolism (PE) in this patient?
   A. Based on her history and examination, she has a < 2% chance of having a PE, and thus no further testing is necessary.
   B. Send a D-dimer on this patient, which, if negative, rules out PE.
   C. Obtain a lower extremity ultrasound, which, if negative, rules out PE.
   D. Go right to CT (computed tomography) angiography, which, if negative, rules out PE.

10. A 72-year-old female smoker with hypertension and history of myocardial infarction (MI) following an percutaneous coronary intervention (PCI) presents with severe RLE (right lower extremity) thigh and leg pain beginning 20 minutes prior to arrival. On examination, she has nonpalpable dorsalis pedis pulses bilaterally and symmetric-appearing skin and no edema in either extremity. Which of the following diagnostic modalities is matched with the correct finding?
    A. Doppler ultrasonography demonstrates triphasic signal.
    B. Ankle-brachial index is 0.9 bilaterally.
    C. Arteriography demonstrates abrupt contrast termination at the popliteal artery without evidence of collateral circulation.
    D. Duplex ultrasound demonstrates uniphasic signal and diffuse, severe arterial stenosis in the common femoral and popliteal arteries.

ANSWERS

1. **B.** The case describes a man with hypertrophic cardiomyopathy (HCM). In this disorder, LVH occurs in the absence of hypertension or valvular disease. The hypertrophy is asymmetric and usually more pronounced in the ventricular septum, causing anterior motion of the mitral valve leaflets and an associated left ventricular outflow obstruction. When performing a Valsalva maneuver, this patient experiences a drop in preload which exacerbates the outflow obstruction and increases the intensity of the murmur. The murmur decreases in intensity when venous return and preload increase during squatting.

2. **C.** In STEMI, fibrinolytics are most effective when given within 3 hours of symptom onset. The patient has had 5 hours of symptoms and should be transferred to a PCI center. There is no benefit to "facilitated PCI," whereby fibrinolytics are given prior to PCI. Therefore, the patient should be transferred without giving fibrinolytics.

3. **D.** Asymptomatic hypertension is a common ED complaint. This patient does not have any symptoms or signs of hypertensive emergency, so no further testing is needed. Moreover, IV medications should not be used to lower blood pressure in patients without hypertensive emergency. This patient can be safely discharged home and referred to his primary care doctor.

4. **C.** The scenario describes a patient with non-ST elevation MIs who suffers one of the acute complications of MI: interventricular septal rupture. Patients with septal rupture can become acutely hypotensive and develop a harsh murmur that can be heard during both systole and diastole (papillary muscle rupture can cause mitral insufficiency, which is a holosystolic murmur). Bedside ultrasonography can be used to identify this diagnosis. Treatment includes inotropic support of blood pressure and emergency consultation with cardiothoracic surgery for operative repair.

5. **C.** Diuretics and digoxin reduce hospitalizations and improved symptoms but provide no mortality benefit in the long-term management of congestive heart failure. In contrast, angiotensin-converting-enzyme (ACE) inhibitors (and angiotensin receptor blockers [ARBs]), β-blockers, and nitrates + hydralazine all improve survival.

6. **B.** This is a case of aortic dissection as is suggested by the patient's age, history, presenting symptoms, and vital signs. The rate of dissection is related to blood pressure and heart rate. Blood pressure should be reduced to 100-120 mm Hg systolic and heart rate to < 60 bpm. Esmolol is a great choice because of its short half-life, ease of titration, and in the case of this patient with COPD, a selective β_1-blocker that minimizes the chance of causing bronchospasm.

7. **C.** This patient has a normal chest x-ray, which occurs in 15% of patients with a dissection. The diagnostic test of choice is CT angiography. D-dimers will often be elevated but because of poor specificity cannot rule out the diagnosis in such a high-risk patient. Transthoracic echocardiography is specific but poorly sensitive, particularly for type B dissections. Aortography has long been considered the "gold standard," but is not often readily available.

8. **D.** This patient is likely symptomatic from her AAA (syncope). It is reasonable to resuscitate a significantly hypotensive patient in the ED prior to operating room (OR) transfer, but the blood pressure goal is 80-100 mm Hg (permissive hypotension). This patient is mildly hypotensive but within this blood pressure range and thus should be transferred to the OR immediately.

9. **A.** This patient satisfies the PERC rule, which is nearly as good as a negative D-dimer, and low enough to rule out PE in a low-risk patient. A negative D-dimer would also rule out PE in this low-risk patient, but you risk obtaining a false-positive result because of the test's poor specificity.

10. **D.** This patient has thrombosis in situ. Her comorbidities are highly suggestive of atherosclerosis, which likely gave rise to thrombosis in situ, either through acute plaque rupture or by causing turbulent and/or sluggish blood flow. Her relatively symmetric and benign examination is more consistent with thrombotic occlusion than thromboembolism, which would likely present with asymmetric pulses and skin temperature and color asymmetry. All the diagnostic tests listed can be utilized when evaluating peripheral arterial disease, but only duplex ultrasound is matched with the expected findings in thrombotic occlusion.

CHAPTER 3

Trauma

Jenny L. Chua-Tuan, MD, MBA and
Elaine M. Reno, MD

Initial Trauma—Stabilization and Resuscitation

Injuries remain the leading cause of death among persons 1-44 years of age.

EXAMINATION/DIAGNOSIS

As with any critically ill patient, the initial assessment of a trauma patient begins with ABCs. Further assessment and treatment should be directed to specific complaints or injuries. In a patient with multiple injuries, the ABCDE approach described by the Advanced Trauma Life Support (ATLS) guidelines provides a methodical approach to patient assessment and treatment. The goal of the primary survey is to identify immediate life threats, with the emphasis on simultaneous assessment and intervention (eg, intubating a patient airway for protection) at each step.

PRIMARY SURVEY

Do not move onto the next step unless the first step is secure. If the patient's clinical status worsens or changes during your assessment, restart at Airway.

- **A**irway, with C-spine stabilization
- **B**reathing and ventilation
- **C**irculation and control of bleeding
- **D**isability (mental status)
- **E**nvironment/**E**xposure of patient

AIRWAY

- Examine face/oropharynx/neck for signs of trauma or obstruction.
- Administer O_2 to maintain $Pao_2 > 60$ mm Hg.
- Perform airway maneuvers (chin-lift/jaw-thrust, nasopharyngeal airway, suction, etc).
- Maintain C-spine immobilization during intubation
- Intubate for:
  - Glasgow Coma Scale (GCS) ≤ 8 (see Table 3.2)
  - Loss of airway reflexes in setting of intoxication
  - Severe facial or airway trauma, burns or smoke inhalation with *potential* for swelling and obstruction Intubate early!

BREATHING

- Look for adequate chest rise and external signs of trauma.
- Listen to breath sounds bilaterally to assess symmetry and an appropriate volume of air movement.
- Feel for crepitus and tracheal deviation.
- Look for prominent neck veins.
- Life-threatening injuries that should be identified *and* treated here include:
  - Tension pneumothorax
  - Open pneumothorax (sucking chest wound)
  - Flail chest
  - Massive hemothorax

CIRCULATION

- Evaluate circulation, including level of consciousness, skin color, pulses, capillary refill, blood pressure, and heart rate.
- ATLS guidelines separate hemorrhage into 4 classes based on physiologic parameters (Table 3.1). It is important to keep in mind that increased age, medication use (eg, β-blockers), comorbidities, and type of injury (eg, blunt cardiac injury, tension pneumothorax) can alter these parameters causing misleading results.

KEY FACT

Head injury and hemorrhage are the two most common causes of death in trauma patients.

KEY FACT

Glasgow Coma Scale (GCS) of 8? Intubate! Avoid both hypoxia and extreme hyperoxia in the head injured patient.

KEY FACT

Before intubation, perform a brief neurologic examination consisting of GCS, pupils, and motor function of extremities.

KEY FACT

Five types of shock in trauma:

Hypovolemic (hemorrhage)

Neurogenic (spinal cord injury)

Cardiogenic (direct cardiac injury)

Obstructive (tamponade, tension pneumothorax)

Dissociative (CO or CN)

TABLE 3.1. Classes of Hemorrhage

	Class I	Class II	Class III	Class IV
Blood loss	< 750 mL (< 15%)	750-1500 mL (15%-30%)	1500-2000 mL (30%-40%)	> 2000 mL (> 40%)
BP	Normal	Normal	**Decreased**	Decreased
HR	< 100	**100-120**	120-140	> 140
RR	14-20	**20-30**	30-40	> 35
Pulse pressure	Normal or increased	**Decreased**	Decreased	Decreased
Mental status	Slightly anxious	Mildly anxious	**Anxious and confused**	Confused, lethargic

BP, blood pressure; HR, heart rate; RR, respiratory rate.

- Look for evidence of external or internal bleeding. The eFAST examination should be considered an assessment of circulation.
- Ensure patient has adequate intravenous (IV) access (2 large-bore IVs). Treat hypotension with an initial challenge of 1-2 L of isotonic fluid.
- If the patient remains hypotensive, transfuse with O positive (O negative if female of child-bearing age) or type-specific blood.
- In patients requiring massive blood transfusion (the patient's total blood volume, or ~10 units), give packed red blood cells (RBCs), platelets, and fresh frozen plasma (FFP) in a unit ratio of 1:1:1.
- Studies have shown that **tranexamic acid** given within 3 hours of injury in the polytrauma or bleeding trauma patient reduces mortality.
- Treatment should be concurrent with efforts to identify and control sources of hemorrhage as well as other possible causes of hypotension, including cardiac, chest, and spinal injury.

KEY FACT

1:1:1 ratio for transfusion in uncontrolled hemorrhage: For every unit of RBCs, give one unit of platelets and one unit of FFP.

Disability

- Perform rapid neurologic evaluation to assess patient's level of consciousness.
- The GCS is a score of mental status that measures 3 attributes: Eye opening, verbal response, and motor response (Table 3.2).
- Assess bilateral pupil size and reaction.
- Assess extremity motor and sensory function to screen for potential spinal cord injury.

KEY FACT

GCS was designed for use specifically in the setting of trauma.

TABLE 3.2. The Glasgow Coma Scale

Eye Opening	Score	Verbal Response	Score	Motor Response	Score
Spontaneous	4	Oriented	5	Follows commands	6
To voice	3	Confused	4	Localizes pain	5
To painful stimuli	2	Inappropriate words	3	Withdraws from pain	4
Never	1	Unintelligible sounds	2	Flexor response	3
		None	1	Extensor response	2
				None	1

Q

A 40-year-old woman is brought in by ambulance after a high-speed rollover motor vehicle crash. She has signs of injury to the head, chest, and abdomen. What are the first steps in assessing this patient?

KEY FACT

Highest GCS: 15

Lowest GCS: 3

Four eyes

Jackson 5: verbal

V6 engine: motor

Exposure/Environment

- Undress the patient completely to look for additional torso and extremity injuries.
- While maintaining C-spine immobilization, roll the patient off the backboard as soon as possible. Lying on a backboard can lead to soft tissue injury. Evaluate the spine and soft tissue of the back and perineum.
- Cover the patient in a warm blanket or external warming device to prevent hypothermia. Check a core temperature in patients who may be cold or hot.

Secondary Survey

- The secondary survey includes a directed history and a detailed physical examination of the entire body.
- The eFAST examination should be performed, if not already done.

Emergency Department Thoracotomy

Goals of emergency department (ED) thoracotomy include:

- Relieve tamponade (pericardotomy)
- Control active bleeding from cardiac or pulmonary injuries
- Compress descending aorta to maximize coronary/cerebral perfusion
- Perform open cardiac massage

For resuscitative purposes, **signs of life** include: palpable pulse, spontaneous movement, spontaneous respiratory effort, cardiac activity on electrocardiogram (ECG), and pupillary response to light.

ED Thoracotomy for Blunt Trauma

ED thoracotomy following blunt trauma with cardiac arrest has a survival of < 2%. Accepted indications for ED thoracotomy in blunt trauma are:

- Prehospital/hospital signs of life with loss for LESS than 10 minutes
- Unresponsive hypotension (blood pressure [BP] < 70 mm Hg) despite resuscitation with echo evidence of cardiac tamponade
- Rapid exsanguination from a chest tube (> 1500 cc output upon insertion)

Contraindications include:

- Prehospital cardiopulmonary resuscitation (CPR) > 10 minutes without response
- Asystole as presenting rhythm and no echo evidence for cardiac tamponade
- Significant head trauma

ED Thoracotomy for Penetrating Trauma

Survival rates are much higher with ED thoracotomy in penetrating trauma. Accepted indications for ED thoracotomy in penetrating trauma are:

- Prehospital/hospital signs of life
- Echo evidence of cardiac activity with cardiac tamponade
- Unresponsive hypotension (BP < 70 mm Hg) despite resuscitation with penetrating chest wound

Contraindications include:

- Prehospital CPR > 15 minutes without response
- Asystole as presenting rhythm and no echo evidence for cardiac tamponade
- Significant head trauma

A

ABCDE—assess **A**irway, **B**reathing, **C**irculation, and **D**isability (neurologic status). **E**xpose patient completely, then cover to prevent hypothermia.

Head Trauma

TRAUMATIC BRAIN INJURY

The goals of care for the patient with head trauma are to determine what (if any) degree of traumatic brain injury exists and to maximize neurologic outcomes. Traumatic brain injury (TBI) is typically classified as mild, moderate, or severe based on GCS score (Table 3.2 and Table 3.3). The term **concussion** is used to describe a subset of patients with mild TBI. The challenge is identifying patients with mild TBI who have injuries that require neurosurgical intervention to prevent future decompensation.

Pathophysiology

Direct injury or shearing force → brain edema or hemorrhagic mass effect → cerebral ischemia (ICP [intracranial pressure] > CPP [cerebral perfusion pressure]) and/or herniation of brain tissue.

Symptoms

Symptoms may include headache, nausea/vomiting, loss of consciousness, visual disturbances, confusion, sleepiness, vertigo, amnesia, focal neurological deficits, and seizures.

Examination

- GCS score to quantify level of consciousness
- Hypertension, bradycardia, and irregular respirations (**Cushing reflex**) should raise concern for life-threatening elevation in ICP.
- Examine head and neck for evidence of bruising, lacerations, leakage of fluid, etc.
- **Pupillary response:**
  - In a comatose patient, a single fixed and dilated pupil may be a sign of ipsilateral uncal herniation. In awake patients, it usually indicates ocular trauma (eg, traumatic mydriasis).
  - Bilateral fixed and dilated pupils may indicate complete uncal herniation, poor brain perfusion, or stimulant use.

Q

A young man arrives in the ED following isolated head trauma with loss of consciousness (LOC). His mental status has returned to baseline, but he has been vomiting and complains of persistent headache. What should you do next?

KEY FACT

Severe TBI: GCS < 9

Moderate TBI: GCS 9-13

Mild TBI: GCS 14-15

KEY FACT

Loss of consciousness is not required in mild TBI

KEY FACT

CPP = MAP (mean arterial pressure) – ICP

Ideal CPP: > 60 mm Hg

Ideal MAP: > 80 mm Hg

Ideal ICP: < 15 mm Hg

TABLE 3.3. Categorization of Traumatic Brain Injury

	Mild TBI			Moderate TBI	Severe TBI
GCS	14-15			9-13	< 9
Risk for injury	**Low** No LOC No/mild HA Normal examination	**Moderate** LOC Amnesia Vomiting Diffuse HA	**High** Skull fracture Neuro deficit High-risk patient	High	High
Head CT required?	No	Yes	Yes	Yes	Yes
Incidence of surgical intervention	0.1%	1%-3%	Up to 10%	8%	
Mortality				20%	60%

CT, computed tomography; GCS, Glasgow Coma Scale; HA, headache; LOC, loss of consciousness.

A

This patient has a moderate risk for intracranial injury based on his presenting symptoms. Administer antiemetics and obtain a head computed tomography (CT) with or without C-spine imaging.

- **Motor examination:**
  - **Decorticate posturing**: Abnormal flexion of the upper extremities with extension of lower extremities. Indicates damage to corticospinal tract above brainstem.
  - **Decerebrate posturing**: Extension/adduction and internal rotation of arms and legs with flexion of wrist, fingers, feet (plantar), and toes. Indicates injury to brainstem.
- **Brainstem testing:**
  - **Oculocephalic response** (pontine gaze centers): Conjugate deviation of eyes in direction *opposite* to passive head rotation (once C-spine cleared) indicates intact brainstem function in a comatose patient (positive "doll's eyes" response).
  - **Oculovestibular response**: Instillation of 30-mL *cold* saline into the ear; horizontal nystagmus with fast component *away* from tested ear indicates intact brainstem function.

KEY FACT

Cushing reflex: Hypertension, bradycardia, and irregular respirations

Uncal Herniation Syndrome

Results from a hematoma, mass or edema compressing the temporal lobe, pushing the medial temporal lobe (uncus) into the tentorium and causing pressure on the brainstem

- Compression of ipsilateral CN III →
  - Ipsilateral pupillary dilation and decreased reactivity
  - "Down and out" position of eye with only lateral rectus (CN VI) and superior oblique (CN IV) functioning
- Eventual compression of ipsilateral peduncle → contralateral hemiparesis

KEY FACT

Decorticate posture: Flexion of upper extremities ("clutch your cortex")

KEY FACT

Kernohan notch phenomenon: Compression of *contralateral* peduncle in uncal herniation leading to *ipsilateral* hemiparesis (false localizing sign)

Diagnosis

- Noncontrast CT is imaging modality of choice and is indicated for all patients with moderate to severe traumatic brain injuries.
- Mild TBI patients need imaging based on risk for injury requiring neurosurgical intervention or close monitoring. Consensus guidelines for CT imaging have been published by the American College of Emergency Physicians (Table 3.4).
- The Pediatric Emergency Care Applied Research Network (PECARN) has created and validated rules to guide CT imaging in children with head injury (Table 3.5).
- Magnetic resonance imaging (MRI) is more sensitive in showing contusions, petechial hemorrhage, axonal injury, and small hematomas, but is rarely indicated in the ED setting.

Treatment

Severe TBI (GCS ≤ 8) patients warrant **aggressive management** to prevent secondary brain injury:

- Secure airway via rapid sequence intubation (RSI) with neuroprotective agents.
- Aggressively treat hypotension with fluids or blood transfusion to maintain systolic blood pressure (SBP) ≥ 90 mm Hg and prevent hypoperfusion to injured brain tissue.
- Elevate head of bed to 30°.
- If evidence for herniation or acute clinical deterioration:
  - Consider hyperventilation as a temporizing measure—to P_{CO_2} of 30-35 mm Hg.

KEY FACT

Beware that prolonged hyperventilation can cause cerebral vasoconstriction and ischemia

TABLE 3.4. ACEP Consensus Guidelines for CT Imaging in Mild TBI

Indications for Noncontrast CT in Adults with Mild TBI
Headache
Vomiting
Age > 60 with LOC or amnesia
Age > 65 without LOC or amnesia
Drug or alcohol intoxication
Short-term memory deficits
Evidence of trauma above clavicles
Post-traumatic seizures
GCS < 15
Focal neurological deficit
Coagulopathy
Dangerous mechanism (ejection, pedestrian struck, fall > 3 ft or 5 stairs)

CT, computed tomography; GCS, Glasgow Coma Scale; LOC, loss of consciousness; TBI, traumatic brain injury.

- Administer mannitol 0.25-1 g/kg IV bolus (adults) or hypertonic saline 3% 0.1-1 mL/kg/h (infants/children) to produce osmotic diuresis.
- Consider emergent cranial decompression with burr hole.

- Provide seizure prophylaxis.
- Administer antibiotics if penetrating injury.
- Reverse any anticoagulation.

KEY FACT

Hypotension, hypoxemia, hyperpyrexia, and hypoventilation can worsen CPP in severe head injury.

KEY FACT

Hypercarbia or Hypoxemia
↓
Cerebral vasodilation
Hypocarbia
↓
Cerebral vasoconstriction

TABLE 3.5. PECARN Indications for Head CT in Pediatric Head Injury

Children < 2 y Old (SCALPS)	Children 2-18 y Old
Scalp hematoma (except frontal)	Palpable skull fracture
Caregiver concern for change in behavior	Altered level of consciousness
Altered level of consciousness	LOC
LOC ≥ 5 s	History of vomiting
Palpable skull fracture	Severe headache
[a]Severe mechanism of injury	*Severe mechanism of injury

LOC, loss of consciousness.

[a]MVC with patient ejection, death of occupant or rollover; pedestrian or bicyclist without helmet struck be vehicle; fall > 3 ft if < 2 years old or > 5 ft if ≥ 2 years, head struck by high-impact object.

Moderate TBI (GCS 9-13) patients (even those with negative CT) require admission for close observation with frequent neurological checks and repeat CT scan for clinical deterioration. The overall morbidity and mortality for these patients remains high.

Minor TBI (GCS 14-15) patients with a negative CT scan can be safely discharged from the ED. Those who are not imaged can be discharged after a 4- to 6-hour period of observation if no worsening symptoms.

- Neurologic, behavioral, and cognitive symptoms (**postconcussive syndrome**) are common after minor TBI. Most patients completely recover, although 30%-80% have symptoms at 3 months out, and 15% have symptoms at 1 year.
- Patients should be prescribed a period of complete physical and cognitive rest with a stepwise return to normal activity as symptoms allow. Patients should not return to contact sports until complete resolution of symptoms. A repeat TBI while still symptomatic can have devastating results.
- Anticoagulated patients with minor head injury are at increased risk for delayed intracranial hemorrhage. CT and anticoagulant levels should be obtained. These patients require admission for close observation regardless of CT results.

KEY FACT

Steroids have no benefit in head-injured patients.

KEY FACT

Beware the risk of delayed hemorrhage in head injured patients taking anticoagulants.

INTRACRANIAL INJURIES

Epidural Hematoma

Usually associated with skull fracture after blunt trauma. Classically in the temporoparietal area with injury to the **middle meningeal artery and temporal bone fracture**, but epidurals may occur in other locations (Table 3.6).

Symptoms/Examination

Classically presents with lucid interval after initial LOC followed by recurrence of unconsciousness from expanding hematoma.

Diagnosis/Treatment

- CT shows biconvex or lens-shaped opacity usually at temporal/temporoparietal area (Figure 3.1).
- A surgical emergency; evacuation is required unless very small.

Subdural Hematoma

Caused by tearing of bridging veins. More common in the **elderly and alcoholics** because of brain atrophy and increased intracranial space, leading to increased movement of the brain and shearing forces on bridging veins; may be associated with minor or no known trauma.

Diagnosis/Treatment

- Crescent-shaped hematoma on CT (Figure 3.2): Bright if acute, dark if chronic (> 14 days)
- Surgical intervention usually required for acute (< 24 hours) and subacute (< 2 weeks) bleeds, and any bleed associated with a change in mental status or significant midline shift.

KEY FACT

In patients who have very low GCS but no findings on CT, consider diffuse axonal injury (DAI), diagnosed on MRI.

TABLE 3.6. Intracranial Hematomas

	Type of Patient	Anatomic Location	CT Findings	Common Cause	Classic Symptoms
Epidural	Young, rare in the elderly and those aged < 2 y	Potential space between skull and dura mater	Biconvex, football-shaped hematoma	Skull fracture with tear of the middle meningeal artery	Immediate LOC with a "lucid" period prior to deterioration (only occurs in about 20%)
Subdural	More risk in the elderly and alcoholic patients	Space between dura mater and arachnoid	Crescent- or sickle-shaped hematoma	Acceleration-deceleration with tearing of the bridging veins	Acute: rapid LOC, lucid period possible Chronic: altered mental state and behavior with gradual decrease in consciousness
Subarachnoid	Any age group after blunt trauma	Subarachnoid	Blood in the basilar cisterns and hemispheric sulci and fissures	Acceleration-deceleration with tearing of the subarachnoid vessels	Mild, moderate, or severe traumatic brain injury with meningeal signs and symptoms
Contusion/intracerebral hematoma	Any age group after blunt trauma	Usually anterior temporal or posterior frontal lobe	May be normal initially with delayed bleed	Severe or penetrating trauma; shaken baby syndrome	Symptoms range from normal to LOC

LOC, loss of consciousness.

(Reproduced, with permission, from Tintinalli JE, Stapczynski S, Ma OJ, et al. *Tintinalli's Emergency Medicine: A Comprehensive Study Guide*. 8th ed. New York, NY: McGraw-Hill, 2015. Table 257-10.)

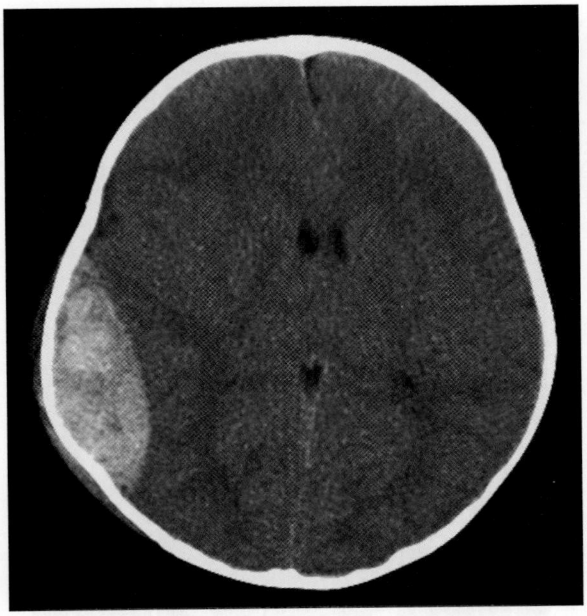

FIGURE 3.1. Epidural hematoma in a 5-year-old. Noncontrast head CT showing epidural hematoma with midline shift. (Reproduced, with permission, from Doherty GM. *Current Diagnosis & Treatment Surgery*. 14th ed. New York, NY: McGraw-Hill Education, 2015. Figure 36.8.)

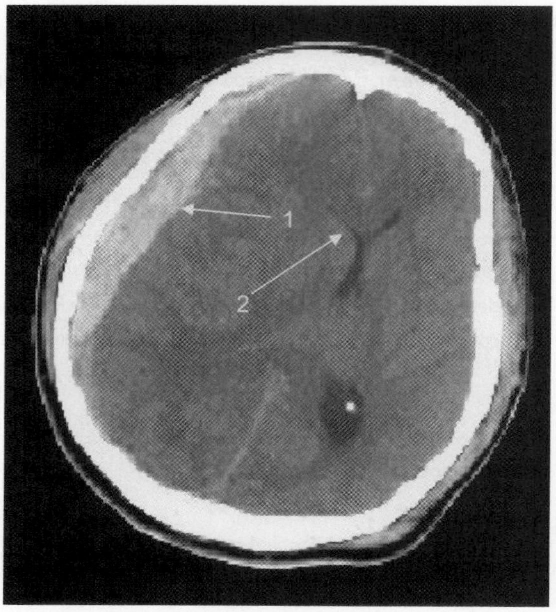

FIGURE 3.2. Subdural hematoma. Noncontrast head CT showing subdural hemorrhage with midline shift. (Reproduced, with permission, from Tintinalli JE, Kelen GD, Stapczynski JS. *Emergency Medicine: A Comprehensive Study Guide.* 6th ed. New York, NY: McGraw-Hill; 2004:1568.)

KEY FACT

Nimodipine is used for treatment of subarachnoid hemorrhage (SAH) from spontaneous ruptured aneurysm but not for traumatic head injury.

Traumatic Subarachnoid

Most common intracranial bleed in moderate to severe TBI. Caused by disruption of subarachnoid vessels.

- Symptoms include headache, photophobia, and/or meningeal signs.
- CT scan may show blood in the ventricles, cisterns, or sulci (Figure 3.3).

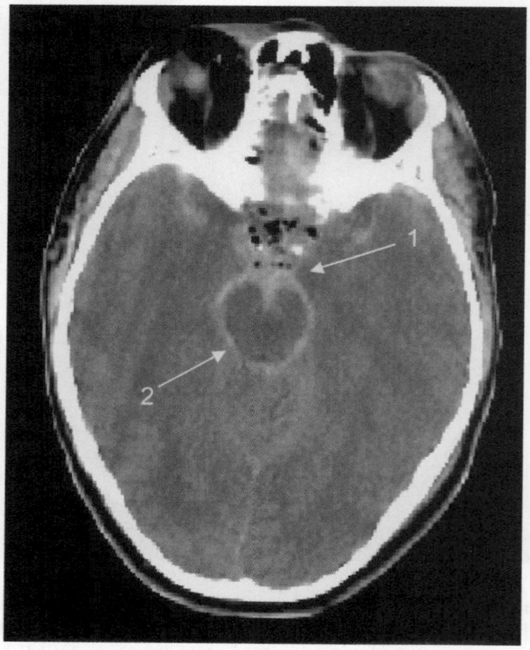

FIGURE 3.3. Traumatic subarachnoid hemorrhage. Noncontast CT showing subarachnoid hemorrhage. Arrows indicate blood in the cisterns. (Reproduced, with permission, from Tintinalli JE, Kelen GD, Stapczynski JS. *Emergency Medicine: A Comprehensive Study Guide.* 6th ed. New York, NY: McGraw-Hill; 2004:1567.)

Cerebral Contusion

Cerebral contusions are seen in **deceleration injuries** and **shaken baby syndrome.**

- Usually frontal or temporal lobes.
- Contusion may be at side of injury ("coup") or opposite to injury ("contrecoup").
- Symptoms and examination vary with location and severity of injury.

BASILAR SKULL FRACTURE

The base of the skull is divided into three parts (anterior, middle, and posterior) and is made of five bones. Basilar skull fracture occurs most commonly in the petrous portion of temporal bone.

Symptoms/Examination

- Patients may present with vertigo, hearing difficulties, hemotympanum, or seventh nerve palsy.
- Cerebrospinal fluid (CSF) otorrhea or rhinorrhea—look for a target lesion on filter paper with a ring of CSF around blood.
- Mastoid ecchymosis (Battle sign) 1-3 days after injury.
- Periorbital ecchymosis (raccoon eyes) 1-3 days after injury.

Diagnosis/Treatment

- Study of choice is noncontrast head CT with thin cuts through temporal bone and base of skull.
- Nasogastric tube (NGT) placement is contraindicated in suspected/confirmed cribriform plate fracture.
- Generally, patients with basilar skull fractures do not require treatment other than pain medications, antiemetics, and observation.
- Consider discharge for adults with simple linear fractures who are neurologically intact.

Complication

Meningitis may occur following basilar skull fracture, requiring antibiotics and neurosurgical consultation. No consensus exists on the use of prophylactic antibiotics.

> **KEY FACT**
>
> **Five bones of skull base:**
>
> Frontal (orbital plate)
>
> Ethmoid (cribriform plate)
>
> Sphenoid
>
> Temporal (petrous and squamous portions)
>
> Occipital

FRACTURE OF SKULL CONVEXITY

Skull convexity fractures are described by their location and type (comminuted, depressed, linear).

Symptoms/Examination

- Symptoms depend on degree of underlying brain injury.
- Overlying hematoma or laceration is a common finding. Look for exposed or depressed bone.

Diagnosis/Treatment

- CT is imaging of choice. The presence of pneumocephalus indicates an open fracture.
- Occipital impression fractures, fractures crossing sutures and multiple "eggshell" fractures suggest abuse in children.

> **Q**
>
> A stable patient has sustained a stab wound to the neck. What should be your first consideration in determining extent of injury?

- The role of antibiotics in patients with open and depressed skull fractures is controversial, discuss with neurosurgery.
- Operative repair is required for fractures depressed beyond one full thickness of the skull because of increased likelihood of direct compression of the brain.

Neck Trauma

BLUNT LARYNGOTRACHEAL INJURY

Most blunt laryngotracheal injury occurs as a result of direct impact from a seat belt, steering wheel, handle bar or clothesline, but it is also seen with strangulation.

Symptoms/Examination

- Patients may present with neck pain and upper airway symptoms ranging from hoarseness and hemoptysis to severe dyspnea with airway compromise.
- Findings include dysphonia, stridor, tenderness, subcutaneous (SQ) emphysema, and loss of anatomic landmarks.

KEY FACT

Consider tracheal injury in patients with blunt neck trauma and subcutaneous (SQ) emphysema.

Diagnosis/Treatment

- Awake direct laryngoscopy or flexible nasopharyngoscopy is the initial study of choice to evaluate laryngeal integrity.
  - Intubate if evidence for injury or edema. Early airway management is critical before swelling causes complete obstruction. **Awake fiberoptic-guided oral intubation** is considered the best approach.
  - Do NOT paralyze the patient or attempt intubation without having neck prepped for **tracheostomy** (not cricothyrotomy, which may worsen the injury).
- After evaluation/management of airway, CT neck with 1-mm cuts can be used to look for fractures. CT is less useful in children as laryngeal structures do not calcify until the teenage years.
- Rigid bronchoscopy is necessary for evaluation of lower airway structures.
- Surgical repair is often required.

KEY FACT

Intubation of patients with laryngotracheal injuries may create a "false lumen" and loss of airway.

BLUNT PHARYNGOESOPHAGEAL INJURY

Pharyngoesophageal injury is most likely to result from penetrating injury, caustic or foreign body ingestions or in the case of Boerhaave, forceful vomiting or retching. It rarely results from blunt trauma.

KEY FACT

Esophageal injuries are rare but are the most commonly missed injuries of the neck.

Symptoms/Examination

- Often asymptomatic initially, but findings include hematemesis, SQ emphysema, and blood in saliva or NGT.
- If left unrecognized, life-threatening mediastinal infection may develop.

Diagnosis

- Plain film chest x-ray (CXR) and neck films may show pneumomediastinum or retropharyngeal air.
- Sensitivity of endoscopy or esophagography alone is poor; together these tests have improved sensitivity.

A

Visual inspection to determine if the platysma has been violated.

TREATMENT

- Broad-spectrum antibiotics with anaerobic coverage.
- Nothing by mouth; do not place NGT blindly.
- Surgical repair is required for full-thickness injuries.

BLUNT CEREBROVASCULAR INJURY

The primary concern in blunt trauma to the neck is intimal tear, pseudoaneurysm, or dissection of the carotid or vertebral arteries. Such injury can lead to secondary thrombosis and occlusion or embolus causing serious morbidity.

Mechanisms include:

- Direct impact to neck from seatbelt, clothesline, strangulation etc, causing compression of carotid.
- Hyperextension with lateral rotation → stretching of carotid across C-spine transverse process; most common.
- Intraoral trauma causing damage to internal carotid at angle of jaw
- Basilar skull fractures causing laceration of the carotid in region of carotid canal
- Hyperextension and/or lateral rotation of neck causing stretching of vertebral artery in region of the more mobile first and second vertebrae

SYMPTOMS/EXAMINATION

- Most patients will complain of pain in region of injury but the vast majority of patients have no neurologic signs or symptoms at the time of initial presentation. Maintaining a high-index of suspicion based on presenting mechanism and injuries is critical.
- Hard signs that suggest injury include expanding hematoma, bruits, active bleeding, transient ischemic attach (TIA)/stroke, airway compromise.
- Horner syndrome: Ptosis, miosis, anhidrosis from disruption of periarterial sympathetic plexus of the carotid.

DIAGNOSIS

The use of computed tomography angiography (CTA) of the head and neck has largely replaced the need for conventional neck angiography.

TREATMENT

- Anticoagulation
- Surgical intervention if neurologic deficit

> **KEY FACT**
>
> **Risk factors for blunt carotid or vertebral artery injury:**
>
> Near hanging
> Clothesline injury
> Seatbelt sign with swelling
> Severe TBI
> Major thoracic injury
> Cervical spine fracture
> Occipital condyle fracture
> Basilar skull fracture
> Mandible fracture
> Displaced mid-face fracture
> Scalp degloving injury

PENETRATING NECK TRAUMA

In regard to penetrating trauma, the neck is anatomically divided into zones that have both anatomic (Table 3.7 and Figure 3.4) and management implications. Trauma to any zone may injure the nervous system, vessels, or aerodigestive structures.

SYMPTOMS/EXAMINATION

- Findings that suggest major injury (**hard signs**) include airway compromise, air bubbling from wound, shock, severe active bleeding, expanding or pulsatile hematoma, neurologic deficit, hematemesis, and massive SQ emphysema.
- Unfortunately, lack of physical findings does not rule out injury.

> **KEY FACT**
>
> **Hard signs in penetrating neck trauma**
>
> Airway compromise
> Air bubbling from wound
> Shock
> Severe active bleeding
> Expanding/pulsatile hematoma
> Neurologic deficit
> Hematemesis
> Massive SQ emphysema

TABLE 3.7. Zones of the Neck

<table>
<tr><th>Zones</th><th>Landmarks</th><th colspan="2">Involved Structures</th></tr>
<tr><td>Zone I</td><td>Clavicles to cricoid cartilage</td><td rowspan="2">Trachea, esophagus, vertebral, and carotid arteries</td><td>Great vessels, lung apices, thoracic duct, spinal cord</td></tr>
<tr><td>Zone II</td><td>Cricoid cartilage to angle of mandible</td><td>Larynx, jugular veins</td></tr>
<tr><td>Zone III</td><td>Angle of mandible to base of skull</td><td colspan="2">Pharynx, jugular veins, vertebral, and internal carotid arteries, skull base</td></tr>
</table>

Diagnosis/Treatment

- Consider early intubation in patients with suspected arterial injury, as expanding hematomas can quickly lead to airway compromise.
- Neck wounds with **intact platysma** can be closed.
- Violation of the platysma indicates a possibility of significant neck injury and requires surgical consultation. Do not probe neck wounds beyond the level of the platysma because of the risk of dislodging a clot.
- **Zones I and III injuries** can be difficult to evaluate surgically and therefore angiography or CTA is usually indicated.
- **Zone I injuries** should also undergo esophageal evaluation with esophagram or endoscopy and tracheal evaluation via laryngoscopy or bronchoscopy.
- **Zone II injuries** with hard signs of injury are typically explored surgically. Those without hard signs may be evaluated as with Zone I injuries.
- Keep in mind that an entrance wound to any zone can represent an internal injury to structures in any or all of the zones.
- With open venous injuries, prevent venous air embolism with direct pressure and Trendelenburg position.

KEY FACT

To remember the neck zones, remember 1, 2, 3, upward, like floors of a building. The neck goes from clavicles to base of the skull, split into thirds at the cricoid and angle of mandible.

Penetrating Neck Trauma Evaluation
Zone I: Angiography, esophageal, and tracheal evaluation
Zone II: Surgery if hard signs, otherwise as per Zone I
Zone III: Angiography

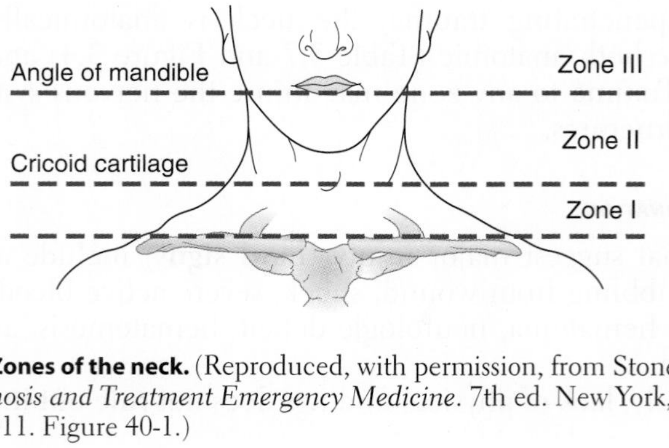

FIGURE 3.4. Zones of the neck. (Reproduced, with permission, from Stone CK, Humphries RL. *Current Diagnosis and Treatment Emergency Medicine*. 7th ed. New York, NY: McGraw-Hill Education, 2011. Figure 40-1.)

Spinal Injuries

Spinal injuries are most commonly caused by blunt trauma, including MVCs, falls and diving into shallow water. They are classified into four categories according to mechanism of injury:

- Flexion fractures (eg, wedge, flexion teardrop, clay shoveler's)
- Vertical compression fractures (eg, burst, Jefferson)
- Flexion-rotation (eg, unilateral facet)
- Extension (eg, Hangman's)

Mechanisms

- Motor vehicle crashes
- Sports, falls, diving into shallow water
- Abrupt flexion during lifting (clay shoveler's fracture)

CERVICAL SPINAL FRACTURES

Cervical spine fractures are divided into stable fractures and unstable fractures based on radiographic imaging.

Symptoms/Examination

- Individuals with C-spine fractures typically complain of posterior midline neck pain, pain with movement of the neck, numbness, or weakness.
- The examination varies with the fracture location and degree of associated spinal cord injury.

Diagnosis

- The decision to image the C-spine is based on the mechanism of injury, pain, tenderness, neurologic findings, and the alertness of the patient.
- The **National Emergency X-Radiography Utilization Study (NEXUS)** has identified 5 criteria that have 99.6% sensitivity of detecting clinically significant C-spine injury (Table 3.8).
- The **Canadian C-spine Rule** adds mechanisms of injury to the assessment (Table 3.9).
- A C-spine series consists of anteroposterior (AP), lateral, swimmer's, and odontoid views.
- On a lateral C-spine x-ray, 3 imaginary lines are identified (Figure 3.5). Disruption to any line suggests injury (Tables 3.10 and 3.11).
  - Anterior contour line: Formed by anterior margin of vertebral body
  - Posterior contour line: Formed by posterior margin of vertebral body
  - Spinolaminar line: Connects the bases of the spinous processes and extends to the posterior aspect of the foramen magnum

TABLE 3.8. NEXUS Criteria

According to NEXUS, cervical spine imaging is NOT required if patient meets all the following low risk criteria:
No posterior midline cervical spine tenderness
No focal neurologic deficits
No evidence of intoxication
Normal level of alertness
No painful distracting injuries

Q

A 71-year-old man presents with bilateral arm weakness after a ground-level fall. He denies neck pain and moves his neck without discomfort. What's the diagnosis and mechanism of injury?

KEY FACT

Most common fracture level is C5. Most common subluxation is C5 on C6.

MNEMONIC

Although posterior neck tenderness is one of the NEXUS criteria, posterior neck pain is not.

Remember NEXUS by NSAID

Neuro deficit?
Spinal tenderness to midline?
Alert?
Intoxicated?
Distracting injury?

A

Central cord syndrome, resulting from hyperextension injury with buckling of the ligamentum flavum against the central cord. X-rays are often normal. MRI is confirmative.

TABLE 3.9. Canadian C-Spine Rule. A "Yes" Answer to all Three Question/Assessment Criteria Means Cervical Spine Imaging is Unnecessary.

Question or Assessment	Definitions
There are no high-risk factors that mandate radiography.	High-risk factors include: ■ Age 65 years or older ■ A dangerous mechanism of injury (fall from a height of > 3 ft; an axial loading injury; high-speed motor vehicle crash, rollover, or ejection; motorized recreational vehicle or bicycle collision) ■ The presence of paresthesias in the extremities
There are low-risk factors that allow a safe assessment of range of motion.	Low-risk factors include: ■ Simple rear-end motor vehicle crashes ■ Patient able to sit up in the ED ■ Patient ambulatory at any time ■ Delayed onset of neck pain ■ Absence of midline cervical tenderness
The patient is able to actively rotate his/her neck.	Can rotate 45° to the left and to the right

ED, emergency department.

(Reproduced, with permission, from *Tintinalli's Emergency Medicine*. 7th ed. Chapter 255, Spine and spinal cord trauma, Table 255-6.)

KEY FACT

Abnormal soft-tissue findings on a lateral C-spine: Remember 6 at 2 and 22 at 6, and adjust up and down by 1 to get 7 mm and 21 mm.

- Up to 80% of C-spine injuries can be detected by the lateral C-spine film. The C7-T1 junction must be visualized as 20% of injuries occur at C7. Swelling of the prevertebral soft tissue suggests injury; a measurement > 7 mm at C2 or > 21 mm at C6 is abnormal.
- Odontoid views are obtained to identify odontoid fractures:
  - Type I: Avulsion of the tip (stable)
  - Type II: Fracture at junction of odontoid and body of C2 (most common)
  - Type III: Fracture at base of dens
- Obtain CT in all patients with abnormal or inadequate C-spine x-rays or high clinical suspicion for injury.
- Obtain MRI if ligamentous injury is suspected and plain film and CT imaging are negative. Flexion-extension views are limited by muscle spasm and pain and therefore have little utility in the immediate postinjury period.

KEY FACT

Instability increases with multicolumn injuries.

Spinal fractures tend to occur at junctions where the spine transitions from more to less mobile, and vice versa (thoracolumbar, cervicothoracic, odontoid, etc).

THORACOLUMBAR FRACTURES

The thoracic spine (to ~T11) is more rigid than the cervical and lumbar spine due to its articulation with the rib cage but its canal is narrow. Injury to the thoracic spine is therefore less common, but is often associated with spinal cord injury.

Symptoms/Examination

- Individuals with thoracolumbar fractures typically complain of pain in the region of injury.
- The examination varies with the fracture location and degree of associated spinal cord injury.

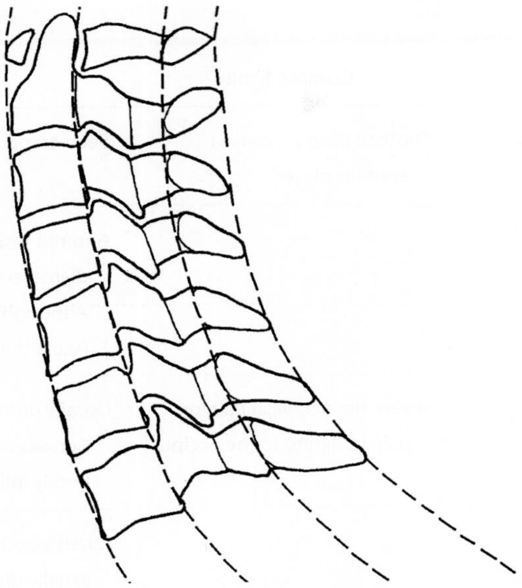

FIGURE 3.5. Diagram of lines on lateral C-spine. (Reproduced, with permission, from Tintinalli JE, Kelen GD, Stapczynski JS. *Emergency Medicine: A Comprehensive Study Guide*. 6th ed. New York, NY: McGraw-Hill; 2004:1703.)

MNEMONIC

Unstable fractures:

Jefferson Bit Off A
Hangman's Thumb (Table 3.11)

KEY FACT

Markers of unstable C-spine injury include damage to anterior 20% of vertebral body and loss of > 50% of body height.

Diagnosis

- Suspect based on clinical presentation and/or plain radiographs.
- CT scan is confirmative and can fully define the injury.
- Injuries are divided into major fractures (Table 3.12) and minor fractures (transverse process, spinous process, and pars interarticularis) based on radiographic imaging.

TABLE 3.10. Stable Fractures of the C-Spine

Type	Mechanism	Notes
Wedge fracture	Flexion	Multiple wedge fracture or loss of > 50% of vertebral body height may be unstable
Transverse process fracture	Flexion	Tend to be benign
Clay shoveler's fracture (spinous process avulsion)	Flexion against contracted posterior muscles	Most commonly at C7; stable fracture
Unilateral facet	Flexion and rotation	Anterior displacement < 50% of width
Burst fracture	Vertical compression	Can be unstable if fragments enter canal
Isolated fractures of articular pillar and vertebral body	Vertical compression	"Double-outline" sign

TABLE 3.11. Unstable Fractures of the C-Spine

Type	Image	Mechanism	Clinical Story	Notes
Jefferson fracture (C1 burst fracture)	Figure 3.6	Axial load with vertical compression	Football player spearing another player	Seen on odontoid view
Bilateral facet dislocation	Figure 3.7	Flexion		Anterior displacement > 50% diameter of vertebral body Although called locked facets the injury is unstable
Odontoid type II/III	Figure 3.8	Flexion	Severe high cervical pain or pain radiating to the occiput	Usually due to major forces Consider other C-spine and bodily injuries
Atlantoaxial or atlanto-occipital		Flexion or extension		Atlanto-occipital dissociation usually dislocations results in death
Hangman's fracture (bilateral C2 pedicle fracture)	Figure 3.9	Extension; C2 displaced anteriorly on C3	Hyperextension injury with fall down stairs	
Teardrop fracture		Flexion (compression fracture) or extension (avulsion fracture)		The teardrop is the anteroinferior portion of the vertebral body

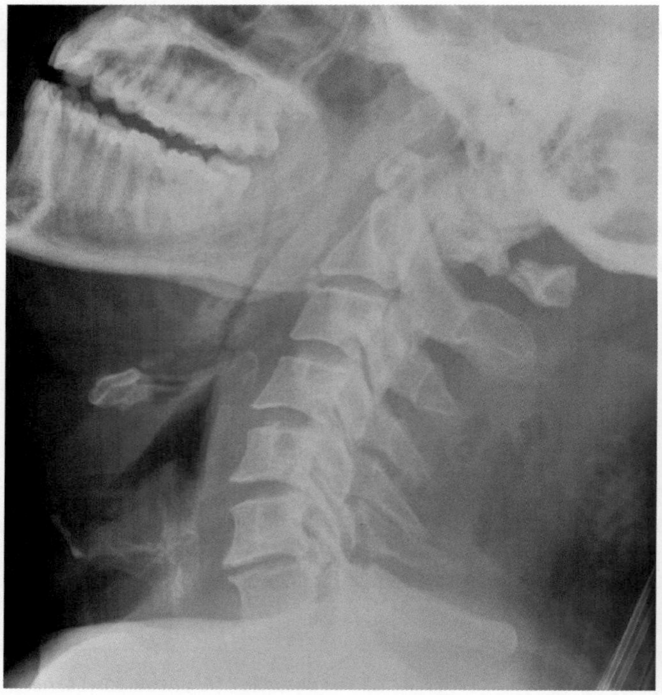

A

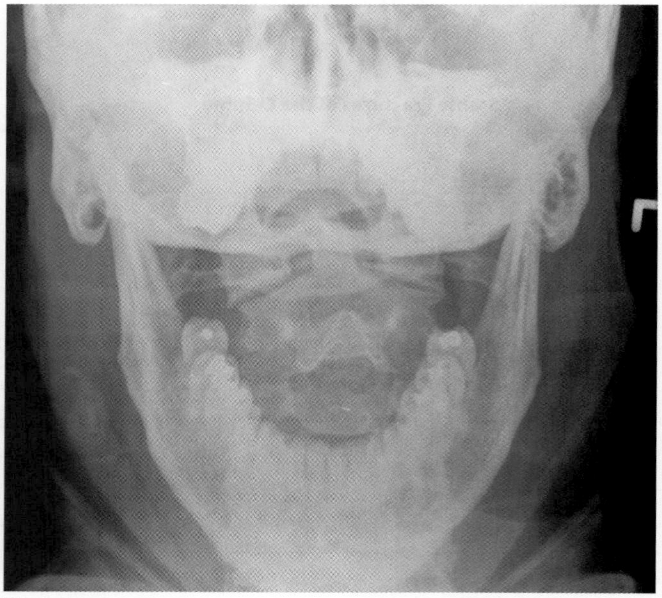

B

FIGURE 3.6. Jefferson fracture. Lateral view showing fracture of the posterior arch of C1 (**A**) and odontoid view showing asymmetry and slight widening of the lateral masses (**B**). (Reproduced, with permission, from Tintinalli JE, Stapczynski S, Ma OJ, et al. *Tintinalli's Emergency Medicine: A Comprehensive Study Guide*. 7th ed. New York, NY: McGraw-Hill, 2011. Figure 255.3BC.)

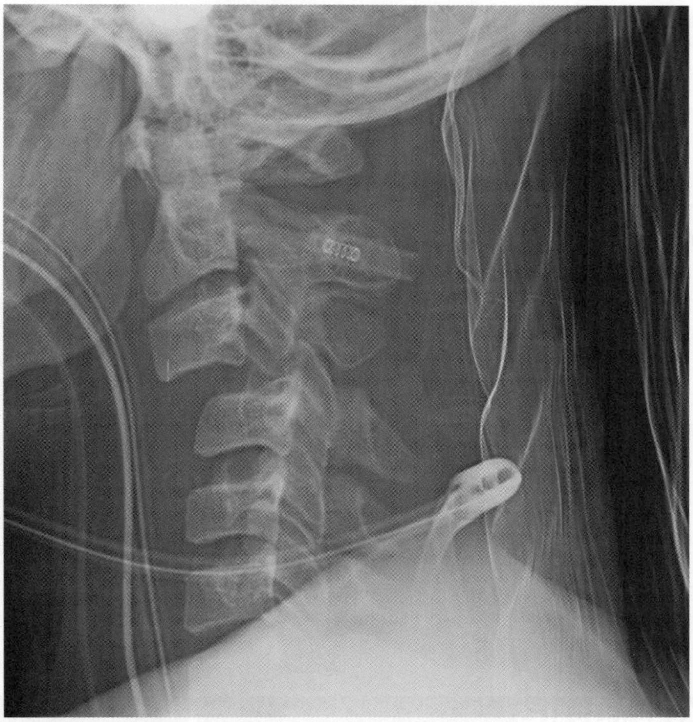

FIGURE 3.7. Bilateral facet dislocation. (Reproduced, with permission, from Tintinalli JE, Stapczynski S, Ma OJ, et al. *Tintinalli's Emergency Medicine: A Comprehensive Study Guide*. 7th ed. New York, NY: McGraw-Hill, 2011. Figure 255.8A.)

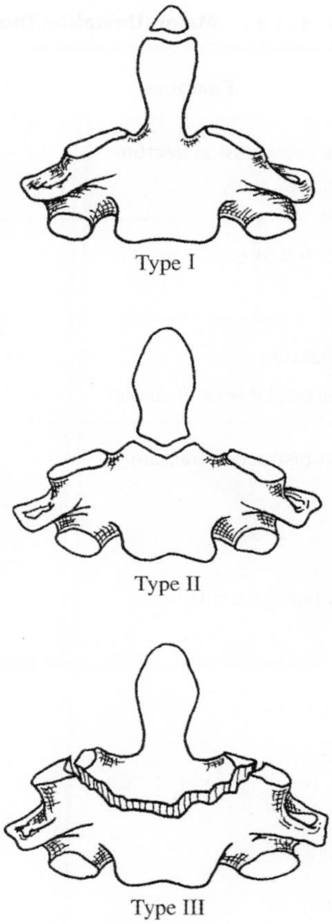

FIGURE 3.8. Odontoid fractures. (Reproduced, with permission, from Tintinalli JE, Kelen GD, Stapczynski JS. *Emergency Medicine: A Comprehensive Study Guide*. 6th ed. New York, NY: McGraw-Hill; 2004:1704.)

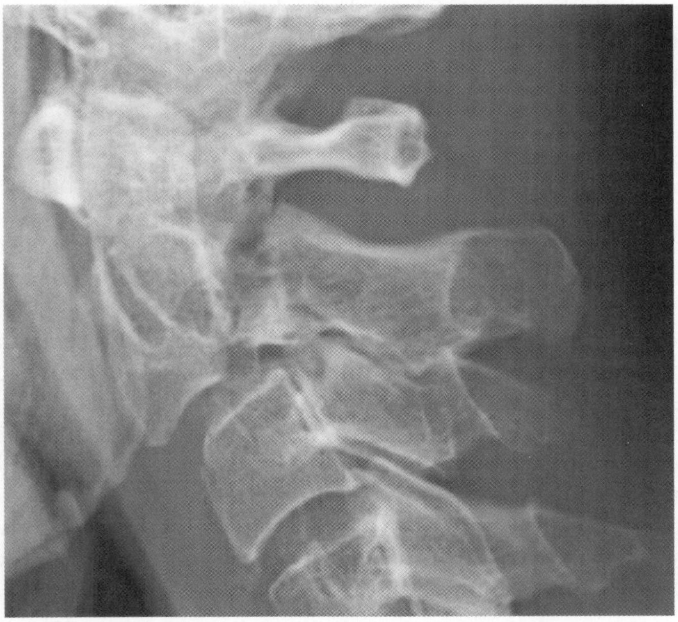

FIGURE 3.9. Hangman's fracture. (Reproduced, with permission, from Tintinalli JE, Kelen GD, Stapczynski JS. *Emergency Medicine: A Comprehensive Study Guide*. 6th ed. New York, NY: McGraw-Hill; 2004:1707.)

TABLE 3.12. Major (Unstable) Thoracolumbar Spine Fractures

Fracture	Mechanism	Radiographic Findings
Wedge compression fracture	Flexion injury	Loss of anterior vertebral body height Neurologic deficit uncommon
Chance fracture	Flexion around an anterior axis usually associated with lap belt	Horizontal fracture through the vertebral body and all posterior elements
Burst fracture (may be stable or unstable)	Vertical compression	Loss of anterior and posterior height
Flexion-distraction fracture	Flexion with compression of anterior elements and distraction of posterior elements	"Fanning"—increased posterior interspinous space
Translational fracture	Shear	Shift of one or more vertebral body causing complete disruption

SPINAL CORD INJURIES

Spinal cord injuries may be complete (total loss of function below lesion) or incomplete (partial loss of function). The most common incomplete lesions include Brown-Séquard syndrome, central cord syndrome, and anterior cord syndrome (Figure 3.10).

Diagnosis

Any patient exhibiting signs of neurologic dysfunction following trauma, with or without vertebral fracture, needs MRI with possible magnetic resonance angiogram (MRA) to evaluate extent of injury to cord and vessels.

Treatment

- Spinal injury at or above C5 usually requires intubation because of weakness of the diaphragm.
- Patients with C-spine fractures, ligamentous instability, or neurologic deficits consistent with a C-spine injury should be immobilized.
- Neurosurgical consultation is mandatory.
- Volume and pressors may be necessary for hypotension secondary to neurogenic shock, but be sure to rapidly evaluate for other causes of hypotension (ie, assume there is hemorrhagic shock).
- Therapy with **high-dose methylprednisolone** remains controversial after spinal cord injury. This therapy should only be given in consultation with the spine specialist who will be caring for the patient.
  - Initial dose of 30 mg/kg IV over 15 minutes; must be given within 8 hours of injury. This is followed by a 45-minute pause, then an infusion of 5.4 mg/kg/h for 23 hours.

KEY FACT

C3, C4, and C5 keep the diaphragm alive (via the phrenic nerve).

Brown-Séquard Syndrome (Good Prognosis)

Hemisection of the cord, usually associated with penetrating trauma. It has the best prognosis for full recovery of all the incomplete spinal cord syndromes.

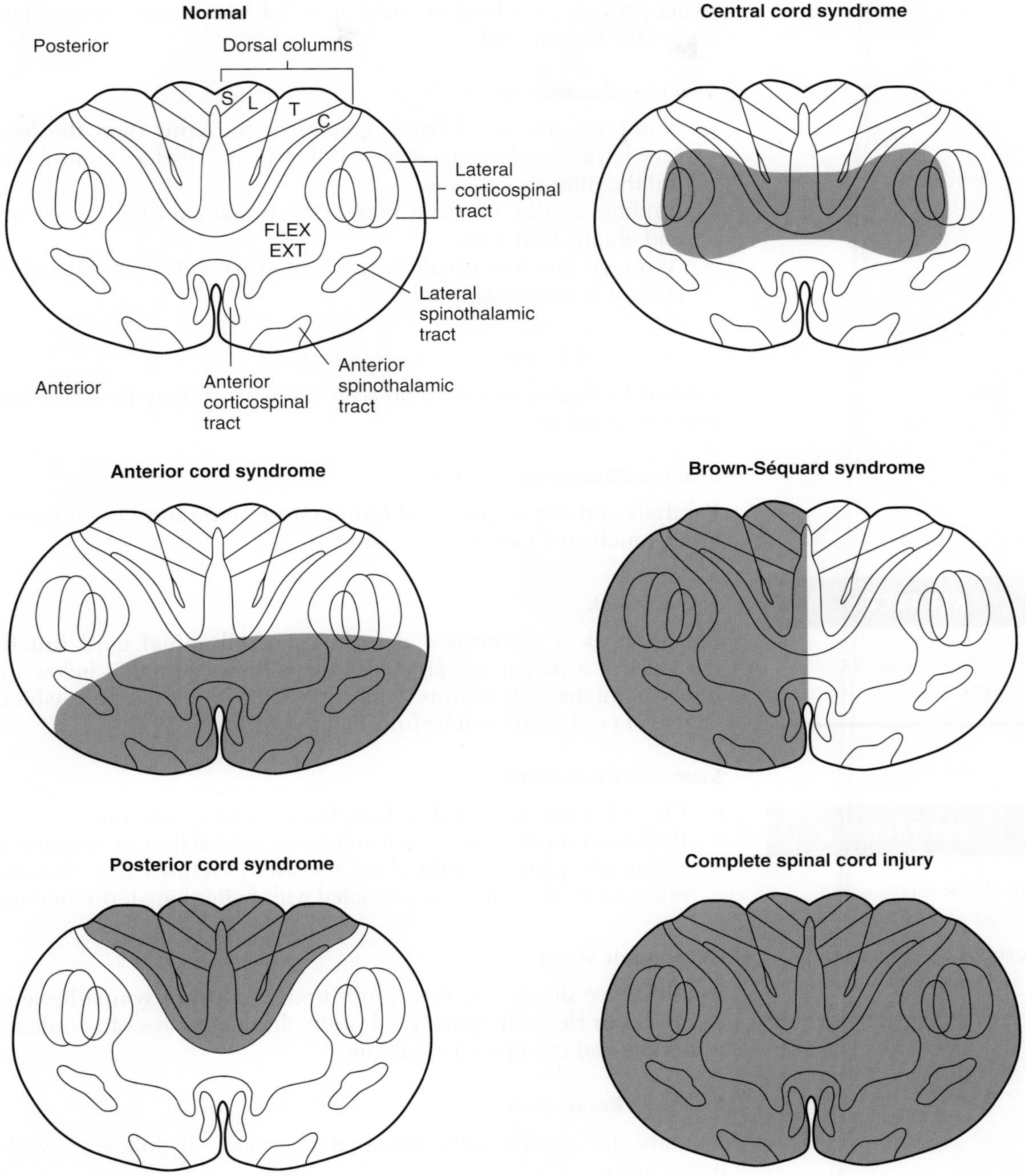

FIGURE 3.10. Cross-sectional views of the normal and injured spine. (Reproduced, with permission, from Skinner HB, McMahon PJ. *Current Diagnosis & Treatment in Orthopedics*. 5th ed. New York, NY: McGraw-Hill Education, 2014. Figure 4.28.)

Symptoms/Examination

Ipsilateral loss of motor, proprioception, and vibratory sensation with contralateral loss of pain and temperature sensation.

Central Cord Syndrome (Fair Prognosis)

The most common incomplete spinal cord lesion. It is caused by a hyperextension injury on a congenitally narrow canal or preexisting cervical spondylosis (older patients), resulting in buckling of the ligamentum flavum and compression of the central cord.

Symptoms/Examination

- Numbness and/or weakness **greater in the arms than the legs** (patients may have complete quadriplegia); bowel and bladder control remain in all but the most severe cases.
- Findings can be subtle at presentation; maintain high index of suspicion and obtain MRI early.
- Although function usually returns, most patients do not regain fine motor control in upper extremities.

Anterior Cord Syndrome (Poor Prognosis)

Caused by flexion or extension with vascular or bony fragment injury of the anterior spinal artery.

Symptoms/Examination

Paralysis and loss of pain and temperature sensation but preserved position, crude touch, and vibration sensation

KEY FACT

Spinal shock can make an incomplete injury appear complete.

Spinal Shock

Spinal shock is a ***transient*** **depression of all spinal cord function** below the level of a partial or complete injury. Reflex function below the level of injury spontaneously returns (typically within 24-48 hours), at which time the degree of cord injury can be fully determined.

Symptoms/Examination

- Flaccid paralysis, including bowel and bladder, priapism.
- Bulbocavernosus reflex (anal sphincter contraction in response to squeezing penile glans or pulling on the Foley) returns first. Presence of this reflex early after injury is associated with better long-term outcomes.

KEY FACT

Hemorrhagic shock: Patient is cold, clammy, pale, tachycardic.

Neurogenic shock: Patient is warm, vasodilated, bradycardic.

Neurogenic Shock

A distributive shock state that results from the **loss of sympathetic outflow** in a **cervical or thoracic** spinal cord injury, leading to loss of peripheral vascular resistance and unopposed vagal tone.

Symptoms/Examination

Patients are peripherally vasodilated, warm, hypotensive with relative bradycardia.

Diagnosis/Treatment

- Clinical diagnosis, but be sure to rule out other causes of hypotension first.
- Treated with intravenous fluid (IVF) resuscitation to correct the relative hypovolemia, then inotropes if this is not effective.

KEY FACT

SCIWORA is defined by neurologic deficits with negative x-ray and CT. MRI is often positive. Occurs mostly in children < 8 years old and in older adults.

Spinal Cord Injury Without Radiographic Abnormality

Trauma patients with neurologic deficits consistent with a spinal cord injury but with **negative plain films and CT. Spinal cord injury without radiographic abnormality** (SCIWORA) is thought to be common in children, but also occurs in older patients. Central cord syndrome, which results from buckling of the ligamentum flavum during hyperextension, is the classic form of SCIWORA in adults (mainly the elderly).

Chest Trauma

SIMPLE PNEUMOTHORAX

Pneumothorax is the accumulation of air within the pleural space, most commonly a result of trauma, though may occur spontaneously (see Chapter 10, Thoracic and Respiratory Disorders).

Symptoms/Examination

Pleuritic chest pain and shortness of breath with tachycardia and decreased or abnormal breath sounds.

Diagnosis

- Upright CXR: Findings that suggest pneumothorax include absent lung markings in the periphery of the lung field, SQ emphysema, or a low lateral diaphragm on the side of the injury (Figure 3.11). An expiratory CXR offers no benefit over an inspiratory film.
- Lateral decubitus CXR is reported to have the highest sensitivity among plain radiographs for detecting pneumothorax.
- **Supine CXR will show air toward the diaphragm—deep sulcus sign.**
- Supine lung ultrasound will show **absence of lung slide and loss of normal vertical comet tail artifact**. Ultrasound has a higher reported sensitivity than CXR and should be performed as part of the eFAST.
- CT has the highest sensitivity and will often detect occult pneumothoraces.

Treatment

- A small traumatic pneumothorax < 15%-25% in a stable patient may be treated with **100% O_2 via non-rebreather (NRB) mask** and repeat CXR.
  - Consider chest tube placement if patient requires intubation. A simple pneumothorax may be converted into a tension pneumothorax under positive pressure ventilation.

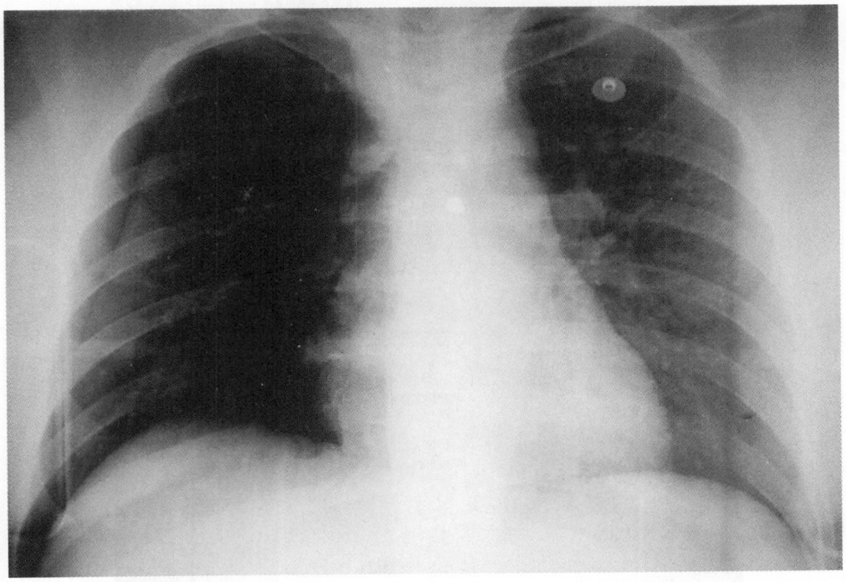

FIGURE 3.11. Right-sided pneumothorax. Note the deep sulcus on the side of injury. (Reproduced, with permission, from Stone CK, Humphries RL. *Current Diagnosis & Treatment: Emergency Medicine*. 7th ed. New York, NY: McGraw-Hill Education, 2011. Figure 13.3.)

Q

A 60-year-old woman is brought into the ED after MVC with hypotension, dyspnea, and tracheal deviation to the right. Lung sounds are absent over the left chest. What should be your first step?

KEY FACT

Pneumothorax heals approximately 1%-2% daily without chest tube.

A

This patient clinically has a tension pneumothorax. Do not wait for x-ray confirmation. Perform immediate decompression by placing a 14-gauge angiocath in the left second intercostal space at the midclavicular line.

KEY FACT

Findings of hypotension with distended neck veins may also occur with cardiac tamponade. The lung examination and cardiac/pleural lung ultrasound should differentiate the two.

KEY FACT

Serious/symptomatic pneumothorax:

- Tension pneumothorax
- Pneumothorax > 40% of a hemithorax
- Concurrent with hemorrhagic shock or preexisting cardiopulmonary disease

- Large pneumothoraces should receive a chest tube (36 French if concern for hemothorax).
- If the lung does not reexpand after chest tube placement and there is no mechanical malfunction, consider the possibility of a large tear in lung parenchyma or a bronchial injury. If placement of a second chest tube doesn't reinflate the lung, then surgical intervention is needed either via bronchoscopy, thoracotomy, or video-assisted thoracoscopy.

TENSION PNEUMOTHORAX

Caused by a 1-way communication from lung parenchyma into pleural space, allowing air into the space but not out (Figure 3.12). The progressive increase in air in the pleural space increases pressure in the hemithorax, causing shifting of the mediastinum, compression of the vena cava, **obstruction of venous return**, and decreased cardiac output.

Symptoms/Examination

- Shortness of breath with marked tachycardia and diminished or absent breath sounds on the affected side
- Distended neck veins and tracheal deviation to opposite side
- **Hypotension**

Diagnosis/Treatment

- Diagnosis is clinical.
- Immediate needle decompression should yield a rush of air and improvement of vital signs.
- All patients require subsequent chest tube placement.

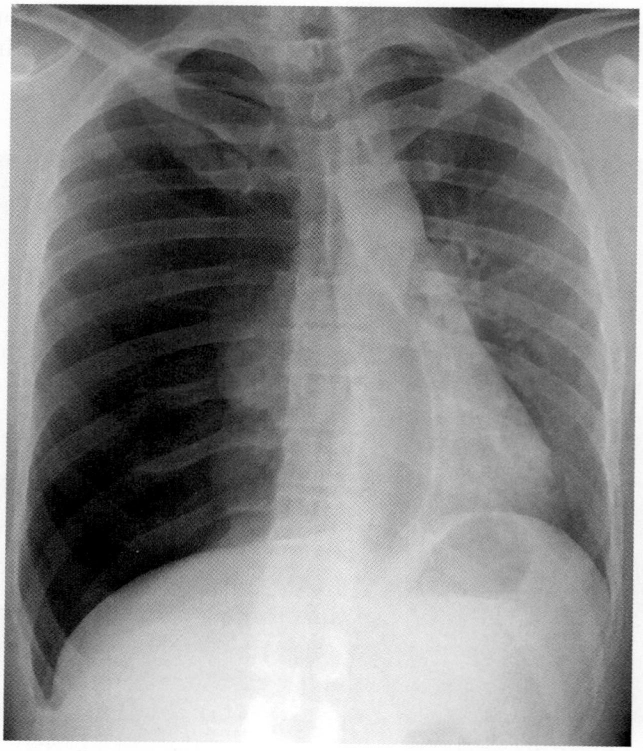

FIGURE 3.12. Right-sided tension pneumothorax. Note the leftward shift of mediastinal structures.

OPEN PNEUMOTHORAX (SUCKING CHEST WOUND)

Open communication between outer chest wall and pleural space with air moving in and out. Usually results from a large chest stab wound or gunshot wound.

Symptoms/Examination

- Shortness of breath with decreased breath sounds and a sucking chest wound.
- SQ emphysema is common.

Diagnosis

Clinical, based on the presence of air movement or bubbles at the site of a chest wound

Treatment

- Place a three-sided dressing to allow air to exit and not enter the pleural space while preparing for placement of a chest tube. A dressing that completely occludes the wound may cause a tension pneumothorax (PTX).
- Do not insert a chest tube through the wound because it may push foreign material into the chest and may also preferentially follow the injury tract into the lung parenchyma or across the diaphragm.

PNEUMOMEDIASTINUM

Pneumomediastinum is air within the mediastinum. It may occur in the absence of trauma from a ruptured alveoli. After trauma, its presence implies injury to air containing structures in the mediastinum such as larynx, trachea, major bronchi, pharynx, or esophagus.

Symptoms/Examination

- Often asymptomatic
- Findings include SQ emphysema of neck and crunching sound over heart during systole (**Hamman sign**).

Diagnosis/Treatment

- Can be seen on CXR but better visualized by chest CT.
- Further testing to **exclude esophageal injury** (such as an x-ray with oral contrast) may be necessary in patients with a history of penetrating trauma, vomiting, or other mechanism that might implicate the esophagus.
- Treat underlying cause.

> **KEY FACT**
>
> Evaluate possible esophageal injury with a contrast esophagram. Consider endoscopy in patients with a high likelihood of injury.

HEMOTHORAX

Results from traumatic injury to the chest with bleeding from lung parenchyma, intercostal arteries, internal mammary artery, and less commonly, hilar or great vessels. An associated pneumothorax is present in 25% of cases.

Symptoms/Examination

- Diminished or absent breath sounds with dullness to percussion over area of effusion (pneumothorax will have resonant percussion)
- Hypotension if large

> **KEY FACT**
>
> **Lung opacification after trauma:**
>
> Massive hemothorax
>
> Diaphragmatic rupture with herniation
>
> Lung collapse
>
> Pulmonary contusion

DIAGNOSIS

- Upright CXR will show blunting of the costophrenic angle when > **250 mL** blood is present.
- Supine films typically just show haziness from the layering effusion.
- Acute whiteout of 1 hemithorax implies a massive hemothorax, usually associated with mediastinal shift **away** from the hemothorax.

DIFFERENTIAL

Differential includes diaphragmatic rupture with herniation, lung collapse and pulmonary contusion. Pulmonary contusion appearance of CXR is often somewhat delayed.

TREATMENT

- Place large-bore chest tube (36-40 Fr) as smaller ones will clot.
- Initial chest tube output of > 1500 mL (> 20 mL/kg) or persistent output of > 200 mL/h (> 3 mL/kg/h) indicates massive hemothorax and need for thoracotomy.
- Persistent hypotension in the setting of hemothorax is also an indication for surgical intervention even if chest tube output does not cross the above threshold.

> **KEY FACT**
>
> In patients with traumatic hemothorax, initial chest tube output of > 1500 mL or subsequent output of > 200 mL/h are indications for operating room.

COMPLICATIONS

- Infection or late pulmonary fibrosis from undrained or insufficiently drained hemothorax
- Chest tubes can also introduce infection into the chest.

RIB FRACTURES

Rib fractures are the most common significant chest injury in adults (usually ribs 4-9). The primary initial concern is associated injury to underlying structures:

- Hemothorax from injury to major or intercostal vessels
- Liver and/or spleen injury with lower rib fractures (9-11)
- Pneumothorax
- Brachial plexus, great vessels, neck, head, and face injuries are associated with first and second rib fractures from the violent forces involved

> **KEY FACT**
>
> Pediatric bony structures are more pliable than adults. As a result, children are less likely to have rib fractures but more likely to have underlying contusion/injury following blunt trauma.

EXAMINATION/DIAGNOSIS

- Typical presentation is chest wall pain with focal tenderness upon palpation of fractured rib.
- CXR is the initial imaging of choice to look for associated pneumothorax, hemothorax, or pulmonary contusion. About 50% of fractures are not evident on CXR.
- CT can reliably detect fractures and is indicated in patients where multiple fractures or associated injuries are suspected.

> **KEY FACT**
>
> The greater the number of rib fractures, the greater the morbidity and mortality.

TREATMENT

- Pain management and pulmonary toilet with incentive spirometry are the mainstay of therapy.
- Patients with 3 or more rib fractures should be admitted to the hospital. Consider intercostal nerve blocks and thoracic epidural analgesia.
- Patients > 65 years old with 6 or more fractures have a high risk of death and should be admitted to the ICU.

> **KEY FACT**
>
> Patients with 3 or more rib fractures should be admitted.

COMPLICATIONS

Include pneumonia, empyema, respiratory failure, chronic pain

FLAIL CHEST

Flail chest is defined by the presence of fractures in more than 1 location on each of 3 or more adjacent ribs causing a free floating segment of ribs and an unstable chest (Figure 3.13). This results in paradoxical movement with the rest of the chest (in with inspiration and out with expiration).

Symptoms/Examination

- Chest pain with tachycardia and tachypnea.
- Paradoxical movements may initially be difficult to detect, but become more apparent as lung compliance worsens from underlying pulmonary contusion, necessitating greater inspiratory effort.

Diagnosis/Treatment

- Diagnosed by CXR or CT scan showing multiple rib fractures and flail segment.
- Primary treatment is analgesia, coughing and chest physiotherapy, and preventing fluid overload and consequent lung edema. These measures maximize tidal volumes and help prevent hypoxia and pneumonia.
- **Continuous positive airway pressure** ventilation may obviate the need for intubation in patients without significant respiratory distress.
- Early ventilatory support can help reduce mortality of severe flail chest from 69% down to 7%.
- Do not wrap the chest as this inhibits chest expansion.

Complications

Anticipate patient fatigue because of decreased mechanical efficiency causing increased work of breathing.

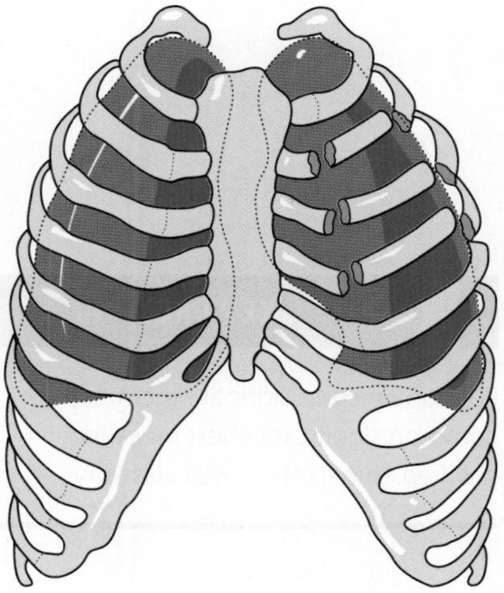

FIGURE 3.13. Diagram of flail chest. (Reproduced, with permission, from Doherty GM. *Current Surgical Diagnosis and Treatment.* 12th ed. New York, NY: McGraw-Hill; 2005:214.)

KEY FACT

In patients with flail chest, pain, hypoexpansion and underlying **lung contusion** are the main causes of hypoxemia.

STERNAL FRACTURE

Typically seen in victims of head-on MVCs, either from anterior chest striking steering wheel or from diagonal part of seat belt restraining upper sternum.

Symptoms/Examination

- Anterior chest pain, often pleuritic.
- Point tenderness.
- Palpable deformity may be present.

Diagnosis/Treatment

- A sternal fracture is usually evident on a **lateral CXR**, but only if you are looking for it. The PA (posteroanterior) or AP film is often normal.
- A CT scan should be obtained to look for associated intrathoracic injuries.
- Pain control and treatment of associated injuries are the mainstay of treatment.
- The presence of an isolated sternal fracture has a low morbidity and mortality and does **not** predict the presence of blunt myocardial injury; patients do not warrant continued monitoring if initial ECG and troponin are normal.

KEY FACT

Restrained passengers are much more likely to have sternal fractures than unrestrained passengers.

PULMONARY CONTUSION

Pulmonary contusion is a compression–decompression injury of the lung parenchyma from blast, blunt, or penetrating injury. It can occur without the presence of rib fracture (especially in children). The uninjured lung may develop pulmonary edema in response to the reflex shunting of blood flow.

Symptoms/Examination

- Hemoptysis is present in up to 50% of pulmonary contusions.
- Other findings include dyspnea, tachypnea, and tachycardia.
- Chest wall bruising or tenderness is usually present.

KEY FACT

Pulmonary contusions are the most common significant chest injury in children, due to chest wall elasticity.

Diagnosis

- Evidence of contusions (patchy infiltrates) appear on CXR **within minutes to 6 hours** (Figure 3.14).
- Appearance on CXR is usually milder than actual extent of damage, which may be better visualized on CT.

Treatment

- Intubate for failure of oxygenation or ventilation.
- Admit all patients to ICU for close monitoring, pain control, and pulmonary toilet.
- There is no benefit to prophylactic antibiotics or steroids.
- Avoid overhydration, when possible.

Complications

The most common complications are pneumonia and acute respiratory distress syndrome (ARDS).

Myocardial Contusion/Blunt Cardiac Injury

Blunt cardiac injury encompasses a spectrum ranging from a minor contusion to myocardial wall rupture. Myocardial contusion is most common, usually affecting the right ventricle. For myocardial wall rupture, 90% of victims die on scene. Other injuries include septal rupture, valvular injuries (aortic most common), coronary artery laceration, or thrombosis. It occurs

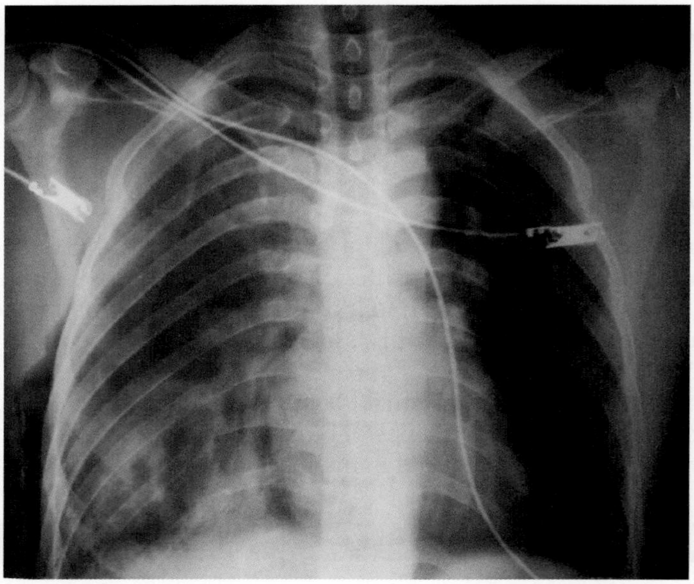

FIGURE 3.14. Pulmonary contusion after blunt chest trauma. (Reproduced, with permission, from Tintinalli JE, Stapczynski S, Ma OJ, et al. *Tintinalli's Emergency Medicine: A Comprehensive Study Guide*. 8th ed. New York, NY: McGraw-Hill, 2015. Figure 261.7.)

most often from high-speed deceleration with blunt impact to chest (often an MVC).

Symptoms/Examination

- Vary with severity of injury.
- Presentation for cardiac contusion includes chest pain, unexplained tachycardia, dysrhythmias (Afib, PACs/PVCs, blocks).

Diagnosis

- There is no diagnostic standard for cardiac contusion.
- ECG and troponin should be obtained for all patients. If both are normal, can effectively rule out blunt myocardial injury.
- Echocardiography is warranted if more serious injury is suspected, especially with unexplained shock, ECG changes (new from prior), or troponin abnormalities.

> **KEY FACT**
>
> A normal ECG and troponin effectively rule out blunt myocardial injury.

Treatment

- Supportive care.
- Evidence of tamponade should raise concern for rupture and warrants surgical intervention.
- Treat hypotension without tamponade with fluids and pressors as needed.
- Patients with suspected myocardial contusion can be safely discharged if initial ECG and troponin are normal. All other patients need admission for continued monitoring.

Complications

- Over half of patients with myocardial contusion will develop a **pericardial effusion,** typically around 2 weeks after injury.

CARDIAC TAMPONADE

Consider cardiac injury in patients with:
- GSW anywhere above the umbilicus
- Stab wound to the left chest, the right chest medial to the midclavicular line, or upper abdomen
- Persistent unexplained hypotension after rapid-deceleration trauma to chest

Symptoms/Examination

Look for signs of tamponade such as Beck's triad and pulsus paradoxus (a reduction in SBP of > 10 mm Hg on inspiration).

> **KEY FACT**
>
> **Beck's triad for cardiac tamponade:**
>
> Hypotension
>
> JVD
>
> Muffled heart sounds

Diagnosis

- A globular cardiac silhouette on CXR may indicate tamponade, but most cases of tamponade have a normal CXR because the pericardium does not have time to expand in the acute setting.
- The cardiac view of eFAST examination is a quick way to detect pericardial blood (Figure 3.15).
- ECG may show electrical alternans - a changing beat to beat changes in QRS amplitude.

Treatment

- Administer fluids to maximize cardiac output.
- For the patient who is not in extremis, start with ultrasound-guided pericardiocentesis. Removal of only 5-10 mL of blood can dramatically improve hemodynamics.

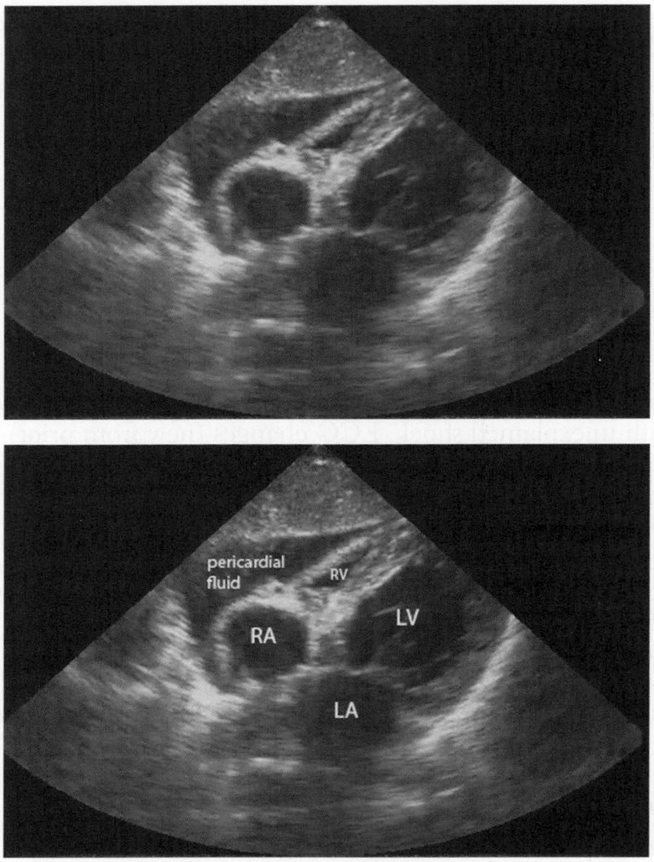

FIGURE 3.15. Positive FAST examination with pericardial fluid. (Reproduced, with permission, from Knoop KJ, Stack LB, Storrow AB, et al. *The Atlas of Emergency Medicine*. 3rd ed. New York, NY: McGraw-Hill Education, 2010. Photographer: Department of Emergency Medicine, Ultrasound Section, Vanderbilt University. Figure 7.9.)

- ED thoracotomy should be performed for patients who have hypotension (BP < 70 mm Hg) unresponsive to resuscitation with ultrasound evidence of cardiac tamponade.

KEY FACT

90% of blunt aortic injuries occur at the isthmus of the aorta, between the left subclavian artery and ligamentum arteriosum.

TRAUMATIC AORTIC INJURY

Consider in the setting of high-speed deceleration, lateral impact MVCs and in presence of multiple rib fractures or flail chest. One-third of blunt aortic injuries have no obvious external thoracic injury. Most injuries occur at the **aortic isthmus** just distal to the left subclavian artery.

SYMPTOMS/EXAMINATION

- Retrosternal or interscapular pain, dysphagia, shortness of breath, hypotension
- Stridor or hoarseness in the absence of laryngeal injury
- Harsh murmur over precordium or space between the scapula
- Signs of superior vena cava syndrome
- Compare BP in upper versus lower extremities: Relative upper extremity hypertension indicates "**pseudocoarctation syndrome**" from a periaortic hematoma

KEY FACT

Symptoms of descending aortic injury include paraplegia (vertebral artery deficits), mesenteric and LE ischemia, and anuria.

DIAGNOSIS

- CXR can show a variety of abnormalities (Table 3.13), but 10% are normal.
  - **Widened mediastinum** to > 8 cm on supine AP film (Figure 3.16) and loss of distinct aortic knob are the most reliable signs.

TABLE 3.13. CXR Findings Suggesting Aortic Injury

Widened mediastinum
Loss of distinct aortic knob
Esophageal or tracheal deviation to right
Widened right paraspinous interface
Widened right paratracheal stripe
Loss of clear space between aortic knob and left pulmonary artery
Left apical cap
Depression of left main stem bronchus 40° below horizontal
Left hemothorax

- CT with contrast is a good test for stable patients.
- Transesophageal echocardiogram can be performed at the bedside in unstable patients.

TREATMENT

- Use β-blockade to control blood pressure (keep SBP < 120 mm Hg and replace fluids carefully to prevent worsening tear/rupture).
- Instruct patient not to Valsalva.
- **Operative repair** is almost always necessary, but there is no clear consensus as to the optimal timing (immediate or delayed) or method (open vs intravascular).

KEY FACT

Half of all patients with traumatic aortic injury who reach the hospital and survive for 1 hour die within 24 hours, and 75% die within 7 days.

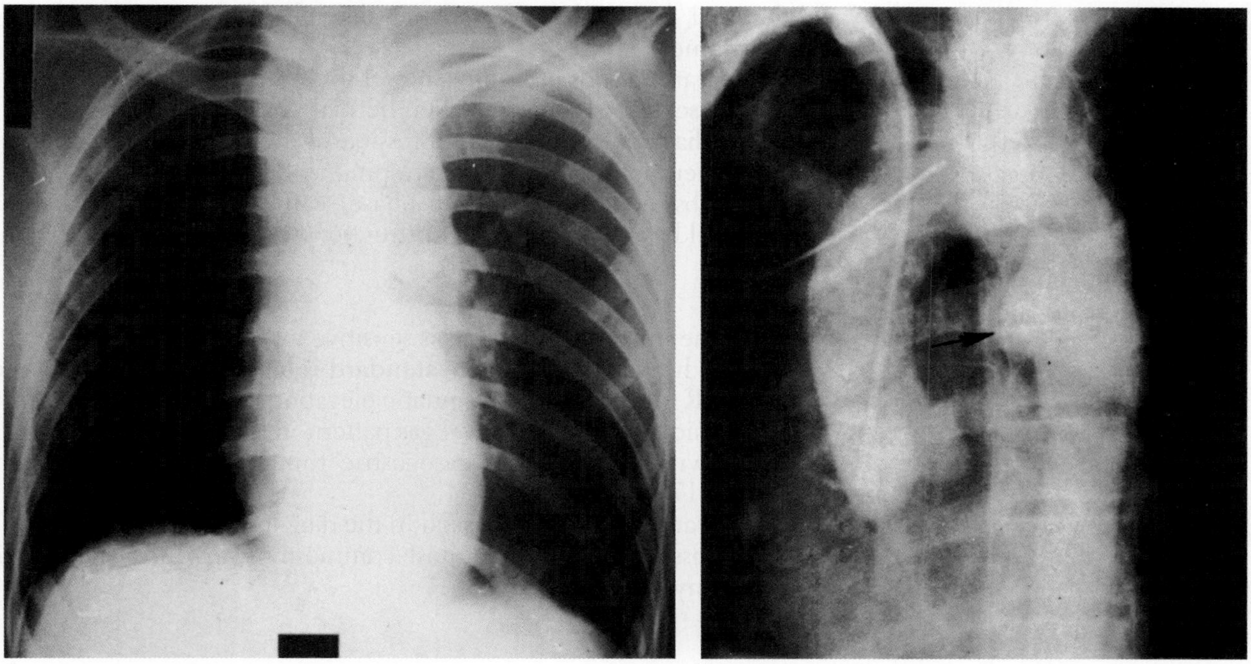

A B

FIGURE 3.16. Traumatic aortic disruption. Anterior-posterior view showing wide mediastinum (**A**). Lateral view with contrast showing defect in the anterior aspect of the descending aorta (**B**). (Reproduced, with permission, from Fuster V, Alexander RW, O'Rourke RA. *Hurst's The Heart.* 12th ed. New York, NY: McGraw-Hill; 2008:2207.)

PENETRATING GREAT VESSEL INJURY

Examination

- The majority of patients with penetrating great vessel injuries will present to ED in extremis from massive blood loss.
- For the stable patient, bruits on auscultation of the chest may be heard.

> **KEY FACT**
>
> Unilateral absence of radial pulse following chest trauma implies subclavian artery occlusion/disruption.

Diagnosis

- Foreign body (eg, bullet) within the chest that appears "fuzzy" on CXR may indicate vascular injury. Blurring of the borders of the foreign body may occur because of movement with cardiac pulsations.
- Diagnosis is typically made in the OR but CTA is indicated for the stable patient.
- Never probe a chest wound or remove an impaled FB because you may dislodge a clot and cause massive hemorrhage.
- Treatment is surgical.

Abdominal Trauma

BLUNT DIAPHRAGMATIC INJURY

Diaphragmatic injury accounts for < 1% of blunt traumatic injuries. It is frequently a missed diagnosis with only 22% of injuries identified initially. The **left diaphragm** is injured three times more often than the right, because of a lack of protection from the liver. Due to low intrathoracic pressures, if a diaphragmatic injury is not repaired abdominal organs can herniate through the defect into the chest.

Symptoms/ Examination

- Abdominal pain radiating to the ipsilateral shoulder (Kehr sign), worse when supine.
- Absent breath sounds or positive bowel sounds in the chest.
- Tension viscerothorax occurs when herniated abdominal contents in chest cause mediastinal shift and compression of the adjacent lung, similar to a tension pneumothorax leading to respiratory distress.
- Visceral obstruction (obstructive phase) can develop, at which time the patient will have signs of bowel obstruction or strangulation.

Diagnosis

- None of the imaging modalities is sensitive for diaphragm injury with minimal or no herniation. The **gold standard is laparoscopy or thoracoscopy.**
- Initial CXR may show diaphragmatic elevation, basilar atelectasis, blurring of left hemidiaphragm, or bowel gas pattern in the hemithorax.
- CXR showing coiling of a nasogastric tube in the chest is diagnostic (Figure 3.17).
- CT, MRI, and contrast studies aid in the diagnosis.
- Look for associated injuries, most commonly liver, lung, spleen, rib, or bowel injury.

Treatment

- Emergent nasogastric decompression is the first step in treatment and should be performed promptly in the ED.
- Definitive treatment is surgical repair.

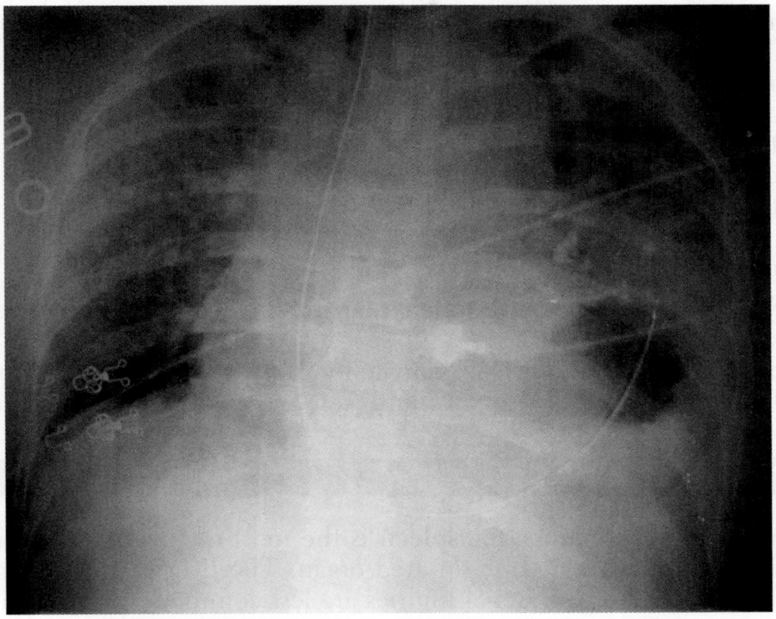

FIGURE 3.17. Diaphragmatic injury with air bubble and nasogastric tube in the L chest. (Reproduced, with permission, from Stone CK, Humphries RL. *Current Diagnosis & Treatment: Emergency Medicine*. 7th ed. New York, NY: McGraw-Hill Education, 2011. Figure 25.3.)

Q

A 14-year-old adolescent boy presents to the ED after falling forward onto the handlebars of his bike. CT scan of the abdomen is negative. The patient complains of persistent pain. What injuries should you be worried about?

Complications

- **Missed injuries tend not to heal** because of the negative intrathoracic pressure promoting upward herniation of abdominal contents. For this reason, all left-sided and most right-sided injuries require surgical repair.
- Diaphragmatic injuries are often **misinterpreted as a hemothorax** and may be treated inappropriately with tube thoracostomy.

BLUNT HOLLOW VISCUS INJURY

Accounts for < 5% of injuries in blunt abdominal trauma and range from hematomas to full thickness lacerations. Blunt hallow viscus injury is often caused by compression of bowel between the spine and a seat belt, steering wheel or handle bar and can be difficult to identify on CT. Injury can occur to the stomach, small or large intestines and when seen with lap belt restraints, is associated with Chance fractures of the lumbar spine.

Symptoms/Examination

- Injury is suggested on physical examination by abdominal wall contusion (seat belt sign) and abdominal tenderness.
- Unlike solid organ injuries, which present with signs of blood loss, hollow viscus injuries tend to cause **delayed peritoneal signs** from developing full-thickness necrosis and subsequent perforation.

Diagnosis

- Free air under the diaphragm on upright CXR or CT is indicative of a full thickness hollow viscus injury with perforation. Additional findings on CT scan concerning for a viscus injury include mesenteric air, discontinuity of bowel wall, extraluminal enteric contrast, free intraabdominal fluid, extravasated IV contrast, bowel wall thickening, and mesenteric hematoma.

KEY FACT

The three abdominal injuries in blunt trauma that are difficult to diagnose with CT imaging are **diaphragm, pancreas, and bowel.**

A

Pancreas and duodenal injuries are classic for this mechanism. An occult diaphragmatic rupture should also be considered.

- Maintain a high index of suspicion in patients that have a seat belt sign with abdominal tenderness and a negative CT.
- Surgical exploration is definitive for the diagnosis, but diagnostic peritoneal lavage (DPL) can also be used to identify perforation (see DPL later in the chapter).
- Focused assessment with sonography for trauma (FAST) examination is not sensitive for hollow viscus injury.

Treatment

- Bowel perforations should undergo laparotomy, while contusions can be observed.
- A period of observation is appropriate for those with negative CT imaging but concerning mechanism for injury.

BLUNT SOLID ORGAN INJURY

In blunt abdominal trauma, the **spleen is the most often injured organ** and two-thirds of the time the only injured organ. The liver is the second most commonly injured organ. Renal injuries are less common. Injury to the pancreas is uncommon and has a similar mechanism to that of blunt hollow viscus injuries, described earlier.

Diagnosis

- A positive FAST is suggestive, although a negative FAST examination does not exclude the possibility of a liver or splenic injury.
- CT with IV contrast is confirmative.
- Lipase and amylase levels are neither sensitive nor specific for pancreatic injury (levels in the injured may be normal, uninjured high); however, they can be used in conjunction with other tests and trended.

KEY FACT

A positive FAST in blunt abdominal trauma is most likely due to splenic injury.

Treatment

- In hemodynamically stable patients, liver and splenic injuries can often be treated expectantly rather than surgically. Hemodynamically unstable patients with a positive FAST examination should undergo an emergent laparotomy.
- Surgery is often required for splenic injuries grade III or higher.
- High-grade liver injuries have a higher likelihood of requiring surgical intervention; however, these can be managed nonoperatively as long as the patient is hemodynamically stable.
- Interventional radiology is taking on an increasingly greater role in the treatment of solid organ injury, using embolization to help delay or prevent surgical intervention.

KEY FACT

Management of solid organ injury is based on hemodynamic status and transfusion requirements rather than injury grade.

Penetrating Abdominal Injury

Around 70% of anterior stab wounds penetrate the peritoneum, and 50% of those cause organ damage. A lower chest stab wound has a 15% chance of causing intra-abdominal injury. The dome of the diaphragm can rise as high as T4 on expiration, so any injury below this may involve the diaphragm or abdomen.

The most commonly injured organs in penetrating trauma are:

- Stab wound: Liver first, then small bowel (both have large surface areas)
- GSW: Small bowel, then colon, then liver

Diagnosis/Treatment

- Penetrating trauma with peritonitis requires immediate surgery.
- Stab wounds to the abdomen may be evaluated using **local wound exploration**. Digital probing or injection of contrast is not recommended.
- Triple contrast CT scans (CT with PO, IV, and rectal contrast) can be used to evaluate a penetrating abdominal injury, especially if direct exploration is not possible or is inconclusive. PO contrast helps identify small bowel injuries, while rectal contrast helps delineate colonic injuries. An extended PO contrast preparation is not required.
- Observation with serial examinations without imaging is an acceptable method of evaluating penetrating abdominal trauma patients with a low clinical suspicion for significant injury.

STUDIES IN ABDOMINAL TRAUMA

Extended Focused Assessment With Sonography for Trauma (eFAST)

Technique

- Visualize the following areas using a low-frequency probe (high frequency/linear probe can be used to visualize the lungs for better resolution):
  - Hepatorenal (Morison) space (Figure 3.18)
  - Splenorenal space
  - Pouch of Douglas/rectouterine space (females) or rectovesicular space (males)
  - Pericardium (see Figure 3.15)
  - Lungs (place probe anteriorly over both third and fourth intercostal spaces)

Interpretation of Results

- Presence of intraabdominal free fluid:
  - Indicates a need for exploratory laparotomy in the hemodynamically unstable patient.

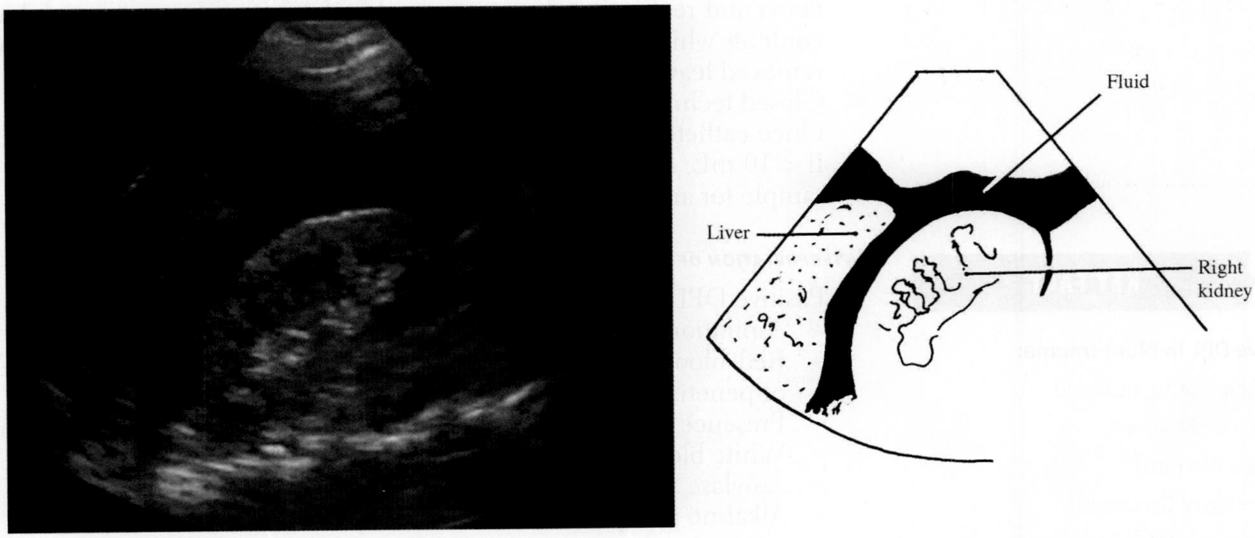

FIGURE 3.18. Positive FAST examination with fluid stripe in hepatorenal space. (Reproduced, with permission, from Knoop KJ, Stack LB, Storrow AB. *Atlas of Emergency Medicine*. 2nd ed. New York, NY: McGraw-Hill, 2002. Photographer: Michael J. Lambert, MD, RDMS.)

- Serves as tool to expedite CT and surgical consultation in the stable patient.
- eFAST is specific for presence of fluid but cannot identify source.
- False-positive eFAST examinations may be found in patients who have ascites and in females who may have a small amount of physiologic free fluid in the pouch of Douglas.
- Presence of pericardial fluid is sensitive and specific for pericardial effusion, but cannot localize source.
- Presence of lung slide (movement of visceral pleura over parietal pleural during inspiration/expiration) is sensitive and specific for the *absence* of a pneumothorax.
- A normal eFAST examination does not *exclude* injury. Observe or obtain further imaging on patients with suspected injuries that have a negative eFAST examination.

KEY FACT

The eFAST examination should be done SLOWLY to ensure an adequate examination.

The eFAST examination can also be serially performed for increased sensitivity.

DIAGNOSTIC PERITONEAL LAVAGE

KEY FACT

DPL has been largely replaced by CT and FAST in the evaluation of blunt abdominal trauma.

Indications

- Blunt abdominal trauma where CT or FAST is not obtainable or is equivocal.
- High suspicion for hollow viscus injury with negative or equivocal CT imaging.

Technique

- Decompression of stomach and bladder is recommended before procedure.
- Always use sterile technique to prevent infection.
- Anesthetize the infraumbilical skin and soft tissue with 1% lidocaine with epinephrine.
- Exceptions to infraumbilical approach:
  - Pelvic fractures: Perform open and above the umbilicus to prevent false-positives due to pelvic hematomas.
  - Pregnant patients: Perform above the level of the uterus.
  - Midline scarring: Perform open and lateral to rectus abdominus in left lowe quadrant
- Semiopen technique: Skin incision is made and subcutaneous tissue dissected down to the linea alba; a small incision is made in the linea alba; fascia and rectus muscles are grasped and raised up away from abdominal contents while trocar and catheter are advanced into peritoneum; trocar is removed leaving catheter in peritoneum.
- Closed technique: Seldinger (guidewire) technique.
- Once catheter is in place, attempt aspiration blood from peritoneal cavity. If < 10 mL, instill warmed 1 L bag of IVF, drain fluid by gravity and send sample for analysis.

Interpretation of Results

- Positive DPL is defined as:
  - Aspiration of 10 mL of free flowing blood
  - Red blood cells (RBC) count >100,000/mm^3; 10,000/mm^3 for GSWs or penetrating injury to lower chest
  - Presence of gastrointestinal (GI) contents (bile, food, fecal material)
  - White blood cell (WBC) > 500/mm^3
  - Amylase > 20 IU/L
  - Alkaline phosphatase ≥ 3 IU/L

KEY FACT

Positive DPL in blunt trauma:

Aspiration of 10 mL blood

>100,000 RBCs/mm^3

WBCs > 500 mm^3

Aspiration of GI contents

Amylase > 20 IU/L

Alkaline phosphatase ≥ 3 IU/L

Complications

- Major complications (eg, bowel injury, bleeding, infection) are uncommon.

INDICATIONS FOR SURGERY

Blunt

- Abdominal injury (free fluid by FAST or DPL) Positive FAST or DPL with hypotension
- Evisceration of abdominal wall contents
- Peritonitis
- Free air under diaphragm on imaging or aspiration of GI contents on DPL
- Injuries to diaphragm, aorta, or kidney injury with urine leaking outside of Gerota fascia
- Persistent blood from NGT, rectum or vagina

Penetrating

- Injury with hypotension
- Peritonitis
- Evisceration of abdominal contents through wound
- Positive FAST or DPL with hypotension
- Any GSW to the abdomen that is believed to have entered the peritoneum based on projectile trajectory
- Local wound exploration that reveals violation of abdominal wall
- Foreign body in abdomen
- Suspected diaphragmatic injury
- Blood from NGT, rectum or vagina

> **KEY FACT**
>
> For penetrating trauma > 10,000 RBCs/mm^3 is considered a positive DPL.

> **KEY FACT**
>
> Initial hemoglobin level may not reveal significant bleeding, as may take time for volume to be replaced by extracellular fluid. Serial values will show a trend.

Trauma in Pregnancy

Trauma affects 6%-7% of pregnancies in the United States and is the leading cause of nonobstetric maternal death. Pregnant women who experience trauma have a higher incidence of serious abdominal injury but a low incidence of chest and head trauma. After 12 weeks of gestation, the maternal uterus and bladder are no longer shielded by the pelvis and are more susceptible to injury. After 16 weeks of gestation, placental abruption is a concern. The most common direct fetal injury is skull fractures, which confers a 42% fetal mortality.

MECHANISMS

- MVCs account for half of trauma in pregnancy. Failure to wear a **seat belt** and placement of the lap belt over the pregnant abdomen increases the risk of fetal death.
- Intimate partner violence during pregnancy is also common with the abdomen being the most common site of injury.

SYMPTOMS/EXAMINATION

- Changes in normal vital signs in pregnant patients may complicate the evaluation of the injured pregnant patient:
  - Baseline heart rate increases by 10-15 bpm.
  - Baseline BP decreases in the first and second trimesters.
  - In the third trimester, supine hypotension may occur due to **uterine compression of the inferior vena cava**. Positioning the patient in the **left lateral decubitus position** may improve venous return.
- The normal fetal heart rate is **120-160 bpm**. An abnormal rate suggests fetal distress.
- The diaphragm rises an extra 4 cm into the thoracic cavity.

KEY FACT

Consider abuse in injured pregnant patients, particularly those with abdominal injury who report a fall or with multiple trauma-related ED visits.

KEY FACT

A Pco_2 of 40 mm Hg during the latter half of pregnancy suggests hypoventilation.

KEY FACT

Fetal viability: 24-week gestation, dome of uterus above umbilicus.

- Signs of placental abruption include spontaneous rupture of membranes, vaginal bleeding and uterine tenderness.
- The presence of vaginal discharge mandates a speculum examination to assess for rupture of membranes (ferning, pH > 7).
- Continuous fetal monitoring should be initiated in patients beyond 24 weeks of gestation, even with minor trauma. Abnormal rates and decelerations after a uterine contraction indicate fetal distress and may also be a marker of occult maternal distress.

Diagnosis

- Changes in normal laboratory values during pregnancy complicate interpretation in the trauma patient:
  - Baseline hematocrit is decreased to 32%-34%.
  - Baseline Pco_2 is decreased to 30 mm Hg.
  - Baseline serum bicarbonate is decreased to 21 mEq/L.
- Physical examination of the abdomen is less reliable in pregnancy due to enlargement of the uterus and realignment of the abdominal organs.
- **Ultrasound** is the initial modality of choice both for evaluating for intra-abdominal bleeding (FAST) and for assessing gestational age and fetal viability.
- Because of concerns about radiation exposure, CT of the abdomen is usually inappropriate in stable patients who can be observed and undergo serial abdominal examinations, but imaging of the abdomen should not be withheld if there is a high clinical concern for injury.
- For women > 20 weeks of gestation, large amounts of fetomaternal hemorrhage may occur and the **Kleihauer-Betke test** should be used to guide the administration of extra vials of RhoGAM.

Treatment

- Tube thoracostomy when indicated, should be performed above the fourth intercostal space (ICS) in the anterior axillary line. DPL should be performed above the level of the uterus.
- Management of an unstable mother with a fetus showing signs of distress should primarily **focus on resuscitating the mother** and stabilizing or repairing her injuries.
- Emergent C-section is indicated if the fetus is viable (> 24 weeks) and shows signs of distress, uterine rupture, placental abruption, or premature labor with fetal malpresentation *and* the mother can tolerate the procedure.
- In the case of maternal cardiac arrest with estimated fetal age > 24 weeks, a perimortem C-section should be performed **if no ROSC by 4 minutes of resuscitative efforts.** (see Chapter 19, Procedures and Skills).

Pelvic Fractures

Pelvic fractures may be divided into major ring fractures, acetabular fractures, and avulsion/single bone fractures.

ACETABULAR FRACTURES

Acetabular fractures have a bimodal distribution. In young patients, they are frequently due to high energy MVCs where the knee is thrust into the dashboard. In elderly patients, acetabular fractures are usually associated with a low energy mechanism such as a fall.

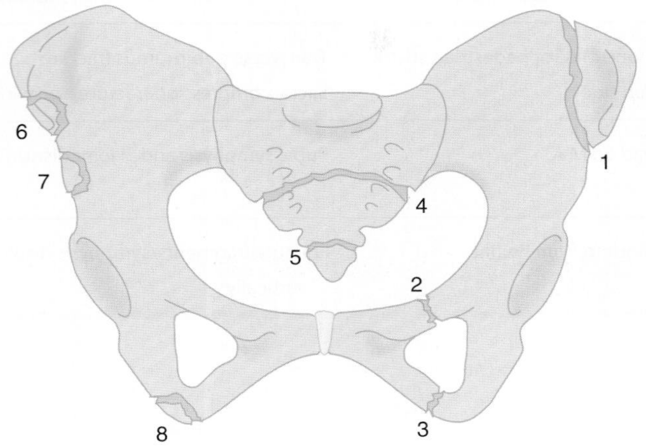

FIGURE 3.19. Avulsion fractures of the pelvis. 1. Iliac wing fracture (Duverney fracture). 2. Superior pubic ramus fracture. 3. Inferior pubic ramus fracture. 4. Transverse sacral fracture. 5. Coccyx fracture. 6. Anterior superior iliac spine avulsion. 7. Anterior inferior iliac spine avulsion. 8. Ischial tuberosity avulsion. (Reproduced, with permission, from Tintinalli JE, Kelen GD, Stapczynski JS. *Emergency Medicine: A Comprehensive Study Guide.* 6th ed. New York, NY: McGraw-Hill;2004:1718.)

Diagnosis/Treatment

- CT is better than x-ray at detecting these fractures.
- Treatment is with operative repair or conservative management based on specific characteristics of the fracture.

AVULSION FRACTURES

Pelvic avulsion fractures occur when a fragment of bone tears away from the main structure. They are most prevalent in the adolescent age group and occur at unfused apophysis at the level of tendon attachment. They commonly occur from rapid, strong muscular contractions during athletic activities, but can also occur from falls (Figure 3.19). Most of these are treated nonoperatively.

MAJOR RING FRACTURES

Major ring pelvic fractures are usually classified by the Young-Burgess Classification System which separates the fractures by vector of force into lateral compression (most common), AP compression and vertical shear fractures (Table 3.14 and Figures 3.20-3.22). Retroperitoneal bleeding is common with these injuries and results from injury to low pressure veins. The vertical shear fracture has the highest incidence of associated severe hemorrhage.

Symptoms

- Pain and tenderness of pelvis; most patients are unable to ambulate.
- Perineal or pelvic edema/ecchymosis/laceration/deformity.
- Hematoma above inguinal ligament or over scrotum (**Destot sign**).

Q

A 27-year-old male is brought in by EMS after a 20-foot fall, landing on his back. He is tachycardic and has a grossly unstable pelvis. eFAST is negative. What bedside maneuver can you perform to help limit ongoing blood loss?

TABLE 3.14. Young-Burgess Classification of Major Pelvic Fractures

Type	Incidence[a]	Mechanism	Radiographic Findings
Lateral compression	45%-50%	T-bone MVC or pedestrian struck on side	Transverse pubic ramus fracture Sacral compression fracture Iliac wing fracture
Anteroposterior compression (open book)	25%	Head on MVC	Pubic symphysis and SI joint disruption
Vertical shear	5%	Fall/jump from height	Fracture fragments/symphysis displaced vertically

MVC, motor vehicle collision; SI, sacroiliac.

[a]The remaining 20%-25% result in a combination of the above types.

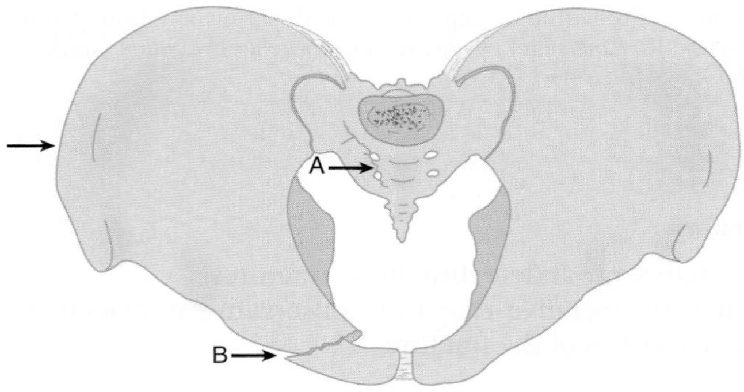

FIGURE 3.20. Lateral compression fracture. Note the horizontal fracture pattern. (Reproduced, with permission, from Tintinalli JE, Stapczynski S, Ma OJ, et al. *Tintinalli's Emergency Medicine: A Comprehensive Study Guide*. 7th ed. New York, NY: McGraw-Hill, 2011. Figure 269.5.)

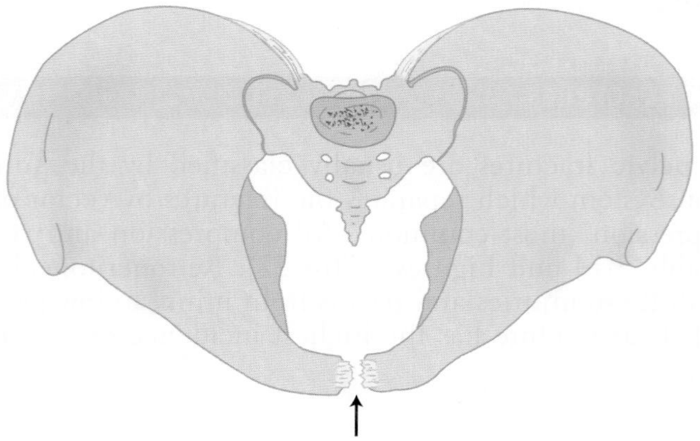

FIGURE 3.21. Anteroposterior compression fracture with opening of the pubic symphysis. (Reproduced, with permission, from Tintinalli JE, Stapczynski S, Ma OJ, et al. *Tintinalli's Emergency Medicine: A Comprehensive Study Guide*. 7th ed. New York, NY: McGraw-Hill, 2011. Figure 269.10.)

A

Apply a pelvic binder at the level of the greater trochanters.

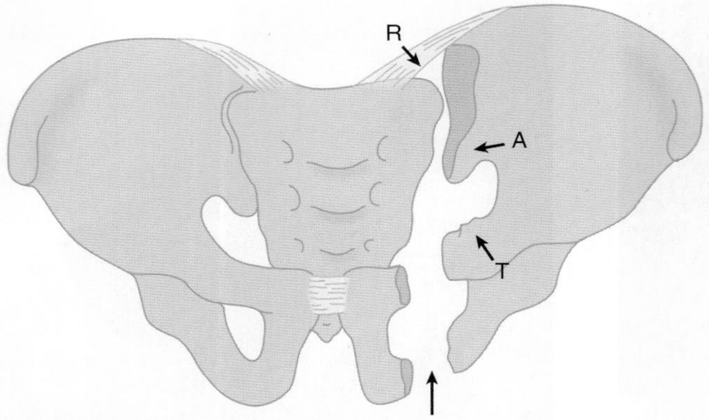

FIGURE 3.22. Vertical shear fracture. Note the vertical fracture pattern. (Reproduced, with permission, from Tintinalli JE, Stapczynski S, Ma OJ, et al. *Tintinalli's Emergency Medicine: A Comprehensive Study Guide*. 7th ed. New York, NY: McGraw-Hill, 2011. Figure 269.13.)

EXAMINATION

- Compress pelvis medially at iliac crests and anteroposteriorly at symphysis pubis. If instability exists, minimize further movement and examinations of the pelvis.
- Perform rectal, perineal, and vaginal examinations for lacerations indicating an open pelvic fracture.
- Palpate prostate for superior or posterior displacement suggesting intraperitoneal or urologic injury. Abnormal prostate position or blood at the urethral meatus requires **urethrogram prior to Foley placement** to assess for urethral injury.

> **KEY FACT**
>
> **Signs of Retroperitoneal Hemorrhage**
>
> Grey-Turner sign (flank ecchymosis)
>
> Cullen sign (bruising around umbilicus).

DIAGNOSIS

- Initial AP plain film of pelvis will show most fractures (Figure 3.23).
- Displacement of ring fractures may be better defined with inlet (superior–inferior) and outlet (anterior–posterior) views.
- Oblique (Judet) views better define acetabular fractures.
- When 1 part of the pelvic ring has been fractured, always look for a second fracture or opening. Double ring fractures are unstable.

> **KEY FACT**
>
> One-third of all pelvic fractures involve individual bones but not the ring.

TREATMENT

- Patients with pubic symphysis widening should be treated with a pelvic binder (such as bed sheets) at the level of the **greater trochanter**, or external fixation to minimize the volume of the pelvis and help control bleeding.
- Signs of ongoing bleeding or hemorrhagic shock without other cause identified is indication for fracture fixation and angiography or pelvic packing.
- Displaced pelvic ring fractures require operative repair.
- Open pelvic fractures require antibiotics, tetanus booster and operative repair.
  - For patients with multiple abdominal/pelvic bleeding sources or open pelvic fractures, operative fixation and extraperitoneal pelvic packing is considered first-line therapy.
  - For patients without other operative injuries, angiography can help control bleeding through arterial embolization, although **the bleeding is often venous**. Indications for embolization include:

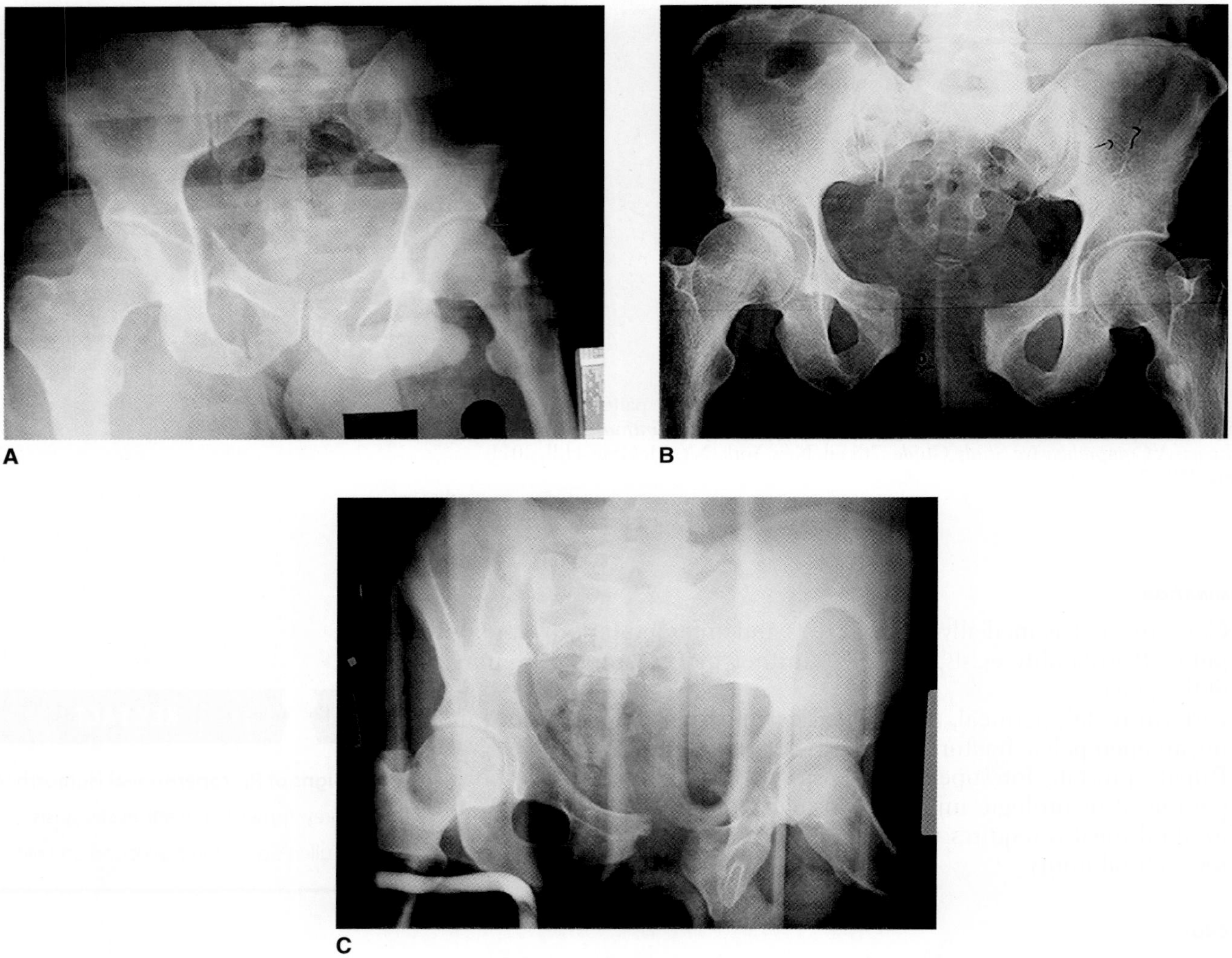

FIGURE 3.23. The 3 types of mechanically unstable pelvic fractures: (A) Lateral compression, (B) Anteroposterior compression, (C) Vertical shear. (Reproduced, with permission, from Brunicardi FC, Andersen DK, Billiar TR, et al. *Schwartz's Principles of Surgery*. 10th ed. New York, NY: McGraw-Hill Education, 2015. Figure 7.30.)

> **KEY FACT**
>
> Perform a bimanual vaginal examination on all women with pelvic fractures. Vaginal lacerations are most commonly seen with anterior pelvic fractures and usually require operative repair.

- Persistent hypovolemia/hypotension after treatment of other sources of bleeding
- Four units packed red blood cells (PRBC)/24 hours or six units PRBC/48 hours
- Large pelvic hematoma on CT

Hip Dislocation

Hip dislocations may be **anterior** (due to an anterior and a medial force applied to the abducted leg), **central** (direct impact through acetabulum) or **posterior** (posterior force through a flexed knee). Posterior dislocations are the most common (80%-90%).

POSTERIOR HIP DISLOCATION

Typically result from a head-on MVC with the knee hitting the dashboard and the body moving forward over a fixed femur; often associated with posterior wall/lip fractures of the acetabulum (Figure 3.24).

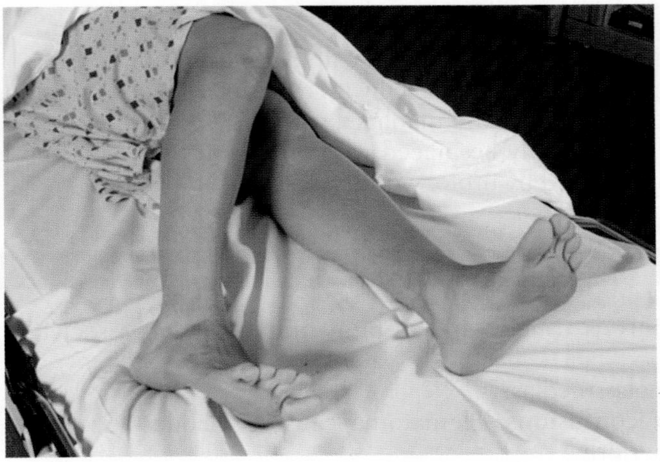

FIGURE 3.24. Right Posterior hip dislocation. (Reproduced, with permission, from Tintinalli JE, Stapczynski S, Ma OJ, et al. *Tintinalli's Emergency Medicine: A Comprehensive Study Guide*. 7th ed. New York, NY: McGraw-Hill, 2011. Figure 269-7B.)

Q

A 30-year-old man arrives in the ED after a 10-foot fall with perineal/pelvic pain and inability to void. Rectal examination reveals a high-riding prostate. What is the most appropriate next step?

EXAMINATION/DIAGNOSIS

- Extremity is shortened, internally rotated, and adducted.
- X-ray is confirmative.

TREATMENT/COMPLICATIONS

- Closed reduction under conscious sedation as soon as possible to restore blood supply to the femoral head
- Sciatic nerve injury may occur
- **Complication to avoid: Avascular necrosis of the femoral head due to prolonged dislocation**

Genitourinary Trauma

URETHRA

Injury to the anterior urethra is commonly due to a straddle injury (most common), direct blow, instrumentation, or penile fracture. Posterior urethral injury typically results from a significant pelvic fracture with associated shearing force to bladder and urethra. Urethral injury is more common in men due to longer urethral length and attachments to the pubis.

SYMPTOMS/EXAMINATION

- Blood at the urethra meatus and an inability to void are common symptoms.
- In females, urethral injury is often associated with vaginal bleeding.
- Anterior urethral injury: "Butterfly" perineal hematoma.
- Posterior urethral injury: Perineal hematoma and high-riding prostate on rectal examination.

DIAGNOSIS

Retrograde urethrogram (RUG) will demonstrate the injury and should always be performed before placing a Foley in the setting of meatal blood or a high-riding prostate and suspected pelvic fracture.

A

Obtain a retrograde urethrogram to rule out the presence of a urethral injury. This should always follow more critical resuscitative procedures, but must be done prior to Foley placement.

Treatment

- Contusions heal with or without catheter placement.
- Partial lacerations are managed with a catheter placed by urology.
- Complete lacerations are managed surgically.
- A Foley should only be placed when the path of the urethra is still intact and is best placed by urology under direct visualization.

BLADDER

Bladder injury is usually due to blunt trauma, often associated with pelvic fractures.

Injuries are classified as:

- **Bladder contusions:** Hematoma causing bladder to change shape and shift superiorly
- **Extraperitoneal bladder rupture:** Tearing and rupture at bladder neck from shearing forces of anterior pelvic fracture; no communication to peritoneum
- **Intraperitoneal bladder rupture:** Rupture of distended bladder at its dome, leading to leakage of urine into peritoneum

KEY FACT

Degree of hematuria does not always correlate with the degree of injury.

KEY FACT

Blood at urethral meatus mandates RUG before Foley placement.

Symptoms/Examination

- Abdominal pain and tenderness
- Gross or microscopic hematuria
- Inability to void
- Peritonitis (if intraperitoneal rupture)

Diagnosis

- Retrograde cystogram (plain film or CT) is test of choice: 400 mL (5 mL/kg in children) of contrast is instilled into bladder via a Foley catheter. The Foley is then clamped. Simply clamping the Foley and allowing the bladder to passively fill will miss half the injuries.
- Extraperitoneal rupture: Contrast will extravasate into surrounding tissue in a flame pattern (Figure 3.25).

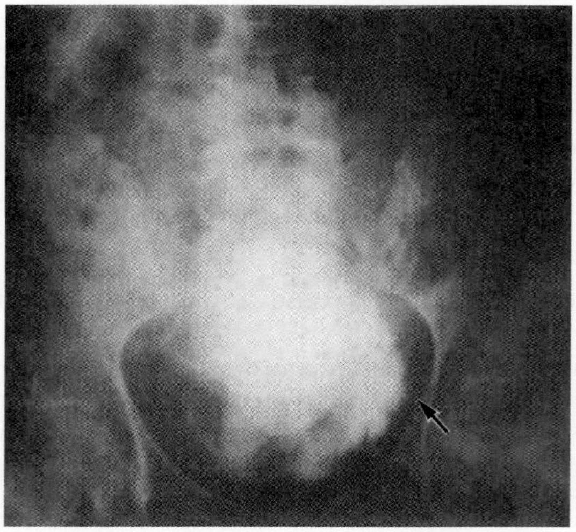

FIGURE 3.25. Extraperitoneal bladder rupture seen on retrograde cystogram with contrast surrounding bladder in pelvis. (Reproduced, with permission, from McAninch JW, Lue TF. *Smith and Tanagho's General Urology*. 18th ed. New York, NY: McGraw-Hill Education, 2013. Figure 18.12.)

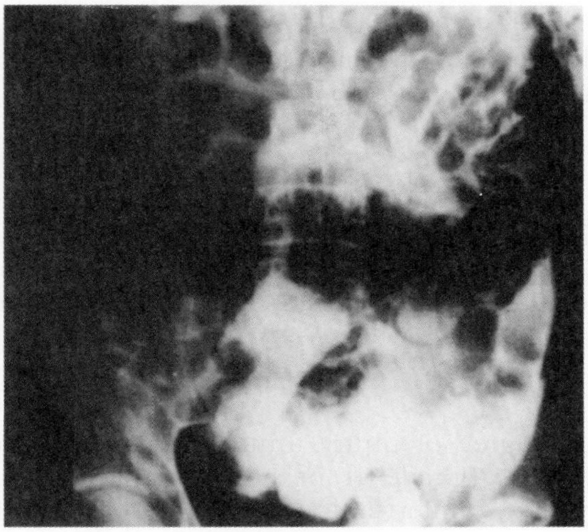

FIGURE 3.26. Intraperitoneal bladder rupture seen on retrograde cystogram with contrast surrounding loops of bowel. (Reproduced, with permission, from Tanagho EA, McAninch JW. *Smith's General Urology*. 17th ed. New York, NY: McGraw-Hill; 2008:290.)

- Intraperitoneal rupture: Contrast will leak into cul-de-sac posterior to bladder and surround loops of bowel (Figure 3.26).

TREATMENT

- **Surgery for intraperitoneal rupture** and penetrating injuries
- Foley catheter decompression for 10-14 days for incomplete lacerations or extraperitoneal rupture
- No intervention necessary for contusions

URETER

Ureteral injury is usually due to penetrating trauma or iatrogenic during abdominal/pelvic surgery.

SYMPTOMS/EXAMINATION

- Hematuria (rarely present with complete tears)
- Flank pain

DIAGNOSIS

CT with IV contrast or intravenous pyelogram (IVP) is initial imaging of choice.

TREATMENT

Most ureteral injuries require intervention via surgical repair or interventional radiology (IR) stenting.

KIDNEY

The kidneys are fairly protected in the retroperitoneal space, so significant forces are typically involved. Injuries are graded I-V based on degree of injury ranging from a minor contusion or subcapsular hematoma (Grade I) to complete avulsion of the renal hilum (Grade V).

KEY FACT

IVP or cystogram in patients who have received oral contrast may be difficult to interpret due to a background of abdominal contrast.

KEY FACT

Significant blunt force is necessary to damage the kidneys because they are so well protected.

> **KEY FACT**
>
> **Isolated microscopic hematuria does not mandate further imaging.**
>
> Exceptions include:
>
> Rapid deceleration injuries where renal pedicles can be damaged
>
> Hematuria in a patient with even transient hypotension
>
> Hematuria following penetrating trauma to the flank

Symptoms/Examination

Patients typically present with flank bruising and/or tenderness along with microscopic or gross hematuria.

Diagnosis

- CT with IV contrast. A one-shot IVP can be performed in the OR for the unstable patient.
- When the CT or IVP fails to demonstrate contrast to kidney, a renal pedicle injury should be suspected. Further imaging with an angiogram and/or venogram should occur.

Treatment

Depends on the degree of injury. Injuries with lacerations of > 1 cm depth into renal cortex (Grade III) or those with vascular injury (Grades IV and V) typically require intervention (IR or OR, depending on stability of patient).

PENILE INJURY

Injury ranges from a simple laceration to a fracture or amputation. Penile fracture results from traumatic rupture of the corpus cavernosum (see also Chapter 18, Renal and Genitourinary Emergencies), most commonly caused by blunt trauma to erect penis during sexual intercourse with penis striking perineum, pubic symphysis, desk, etc.

Symptoms/Examination

- Depend on type of injury.
- With penile fracture, patient often reports cracking sound and pain, with rapid detumescence.

Treatment

- Fractures are treated surgically with immediate hematoma evacuation and **repair of tunica albuginea**.
- Amputations must be reattached within 8-12 hours. The amputated penis should be wrapped in saline-soaked gauze, placed in a sterile bag and then placed on ice. Cooling prolongs viability.
- Skin lacerations can be repaired with 4-0 absorbable suture. Skin avulsions usually require grafting.

TESTICULAR TRAUMA

Trauma to the testicles may result in hematoma, contusion, laceration, fracture, or dislocation into the superficial scrotal pouch, inguinal canal, or abdominal cavity.

Examination/Diagnosis

- A swollen, bruised scrotum with absent testis is c/w traumatic dislocation of testis.
- Color Doppler ultrasound of testis will help determine severity of injury by assessing blood flow and hematoma formation.

Treatment

- Laceration, disruption, and dislocation of testis mandate operative repair.
- All other injuries can be managed with ice, rest, and pain control.

Soft-Tissue Trauma

COMPARTMENT SYNDROME

Occurs when compartment pressure gets high enough to prevent adequate perfusion, resulting in tissue ischemia. It can occur in closed or open fractures. It is most commonly associated with midshaft fractures of the tibia.

Mechanisms

- Constriction around the compartment
  - Cast or external wrapping
  - Deep circumferential burns
- Swelling within the compartment
  - Hemorrhage
  - **Fractures** (tibia, forearm, supracondylar)
  - Crush injury
  - Drug or medication injections
  - Ischemic and/or reperfusion injury

Anatomy

- Two arm compartments: Anterior, posterior
- Two forearm compartments: Dorsal, volar
- Four hand compartments: Thenar, hypothenar, central, interossei
- Three gluteal compartments: Gluteus maximus, gluteus medius and minimus, and tensor fascia latae
- Three thigh compartments: Anterior, medial, posterior
- Four leg compartments: Anterior, lateral, superficial posterior, deep posterior
- Four foot compartments: Medial, lateral, central, interosseous

Pathophysiology

- Normal compartment pressure is 0-10 mm Hg. At 20 mm Hg, capillary blood flow is affected, and at > 30-40 mm Hg muscles and nerves can undergo ischemic necrosis.
- Nerves are the first structure to be affected by compartment syndrome leading to loss of 2-point discrimination.
- Even at elevated compartment pressures, arteries and arterioles are often not affected and therefore loss of pulse is a late finding.

Symptoms/Examination

- Tense compartment/extremity
- Pain out of proportion to injury or physical findings
- Pain with passive stretch of muscle
- Paresthesias with decreased sensation
- Paresis
- Distal pulses, perfusion, and capillary refill are unreliable (arterial insufficiency is a late finding).

Diagnosis

- Primarily a clinical diagnosis.
- Compartment pressure of 30 mm Hg is considered by some to be diagnostic of compartment syndrome. However, both false positives and false negatives are seen and interventions should be based on the whole clinical picture and not just the measurement.

Q

A 24-year-old man presents with severe pain in his left calf after his leg was run over by a car. The calf appears tense. The x-ray is normal. What diagnosis should be considered?

KEY FACT

Most common compartment in compartment syndrome? Anterior compartment of leg.

KEY FACT

Loss of pulse is a late finding in compartment syndrome. Do not exclude the diagnosis based on the presence of a pulse. Severe pain may be your only clue to this diagnosis.

KEY FACT

Pain out of proportion to examination:

- Compartment syndrome
- Mesenteric ischemia
- Necrotizing fasciitis

KEY FACT

The 5 Ps of compartment syndrome are pain, pain, pain, pain, and pain. Waiting for further findings leads to a delay in diagnosis and worse outcomes!

A

Severe pain or pain out of proportion to physical examination findings suggests compartment syndrome.

Treatment

- Always remove any external wrapping or compressive force.
- < 15 mm Hg: No treatment is needed.
- 20-30 mm Hg: Maintain close observation and repeat measurements.
- > 30 mm Hg: Consider fasciotomy.
- **Avoid fasciotomy following snake bites**. Extremity snake bites may cause increased compartment pressure, but animal studies show worse outcomes with fasciotomy.

PERIPHERAL VASCULAR INJURIES

Traumatic peripheral vascular injuries can be due to complete transection of the vessel (most common) or an incomplete injury with resultant thrombosis, spasm, arteriovenous (AV) fistula, or pseudoaneurysm. The degree of distal perfusion varies with type of injury, degree of spasm, etc.

Symptoms/Examination

Hard Signs of Arterial Injury (90% chance of injury; immediate surgery indicated)

- Pulsatile bleeding
- Audible bruit/palpable thrill
- Rapidly expanding hematoma
- Obvious arterial occlusion
- Decreased temperature

Soft signs of arterial injury (further investigation indicated)

- History of arterial bleeding
- Proximity to major artery
- Diminished distal pulse
- Peripheral nerve injury (next to vasculature)
- Small nonpulsatile hematoma
- Abnormal flow velocity on Doppler
- Arterial pressure index of < 0.9 (also known as ankle-brachial index [ABI] for lower extremity)

MNEMONIC

The 6 Ps of arterial occlusion:

Pain
Pallor
Pulselessness
Paresthesia
Paralysis
Poikilothermia

KEY FACT

Arterial pressure index:

Doppler SBP of ankle/forearm on injured extremity (cuff inflated distal to injury)
divided by
Doppler brachial SBP of uninjured extremity

Diagnosis

- In the presence of hard signs for arterial injury the diagnosis is confirmed in the OR.
- With soft signs for arterial injury, observation or further investigation is warranted:
  - Duplex scan—real time B-mode ultrasound with Doppler
  - Arteriography.
- Knee dislocations have a high risk of popliteal artery injury and in the past have required routine angiography. Current thinking suggests, however, that a knee dislocation with normal postreduction ABI may be observed with serial examinations and ABIs.

KEY FACT

In the setting of nerve injury, always consider vascular injury as **nerves and vessels usually travel together.**

KEY FACT

Knee dislocations have a high risk for popliteal artery injury.

Treatment

- Direct pressure to stop bleeding.
- Tourniquet if there is life-threatening bleeding not responsive to direct pressure. Document time placed and do not leave for > 120 minutes. Do not clamp or tie off vessels.
- Hypotensive resuscitation (controversial): Keep SBP around 90 mm Hg prior to surgical repair to prevent dislodging clot and persistent bleeding.
- Major arterial injuries must be repaired within six hours.

- Minor arterial injuries (intact distal circulation, no active hemorrhage, and < 5-mm intimal flap or pseudoaneurysm on angiogram) can be closely observed. Be cautious with children and vasculopaths.
- Major venous injuries usually require repair.

COMPLICATIONS

- As with compartment syndrome, ischemic muscle contracture resulting from nerve and muscle damage may occur.
- Prolonged ischemia may require amputation.

> **KEY FACT**
>
> In penetrating extremity trauma, always perform bilateral ABIs.

AMPUTATION/REPLANTATION

Amputated appendages can tolerate 6-8 hours of warm ischemia and 12-24 hours of cold ischemia at 4°C. Digits tolerate ischemia better than limbs. Fingertip amputation are the most common and fit into 4 categories:

- Zone I: Distal amputation in which the bone and nail bed are intact
- Zone II: **Exposed bone** of distal phalanx
- Zone III: Amputation of entire nail bed
- Zone IV: Amputation near distal interphalangeal joint (DIP) joint

TREATMENT

- To protect amputated body part wash with sterile saline (do not scrub or use antiseptics), wrap in saline-soaked gauze, place in closed plastic bag and then on ice (**do not place directly on ice**).
- Contraindications to replantation include severe crush injury, prolonged ischemia to amputated appendage and the presence of other life-threatening injuries requiring stabilization.
- Toes: Other than great toe, they are not usually replanted.
- Fingers:
  - Zone I injuries require conservative wound management (tetanus prophylaxis, nonadherent sterile dressing, splinting and bulky dressing). For wounds < 1 cm^2, healing by secondary intention should be adequate.
  - Zones II-IV injuries usually require a graft, flap, or replantation by a hand specialist. Do NOT leave bone exposed.
  - Try to save thumb and index finger. Always attempt replantation in children.
- Penis may be replanted up to 12 hours after amputation.

> **KEY FACT**
>
> 5 mm of healthy nail bed is required for nail adherence.

> **KEY FACT**
>
> Cooling extends the duration of viability of the amputated part.

HIGH-PRESSURE INJECTION INJURIES

These injuries are caused by injection of fluid (classically grease or paint) into the skin by a high-pressure injector. The fluid enters the skin and extends along deep tissue planes leading to inflammation with vascular compromise and tissue necrosis. These injuries tend to have a benign appearance, but without prompt treatment, the amputation rate is 30%-48%.

SYMPTOMS/EXAMINATION

- Innocuous examination with small injection wounds.
- Pain at injection site extending up arm is common.

TREATMENT

- Considered a surgical emergency requiring operative exploration and debridement.

KEY FACT

High-pressure injection injuries require immediate surgical consultation.

- Give prophylactic antibiotics, update tetanus, and elevate and splint extremity.
- Do not perform a digital block as this may increase compartment pressure and worsen injury.

Burns

THERMAL BURNS

Burns are described according to depth, with superficial burns involving only the epidermis, partial-thickness burns involving both the epidermis and part of the dermis, full-thickness burns destroying the entire epidermis and dermis, and subdermal burns involving the subdermal tissues (Table 3.15).

The majority of deaths in fire victims are due to smoke inhalation, primarily from carbon monoxide poisoning. Thermal inhalation injuries rarely extend below the vocal cords, but can cause rapid upper airway swelling. Particulate matter and other toxic gases result in lower airway and lung injury.

Evaluation of burns involves five main components:

- Evaluation of airway and breathing
- Consideration of possible carbon monoxide and cyanide exposure (see Chapter 6, Toxicology)
- Estimation of involved total body surface area (TBSA)
- Determination of depth of burned skin (Table 3.16)
- Evaluation for involvement of critical parts and for circumferential burns

Symptoms/Examination

- Suspect inhalation injury for patients presenting after fire in enclosed space or with singed nasal hairs, carbonaceous sputum, or soot in mouth or nose. Direct visualization of the airway showing soot, charring or edema is the gold standard for diagnosis.
- To estimate involved TBSA in adults, the rule of nines is commonly used (Figure 3.27):
  - Nine for each upper extremity
  - 18 for each lower extremity
  - 18 each for front and back of torso
  - Nine for the head
  - One for perineum
- Alternatively, the % burn may be estimated using the patient's palm and fingers = 1% TBSA.

TABLE 3.15. Burn Classifications

New Terminology	Old Terminology	Depth
Superficial	First-degree	Epidermal layer only
Partial-thickness	Second-degree	Epidermis and superficial dermis
Full-thickness	Third-degree	Epidermis and dermis (all structures)
Subdermal	Fourth-degree	Subdermal structures (muscles, nerves, bone)

TABLE 3.16. Burn Clinical Findings and Prognosis

Type	Clinical Findings	Prognosis
Superficial	Similar to sunburn: red, painful, tender, no blistering	Heals without scarring in 1 wk
Superficial partial-thickness	Red, painful, blistering, blanching	Hair follicles and sweat glands are retained Usually heals with minimal scarring in 2-3 wk
Deep partial-thickness	Red to pale white-yellow, blistering with rupture, no blanching Decreased two-point discrimination but can feel pressure	Healing can take 3-8 wk with scarring, and contracture
Full-thickness	Charred, white/black, painless, and leathery	Surgical grafting is required unless < 1 cm diameter
Subdermal	Severe burns	Life and limb threatening

- Estimation of burn depth may be difficult on initial evaluation. For this reason, burns should be reevaluated in 24 hours to determine true depth and extent of tissue damage.

Treatment

- Supplemental oxygen as needed.
- Intubate for:
  - Inhalation injury—intubate early, do not wait for stridor or respiratory distress to develop.
  - Full-thickness face or perioral burns
  - Circumferential neck burns
  - Tachypnea, hypoxia, hypoventilation, or AMS
- The Parkland Formula provides a guide for fluid resuscitation for patients with significant burns:

4 mL × %burn × weight (kg) = fluid requirement (mL) over first 24 hours

  - Multiply by 3 mL instead of 4 mL in children and add maintenance fluids.
  - Use only area of partial- and full-thickness burns to determine % burn for resuscitation.
  - Give half of fluid over first eight hours. The Parkland formula is merely a guide, and adequate fluid must be given to maintain urine output of 0.5-1 mL/kg/h.
- **Circumferential burns** to extremities run the risk of circulatory compromise due to pressure from burn/swelling. Circumferential burns to the torso may interfere with breathing via constriction. Consider early escharotomy for both.

Apply Silvadene to body but not to face because of scarring risk. Use topical agent like bacitracin to face.

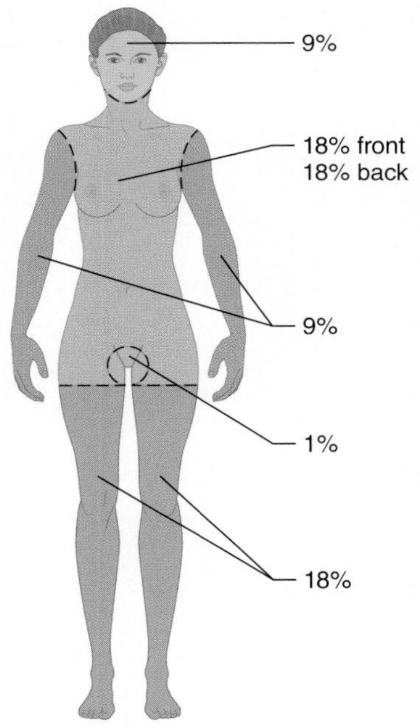

FIGURE 3.27. Rule of nines to estimate percent burn area in adults. (Reproduced, with permission, from Tintinalli JE, Stapczynski S, Ma OJ, et al. *Tintinalli's Emergency Medicine: A Comprehensive Study Guide*. 7th ed. New York, NY: McGraw-Hill, 2011. Figure 210.2.)

KEY FACT

For estimation of TBSA in children, use the Lund-Browder chart, not the rule of nines.

KEY FACT

Area of the patient's palm is approximately 1% TBSA, which is useful when evaluating children.

TABLE 3.17. American Burn Association Criteria for Transfer to Burn Unit

Partial-thickness burns > 10% total body surface area (TBSA)
Burns that involve the face, hand, feet, genitalia, perineum, or major joints
Full thickness burns in any age group
Electrical burns, including lightning injury
Chemical burns
Inhalation injury
Burn injury in patients with preexisting medical disorders that could complicate management, prolong recovery, or affect mortality
Any patients with burns and concomitant trauma (such as fractures) in which the burn injury poses the greatest risk of morbidity or mortality
Burned children in hospitals without qualified personnel or equipment for the care of children
Burn injury in patients who will require special social, emotional, or long-term rehabilitative intervention

DISPOSITION

- Major: Admission to Burn Center (Table 3.17)
- Moderate: Hospitalization
  - Partial thickness burns 10%-20% TBSA for adults, 5%-10% TBSA in children and the elderly
  - Full thickness burns 2%-5% TBSA, circumferential, comorbid conditions, inhalation injury
- Minor: Outpatient
  - Partial thickness < 10% TBSA for adults, < 5% TBSA in children/elderly
  - Full thickness < 2% TBSA

CHEMICAL BURNS

> **KEY FACT**
>
> Common alkalis ("lyes") include drain and toilet cleaners, detergents, cement, and paint removers. Treat with copious irrigation.

The classes of burning chemicals include acids, alkalis, oxidizing agents, corrosives, reducing agents, desiccants, vesicants and protoplasmic poisons (Table 3.18).

- **Acids cause coagulative necrosis,** creating a tough eschar preventing deep penetration of burn.
- **Alkalis cause liquefactive necrosis**, a poor barrier, so burns travel much deeper. For this reason, alkali burns tend to be worse than acid burns.
- **Cement** contains lime, which is converted with water to the alkali calcium hydroxide.

TREATMENT

- The first line in chemical-burn therapy is ample irrigation to remove the offending agent, except with:
  - Dry powder (lime): Brush away before hydration.
  - Sodium metals: Use oil, not water.
  - Phenol (carbolic acid): Use polyethylene glycol 300 and industrial methylated spirits in 2:1 mixture or more simply, use isopropyl alcohol or glycerol.
- Be careful of heat production when chemicals react with water or their neutralizing agents.
- Lacrimators (tear gas and pepper spray) irritate mucosa and are treated with copious water irrigation.

TABLE 3.18. Chemical Burns

	Where Found	Damage	Treatment	Special
Acids				
Carbolic acid (Phenol)	Industry and medicine	Painless white/brown coagulum—**may prevent penetration of water irrigation**	Polyethylene glycol Water irrigation is second line if PEG not available	**Penetrates more deeply when dilute than when concentrated**
Chromic acid	Chromium plating Glass cleaning	Chronic penetrating ulcerating lesions	Water irrigation and surgical excision to **prevent systemic toxicity**	**High systemic toxicity following skin absorption**
Formic acid	Industry and agriculture	Coagulative necrosis	Water irrigation	Acidosis, hemolysis, hemoglobinuria
Hydrochloric/Sulfuric acid	Toilet bowl/drain cleaners Battery acid Bleach Industrial	Dark brown or black burns	Water irrigation	
Hydrofluoric acid	High-octane fuel Etching Semiconductors Rust remover	Deep painful burns with possible blue-gray skin and erythema	Irrigation Calcium gluconate (topical/IM/SQ/intra-arterial) Treat until pain is gone	**Concentration effect not duration effect** Ca ↓, Mg ↓, K ↑, myocardial instability **Pain parallels extent of injury**
Methacrylic acid	Nail cosmetics	Dermal burns	Water irrigation	Preschoolers
Nitric acid	Metal work Fertilizers	Yellowish burns	Water irrigation	
Oxalic acid	Leather and blueprint		Water irrigation and IV calcium	Binds Ca^{++}, inhibits muscle contraction
Alkalis				
Lyes Ammonium hydroxide KOH, NaOH	Drain cleaners Detergents Paint removers	Deep burns	Prolonged water irrigation	**Ingestion can cause airway occlusion and/or esophageal trauma**
Lime (calcium oxide)	Cement	Exothermic reaction when neutralized with water	Profuse water via strong stream to prevent burn	First, brush away dry particles
Elemental Metals	Agriculture	Molten metal burns	**Mineral oil and excision NO water**	**Metal can ignite when in contact with air or water**
Hydrocarbons	Gasoline and tar	Fat-dissolving corrosive injury	Decontamination Polysorbate to remove tar	Frostbite and dehydration from skin contact
Vesicants	DMSO Cantharides Mustard gas	Deep penetration, blisters, ulcers	Water irrigation or adsorbent powder	Anoxic necrosis
Alkyl mercury	Disinfectants Fungicides Wood preservatives	Erythema and blistering	Debride and drain blisters Water irrigation	Blisters contain mercury
White phosphorus	Explosives	Deep and superficial	Irrigation with normal saline	May ignite when dry; keep wet

DMSO, dimethyl sulfoxide; IM, intramuscular; SQ, subcutaneous.

- Airbag deployment utilizes an exothermic reaction that can cause burns (sodium azide) and keratitis (sodium hydroxide). These are treated with copious water irrigation.
- Ophthalmic chemical burns should be copiously irrigated using a Morgan lens or similar device until pH of affected eye is neutralized. Prophylactic topical antibiotics are warranted when corneal epithelium is damaged. Additionally, the intraocular pressure of affected eye should be monitored.

> **KEY FACT**
>
> **Glass etching = > hydrofluoric acid burn** = > treat with **calcium gluconate**. The skin often looks normal and pain may not begin for hours after exposure.

> **KEY FACT**
>
> The primary treatment for almost all chemical exposures except metals, dry powder lime, and phenol is water irrigation.

Ballistics

Bullets cause injury by direct crush or laceration of tissue (permanent cavitation) and the associated pressure-wave damage to adjacent tissue (temporary cavitation). The temporary cavitation injury can be 10 times the size of permanent cavitation.

Characteristics that determine injury pattern:

- Bullet mass: Determines depth of penetration and diameter of crush or laceration injury.
- Bullet construction: Increased bullet deformity or fragmentation as with hollow point bullets and lead bullets without a cap yields greater crush or laceration injury.
- Bullet yaw (tilt off long axis): Greater yaw yields greater crush or laceration injury.
- Bullet velocity: Higher velocity yields a greater pressure wave and therefore greater **temporary cavitation**.
  - Shorter gun barrels produce lower velocity because the expanding gases are released into the atmosphere sooner.
  - As a result, **handguns fire low-velocity bullets** and do not produce significant temporary cavitation. Injury results from direct crush/laceration of vital tissues.
- Tissue type: Inelastic tissue (brain, liver, spleen, and bone) is more prone to temporary cavitation. By contrast, highly elastic tissue such as muscle may be injured by crush or laceration but not by temporary cavitation.
- Shotgun pellets tend to produce less damage owing to small size and spherical shape, unless fired at close range. At close range the pellets clump together and cause much deeper tissue penetration.

> **KEY FACT**
>
> GSWs to the head result in cavitation injury 3-4 times the bullet's diameter.

> **KEY FACT**
>
> **Determinants of injury:**
>
> Degree of crush or laceration—bullet mass, deformation, and yaw
>
> Amount of temporary cavitation—bullet velocity, tissue elasticity

Examination

Determination of entrance and exit sites is prone to error and has potential legal implications.

Treatment/Complications

- To preserve evidence in gunshot, victims do **NOT**:
  - Cut through bullet holes on clothing
  - Cut through bullet holes on skin unless medically necessary
  - Handle bullets/fragments with metal instruments so as not to disturb/cause markings
  - Describe wounds as entrance or exit
- **Bullets can embolize.**
  - If bullet is not found in its expected location, further workup is warranted.
  - In general embolized bullets must be removed.

- A bullet lodged within the spinal canal may migrate and cause further damage. Consult Neurosurgery. Removal should be considered.
- Lead poisoning is not usually a concern since bullets typically become encapsulated in fibrous tissue. However, bullets resting in synovial fluid (intraarticular, disk space and bursa) may dissolve and release lead into the body. Bullets must be removed from joints to prevent mechanical and lead damage to joints and lead poisoning.

KEY FACT

Handguns fire low-velocity bullets.

KEY FACT

Bullets are not sterilized by the heat of firing, and they can track in skin/clothing/foreign bodies.

REVIEW QUESTIONS

QUESTIONS

1. A 24-year-old man presents after a high speed motor vehicle accident. He has obvious head trauma and was intubated for a Glasgow Coma Scale of 6. While looking at the chest x-ray to confirm endotracheal tube placement, it looks like the nasogastric tube (NGT) is in the lungs even after seeing gastric contents in the tube. Which of the following is the most likely diagnosis?
   A. Hemothorax
   B. Diaphragmatic rupture
   C. Pneumothorax
   D. Splenic rupture
   E. Rib fracture

2. Which of the following is considered a stable cervical spine fracture?
   A. Jefferson fracture
   B. Hangman's fracture
   C. Teardrop fracture
   D. Transverse process fracture
   E. Odontoid fracture

3. A 27-year-old man presents one day after a fist fight. He has Battle sign and raccoon eyes? What type of head injury is most suspected?
   A. Subdural hematoma
   B. Epidural hematoma
   C. Basilar skull fracture
   D. Diffuse axonal injury
   E. Cerebral contusion

4. A 35-year-old man presents to the emergency department (ED) with a stab wound to the right chest. He has no breath sounds on the right side of his chest and has progressive dyspnea and hypotension. What is your next step?
   A. Intubation
   B. Large bore chest tube
   C. Pigtail catheter
   D. 3-way dressing over stab wound
   E. Needle decompression in the second intercostal space at the midclavicular line

5. A 24-year-old 70-kg man presents to the ED via EMS after being caught in a house fire. He is awake and alert with examination showing partial-thickness to full-thickness burns to the front and back of his torso as well as his left arm. He also has superficial burns to his right forearm and hand. According to the Parkland formula, what is his fluid requirement?
   A. 6.3 L over first 12 hours, 12.6 L total over 24 hours.
   B. 6.3 L over first 8 hours, 12.6 L total over 24 hours.
   C. 7.5 L over first 24 hours, 6.2 L total over 48 hours.
   D. 7.5 L over first 8 hours, 15 L total over 24 hours.

6. Your patient is a 22-year-old woman who presents to the ED after spilling about 5 mL of solution on her foot while etching glass. She complains of severe pain. Examination reveals a 3 × 3 cm area of slight redness. What is your next step?
   A. Remove soiled clothing, irrigate, apply topical antibiotic cream, and discharge home
   B. Remove soiled clothing, irrigate, and consult burn surgery team
   C. Remove soiled clothing, irrigate, and apply 2.5% calcium gluconate gel
   D. Remove soiled clothing, irrigate, and apply 4% calcium chloride gel

7. A 44-year-old man presents to the ED with a small puncture wound to his hand. He has minimal pain but reports that about 15 minutes prior he was using a pressurized paint gun when he accidentally injected himself. He denies any medical problem, has an up to date tetanus shot, and is hoping to head home to pick his children up from school. What is your next best step?
   A. Clean the wound, discharge home
   B. Clean the wound, emergently consult surgery and get the patient ready for the operating wound
   C. Clean wound, dress wound, and observe patient for six hours
   D. Clean wound, discharge patient, and request he return in 24 hours for a wound recheck

8. A 34-week pregnant patient presents to the ED after a major car accident. On evaluation of the patient, you note that she is struggling to breathe and you cannot hear any breath sounds on the right side. What is your next step?
   A. CXR
   B. Needle decompression of right chest followed by chest tube placement at the fifth intercostal space (ICS) in the anterior axillary line
   C. Needle decompression of the right chest followed by chest tube placement at the fifth ICS in the midaxillary line
   D. Needle decompression of right chest followed by chest tube placement at the third ICS in the anterior axillary line

ANSWERS

1. **B.** The presence of a gastric bubble or NGT in the thoracic cavity indicates a diaphragmatic rupture. This can occur after blunt or penetrating trauma. It is thought that the left side of the diaphragm is usually more affected because the liver has a protective effect. These patients will need surgical repair.

2. **D.** Spinal injuries are classified as stable versus unstable. Unstable fractures have high risk of spinal cord injury and usually require surgery to stabilize the fracture. Remember: Jefferson Bit Off A Hangman's Thumb. A Jefferson fracture is blowout/burst fracture of C1, usually from an axial load. Bilateral-faced dislocation has high risk for spinal cord injury. Odontoid fracture of C2 is caused by a flexion injury with shearing force. A hangman's fracture involves bilateral pedicles of C2, usually caused by significant hyperextension. A teardrop fracture usually involves C2 and is associated with central cord syndrome.

3. **C.** These signs are present 1-3 days after injury and should make you highly suspicious of a basilar skull fracture. Battle sign is ecchymosis of the mastoid, usually due to a temporal bone fracture. Raccoon eyes are described as nontender periorbital ecchymosis. You may also see hemotympanum or a ring sign when CSF from the ears or eyes forms a ring of CSF around a central target of blood.

4. **E.** The patient is suffering from a tension pneumothorax. This is essentially a 1-way valve that allows air to move in with inspiration, but does not allow air to leave with expiration. This causes significantly increased intrathoracic pressure leading to hypotension, tachycardia, and tracheal deviation away from injured lung. Intubation can increase the positive pressure in the thoracic cavity worsening his symptoms. A patient with a sucking wound can initially be treated with a 3-way dressing, but once they develop a tension pneumothorax, remove the dressing immediately. A tension pneumothorax requires time sensitive treatment, while a chest tube is the ultimate treatment, it is more important to relieve the pneumothorax with needle decompression first.

5. **B.** For calculating resuscitation with the Parkland formula, use only partial- and full-thickness burns. Give half of the fluid over the first eight hours, the rest over the subsequent 16 hours. The ultimate goal is a urine output of 0.5-1 mL/kg/h. The calculations are as follows:

$$\text{TBSA for resuscitation} = 18 \text{ (front torso)} + 18 \text{ (back torso)} + 9 \text{ (left arm)} = 45\%$$

$$\mathbf{4\ mL \times \%burn \times weight\ (kg) = fluid\ requirement\ (mL)\ over\ first\ 24\ hours}$$

$$4 \text{ mL} \times 45\% \times 70 \text{ kg} = 12.6 \text{ L}$$

6. **C.** Hydrofluoric acid is found in common industrial products used for glass etching, metal cleaning and electronic manufacturing. Initially, burns can appear mild but hydrofluoric acid is unique in that dilute solutions can penetrate deeply, causing severe burns. Burns should be copiously irrigated and calcium gluconate gel should be applied. If ongoing pain occurs, consider subcutaneous or IV administration of calcium gluconate. Additionally, hydrofluoric acid can cause severe metabolic abnormalities, so consider checking a basic metabolic panel (BMP), magnesium, and calcium level in large exposures.

7. **B.** High-pressure injection injuries occur when a high-pressure injection device injects a substance such as grease or paint. Normally, an examination shows only a small puncture wound, which can appear fairly benign. Unfortunately, high-pressure injection injuries are considered a surgical emergency. Without decompression and cleaning of offending agent from tissue, necrosis and amputation can result.

8. **D.** In pregnant women, especially late in the pregnancy, a chest tube should be placed 1-2 intercostal spaces higher than the usual fourth to fifth ICS.

CHAPTER 4

Orthopedics

Sarah Leeper, MD

Evaluation Of Orthopedic Injuries

DEFINITIONS OF FRACTURES AND THE ORTHOPAEDIC TRAUMA ASSOCIATION CLASSIFICATION SYSTEM

- **Closed fractures:** Break in the bone or cartilage with skin intact
- **Open fractures:** Any fracture where there is a traumatic wound allowing the outside to communicate with the bone
  - **High risk of infection**
  - Treatment includes irrigation and debridement, prophylactic antibiotics with first-generation cephalosporin (add aminoglycoside if crush injury, contamination, or wound > 5 cm), tetanus prophylaxis, and emergent orthopedic consultation

KEY FACT

All open fractures require emergent orthopedic consultation because of high risk of infection.

Components of the Orthopaedic Trauma Association (OTA) classification system of fractures (Figure 4.1):

1. **Bone:** Describes the bone(s) that is/are involved, eg, radius.
2. **Segmental location:** Anatomic location of a fracture in terms of bone segments: In adults, this is either proximal, diaphyseal (shaft), or distal. In children, the Salter-Harris classification (see Chapter 5, Pediatrics) describes fractures through the physis or growth plate.
3. **Type:** Describes how many fragments are present (simple, wedge, or complex) and whether articular surfaces are involved (extra-articular, partial articular, or complete articular).
4. **Group:** Describes the orientation of the fracture line, eg, transverse (perpendicular to long axis of the bone), oblique (oblique to long axis of the bone), or spiral (encircles the shaft in two different oblique directions).

   Torus (buckling injury without a break in the cortex), and greenstick (a bend in the bone on one side and a break in the cortex on the other) are terms applied to growing bones.

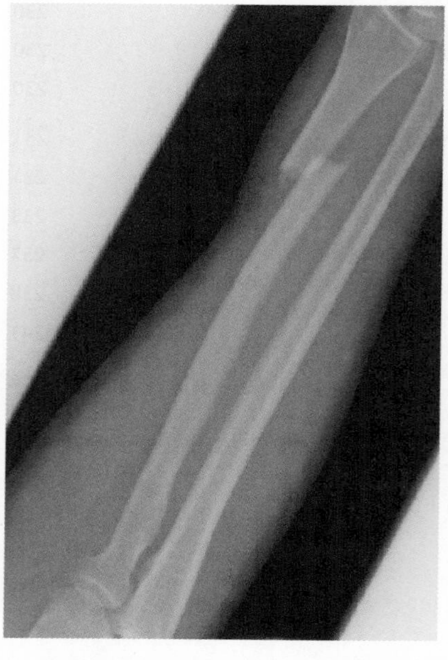

FIGURE 4.1. The AP view of the forearm shows a simple, transverse distal radial shaft fracture with approximately 90% displacement.

5. **Subgroup:** Describes the relationship of fracture fragments to one another, eg, displacement (described in terms of the distal fragment relative to the proximal fragment), separation, shortening, angulation (described in terms of which direction the apex of the angle formed by the fracture fragments is pointing), and rotation.

ASSESSMENT OF NEUROVASCULAR STRUCTURES

See Table 4.1 for common injuries and their associated neurovascular complications.

TABLE 4.1. Common Injuries and Associated Neurovascular Complications

Types of Fractures or Dislocations	Neurovascular Complications	Clinical Signs
Anterior shoulder dislocation	Axillary nerve injury	Deltoid muscle paralysis—check by asking patient to abduct shoulder against resistance
	Axillary artery injury	Diminished pulse, expanding hematoma
Humeral shaft injury	Radial nerve injury	Loss of wrist extension, inability to give "thumb's up" Numbness of dorsal web space
Medial epicondylar fracture	Ulnar nerve injury	Inability to spread fingers against resistance Numbness over dorsal and palmar surfaces of fourth/fifth digits
Supracondylar fracture/elbow dislocation	Brachial artery injury	Diminished pulses at wrist, delayed cap refill or cyanosis of nail beds
	Radial, ulnar, and median nerve injury	**Radial and ulnar nerve injuries:** (see above) **Median nerve injury:** Inability to make "ok sign" Numbness over palmar aspect of index finger
Hip dislocation	Femoral nerve injury	Weakened extension at knee Numbness over anterior/medial thigh, medial shin, arch of foot
Knee dislocation	Popliteal artery injury	"Hard signs" of vascular injury include expanding hematoma, absent distal pulses, distal ischemia, bruit/thrill
	Peroneal and tibial nerve injury	**Peroneal nerve injury:** Weakened dorsiflexion at ankle ("foot drop") Numbness over anterior shin, dorsal foot **Tibial nerve injury:** Weakened plantarflexion, dorsiflexion, and eversion of foot at ankle Numbness over lateral aspect of calf and foot
Lateral tibial plateau fracture	Peroneal nerve injury	Weakened dorsiflexion at ankle ("foot drop") Numbness over anterior shin, dorsal foot

MNEMONIC

Neurovascular evaluation:

CMS

Circulation (pulse, cap refill)
Motor
Sensation

MANAGEMENT OF ORTHOPEDIC INJURIES

- Analgesia
- Reduction if necessary (assess and document neurovascular status before and after reduction)
- Antibiotic prophylaxis for open or contaminated fractures
- Tetanus booster
- Splint (should immobilize joints above and below injury to prevent rotation)
- Orthopedic consultation or referral

COMPLICATIONS OF ORTHOPEDIC INJURIES

- Malunion or nonunion
- **Avascular necrosis (AVN)**
  - Most common with femoral head, proximal scaphoid, capitate, and talus fractures
- Infection
- Vascular injury or hemorrhage
- Nerve injury: Pain, paresthesias, weakness, or paralysis
- Soft-tissue or organ injury
- Deformity
- **Compartment syndrome**
  - Most commonly seen with tibia fractures in the anterior compartment
  - Clinical diagnosis: Excessive or increasing pain, pain on passive stretch, paresthesias, tender/tight compartment
  - Surgical fasciotomy indicated for compartment pressure > 30 or within 30 mm Hg of mean arterial pressure (MAP)
- **Fat embolism syndrome**
  - Fat emboli travel from fracture site to pulmonary capillary beds → endothelial damage → lung injury, platelet aggregation, and mediator release.
- Most common 1-2 days after **long bone and pelvic fractures** or surgical repair.
- Triad of respiratory distress/hypoxemia, petechiae, altered mental status.
- Treatment is supportive.
- **Volkmann ischemic contracture**
  - Flexion contracture of hand/wrist due to untreated forearm compartment syndrome or brachial artery injury and resultant muscle ischemia
- Reflex sympathetic dystrophy (complex regional pain syndrome)

MNEMONIC

The 6 Ps of compartment syndrome:

Pain (most common symptom)

Paresthesias
Poikilothermia
Paralysis
Pallor
Pulselessness **(late finding!)**

Injuries to the Upper Extremities

SHOULDER INJURIES

Anterior Shoulder Dislocation

Most commonly **subcoracoid** (> 90%). **Also can be subglenoid, subclavicular, and intrathoracic (though rare).**

Mechanism

Blow to abducted, externally rotated arm, or less commonly fall on the outstretched hand (**FOOSH**).

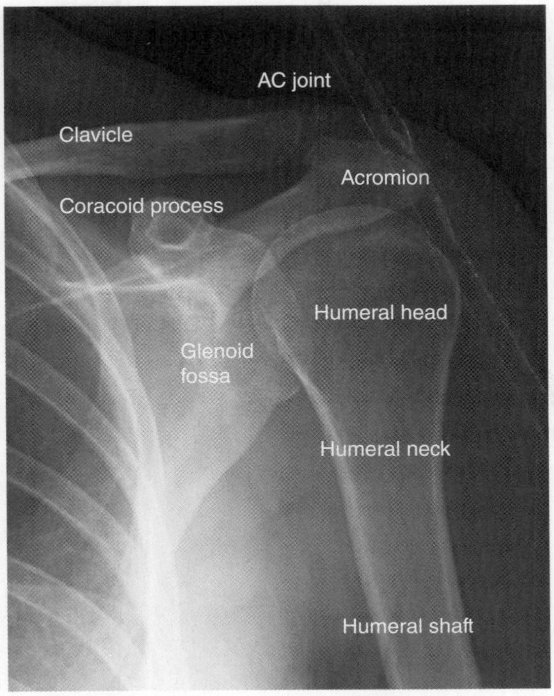

FIGURE 4.2. Normal x-ray of the shoulder. (Used with permission from, David Berkoff, MD, FAAEM, CAQSM.)

Diagnosis

- Outer round contour of shoulder is flattened. Displaced humeral head is palpated inferiorly. Arm is **abducted and slightly externally rotated.**
- Two-view x-ray of the shoulder, including anteroposterior (AP) view and axillary or Y view (Figure 4.3), shows dislocation.

Treatment

Reduction methods for anterior dislocations:

- (Hanging weight Stimson technique), scapular manipulation, external rotation (Hennepin technique), forward elevation (Cooper and Milch), traction-countertraction.
- Analgesia may be obtained from procedural sedation or intra-articular injection of local anesthetic.
- **Not recommended:** External rotation, forward elevation, followed by internal rotation (Kocher) and foot in the axilla for countertraction (Hippocratic) techniques because of higher complication rates.

Postreduction, recheck pulse, motor, sensation, and apply sling and swathe or shoulder immobilizer. Patients should be discharged with recommendation for orthopedic follow-up.

Complications

- Axillary nerve injury: Loss of sensation at "badge" area of shoulder, weak abduction due to deltoid paralysis.
- **Bankart lesion:** An avulsion of the anteroinferior glenoid labrum (often diagnosed on magnetic resonance imaging [MRI], but may have bony component). If present, high incidence of instability and may require surgery.
- **Hill-Sachs deformity:** An impaction fracture of the posterolateral aspect of the humeral head (Figure 4.4). Generally not clinically significant unless large enough to cause instability.

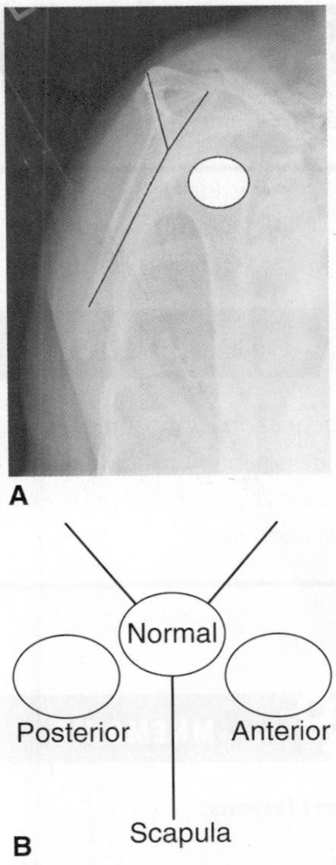

FIGURE 4.3. On the scapular Y-view shoulder radiograph for an anterior dislocation, the humeral head will often appear anterior to the glenoid (as pictured in [A] and for a posterior dislocation the humeral head will usually appear posterior [B]).

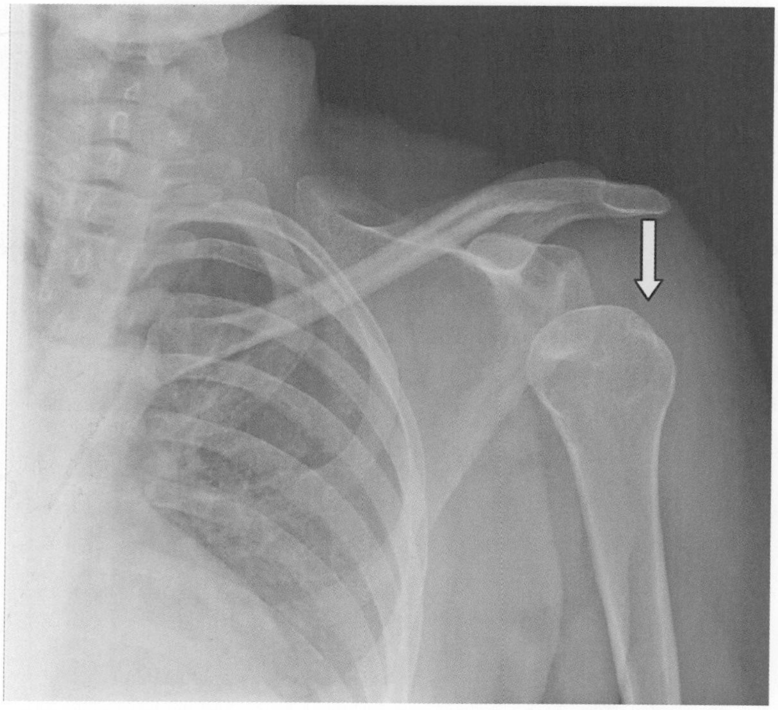

FIGURE 4.4. Anterior shoulder dislocation with a small Hill-Sachs deformity (arrow).

- Recurrent dislocation.
- Adhesive capsulitis from shoulder immobilization; incidence reduced with early shoulder range of motion activities.

Posterior Shoulder Dislocation

Mechanism

Requires significant direct force to the anterior shoulder classically from a **seizure, electrocution,** or **high-speed injury—fall from height or grabbing dashboard during motor vehicle collision (MVC).**

Diagnosis

- Clinical: Arm is usually **adducted** and slightly **internally rotated (patient cannot externally rotate the arm)**. The coracoid process is prominent anteriorly.
- Standard AP x-rays can appear deceptively normal—50% of posterior dislocations are initially missed. Proximal humerus may look like a **lightbulb or drumstick** (due to internal rotation). The Y or axillary view can confirm the diagnosis—the humeral head is displaced posteriorly.

Treatment

Closed reduction using in-line traction and gentle anterior manipulation of humeral head. If unsuccessful, orthopedic consultation for closed vs open reduction.

Complications

Impaction fracture of anteromedial humeral head (**reverse Hill-Sachs deformity**).

MNEMONIC

Hill-Sachs = **H**umeral **H**ead deformity

KEY FACT

The Kocher and Hippocratic techniques for reducing anterior shoulder dislocations have unacceptably high complication rates.

MNEMONIC

Bankart lesions:

TUBS

Traumatic
Unilateral
Bankart
Surgery

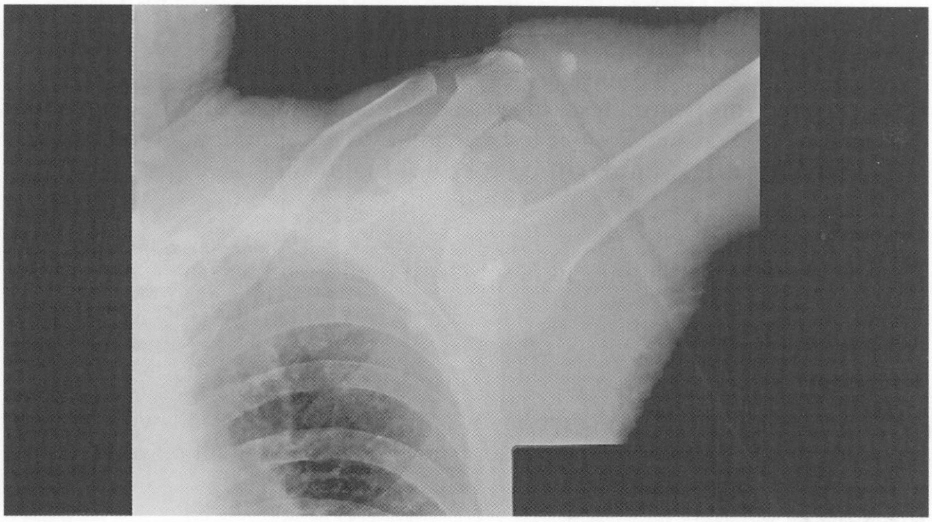

FIGURE 4.5. Inferior shoulder dislocation (luxatio erecta).

Inferior Shoulder Dislocation (Luxatio Erecta)

Mechanism

Results from **hyperabduction** of the shoulder levering the humeral head out inferiorly. It is uniformly associated with serious injury to the shoulder complex.

Diagnosis

Arm is held in a fixed position up over head (180° of elevation). X-ray is confirmative (Figure 4.5).

Treatment

Procedural sedation and closed reduction via traction-countertraction.

Complications

- Almost always accompanied by disruption of the rotator cuff and tear through the inferior capsule. Often associated with fractures of the proximal humerus.
- High incidence of neurovascular compromise, including axillary nerve, brachial plexus, and axillary artery injuries.

Rotator Cuff Injuries

Continuum of injury: Mechanical impingement → rotator cuff tendonitis (repetitive microtrauma) → rotator cuff tear.

Mechanism

Impingement of subacromial space by humeral head due to repeated elevation of arms above shoulders.

Diagnosis

- Shoulder pain (initially only with activity) and eventual loss of motion.
- Typically have pain between 60° and 120° of shoulder abduction **(painful arc).**
- **Rotator cuff tendonitis:** Preserved strength of rotator cuff **SITS** (supraspinatus, infraspinatus, teres minor, subscapularis) muscles especially after **lidocaine injection.**

KEY FACT

Most common **shoulder** dislocation = **anterior** dislocation

KEY FACT

Most common **elbow** dislocation = **posterior** dislocation

MNEMONIC

Most common types of dislocations:

PEAS

Posterior for
Elbow
Anterior for
Shoulder

- **Rotator cuff tear:** Most are acute injuries to a tendon weakened from chronic impingement.
  - Weakness of SITS muscles.
  - Positive **drop arm test:** Have patient abduct arm to 90°, then lower slowly to her side. Positive test = inability to lower in slow, controlled arc.
  - MRI or ultrasound can be used for diagnosis.

TREATMENT

Physical therapy, steroid injection, surgery if rotator cuff tear.

Acromioclavicular Separation

MECHANISM

Acromioclavicular (AC) separation usually results from a fall with a direct blow downward on the outer shoulder (snowboarders, football players).

DIAGNOSIS

The diagnosis can usually be made clinically by reproducing the pain with palpation of the AC joint.

TREATMENT

Depends on the degree of separation (Table 4.2).

Clavicular Fractures

Most commonly due to fall on affected shoulder. Classified by segment (distal third, middle third, or medial third).

TREATMENT/COMPLICATIONS

- Immediate orthopedic consult for open fractures, skin tenting, or associated neurovascular injury.
- **Middle third (80% of clavicle fractures):** Reduction, immobilization with sling; orthopedic consultation if severely comminuted (> 20 mm of shortening or 100% displacement).

TABLE 4.2. Types of Acromioclavicular Separation

TYPE OF AC SEPARATION	DESCRIPTION	TREATMENT
1	Sprain of the AC ligament. Radiograph is normal.	Sling, 1-2 wk
2	Disruption of AC ligament with CC ligament sprain. Distance between acromion and clavicle is increased by less than or equal to **half clavicle width**.	Sling and orthopedic referral; rehab
3	Both AC and CC are disrupted. Distance between acromion and clavicle is increased by **full width** of clavicle.	Sling and orthopedic referral; surgical fixation may be needed if conservative treatment fails.
4	Clavicle displaced ***posteriorly***.	For Types 4-6, sling and orthopedic referral with likely surgical fixation
5	Clavicle displaced far ***superiorly and anteriorly***.	
6	Clavicle displaced ***inferiorly***.	

AC, Acromioclavicular; CC, coracoclavicular.

- **Distal third (15%):** Immobilization with sling; may require surgery to avoid nonunion if associated rupture of coracoclavicular ligament
- **Medial third (5%):** Immobilization with sling; may be associated with intrathoracic injuries and can be life threatening if there is injury to underlying vascular structures

Sternoclavicular Dislocations

MECHANISM

- Usually the result of MVC or sports injury.
- **Anterior dislocations** (most common) result from a force applied to the anterolateral shoulder, rolling the shoulder backward, and forcing the medial clavicle anteriorly.
- **Posterior dislocations** may be due to direct blow to the medial clavicle or from a force applied to the posterolateral shoulder, rolling the shoulder forward, and forcing the medial clavicle posteriorly.

DIAGNOSIS

- Patient typically has severe pain that is exacerbated by shoulder movement. X-rays often miss this diagnosis. Computed tomography (CT) is the most useful imaging study, especially in posterior dislocations to help visualize underlying structures.
- **First-degree dislocation:** Sprain, mild pain/swelling.
- **Second-degree dislocation:** Rupture of sternoclavicular ligament with clavicle subluxation.
- **Third-degree dislocation:** Rupture of sternoclavicular and costoclavicular ligaments with clavicle dislocation.

TREATMENT

- **First-degree dislocation:** Arm sling
- **Second-degree dislocation:** Figure-of-eight clavicular strap or sling
- **Third-degree dislocation:**
  - Anterior: Reduction attempt and sling
  - Posterior: Neurovascular assessment, with emergent orthopedic and thoracic surgery consults and rapid reduction

> **KEY FACT**
>
> Posterior sternoclavicular dislocations have a high incident of underlying esophageal and great vessel injuries.

COMPLICATIONS

With third-degree posterior dislocations, there is a 25% chance of life-threatening injuries, including esophageal rupture, carotid artery injury, and injury to the great vessels.

Scapular Fractures

MECHANISM

Require a significant amount of blunt force and are **frequently associated with injury to the ipsilateral lung, chest wall, and shoulder.**

DIAGNOSIS

Shoulder x-ray **and chest x-ray (CXR).**

TREATMENT

- Most are treated with sling and immobilization.
- Open reduction internal fixation (ORIF) is required for severely displaced or angulated fractures, particularly if fracture includes scapular neck or glenoid fossa.

KEY FACT

Scapula fractures are often associated with injury to the ipsilateral lung, chest wall, and shoulder.

Complications

Rib fractures, pneumothorax, hemothorax, pulmonary contusion, clavicular fractures, shoulder dislocation with associated rotator cuff tears, neurovascular injuries, and vertebral compression fractures.

HUMERUS INJURIES

Proximal Humerus Fracture

Mechanism

Most common is fall onto outstretched extremity. 75% occur in adults > 60 years.

NEER CLASSIFICATION

The proximal humerus is made up of four anatomic parts: Humeral head, greater tuberosity, lesser tuberosity, and humeral shaft. Neer classification is a descriptive system based on the number of displaced (> 1 cm) or angulated (> 45°) parts visible on radiograph:

- 1-part fracture (most common): Fractures present, but none are displaced or angulated.
- 2-part fracture: 1 displaced/angulated part (eg, anatomic neck fracture or greater tuberosity fracture).
- 3-part fracture: 2 displaced/angulated parts (eg, surgical neck fracture with greater tuberosity fracture).
- Other descriptors include 4-part fracture, intra-articular fracture, fracture dislocation.

Treatment

- No or minimal displacement: Immobilization and early range of motion
- More than minimal displacement: Refer to orthopedics for consideration of operative management

Complications

- Most common is adhesive capsulitis. Less common are brachial plexus injury, axillary nerve or artery injuries, nonunion/malunion. AVN of humeral head is rare except with significant displacement/angulation.

Humeral Shaft Fracture

Mechanism

Usually due to direct blow or MVC.

Treatment

- Nondisplaced humeral shaft fractures require stabilization with coaptation splint with sling and swath or hanging cast (cast extending from one in proximal to fracture line to distal palmar crease, elbow in 90° flexion; arm hangs from forearm sling, allowing gravity to align bones).
- Displaced or comminuted fractures or those with neurovascular compromise require orthopedic consultation.

KEY FACT

Radial nerve injury causes weakness of the extensors of the wrist and digits and numbness of the dorsoradial aspect of the hand.

Complications

- Most common complication (20%): Radial nerve injury; often a neuropraxia that resolves spontaneously after weeks to months. Radial nerve injury causes weakness of the extensors of the wrist and digits and numbness of the dorsoradial aspect of the hand.

- Others include adhesive capsulitis of shoulder, delayed union, brachial artery injury, ulnar and median nerve injury

ELBOW INJURIES

Supracondylar Fracture

Distal humerus fracture proximal to the condyles. Almost exclusively seen in children where strong collateral ligaments and joint capsule prevent dislocation of elbow. Peak age is 5-10 years.

Mechanism/Diagnosis

- The vast majority are due to a FOOSH with hyperextension of elbow.
- X-ray shows presence of posterior fat pad sign and anterior displacement of the anterior humeral line (Figure 4.8).

Treatment

Gartland classification guides treatment:
- Type I (nondisplaced) may be immobilized in posterior splint with orthopedic follow-up in 48 hours.
- Type II (some displacement but intact posterior cortex) and type III (completely displaced, no cortical contact require urgent operative management.

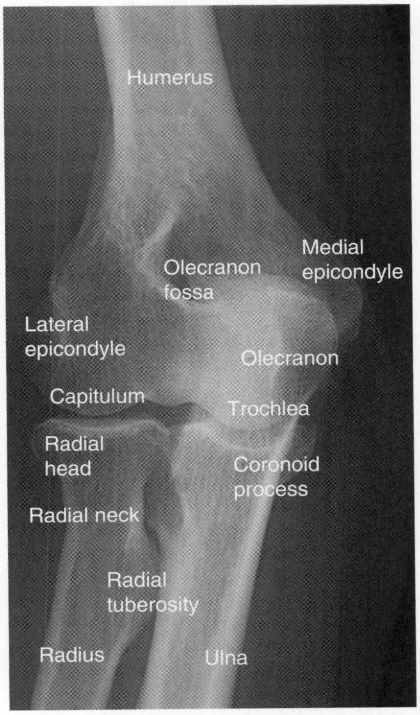

FIGURE 4.6. Normal x-ray of elbow. (Used with permission from, David Berkoff, MD, FAAEM, CAQSM.)

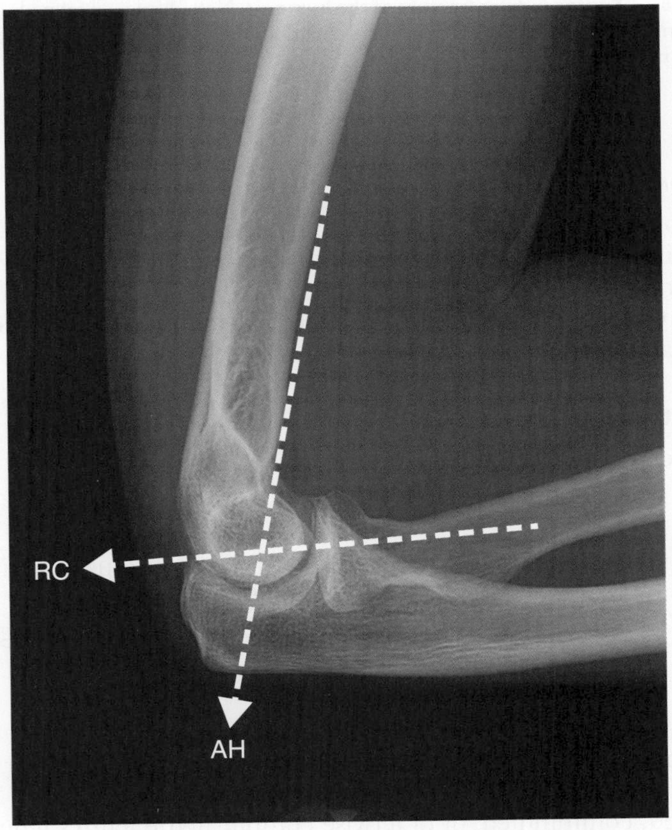

FIGURE 4.7. Normal x-ray of elbow with radiocapitellar (RC) and anterior humeral (AH) lines. A line drawn through the center of the radial neck (RC) should pass through the center of the capitellum. A line drawn along the anterior surface of the humerus (AH) should pass through the middle third of the capitellum. (Used with permission from, David Berkoff, MD, FAAEM, CAQSM.)

Q

A 6-year-old boy presents with elbow pain after falling off the jungle gym at school. The x-ray reveals a supracondylar fracture. The boy's arm is splinted with pulse, motor, and sensation intact, and he is sent home with instructions to follow up with orthopedics in 48-72 hours. When Mom presents to the orthopedist, she states that he has been crying almost nonstop since the accident. What complication might have occurred?

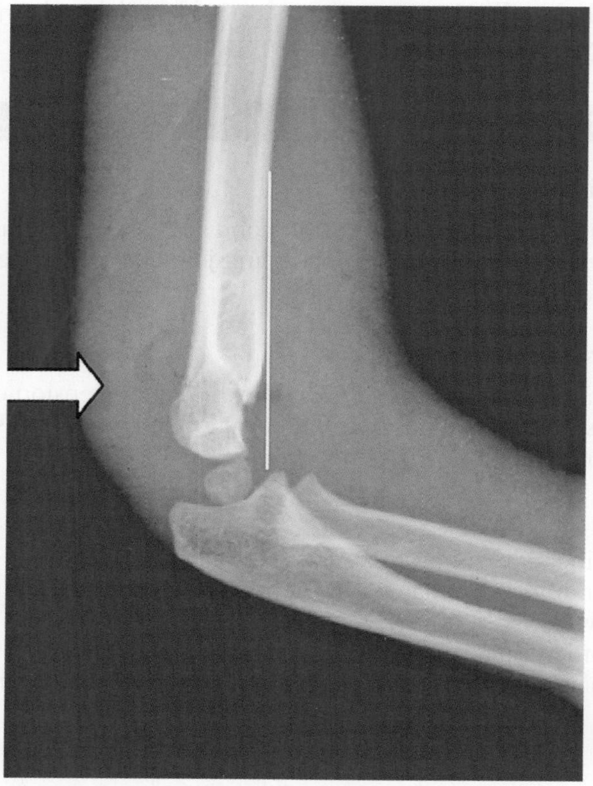

FIGURE 4.8. Supracondylar fracture of the humerus. Note displaced fat pads (arrow) signifying joint effusion. The anterior humeral line does not pass through the middle third of the capitellum.

Complications

- Most common, overall: Loss of carrying angle
- Nerve injury: Median/anterior interosseus nerve (most likely) but also radial and ulnar nerves
- Forearm compartment syndrome and **Volkmann ischemic contracture** from brachial artery compromise

KEY FACT

Volkmann ischemic contract is a result of untreated forearm compartment syndrome.

Condylar Fractures

Include lateral condyle, medial condyle, or intercondylar.

Mechanism

- Intercondylar fracture (most common distal humerus fracture): Force applied to 90° flexed elbow driving ulna into trochlea
- Medial/lateral condyle fracture: FOOSH with varus/valgus stress, respectively

Treatment

- Nondisplaced condylar fractures can be stabilized with posterior splint and early orthopedic follow-up.
- Displaced, comminuted, or otherwise complicated fractures require immediate orthopedic consultation.

A

Always consider compartment syndrome with supracondylar fractures and any fracture involving the forearm. If untreated, forearm ischemia can lead to Volkmann ischemic contracture.

Complications

Nonunion, ulnar nerve palsy, AVN, compartment syndrome, arthritis.

Epicondylar Fractures

Mechanism

In adults, these fractures are uncommon and usually result from a direct blow. In children, **medial epicondyle fractures** are much more common and are associated with repeated valgus stress (**little leaguer's elbow**) or posterior elbow dislocation.

Treatment/Complications

- Nondisplaced medial epicondylar fractures can be stabilized with a posterior splint with the elbow in 90° flexion and the forearm in pronation.
- Fractures with > 3-5 mm displacement or intra-articular fractures require orthopedic consultation.
- 60% of epicondylar fractures will have an associated ulnar nerve injury.

Elbow Dislocations

Classified according to position of ulna relative to humerus: Posterior are far more common than anterior.

Mechanism

- Posterior: FOOSH with elbow hyperextended
- Anterior: Direct posterior blow to flexed elbow

Diagnosis/Treatment

- Posterior: Posterior prominence of the olecranon with swelling, shortened forearm held in 45° flexion
- Anterior: Elongated forearm, arm held in full extension
- AP and lateral x-ray confirm dislocation, may identify associated fractures
- Treatment is reduction, immobilization in 90° flexion in posterior splint, ortho referral

Complications

- Most serious complication: Brachial artery injury.
- Other complications include elbow fracture (30%-60% of cases), medial nerve traction injury and/or entrapment, and triceps avulsion.

Olecranon Fracture

Mechanism

Direct blow to tip of elbow.

Treatment/Complications

- For a nondisplaced olecranon fracture, stabilize with a posterior splint.
- For an olecranon fracture with > 2 mm displacement, obtain orthopedic consult for ORIF.
- Ulnar nerve injury, loss of triceps function (inability to actively extend elbow).

Radial Head Fracture

Mechanism/Diagnosis

- Most isolated fractures are due to FOOSH.
- Tenderness over the radial head (over lateral elbow) with a posterior fat pad sign on x-ray in the adult patient.
- Nondisplaced fracture may not be visible on initial radiograph.

KEY FACT

Elbow fractures (particularly of the radial head) can be occult on radiograph, so look for a **posterior** fat pad sign, which is always **pathologic**. A large anterior fat pad (**sail sign**) can also sometimes be pathologic. In adults suspect an occult radial head fracture; in pediatrics a supracondylar fracture is more likely.

KEY FACT

Posterior fat pad sign without visible fracture after FOOSH?

Adult patient = radial head fracture

Pediatric patient = supracondylar fracture

Treatment

- Nondisplaced fracture can be treated with sling and early range of motion.
- More complicated fractures require operative intervention.

FOREARM INJURIES

Eponym	Description	
Colles	Distal radius fracture, dorsal displacement	R
Smith	Distal radius fracture, volar displacement	A
Barton	Distal radius rim fracture, intra-articular	D I
Essex-Lopresti	Radial head fracture + dislocation of distal radioulnar joint	U
Galeazzi	Radial shaft fracture + dislocation of distal radioulnar joint	S
Nightstick	Midshaft ulnar fracture	U
Monteggia	Ulnar shaft fracture + radial head dislocation	L N A

Colles Fracture

Mechanism/Diagnosis

- FOOSH.
- X-ray shows transverse fracture of distal radial metaphysis with dorsal displacement (“**dinner fork deformity**”) (Figure 4.10).

Treatment/Complications

- Closed reduction should be performed if there is:
  - Dorsal angulation of fracture fragment (distal radius is normally tilted 15° volarly). Goal is neutral volar tilt.
  - Intra-articular step-off > 1 mm.
  - Radial length shortened > 2-3 mm compared to opposite wrist.
  - Radial inclination < 15°.
- Goals of reduction are to restore volar tilt, inclination, and length to radius.
- Sugar-tong splint, orthopedic follow-up.
- Complications include: Early arthritis (if intra-articular), malunion, median nerve injury, 60% associated with ulnar styloid fracture.

Goals of reduction for Colles fracture:

Neutral volar tilt
< 5° loss of volar inclination
< 2-3 mm loss of length
Step-off < 2 mm

Smith Fracture (Reverse Colles Fracture)

Mechanism/Diagnosis

- Direct blow to dorsum of hand or fall onto dorsum of hand
- Transverse fracture of distal radial metaphysis with volar displacement (“**garden spade deformity**”) of the distal fragment (see Figure 4.11)

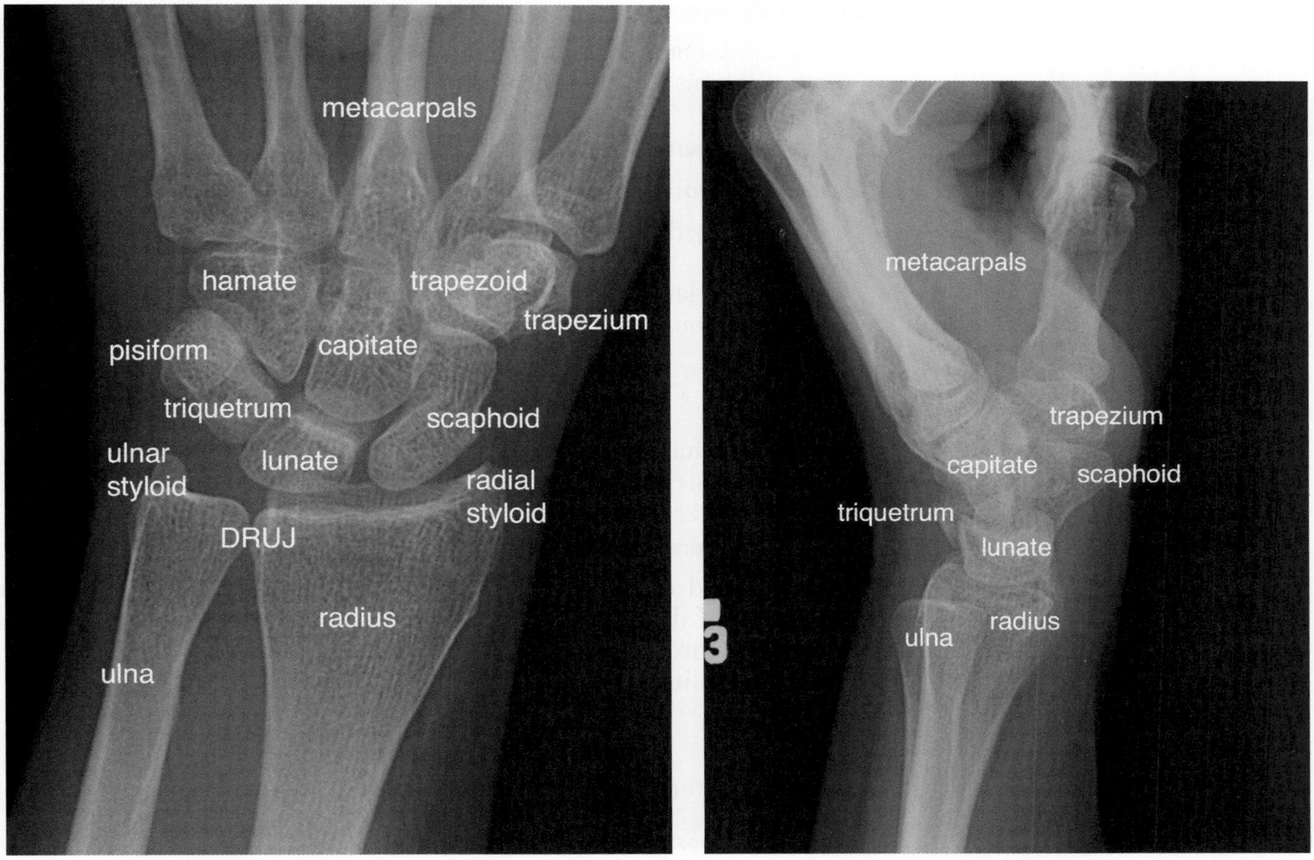

FIGURE 4.9. Normal x-rays of the wrist. (Used with permission from, David Berkoff, MD, FAAEM, CAQSM.)

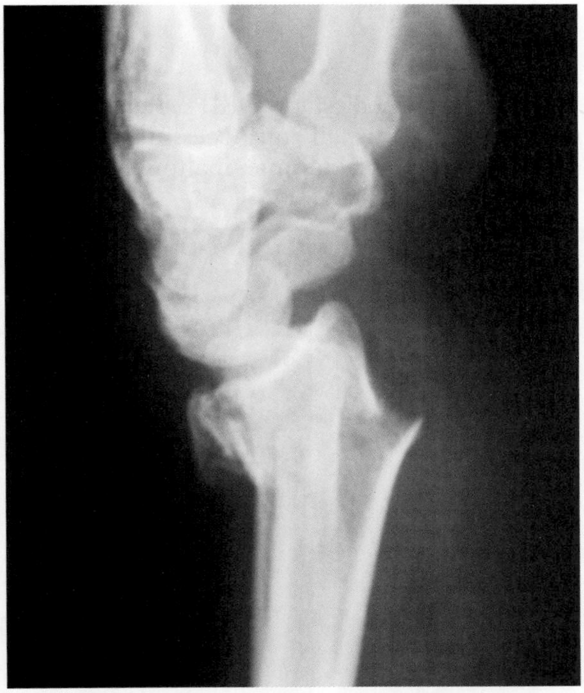

FIGURE 4.10. Lateral wrist radiograph of a Colles fracture demonstrating significan't dorsal tilt requiring reduction. (Reproduced, with permission, from Simon RR, Sherman SC, Koenigsknecht SJ. *Emergency Orthopedics, the Extremities*. 5th ed. New York, NY: McGraw-Hill; 2007.)

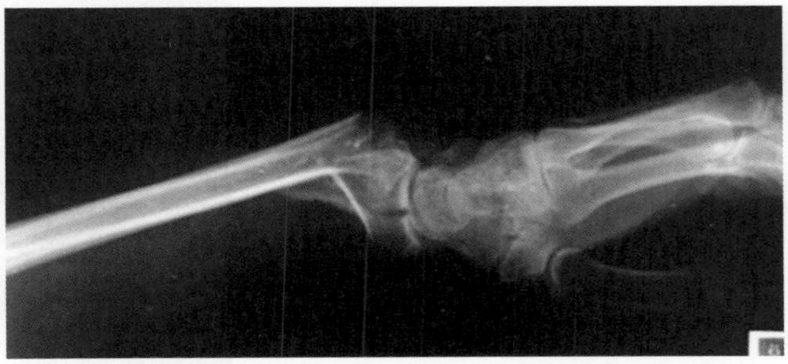

FIGURE 4.11. Severely displaced Smith fracture on lateral radiograph. (Reproduced, with permission, from Simon RR, Sherman SC, Koenigsknecht SJ. *Emergency Orthopedics: the Extremities*. 5th ed. New York, NY: McGraw-Hill; 2007.)

Treatment/Complications

- Closed reduction, long arm or sugar-tong splint, orthopedic follow-up
- Complications include: Median nerve injury, arthritis

Barton Fracture (Figure 4.12)

Mechanism/Diagnosis

- Usually caused by high speed, direct injury to the wrist, eg, motorcycle accident
- Dorsal or volar rim fracture of the distal radius, intra-articular, disrupts radiocarpal joint
- **Unstable**

Treatment

Typically these fractures require ORIF for joint stabilization. Initial management may include long arm sugar-tong splint, close orthopedic follow-up.

Essex-Lopresti Fracture

- A radial head fracture with dislocation of the distal radioulnar joint and disruption of the interosseous membrane (similar to Galeazzi, but radial **head** is fractured instead of **shaft**).
- Treat with splint and referral to orthopedics for ORIF.

Galeazzi Fracture

Radial shaft fracture with dislocation of distal radioulnar joint.

Mechanism/Diagnosis

- FOOSH in forced pronation or direct blow.
- X-ray shows distal radial shaft fracture and distal radioulnar joint injury (eg, widening of joint space) (Figure 4.13).

Treatment/Complications

- Sugar-tong splint, referral to orthopedics for ORIF. Because this is an unstable fracture, closed reduction is usually unsuccessful.
- Complications include: Compartment syndrome, malunion, chronic pain.

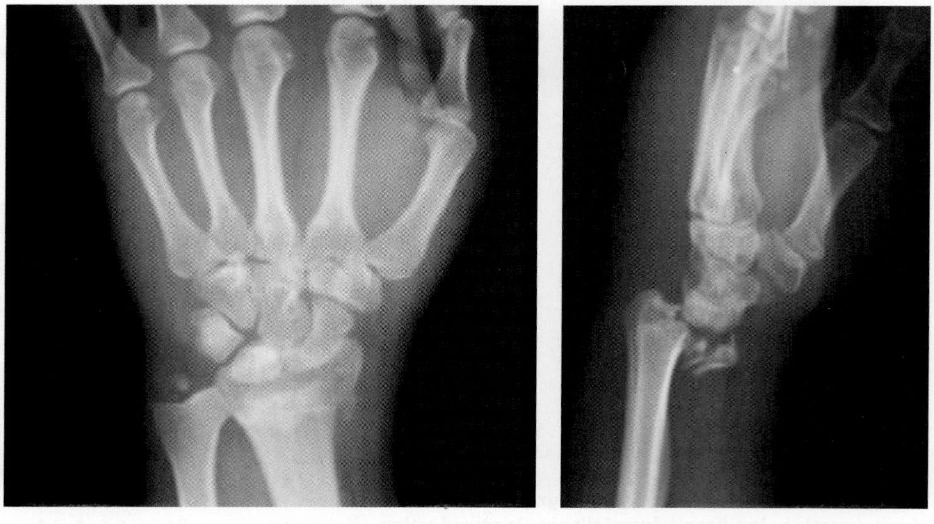

FIGURE 4.12. Volar Barton fracture with associated dislocation. (Reproduced, with permission, from Simon RR, Sherman SC, Koenigsknecht SJ. *Emergency Orthopedics: the Extremities*. 5th ed. New York, NY: McGraw-Hill; 2007.)

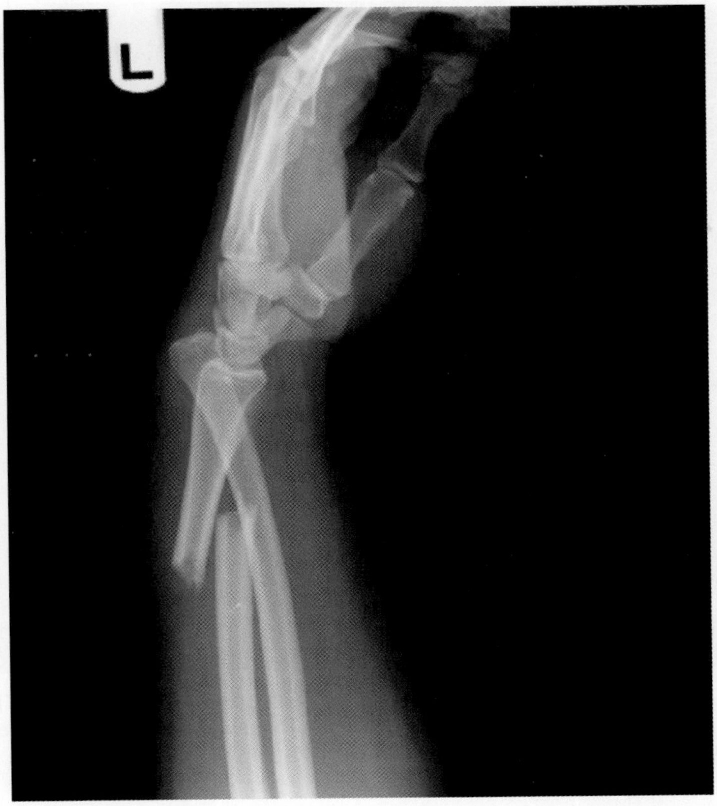

FIGURE 4.13. Galeazzi fracture. (Reproduced, with permission, from Shah B, Lucchesi M. *Atlas of Pediatric Emergency Medicine*. New York, NY: McGraw-Hill; 2006.)

Monteggia Fracture

Ulna fracture (usually proximal shaft) with radial head dislocation (Figure 4.14).

Mechanism/Diagnosis

- FOOSH or direct blow to ulna.
- Suspect if patient has significant pain and swelling to the elbow.
- X-ray shows proximal ulnar shaft fracture with radial head dislocation.

Treatment/Complication

- Reduction, long arm splint, ORIF.
- Radial nerve injury is a frequent complication.

> **KEY FACT**
>
> **GRUM**ble, **GRUM**ble, how do I remember these forearm fractures?
>
> **G**aleazzi = **R**adial fracture and radioulnar dislocation
>
> **M**onteggia = **U**lnar fracture with radial dislocation

Nightstick Fracture

Mechanism/Diagnosis

- This isolated ulnar shaft fracture typically results from a direct blow to the forearm.
- X-ray shows midshaft ulnar fracture. Always examine the proximal radius to exclude a Monteggia fracture.

Treatment

- Long arm splint for simple nightstick fractures.
- If displaced > 50% or angulated > 10°, obtain orthopedic referral for possible ORIF.

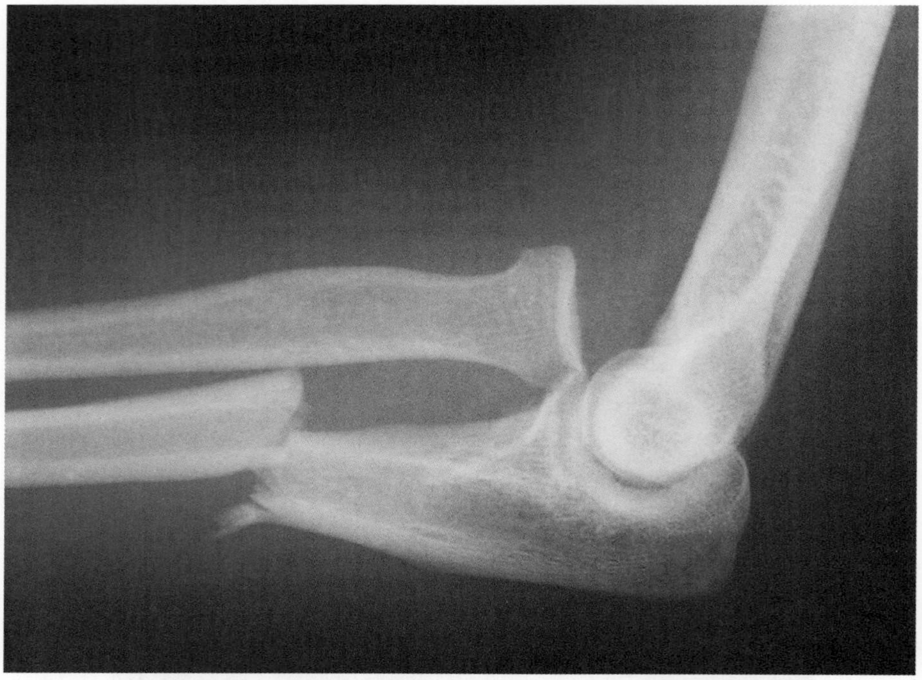

FIGURE 4.14. Monteggia fracture. (Reproduced, with permission, from Knoop KJ, Storrow AB, Stack LB, and Thurman RJ. *The Atlas of Emergency Medicine*. 3rd ed. New York, NY: McGraw-Hill; 2010. Photo contributor: Alan B. Storrow, MD.)

MNEMONIC

Carpal bones (starting at articulation with radius and ending at articulation with fifth metacarpal):

Some **L**overs **T**ry **P**ositions **T**hat **T**hey **C**an't **H**andle

Scaphoid
Lunate
Triquetrum
Pisiform
Trapezium
Trapezoid
Capitate
Hamate

CARPAL INJURIES

Scaphoid Fracture

Most common carpal fracture.

Mechanism/Diagnosis

- FOOSH.
- Suspect diagnosis if **snuff box tenderness** is present. Wrist and scaphoid x-rays should be obtained, but may be negative in the setting of acute fracture (Figure 4.15).

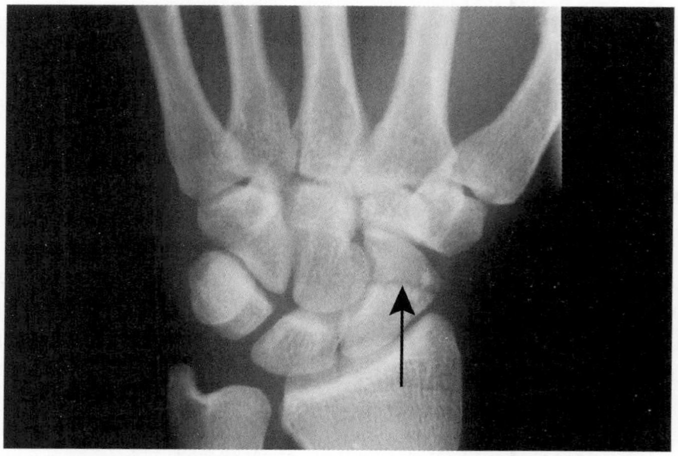

FIGURE 4.15. Scaphoid fracture in the middle third or waist (arrow). (Reproduced, with permission, from Tintinalli JE, Stapczynski JS, Ma OJ, et al. *Tintinalli's Emergency Medicine*. 7th ed. New York, NY: McGraw-Hill; 2011:1815.)

- CT and MRI can identify fractures not seen on x-ray. Consider using these modalities early for patients who might suffer from unnecessary prolonged immobilization (athletes, laborers).

TREATMENT/COMPLICATIONS

For fractures **and** suspected fractures with normal x-ray: Place in thumb spica splint, orthopedics follow-up in 7-10 days for reexamination and reimaging.

Complications include AVN (only distal scaphoid is supplied by radial artery). The more proximal the fracture, the greater likelihood of AVN and the longer the fracture needs to be immobilized.

Triquetral Fracture

Fracture of the triquetrum is the **second most common carpal fracture**. It is usually a dorsal chip fracture but can also occur through the body of the triquetrum (which is associated with perilunate and lunate dislocations).

MECHANISM/DIAGNOSIS

- Usually fall on hyperextended wrist with ulnar deviation. Can also occur with hyperflexion of the wrist.
- Point tenderness about 2 cm distal to ulnar styloid.
- X-ray is usually diagnostic (Figure 4.16).

TREATMENT

Volar splint.

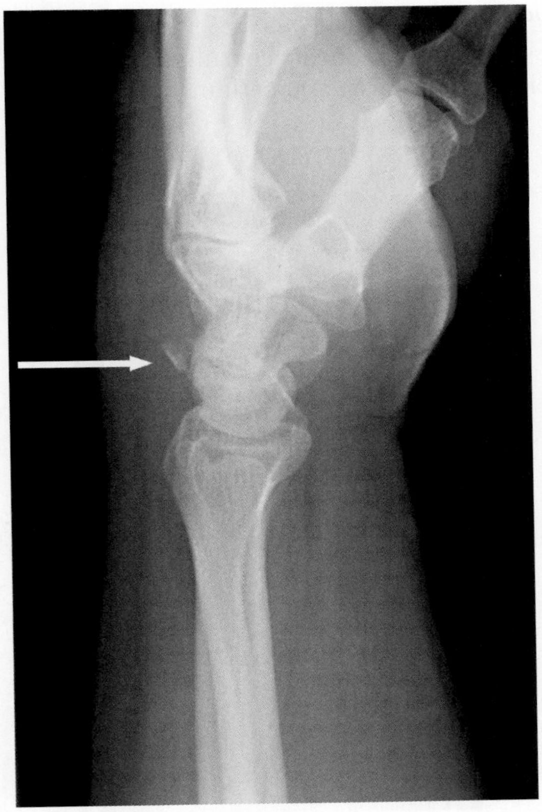

FIGURE 4.16. **Triquetrum fracture.** Triquetrum fracture seen at tip of arrow. (Used with permission from Jeffrey Kanne, Radiologist, Vancouver General Hospital, Vancouver, Canada.)

Lunate Fracture

Lunate fracture is the third most common carpal fracture. It usually occurs in association with other injuries (rare to have isolated lunate fracture).

Mechanism/Diagnosis

- FOOSH.
- Suspect diagnosis if there is tenderness over middorsum of the wrist, worse with axial compression of the middle finger. X-rays are often negative in acute injury.
- CT/MRI can identify fractures not seen on x-ray.

Treatment/Complications

- Thumb spica, referral.
- **Kienbock disease** (AVN of the lunate).

Scapholunate Dissociation

The most common carpal ligamentous wrist injury, typically resulting from an acute tear of the scapholunate ligament.

Mechanism/Diagnosis

- FOOSH is most common, though may result from chronic overuse.
- **Signet ring sign** on AP radiograph: Loss of ligamentous support results in rotary subluxation and palmar tilt of the scaphoid, causing the circular cortex to appear as a ring.
- **Terry Thomas sign** (widening of the scapholunate joint space) on AP x-ray (Figure 4.17): Terry Thomas was a comedian with a large space between his two front teeth. The space between the scaphoid and lunate is normally the same as between the other carpal bones (< 2 mm).

Treatment/Complications

- Radial gutter splint and orthopedic consultation
- May be associated with lunate and perilunate dislocations

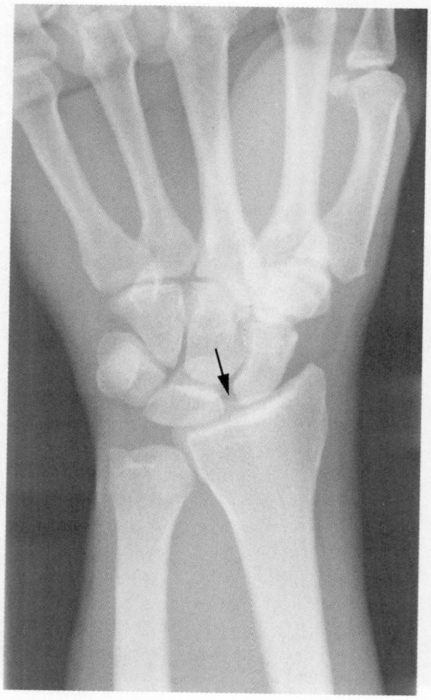

FIGURE 4.17. Scapholunate dissociation. There is widening of the scapholunate space (arrow). The signet ring sign is not well seen on this radiograph.

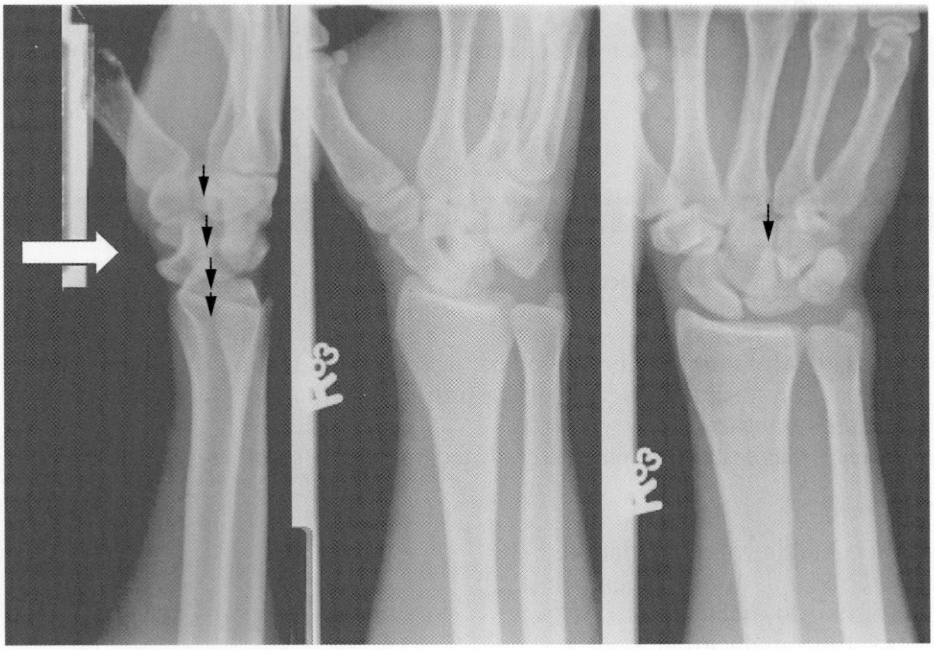

FIGURE 4.18. Lunate dislocation. "Piece-of-pie-shaped" lunate on the frontal view (black arrow) is a clue but the "spilled teacup" (white arrow) on lateral view is diagnostic. Normally the axis of the lunate should line up with that of the distal radius and the capitate on the lateral view (white dotted line).

Lunate and Perilunate Dislocations

Mechanism/Diagnosis

- FOOSH (of significant force, eg, fall from height) with wrist hyperextension and disruption of carpal ligaments.
- **Lunate:** X-ray findings include the **spilled teacup sign** (lateral view) and **piece-of-pie sign** (AP view) (lunate normally has a quadrangular shape on AP x-ray but when dislocated, it looks triangular; see Figure 4.18).
- **Perilunate:** Teacup is upright but the capitate does not sit on top of the lunate (capitate is most frequently found **dorsally** displaced sitting on top of radius; Figure 4.19).

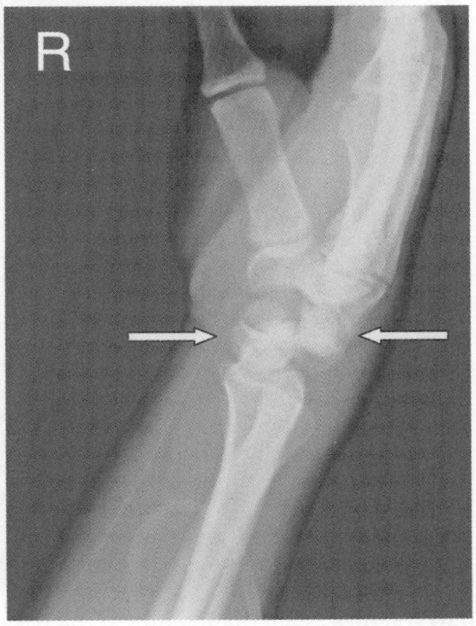

FIGURE 4.19. Perilunate dislocation. The "teacup" (lunate) is upright but the capitate is positioned posterior to the lunate.

TREATMENT/COMPLICATIONS

- Most require emergent orthopedist evaluation due to high incidence of complications.
- Complications include: Median nerve injuries, acute carpal tunnel syndrome, early arthritis, AVN.

METACARPAL AND OTHER DIGITAL INJURIES

Second to Fourth Metacarpal Fractures

MECHANISM/DIAGNOSIS

- Usually dominant hand involved from an altercation involving direct impaction forces. A fracture of the fifth metacarpal neck is referred to as a **boxer's fracture**.
- X-ray is diagnostic. Examine carefully for angulation, shortening, comminution.

TREATMENT

- Acceptable volar angulation:
  - Second, third metacarpal: < 10°
  - Fourth metacarpal: < 30°
  - Fifth metacarpal: < 40°
- Fractures without significant angulation may be treated with an ulnar gutter splint.
- Fractures with unacceptable degrees of volar angulation or with rotational deformity require closed vs open reduction.

KEY FACT

A boxer's fracture with angulation > 40° may result in functional impairment and must be reduced.

First Metacarpal Fractures

MECHANISM/DIAGNOSIS

- Axial load on thumb, often during a fistfight, or fall on hand.
- X-ray is diagnostic. May be intra- or extra-articular.
- Bennett fracture: **Intra-articular** fracture of thumb at the base of the metacarpal with associated **subluxation or dislocation** at the carpometacarpal joint (Figure 4.20).

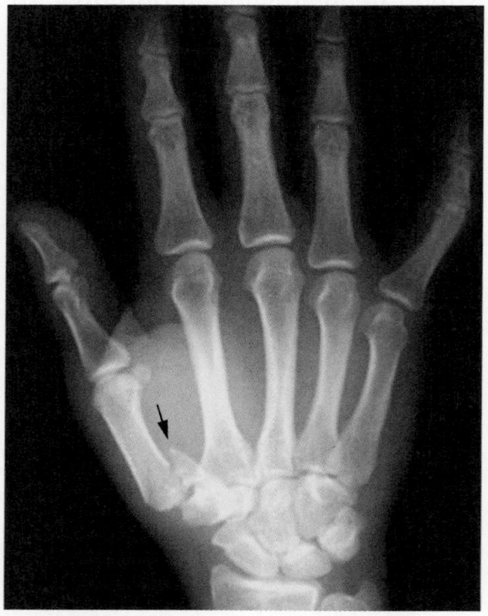

FIGURE 4.20. Bennett fracture. Note the fracture at the base of the first metacarpal (black arrow) with joint subluxation (white arrow). (Reproduced, with permission, from Simon RR, Sherman SC, Koenigsknecht SJ. *Emergency Orthopedics, the Extremities*. 5th ed. New York, NY: McGraw-Hill; 2007.)

- Rolando's fracture: **Comminuted intra-articular** fracture of the thumb at the base of the metacarpal.

TREATMENT/COMPLICATIONS

- Treat with thumb spica, orthopedic consult.
- Worse outcome for Rolando's fracture.

FINGER INJURIES

Proximal and Middle Phalanx Fractures

- Fractures of digits are most often stable and nondisplaced. Treat with buddy taping.
- Fractures that cannot be reduced, spiral fractures, and intra-articular fractures should be splinted (immobilizing wrist and injured finger) and referred to orthopedic surgery for fixation.

LIGAMENT AND TENDON INJURIES

Gamekeeper's Thumb

Rupture of the ulnar collateral ligament (UCL), also known as **skier's thumb.**

MECHANISM

- The UCL runs along the ulnar aspect of the metacarpophalangeal (MCP) joint of the thumb, and helps stabilize the joint.
- Hyperabduction of the thumb (eg, fall on the hand while holding a ski pole) leads to a tear of this ligament or avulsion from its insertion site on the base of the proximal phalanx.

DIAGNOSIS

- X-ray can identify associated avulsion fractures (25%-30%).
- Swelling and tenderness over the ulnar side of the MCP joint of the thumb. Pinch strength is markedly reduced and causes pain.
- Stress testing may differentiate incomplete (< 30° laxity) vs complete (≥ 30°-45° laxity) tears.

TREATMENT

- Incomplete tear: Thumb spica, follow up with orthopedic surgeon
- Complete tear: Surgical repair

FLEXOR TENDON INJURIES

These include injuries to the flexor digitorum superficialis (FDS) and flexor digitorum profundus (FDP). Both tendons start in the forearm and pass through the hand. In the digits, the FDS divides into two slips that insert on either side of the middle phalanx. The FDP tendon passes through these slips to insert on the base of the distal phalanx.

MECHANISM

- Commonly associated with lacerations to the palmar surface.
- Closed injuries are associated with **rheumatoid arthritis** and **athletic injury**.
  - Classic athletic injury occurs when a football player grabs another player's jersey (thus the term "**jersey finger**"), avulsing the FDP from its bony insertion.

Q

A 19-year-old man presents to a university health clinic with a swollen and tender hand over the fourth and fifth metacarpal and a laceration over the fifth knuckle. What fracture is most likely and how should the laceration be treated?

A boxer's fracture and the laceration are probably due to a tooth. Do not suture these lacerations, irrigate well, and provide prophylactic antibiotics.

KEY FACT

If the FDS is cut, the patient can still flex both the DIP and PIP joint.

Diagnosis

Injury to both FDS and FDP: Loss of flexion of the PIP and DIP joint.
Isolated FDP injury: Loss of flexion at DIP joint only.
Isolated FDS injury: Patients can still flex both joints.

Treatment/Complications

Both open and closed injuries usually require surgical repair.
Laceration injuries may cause damage to the digital arteries and nerves.

EXTENSOR TENDON INJURIES (FIGURE 4.21)

Most common site of tendon injuries due to their superficial location over the dorsum of the hand. "Zones" are used to guide management.

Zone 1: Distal phalanx and DIP joint (eg, Mallet finger)
Zone 2: Middle phalanx
Zone 3: PIP joint (eg, Boutonniere injury)
Zone 4: Proximal phalanx
Zone 5: MCP joint (eg, fight bite)
Zone 6: Dorsum of the hand
Zone 7: Wrist
Zone 8: Distal forearm

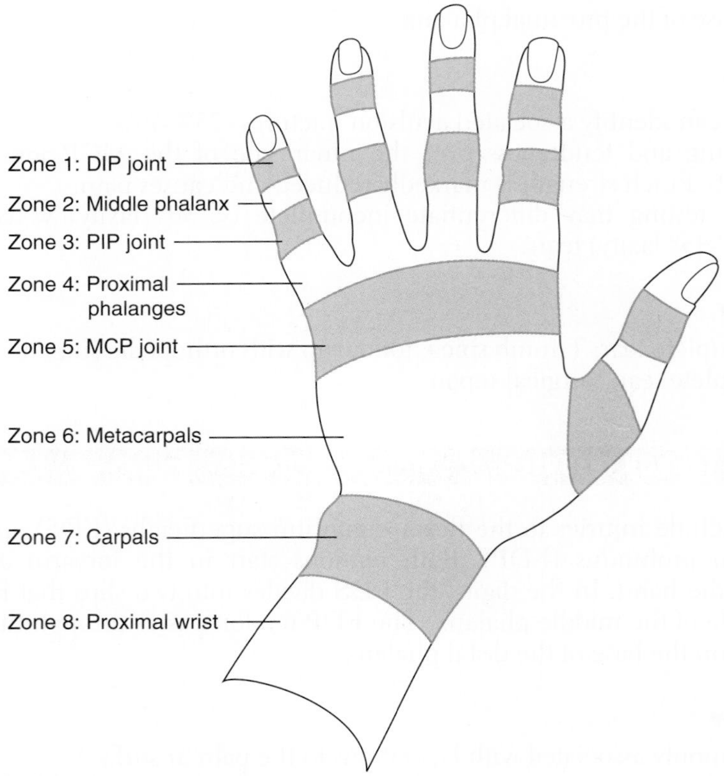

FIGURE 4.21. Extensor tendon injuries by zone. (Reproduced, with permission, from Stone CK, Humphries RL. *Current Diagnosis and Treatment: Emergency Medicine*. 7th ed. New York, NY: McGraw-Hill Education; 2011. Figure 29.12.)

MECHANISM/DIAGNOSIS

- Injuries may be open (due to laceration) or closed (crush, avulsion).
- X-ray to exclude associated fractures.

TREATMENT/COMPLICATION

See "Procedures" Chapter 19, Procedures and Skills for details.

MALLET FINGER

Most common closed tendon injury to hand in athletes.

MECHANISM/DIAGNOSIS

- Forced flexion of the DIP ("jammed finger"), leading to extensor tendon rupture or bony avulsion of the tendon at its insertion on the base of the distal phalanx.
- Unable to extend DIP.
- X-ray may reveal avulsion fracture.

TREATMENT/COMPLICATIONS

- Splint DIP in strict extension for 6-8 weeks (with a Stack-type splint): Watch for development of pressure sores!
- If untreated, a swan-neck deformity (hyperextension of PIP, flexion of DIP) may result (Figure 4.22).

BOUTONNIÈRE INJURY (CENTRAL SLIP INJURY) (FIGURE 4.23)

MECHANISM/DIAGNOSIS

- Disruption of the extensor tendon at the central slip over the PIP.
- May also be caused by chronic synovitis of PIP joint (eg, rheumatoid arthritis).
- Unable to fully extend PIP with the wrist and MCP joints fully flexed.

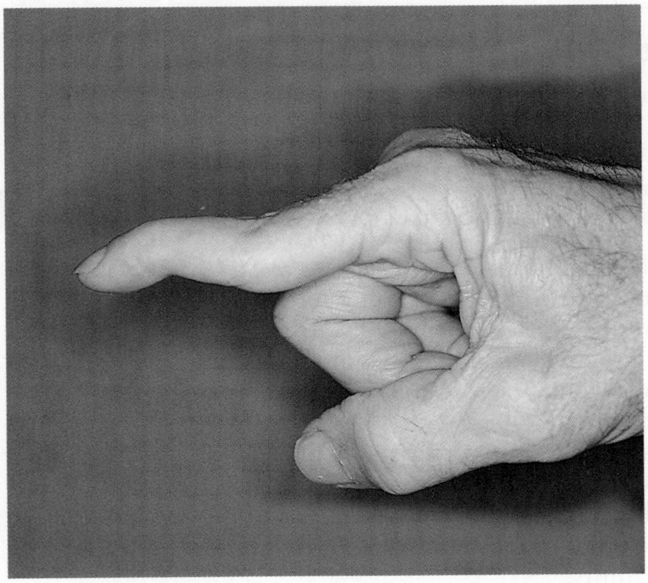

FIGURE 4.22. Swan-neck deformity. A swan-neck deformity of the index finger. Note the hyperextension of the PIP joint and the flexion of the DIP joint. (Used with permission, from Cathleen M. Vossler, MD.)

Q

A football player snags his index finger in another player's jersey and finds it difficult to catch the football for the rest of the game. When you immobilize the proximal interphalangeal (PIP) and MCP joints in extension, he is no longer able to flex the distal interphalangeal (DIP) joint. What is injured and how is it treated?

KEY FACT

An untreated mallet finger can result in a **swan-neck deformity**.

A

The football player has a flexor digitorum profundus (FDP) tendon avulsion, or "**jersey finger**," which is treated by splinting the finger in a comfortable position and referral to orthopedics as soon as possible.

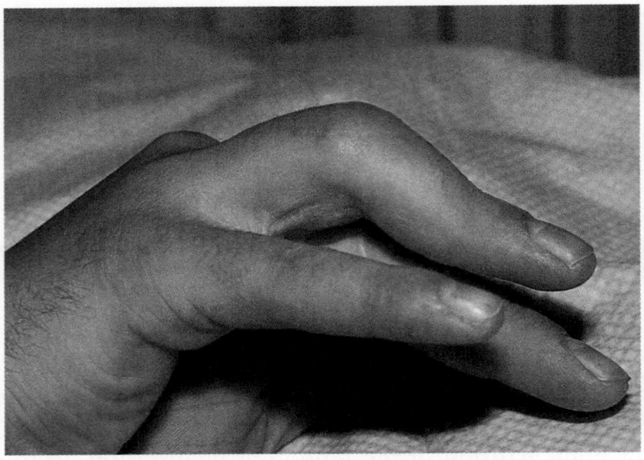

FIGURE 4.23. **Boutonnière deformity.** A boutonnière deformity of the fourth digit. Note the flexion of the PIP joint and the extension of the DIP joint. (Used with permission from E. Lee Edstrom, MD.)

Treatment

- Traumatic: Treat by splinting PIP in extension for 4-6 weeks.
- Atraumatic: Often requires surgical intervention.

AMPUTATED DIGITS

- Require immediate hand surgery consultation.
- Wrap in sterile gauze soaked in normal saline (NS) and surround with plastic bag, then place bag with digit(s) in ice water.
- Absolute contraindications to reimplantation: Unstable patient or severe crush injury. Amputations distal to DIP are difficult to reimplant.

FINGERTIP INJURY/PARTIAL AMPUTATION

Mechanism/Diagnosis

- May result from crush injury or laceration
- Clinical examination and x-ray

TREATMENT

- Distal phalanx fracture:
  - Most can be treated with splint for comfort.
  - Open fractures require copious irrigation and debridement prior to closure. Prophylactic antibiotics are not beneficial.
  - Nonreducible fractures require surgical repair.
- Tip amputation:
  - Conservative wound management for small soft-tissue injuries
  - Close soft tissue and skin over any exposed bone; this may require cutting bone back
  - Orthopedic surgery consultation for more complex injuries
- Nailbed injury:
  - Trephinate large, painful subungual hematomas.
  - Remove nail and repair nailbed with 5-0 to 6-0 absorbable suture if nail is disrupted; use removed nail as temporary splint after repair.

Injuries to the Lower Extremities

FEMUR INJURIES

Femoral Head Fractures

Mechanism/Diagnosis

- Almost always associated with hip dislocations.
- AP and Judet views of the pelvis may demonstrate fracture fragments in the acetabular fossa.
- Hip CT is almost always needed following reduction to help further delineate the extent of fracture as well as to evaluate for intra-articular fragments.

Treatment/Complications

- For specific treatments, see the section "Hip Dislocation" in Chapter 3, Trauma.
- Other common concomitant injuries include acetabular fractures, knee ligament injuries, patella fractures, and femoral shaft fractures.
- Long-term complications include osteonecrosis and posttraumatic osteoarthritis.

Femoral Neck Fractures

Mechanism

- Most commonly an insufficiency fracture in the elderly and often with minimal or no report of trauma
- In younger patients are due to high-energy trauma, including motor vehicle accidents and falls from a significant height
- Stress fractures: Seen with repeated loading such as in athletes, military recruits, and ballet dancers

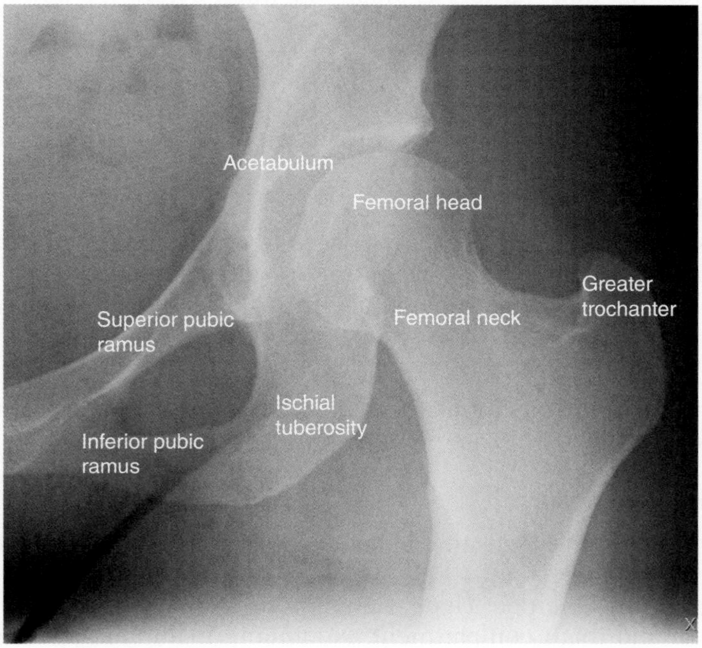

FIGURE 4.24. Normal x-ray of the hip. (Used with permission from David Berkoff, MD, FAAEM, CAQSM.)

Q

A 30-year-old woman is complaining of knee pain after an MVC. Examination shows a moderate knee effusion, positive posterior drawer test with marked joint instability. What else do you need to evaluate in this patient and how will you do so?

A

The patient likely had a posterior knee dislocation that spontaneously relocated. It is important to check pulses, motor, and sensation, especially investigating for injury to the popliteal artery and peroneal nerve. Ankle-brachial index (ABI) or ankle-ankle index < 0.9 is an indication for arteriogram. For evaluation of the peroneal nerve, check sensation of the dorsum of the foot and strength of dorsiflexion.

Diagnosis

- Pain with palpation of joint, axial compression, and range of motion.
- Displaced fractures: Patient nonambulatory with limb **shortened and externally rotated**; x-rays of the pelvis and femur are diagnostic.
- Occult or stress fracture: Suspect if significant or persistent pain with ambulation; MRI (gold standard) may be required to visualize. CT has an unacceptably high misdiagnosis rate.

Treatment/Complications

- Urgent orthopedic consultation for reduction and surgical repair.
- **AVN** occurs in up to 25% of displaced fractures.
- Nonunion and postoperative septic arthritis can also occur.

Intertrochanteric Fractures

Fracture line runs between greater and lesser trochanters.

Mechanism

90% of intertrochanteric fractures in elderly are secondary to falls. In younger patients, high-energy trauma is usually required.

Diagnosis

- Pain with range of motion and axial loading of the hip.
- Displaced fracture: Patient nonambulatory with limb **shortened and externally rotated;** x-rays of pelvis and femur are diagnostic.
- Nondisplaced or occult fracture: Patients may be ambulatory and experience minimal pain; MRI may be required to visualize.

Treatment/Complications

- Urgent orthopedic consult for reduction and surgical repair.
- Hypovolemia from up to 3 L blood loss into fracture site and thigh compartment.

Subtrochanteric Fractures

Includes fractures between the lesser trochanter and proximal 5 cm of femur.

Mechanism

- Bimodal distribution: Typically low-energy mechanisms in the elderly (minor falls), high-energy mechanisms in young adults.
- Pathologic fractures are (metastatic disease, Paget disease) also seen.

Diagnosis

- Patient is usually nonambulatory with varying degrees of gross deformity.
- X-rays of the pelvis, hip, and femur with visualization of the knee.

Treatment/Complications

- Urgent orthopedic consult for traction pinning, reduction, and surgical repair.
- Complications include: Hypovolemia from up to 3 L blood loss into fracture site and thigh compartment. Nonunion, malunion, and leg shortening are other potential complications.
- Neurovascular compromise is uncommon.

Femoral Shaft Fractures

Mechanism

- Most commonly occurs in young adults after high-energy trauma but can also be seen in elderly (mostly women) after low-energy fall.
- Stress fractures may be seen in military recruits or runners with a report of recent increase in the intensity of training.

Diagnosis

- Clinical: Usually obvious; patient nonambulatory with a gross deformity, pain, swelling, and extremity shortening.
- X-rays are diagnostic in most cases. MRI may be required if stress fracture is suspected.

Treatment

- Traction splinting may help with pain control and fracture reduction; however, avoid **prolonged** traction which can cause nerve injury and skin breakdown. Contraindications include pelvic fracture, and injuries to knee and lower leg.
- Emergent orthopedic consult for reduction and surgical repair.

Complications

- Watch for hypovolemia from up to 3 L blood loss into fracture site and thigh compartment.
- Patients often have concomitant ligamentous injury to knee and other orthopedic fractures.
- Neurovascular injuries are uncommon in closed fractures.

Distal Femur Fractures

Mechanism/Diagnosis

- Generally requires high-energy mechanism, such as direct blow to flexed knee.
- Patient is nonambulatory with pain, swelling, and deformity to lower thigh or knee.
- X-rays are confirmative. Assess proximity of fracture to neurovascular structures.
- If vascular injury suspected by examination or ABIs, exploration or angiography is indicated.

Treatment/Complications

- Immobilization, urgent orthopedic consultation.
- Open fractures occur in 5%-10%, require joint injection to rule out joint space involvement.
- Loss of knee mobility is the most common complication.

KNEE AND LOWER LEG INJURIES

Patella Fracture

Mechanism

Transverse fractures are most common and may result from blunt trauma or from the pull of the quadriceps muscle (quadriceps avulsion fracture).

KEY FACT

Always check for an intact extensor mechanism if a patient has a patella fracture.

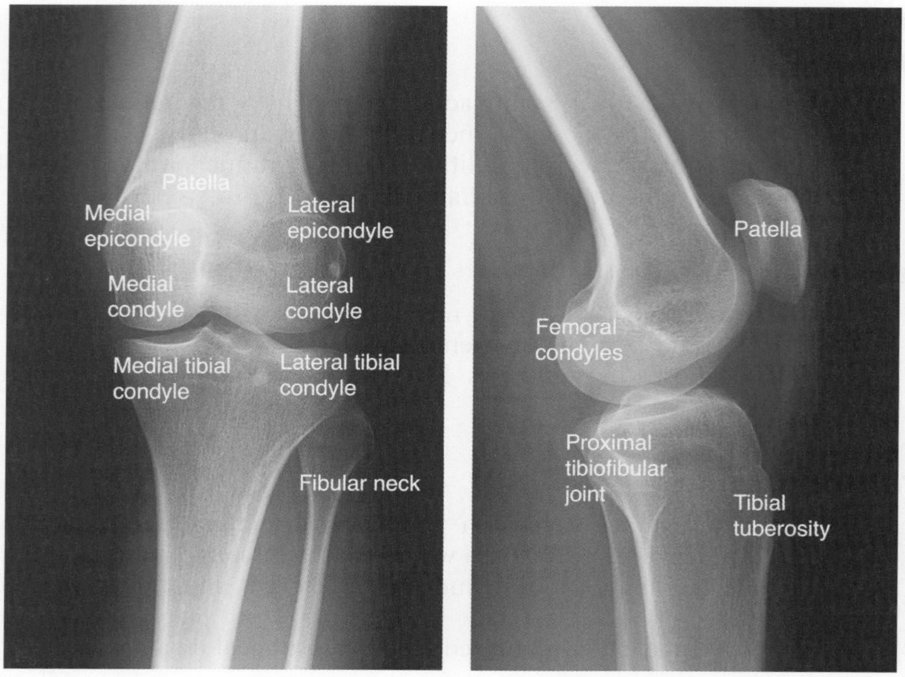

FIGURE 4.25. Normal x-ray of the knee. (Used with permission from David Berkoff, MD, FAAEM, CAQSM.)

Diagnosis

- Patellar tenderness and swelling: With a transverse fracture, the patient may be unable to extend the knee.
- X-rays of the knee: AP, lateral, and sunrise views should be obtained.
- **Bipartite patella** is a normal variant and can be differentiated from a true fracture by its smooth cortical margins. If in doubt, x-ray the other knee as this condition is often bilateral.

Treatment

- Nondisplaced patella fractures require immobilization in full extension with weight bearing as tolerated and orthopedic referral.
- Patella fractures with > 3 mm displacement or loss of extensor function mandate orthopedic referral for surgical intervention.

> **MNEMONIC**
>
> ***Ottawa Knee Rules***
>
> **Obtain radiographs if at least one of the following is true after knee trauma:**
>
> - Age > 55
> - Fibular head tenderness
> - Isolated tenderness of patella
> - Inability to flex knee to 90°
> - Inability to bear weight in the emergency department (ED) for 4 steps after injury

Patella Dislocation

The patella usually displaces laterally over the lateral femoral condyle, most often from a direct blow.

Treatment

- ED reduction is accomplished by placing the knee in full extension, the hip in some flexion, and pushing on the patella in a medial direction up and over the lateral condyle. Procedural sedation aids reduction.
- Once reduced, immobilize in full extension for orthopedics follow-up.

Knee Dislocation

Displacement of tibia relative to femur. Anterior is most common, posterior is second most common.

Mechanism

- Always requires significant force and is universally associated with significant ligamentous injury.
- About half self-reduce prior to presentation, therefore based on mechanism and forces required, **fractures with significant ligamentous laxity (eg, anterior cruciate ligament [ACL] and posterior cruciate ligament [PCL] rupture) should be treated as a dislocation**.

Treatment

- **Immediate** reduction.
- Assess status of popliteal artery:
  - Immediate surgical exploration when hard signs of vascular injury are present (absent pulses, expanding popliteal hematoma, cool mottled foot).
  - Angiogram or duplex ultrasound for soft signs of vascular injury (paresthesias, asymmetrical pedal pulses).
  - If none of the above, check ABIs. ABI < 0.9 on injured leg, proceed with arteriogram, color-flow Doppler studies, or surgical exploration. If ABI is > 0.9, perform serial examinations and ABIs.
- Evaluate for injury to peroneal nerve (dorsiflexion of ankle, sensation to dorsum of foot).
- Posterior splint with immobilization in 15° of flexion.
- Obtain orthopedics ± vascular surgery consultation.

Complications

- **Peroneal nerve injury** (foot drop)
- **Popliteal artery injury** especially with anterior and posterior dislocations
- Less commonly, tibial nerve injury and meniscal injury

Tibial Plateau Fracture

- **Most common fracture of the knee**
- Most involve the lateral plateau

Mechanism/Diagnosis

- Impact that drives the femoral condyles into the tibial plateau, such as fall from height or impact with automobile bumper.
- Maintain a high index of suspicion. X-rays (AP, lateral, and oblique views) often reveal the fracture, but sometimes only show an effusion. CT is occasionally needed to diagnose the fracture.

> **KEY FACT**
>
> Arthrocentesis may be performed to relieve some of the pressure associated with a large joint effusion. If **lipohemarthrosis** is present, this is indicative of an **intra-articular knee fracture**.

Treatment

Nondisplaced fractures can be treated with knee-immobilizer and non–weight bearing. Displaced fractures require ORIF.

Complications

- Popliteal and anterior tibial artery injuries can occur.
- Associated ligamentous injuries are present in one-third of cases.
- Early arthritis can occur if the fracture is intra-articular.

Rupture of Extensor Mechanism of the Knee

- Quadriceps tendon rupture (> 40 years old)
- Patellar tendon rupture (< 40 years old)
- Patella fracture
- Avulsion of the tibial tuberosity (young adolescents)

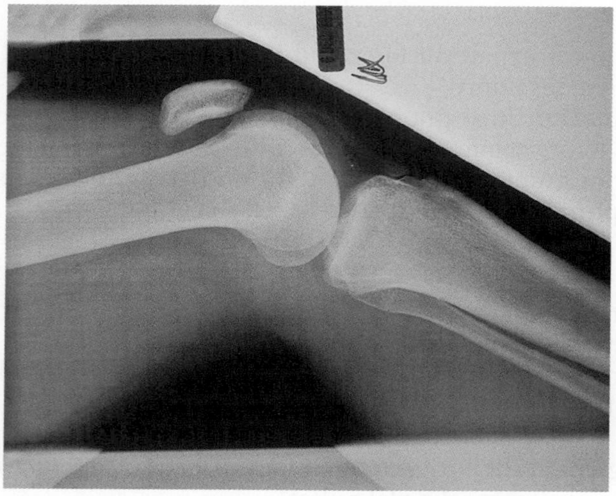

FIGURE 4.26. Patellar tendon rupture. A lateral radiograph reveals the proximal patellar displacement seen with complete patellar tendon rupture. (Used with permission from Kevin J. Knoop, MD, MS.)

Mechanism/Diagnosis

- Forceful contraction of quadriceps muscle or fall on a flexed knee.
- Knee pain and swelling with inability to extend knee.
- Patella may be low riding (quadriceps tendon rupture) or high riding (patellar tendon rupture) (Figure 4.26).

Treatment

Orthopedic consult for surgical repair.

Chondromalacia Patella (Patellofemoral Pain Syndrome)

Anterior knee pain localized to the patellofemoral joint. Precise pathophysiology is poorly defined. It is the **most common cause of knee pain** (frequently seen in female athletes) and is often bilateral.

Symptoms/Examination

- Pain worsens after prolonged sitting, climbing stairs, or squatting. Sticking or buckling of the knee may occur. There is usually no history of trauma.
- **Patella compression test:** Pain and crepitus occur with compression of the patella into the femoral groove when the knee is extended and quadriceps muscle tightened.

Treatment

Initial treatment includes: Nonsteroidal anti-inflammatory drugs (NSAIDs), hip-abductor and quadriceps-strengthening exercises.

Patellar Tendinitis (Jumper Knee)

Overuse injury of patellar tendon and extensor mechanism from stress of running and jumping.

Symptoms/Examination

- Anterior knee pain; night pain; pain with sitting, standing up, squatting, kneeling, climbing stairs.
- **Tenderness to palpation over proximal patellar tendon:** There is normal range of motion but can be painful at full extension and with resisted extension.

TREATMENT

Heat, NSAIDs, hip-abductor and quadriceps-strengthening exercises.

LIGAMENTOUS AND MENISCAL INJURIES OF THE KNEE

Anterior Cruciate Ligament Injury

The most common knee ligamentous injury; it results from **high-speed, traumatic twisting movements (especially if accompanied by a valgus stress)** and can occur from a noncontact injury ("plant and pivot").

SYMPTOMS/EXAMINATION

- A "**pop**" is frequently felt at the time of injury.
- Hemarthrosis is common (75% of all knee hemarthroses are caused by ACL [anterior cruciate ligament] tears).

DIAGNOSIS

Positive **Lachman test** (most sensitive) and **anterior drawer sign** are suggestive (Table 4.3). MRI or arthroscopy is diagnostic.

TREATMENT

Rest, ice, elevate, NSAIDs, immobilization, orthopedics referral, physical therapy.

COMPLICATIONS

If resulting from lateral blow to knee, it is often associated with **medial collateral ligament tear and medial meniscus injury (terrible triad).**

KEY FACT

ValGus: Gum sticking your knees together

VARus: Air between your bowed knees

TABLE 4.3. Physical Examination of the Knee

Test	Maneuver	Abnormality
Valgus stress	Instability with valgus stress in 30° flexion	Tear of the MCL
Varus stress	Instability with varus stress in 30° of flexion	Tear of the LCL
Anterior drawer sign	Instability with anterior stress with knee in 90° of flexion	Tear of the ACL
Lachman test	Instability with anterior stress in 15°-30° of flexion; more sensitive than drawer signs	Tear of the ACL
Posterior drawer sign	Instability with posterior stress in 90° of flexion	Tear of the PCL
McMurray test	Pain as the knee is brought from full flexion to 90° flexion while the leg is externally rotated with compression over the medial joint line **and/or** when the leg is internally rotated with compression over the lateral joint line	Medial joint line pain = medial meniscus injury Lateral joint pain = lateral meniscus injury
Apley test	In prone position with knee flexed 90°, pain as knee is internally/externally rotated with downward pressure to heel	Meniscal injury
Ege test	In squatting position, pain, and/or click on maximum rotation of knee	External rotation = medial meniscus tear Internal rotation = lateral meniscus tear

ACL, anterior cruciate ligament; LCL, lateral collateral ligament; MCL, medial collateral ligament; PCL, posterior cruciate ligament.

> **KEY FACT**
>
> The Lachman test is better than the anterior drawer test for detecting ACL injuries. Diagnoses for meniscal and ligamentous injuries are improved when tests are used in combination.

Posterior Cruciate Ligament Injury

Far less common than ACL tears and usually occurs in combination with other injuries. Associated with blow to flexed knee (as in dashboard injury).

DIAGNOSIS

Positive posterior drawer test is suggestive. MRI or arthroscopy is diagnostic.

TREATMENT

Rest, ice, elevate, NSAIDs, immobilization, orthopedics referral, physical therapy.

Medial Collateral Ligament and Lateral Collateral Ligament Injuries

Medial collateral ligament (MCL) is the most common isolated knee injury.

Common mechanisms include MCL valgus stress from lateral blow or (lateral collateral ligament [LCL]) hyperextension with varus stress.

DIAGNOSIS

Positive varus (medial) stress test for LCL injury or valgus (lateral) stress tests for MCL injury are suggestive. MRI or arthroscopy is diagnostic.

TREATMENT

Rest, ice, elevate, NSAIDs, immobilization, orthopedics referral, physical therapy.

> **MNEMONIC**
>
> ***Match the Mechanism to the Injury:***
>
> 1. Two skiers collide. One sustains a blow to the outside of her left knee, causing a tearing sensation and pain along the medial aspect of her knee.
> 2. While running downfield during a soccer match, a defender plants her foot to decelerate and change directions, causing a pop in her knee. A large effusion is seen shortly afterward.
> 3. While bending down to pick up a heavy box with his right knee externally rotated, a man feels a pop in his knee. He has had problems with his knee locking since the incident.
> 4. The patient's knee hit the dashboard in an MVC. No fracture is found, but patient is complaining of knee pain.
>
>   a. PCL injury
>   b. ACL injury
>   c. LCL injury
>   d. MCL injury
>   e. Lateral meniscus injury
>   f. Medial meniscus injury
>
> **Answers: 1. d 2. b 3. f 4. a**

Medial and Lateral Meniscus Injuries

Medial meniscus is injured twice as often. Injury usually results from quickly changing directions, squatting, or twisting knee while weight-bearing.

SYMPTOMS/EXAMINATION

Pain and swelling (acute injury), clicking, or locking of the knee.

DIAGNOSIS

Positive **McMurray** and Ege tests are suggestive. MRI or arthroscopy is diagnostic.

TREATMENT

Rest, ice, elevate, NSAIDs, orthopedics referral.

ANKLE INJURIES

Ligamentous Injury (Ankle Sprain)

Three groups of ligaments stabilize the ankle joint: medial, lateral, and syndesmotic (interosseous between the distal tibia and fibula).

Ankle sprains can be graded based on degree of functional impairment and presumed pathologic findings:

- Grade I (first-degree) sprain:
  - Ligamentous stretching without tear or rupture. No joint instability. Able to bear weight.
- Grade II (second-degree) sprain:
  - More significant ligament damage (partially torn), but no joint instability. Limp with walking.
- Grade III (third-degree) sprain:
  - Torn ligament with joint instability. Unable to bear weight, severe swelling.

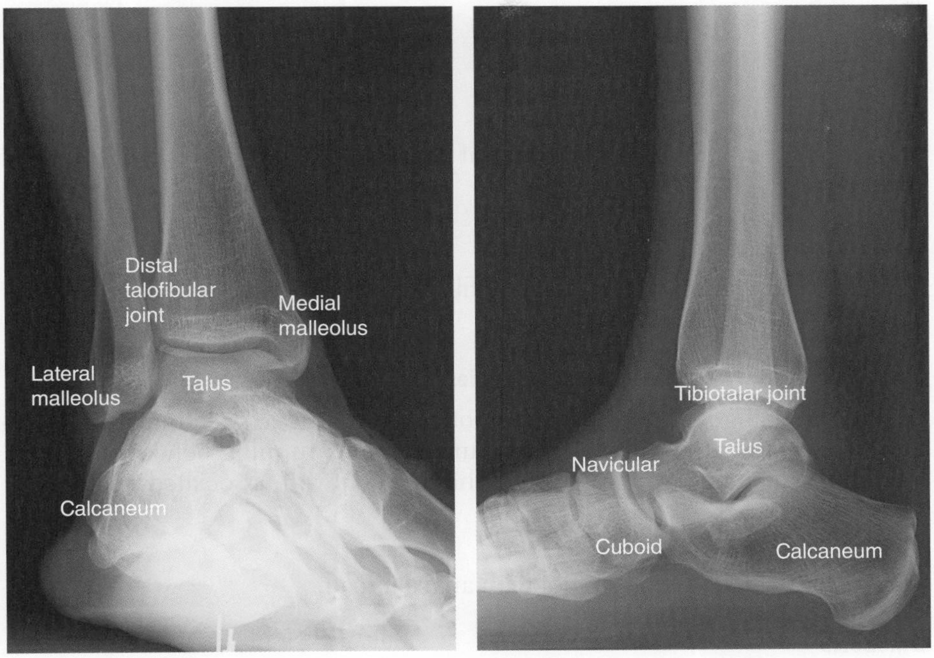

FIGURE 4.27. Normal x-ray of ankle. (Used with permission from David Berkoff, MD, FAAEM, CAQSM.)

Treatment

- If ankle is unstable, consider posterior splint and urgent orthopedic referral.
- If ankle is stable but patient is unable to bear weight, rest, ice, compression, elevation, crutches, apply ankle brace, and follow-up in one week with orthopedics.

Lateral Ligamentous Ankle Injury

Ankle inversions with lateral ankle sprains are far more common than medial injuries. The **anterior talofibular ligament is the most commonly injured ligament** (runs anteriorly/medially from fibula at the lateral malleolus to the talus) followed by the calcaneofibular ligament and the posterior talofibular ligament.

Mechanism

Inversion with internal rotation of a plantar-flexed foot.

Diagnosis

- Abnormal **anterior drawer test** (knee in 90° flexion, ankle neutral, one hand pushing posteriorly on base of tibia, instability when pulling heel forward) with anterior talofibular ligament rupture
- Abnormal **talar tilt test** (knee in 90° flexion, ankle neutral, > 5° rotation with inversion of heel) with presence of both anterior talofibular **and** calcaneofibular ligament ruptures

Medial Ligamentous Ankle Injury

Far less common because the **medial deltoid** ligament is much stronger.

MNEMONIC

Ottawa Ankle and Midfoot Rules

Get ankle films if there is malleolar pain and any of the following:

1. Tenderness on the posterior edge, tip, or distal 6 cm of lateral or medial malleolus
2. Inability to complete 4 steps now and at the scene of the injury

Get foot films as well if midfoot pain and any of the following:

1. Navicular tenderness
2. Base of fifth metatarsal tenderness
3. Inability to complete 4 steps

Mechanism

Eversion and external rotation of foot.

Diagnosis

Significant tenderness and swelling at the level of and distal to the medial malleolus.

Complications

Sometimes associated with a proximal fibula fracture, ie, Maisonneuve fracture.

Distal Tibiofibular Syndesmotic Ligament Injuries

Injuries can range from mild syndesmotic sprains due to stretching of the syndesmotic ligament (a collection of four ligaments running between the tibia and fibula) to complete disruption of the ligament with associated fractures.

Mechanism

Dorsiflexion and eversion of foot with an axial load.

Diagnosis

- If minor sprain, patient will have localized pain and swelling to area of injury.
- Positive **squeeze test** in which the examiner firmly grasps the patient's lower leg and "squeezes" the distal tibia and fibula together, causing pain if the injury is present.
- Abnormal external rotation stress test (knee in 90° flexion, ankle neutral, pain at syndesmosis, or sensation of lateral talar motion with external rotation of foot).

Peroneal Tendon Subluxation/Dislocation

Often mistaken for ankle sprain, but often requires surgical repair to prevent chronic pain and ankle instability.

Peroneal muscles assist with foot eversion/plantar flexion. Tendons run around lateral malleolus and attach at the midfoot.

Mechanism

Forced dorsiflexion with peroneal muscle contraction causing tear of the superior peroneal retinaculum (holds tendon in place). Often associated with **skiing injuries.**

Diagnosis

- Swelling posteriorly/inferiorly to lateral malleolus **in absence of** tenderness over anterior talofibular ligament (anteriorly).When held in dorsiflexion, patients are unable to evert their foot.
- 50% have a small avulsion fracture of the lateral ridge of distal fibula.

Treatment

Splint in midplantar flexion, orthopedic referral for possible surgical repair.

Achilles Tendon Rupture

Commonly seen in older athletes (eg, "weekend warriors"), patients with rheumatoid arthritis, lupus, and recent **fluoroquinolone use.** 25% are initially misdiagnosed as ankle sprains.

Mechanism

Forceful plantar flexion against resistance.

Symptoms/Examination

Often hear a "pop" during the acute injury; tenderness and a possibly a defect 2-6 cm above the insertion site to the calcaneus.

Diagnosis

Abnormal **Thompson test** (position the patient prone with knee bent to 90°. With tibia pointing perpendicular to the ground, squeeze the calf, and if tendon is intact, the foot should plantarflex.

Treatment

Apply posterior splint in plantar flexion and orthopedic consult. If indicated, early surgical repair leads to a better outcome.

Ankle Fractures

Mechanism

Ranges from simple inversion/eversion twisting injury to falls from height or high-energy MVCs.

Treatment

Fractures that require orthopedic consultation in the ED include:

- Any injuries that produce instability of the ankle joint, including medial malleolar fractures with lateral collateral ligament rupture, lateral malleolar fractures with deltoid ligament rupture, bi- or trimalleolar fractures, etc.
- Intra-articular fractures
- Open fractures
- Fracture dislocations (reduce before radiographs if skin tenting or neurovascular compromise)

Maisonneuve Fracture

- Ankle-eversion injury with forces transmitted along interosseous membrane causing proximal fibula fracture.
- May also be associated with avulsion fracture of the medial malleolus, rupture of the deltoid ligament, or distal tibiofibular syndesmosis.

Diagnosis

X-rays of the entire lower leg in addition to the ankle if any pain with palpation over proximal fibula.

Treatment

Often requires ORIF to stabilize the tibiofibular syndesmosis.

FOOT INJURIES

Calcaneus Fracture

Most commonly fractured tarsal bone. Often bilateral, or associated with other injuries to lower extremities or spine.

Mechanism

Usually severe axial load caused by a fall from a significant height.

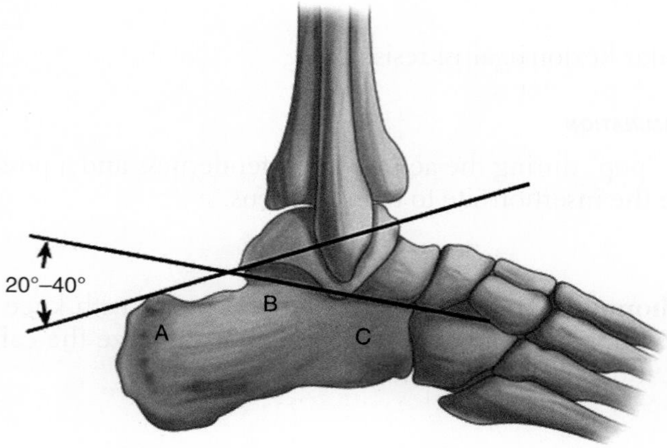

FIGURE 4.28. Bohler's angle to detect compression fractures of the calcaneus may be useful in adolescents, but it is unreliable in younger children. (Reproduced, with permission, from Strange GR, Ahrens WR, Schafermeyer RW, Wiebe RA. *Pediatric Emergency Medicine*. 3rd ed. New York, NY: McGraw-Hill; 2009.)

DIAGNOSIS

- On plain film, **Bohler's angle** < 20° (angle between a line formed from the posterior tuberosity of the calcaneus and the apex of the posterior facet and a line between the apex of the posterior facet and anterior process of the calcaneus) suggests compression fracture. A Bohler's angle of 20°-40° is normal (Figure 4.28).
- CT scan may be needed to determine if injury is extensive enough to require surgery.

TREATMENT

- Bulky Jones dressing, posterior splint, non–weight bearing; orthopedic consult.
- Surgical repair (when needed) is delayed up to three weeks until swelling is improved.

COMPLICATIONS

- Comminuted fractures have a high rate of **compartment syndrome.**
- Chronic pain and disability.

TALAR FRACTURE

Second most common tarsal fracture. The talar neck is the most common location.

TREATMENT

- Minor avulsion fractures can be treated with a posterior splint and crutches.
- Major fractures of the neck and body require orthopedic consultation as these fractures often require ORIF.

COMPLICATION

High rates of **AVN** and chronic arthritis.

LISFRANC (TARSOMETATARSAL) FRACTURE

The Lisfranc joint is the tarsometatarsal complex made up of the 5 metatarsals and their adjoining tarsal bones (3 medial cuneiforms and 2 lateral cuboids).

MNEMONIC

Lover's triad*:

Calcaneal fractures
Lumbar compression fractures
Forearm fractures

*Lover jumps out of bedroom window to avoid discovery.

KEY FACT

Midpart (navicular, cuboid, cuneiforms).

Separated from hindpart by **Chopart** joint.

Separated from forepart by **Lisfranc** joint.

Mechanism

Can be quite varied (axial load, crush injury, or rotational stress); may occur with relatively minor trauma.

Diagnosis

- Inability to stand on toes, severe pain in midfoot, or **Plantar ecchymosis sign** (bruise over the plantar aspect of the midfoot) should raise clinical suspicion.
- Weight-bearing, bilateral plain films are required and will increase diagnostic yield.
- Suspect Lisfranc injury if there is gap > 1 mm between the base of the first and second or second and third metatarsals (Figure 4.29) or any fractures around the Lisfranc joint.
- **Fleck sign** is an avulsion fracture of the base of the second metatarsal on the medial side. It is pathognomonic of a Lisfranc fracture.

KEY FACT

"Sprained foot"?
Think Lisfranc injury!

Treatment/Complications

- Emergent orthopedic referral.
- Frequently associated with dorsalis pedis artery injury, early arthritis, and chronic pain. Delayed or missed diagnosis is common and associated with increased complications.

Jones Fracture

Diagnosis

Jones fracture is a transverse fracture through the **metaphyseal-diaphyseal junction** of the fifth metatarsal. The fracture line will be at least 1.5 cm distal to the base of the fifth metatarsal (Figure 4.30).

KEY FACT

A fracture of the base of the second metatarsal on the medial side is pathognomonic of a Lisfranc fracture.

Treatment

Cast/splint, non–weight bearing, and orthopedic referral for ORIF evaluation.

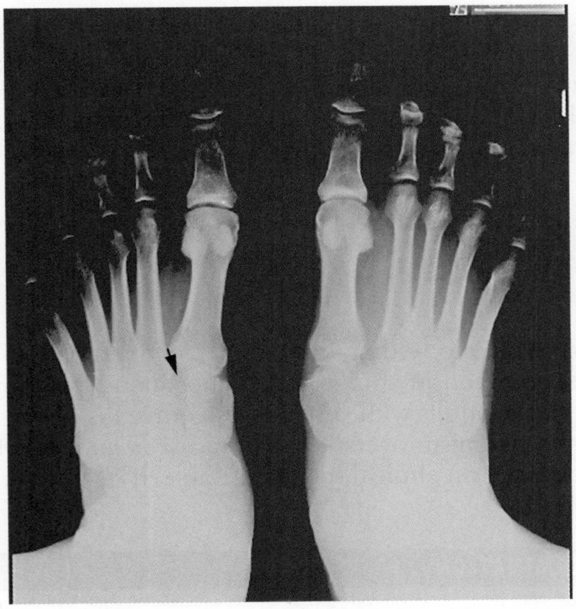

FIGURE 4.29. Lisfranc fracture. The space between the base of the first and second metatarsal is widened (black arrow), which indicates disruption of the tarsometatarsal joint.

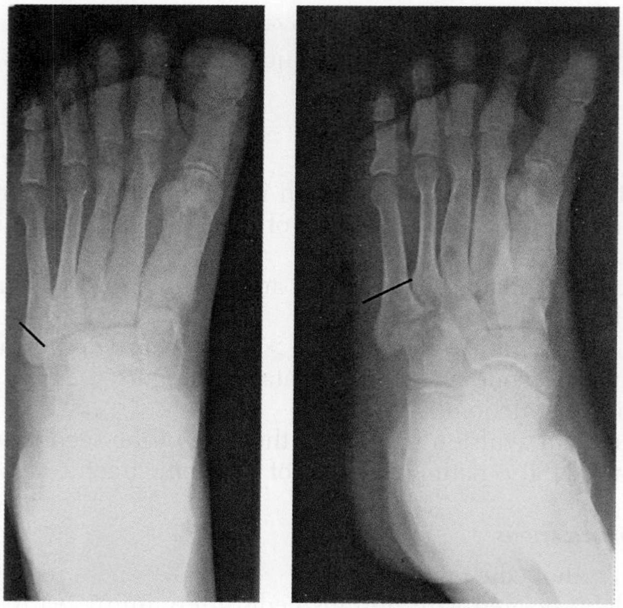

FIGURE 4.30. Jones and pseudo-Jones fracture. The lines indicate the general appearance of the location of fracture sites, with a pseudo-Jones as a very proximal avulsion-type fracture (left) and a Jones as a proximal shaft fracture (right).

KEY FACT

The Jones fracture is frequently complicated by nonunion or malunion.

Complication

Frequent nonunion or malunion.

Pseudo-Jones Fracture

More common than the Jones fracture.

Diagnosis

Avulsion fracture of the base of the fifth metatarsal (see Figure 4.30).

Treatment

- Ankle stirrup splint, hard post-op shoe, or rocker walker.
- See Table 4.4 for indications for emergent and urgent (< 72 hours) orthopedic referral in ankle and foot injuries.

Osteomyelitis

- Infection of the bone, either from direct contamination or contiguous spread (most common in adults) or hematogenous spread (most common in children and in adults with vertebral osteomyelitis).
- Most common organism overall: *Staphylococcus aureus*. Other pathogens possible depending on clinical scenario (Table 4.5).

SYMPTOMS/EXAMINATION

- Can be relatively nonspecific: Fever, fatigue, anorexia
- Local swelling, erythema, and tenderness over the affected bone

TABLE 4.4. Indications for Emergent Ankle or Foot Orthopedic Intervention and Injuries for Orthopedic Referral

ORTHOPEDIC EMERGENCIES	ORTHOPEDIST REFERRAL (< 72 H)
Major talar neck and body fractures	Extra-articular calcaneal fractures
Intra-articular calcaneus fractures	First metatarsal fracture
All open fractures	Displaced metatarsal shaft
All fracture dislocations	Unstable ligamentous injuries
Maisonneuve fractures with neurovascular compromise Bimalleolar and trimalleolar fractures with neurovascular compromise Lisfranc injuries	Stable unimalleolar fracture Peroneal dislocations Maisonneuve, bimalleolar, and trimalleolar fractures with good reduction, no neurovascular compromise
Compartment syndromes	Jones fracture

TABLE 4.5. Common Organisms and Recommended Antibiotics for Osteomyelitis

GROUP	COMMON ORGANISM	ANTIBIOTIC
Neonates	Group B streptococci, Enterobacteriaceae, *Staphylococcus epidermidis*	Penicillinase-resistant penicillin (PRP) + ceph 3
Younger children	*Staphylococcus aureus*, group A streptococci, *Kingella kingae*	PRP + ceph 3
Puncture through sole of shoe	***Pseudomonas aeruginosa***	Antipseudomonal ceph
Sickle cell disease	*S. aureus*, ***Salmonella sp.***	PRP + ceph 3
Human or animal bite	*Eikenella corrodens*, *Pasteurella multocida*	Penicillin ± Augmentin
Chronic infection or diabetic foot infection	*S. aureus*, Enterobacteriaceae, anaerobes	PRP + fluoroquinolone + flagyl
Injection drug use	*S. aureus*, *P. aeruginosa*, Enterobacteriaceae	PRP + antipseudomonal aminoglycoside

PRP: CONDOM—cloxacillin, oxacillin, nafcillin, dicloxacillin, methicillin.

Antipseudomonal cephalosporin: Ceftazidime, cefepime.

Ceph 3 (many): Ceftriaxone, cefotaxime, ceftazidime.

Antipseudomonal aminoglycoside: TAG—tobramycin, amikacin, gentamycin.

DIAGNOSIS

- Erythrocyte sedimentation rate (ESR) and C-reactive protein (CRP) are elevated in most cases, but these are nonspecific.
- X-ray may reveal periosteal elevation or soft-tissue edema. Later, bony lucencies may be apparent. Most often, no x-ray abnormalities are seen, particularly early in the course of disease.
- Bone scan or MRI is usually diagnostic.
- Getting an exact microbiologic identification in the ED is challenging, but it can involve aspiration of affected bone/joint and blood cultures (positive in half).

TREATMENT

- Early antibiotics (see Table 4.5). If methicillin-resistant *S. aureus* (MRSA) is likely, add vancomycin.
- Surgical debridement of wound or removal of bone may be necessary.

COMPLICATION

Sepsis, bone abscess, pathological fracture, nonhealing wound.

Disorders of the Spine

LOW BACK PAIN

The causes of low back pain are varied and often impossible to pinpoint in the ED. It is more important to determine if an emergency exists that requires neurosurgical intervention or a condition, eg, osteomyelitis that requires specific treatment. Patients at high risk for a serious cause of back pain include injection drug users, the elderly, immunocompromised, and those with a history of cancer or recent trauma.

Causes

Range from minor musculoskeletal pain to can't miss emergencies, including aortic dissection, cauda equina, epidural abscess or hematoma, and spinal fracture with cord impingement.

Symptoms

Symptoms that indicate a potential neurosurgical emergency include: Fever, severe pain (may be radicular), neurologic impairment, bladder or bowel retention or incontinence.

Examination

- Findings that indicate a neurosurgical emergency, including motor weakness, saddle anesthesia, loss of deep tendon reflexes, and decreased rectal tone.
- **Straight leg raise (SLR) test:** A positive SLR is back pain that radiates PAST the knee at an elevation < 60°. **A positive contralateral SLR is *highly specific* for sciatica.**

KEY FACT

A straight leg raise test is positive when it elicits back pain that radiates past the knee at an elevation < 60°. **A positive contralateral straight leg raise is highly specific for sciatica**.

DIFFERENTIAL

- Aortic aneurysm
- Kidney stone/infection

DIAGNOSIS

- History and examination are critical!
- More extensive workup starting with lumbosacral x-rays should be done if:
  - Age < 18 or > 50 years
  - Trauma with vertebral tenderness
  - Pain lasting longer than 1 month
  - History of IDU
  - Suspicion for cancer or infection such as fever or weight loss
  - Neurologic deficits
- CT scan is best for identifying fractures.
- MRI is better for herniated disks, infection, malignancy, and neurological impairment.

TREATMENT

- Treat the underlying cause (see also the section "Spinal Cord Disorders," Chapter 15, Neurology).
- If musculoskeletal in origin:
  - Ice in first 24-72 hours; afterward, heat may be helpful.
  - Pain medication.
  - Muscle relaxants.
  - Activity as tolerated: **Neither complete bedrest nor active physical therapy that causes pain is helpful.**
- Immediate neurosurgical or spine specialist consultation if any neurologic impairment.

COMPLICATION

Chronic pain, neurological impairment, disability, opiate addiction

CAUDA EQUINA SYNDROME

Usually stems from a herniated disk that protrudes midline and compresses the nerve roots of the cauda equine; can also be caused by tumor and infection. Acute cauda equina is a medical/surgical emergency.

SYMPTOMS

Back pain, leg weakness, numbness, and bladder and/or bowel retention (followed by overflow incontinence)

EXAMINATION

Findings may include loss of sensation in the "saddle distribution," loss of rectal tone, loss of bulbocavernosus and deep tendon reflexes, and a distended bladder.

DIAGNOSIS

Emergent MRI or CT myelogram

TREATMENT

Emergent spine consultation.

Q

A 26-year-old man comes into the ED with a fever; a swollen, painful right knee and left elbow; and a vesiculopustular lesion on his fingers. He had been treated for *Chlamydia* 2 weeks earlier. What is his diagnosis?

Complications

- Permanent loss of bladder/bowel function
- Leg weakness

Joint Abnormalities

ARTHRITIS

Arthritis is joint damage as a result of degeneration (eg, osteoarthritis), inflammation (eg, rheumatoid arthritis, gout), or infection. It is characteristically divided into monoarticular and polyarticular causes (Tables 4.6 and 4.7), although overlap exists and virtually any arthritic disorder can present as one swollen joint.

Causes

KEY FACT

A monoarticular arthritis should be presumed to be septic until proven otherwise.

For monoarticular arthritis, the most common etiologies are septic arthritis, crystalline arthritis, and trauma.

Oligo-/polyarticular arthritis is a broad group, but can typically be divided into systemic rheumatic disease (very broad group of disorders) or viral arthritis, although both infectious and crystalline arthritis may occasionally present with multiple joint involvement.

Systemic rheumatic diseases are sometimes further classified into symmetric (rheumatoid arthritis, SLE, viral, inflammatory bowel disease, ankylosing spondylitis) and asymmetric (psoriatic arthritis, reactive arthritis).

TABLE 4.6. Most Common Causes of Monoarticular Arthritis

Condition	Joints Involved	Unique Features	Treatment
Septic	Knee and hip; unique sites in IDU patients include sacroiliac, sternoclavicular, and intervertebral joints	***Staphylococcus aureus*** (overall) ***Neisseria gonorrhoeae*** in teenagers and young adults	Antibiotics starting with vancomycin; ceph 3 if GC suspected; surgical drainage
Gout	First MTP, knee	**Needle-shaped; negatively birefringent** crystals; yellow when parallel and blue when perpendicular to polarizing light	NSAIDs, steroid injection, colchicine. **Do not use allopurinol for acute attacks**
Pseudogout (chondrocalcinosis)	Knee, first MTP, wrist	**Rhomboid-shaped; positively birefringent** crystals; blue when parallel and yellow when perpendicular to polarizing light	NSAIDs, steroid injection
Trauma	Knee	Hemarthrosis associated with intra-articular fractures and ligamentous injury	Compression dressing and aspiration if necessary for symptomatic relief
Osteoarthritis	Hip, knee, hand (DIP and first carpometacarpal)	Older age group, weight-bearing joints	Rest, NSAIDs, joint replacement surgery

DIP, distal interphalangeal; IDU, intravenous drug user; MTP, metatarsal phalange; NSAIDs, nonsteroidal anti-inflammatory drugs.

TABLE 4.7. Common Causes of Polyarthritis

CONDITION	JOINTS INVOLVED	UNIQUE FEATURES	TREATMENT
Viral	All joints	Parvovirus, hepatitis A, B, C most common; classic "slapped cheek" and lacey rash may be seen with parvovirus	NSAIDs
Rheumatoid arthritis	Hand (MCP and PIP joints), wrist	Women in their 20s and 30s; associated with HLA-DR4 haplotype; early morning stiffness; sparing of DIP joints; multisystem involvement common	Anti-inflammatory agents, disease-modifying antirheumatic drugs, TNF-inhibitors, immunosuppressants
Systemic lupus	All. Usually PIP and MCP joints of the hand	Women 15-40 y old; can be migratory; associated with rash: malar, discoid, or photosensitivity	NSAIDs, immunosuppressants
Acute rheumatic fever	Large joints (knees, ankles, elbows, wrists)	Migratory; 2-3 wk after Group A strep infection; use Jones criteria for diagnosis	ASA or NSAIDs, penicillin IM/PO
Henoch-Schönlein purpura	Ankle, knee	Children 4-12 y old; **triad: migratory arthritis, palpable purpuric rash on lower extremities, abdominal pain**	NSAIDs and supportive care
Ankylosing spondylitis	Sacroiliac and other weight-bearing joints (hip, knee, ankles, feet)	Onset between ages 20 and 40 with back pain that gradually worsens; uveitis, plantar fasciitis, Achilles tendinitis common	NSAIDS, steroids, TNF-inhibitors
Reiter syndrome	Weight-bearing joints	Males 15-30 y old; **triad: conjunctivitis, urethritis, arthritis;** 80%-90% are HLA-B27 positive; often preceded 2-6 wk by viral illness, diarrhea, or infection with *Chlamydia* or *Ureaplasma*	NSAIDs; **antibiotics not helpful**

DIP, distal interphalangeal; IM/PO, intramuscular/by mouth; MCP, metacarpophalangeal; NSAIDs, Nonsteroidal anti-inflammatory drugs; PIP, proximal interphalangeal; TNF, tumor necrosis factors.

Symptoms/Examination

- Swollen, tender joint(s)
- Morning stiffness or pain worse with rest indicates an inflammatory process; AM stiffness lasting > 1 hour = rheumatoid arthritis
- Associated symptoms: Depending on etiology, look for urethritis, eye pain/discharge, rash, gastrointestinal (GI) symptoms
- Fever, most commonly with septic arthritis

KEY FACT

Reiter syndrome: Can't see (conjunctivitis), can't pee (urethritis), can't bend my knee (arthritis).

Differential

Includes arthralgias, enthesitis, bursitis, tendinitis, fracture, cellulitis.

Diagnosis

- **Joint aspiration is the key!**
- Send joint fluid for cell count, crystals, Gram stain, and culture.
- Considerable overlap of white blood cell (WBC) count exists between inflammatory and infectious etiologies of arthritis. In particular, gout and pseudogout can have WBC counts > 70,000 (Table 4.8) and gonococcal septic arthritis may have WBC counts < 50,000.

KEY FACT

Do not use allopurinol for acute gout attacks.

A

Gonococcal arthritis.

TABLE 4.8. Features of Synovial Fluid

Type	WBC/mL[a]	Viscosity	Color
Noninflammatory	< 2000	High	Clear
Inflammatory	2000-100,000	Variable	Yellow
Infectious	> 100,000	Low	Opaque

WBC, white blood cell.

[a]Considerable overlap may exist between cell counts for infectious and inflammatory arthritis; only synovial fluid culture is definitive.

- Peripheral WBC, ESR, and CRP are neither sensitive nor specific but should be obtained, as they can help with monitoring effectiveness of treatment.
- X-ray may be helpful to diagnose trauma, tumor, AVN, or osteomyelitis.

SEPTIC ARTHRITIS

Most commonly results from hematogenous spread of bacteria, but may result from contiguous spread of infection or direct inoculation. Large joints of lower extremity (hip and knee) are most common locations.

Causes

The most common cause overall is *S. aureus*. In teenagers or young adults, *Neisseria gonorrhoeae* is most common. Monoarticular arthritis may develop in patients with **Lyme disease** during the late disseminated stage. Other identified pathogens match those seen in osteomyelitis (see Table 4.5).

KEY FACT

Suspect septic arthritis in the pediatric patient who is unable to bear weight.

Symptoms/Examination

- Significant joint pain with passive and active range of motion (ROM).
- Swelling, warmth, and redness in the affected joint.
- Infants may present with "pseudoparalysis" of involved extremity, ie, refusal to use it.

Diagnosis

- Diagnosed by joint fluid aspirate. Send for Gram stain, culture, cell count, crystal analysis.
- Traditionally WBC > 50,000 = septic arthritis; however, mounting evidence shows that Gram stain and cell count alone cannot be used to confirm or exclude septic arthritis especially in patients with suppressed immune responses. **Joint fluid culture is the only definitive test**.
- Bloodwork: WBC, ESR, CRP usually elevated but nonspecific. Blood cultures may identify pathogen in up to 50% of cases. If Lyme endemic area, send serum antibody titers.
- For teenagers or sexually active adults: Swab samples from cervix/urethra, rectum, and pharynx should also be cultured to increase diagnostic yield (joint fluid culture is negative in ~50% of gonococcal arthritis).

Treatment

- Surgical drainage is needed in most cases.
- Empiric antibiotics should be directed at suspected underlying pathogen (see Table 4.6), but include penicillinase resistant penicillin (vancomycin if MRSA suspected) and third-generation cephalosporin.

BURSITIS

Bursitis is inflammation of the synovial-lined sacs that allow free movement of soft tissues over areas of friction or potential impingement. Common locations include the olecranon and prepatellar bursae.

CAUSES

Causes include infection (most commonly S. *aureus*), trauma, and rheumatologic disorders. Predisposing factors for infectious (or "septic") bursitis include: diabetes mellitus (DM), ethyl alcohol (ETOH) abuse, overlying skin disease, trauma (most common), and steroid use.

SYMPTOMS/EXAMINATION

- Pain and tenderness over affected bursa.
- Findings that are suggestive of septic bursitis include: Fever, tenderness, redness, and warmth.

DIAGNOSIS/TREATMENT

- Aspiration should be done in all cases of suspected septic bursitis; fluid WBC counts > 5000/μL suggest infection.
- Treatment for septic bursitis: Oral antistaphylococcal antibiotic (eg, oxacillin) along with bursal drainage via needle aspiration; aspiration may be repeated at 1- to 3-day intervals as needed.
- Treatment for noninfectious bursitis: Rest, elevation, ice, NSAIDs; aspiration and steroid injections may also be helpful.

SACROILIITIS

Sacroiliitis is an inflammation of one or both of the sacroiliac joints.

CAUSES

- Trauma or overuse, infection (injection drug use), pregnancy, degenerative arthritis.
- May be a part of a larger inflammatory arthritis, ie, ankylosing spondylitis, which is a seronegative spondyloarthropathy typically found in young males with prolonged (> 3 months) back pain.

SYMPTOMS/EXAMINATION

- Generally vague with low-grade fever and pain in back, thighs, or buttocks, especially in the morning or after prolonged rest.
- Tender sacroiliac joint.

DIFFERENTIAL

- Septic hip, psoas abscess, sciatica, herniated disk, pyelonephritis, ankylosing spondylitis

DIAGNOSIS

- X-rays show symmetric erosion and sclerosis of the sacroiliac joint (SI) joint. Squaring off of the lumbar vertebral bodies (**bamboo spine**) will be visible if the patient has ankylosing spondylitis. MRI of SI joint can detect inflammation before structural damage occurs.
- Aspiration and blood cultures if infection suspected.

TREATMENT

Depends on underlying cause (eg, anti-inflammatory agents for inflammatory causes, antibiotics if infection suspected).

Rhabdomyolysis

Breakdown of muscle cells with release of contents into the bloodstream.

CAUSES

- Trauma or compression: Crush syndrome, prolonged immobilization, electrical current, ischemia
- Nontraumatic, exertional: Hyperthermia, excessive muscle activity
- Nontraumatic, nonexertional: Electrolyte abnormalities (especially hypophosphatemia), toxins/drugs (ethanol, cocaine, stimulants, carbon monoxide, statins), infection

COMPLICATIONS

- Renal failure: Myoglobin blocks renal tubules and also has direct toxic effect
- Electrolyte abnormalities: **Hyperkalemia, hypocalcemia** (early) or hypercalcemia (late), hyperphosphatemia, hyperuricemia
- Hypovolemia: Fluid shifts out of intervascular space into damaged muscle compartments
- Compartment syndrome: Fluid shifts into damaged muscle compartments, increasing intracompartmental pressures
- Disseminated intravascular coagulation (DIC)

SYMPTOMS/EXAMINATION

- Symptoms are often very subtle; maintain a high index of suspicion.
- Only half of patients complain of muscle pain, and only a small fraction complain of dark urine.
- Tender or focal muscle swelling is rare. If present, must consider compartment syndrome!

KEY FACT

Hypocalcemia is the most common electrolyte abnormality. Hyperkalemia is the most lethal.

DIAGNOSIS

- Creatine kinase (CK) > 5 times normal (~1000 U/L). Serial CKs can be useful (peaks during first 3 days).
- Urine dipstick test is **positive for blood (globin) but there are no red blood cells (RBCs)** in the urine microscopic examination.
- Serum myoglobin (the causative factor for renal failure) is cleared rapidly from plasma and is therefore not a useful marker.
- Lactate dehydrogenase (LDH) and aspartate transaminase/alanine aminotransaminase (AST/ALT) may be elevated due to muscle necrosis.
- Potassium, phosphate, and uric acid are elevated due to release from injured cells.
- The most common electrolyte abnormality is **hypocalcemia**. Hypercalcemia may develop later in course.

- Monitor platelets, **prothrombin time/partial thromboplastin time** (PT/PTT) for early DIC.
- Measure compartment pressures if compartment syndrome is suspected.

KEY FACT

Suspect rhabdomyolysis when the urine dipstick test is positive for blood but there are no RBCs in the urine microscopic examination.

TREATMENT

- **Aggressive IV hydration.** Administer isotonic fluid with target urine output of 3 mL/kg/h.
- No clear evidence for concomitant administration of sodium bicarb exists, but it remains recommended practice. Goals: Urine pH > 6.5, blood pH 7-7.5. **Watch for worsening hypocalcemia.**
- Diuretic use is controversial: No evidence of benefit, clear potential for harm.
- Treat associated electrolyte abnormalities, especially hyperkalemia.
- Dialysis for uncorrectable metabolic acidosis, life-threatening electrolyte abnormalities, fluid overload (does **not** filter myoglobin).
- Admit to telemetry unit for continued treatment and monitoring of fluids, electrolytes, and renal function.

Overuse Syndromes

EPICONDYLITIS

Inflammatory process of the lateral epicondyle (tennis elbow) or medial epicondyle (golfer's elbow, climber's elbow) of the humerus, felt to be a result of repeated strain at the epicondylar tendon insertion sites.

Symptoms/Diagnosis

- Pain over lateral or medial aspect of elbow. May be acute or subacute.
- Medial epicondylitis pain elicited with flexion at the elbow or hand pronation against resistance.
- Lateral epicondylitis pain elicited with extension of wrist against resistance.
- Clinical diagnosis based on characteristic history and examination. X-ray generally unhelpful, MRI not indicated urgently.

Treatment

- Rest, ice, NSAIDs, then gradual strengthening exercises.

BICEPS TENDON RUPTURE

Occurs more commonly in men, generally athletes or laborers. Can be proximal (long head of the biceps) or distal (at insertion on radial tuberosity).

Symptoms/Examination

- Mechanism c/w injury: Sudden heavy loading of flexed arm.
- Visible defect at top of bicipital groove with bunching of muscle distally (proximal rupture) or palpable deformity and superior migration of biceps muscle belly (distal rupture).
- Flexion remains intact due to intact short head of biceps.

Diagnosis

Clinical diagnosis based on characteristic history and examination. X-ray not helpful. MRI may assist with diagnosis of partial rupture.

TREATMENT

- Splinting, ice, rest, NSAIDs
- Referral to orthopedic surgeon for possible surgical repair

CARPAL TUNNEL SYNDROME

A compressive neuropathy of the median nerve at the level of the carpal tunnel in the volar aspect of the wrist. It is more common in females.

MECHANISM

- Most common causes are repetitive strain of the hands and wrists (eg, typists, musicians) and distal radius fracture.
- Patients often have associated trauma, obesity, collagen vascular disease, renal failure, hypothyroidism, congestive heart failure (CHF), or diabetes.

SYMPTOMS

- Gradual onset and progression. Often bilateral but may begin first in dominant hand
- Early: Paresthesias in median nerve distribution (palmar aspect of first three digits and radial half of the fourth digit)
- Late: Persistent pain present, atrophy of thenar muscles

DIAGNOSIS

- Usually a clinical diagnosis. Electromyography (EMG) and nerve conduction studies establish severity of disease.
- **Durkin compression test**: Reproduction of symptoms with compression of carpal tunnel for 30 seconds.
- **Phalen sign**: Reproduction of symptoms with hyperflexion of wrists at 90° for 1 minute.
- **Tinel sign**: Pins-and-needles sensation in the median nerve distribution with tapping on the carpal tunnel.
- **Flick sign**: Shaking or "flicking" the hands provides relief of symptoms during episodes.

DIFFERENTIAL

Brachial plexus compressive neuropathy, peripheral neuropathy of other causes.

> **KEY FACT**
>
> Positive Durkin compression test, Phalen sign, Tinel sign, and Flick sign are all indicative of carpal tunnel syndrome.

DIAGNOSIS

- Treatment.
- Initial medical management includes volar splint in neutral position, local steroid injection. NSAIDs have not proven beneficial.
- Patients who fail the above may need surgery for release of the flexor retinaculum.

COMPLICATION

Chronic pain, weakness, paresthesias, and disability.

DE QUERVAIN TENOSYNOVITIS

Synovitis of the tendons in the first dorsal wrist compartment (abductor pollicis longus and extensor pollicis brevis) due to thickening of the extensor retinaculum of the wrist from repetitive trauma or wrist movement.

Symptoms/Examination

Pain over radial styloid that radiates proximally or down thumb

Diagnosis/Treatment

- **Finkelstein test** is pathognomonic: Pain near radial styloid upon ulnar deviation of wrist with hand in fist position (thumb against palm)
- Rest, ice, NSAIDs, thumb spica splint

PLANTAR FASCIITIS

Plantar fasciitis is a common cause of plantar heel pain that occurs where the plantar fascia arises from the medial calcaneal tuberosity. Inflammation in both the bone and plantar fascia occurs from chronic degeneration in the fascia fibers that arise from the bone.

Symptoms/Examination

- Pain worse upon awakening or after prolonged rest that is localized to the heel or arch of the foot, and, occasionally, over the Achilles tendon.
- Patients often have point tenderness over the plantar medial calcaneal tuberosity (anterior medial aspect of the calcaneus).

Differential

Calcaneal stress fracture/tumor, fat pad atrophy, sciatica, tarsal tunnel syndrome, ruptures of the plantar fascia.

Diagnosis

Clinical diagnosis (characteristic pain after rest and localized heel tenderness).

Treatment

Conservative management with rest, orthotics, stretches. Surgery is rarely needed.

Soft-Tissue Infections

FELON

Felon is infection of the fingertip pulp. The fingertip is separated into small closed spaces by vertical septae. Infection can easily spread along these compartments and cause an abscess. *S. aureus* is the most common agent.

Symptoms/Examination

- Swollen, tender fingertip, usually thumb or index finger
- Previous finger trauma or splinter

Diagnosis

- Clinical diagnosis
- X-ray if foreign body, fracture, or osteomyelitis suspected

Treatment

- If early, warm soaks and antibiotics may be sufficient.
- Incision and drainage (longitudinal incision in midline of volar surface vs lateral incision), loose packing, antibiotics to cover *S. aureus*.
- Culture if MRSA is prevalent in the area.

Complication

Osteomyelitis, tenosynovitis, septic joint, neurovascular injury.

PARONYCHIA

The most common hand infection, paronychia is a soft-tissue infection along the border of the fingernail or paronychium that results from the breakdown of the skin (minor trauma, nail biting) and entry of bacteria or fungi into the nail fold. It can be acute or chronic in nature:

- Acute: *S. aureus* is the most often implicated organism, may be polymicrobial.
- Chronic: A chronic inflammatory condition, often due to chronically moist hands (eg, bartenders, housekeepers, marine workers). *Candida albicans* is implicated pathogen.

Symptoms/Examination

- Acute: Swollen, tender, erythematous nail fold.
- Chronic: Symptoms > 6 weeks. It can be episodic. There is usually no fluctuance. Patient may have thickened and discolored nail plates.

Differential

Herpetic whitlow (clear vesicles on an erythematous base), skin cancers, warts, chancres, granulomas.

Diagnosis

- Clinical diagnosis of acute paronychia is sufficient.
- KOH prep may be helpful to distinguish chronic cases caused by *C. albicans*.
- Tzanck smear or viral culture if herpetic whitlow suspected.

Treatment

Acute:

- If early, warm soaks and antibiotics may suffice.
- If an abscess has developed, drainage can usually be accomplished by elevating the paronychium with a blunt instrument. More advanced abscesses must be incised with a No. 11 blade and drained. Occasionally, a portion of the nail plate must be removed.
- If complex abscess or surrounding cellulitis, treat with antibiotics for 5-7 days.
- **Do not incise the lesion if herpetic whitlow is suspected**.

Chronic:

- Avoid water and irritating substances; treat with topical antifungals for persistent cases.

Complication

Osteomyelitis, bacteremia.

FLEXOR TENOSYNOVITIS

The flexor tendons of the fingers are covered by a double layer of synovium to promote gliding of the tendon underneath. Infection of these flexor tendon sheaths presents a true surgical hand emergency. It is usually associated with penetrating trauma, although the patient may not recall the injury. *S. aureus* and streptococci are the most common organisms identified.

Symptoms/Examination (Kanavel Cardinal Signs)

- Flexed posture of the involved digit
- Fusiform swelling of the finger ("sausage digit")
- Tenderness over the flexor tendon sheath
- Pain with passive extension

Diagnosis

- Clinical diagnosis: X-ray may reveal air or a foreign body.

Treatment

- Immobilize and elevate the affected hand.
- Administer IV antibiotics with ampicillin/sulbactam, first-generation cephalosporin, or vancomycin.
- Consult hand surgeon for possible surgical drainage.

Complications

Osteomyelitis, septic arthritis, loss of digit, chronic stiffness.

KEY FACT

Kanavel cardinal signs of flexor tenosynovitis:

1. Flexed posture of the involved digit
2. Fusiform swelling of the entire digit
3. Tenderness over the flexor tendon sheath
4. Pain with passive extension

HIGH-PRESSURE INJECTION INJURIES

These injuries are caused by injection of fluids (classically grease or paint) into the skin by a high-pressure injector. The fluid enters the skin and extends along deep tissue planes. The fluid and resultant inflammation leads to vascular compromise and tissue necrosis. Prognosis is poor even with aggressive early intervention.

Important factors to consider:

- Substance injected: **Low** viscosity **corrosives** are the most damaging (eg, paint solvent)
- Velocity of injection: **Higher** velocity = greater penetration
- Duration of exposure: **Longer** exposure = worse prognosis

Symptoms/Examination

- Generally innocuous examination on presentation with 1- to 3-mm injection wounds
- Pain at the injection site extending up the injection track (typically along tendons)

Diagnosis

- Historical diagnosis
- X-ray: May be able to see extent of spread if radiopaque

Treatment

- These injuries are considered true surgical emergencies.
- Splint and elevate extremity, administer parenteral broad-spectrum antibiotics and update tetanus prophylaxis as needed.

- Provide analgesia (**NO** digital blocks—can increase tissue pressure leading to vascular compromise).
- Obtain emergent orthopedic consultation for operative debridement.

Complications

- There is a 30%-50% amputation rate, extreme morbidity even with aggressive early management.
- For a quick summary of key points and board review facts for each injury, see Table 4.9.

TABLE 4.9. Quick Review Study Chart

Injury Name	Injury Description/ Exam Findings	Unique Complications	Treatment	Board Pearls
Anterior shoulder dislocation	> 90% subcoracoid	Axillary nerve injury	Reduction (not Kocher or Hippocratic)	"Badge" anesthesia Bankart lesion Hill-Sachs deformity
Posterior shoulder dislocation		Humerus fx common	Reduction	High-energy injury AP XR: lightbulb or drumstick humerus
Luxatio erecta	Inferior shoulder dislocation	Neurovascular injury (axillary artery and nerve, brachial plexus) Humerus fx	Traction-countertraction reduction	Rare High-energy injury
Clavicle fracture	Distal, middle (80%), or medial	10% rib fx Vascular injury Brachial plexus injury	Sling	
Proximal humerus fracture	85% surgical neck	Brachial plexus injury Axillary nerve or artery A vascular necrosis	Displaced: Ortho Nondisplaced: Sling and early ROM	
Humeral shaft fracture		Radial nerve injury Brachial artery injury	Sugar tong splint Ortho if displaced	
Distal humerus condylar fracture	Usually involves both the articular and nonarticular surfaces	Ulnar nerve palsy Avascular necrosis Compartment syndrome	ORIF if > 3 mm displacement	Lateral fx more common Medial fx in kids
Little leaguer's elbow	Medial epicondyle fx	60% ulnar nerve injury	Posterior splint Refer to ortho if > 3-5 mm displacement	
Supracondylar fracture	Distal humerus	Injuries to: Brachial artery, median nerve (AIO), radial and ulnar nerve Volkmann ischemic contracture Compartment syndrome	Posterior splint Ortho referral if displaced	Posterior fat pad sign

TABLE 4.9. Quick Review Study Chart (*Continued*)

Injury Name	Injury Description/ Exam Findings	Unique Complications	Treatment	Board Pearls
Posterior elbow dislocation		30%-60% elbow fx Brachial artery injury	Reduction	Most common elbow dlx
Anterior elbow dislocation		Triceps avulsion Vascular injury common (esp brachial artery)	Reduction	
Olecranon fracture		Ulnar nerve injury	Posterior splint ORIF if > 2 mm displacement	
Colles fracture	Distal radius fx Dorsal displacement	Median nerve injury 60% ulnar styloid fx	Reduce PRN Sugar-tong splint Ortho referral	XR: Dinner fork deformity
Smith fracture	Distal radius fx Volar displacement	Median nerve injury	Reduce Long arm splint Ortho referral	XR: Garden spade deformity
Barton fracture	Distal radius rim fx		Long arm splint ORIF if > 50% articular	
Nightstick fracture	Isolated ulnar fx		Long arm splint ORIF if > 50% displaced or > 10° angulated	Always r/o Monteggia fx
Essex-Lopresti fracture	Radial head fx w/ dislocation of distal rad/uln joint		Sugar-tong splint ORIF	
Galeazzi fracture	Distal radial shaft fx and radioulnar dislocation	Ulnar nerve injury Compartment syndrome	Sugar-tong splint ORIF	Suspect with both wrist and elbow pain
Monteggia fracture	Ulnar fx and radial dislocation	Radial nerve injury Compartment syndrome	Reduce Long arm splint ORIF	Suspect w/ significant elbow pain and swelling
Scaphoid fracture	Snuff box tenderness	Avascular necrosis (> w/ proximal fx)	Thumb spica	Most common carpal fx
Triquetral fracture	Usually dorsal chip Tenderness distal to ulnar styloid	Body fx associated with perilunate and lunate dislocations	Volar splint	
Lunate fracture	Tender over middorsum of wrist and with axial compression of middle finger	Kienbock disease (lunate avascular necrosis)	Thumb spica Ortho referral	Often XR negative Rarely isolated fx

(*Continued*)

TABLE 4.9. Quick Review Study Chart (*Continued*)

Injury Name	Injury Description/ Exam Findings	Unique Complications	Treatment	Board Pearls
Scapholunate dissociation	Tear of scapholunate ligament	Associated with perilunate and lunate dislocations	Radial gutter splint Ortho referral	AP XR findings: Signet ring sign Terry Thomas sign
Lunate dislocation	Significant force FOOSH Disruption of carpal ligaments	Median nerve injury Avascular necrosis Acute carpal tunnel syndrome	Ortho reduction	Lateral XR finding: Spilled teacup sign AP: piece-of-pie sign
Perilunatecarpal dislocation	Same as above	Same as above	Ortho reduction	Lateral XR finding: Upright teacup with lunate sitting posterior
Mallet finger	DIP at base of distal phalanx	Swan-neck deformity	Splint DIP in extension	
Boutonniere deformity	Tear of extensor tendon at PIP	Boutonniere deformity	Splint PIP in extension	
Jersey finger	FDP rupture		Surgical repair	Commonly ring finger
Gamekeeper's or skier's thumb	Rupture of ulnar collateral ligament	30% have associated fx	Thumb spica Surgical repair	Have decreased pinch strength
Bennett fracture	Intra-articular fx at thumb base	Associated CMC dislocation	Thumb spica Ortho referral	
Rolando's fracture	Comminuted intra-articular fx at thumb base		Thumb spica Ortho referral	Worse prognosis than Bennett
Boxer's fracture	Fifth MC neck fx		Ulnar gutter splint	Check for fight bite Angulation allowed radial → ulnar 10°/10°/30°/40°
Femoral head fractures		Hip dislocations Osteonecrosis	Surgical repair	Judet views
Femoral neck fractures		Osteonecrosis	Surgical repair	
Intertrochanteric fractures		Superficial femoral artery injury	Surgical repair	Most common femur fx
Subtrochanteric fractures	> 5 cm distal to lesser trochanter	Compartment syndrome	Surgical repair	Common site of pathologic fx
Femoral shaft fractures		Femoral artery injury Compartment syndrome	Traction Surgical repair	Check ABIs

TABLE 4.9. Quick Review Study Chart (*Continued*)

Injury Name	Injury Description/ Exam Findings	Unique Complications	Treatment	Board Pearls
Distal femur fractures		Neurovascular injury Knee immobility Joint involvement	Nondisplaced: Hinged knee brace All others: surgery	Check ABIs
Patella fracture		Extensor mechanism injury	Nondisplaced: Knee immobilizer Refer to ortho if: > 3 mm displaced or lost ext function	
Knee dislocation	Any direction	Popliteal artery injury Peroneal nerve injury (foot drop) Tibial nerve injury	Immediate reduction	Check ABIs
Tibial plateau fracture	Usually lateral	Popliteal or anterior tibial artery injury 33% ligament inj	Nondisplaced: Knee immobilizer Displaced: Ortho	XR often negative
Extensor mechanism rupture		> 40 y old: Quad tendon rupture < 40 y old: Patellar tendon rupture Patella fx Tibial tuberosity avulsion	Surgical repair	Suprapatellar gap or high-riding patella Unable to extend leg
Patellofemoral syndrome	Chondromalacia of the patella		NSAIDs Quad strengthening	Most common cause of knee pain Patella compression test Apprehension test Increased Q angle
Achilles tendon rupture			Posterior splint in plantar flexion Early ortho referral	Thompson test Common in "weekend warriors" Associated with quinolone use
Maisonneuve fracture	Medial malleolus or deltoid ligament injury + proximal fibula fx		ORIF	
Calcaneus fracture		Compartment syndrome Lumbar fx	Bulky Jones dressing with posterior splint Ortho referral	Bohler's angle < 20° Most common tarsal fx
Talus fracture	Usually neck	Avascular necrosis	Posterior splint Ortho referral	

(*Continued*)

TABLE 4.9. Quick Review Study Chart (*Continued*)

Injury Name	Injury Description/ Exam Findings	Unique Complications	Treatment	Board Pearls
Lisfranc fracture	Tarsometatarsal fx	Dorsalis pedis artery injury	Emergent ortho referral	Plantar ecchymosis sign > 1 mm between first and second MT Fleck sign—pathognomonic
Jones fracture	Fifth MT transverse fx through metaphyseal-diaphyseal junction	Non- or malunion	Splint, Non–weight bearing Ortho referral	Fx 1.5 cm distal to base of fifth MT
Pseudo-Jones fracture	Avulsion fx of base of fifth MT		Hard sole shoe or CAM boot, weight bearing as tolerated.	More common than Jones

ABI, ankle brachial index; AP, anteroposterior; DIP, distal interphalangeal; dlx, dislocation; FDP, flexor digitorum profundus; FOOSH, fall on the outstretched hand; fx, fracture; fxn, function; inj, injuries; MC, metacarpal; MT, metatarsal; PIP, proximal interphalangeal; PRN, as needed; ORIF, open reduction internal fixation; XR, x-ray.

REVIEW QUESTIONS

QUESTIONS

1. Patient presents with gradual onset numbness and tingling in the thumb, and second and third fingers, worse at night and with repetitive activity. Which of the following is **not** a risk factor for development of this syndrome?
   A. Male gender
   B. Hypothyroidism
   C. Diabetes
   D. Obesity

2. Patient is a 40-year-old right hand–dominant man who presents from his job site after an injury. He states he was working with a paint gun and accidentally discharged it against his left hand. On examination, you note a small puncture on the palm in the area of the second metacarpophalangeal joint. He has brisk capillary refill in his index finger, sensation intact to light touch, and full range of motion (ROM) at all joints although this is painful in his index finger. Unsure of his last tetanus shot. What are the best next steps in emergency medicine management of this patient?
   A. Update tetanus, broad-spectrum antibiotics, splint and elevate extremity, emergent orthopedic consultation.
   B. Update tetanus, splint DIP joint in full extension, orthopedics follow-up in 7-10 days.
   C. Update tetanus, digital block for pain control, 3-view x-ray of affected hand.
   D. Update tetanus, thoroughly irrigate affected area, discharge home without scheduled follow-up.

3. A rodeo cowboy presents to your emergency department (ED) after a fall from a bull just prior to arrival, landing on his left shoulder. He is complaining of severe pain over his clavicle medially, worse with any movement. He is tender to palpation with slight dimpling of his skin over his left sternoclavicular joint. X-ray of chest and shoulder are read as normal. What is the next best step in the evaluation and management of this patient?
   A. Computed tomography angiography (CTA) chest to evaluate great vessels and mediastinal structures
   B. Sling and swath for 3 weeks, early range of motion exercises
   C. Follow-up with orthopedics in 7-10 days for magnetic resonance imaging (MRI) shoulder to evaluate rotator cuff injury
   D. Outpatient referral for surgical correction of acromioclavicular (AC) separation

4. An adult woman presents to your ED after slipping on an icy patch and falling backward onto her left outstretched arm. She is complaining of pain and swelling around the L elbow. Wrist and shoulder examinations are unremarkable. You obtain an x-ray that shows anterior and posterior fat pads but no obvious fracture. What is the most likely diagnosis?
   A. Radial head fracture
   B. Supracondylar fracture
   C. Nightstick fracture
   D. Monteggia fracture

5. An 89-year-old man slips on his front porch and falls on his left hip. He presents complaining of pain primarily in his left groin, worse with any movement of his left femur. X-rays of hip and femur are read as unremarkable, but after postoperative pain control patient is still unable to ambulate. What is the gold standard for ED diagnosis of the most likely injury?
   A. MRI hip/pelvis
   B. CT hip/pelvis
   C. Bone scan hip/pelvis
   D. X-ray hip/pelvis

6. A 50-year-old woman steps awkwardly on the lateral aspect of her left foot while ballroom dancing just prior to arrival, and presents complaining of pain and swelling in that area. X-ray is shown in Figure 4.31. What is the best next step in ED evaluation and management?

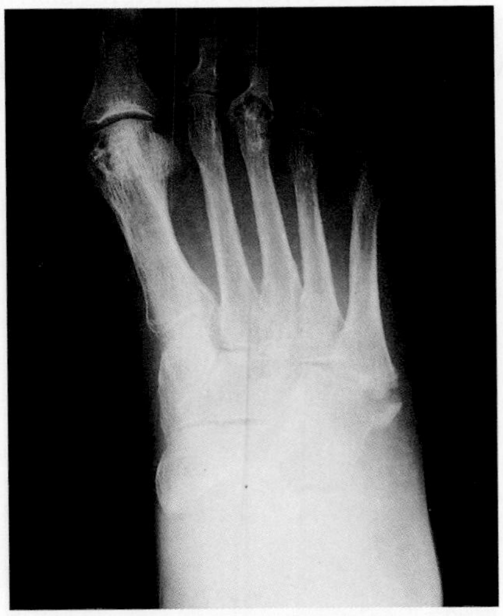

FIGURE 4.31. (Reproduced, with permission, from Knoop KJ, Storrow AB, Stack LB, and Thurman RJ. *The Atlas of Emergency Medicine*. 3rd ed. New York, NY: McGraw-Hill; 2010. Figure 11.92. Photo contributor: Alan B. Storrow, MD.)

A. Hard post-op shoe, weight bearing as tolerated
B. Cast/splint, non–weight bearing, orthopedic follow-up in 7-10 days
C. Urgent orthopedic consultation in the ED for internal fixation
D. Bilateral weight-bearing foot x-rays to further describe injury

7. *Staphylococcus aureus* is the most common cause of osteomyelitis in all of the following groups *except*:
A. Neonates
B. Injection drug users
C. Diabetics
D. Adults with sickle cell disease

8. An injection drug user is brought to the ED after being found on her kitchen floor by family members. Her mental status is altered, and creatine kinase (CK) is 15,000. What is the most common electrolyte abnormality in this condition?
A. Hypocalcemia
B. Hypokalemia
C. Hyperphosphatemia
D. Hyperuricemia

9. A 75-year-old woman was the restrained driver in a motor vehicle collision (MVC), presenting to the ED with pain and deformity over her left upper arm. X-ray is shown in Figure 4.32. She develops the most common complication associated with this injury. What examination findings are most consistent with this?
A. Weakness of extensors of her wrist and hand and numbness over dorsoradial aspect of hand
B. Decreased pinch strength in hand
C. Numbness in a "shoulder patch" distribution over her left deltoid
D. Claw-like deformity of hand and fingers

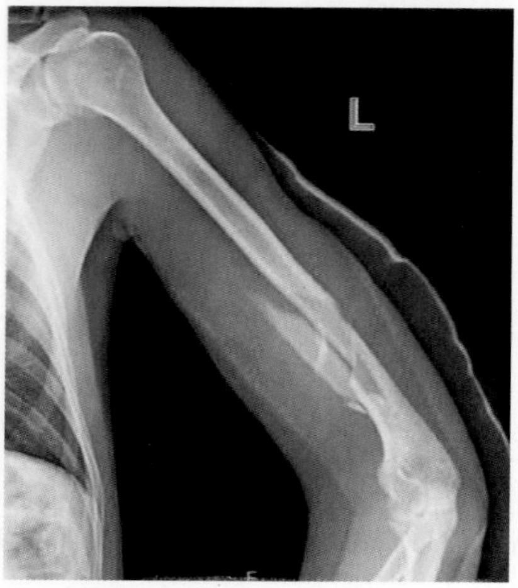

FIGURE 4.32. (Reproduced, with permission, from Sherman S. *Simon's Emergency Orthopedics*. 7th ed. New York, NY: McGraw-Hill Education, 2015. Figure 15.6.)

10. A 25-year-old right hand–dominant man presents intoxicated to your emergency department after punching a wall. Skin is intact over the affected hand. X-ray shows a metacarpal fracture. Which is an indication for closed reduction of this injury?
A. Second metacarpal 5° volar angulation
B. Third metacarpal 5° volar angulation
C. Fourth metacarpal 35° volar angulation
D. Fifth metacarpal 35° volar angulation

11. A 30-year-old man presents with eye pain, pain with urination, right knee pain, and left heel pain. He recalls an episode of diarrhea about 2 weeks ago that has since resolved. He was seen at the health department last week and had negative swabs for Gonorrhea and *Chlamydia*. The best initial treatment for his condition includes which of the following?
A. High-dose NSAIDs
B. Ciprofloxacin + flagyl
C. Rocephin IM + azithromycin 1 g PO once
D. Oral corticosteroids

ANSWERS

1. **A.** Male gender. The prompt describes carpal tunnel syndrome, a compressive neuropathy of the median nerve. Females are at higher risk for development of carpal tunnel. Other risk factors include hypothyroidism, diabetes, obesity, chronic heart failure (CHF), collagen vascular disease, trauma, and renal failure.

2. **A.** Update tetanus, broad-spectrum antibiotics, splint and elevate extremity, emergent orthopedic consultation. High-pressure injection injuries are true emergencies despite what might be an initially benign physical examination. Emergency consultation in the ED is indicated. Digital blocks should be avoided as they may contribute to vascular compromise.

3. **A.** CTA chest to evaluate great vessels and mediastinal structures. Sternoclavicular dislocations are frequently missed on initial examination, but when dislocated posteriorly (as in this case) can be associated with life-threatening injuries, including esophageal rupture, carotid artery injury, and injury to the great vessels. CTA is indicated to evaluate these structures.

4. **A.** Radial head fracture. Anterior fat pad may be normal but posterior fat pad is always pathological and usually indicates an occult fracture or dislocation. In adults the most common occult fracture associated with a posterior fat pad is a radial head fracture. In pediatrics it is a supracondylar fracture.

5. **A.** MRI hip/pelvis. Inability to ambulate with hip/groin pain in elderly adults after trauma is concerning for an occult hip/pelvic fracture. MRI is the gold standard for this diagnosis. CT is more sensitive than x-ray, but has an unacceptably high miss rate.

Bone scan is most sensitive about 48-72 hours after the initial injury, but if performed earlier can result in false negatives.

6. **A.** Hard post-op shoe, weight bearing as tolerated. The x-ray shows a Pseudo-Jones fracture, an avulsion fracture through the base of the fifth metatarsal. Management includes ankle stirrup splint, hard post-op shoe, or rocker walker, weight bearing as tolerated. It is important to differentiate this from a Jones fracture, where the fracture line passes through the metaphyseal-diaphyseal joint. Management for a Jones fracture (frequently complicated by nonunion) includes cast/splint, non–weight bearing, and orthopedic follow-up.

7. **A.** Neonates. The most common organisms in this age group include Group B streptococci, Enterobacteriaceae, and *Staphylococcus epidermis*. In adults with sickle cell disease, *Salmonella* species are a common organism but S. *aureus* still predominates.

8. **A.** Hypocalcemia. The prompt describes rhabdomyolysis, which is complicated by multiple electrolyte abnormalities, including hyperkalemia, hyperphosphatemia, and hyperuricemia. Hypocalcemia is the most common and is present early in the course. Later in the course, hypercalcemia may be seen.

9. **A.** Weakness of extensors of her wrist and hand and numbness over dorsoradial aspect of hand. The x-ray shows a midshaft fracture of the humerus. The most frequent complication associated with this injury is a radial nerve palsy, as described in answer A. Answer B may be associated with gamekeeper's thumb; Answer C with axillary nerve injury after shoulder dislocation. Answer D, associated with Volkmann ischemic contracture, is a devastating condition that can be associated with brachial artery disruption in humeral shaft fractures; however, radial nerve palsy is significantly more common.

10. **C.** Fourth metacarpal 35° volar angulation. Acceptable volar angulation in these injuries: $< 10°$ in second/third metacarpals, $< 30°$ in fourth metacarpal, $< 40°$ in fifth metacarpal.

11. **A.** High-dose nonsteroidal anti-inflammatory drugs (NSAIDs). The clinical scenario is consistent with Reiter syndrome, which is frequently preceded by viral illness, diarrheal illness, or sexually transmitted diseases (STDs). In sexually active young adults consideration should be given to STD testing. If negative, antibiotics are not helpful, and NSAIDs are the mainstay of treatment.

CHAPTER 5

Pediatrics

Christina L. Shenvi, MD, PhD

Common Pediatric Problems

FEVER

Fever is the most common pediatric chief complaint in the emergency department (ED). Fever that is concerning for serious illness is typically defined as a **rectal temp > 38°C (100.4°F)** in infants < 3 months and 39°C (102.2°F) in children > 3 months. However, serious illness can certainly occur at temperatures below this range and have been associated with hypothermia as well. Evaluation and disposition of patients with fever are determined by age at presentation in conjunction with other factors such as underlying medical conditions (eg, cancer, immunosuppression) and coexisting factors (eg, immunization status). The emergency medicine (EM) physician's primary role in evaluating fever is to rule out serious infections, the majority of which tend to be serious bacterial infections (SBIs) (Table 5.1).

TABLE 5.1. Bacterial Causes of Fever in Children

Age	Bacterial Causes
0-28 d	Group B *Streptococcus* *Escherichia coli* *Klebsiella pneumoniae* *Listeria monocytogenes* *Chlamydia trachomatis* *Neisseria gonorrhea*
1-3 mo	*Streptococcus pneumoniae* *Neisseria meningitidis* *E coli* *Haemophilus influenzae*
3 mo-3 y	*S pneumoniae* *E coli* *N meningitidis*

KEY FACT

SBIs = Meningitis, pneumonia, urinary tract infection (UTI), bacteremia, sepsis

Fever 0-28 Days

The most common causative organisms of SBI arise from maternal vaginal flora in this age group. An immature immune system and unvaccinated status place children < 28 days at higher risk for SBI.

Symptoms/Examination

- Fever > 38°C (100.4°F) indicates need for full sepsis evaluation in infants < 28 days.
- Evaluation in this age range is based on the premise that the history and physical examination can be difficult to interpret. SBI can be present in the absence of any significant historical or physical examination findings. SBI can also be present in child with hypothermia or even in the absence of fever.

Diagnosis

- All patients should have a complete blood count (CBC) with differential, blood cultures, catheterized urinalysis, urine culture, lumbar puncture (LP) with culture, and chest x-ray if lower respiratory symptoms are present.
- Consider testing for herpes simplex virus (HSV) if any signs suggestive of disseminated HSV (vesicular rash, bloody LP not attributable to traumatic LP, elevated transaminases, seizures) or if the patient's mother has a history of HSV (especially if vaginal delivery with active lesions).
- Stool for white blood count (WBC) and culture should be obtained for those with diarrhea.

Treatment

- Empiric intravenous (IV) antibiotics with ampicillin plus cefotaxime (gentamicin is an alternative) (Table 5.2).
- IV acyclovir should be started immediately for those in whom HSV is suspected. This should be coupled with adequate IV hydration.
- Admit all patients for IV antibiotics until cultures have resulted. In the event that cultures cannot be obtained, use clinical judgment to start antibiotics or admit and observe without antibiotics.

KEY FACT

Start empiric IV antibiotics (ampicillin and cefotaxime OR ampicillin and gentamicin) and admit all patients < 28 days with fever until cultures are resulted.

Fever 29-90 Days

While the evaluation of febrile infants < 28 days is standardized, the evaluation of infants 29 days to 3 months is more controversial. Multiple studies have attempted to determine which infants can be managed as outpatients

TABLE 5.2. Summary: Fever 0-28 Days

BACTERIAL PATHOGENS	EVALUATION	TREATMENT AND DISPOSITION
Group B *Streptococcus* *Klebsiella pneumoniae* *Neisseria gonorrhea* *C trachomatis* *Listeria monocytogenes*	CBC with differential Urinalysis + culture Blood cultures CSF analysis + culture CXR if suggested Stool studies if suggested	Ampicillin + cefotaxime (or gentamicin) Admit all to hospital for IV antibiotics until cultures are resulted

CBC, complete blood count; CSF, cerebrospinal fluid; CXR, chest x-ray; IV, intravenous.

in this age group. If the infant is septic appearing or high risk, they should be evaluated with a full sepsis workup (blood, urine, and cerebrospinal fluid [CSF] cultures), treated with empiric IV antibiotics, and admitted to the hospital. If the infant is well appearing, has no obvious source of infection, has reliable caregivers, and has had all appropriate immunizations, then outpatient management can be considered following risk stratification with laboratory tests (Table 5.3).

SYMPTOMS/EXAMINATION

While the immune system has improved in this age group compared with neonates, infants < 3 months can still have SBI without any sign other than fever.

DIAGNOSIS

- Well-appearing infants without focus of infection often only need a limited evaluation, to include CBC with differential, blood cultures, catheterized urinalysis, and urine culture.

TABLE 5.3. Management Strategies for Well-Appearing Febrile Infants 29 Days-3 Months

	BOSTON	PHILADELPHIA	ROCHESTER
Age	29-90 d	28-60 d	≤ 60 d
Temperature	≥ 38.0°C (100.4°F)	≥ 38.2°C (100.8°F)	≥ 38.0°C (100.4°F)
Definition of low risk	WBC < 20,000/mm³ and > 5000/mm³ UA < 10 WBCs/hpf CSF < 10 WBCs/hpf CXR negative (if obtained)	WBC < 15,000/mm³ Bands: Neutrophils < 0.2 UA < 10 WBCs/hpf CSF < 8 WBCs/hpf CXR negative (if obtained)	WBC 5-15,000/mm³ Abs bands < 1500 UA ≤ 10 WBCs/hpf Stool < 5 WBCs/hpf (if obtained)
Management of high risk	Full sepsis workup Admit + IV antibiotics	Full sepsis workup Admit + IV antibiotics	Full sepsis workup Admit + IV antibiotics
Management of low risk	Home Empiric antibiotics (ceftriaxone 50 mg/kg) Reevaluation in 24 h	Home No antibiotics Reevaluation in 24 h	Home No antibiotics Reevaluation in 24 h

CSF, cerebrospinal fluid; CXR, chest x-ray; IV, intravenous; UA, urinanalysis; WBC, white blood count.

TABLE 5.4. Summary: Fever 29 Days-3 Months

Bacterial Pathogens	Evaluation	Treatment and Disposition
S pneumoniae	CBC with differential	High risk: IV antibiotics and admission
E coli	Urinalysis + culture	Low risk: Home with reevaluation in 24 h ±
Neisseria meningitidis	Blood cultures	IM ceftriaxone (only if CSF obtained first)
Haemophilus influenza	Optional: CSF, CXR, stool studies	

CBC, complete blood count; CSF, cerebrospinal fluid; CXR, chest x-ray; IM, intramuscular; IV, intravenous.

- If there is any concern for SBI based on young age, prematurity, toxicity, or incomplete vaccination status, then CSF cultures should also be obtained.

KEY FACT

All children < 3 months with fever discharged from the ED require reevaluation in 24 hours.

Treatment

- All septic-appearing or high-risk infants need a full sepsis workup, empiric antibiotics, and admission to the hospital.
- Well-appearing, fully immunized, and low-risk infants can be considered for outpatient management if 24-hour follow-up is available. The definition of a "low-risk infant" varies based on the criteria used (Boston, Philadelphia, or Rochester, see Tables 5.3 and 5.4). The Rochester criteria are the least sensitive of the 3 strategies (92%) and have the potential to miss patients with SBI.

Fever 3 Months-3 Years

Fever in infants 3 months to 3 years is more commonly due to viral rather than bacterial pathogens. Given the improved immune system and subsequent decreased risk of SBI in this age group, evaluation is tailored to clinical presentation, vaccination status, and temperature.

Symptoms/Examination

- Physical examination findings and historical clues are usually more reliable for pinpointing the diagnosis in this age range.
- **Urinary tract infection (UTI) is still the most common bacterial infection** in this age group, especially girls < 2 years and uncircumcised boys < 1 year.
- Immunization status is extremely important to note. Infants < 6 months have not completed the appropriate initial 3 rounds of *S pneumoniae* and *H influenzae* vaccinations typically given at 2, 4, and 6 months and are still at risk for SBI, albeit significantly lower risk after 1 round of vaccines.
- Fever ≥ 39°C without an obvious source should prompt further evaluation based on immunization status and age.

Diagnosis

- Children with focal symptoms/signs (ie, otitis media, pneumonia, meningitis, cellulitis) should have workup and treatment directed at these specific diseases.
- Children with fever ≥ 39°C who are between the ages of 3 and 6 months without focal findings, or are > 6 months but are not fully vaccinated should have:
  - CBC with differential
  - Blood culture

TABLE 5.5. Summary: Fever 3 Months-3 Years

Bacterial Causes	Evaluation	Treatment and Disposition
S pneumoniae	Ill appearing:	IV antibiotics and admission
E coli	Full sepsis workup	Consider empiric antibiotics if WBC > 15,000/mm³
Neisseria meningitidis	Well appearing and no obvious source, but not fully immunized and fever ≥ 39°C (102.2°F):	Discharge home with follow-up in 24 h
	UA + culture	No antibiotics unless UA positive
	Consider CBC w/ differential	Discharge home
	Consider blood cultures	
	Well appearing, no obvious source, fully immunized but fever ≥ 39°C (102.2°F):	No antibiotics
	UA + culture based on gender and circumcision status	Discharge home
	Well appearing, no obvious source, fully immunized and fever < 39°C (102.2°F):	
	No further workup	

CBC, complete blood count; IV, intravenous; UA, urinanalysis; WBC, white blood count.

    - Chest x-ray (CXR) for WBC > 20,000/mm³
    - Catherized UA and urine culture
- Children with fever ≥ 39°C who are > 6 months and vaccinated should have:
    - Catherized UA and urine culture for girls up to age 2 years and for uncircumcised boys up to age 1 year and circumcised boys up to 6 months, or any child with previous UTI

Treatment

- Therapy is directed at the likely causative organisms.
- Patients who are well appearing can generally be followed as outpatients (Table 5.5).

COLIC

Parents often seek medical attention for their infant when they cannot identify the cause of excessive or disturbing crying. While no standard definition of colic exists, the most widely accepted definition is the Wessel criteria; otherwise known as "the rule of three." Given crying must have occurred for 3 weeks, the diagnosis of colic is rarely made in the ED.

> **KEY FACT**
>
> Colic rule of three: Crying at least 3 hours a day, at least 3 days a week, for at least 3 weeks.

Symptoms/Examination

Beyond the Wessel criteria, other characteristics of infantile colic have been described, including the inability to be consoled, an alarming quality to the crying, paroxysms of crying, and hypertonic activity such as drawing the legs up, arching the back, and distending the abdomen.

MNEMONIC

Differential diagnosis of colic:

CAN'T FART

Corneal abrasion, **C**onstipation, **C**ongenital anomalies (cardiac and metabolic)
Anal fissure, **A**ppendicitis
I**N**tussusception, i**N**fection (meningitis, otitis, UTI)
Tourniquet (around digit or penis)
Formula intolerance, **F**oreign body in eye
Abuse (shaken-baby syndrome, fractures)
Recent immunization (particularly pertussis)
Testicular torsion

KEY FACT

While episodes of pulling the knees to the chest can occur with colic, also consider intussusception.

Differential

The differential diagnosis for colic is extensive and is ultimately a diagnosis of exclusion. The infant must be otherwise healthy with appropriate weight gain and growth for their age.

Diagnosis

- The EM physician's role is to determine if the presentation represents benign crying or excessive crying secondary to a life-threatening etiology. The vast majority of etiologies can be determined based on the history and physical alone.
- A careful history regarding to the crying itself should be elicited from the parents, including onset, duration, frequency, and associated events such as fever, feeding patterns, and vaccinations.
- A thorough head-to-toe examination must also be done.
- Further evaluation for child abuse, sepsis, and cardiac or abdominal pathology should be done if suggested by the history or physical examination.

Treatment

- Many studies have attempted to provide evidence for specific treatments. However, these studies have mixed results. Some infants may benefit from a protein hydrolysate formula. Dicyclomine (Bentyl) is contraindicated in infants < 6 months given increased risk of seizure, apnea, and coma.
- Attention should be paid to answering parental questions and alleviating their fears, because colic can exacerbate family stress and promote child abuse.

NEONATAL JAUNDICE

Neonatal hyperbilirubinemia can be either a physiologic or a pathologic process depending on the time of onset and the type of bilirubin elevated. Elevated serum bilirubin can damage the infant's brain, causing irreversible **kernicterus**, a rare but preventable form of cerebral palsy.

Causes

- Table 5.6 lists the causes of neonatal jaundice based on age of onset.
- **Unconjugated hyperbilirubinemia is the most common form of neonatal jaundice**. Causes include physiologic jaundice, breast milk, hemolysis, and bruising from birth trauma.
- Conjugated hyperbilirubinemia is always pathologic. Causes include sepsis, biliary obstruction, toxoplasmosis, rubella, cytomegalovirus, and herpes simplex (TORCH) infections, and metabolic/genetic abnormalities.
- Physiologic jaundice occurs in the first few days of life secondary to a number of factors that increase unconjugated bilirubin production, impair conjugation of bilirubin, and increase enterohepatic circulation of bilirubin. Physiologic jaundice peaks during the second to fourth days of life (< 6 mg/dL) and falls to < 2 mg/dL within 1 week.

KEY FACT

All forms of hyperbilirubinemia are pathologic in the first 24 hours of life.

Symptoms/Examination

As serum bilirubin levels increase, jaundice will become more detectable, starting at the infant's head and progressing toward the feet (Table 5.7). Estimates of bilirubin levels based on physical examination are unreliable and should always be confirmed with serum levels.

Symptoms of bilirubin toxicity include:

- Extensor rigidity
- Tremor

KEY FACT

Jaundice is often the only sign of hyperbilirubinemia in infants.

TABLE 5.6. Causes of Neonatal Jaundice

Age	Etiologies
< 24 h	Hemolysis due to ABO, Rh incompatibility Congenital infection (rubella, toxoplasmosis, CMV) Excessive bruising from birth trauma (cephalohematoma or intramuscular hematoma) Acquired infection
2-3 d	Physiologic (most common cause overall)
3 d-< 1 wk	Acquired infection Congenital decrease in glucuronyl transferase (Crigler-Najjar syndrome, Gilbert syndrome) Congenital infections (syphilis, toxoplasmosis, CMV)
> 1 wk	Breast milk jaundice (common) Acquired infection Biliary atresia Congenital and acquired hepatitis Red cell membrane defects (sickle cell, spherocytosis, elliptocytosis) Red cell enzyme defects (G6PD deficiency) Hemolysis due to drugs Endocrine disorders (hypothyroidism) Metabolic disorders (galactosemia, fructosemia)

CMV, cytomegalovirus.

(Modified, with permission, from Tintinalli JE, Stapczynski JS, Ma OJ, et al. *Tintinalli's Emergency Medicine*. 7th ed. New York, NY: McGraw-Hill; 2011:743.)

- Loss of suck reflex
- Lethargy
- Seizures

Diagnosis/Treatment

Diagnosis and treatment options are based on **total serum bilirubin level** and other risks such as prematurity, risks of hemolysis, sepsis, asphyxia, hypoalbuminemia, and acidosis.

- Serum bilirubin levels should be interpreted relative to the infant's age in **hours**, not **days**.
- Additional laboratory studies such as Coombs test, reticulocyte count, peripheral blood smear, and sepsis workup may be indicated.

TABLE 5.7. Clinical Jaundice and Serum Bilirubin Levels

Face/eyes	7-8 mg/dL
Shoulder/torso	8-10 mg/dL
Lower body	10-12 mg/dL
Generalized	> 12 mg/dL

- The American Academy of Pediatrics (AAP) publishes nomograms for when to start phototherapy and exchange transfusion. Phototherapy can be performed at home, if the neonate is at low risk and reliable follow-up is arranged within 24 hours to ensure bilirubin levels are improving. Higher-risk neonates may require inpatient management. This includes those born preterm, those with jaundice in the first 24 hours, those with ABO incompatibility with a positive direct Coombs test, those with hemolytic disease, easy bruising or hematomas, poor feeding or weight loss, lethargy, or high respiratory rate.
- Consider **phototherapy** if total serum bilirubin is > 5 × the birth weight in kilograms (usually 15-25 mg/dL).
- Consider **exchange transfusion** if total serum bilirubin is > 10 × the birth weight in kilograms (usually 25-30 mg/dL).
- All patients with conjugated hyperbilirubinemia require admission and evaluation for the cause of jaundice.

COMPLICATIONS

Acute bilirubin encephalopathy and chronic brain injury (kernicterus).

DIARRHEA

> **KEY FACT**
>
> **Norovirus has replaced rotavirus as the most common cause of diarrhea** in children < 5 years in the United States because of the rotavirus vaccine introduced in 2006.

Diarrhea is the passage of increased volume of loose or watery stools. There is no consensus on the absolute number of stools per day that defines diarrhea. An increase in frequency, volume, or liquidity should prompt evaluation. Diarrheal illnesses continue to be a major cause of morbidity and mortality around the world. In the United States, the majority of diarrheal illnesses are due to viruses with < 25% caused by bacteria.

SYMPTOMS/EXAMINATION

- Important history includes the presence of blood or mucus in the stool, recent antibiotic use, recent travel, sick contacts (daycare, siblings), and exposure to unsanitary water. These risk factors are associated with bacterial or parasitic etiologies.
- Typically, viral enteritis is associated with community-acquired nonbloody diarrhea, without mucus (< 5 PMNs/hpf on microscopic examination of the stool). Diarrheal diseases caused by viruses usually last around 5 days and occur most frequently in the late winter or spring.
- Bacterial enteritis may present with severe abdominal pain, tenesmus, bloody/mucoid stool, fever, and possibly altered mental status.
- Fluid intake, urine output, alertness, activity level, capillary refill, skin turgor, and mucus membranes should also be assessed for evaluation of dehydration (Table 5.8).

DIFFERENTIAL

Perform a careful physical examination to evaluate for dehydration and the presence of intra-abdominal emergencies, such as intussusception and necrotizing enterocolitis (NEC) (Table 5.9).

DIAGNOSIS

- Based on history and physical examination.
- Stool guaiac and fecal leukocytes may support a bacterial etiology.
- Laboratory studies are not routinely needed unless a child is moderately to severely ill or the diarrhea is persistent.
- Diarrhea may lead to severe dehydration, as well as a nonanion gap metabolic acidosis due to loss of bicarbonate in the stool. There are numerous infectious causes of diarrhea (Table 5.10).

TABLE 5.8. Clinical Assessment of Dehydration

Findings	Mild (3%-5%)	Moderate (6%-9%)	Severe (≥ 10%)
Pulse	Normal	High	High, weak pulse
Blood pressure	Normal	Normal to low	Low
Mental status	Normal	Normal to listless	Lethargic
Anterior fontanelle	Normal	Sunken	Markedly sunken
Eyes	Normal	Sunken	Markedly sunken
Tears	Present	Decreased	Absent
Mucous membranes	Normal	Dry	Parched
Capillary refill/skin	Normal	Delayed, cool	Delayed, cool, mottled
Urine output	Slight decrease	Decreased	Anuric
Thirst	Slight increase	Moderate increase	Marked increase

TABLE 5.9. Differential Diagnosis of Diarrhea

Infection—viral	*Rotavirus*: Most common *Enterovirus* Norwalk virus
Infection—bacterial	*Salmonella* *Shigella* *E coli* Others: *Campylobacter, Yersinia, Vibrio cholera, Staphylococcus aureus, Bacillus cereus*
Infectious colitis	*Clostridium difficile* colitis; typically associated with antecedent antibiotics
Inflammatory bowel disease	Crohn disease or ulcerative colitis
Intussusception	Classically associated with bloody diarrhea, intermittent crying, and lethargy
Other infections	UTI, otitis media, pneumonia
Malabsorption	Cystic fibrosis, celiac disease
Other	Overflow with chronic constipation, endocrine, drugs

UTI, urinary tract infection.

TABLE 5.10. Mechanisms of Infectious Diarrheal Disease

Pathogen Type	Characteristic Examples	Mechanism	Pathologic Impact	Clinical Impact
Viral enteropathogens	Rotaviruses Adenoviruses	Invade small intestinal mucosa villous epithelium	Loss of mature absorptive cells, producing a proliferative response, resulting in repopulation of intestinal epithelial lining with poorly differentiated cells	Salt and water absorption is decreased Carbohydrate malabsorption and osmotic diarrhea
Bacterial enteropathogens	Invasive *Shigella* *Salmonella* *Yersinia enterocolitica* *Campylobacter jejuni* *Vibrio parahaemolyticus*	Adhere to mucosal cells followed by invasion and multiplication, primarily in large intestine	Intramucosal multiplication elicits an acute mucosal inflammatory reaction, resulting in ulceration and synthesis of a variety of secretagogues	Salt and water absorption is decreased (secretory diarrhea)
	Cytotoxic *Shigella* Enteropathogenic *E coli* Enterohemorrhagic *E coli* *Clostridium difficile*	Elaboration of cytotoxins	Cause cell damage and death by inhibiting protein synthesis or by inducing the secretion of one or more inflammatory mediator substances	Decreased intestinal absorptive surface
	Toxigenic *Shigella* Enterotoxigenic *E coli* *Y enterocolitica* *Aeromonas* *Vibrio cholerae*	Colonize small intestine and secrete enterotoxins	Enterotoxin binds to specific mucosal receptors, increasing the concentration of an intracellular mediator (adenosine 3′,5′-cyclic phosphate or cyclic guanosine monophosphate)	Alter intestinal salt and water transport without affecting mucosal morphology
	Adherent Enteropathogenic *E coli* Enterohemorrhagic *E coli*	Colonization and adherence to intestinal surface of small and large intestines	Binding to epithelial cells indents the surface, causes glycocalyx dissolution and microvilli flattening	Decreased intestinal absorptive surface

(Reproduced, with permission, from Tintinalli JE, Stapczynski JS, Ma OJ, et al. *Tintinalli's Emergency Medicine*. 7th ed. New York, NY: McGraw-Hill; 2011:831.)

TREATMENT

- Therapy should focus on two phases: **rehydration** and **maintenance** of hydration.
- Oral rehydration therapy is effective for mild-to-moderate dehydration.
- IV fluids of normal saline or lactated Ringer in multiple boluses of 20 cc/kg may be required to treat severe dehydration or if the child is unable to tolerate oral intake. Glucose containing fluids such as D_5NS may also be used as one of the boluses to expedite improvement in some children.
- Antidiarrheal agents should not be used routinely.

VOMITING

Vomiting is a nonspecific sign that may be caused by a wide variety of conditions ranging from the benign to the catastrophic. Vomiting may arise from gastrointestinal (GI) processes (infection, inflammation, obstruction), central nervous system (CNS) processes (infection, increased pressure), renal processes (uremia), or metabolic processes (inborn errors of metabolism [IEM], diabetic ketoacidosis [DKA], adrenal insufficiency). Differential diagnosis is largely age dependent.

SYMPTOMS/EXAMINATION

The history should first define whether the vomiting is bilious or nonbilious. Bilious vomiting should prompt concern for a surgical emergency secondary to an obstructive pathology. History should also elicit whether vomiting is present alone or with diarrhea. Physical examination should be focused on signs of dehydration, surgical abdomen, and systemic toxicity such as altered mental status and shock.

DIFFERENTIAL

Table 5.11 lists causes of vomiting in the pediatric population.

DIAGNOSIS

Diagnosis is based on a careful history and physical examination. Ancillary studies such as laboratory tests and imaging should be used only if the patient appears toxic or the diagnosis is uncertain.

TREATMENT

- Stabilization and diagnosis are paramount, with specific treatment directed toward the underlying condition.
- **Ondansetron (for patient > 6 months)** improves the success of oral rehydration therapy and may be employed for patients with vomiting and diarrhea.

CONSTIPATION

Constipation in the newborn can be a true emergency, but beyond this stage constipation is less emergent. In general, newborns have approximately four stools a day with breast-fed newborns having more than bottle-fed newborns. The number of stools per day decreases over time. By age 3, children should have one stool per day. However, stool patterns can vary significantly with many children having only one stool every 3-4 days.

SYMPTOMS/EXAMINATION

- Newborns should pass meconium stool within the first 24-48 hours. If they have not, they may present to the ED for constipation, abdominal distention, and/or vomiting.

Q

A full-term infant vomits after her initial feeding and subsequently develops bilious emesis after each feeding. Physical examination reveals a lethargic infant with absent bowel sounds. Plain abdominal radiographs reveal a paucity of air in the distal bowel. What is the most likely diagnosis and what is the appropriate management?

KEY FACT

A young infant with bilious vomiting must be assumed to have malrotation with volvulus until proven otherwise.

KEY FACT

Gastroenteritis should only be diagnosed in patients with both vomiting and diarrhea in whom other more serious causes are unlikely.

A

Malrotation with volvulus. Management should include IV fluid resuscitation, nasogastric tube (NGT) placement, and emergent surgical consultation. Malrotation cannot be ruled out on the basis of plain films alone. If plain films are negative, an upper GI series can be obtained in the stable patient. However, patients who are unstable or in whom there is a high suspicion for malrotation warrant a surgical consultation for possible exploratory laparotomy.

TABLE 5.11. Causes of Vomiting, by Age

NEWBORN	
Obstructive intestinal anomalies	Esophageal stenosis/atresia, pyloric stenosis, intestinal stenosis/atresia, malrotation ± volvulus, incarcerated hernia, meconium ileus/plug, Hirschsprung disease, imperforate anus, enteric duplications
Neurologic	Intracranial bleed/mass, hydrocephalus, cerebral edema, kernicterus
Renal	Urinary tract infection, obstructive uropathy, renal insufficiency
Infectious	Viral illness, gastroenteritis, meningitis, sepsis
Metabolic/endocrine	Inborn errors of metabolism (urea cycle, amino/organic acid, carbohydrate), congenital adrenal hyperplasia
Miscellaneous	Ileus, gastroesophageal reflux, necrotizing enterocolitis, milk allergy, GI perforation
INFANT (< 12 MO)	
Obstructive intestinal anomalies	Pyloric stenosis, malrotation ± volvulus, incarcerated hernia, Hirschsprung disease, enteric duplications, intussusception, foreign body, bezoars, Meckel diverticulum
Neurologic	Intracranial bleed/mass, hydrocephalus, cerebral edema
Renal	Urinary tract infection, obstructive uropathy, renal insufficiency
Infectious	Viral illness, gastroenteritis, meningitis, sepsis, otitis media, pneumonia, pertussis, hepatitis
Metabolic/endocrine	Inborn errors of metabolism, adrenal insufficiency, renal tubular acidosis
Miscellaneous	Ileus, gastroesophageal reflux, post-tussive, peritonitis, drug overdose
CHILD (> 12 MO)	
Obstructive intestinal anomalies	Malrotation ± volvulus, incarcerated hernia, Hirschsprung disease, intussusception, foreign body, bezoars, Meckel diverticulum, acquired esophageal stricture, peptic ulcer disease, adhesions, superior mesenteric artery syndrome
Neurologic	Intracranial bleed/mass, cerebral edema, postconcussive, migraine
Renal	Urinary tract infection, obstructive uropathy, renal insufficiency
Infectious	Viral illness, gastroenteritis, meningitis, sepsis, otitis media, pneumonia, hepatitis, streptococcal pharyngitis
Metabolic/endocrine	Inborn errors of metabolism, adrenal insufficiency, renal tubular acidosis, diabetes mellitus, Reye syndrome, porphyria
Miscellaneous	Ileus, gastroesophageal reflux, post-tussive, peritonitis, drug overdose, appendicitis, pancreatitis, gastritis, Crohn disease, pregnancy, psychogenic, cyclic vomiting syndrome

GI, gastrointestinal.

(Reproduced, with permission, from Tintinalli JE, Stapczynski JS, Ma OJ, et al. *Tintinalli's Emergency Medicine.* 7th ed. New York, NY: McGraw-Hill; 2011:830.)

- Older infants and children may present because the parents are concerned about constipation and/or the child is complaining of abdominal pain. If the child is retaining stool, an abdominal mass and fecal impaction in the rectum may be present on examination.
- With Hirschsprung disease, the patient will often not have any stool in the rectal vault.
- Inspection for anal fissures should also be done because pain can lead to fecal retention.

DIFFERENTIAL DIAGNOSIS

See Table 5.12.

DIAGNOSIS

History and physical examination are usually sufficient to make the diagnosis. When in doubt, an abdominal x-ray can help confirm the diagnosis. Electrolytes and thyroid testing can be done in cases of severe constipation.

TREATMENT

- Disimpaction should be done if fecal impaction is present.
- Oral medication options include polyethylene glycol (MiraLAX), milk of magnesia, lactulose, senna, and bisacodyl.
- Rectal medication options include suppositories (glycerin for infants and bisacodyl for adolescents) and enemas (soap suds and fleets).
- Stool softeners should be given to patients with anal fissures.
- Admit newborns who fail to pass meconium.
- Admit all who are completely obstructed secondary to constipation.

KEY FACT

The most common causes of constipation in all age groups are functional and dietary.

KEY FACT

Hypertonic phosphate enemas (fleets) can cause acute hypocalcemia in young infants and should be avoided.

TABLE 5.12. Differential Diagnosis for Constipation

AGE	ETIOLOGY
Newborn	Imperforate anus Anal stenosis Meconium plug Meconium ileus (associated with cystic fibrosis) Hirschsprung disease (associated with Down syndrome) Volvulust Hypothyroidism
Infant	Functional Dietary (too much cow's milk, low fiber) Dehydration Anal fissure and resultant fecal retention Cerebral palsy Others: Neuromuscular disorders, spinal cord abnormalities, hypothyroidism, hypocalcemia, medications
Older Children	Functional Dietary Dehydration Medications: Opiates, anticholinergics, antihistamines

COMPLICATIONS

- Hirschsprung-associated enterocolitis: Infants with Hirschsprung disease may present with (in decreasing order of frequency) abdominal distention, explosive diarrhea, vomiting, fever, lethargy, rectal bleeding, and shock.
- Intestinal obstruction.
- **Chronic constipation**.

Gastroenterology

CONGENITAL DISORDERS

Hirschsprung Disease

> **KEY FACT**
>
> Unlike functional constipation, children with Hirschsprung will have a history of lifelong stooling difficulties, no abdominal pain, and an empty rectal vault on rectal examination.

Patients with Hirschsprung disease have a segment of bowel that lacks normal ganglion cell innervation in the myenteric and submucosal tissue. Ganglion cells normally oppose the tonic contractions of the bowel; when they are missing there are increased spasms and poor gut motility. This can lead to obstruction or constipation. Males are affected more frequently than females (4:1).

SYMPTOMS/EXAMINATION

- Wide spectrum of disease presentation, depending on the length of affected bowel.
- Symptoms typically develop in the first few days to weeks of life.
- The diagnosis should be considered in neonates who have delayed passage of meconium or failure to pass meconium.
- Hirschsprung disease may cause typical symptoms of colonic obstruction.

DIAGNOSIS

- Barium enema may demonstrate a **cone-shaped transition zone** between the dilated proximal bowel and the abnormally contracted distal bowel. The rectum should not be stimulated with a rectal examination prior to the enema, because it may cause temporary loss of the transition zone.
- Anorectal manometry.
- Rectal suction biopsy (gold standard).

TREATMENT

- Patients who are suspected of having Hirschsprung disease with enterocolitis or who have evidence of colonic obstruction should receive:
  - IV fluid
  - IV antibiotics
  - NGT
  - Rectal tube
  - Emergent surgical consultation
- Well-appearing children without signs of colitis or obstruction can be referred for outpatient evaluation if there is low suspicion for Hirschsprung disease.

COMPLICATIONS

Failure to thrive, constipation, enterocolitis

Tracheoesophageal Fistula

Tracheoesophageal fistula (TEF) is the **most common cause of esophageal obstruction** in neonates. During embryonic development, the trachea and esophagus normally separate and develop in a linear fashion. When a TEF is present, there is an abnormal communication between the trachea and the esophagus. The most common type of TEF (90%) results in the proximal esophagus terminating in a blind pouch, while the distal esophagus communicates with the trachea (Figure 5.1). A more rare form, the H type, consists of an intact esophagus and trachea with a fistula between them. Because this type presents later in life, it is the most common form encountered in the ED.

Symptoms

- Respiratory distress.
- Drooling, with difficulty handling oral secretions.
- Choking with each feed.
- Nonbilious vomiting immediately after/during feeding.
- H-type fistulas present later in childhood with recurrent aspiration events.
- After repair, patients can present with food impaction due to stricture formation at the site of repair.

Examination

Physical examination may be normal, or there may be associated abnormalities, including the **VATER complex**.

Diagnosis

- Inability to pass an NGT into the stomach (except with the H type). The blind proximal esophageal pouch can often be demonstrated on plain radiographs by injecting a small amount of air into the NGT when the chest radiograph is taken.
- Contrast esophagram can also be employed.
- Surgical exploration confirms the diagnosis.

Treatment

- Fluid and nutritional resuscitation
- Surgical correction

Complications

- Chemical pneumonitis if gastric contents reflux into the distal esophagus, enter the TEF, and go into the lungs
- Dehydration

Malrotation With Volvulus

During the first 3 months of gestation, there is normally a 270° counterclockwise rotation of the midgut, with subsequent fixation of the small bowel in the left upper quadrant (LUQ) (ligament of Treitz) and right upper quadrant (RLQ). When malrotation occurs, the small bowel is not anchored in the LUQ or RLQ. Bands of tissue (Ladd bands) form between the cecum and duodenum, potentially causing duodenal obstruction. The malrotation of the midgut also predisposes the bowel to twisting on itself, leading to bowel obstruction and vascular compromise. This compromise can lead to bowel necrosis **within 1 hour**. Of patients with malrotation, 33% present with symptoms within the first week of life, 50% present within the first month, and 85% present within the first year.

Symptoms/Examination

- Symptoms depend on the degree of bowel obstruction.
- Bilious emesis in an infant should always raise concern for malrotation.

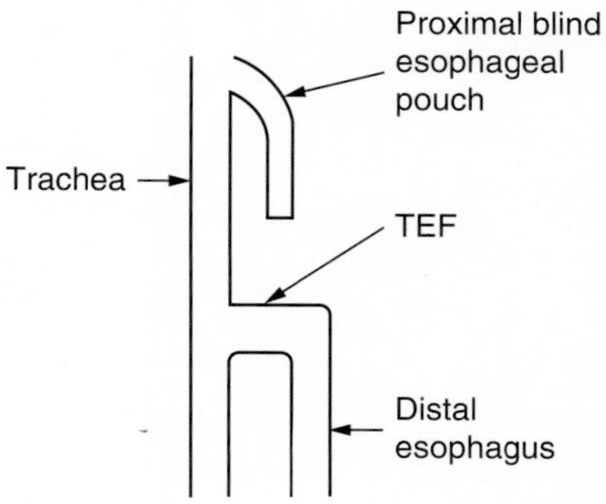

FIGURE 5.1. Most common type of tracheoesophageal fistula (TEF).

MNEMONIC

The VATER complex:

Vertebral anomalies
Anus (imperforate)
TE Fistula
Renal defects

KEY FACT

Bilious emesis in a neonate is malrotation until proven otherwise.

KEY FACT

Plain films alone are insufficient to rule out malrotation in an infant with bilious emesis. Infants require surgical evaluation or a more definitive study, such as an upper GI series.

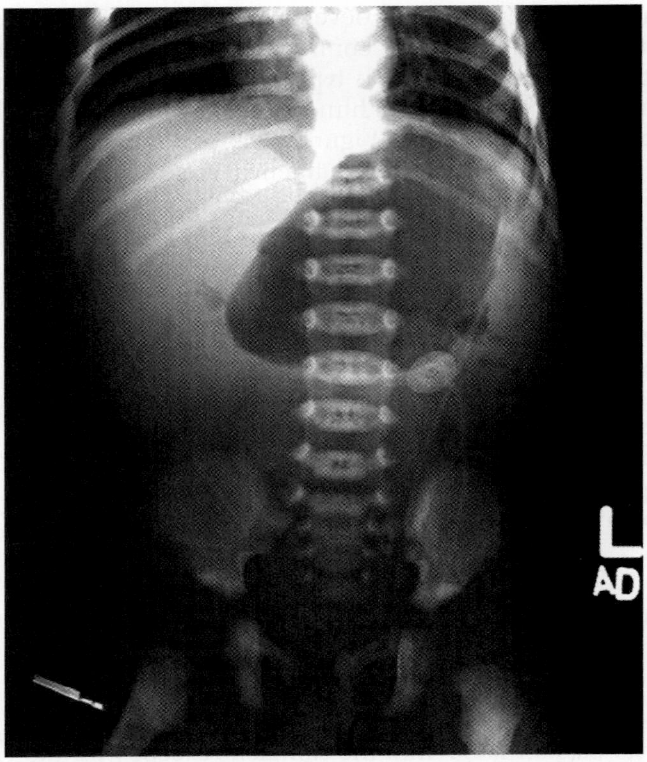

FIGURE 5.2. Malrotation with volvulus. (Reproduced, with permission, from Brunicardi CF, Andersen DK, Billiar TR, et al. *Schwartz's Principles of Surgery*. 9th ed. New York, NY: McGraw-Hill; 2010.)

- Other common symptoms include abdominal pain, hematochezia, or abdominal distention.
- Half of patients will have normal abdominal examinations.

Diagnosis

- Abdominal radiograph (AXR) findings include dilated proximal bowel with little distal bowel gas (Figure 5.2). The classic AXR for duodenal obstruction is the "double bubble" sign of air fluid level in the stomach and proximal duodenum. This can be seen in patients with malrotation and volvulus as well as those with duodenal atresia. However, the AXR can be negative.
- Upper GI series is the gold standard and classically shows obstruction at the level of the duodenum with the duodenojejunal junction at the ligament of Treitz positioned to the right of the vertebral column and a "corkscrew" appearance of the small bowel.
- Barium enema may show a mobile cecum present in the RUQ, although this is not a reliable finding.

Treatment

- IV fluid resuscitation
- IV antibiotics
- NGT to decompress proximal bowel
- Emergent surgical consultation

> **KEY FACT**
>
> Classic AXR finding for duodenal obstruction: Double bubble sign.

Meckel Diverticulum

Meckel diverticulum is a remnant of the omphalomesenteric duct in children that forms a short, blind pouch extending from the ileum. Sixty percent contain heterotopic gastric, pancreatic, or endometrial tissue, which may ulcerate and bleed, leading to painless lower GI bleeding in children. Fifty percent of severe lower GI bleeding is due to Meckel diverticulum.

SYMPTOMS/EXAMINATION

- May be asymptomatic.
- If the diverticulum ulcerates, the child may present with painless lower GI bleeding.
- Abdominal pain should raise concern for intussusception.

DIAGNOSIS

A labeled Technetium-99m scan (**Meckel scan**) may demonstrate the presence of ectopic gastric mucosa within the Meckel diverticulum.

TREATMENT

- Patients may require fluid/blood resuscitation.
- If the Technetium scan is positive, surgical excision is indicated.

COMPLICATIONS

- Massive lower GI bleeding, with resulting anemia and hemorrhagic shock.
- Meckel diverticulum can act as the lead point for intussusception or obstruction.
- Perforation and peritonitis.

> **KEY FACT**
>
> **Rule of 2s for Meckel diverticulum:** **2%** prevalence, **2:1** male-to-female ratio, **2 ft** proximal to ileocecal valve and half of those symptomatic are < **2 years** old

ACQUIRED DISORDERS

Pyloric Stenosis

Pyloric stenosis is the **most common cause** of gastric obstruction in infants. Typically infants present with symptoms after 2 weeks of age and typically around 3-4 weeks of life, but symptoms may occur anytime up to 3-4 months of age. The etiology of pyloric stenosis is unknown, but the end result is hypertrophy of the pyloric muscle with resulting gastric outlet obstruction. The incidence is roughly 1 in 250 live births, with males affected more than females (4:1). First-born males are at highest risk.

SYMPTOMS

- **Nonbilious, projectile vomiting** that typically occurs after feedings and begins after infant feeds without difficulty for the first 1-2 weeks of their life.
- Hematemesis has also been described.
- Until late in the disease, affected infants have a vigorous suck and appear hungry.

> **KEY FACT**
>
> Pyloric stenosis can be differentiated from other causes of vomiting because the vomiting is typically nonbilious and the patients remain hungry and vigorous after feeding.

EXAMINATION

- Infants may have a palpable mass ("**olive**") in the RUQ, although this finding may be difficult to elicit in an agitated infant. In addition, as children are now presenting earlier in the course of this disease, often the olive has not hypertrophied enough or the child is not cachectic enough for the olive to be palpable.
- With prolonged disease, signs of dehydration and weight loss may develop.
- Infants may develop a hypochloremic metabolic alkalosis. In severe cases, this can lead to respiratory compensation for the alkalosis with a decreased respiratory rate.

DIAGNOSIS

- An ultrasound should be obtained. Pyloric stenosis is confirmed if the ultrasound reveals a pylorus > 4 mm thick and longer than 16 mm. The pylorus must be imaged twice over a period of at least 30 minutes if the initial ultrasound shows an enlarged pylorus to ensure it was not due to normal pylorospasm. Conversely it is important to remember than a normal pylorus ultrasound at an early age, especially around 2 weeks of life, does not exclude the diagnosis. If symptoms persist, the infant should have a repeat ultrasound in 24-48 hours as the diseases is progressive.
- If ultrasound is not available, an upper GI series will reveal a narrowed pylorus ("**string sign**").
- If the infant has been vomiting for a few days, serum chemistries will reveal the classic hyponatremic, hypochloremic, and hypokalemic metabolic alkalosis.

TREATMENT

- Isotonic IV fluid resuscitation
- Electrolyte repletion once urine output has been observed
- Surgical consultation for pyloromyotomy

COMPLICATIONS

Weight loss, dehydration, electrolyte abnormalities

GASTROESOPHAGEAL REFLUX

> **KEY FACT**
>
> Sandifer syndrome is associated with reflux after eating—the child arches his or her back with tonic posturing that is often confused for seizures. It does not require treatment.

Nearly all infants experience reflux but most outgrow it without incident.

SYMPTOMS/EXAMINATION

- Spitting up after feeding
- Nonbilious emesis

DIAGNOSIS

- An upper GI series can be helpful to rule out other etiologies of vomiting.
- pH probe should not be used in the ED but is a helpful outpatient study.

DIFFERENTIAL

- Pyloric stenosis
- Hiatal hernia
- Gastroenteritis
- Duodenal or esophageal web

TREATMENT

- Initial therapy is nonpharmacologic—elevate head of bed, thicken feeds, decrease volume of feeds.
- Secondary therapy—H_2 blockers, proton pump inhibitors (PPIs), or promotility agents such as metoclopramide should only be initiated if nonpharmacologic therapy is unsuccessful.
- If these measures fail and the child is experiencing significant morbidity, consult surgery for possible fundoplication.

Necrotizing Enterocolitis

Necrotizing enterocolitis (NEC) occurs due to bacterial overgrowth in the bowel with translocation of bacteria into the bowel wall and the production of bacterial endotoxin and gas. A combination of factors is thought to predispose an infant to NEC, including:

- Prematurity (seen in 90% of cases)
- Ischemia, with perfusion–reperfusion injury to the bowel
- Infection
- Introduction of parenteral feeding
- Reduced immune response

Infants typically develop NEC in the first few days of life, but NEC can appear as late as 1 month of age.

Symptoms/Examination

- Abdominal distention at < 1 month
- Nonbilious emesis
- Grossly bloody or guaiac positive stools
- Sepsis (lethargy, temperature instability, apnea, bradycardia)
- Abdominal wall erythema and firm loops of bowel (if bowel necrosis develops)

Diagnosis

- Confirmed by AXR showing **pneumatosis intestinalis** (gas in the wall of the bowel) or portal venous air (Figure 5.3).
- Pneumoperitoneum may be present if perforation has occurred.

Treatment

- Nothing by mouth
- IV fluid resuscitation
- NGT decompression of bowel
- Broad-spectrum IV antibiotics
- Surgical consultation; emergent bowel resection only if bowel is necrotic or perforated

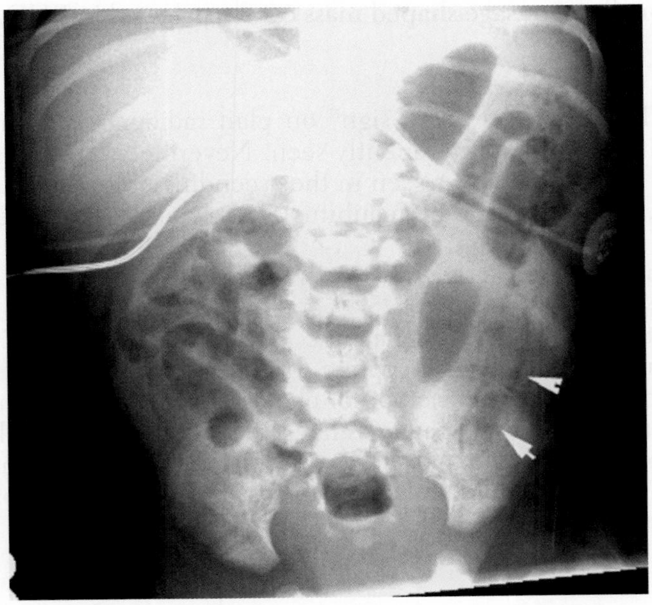

FIGURE 5.3. Necrotizing enterocolitis. (Reproduced, with permission, from Brunicardi CF, Andersen DK, Billiar TR, et al. *Schwartz's Principles of Surgery*. 9th ed. New York, NY: McGraw-Hill; 2010.)

COMPLICATIONS

- Intestinal perforation.
- Infants who recover from NEC may have bowel strictures and postoperatively may develop short gut syndrome.

Intussusception

Intussusception occurs when a proximal portion of bowel telescopes into a more distal portion, typically with the ileum inserting through the ileocecal valve. Intussusception is the most common cause of bowel obstruction in infants between the ages of 3 and 12 months (peak incidence between the ages of 5 and 9 months) but may occur anytime from birth through childhood. Males are affected more frequently than females.

PATHOPHYSIOLOGY

- In children > 2 years old, an abnormal lead point such as a tumor, Meckel diverticulum, or polyp is much more likely.
- In infants, inflamed Peyer patches often serve as the lead point.

SYMPTOMS

- Classic triad:
  - 85%, colicky abdominal pain with child appearing well between episodes.
  - 75%, vomiting.
  - 40%, rectal bleeding (**"currant jelly stools"** is a late finding due to sloughing of the bowel mucosa). Most cases of intussusception are diagnosed prior to bowel necrosis.
- 80% of children will **not** have the classic triad.
- Children may also present with altered mental status or lethargy.

> **KEY FACT**
>
> Currant jelly stools is a late finding of intussusceptions and is not required for initiation of the workup. Earlier in the disease children often have occult blood in their stool.

EXAMINATION

- Variable physical examination, ranging from well appearing and asymptomatic to toxic and lethargic.
- Occasionally, a **sausage-shaped mass** can be palpated in RUQ.

DIAGNOSIS

- AXR: The classic "crescent sign" on plan radiography from the intussuscepting mass is not frequently seen. Nevertheless, AXR is helpful in low-risk cases; when air is seen in the ascending colon on all three views (supine, prone, and lateral decubitus), it substantially reduces the likelihood of intussusception.
- Ultrasound is noninvasive and easily obtained (Figure 5.4). It is highly sensitive (> 95%), specific (> 95%), and has no side effects.
- Contrast or air enema: Therapeutic as well as diagnostic. Enemas may successfully reduce intussusception for 70%-95% of patients. Air-contrast enema has become the method of choice because of the reduced risk of complications and higher success rate. Reductions tend to be less successful in younger children and those with longer duration of symptoms. Surgery should be available for backup in case the enema leads to perforation or is unsuccessful.

TREATMENT

- NGT decompression, IV fluids if dehydrated, nothing by mouth, and IV antibiotics.
- Air contrast/barium enema.

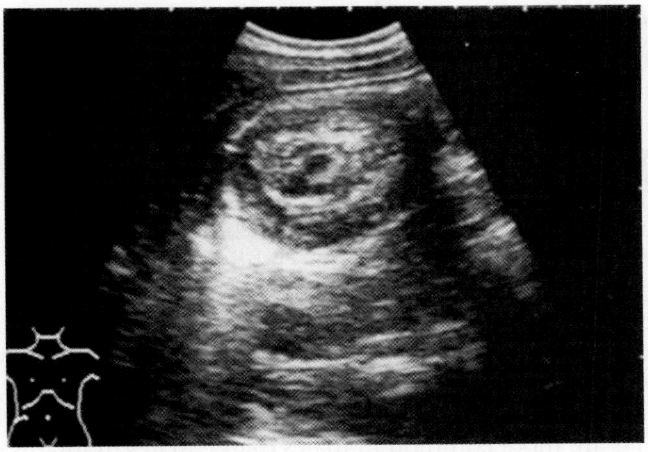

FIGURE 5.4. An ultrasound image of intussusceptions showing classic target appearance of bowel-within-bowel. (Reproduced, with permission, from Ma OJ, Mateer JR, Blaivas M. *Emergency Ultrasound*. 2nd ed. New York, NY: McGraw-Hill; 2008.)

- Surgical intervention is indicated if the two attempts at reduction via enema fail or if the patient is toxic or has signs of peritonitis.
- If perforation occurs during attempted reduction, general resuscitative measures should be instituted with antibiotics and fluids, and an emergent surgical consult should be called.

Complications

Bowel perforation and peritonitis

KEY FACT

Up to 10% of patients will have recurrence of intussusception within the first 24 hours after reduction, and therefore patients should be admitted for observation or given strict return precautions on discharge. Patients may be discharged if they have close follow-up, reliable means to return, are taking PO well, have a benign abdomen after reduction, and have no other comorbid medical problems.

Genitourinary

WILMS TUMOR

Wilms tumors are the **most common** renal tumors in children, with a peak incidence at 3-4 years of age.

Symptoms/Examination

- Abdominal mass without abdominal pain until it has expanded in size significantly.
- Hematuria (25%).
- Hypertension (25%).
- Congenital **W**ilms tumor is associated with **A**niridia, **G**enitourinary (GU) anomalies, and mental **R**etardation (WAGR syndrome).

Diagnosis

- Ultrasound—must include evaluation of surrounding vasculature to evaluate for tumor infiltration.
- Computed tomography (CT) abdomen with contrast; CT chest to evaluate for metastases in the lungs may be required but can generally be deferred until inpatient oncological evaluation.

Treatment

- Admission and surgical consultation for potential excision
- Adjuvant chemotherapy, sometimes with addition of radiation

COMPLICATIONS

- Metastatic spread of tumor
- Recurrent disease after treatment

URINARY TRACT INFECTION

The term urinary tract infection (UTI) includes lower tract infections of the urethra and bladder (urethritis or cystitis), and upper tract infections of the kidney (pyelonephritis). Most UTIs are due to infection by ascending gram-negative enteric bacteria, typically *E coli* (90%). However, the incidence of gram-positive pathogens such as *Enterococcus* is increasing. Infants often become infected by group B *Streptococcus* and adolescents with *S saprophyticus*. The overall incidence of UTIs before puberty is 3% of girls and 1% of boys. However, UTIs are more common in males than females in infants < 6 months. **There is a higher incidence of UTI in Caucasians, infants, uncircumcised males, and sexually active females.**

SYMPTOMS/EXAMINATION

- Depends on the age of the child and severity of infection
  - Neonates: Sepsis or fever
  - Infants: Fever, vomiting, irritability
  - > 2 years: Dysuria, suprapubic pain with cystitis, progressing to back pain, fever, and vomiting with pyelonephritis

KEY FACT

A negative bag urine sample rules out UTI in infants, but a positive sample requires confirmation with urine obtained by catheterization.

DIAGNOSIS

- The diagnosis of UTI depends on obtaining an appropriate sample. **In children < 2 years, the bladder should be catheterized.**
  - + Nitrite
  - Moderate (or greater) leukocyte esterase
  - + Gram stain for bacteria
  - > 10 WBC/hpf
  - The sensitivity of urinalysis is 82% and the specificity is 92%
- Urine culture should be obtained on catheterized samples. Colony count > 10,000 indicates likely infection.

DIFFERENTIAL

The differential diagnosis includes urethritis, vaginitis, chemical irritation, urethral injury, and labial adhesions.

TREATMENT

- Infants < 2 months and all toxic/septic children: Obtain blood cultures and admit for IV antibiotics. If < 30 days, must obtain CSF culture prior to starting antibiotics and consider in child < 60 days.
- Mild infection (cystitis): Consider oral antibiotics. Third-generation cephalosporins such as cefdinir, cefpodoxime, and cefixime can be used, as well as aminoglycosides such as gentamicin. These medications do not treat *Enterococcus* infections, however, so should not be used in patients who have anatomical abnormalities, indwelling urinary catheters, or recent instrumentation.
- Severe infection (pyelonephritis): Oral antibiotics unless toxic or cannot tolerate oral medications.
- Children < 3 years old with the first UTI should be referred to their pediatrician for potential imaging of the GU tract based on current clinical guidelines.

COMPLICATIONS

- Reflux is present in up to 50% of infants who have a UTI.
- Children with reflux are at risk for renal damage, resulting in chronic renal insufficiency, and at a risk of hypertension.

TESTICULAR TORSION

Torsion is the most concerning cause of scrotal pain. Testicular torsion occurs when the testicle rotates in the tunica vaginalis, decreasing blood flow. In general the longer a testicle is torsed, the less likely it is salvageable. ANY torsion should be considered an emergency and immediate urological consultation initiated. After 12 hours of torsion, the testicle is typically no longer salvageable, though intermittent or incomplete torsion may prolong survival of the testis beyond this. Torsion peaks in the neonatal and early adolescent periods.

> **KEY FACT**
>
> For patients with a high clinical probability of testicular torsion, the next step is immediate surgical consultation.

SYMPTOMS/EXAMINATION

- Sudden onset of severe scrotal pain, often upon awakening or with sports
- Nausea, vomiting
- High-riding testicle with horizontal lie
- Decreased cremasteric reflex, although this is unreliable and presence is not reassuring

> **KEY FACT**
>
> **Testicular torsion often presents as abdominal pain or vomiting** in younger children. Therefore, all males with abdominal pain or isolated vomiting should have a GU examination performed.

DIAGNOSIS

Color Doppler ultrasound showing decreased arterial blood flow.

DIFFERENTIAL

- Torsion of appendix testes: Symptoms are often less severe than in testicular torsion. Tenderness is greatest over superior lateral aspect of testis, a blue dot can often be seen with transillumination, the cremasteric reflex is intact, and the testicle has a normal lie. Patients with likely torsion of appendix testes still require ultrasound imaging to differentiate this condition from testicular torsion. However, it does not require surgery.
- Testicular hematoma: Ultrasound evaluation; surgical exploration if any concern for testicular rupture.
- Epididymitis/orchitis.
- Hernia.

TREATMENT

- If there is clinical concern, treatment should not be delayed while awaiting diagnostic studies. Urology or surgery should be consulted immediately for surgical exploration.
- If surgery is not readily available, manual detorsion can be performed by rotating the testis outward toward the thigh (in the direction of opening a book). Patients should receive analgesia prior to performing this procedure.

HYDROCELE

A hydrocele is a collection of fluid around the testicle that leads to painless testicular swelling. There are three categories of hydroceles:

- **Primary hydrocele**: Infants born with excess fluid in scrotum—typically resolves spontaneously by 1 year of age; not significant
- **Secondary hydrocele**: Reactive fluid collection within scrotum due to infection, trauma, testicular torsion, or tumor

- **Communicating hydrocele**: Fluid collection due to the presence of an indirect inguinal hernia, which allows fluid to communicate between the peritoneum and scrotum

Symptoms/Examination

- **Primary hydrocele**: Nontender fluid collection in scrotum, typically transilluminates, does not change in size
- **Secondary hydrocele**: May be an incidental finding in the setting of infection, trauma, testicular torsion, or tumor
- **Communicating hydrocele (indirect hernia)**: Typically nontender, with size of hydrocele increasing with crying or positioning

Differential

Inguinal hernia, testicular tumor

Diagnosis

- Hydroceles can usually be diagnosed clinically.
- A testicular ultrasound should be obtained in patients with a hydrocele and scrotal pain or tenderness to look for an acute pathologic process. If there is clinical concern for incarcerated inguinal hernia, a pediatric surgeon should be emergently consulted.

> **KEY FACT**
>
> A scrotal mass that transilluminates does not rule out an incarcerated inguinal hernia.

Treatment

- **Primary hydrocele**: Observation only. If a 1° hydrocele persists beyond 2 years of age, consider referral to a pediatric surgeon for a possible communicating hydrocele.
- **Secondary hydrocele**: Management of the underlying process.
- **Communicating hydrocele**: Outpatient surgical referral because it may lead to formation of a hernia.

POSTINFECTIOUS GLOMERULONEPHRITIS

Glomerulonephritis is the **most common cause** of acquired renal failure in children. It most commonly arises after infections, particularly streptococcal infections of the throat or skin. It also can arise from primary causes or with other diseases such as Henoch-Schönlein purpura (HSP), hemolytic-uremic syndrome (HUS), and systemic lupus erythematosus (SLE).

Pathophysiology

Immune response to underlying disease process ± immune complex deposition within glomeruli → production of inflammatory mediators → sclerosis and fibrosis of glomeruli.

Symptoms/Examination

- Symptoms arise 1-2 weeks after the original strep infection.
- Asymptomatic hematuria most common presentation.
- Edema can occur with nephrotic syndrome.
- Hypertension.

Diagnosis

- Hematuria, pyuria, proteinuria.
- Low C3, normal C4 (if complement levels are normal, consider noninfectious causes).
- Antistreptolysin O (ASO) documents preceding strep but does not prove strep is the cause of symptoms.

TREATMENT

- Salt and fluid restriction
- Diuretics or blood pressure medications after consultation with nephrologist
- Admit if hypertensive or impaired renal function

COMPLICATION

Hypertension.

NEPHROTIC SYNDROME

Causes excessive proteinuria and can be primary (due to minimal change disease, focal segmental glomerulosclerosis, or membranoproliferative nephritis) or secondary (due to HSP, SLE, human immunodeficiency virus [HIV], or in the setting of glomerulonephritis). It is most common in children between 2 and 6 years but can also present later in childhood.

SYMPTOMS/EXAMINATION

Edema—initially bilateral periorbital and worse in the morning that may become generalized.

DIAGNOSIS

- Proteinuria—urine protein to creatinine ratio > 2
- Hypoalbuminemia
- Hyponatremia

TREATMENT

- Assess volume status: If volume overload, restrict sodium. If hypovolemic, administer isotonic saline.
- Diuretics only after consultation with nephrologist.
- Primary nephrotic syndromes are often responsive to oral corticosteroids, which could be administered in consultation with a nephrologist.

COMPLICATIONS

- Infection
- Ascites
- Pleural effusion
- Thromboembolism

HEMOLYTIC UREMIC SYNDROME

Hemolytic uremic syndrome (HUS) is a disease characterized by microangiopathic hemolytic anemia, thrombocytopenia, and acute renal failure. It is one of the leading causes of renal failure in children in the United States. Most cases occur in children < 5 years.

PATHOPHYSIOLOGY

- **Shiga toxin–producing *E coli* of the 0157:H7 strain** (most common) invades intestinal epithelial cells → hemorrhagic colitis and toxin-mediated microvascular and renal injury → inflammation and platelet aggregation
- Less commonly due to other enteric pathogens that produce Shiga-like toxins and noninfectious causes

KEY FACT

HUS triad:

1. Microangiopathic hemolytic anemia
2. Thrombocytopenia
3. Renal insufficiency

Symptoms/Examination

- Prodrome of bloody diarrhea ± abdominal pain
- HUS develops 1-2 weeks after start of symptoms, usually as diarrhea resolves
- Onset of pallor with petechial or purpuric rash

Diagnosis

- Anemia (Hb < 8 g/dL) and thrombocytopenia.
- Unlike disseminated intravascular coagulation (DIC), coagulation studies are normal.
- Renal failure.
- Peripheral smear: Schistocytes.
- Hematuria often present.

> **KEY FACT**
>
> Avoid antibiotics and antidiarrheal agents in children who have hemorrhagic diarrhea; they may increase risk of HUS. While HUS is typically associated with a prodrome of diarrhea and outbreaks of E coli, it does not always occur in epidemics.

Treatment

- **Avoid antibiotics and antidiarrheal agents in children who have hemorrhagic diarrhea** (both agents may increase subsequent risk of developing HUS).
- Supportive care.
- IV fluids until euvolemic.
- Consider packed red blood cell (PRBC) transfusion if hemoglobin < 6 g/dL.
- Avoid platelet transfusion unless active bleeding or a surgical procedure is required, because platelets will be consumed.
- Consult nephrologist for potential early dialysis if hyperkalemia, fluid overload, or persistent anuria.
- Plasma exchange if CNS symptoms.

Complications

- About half of children with HUS develop renal failure and require dialysis (up to 70% of those who require dialysis eventually recover normal renal function). Renal failure is more common in younger patients.
- About 15%-20% have seizure, stroke, or coma.
- Mortality is 3%-5%.

UROLITHIASIS

While not as common as in adults, the incidence of stones is increasing in children. As in adults, most stones are calcium based. Most children with stones have an anatomic abnormality of the GU tract or metabolic problems leading to hypercalciuria.

Symptoms/Examination

- Flank pain
- Hematuria

Diagnosis

- Evaluate for causes of hypercalciuria, including periods of immobility and vitamin D supplementation.
- Urinalysis.
- Serum electrolytes, including calcium, magnesium, uric acid.
- Noncontrast CT identifies size and location of stone and may identify other structural abnormalities of the GU tract.
- Ultrasound is an alternative to CT, but may miss small stones.
- Consider a kidneys, ureters, and bladder (KUB) scan, which may allow visualization of the stone.

Treatment

- Nonsteroidal anti-inflammatory drugs (NSAIDs).
- Consult urology if stone > 5 mm, evidence of infection, obstruction, kidney damage, or severe symptoms.
- Medications utilized in adults such as calcium channel or α-blockers have not been studied in children.

Complication

Approximately 50% recurrence rate.

Cardiology

CONGENITAL HEART DISEASE

The incidence of congenital heart disease (CHD) is approximately 1% of live births. **The most common congenital heart defect is a ventricular septal defect (VSD)** (20%-25%). In general, the more severe a congenital heart defect, the earlier the newborn presents with complications of cyanosis and shock. However, even severe forms of CHD may not present until 1-2 weeks of life, when the ductus arteriosus closes.

Symptoms/Examination

Depending on the type of defect, a newborn or infant may present with cyanosis, signs of poor perfusion, and/or congestive heart failure (CHF) (Table 5.13). The timing of presentation and the presence or absence of

TABLE 5.13. Presentation of CHD

Defect	Timing of Onset	Cyanosis	Shock	CHF
Transposition	Birth to 2 wk	Yes	—	—
Tetralogy	Birth to 12 wk	Yes	—	—
Total anomalous PVR	Birth to 2 wk	Yes	—	—
Truncus arteriosus	Birth to 2 wk	Yes	—	—
Tricuspid atresia	Birth to 2 wk	Yes	—	—
Pulmonary atresia	Birth to 2 wk	Yes	—	—
Ebstein anomaly	Birth to 2 wk	Yes	—	—
Hypoplastic left heart	1 wk on	—	Yes	—
Coarctation	1 wk on	—	Yes	—
Critical aortic stenosis	1 wk on	—	Yes	—
VSD	4 wk on	—	—	Yes
PDA	4 wk on	—	—	Yes

CHD, congenital heart diseases; CHF, congestive heart failure; PDA; PVR, peripheral vascular resistance; VSD, ventricular septal defect.

Q

A 4-day-old infant born via uncomplicated vaginal delivery presents to the ED with tachypnea and mild cyanosis. Cardiac examination reveals a single second heart sound and increased precordial activity but no murmurs. Pulse oximetry reveals an O_2 saturation of 85%. What are the differential considerations and next steps in diagnosis?

A

Cyanotic congenital heart disease (CHD). A hyperoxia test, chest x-ray, electrocardiogram (ECG), and urgent echocardiogram are needed.

TABLE 5.14. Characteristic CXR Findings With CHD

CHD	Heart Size and Shape	Pulmonary Vascular Markings
TOF	Boot-shaped heart	Decreased
TGA	Egg-on-a-string	Increased (if no VSD/ASD)
TAPVR	Snowman	Increased (if no VSD/ASD)

ASD, atrial septal defect; CHD, congenital heart disease; CXR, chest x-ray; TAPVR, total anomalous pulmonary venous return; TGA, transposition of the great arteries; TOF, tetralogy of Fallot; VSD, ventricular septal defect.

KEY FACT

Cyanotic congenital heart defects worsen with crying.

KEY FACT

Congenital heart defects causing CHF cause diaphoresis with feeding, poor feeding habits, or poor weight gain.

MNEMONIC

Cyanotic CHD = "Five terrible Ts":

Tetralogy
Transposition
Total anomalous pulmonary venous return (TAPVR)
Tricuspid atresia
Truncus arteriosus

cyanosis and shock provide clues to the type of defect present. Additional clues can be obtained by ascertaining a newborn's characteristics during crying and feeding. Physical examination should focus on the presence and location of cyanosis, the presence of murmurs/gallops/additional heart sounds, and the quality of **pulses and blood pressures in all extremities.**

- Central cyanosis is more consistent with a cardiac etiology, whereas a peripheral cyanosis is more consistent with a respiratory etiology.
- A history of diaphoresis, poor feeding, or failure to thrive suggests a congenital heart defect causing CHF.
- A newborn with a cyanotic heart defect will have worsening cyanosis when crying or eating.
- A newborn with a congenital heart defect who presents with sudden decompensation within the first 1-2 weeks is likely to have a ductal-dependent defect.
- Decreased pulses and blood pressure in the lower extremities suggest **aortic coarctation**.

Differential Diagnosis

- History and physical examination as well as chest x-ray and electrocardiogram (ECG) are essential first steps in ED evaluation. See also Table 5.14 and Figure 5.5.
- Measure pre- and postductal oxygen saturations. Echocardiogram when available is also useful in determining the anatomy.

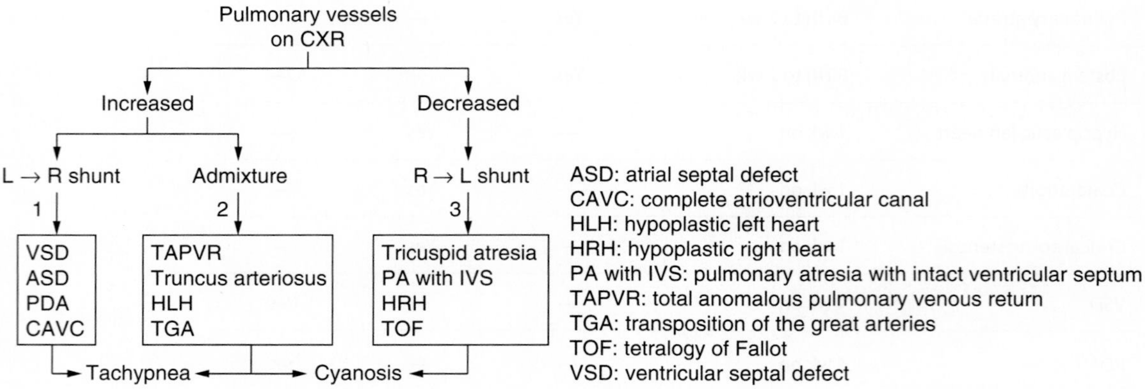

FIGURE 5.5. Classification system for congenital heart disease lesions based on CXR findings and associated symptomatology.

- **Hyperoxia test**: Obtain a room air arterial blood gas (ABG) and then repeat the ABG after several minutes of 100% oxygen. Check the oxygen saturation before and after administration of oxygen. After administration of 100% oxygen:
  - $Pao_2 > 220$ mm Hg suggests pulmonary etiology.
  - Pao_2 100-220 mm Hg suggests intracardiac mixing of blood → evaluate for CHD.
  - $Pao_2 < 100$ mm Hg suggests cyanotic CHD.

Treatment

- Depends on the defect.
- If a ductal-dependent lesion is suspected:
  - Prostaglandin E_1 infusion should be started (0.05-0.1 μg/kg/min).
  - While oxygen should not be withheld from a hypoxic newborn, 100% oxygen will accelerate ductal closure by decreasing pulmonary vascular resistance. Consequently, if a ductal dependent defect is suspected, oxygen should be turned down until PGE_1 can be started.
- Dobutamine and dopamine may be needed to temporize a CHF exacerbation secondary to congenital heart defect until surgery can be arranged.
- Definitive surgical correction is required for most congenital heart defects.
- Treatment of Tet spells involves maneuvers to decrease the right-to-left shunt across the VSD:
  - Place the infant in the knee-to-chest or squatting position. This will increase the systemic vascular resistance.
  - Give supplemental oxygen to improve hypoxia.
  - Give morphine.
  - Consider sodium bicarbonate to correct metabolic acidosis and thereby suppress respiratory compensation (tachypnea).

> **KEY FACT**
>
> Coarctation has characteristic "rib notching" on CXR due to increased collateral blood flow.

> **KEY FACT**
>
> PGE1 may cause apnea. Intubation should be considered prior to starting PGE1, especially if transfer is needed after PGE1 is administered.

MURMURS

Heart murmurs are most often an incidental finding. More than 80% of children have "innocent" murmurs. The EM physician needs to be able to differentiate an innocent from a pathologic murmur. Innocent murmurs are associated with a normal ECG and CXR.

> **KEY FACT**
>
> Innocent murmurs will be accentuated by anemia and fever.

Symptoms/Examination

- Patients are unlikely to have any symptoms unless there is an associated congenital heart defect or CHF.
- Previous cardiac evaluation, underlying Down syndrome or Marfan syndrome, family history of sudden death in young people are all relevant pieces of history.
- Pertinent findings on examination, outside the murmur itself, are signs of cyanosis and CHF such as jugular venous distention (JVD), hepatosplenomegaly, and peripheral edema.

Features concerning for pathologic murmurs:

- Diastolic murmurs
- Systolic murmurs louder than grade 3/6
- Continuous murmurs
- Presence of cyanosis
- Decreased lower extremity pulses/blood pressures
- Single S_2
- Abnormal sounds—clicks, gallops, rubs, thrills
- Abnormal ECG
- Abnormal CXR

TABLE 5.15. Pediatric Murmurs

Murmur	Type	Characteristics	Location
ASD	Systolic	Ejection, split S_2	LUSB
VSD	Systolic	Regurgitant/holosystolic	LLSB
PDA	Systolic/ continuous	Crescendo–decrescendo, machine-like	LUSB
Tetralogy	Systolic	Ejection, cyanosis	LUSB
Coarctation	Systolic	Ejection, weak lower extremity pulses	LUSB
TAPVR	Systolic	Ejection	LUSB
Hypertrophic cardiomyopathy	Systolic	Ejection, increases with maneuvers that ↓ LV filling (standing, Valsalva)	LLSB/Apex
Still's (Innocent)	Systolic	Ejection, vibratory and "musical"	LLSB/Apex
Pulmonary flow murmur (innocent)	Systolic	Ejection, radiates to axilla and back	LUSB

ASD, atrial septal defect; LLSB, left lower sternal border; LUSB, left upper sternal border; PDA, patent ductus arteriosus; TAPVR, total anomalous pulmonary venous return; VSD, ventricular septal defect.

Differential

Differential is broad and can be separated based on the location of the murmur and whether the murmur is systolic, diastolic, or continuous (Table 5.15). Murmurs present in adults will not be discussed here.

Diagnosis/Treatment

- Unless pathologic characteristics are present or there are signs of cyanosis or CHF, the patient does not need to be admitted to the hospital.
- If the patient looks well and the murmur is an incidental finding, but pathologic characteristics are present without signs of cyanosis or CHF, then a CXR and ECG can be obtained to screen for obvious abnormalities.
- If both are normal, referral to a cardiologist rather than admission to the hospital may be appropriate.

CHEST PAIN

Chest pain is rarely life threatening in children. The vast majority of chest pain in children is due to noncardiac causes. However, cardiac causes of chest pain do exist in children, so the complaint should be taken seriously and the child appropriately evaluated with a detailed history and physical examination.

Symptoms/Examination

Concerning historical clues for cardiac chest pain in children:

- Exertional chest pain
- Associated syncope

- Family history of sudden death or unexplained single car accidents or other suspicious accidents
- Personal or family history of Marfan syndrome
- Previous history of Kawasaki disease
- History of lupus
- History of sickle cell disease
- Recent upper respiratory infection (URI) or viral syndrome
- Cocaine abuse
- Pregnancy

Concerning examination findings for cardiac chest pain in children:
- Aortic or pulmonic stenosis murmurs
- Rub
- Distant heart sounds
- Arrhythmia
- Tachycardia

DIFFERENTIAL

See Table 5.16.

DIAGNOSIS

- A careful history and physical examination can largely differentiate chest pain that needs further evaluation from benign causes.
- If any concerning features for cardiac chest pain, a chest x-ray and ECG are warranted.
- If any concern for trauma or there is shortness of breath, a CXR should be ordered to evaluate for pneumothorax.
- Additional laboratory tests and imaging may be appropriate if the history is concerning or the physical examination is abnormal.

TREATMENT

- Treatment depends on the likely etiology of the chest pain.
- For musculoskeletal chest pain, acetaminophen or ibuprofen and reassurance are likely all that is needed.
- A GI cocktail or H_2 blocker may help with reflux.
- Counseling, reassurance, and psychiatric referral or evaluation may be needed for stress-induced chest pain.

KEY FACT

In a young toddler, chest pain may be the only clue to an ingested esophageal foreign body or may represent referred pain from the abdomen.

TABLE 5.16 Differential Diagnosis of Chest Pain in Children

CARDIAC CHEST PAIN	NONCARDIAC CHEST PAIN
Ischemia	**Respiratory**
Anomalous coronary arteries	Pneumonia
Kawasaki disease	Asthma
Structural abnormality	Pulmonary embolism
Aortic stenosis	Pneumothorax
Pulmonic stenosis	**Musculoskeletal**
Hypertrophic cardiomyopathy	**Psychological:** Stress/anxiety
Infection	**Esophageal:** Reflux, foreign body
Pericarditis	**Sickle cell disease**
Myocarditis	Acute chest syndrome
Arrhythmia	**Idiopathic**

TABLE 5.17. Differential Diagnosis of Pericarditis

Infectious	Noninfectious
Viral	Acute rheumatic fever
Coxsackievirus	Lupus
Adenovirus	Leukemia
ECHO virus	Lymphoma
EBV	Uremia
Influenza	
Bacterial	
Pneumococcus	
S aureus	
Meningococcus	
H influenzae	
Tuberculosis	

EBV, Epstein-Barr virus; ECHO, enteric cytopathic human orphan.

PERICARDITIS

Pericarditis is an inflammatory condition of the pericardium. Both infectious and noninfectious causes of pericarditis exist in children (Table 5.17).

Symptoms/Examination

- Symptoms are often preceded by a URI.
- Chest pain that worsens when supine and improves when leaning forward is classic.
- Decreased heart sounds and a friction rub may be heard on examination indicating the presence of a pericardial effusion.
- Hypotension, tachycardia, and distended neck veins should raise the possibility of tamponade.

Differential

See Table 5.17.

Diagnosis

- ECG classically shows PR segment depression and diffuse ST elevations.
- CXR maybe normal or it may show an enlarged heart (water bottle heart) signifying pericarditis with the presence of a large pericardial effusion.
- An echocardiogram is the diagnostic procedure of choice to evaluate for an associated pericardial effusion.

Treatment

- Most cases are self-limiting and can be treated by outpatient management with NSAIDs with close follow-up.
- Antibiotics should be initiated if a bacterial cause is suspected.
- If signs of acute cardiac tamponade, an emergent pericardiocentesis should be performed and fluid sent for analysis and cultures. Give the patient a bolus of IV fluid to improve preload.

TABLE 5.18. Differential Diagnosis of Myocarditis

Infectious	Noninfectious
Virus	Kawasaki disease
Cocksackievirus	Lupus
Adenovirus	
Parvovirus	
Echovirus	
Influenza	
EBV	
Bacterial	
S aureus	
Corynebacterium diphtheriae	
Streptococcus pyogenes	
Mycoplasma pneumoniae	
Borrelia burgdorferi	

EBV, Epstein-Barr virus.

MYOCARDITIS

Myocarditis is an inflammatory condition of the myocardium. The majority of cases in the United States are caused by viruses, most notably, **coxsackievirus B**, echovirus, or influenza (Table 5.18).

Symptoms/Examination

- Symptoms are usually gradual in onset and preceded by a URI.
- Presenting signs and symptoms include fever, fatigue, tachypnea, and chest pain.
- Tachycardia out of proportion to fever that fails to improve, or even worsens, with IV fluids should alert the EM physician of the possibility of myocarditis.
- Physical examination may reveal a new murmur, friction rub, gallop wheezing, or signs of CHF.

Differential

See Table 5.18.

Diagnosis

- CXR will likely show cardiomegaly or pulmonary edema but may be normal in mild cases.
- ECG may show low voltage or nonspecific ST changes or multiple types of dysrhythmias.
- Troponin will often be elevated.
- Echocardiogram is useful for the detection of a pericardial effusion as well as evaluation of left ventricular function.

Treatment

- Treatment depends on the etiology. Antibiotics should be started if a bacterial etiology is present.

- In general, the goals of treatment are to maintain cardiac output with medications such as furosemide, digoxin, or pressors.
- Pressors should be used with caution given the propensity for cardiac dysrhythmias in the setting of myocarditis.
- High-dose IV immunoglobulin may also improve ventricular function.
- In certain cases, extracorporeal membrane oxygenation (ECMO) support may be lifesaving and patients with myocarditis should typically be managed in facilities with ECMO capabilities.

COMPLICATION

Chronic dilated cardiomyopathy.

SYNCOPE

> **KEY FACT**
>
> Breath-holding spells and seizures may mimic syncope in young children.

Syncope is a common chief complaint in both the pediatric and adult patient populations. Syncope is more common in adolescents than young children. While the vast majority of cases are secondary to benign etiologies, care must be taken to rule out life-threatening etiologies. (See also Chapter 2, **Cardiovascular Emergencies**)

SYMPTOMS/EXAMINATION

- Transient loss of consciousness and postural tone with complete recovery.
- Other symptoms or findings vary with underlying cause.
- Features that are concerning for serious underlying cause:
  - Occurring with exertion (aortic stenosis, hypertrophic cardiomyopathy)
  - Occurring with no prodrome
  - Resulting injuries
  - Occurring while supine
  - Patient with known cardiac disease
  - Family history of sudden cardiac death
  - Recurrent episodes
  - Occurring with chest pain or palpitations
  - Prolonged loss of consciousness (suggests cardiac dysfunction or dysrhythmia)
  - Presence of abnormal heart sounds or murmur

DIFFERENTIAL

- Breath-holding spells cause transient cerebral anoxia through cerebral artery vasoconstriction from hypocapnia (children < 6 years).
- Hypoglycemia.
- Seizures (children < 6 years).
- Carbon monoxide poisoning.
- Psychiatric.

DIAGNOSIS

- Complete history, family history, and examination are critical.
- ECG should be obtained in most cases.
- Order laboratory test results based on clinical suspicion for underlying disease process.
- Echocardiogram if suspicion for underlying cardiac cause or disease based on presentation, examination, or ECG findings.

TREATMENT

Treatment depends on the etiology. Patients with symptoms concerning for cardiac cause of their syncope or those with history of CHD, especially those with prior cardiac surgery, warrant further evaluation by a cardiologist prior to deciding disposition.

COMPLICATION

Sudden cardiac death.

DYSRHYTHMIAS

Bradydysrhythmias

Clinically significant bradycardia is defined as a heart rate (HR) < 60 bpm. An exception is athletic adolescents who may have resting heart rates of < 60 bpm.

CAUSES

- The **most common cause** of bradycardia in children is **hypoxia**.
- Cardiac abnormalities including heart block, denervated heart following cardiac surgery, sick sinus syndrome.
- Hypothermia.
- Increased intracranial pressure (ICP).
- Hypothyroidism.
- Medications/toxins such as β-blockers or calcium channel blockers.

TREATMENT

- Ensuring adequate oxygenation and ventilation should be the first step.
- Treatment otherwise depends on the etiology.
- If HR < 60 bpm and evidence of poor perfusion, begin cardiopulmonary resuscitation (CPR).
- Unlike in adults, symptomatic bradycardia is first treated with **epinephrine** (0.01 mg/kg), not atropine. Atropine and cardiac pacing should be considered if heart block is present.

Supraventricular Tachycardia

Supraventricular tachycardia (SVT) is the **most common tachydysrhythmia** in infants and children. A narrow-complex (≤ 0.09 second), regular tachycardia with no normal beat to beat respiratory variation with rate > 220 bpm in an infant or > 180 bpm in a child is likely SVT.

CAUSES

A reentry mechanism secondary to an accessory pathway is the **most common cause** of SVT in children < 12 years. Most are idiopathic (~50%). However, Wolff-Parkinson-White (WPW) syndrome and CHD are considerations as well.

TREATMENT

- If hemodynamically stable, begin with vagal maneuvers. **Apply ice to the face** of infants/young children. Have the older child blow through a narrow straw.
- If vagal maneuvers are unsuccessful, adenosine (0.1 mg/kg, max 6 mg) should be used. If this fails to convert SVT, the dose can be doubled to 0.2 mg/kg (max 12 mg). A continuous ECG should be obtained while adenosine is administered because capturing the conversion can provide valuable diagnostic information for the cardiologist.
- If adenosine is unsuccessful, consider IV procainamide or amiodarone in consultation with a cardiologist. If the child is hemodynamically unstable, cardioversion (0.5-2 J/kg) should be used.

KEY FACT

Differential for sudden cardiac death in young athletes: Hypertropic cardiomyopathy, long QT, Wolff-Parkinson-White (WPW) syndrome, anomalous coronary arteries, aortic stenosis, Marfan (aortic dissection) syndrome.

KEY FACT

First-line medication for symptomatic bradycardia in children is epinephrine (not atropine).

Atrial Flutter and Fibrillation

Both atrial flutter and fibrillation are rare in infants and children. When present, they are likely associated with underlying heart disease, particularly in the postoperative period, or WPW.

Treatment

- If hemodynamically stable and WPW is not suspected, IV β-blockers or calcium channel blockers (for children > 1 year) may be used. Consult cardiology prior to initiating medications.
- If hemodynamically unstable, cardioversion should be used.
- If WPW is suspected, amiodarone, procainamide, or cardioversion should be used.

Wide Complex Tachycardia

All wide complex (QRS > 90 milliseconds) tachycardias in the pediatric patient should be treated as ventricular tachycardia.

Causes

- Structural heart disease
- Prior heart surgery
- Hypomagnesemia
- Long QT syndrome
- Medications (eg, tricyclic antidepressants [TCAs])

Treatment

- If hemodynamically stable and no suspicion for underlying long QT, consult a pediatric cardiologist and consider administering amiodarone or procainamide.
- Treat the underlying condition, when present (eg, bicarbonate for TCA ingestion).
- If unstable, cardioversion (0.5-2 J/kg) should be used.

Endocrine and Metabolic Disorders

CONGENITAL ADRENAL HYPERPLASIA

Congenital adrenal hyperplasia (CAH) refers to a group of autosomal recessive disorders leading to cortisol deficiency. Deficiency of the enzyme **21-hydroxylase** accounts for 95% of cases and leads to low aldosterone and elevated androgens and adrenocorticotropin hormone (ACTH). These changes result in virilization, adrenal hypertrophy, and skin hyperpigmentation.

> **KEY FACT**
>
> Females will usually present with ambiguous genitalia due to virilization; males have normal genital development and usually present with salt wasting during infancy or in the case of nonclassic salt wasting variant, precocious puberty during childhood.

Symptoms/Examination

Affected newborns with the salt-wasting form present in crisis at approximately 2 weeks of age with lethargy, vomiting, poor feeding, poor weight gain, and hypovolemic shock.

Diagnosis

- Electrolytes and blood glucose testing reveal hyponatremia, hyperkalemia, and hypoglycemia.
- While unusual in CAH, an ECG should be obtained to screen for evidence of cardiac dysfunction secondary to hyperkalemia.

- ACTH stimulation testing confirms the diagnosis of adrenal insufficiency.
- Specific enzyme testing should reveal the specific enzymatic deficiency.

TREATMENT

- Initial management is focused on fluid resuscitation with isotonic saline and administration of stress doses of IV hydrocortisone.
- Supplement glucose as needed.
- Consult endocrinology.
- Treat hyperkalemia if ECG changes are present. Saline and steroids are usually all that is needed to treat hyperkalemia.

DIABETIC KETOACIDOSIS

Syndrome of hyperglycemia, dehydration, and metabolic acidosis resulting from insulin deficiency.

CAUSES

- Noncompliance with medications (**most common cause** in adolescents)
- Infection—UTI, appendicitis, gastroenteritis, pneumonia (**most common cause** in younger children)
- Pregnancy
- Trauma
- IEM

SYMPTOMS/EXAMINATION

- Abdominal pain, nausea/vomiting, polyuria, polydipsia, weight loss, and lethargy are common presenting symptoms.
- Physical examination is often significant for tachycardia, tachypnea with Kussmaul respiration, ketotic breath, dehydration, and lethargy.

DIAGNOSIS

- Hyperglycemia and increased anion gap metabolic acidosis with presence of serum ketones confirm the diagnosis.
- Potassium levels often appear normal or high despite **total body potassium deficits.**
- Obtain venous blood gas to assess pH.

TREATMENT

- Fluid replacement and insulin are the cornerstones for treatment of DKA. However, if the potassium is < 3.3, potassium should be repleted before giving insulin. If the potassium is < 5, then potassium chloride should be included in the fluid.
- While fluids in adults are often given in rapid boluses, in children fluids are given less aggressively because of concern for cerebral edema. A 10-mL/kg bolus of normal saline is usually recommended in the first hour and then followed by a second bolus of 10 mL/kg and then normal saline at a twice maintenance rate with the addition of potassium chloride and/or potassium phosphate. Once the blood glucose level has fallen to < 300 mg/dL, then administer D_5NS for maintenance fluids.
- Insulin drip (0.05-0.1 units/kg/h) should be started after the initial fluid bolus is administered. Bolus insulin is no longer recommended.

COMPLICATIONS

Cerebral edema: Once clinically present, mortality approaches 60%-80%. Risk factors include young age, severe acidosis, persistent hyponatremia

Q

A 1-week-old male infant presents to the ED with a history of poor feeding, poor weight gain since birth, lethargy, irritability, and occasional vomiting. Laboratory evaluation shows a Na of 128, a K of 7, and glucose of 52. What is the likely diagnosis?

KEY FACT

If there is any clinical concern for CAH in a sick infant, steroids should be given without delay, because treatment is often lifesaving.

KEY FACT

Patients with adrenal insufficiency, who require chronic steroid supplementation, should be given supplemental glucocorticoids at 2-3 times × their daily dose when stressed from infection or other illness.

KEY FACT

Sodium levels often appear low due to hyperglycemia. Corrected sodium levels are determined by adding 1.6 mEq/L sodium for every 100 mg/dL of glucose over glucose level of 100 mg/dL.

While potassium levels often appear normal initially, patients with DKA have total body potassium deficits and require potassium repletion in their maintenance fluids.

KEY FACT

Bicarbonate should not be given to patients with DKA, because it increases the risk of cerebral edema.

A

Congenital adrenal hyperplasia (CAH).

KEY FACT

Patients with signs of cerebral edema should receive mannitol or hypertonic saline.

(with correction of glucose), and severe hyperosmolarity. Early (first hour) insulin administration and aggressive fluid resuscitation were associated factors in one study. Mannitol should be given at the first sign of altered mental status in the patient under treatment for DKA. Steroids are ineffective.

INBORN ERRORS OF METABOLISM

Disorders involving inborn errors of metabolism (IEM) are numerous. In general, these disorders result in impaired metabolism and accumulation of a toxic metabolite resulting in a picture of acute encephalopathy. Determining the individual inborn error of metabolism is not the responsibility of the EM physician. Rather, the EM physician should know when to be clinically suspicious of such a disorder and how to stabilize and treat it.

Symptoms/Examination

- Nonspecific symptoms of poor feeding, lethargy, vomiting, dehydration, and irritability.
- Patients present at different ages depending on the disorder, but in general, newborns in the first few days are usually asymptomatic because toxic metabolites cross the placenta and are cleared by maternal enzymes.
  - Some IEM present outside the newborn period and do not present unless the patient is stressed with an illness such as gastroenteritis.
- If severe, altered mental status and seizures may be present.
- Examination may be largely unremarkable except for lethargy, but certain findings point to particular IEM.
  - Hepatomegaly and jaundice—galactosemia and glycogen storage disease
  - Tachycardia and tachypnea—organic acidemia
  - Abnormal odor—organic acidemia

Differential Diagnosis

- Sepsis
- CAH
- CHD
- Neonatal thyrotoxicosis

Diagnosis

- Diagnosis largely depends on a high clinical suspicion and laboratory evaluation. See Table 5.19.
- Laboratory evaluation includes:
  - Bedside glucose
  - Ammonia
  - Basic metabolic panel (look for anion gap acidosis)
  - Urinalysis (urine ketones)
  - Venous blood gas with lactate
- Liver function tests (LFTs)
  - Additional laboratory studies may include pyruvate, thyroid-stimulating hormone (TSH), and blood cultures.

Treatment

- Hyperammonemia should be treated with arginine with or without sodium benzoate-sodium phenylacetate which exists as a combined drug preparation. Hemodialysis may also be required.

TABLE 5.19. Diagnostic Findings for Inborn Errors of Metabolism

IEM	Ammonia	Acidosis	Urine Ketones	Other Findings
Urea cycle defect	Elevated	No	N/A	
Organic acidemia	Elevated	Yes	Elevated	
Energy metabolism defects	Elevated	Yes	Yes	Elevated lactate
Carbohydrate metabolism defects	Elevated	Yes	Yes	Hypoglycemia, liver dysfunction
Fatty acid oxidation defects	No	Yes	No	Hypoglycemia without ketosis after fasting
Amino acid metabolism defect	No	No	No	

- Acidosis should be treated with IV fluids. The use of sodium bicarbonate is controversial and is not without side effects, so should only be used in severe refractory metabolic acidosis (pH < 7).
- All food should be stopped and IV dextrose given for substrate typically in the form of D_{10}.
- If refractory seizures are present, administration of pyridoxine can be tried.
- If sepsis is suspected, antibiotics should be administered.

Q

A 6-month-old infant presents in the morning to the ED with mild lethargy. The mother states that he has had a minor URI recently and has not fed since late last night. Laboratory evaluation reveals a glucose of 39; UA shows absent glucose and absent ketones. What is the likely diagnosis?

Dermatology

DIAPER DERMATITIS

Diaper dermatitis is the **most common dermatologic problem** seen in infants and young children. The most common causes of diaper dermatitis are *Candida* and contact irritation (Table 5.20 and Figure 5.6).

SEBORRHEA ("CRADLE CAP")

Seborrheic dermatitis in infants is an inflammatory disease of unclear etiology affecting the hairy scalp and intertriginous folds. Peak incidence is at 2 weeks of age and symptoms typically resolve spontaneously by 1 year.

Symptoms/Examination

Nonpruritic, greasy scale accumulation on the face, scalp, and sometimes diaper area (Figure 5.7).

Treatment

- In severe cases, 1% ketoconazole shampoo can be used.
- Other areas: Topical steroids (1% hydrocortisone).

A

Inborn error of metabolism.

TABLE 5.20. Common Etiologies of Diaper Dermatitis

Etiology	Characteristics	Treatment
Contact dermatitis Allergic Irritant	**Allergic:** Tiny erythematous vesicles that may rupture and look eczematous. Occurs in areas in contact with then diaper. **Irritant:** Erythema of skin in contact with urine or feces.	Increase frequency of diaper changes. Expose skin to air. Use water-based emollient to create a barrier (zinc oxide).
Candida albicans	"Satellite" lesions: Red papules that coalesce and spread outward forming satellite lesions (see Figure 5.6). Skin folds usually involved.	Topical antifungal (nystatin).
Miliaria (prickly heat)	Newborn: Clear vesicles. Infant: Erythematous papules and pustules.	Increase frequency of diaper changes. Expose skin to air. Use water-based emollient to create a barrier (zinc oxide).
Intertrigo	Red denuded skin in areas of apposed skin.	Increase frequency of diaper changes. Expose skin to air. Use water-based emollient to create a barrier (zinc oxide). 1% hydrocortisone cream for no more than 2 wk.

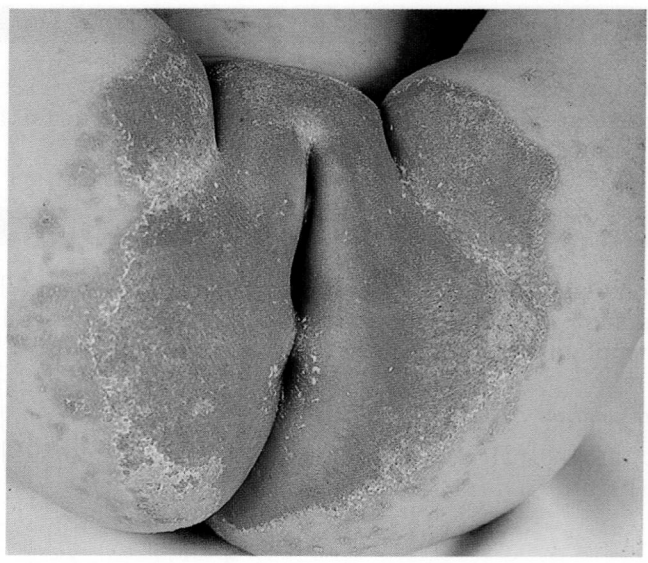

FIGURE 5.6. Candidal diaper dermatitis. (Reproduced, with permission, from Wolff K, Johnson RA. *Fitzpatrick's Color Atlas and Synopsis of Clinical Dermatology*. 6th ed. New York, NY: McGraw-Hill; 2009.)

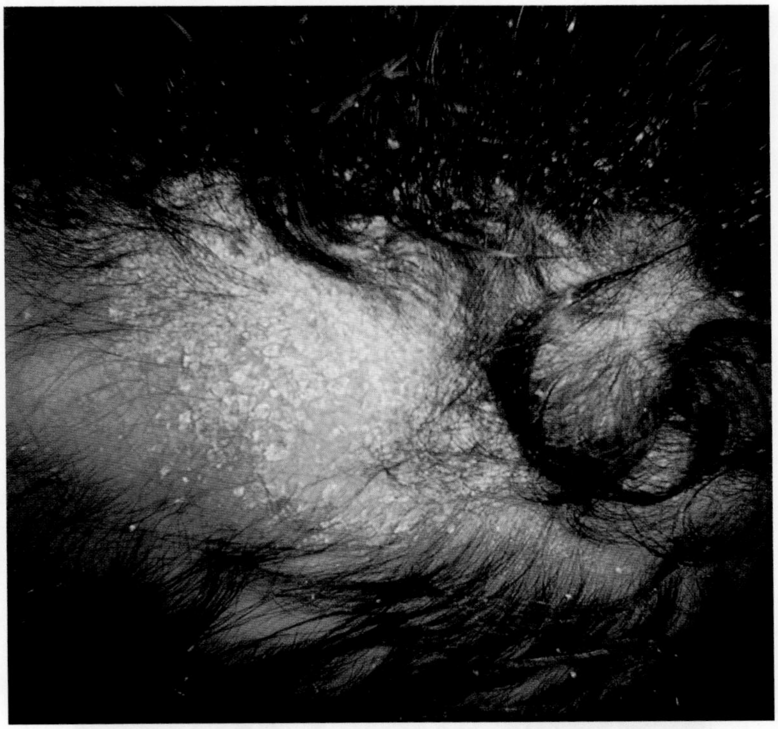

FIGURE 5.7. Seborrhea. (Reproduced, with permission, from Shah BR, Lucchesi M. *Atlas of Pediatric Emergency Medicine*. New York, NY: McGraw-Hill; 2006:295.)

ATOPIC DERMATITIS (ECZEMA)

Atopic dermatitis or eczema is a highly pruritic chronic inflammatory skin disease. There is a clear association between other atopic diseases like asthma and allergic rhinitis.

KEY FACT

Eczema = The itch that rashes

SYMPTOMS/EXAMINATION

- Pruritic, scaly, erythematous lesions (Figure 5.8)
- Typical distribution varies by age:
  - Infants: Face
  - Children (< 12 years old): Extensor surfaces
  - Adolescents: Flexor surfaces

TREATMENT

- Skin moisturizers.
- Topical steroids (1% hydrocortisone): Do not use > 1% hydrocortisone on the face.
- Stronger steroids may be used on the trunk and extremities for brief (1 week) periods.
- Avoid oral steroids even in severe cases because it can lead to rebound.
- Systemic antihistamines for pruritus may be helpful.
- Oral antibiotics if superimposed skin infection.

KEY FACT

Eczema can become infected.

Eczema herpeticum is a systemic rash often due to HSV superinfection.

COMPLICATIONS

- Complications include increased risk for bacterial or viral skin infections.

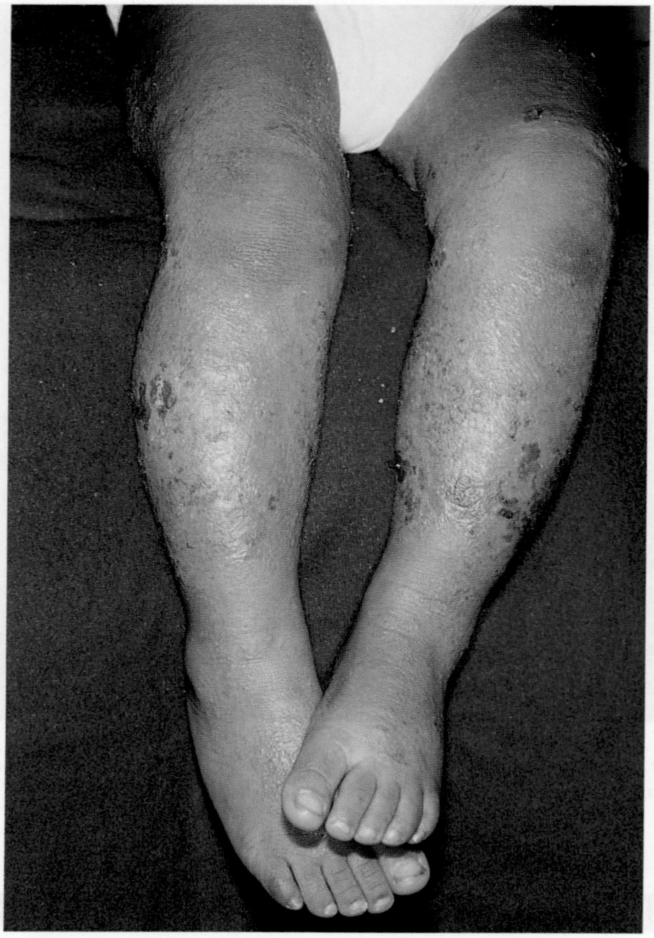

FIGURE 5.8. Eczema. (Reproduced, with permission, from Shah BR, Lucchesi M. *Atlas of Pediatric Emergency Medicine*. New York, NY: McGraw-Hill; 2006:303.)

- **Eczema herpeticum:** Superinfection with HSV or other viruses leading to a systemic rash. Characterized by development of vesicular lesions or erosions in areas of prior eczema, can be life threatening, *S aureus* or streptococcal superinfection frequently occurs, requires acyclovir ± bactrim or clindamycin.
- Prolonged steroid use or high-potency steroids can cause skin atrophy and superinfection.

VIRAL EXANTHEMS

See Table 5.21 for summary of viral exanthems.

Measles (Rubeola)

Measles is rare in United States due to universal vaccination and most cases are imported (or contacts of imported cases).

- Caused by paramyxovirus
- Transmitted by respiratory droplets
- Incubation 10-12 days between exposure and onset of symptoms

TABLE 5.21. Summary of Viral Exanthems

Disease	Virus	Rash	Associated Signs/Symptoms	Complications
Rubeola (measles)	Paramyxovirus	Maculopapules spreading from face down Usually starts on day 3-4	3Cs: Cough, coryza, and conjunctivitis Koplik spots	Encephalitis Pneumonia
Rubella (German measles)	Rubivirus	Maculopapules spreading from face down Usually starts on day 1	Mild fever Lymphadenopathy	Rare Prenatal infections cause congenital anomalies, still birth, and miscarriage
Roseola (exanthem subitum)	HHV-6	Discrete pink maculopapules on trunk with subsequent spread	High fever with onset of rash after defervescence	Febrile seizures
Erythema infectiosum (fifth disease)	Parvovirus B19	"Slapped cheeks" followed by maculopapular rash on trunk and extremities with "lacy" appearance	7-10 d of nonspecific viral symptoms	Aplastic anemia
Varicella (chickenpox)	Varicella-zoster virus	Rash appears in crops at all stages Macules → Papules → Vesicles → rupture and crust "Dew drop on a petal": Clear vesicle on an erythematous base	Pruritus	Infection with staph or GABHS Encephalitis Transverse myelitis Reye syndrome

GABHS, Group A beta-hemolytic streptococci; HHV, human herpesvirus.

Symptoms/Examination

- High fever (up to 40°C or 104°F).
- Cough, conjunctivitis, coryza (nasal congestion).
- Exanthem: Erythematous, nonblanching, maculopapular rash that starts at the hairline, then spreads down face, to trunk/extremities (Figure 5.9).
- Enanthem: **Koplik spots** (pinpoint-sized white spots with red background which appear on the buccal mucosa opposite molars; see Figure 5.10).
- Rash may coalesce into salmon-colored patches, then disappear typically within 1 week of onset.

KEY FACT

Measles (rubeola): Fever and rash with cough, conjunctivitis, coryza, and Koplik spots.

Diagnosis

- Clinical diagnosis may be challenging, particularly because many physicians rarely see patients with the diagnosis.
- Laboratory studies can confirm clinical suspicion. Presence of IgM to measles or rise in antibody titers during course of illness is diagnostic. Viral cultures can also be performed.
- Lymphopenia is common.

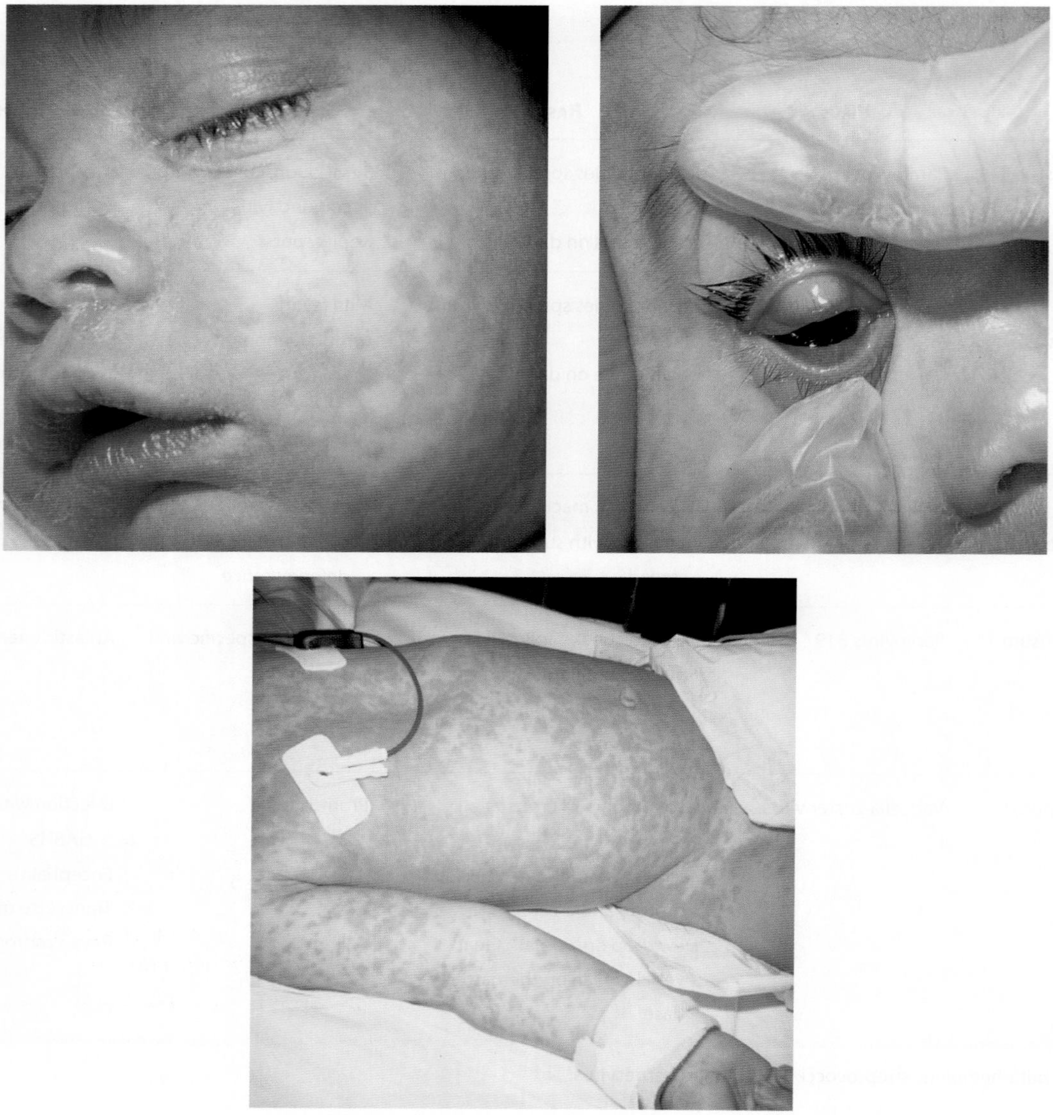

FIGURE 5.9. Measles (rubeola). (Reproduced, with permission, from Shah BR, Lucchesi M. *Atlas of Pediatric Emergency Medicine*. New York, NY: McGraw-Hill; 2006:135.)

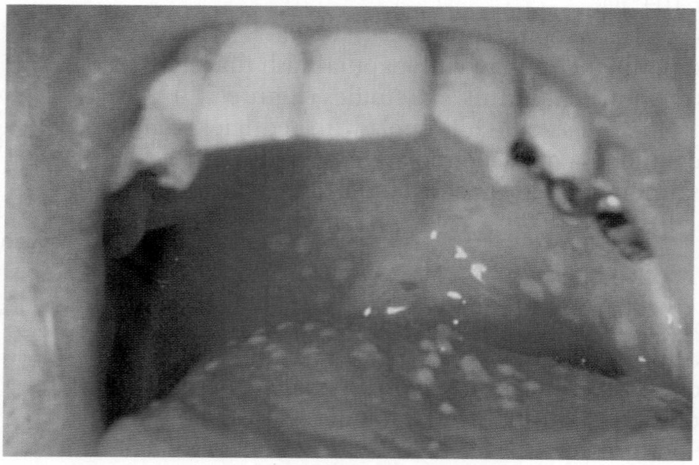

FIGURE 5.10. Measles (rubeola). (Reproduced, with permission, Kane K S-M, Ryder JB, Jonson RA, et al. *Color Atlas & Synopsis of Pediatric Dermatology*. New York, NY: McGraw-Hill; 2002:585.)

TREATMENT

- Supportive care: Antipyretics, prevention of dehydration.
- Treat secondary bacterial superinfections with antibiotics.
- Respiratory isolation.
- Immunize unvaccinated close contacts within 72 hours. (*Note:* Measles, mumps, and rubella (MMR) vaccine is contraindicated in patients who are pregnant or who have significant immunosuppression. Patients who cannot receive MMR should receive immunoglobulin within 6 days of exposure.)
- Report disease to state health authorities.

COMPLICATIONS

- Bacterial superinfection with **acute purulent otitis media** is the most common complication.
- Pneumonia is most common reason for admission.
- Encephalitis (1/1000 cases).
- Death (2/1000 cases in the United States).
- Measles infection during pregnancy may cause spontaneous abortion.

Rubella (German Measles)

Rubella is typically a mild illness, except for congenital infection, which can cause major birth defects.

- Caused by *Rubivirus*
- Transmitted by respiratory droplets

SYMPTOMS/EXAMINATION

- Low-grade fever.
- Exanthem: Erythematous papular rash begins on face, spreads to trunk (Figure 5.11).
- Tender lymphadenopathy is common and usually involves the postauricular, suboccipital, and posterior cervical chains.
- Arthritis or arthralgia (particularly in young women).

KEY FACT

Rubella (German measles): Rash with tender postauricular lymphadenopathy.

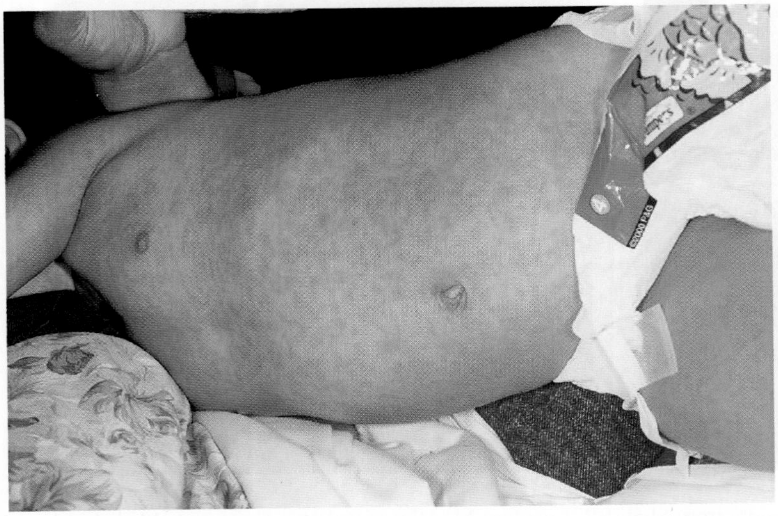

FIGURE 5.11. Rubella (German measles). (Reproduced, with permission, from Shah BR, Lucchesi M. *Atlas of Pediatric Emergency Medicine*. New York, NY: McGraw-Hill; 2006:137.)

DIAGNOSIS

- Primarily a clinical diagnosis.
- Presence of IgM to rubella **or** rise in antibody titers during course of illness is confirmative.

TREATMENT

- Supportive.
- Immunity is conferred by MMR vaccination. Pregnant women cannot be vaccinated, but may benefit from administration of immune globulin within 72 hours of exposure.

COMPLICATIONS

Congenital infection is a major concern, and can lead to fetal viremia and **major birth defects.**

Roseola Infantum

- Caused by human herpes virus (HHV-6)
- Peak incidence: 6 months-2 years; most common in spring and fall
- Transmitted by respiratory droplets

SYMPTOMS/EXAMINATION

- High fever lasting 3-5 days with sudden resolution of fever and onset of rash.
- Exanthem: Pale pink macules, typically located on the neck and trunk, rash usually appears as the fever resolves, with rash persisting 1-2 days (Figure 5.12).

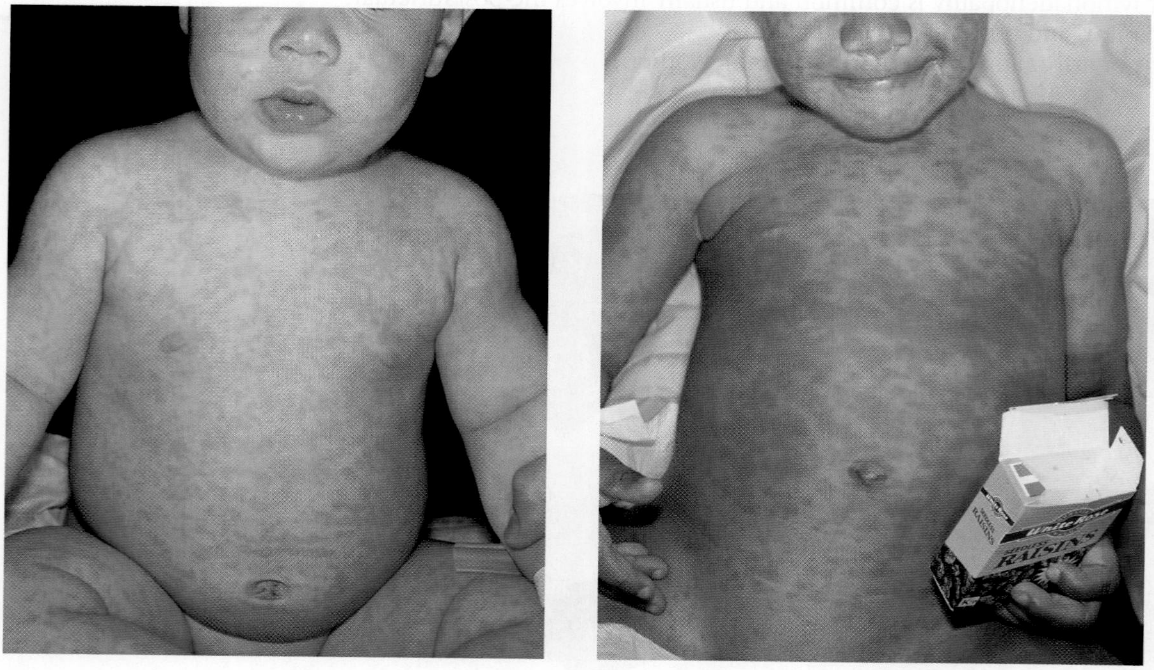

FIGURE 5.12. Roseola. (Reproduced, with permission, from Shah BR, Lucchesi M. *Atlas of Pediatric Emergency Medicine*. New York, NY: McGraw-Hill; 2006:137.)

DIFFERENTIAL

Can mimic other very serious infections, including pneumococcal sepsis or meningitis and bulging fontanel has been described.

DIAGNOSIS/TREATMENT

- Diagnosis is clinical.
- Treatment is supportive.

COMPLICATIONS

- Complications are very rare, but hepatitis or encephalitis can occur.
- Febrile seizures occur in up to 6% of patients.

> **KEY FACT**
>
> Roseola infantum: Onset of rash with resolution of fever.

Erythema Infectiosum (Fifth Disease)

- Caused by parvovirus B19
- Peak incidence: 4-15 years of age, most common during winter and spring
- Transmission: Respiratory droplets

SYMPTOMS/EXAMINATION

- Prodrome (lasts 2-3 days): Mild coryza, headache, fever
- Facial rash (bright red) develops 7 days later: **"slapped cheeks"** appearance (Figure 5.13)

> **KEY FACT**
>
> Erythema infectiosum (fifth disease): "Slapped cheeks" appearance.

DIAGNOSIS/TREATMENT

- Diagnosis is clinical.
- Treatment is supportive.

COMPLICATIONS

- **Aplastic anemia** may develop in patients who have an underlying hemoglobinopathy (such as sickle cell disease). Anemia may be severe, requiring red blood cell (RBC) transfusion.
- **Pregnant women who are infected with parvovirus B19 can** experience intrauterine fetal death **and** hydrops fetalis, **and should be referred to their providers for serologic testing if exposed.**

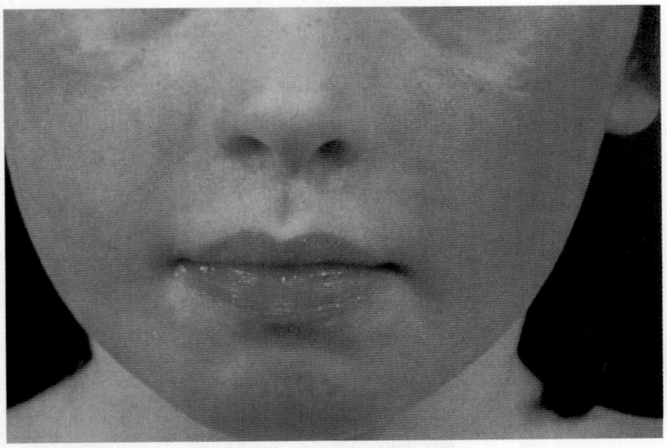

FIGURE 5.13. Erythema infectiosum. (Reproduced, with permission, from Kane KS-M, Ryder JB, Jonson RA, et al. *Color Atlas & Synopsis of Pediatric Dermatology*. New York, NY: McGraw-Hill; 2002:579.)

Varicella-Zoster Virus

Primary infection with varicella-zoster virus results in varicella (chickenpox). The virus subsequently remains latent in sensory ganglia. Reactivation of latent virus (herpes zoster or shingles) occurs in 30% of individuals at some time later in life.

- Peak incidence of varicella: Unvaccinated children < 10 years; most commonly late winter, early spring.
- Transmission of varicella is via direct contact or airborne droplets.
- Highest incidence of herpes zoster: Elderly or immunocompromised individuals.
- Transmission of virus can occur from direct contact with herpes zoster lesions.
- Reactivation (zoster) is not acquired through contact with persons who have chicken pox or zoster.

KEY FACT

In smallpox, all lesions are in the same stage of healing, while in varicella there are often papules, vesicles, and pustules.

Symptoms/Examination

Chickenpox

- Fever precedes rash by 1-2 days.
- Rash typically starts at hairline, with initial formation of macules, which progress to fluid-filled vesicles (**"dew drops on a rose petal"**). Crops of lesions typically appear at the same time with vesicles in various stages of healing on body (Figure 5.14).

Zoster

Rash and pain in dermatomal distribution, typically on trunk or face. Pain may precede rash.

Diagnosis

Clinical diagnosis.

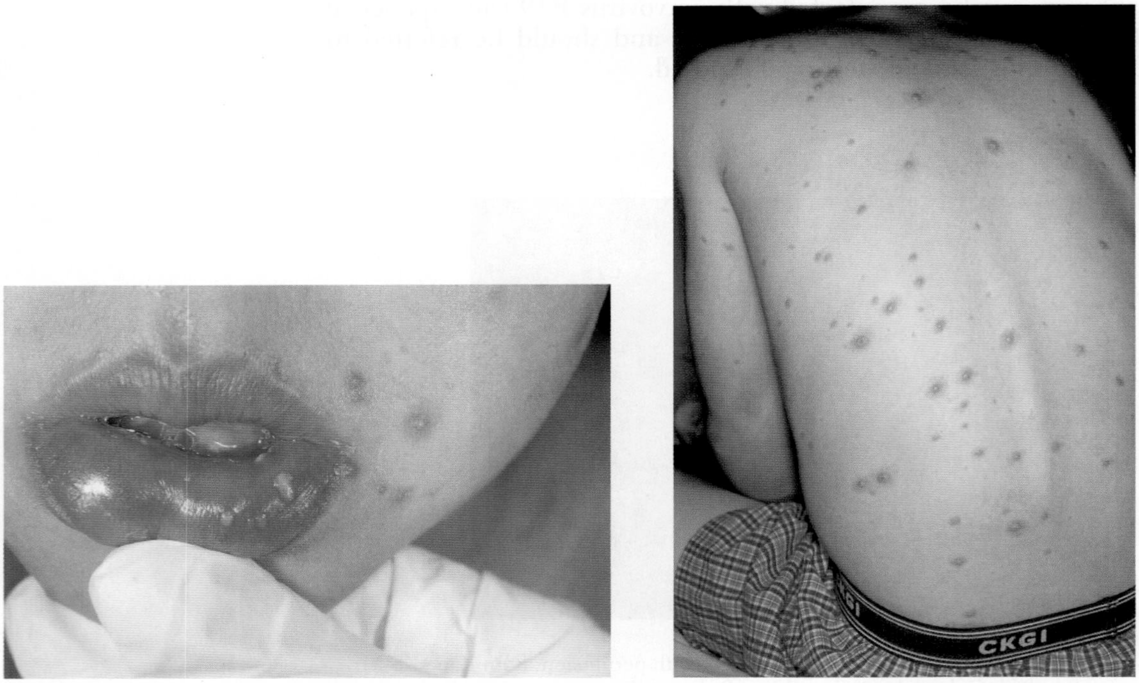

FIGURE 5.14. Varicella. (Reproduced, with permission, from Shah BR, Lucchesi M. *Atlas of Pediatric Emergency Medicine*. New York, NY: McGraw-Hill; 2006:119.)

TREATMENT

Chickenpox

- In healthy children < 12 years, chickenpox is usually a self-limited illness, requiring supportive care (oral antihistamines to treat itching, and antipyretics).
- **Avoid aspirin due to the risk of Reye syndrome.**
- Patients > 12 years are at higher risk for severe disease and should receive oral acyclovir.
- Immunocompromised patients should receive IV acyclovir.
- Immunize unvaccinated close contacts within 72 hours. (*Note*: Varicella vaccine is contraindicated in patients who are pregnant or have significant immunosuppression. These patients should receive varicella zoster immune globulin [VZIG].)

Zoster

- Treat with oral acyclovir if within 72 hours of eruption onset.
- Postexposure prophylaxis as with chickenpox.

COMPLICATIONS

Chickenpox

- Bacterial skin infections are most common complication.
- Children who are immunocompromised are at higher risk for disseminated disease, potentially resulting in meningoencephalitis, pneumonia, hepatitis.
- **Maternal infection during first or second trimester can result in congenital varicella, leading to fetal scarring, limb atrophy, and CNS abnormalities.**
- **Maternal varicella infection at delivery is associated with up to 30% fetal mortality.**

Zoster

Postherpetic neuralgia (uncommon in children), which can last months to years

OTHER VIRAL RASHES

Molluscum Contagiosum

- Caused by **Poxvirus**
- Self-limited skin lesions, typically lasting weeks to months
- Peak incidence: School-age children
- Transmission: Direct contact

SYMPTOMS/EXAMINATION

- **Small, flesh-colored papules that have a centrally depressed area (umbilicated papule,** see Figure 5.15)
- Painless and usually asymptomatic
- Typically affect face, torso, and extremities (sparing palms, soles, and scalp)
- No systemic symptoms

DIAGNOSIS/TREATMENT

- Clinical diagnosis is based on the morphology of the lesions.
- Generally, no treatment is indicated because the lesions are self-limited and resolve without scarring.
- May be referred to dermatologist for treatment if needed.

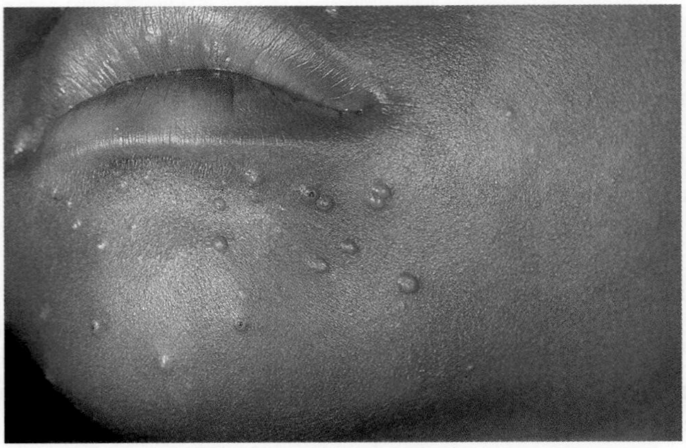

FIGURE 5.15. Molluscum contagiosum. (Reproduced, with permission, from Shah BR, Lucchesi M. *Atlas of Pediatric Emergency Medicine*. New York, NY: McGraw-Hill; 2006:342.)

Pityriasis Rosea

- Etiology is unknown, but possibly a viral agent (HHV-7)
- Highest incidence in adolescents

Symptoms/Examination

- **Herald patch** precedes other symptoms in 50% of patients. The herald patch is a scaly, erythematous, oval lesion typically on the torso.
- 1-2 weeks after appearance of herald patch there is a development of generalized rash, with oval, pink macules aligned along the skin dermatomes of the torso ("**Christmas tree**" distribution; see Figure 5.16).
- Typically, palms and soles are spared.
- Rash may last up to several months.

Differential

- Secondary syphilis (especially if palms and soles are involved).
- Acute drug reaction.
- Reaction to recent immunization.
- Herald patch may resemble tinea corporis.

Diagnosis

Clinical diagnosis.

Treatment

- No treatment is known to shorten length of rash.
- Symptomatic treatment for pruritus: Skin moisturizers, oral antihistamines, possibly topical steroids.

Complications

Hyperpigmentation can occur (especially in patients with dark skin color) due to chronic skin inflammation.

Hand-Foot-Mouth Disease

- Coxsackie virus A16
- Peak US incidence: Summer
- Fecal–oral and respiratory transmission
- Typically affects children < 5 years

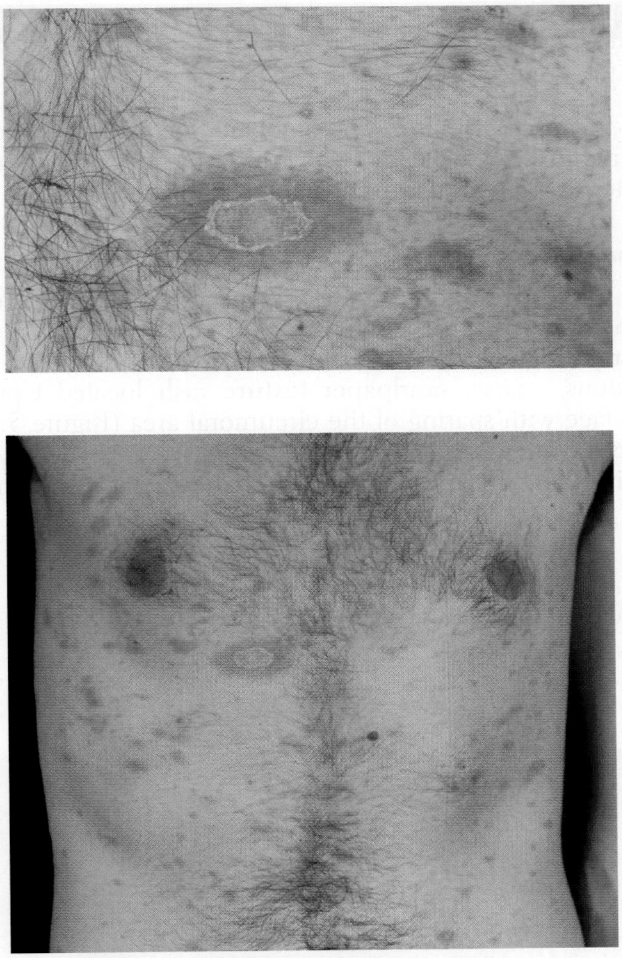

FIGURE 5.16. Pityriasis rosea. (Reproduced, with permission, from Wolff K, Johnson RA, Suurmond D. *Fitzpatrick's Color Atlas & Synopsis of Clinical Dermatology*. 5th ed. New York, NY: McGraw-Hill; 2005:119.)

SYMPTOMS/EXAMINATION

- Fever
- Painful vesicles/ulcers on tongue and palate
- Vesicles on palms and soles and possibly buttocks

DIFFERENTIAL

Other viral infections: Varicella, herpes, herpangina (which is typically caused by other serotypes of Coxsackie virus)

DIAGNOSIS/TREATMENT

- Diagnosis is clinical.
- Treatment is supportive with antipyretics and topical oral analgesics such as nonlidocaine containing "magic mouthwash" preparations.
- Lidocaine mouthwashes should be avoided due to the potential toxicity of lidocaine and resultant seizures.

COMPLICATIONS

- Myocarditis may develop in 2% of patients who have hand-foot-mouth disease.
- Meningoencephalitis is a rare complication.
- Dehydration from decreased oral intake.

BACTERIAL RASHES

Scarlet Fever

Scarlet fever is caused by group A β-hemolytic *Streptococcus*, which produces an erythrogenic toxin. It typically follows a streptococcal pharyngitis, but has been seen after streptococcal skin infections, such as impetigo or cellulitis.

Symptoms/Examination

- Typically sore throat and fever are present for 1-2 days before the appearance of the rash.
- "**Strawberry tongue.**"
- Erythematous, coarse, **sandpaper texture rash** located typically on the torso and face with sparing of the circumoral area (Figure 5.17). Desquamation occurs after the rash fades.
- "**Pastias lines**" are linear nonblanching erythema of the skin folds in joints.

KEY FACT

Scarlet fever: Strawberry tongue, sandpaper rash, Pastia lines.

Differential

- Toxic shock syndrome
- Secondary syphilis
- Infectious mononucleosis

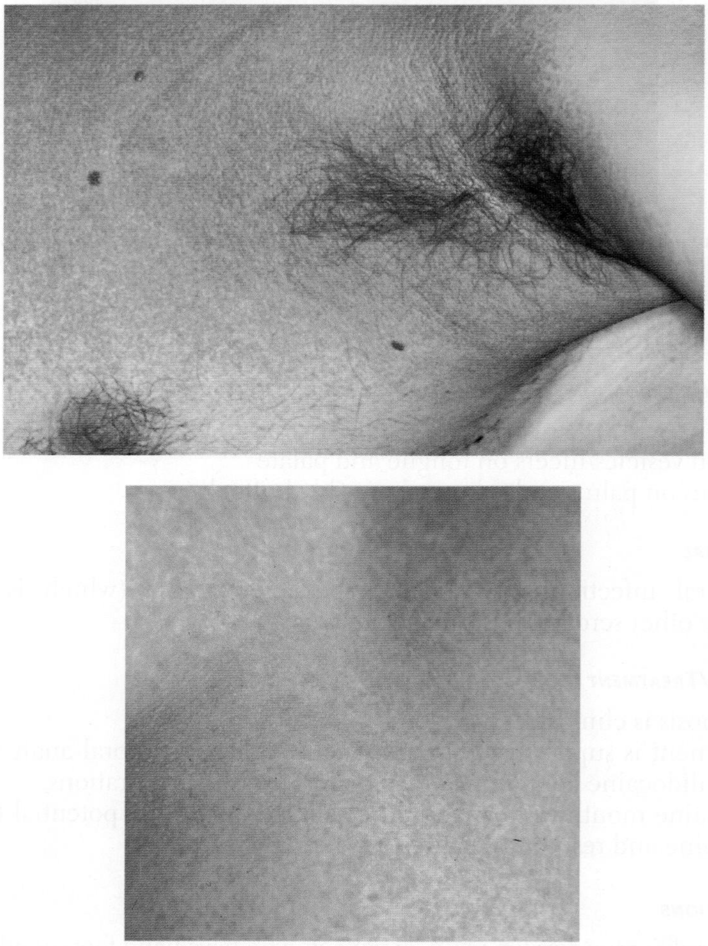

FIGURE 5.17. Scarlet fever. (Reproduced, with permission, from Wolff K et al. *Fitzpatrick's Dermatology in General Medicine*. 7th ed. New York, NY: McGraw-Hill; 2008:1718.)

Diagnosis

Clinical suspicion, confirmed by throat culture positive for strep or a rising ASO titer

Treatment

Penicillin, cephalosporins, or erythromycin for 10 days.

Complications

- Rheumatic fever (can be prevented by treating scarlet fever with antibiotics)
- Glomerulonephritis (**not prevented** by treating scarlet fever with antibiotics)

Staphylococcal Scalded Skin Syndrome

Staphylococcal scalded skin syndrome is because of colonization or infection with an **exfoliative toxin**–producing strain of *S aureus*. The site of colonization/infection may be minor (eg, following a pharyngitis or conjunctivitis). It typically affects children < 5 years.

Symptoms/Examination

- Generalized tender erythema, followed by development of fragile, fluid-filled bullae, and loss of epidermis. Patient is often otherwise well appearing.
- **Nikolsky sign**: Pressure on affected skin leads to separation of the outer portion of epidermis.
- **Mucus membranes are not involved**.

Differential

- Toxic epidermal necrolysis and Stevens-Johnson syndrome may have similar appearance, but often involve mucus membranes.
- Bullous impetigo.

Diagnosis

Clinical diagnosis.

Treatment

- Antibiotics to treat staph infection. Clindamycin may also be given to help decrease toxin release.
- IV fluid resuscitation.
- Isolation.

Complications

- Dehydration.
- Secondary bacterial infection can occur.

Toxic Shock Syndrome

Toxic shock syndrome is caused by release of a specific exotoxin that triggers an inflammatory cascade similar to that seen in sepsis. It is characterized by two distinct syndromes:

- **Staphylococcal toxic shock syndrome (StTSS)**: Because of colonization with exotoxin-producing strain of *S aureus*. Traditionally associated with tampon use or nasal packing.
- **Streptococcal toxic shock syndrome (STSS)**: Typically due to infection with exotoxin-producing strain of group A *Streptococcus* (GAS).

SYMPTOMS/EXAMINATION

- Characterized by the sudden onset of fever, chills, nausea, vomiting, diarrhea, and generalized rash with rapid progression to hypotension and shock.
- In STSS, a severe soft tissue infection may be present.
- Desquamation of rash occurs 1-2 weeks later.

DIAGNOSIS

Based on established clinical criteria (see Table 1.21).

TREATMENT

- Treatment strategy is the same as for patients with sepsis.
- Antibiotics used should cover methicillin-resistant *S aureus* (MRSA) as well as GAS. Clindamycin can also be given to reduce toxin release.

Meningococcal Infections

Caused by organism *Neisseria meningitidis*, a gram-negative diplococcus. Meningococcal infections present with a spectrum of disease ranging from occult bacteremia to fulminant sepsis.

- Infections occur year round, with peak incidence in winter and spring.
- Peak incidence < 4 years, with a second peak between the ages of 15 and 18 years.
- Transmission is via airborne droplets.

SYMPTOMS/EXAMINATION

- Fever is uniformly present.
- Symptoms are often sudden onset and rapidly progressive.
- May exist as isolated sepsis with or without meningitis.
- Headache, vomiting, irritability ± rash are characteristic of meningococcal meningitis.
- Shock and rash (classically petechial/purpuric, but may be maculopapular at onset) are seen with meningococcal sepsis.

DIAGNOSIS

- Culture of organism from sterile body fluid (blood, CSF).
- Gram stain demonstrating gram-negative diplococci supports the presumptive diagnosis of infection.
- DIC may be present.

TREATMENT

- Antibiotics (penicillins or cephalosporins): Give early!
- Intensive supportive care and ICU admission with respiratory isolation are indicated in most cases.
- Children with occult *N meningitidis* bacteremia (+ blood culture obtained as part of fever workup) need LP and admission for early IV antibiotics, even if well appearing.
- Chemoprophylaxis for close contacts (rifampin or ceftriaxone for children; ciprofloxacin for adults).
- Report diagnosis to local health department.

> **KEY FACT**
>
> Petechiae in setting of fever should raise concern for meningococcemia. These patients should be placed on droplet precautions and managed aggressively, because this infection can lead to rapid decompensation.

COMPLICATIONS

- Fatality rate 10% for all ages (fatality rate up to 25% in adolescents).
- Bilateral sensorineural deafness is the **most common complication** in survivors of meningitis caused by *N meningitidis*.
- Myocarditis, pericarditis, or pneumonia can also occur.

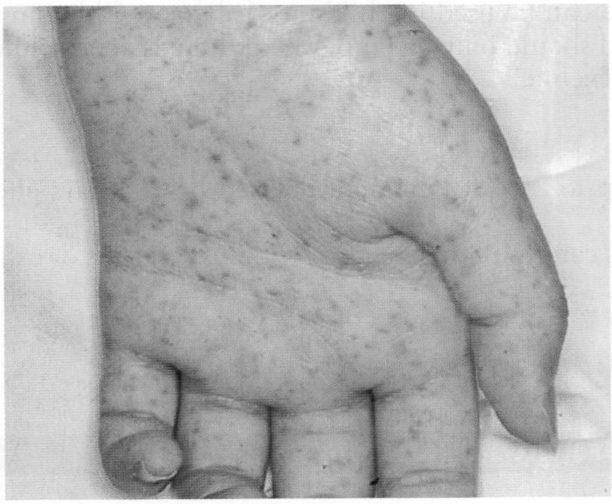

FIGURE 5.18. Rocky Mountain spotted fever. (Reproduced, with permission, from Weinberg S, Prose NS, Kristal L. *Color Atlas of Pediatric Dermatology*. 4th ed. New York, NY: McGraw-Hill; 2008:56.)

Rocky Mountain Spotted Fever

Rocky Mountain spotted fever (RMSF) is a rickettsial infection caused by the gram-negative, obligate intracellular organism *Rickettsia rickettsii*.

- Transmitted via wood or dog tick bite (*Dermacentor andersoni* or *variabilis*)
- Occurs throughout the United States, but primarily in the southeast (not the Rocky Mountains)
- Peak season: April to October
- Peak incidence: 5-9 years of age

KEY FACT

RMSF Triad (present in 60% of cases):

1. Fever
2. Rash
3. Headache

SYMPTOMS/EXAMINATION

- Acute onset of flu-like symptoms of **fever,** headache, nausea, vomiting, myalgias.
- Rash appears 3-5 days after onset of other symptoms. Initially, presents as macular rash on palms, wrists, soles, and ankles. Rash spreads centrally and may become petechial (Figure 5.18).
- Severe headache and signs of meningeal irritation signal CNS involvement.

DIFFERENTIAL

The differential diagnosis is extensive, including meningococcal infection, ehrlichiosis, Kawasaki disease, toxic shock syndrome, secondary syphilis, HSP, drug reactions, and viral infections.

KEY FACT

Treatment of RMSF should be based on clinical suspicion. Do not exclude the diagnosis of RMSF because the patient lacks a rash or known tick exposure.

DIAGNOSIS

- High clinical suspicion in the febrile child is needed to make the diagnosis because patients often present with symptoms prior to onset of rash.
- LP is necessary in any patient with signs of meningitis or altered mental status to rule out other causes.
- CBC may show anemia and thrombocytopenia with normal number of leukocytes but elevated bands.
- Confirmed by antibody testing.

KEY FACT

If there is concern for RMSF, antibiotics should be started in the ED without waiting for the results of serologic testing.

TREATMENT

- Prompt removal of ticks (RMSF unlikely if tick attached < 12 hours).
- Treatment of suspected RMSF should begin based on clinical suspicion alone (prior to confirmatory testing).

- Doxycycline can be used in children of all ages. Chloramphenicol is less effective and should only be employed if there is an absolute contraindication to doxycycline.

COMPLICATIONS

- Mortality up to 25% if treatment delayed by > 5 days after the onset of symptoms.
- Severe cases can result in gangrene, with loss of digits or extremities.

Immunology

JUVENILE IDIOPATHIC ARTHRITIS

Juvenile idiopathic arthritis (JIA), formerly called juvenile rheumatoid arthritis, encompasses a variety of conditions (Table 5.22), which all share the common feature of joint pain or swelling lasting longer than 6 weeks. Affected joints are painful, swollen, stiff, warm to the touch, often have reduced range of motion, and may be erythematous. The etiology of JIA is unknown, with possible connections to antecedent viral infections or to host immune characteristics.

SYMPTOMS/EXAMINATION

- Variable, often with several of the following:
  - Warm, swollen joint
  - Morning stiffness that improves with activity
  - Increased pain after periods of rest
  - Low-grade fever
  - Fatigue
  - Anorexia and weight loss
- Systemic onset JIA is the least common and typically includes several of the following:
  - Daily, spiking high fever.
  - Rash (pink maculopapular on torso, proximal extremities).
  - Hepatosplenomegaly.
  - Pleuritis or pericarditis.

KEY FACT

The methotrexate dose for JIA is much lower and avoids many of the side effects seen with the higher doses for chemotherapy. Side effects can be limited by supplementation with folic acid.

TABLE 5.22. Types of JIA

	POLYARTICULAR ONSET	PAUCIARTICULAR ONSET	SYSTEMIC ONSET
Number of joints	Usually ≥ 5	< 5; mostly knees, ankles, elbows	Variable
Systemic symptoms	Fever, malaise	Few; iridocyclitis (anterior uveitis)	Fever, rash
Age at onset	Early and late childhood	Early childhood	Any age
Sex	♀ > ♂	♀ > ♂	♂ > ♀
ANA	Positive 25%	Positive 60%	Negative

ANA, anti-nuclear antibodies; JIA, juvenile idiopathic arthritis.

- Lymphadenopathy.
- Arthritis may be minimal initially but later systemic symptoms become less apparent and arthritis more prominent.

DIFFERENTIAL

- Infection: Septic arthritis, osteomyelitis, Lyme disease
- Malignancy: Either systemic (such as leukemia) or bone
- Trauma
- Avascular necrosis

DIAGNOSIS

- Diagnosis of JIA is clinical, because no studies are diagnostic.
- Laboratory test results often reveal a mild anemia, leukocytosis, thrombocytosis, and elevated erythrocyte sedimentation rate (ESR), C-reactive protein (CRP).
- Synovial fluid: WBC 10,000-100,000/mm^3, low glucose.
- Rheumatoid factor is positive in polyarticular subtype.
- X-ray of involved joints shows osteopenia and later narrowing or erosion of the joint space.
- If septic arthritis cannot be excluded based on examination, then joint aspiration is required.

TREATMENT

- NSAIDs are first-line therapy.
- For patients who do not respond to NSAIDS, disease-modifying or biologic agents are indicated. Methotrexate is the most commonly used and can cause hepatic fibrosis, lymphopenia, or pulmonary hypersensitivity.
- Systemic steroids should be reserved for severe symptoms and administered in the ED only after consultation with a rheumatologist.
- For patients with pauciarticular disease, regular slit lamp examinations are important to detect the onset of iridocyclitis and begin specific therapy before vision is compromised. Acute iridocyclitis requires immediate consultation with an ophthalmologist.

COMPLICATIONS

- Deformity of limbs and joints in a minority of patients.
- Recurrent arthritis.
- Pericarditis: Complication of systemic JIA.
- Cricoarytenoid arthritis.
- Macrophage activation syndrome: Complication of systemic JIA that presents similarly to sepsis with DIC but progresses to seizures, coma, and death if untreated.
- Blindness may develop in patients with iridocyclitis if treatment is not started promptly.

KEY FACT

Patients with severe JIA are at risk for cervical instability; their C-spine should be immobilized during intubation.

JUVENILE DERMATOMYOSITIS

Autoimmune inflammation of the skin and muscle that typically affects females < 10 years.

SYMPTOMS/EXAMINATION

- Prodrome of gradual onset of myalgias and malaise with edema of hands, feet, and eyelids.
- This is followed by development of symmetric proximal muscle weakness, violaceous heliotrope rash around the eyes, and Gottron papules (red lesions on extensor surface of knees, elbows, and knuckles).

DIAGNOSIS

- Laboratory tests are nonspecific but include elevated creatine kinase (CK), lactate dehydrogenase (LDH), LFTs.
- WBC, ESR, CRP are normal.
- Definitive diagnosis is via magnetic resonance imaging (MRI) of involved muscles.

TREATMENT

- Corticosteroids ± disease-modifying agents.
- Admission.
- Monitor for involvement of respiratory muscles.

COMPLICATIONS

- Muscle atrophy, contractures
- Respiratory failure, aspiration

HENOCH-SCHÖNLEIN PURPURA

Henoch-Schönlein purpura (HSP) is a small vessel vasculitis of the kidney, GI tract, joints, and skin that often develops after a URI. It typically affects children 3-7 years of age but can be seen in older children and adults, with males affected more frequently than females.

SYMPTOMS/EXAMINATION

- Palpable purpura, usually starting on lower extremities and buttocks, progressing toward the torso (Figure 5.19).
- Joint pain, most commonly in the knees.
- Swelling at ankles which can cause difficulty walking.
- Crampy abdominal pain with vomiting and diarrhea. Guaiac positive stool is present in up to 56% of patients.

KEY FACT

Triad of symptoms for HSP: Purpura, abdominal pain, arthritis.

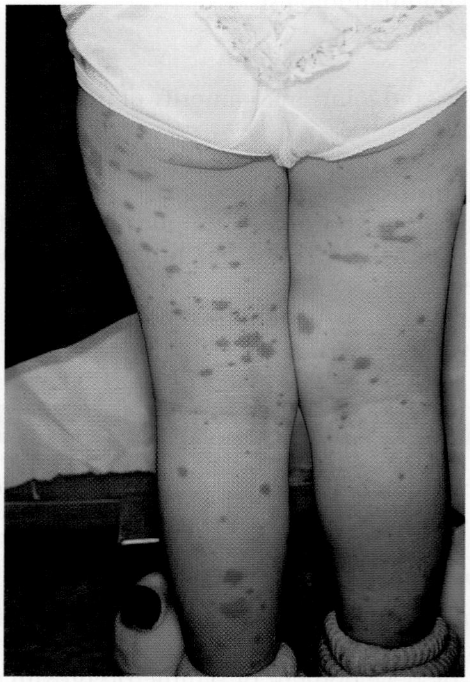

FIGURE 5.19. Henoch-Schönlein purpura. (Reproduced, with permission, from Shah BR, Lucchesi M. *Atlas of Pediatric Emergency Medicine*. New York, NY: McGraw-Hill; 2006:109.)

- Hematuria.
- Additional symptoms can include nonpitting edema of the extremities and face, melena, hematemesis, fever, hepatomegaly, headache, seizures, and testicular pain.

DIFFERENTIAL

- Abdominal pain can mimic acute appendicitis.
- Rash: Consider meningococcal sepsis, bleeding disorder, or drug reaction.
- Arthritis: JIA or SLE.

DIAGNOSIS

- Diagnosis can usually be made clinically.
- Can look and test for infectious triggers and associations such as streptococcal pharyngitis.
- Laboratory tests are nonspecific but may reveal a leukocytosis, anemia, and elevated ESR.
- Urine should be obtained to look for hematuria and proteinuria indicating renal involvement.
- Contrast enema may miss ileoileal intussusception. Ultrasound is the first-line imaging modality, followed by upper GI series with small bowel follow through.

TREATMENT

- Treatment is mostly supportive and can include IV fluid if dehydrated.
- Most patients diagnosed with HSP who do not have significant renal involvement on testing in the ED can be discharged to home with follow-up through their primary care physician.
- Patients who have severe abdominal pain or GI bleeding should be admitted. Limited studies suggest these patients may benefit from steroids.
- Steroids should be given after consultation with nephrologist if there is evidence of nephritis.

COMPLICATIONS

- Intussusception (70% are ileoileal) due to lead point caused by edema or hemorrhage into the bowel wall.
- Nephrotic syndrome with chronic renal disease can develop up to 6 months after initial presentation.
- Recurrent episodes of HSP.

> **KEY FACT**
>
> - Uncommon complications include bowel perforation, pancreatitis, hypertension.
>
> Consider intussusceptions in patients with HSP and episodic intermittent abdominal pain or vomiting.

KAWASAKI DISEASE

Kawasaki disease (initially called mucocutaneous lymph node syndrome) is an idiopathic, acute, small- and medium-vessel vasculitis with predilection for coronary arteries. **It is the leading cause of acquired heart disease in children in the United States**. The peak incidence is between the ages of 18 and 24 months, with the majority of patients < 5 years old.

SYMPTOMS/EXAMINATION

There are three phases to Kawasaki disease (Table 5.23).

DIFFERENTIAL

- Infections (viral or bacterial, including rickettsial)
- Toxic shock syndrome may have similar appearance, but has no lymphadenopathy or arthritis
- Stevens-Johnson syndrome (again, no lymphadenopathy)

TABLE 5.23. Phases of Kawasaki Disease

Acute phase (1-2 wk)
■ Fever
■ Lymphadenopathy (usually anterior cervical; not diffuse)
■ Conjunctivitis (bilateral, painless, without exudates, limbic sparing)
■ Oropharynx: Cracked red lips, "**strawberry tongue**" (prominent papillae on tongue), pharyngeal erythema
■ Rash on perineum, often progressing to torso
■ Erythema/edema of hands and feet
■ Vasculitis may affect virtually any organ system: Pneumonitis, myocarditis, enteritis, meatitis, hepatitis, uveitis
Subacute phase (2-4 wk)
■ Thrombocytosis (platelets up to 500,000-1,000,000/mm^3)
■ Resolution of fever
■ Desquamation of hands and feet
Convalescent phase (> 2 mo)
■ Scarring and calcification of affected coronary arteries

- Rheumatologic conditions (rarely present with mucus membrane involvement)
- Scarlet fever (no ocular involvement)

KEY FACT

Not all patients with Kawasaki disease will meet the full diagnostic criteria. The diagnosis should be entertained in patients with fever ≥ 5 days and any two clinical criteria. In these patients, obtain inflammatory markers and consult a rheumatologist if markers are elevated.

DIAGNOSIS

- Based on a series of criteria (Table 5.24), Kawasaki disease should be entertained for children who have a prolonged, unexplained fever, particularly those with evidence of mucocutaneous inflammation.
- Laboratory findings are nonspecific, but may include leukocytosis with left shift, normocytic anemia, thrombocytosis, elevated ESR/CRP, elevated LFTs, and hyponatremia.
- Clean catch urinalysis with WBCs (WBCs are not detected on cath specimens because they originate in the urethra).
- If Kawasaki disease is strongly suspected, echocardiogram should be performed.

TREATMENT

- Hospitalize.
- If Kawasaki disease is confidently diagnosed, start **intravenous gammaglobulin** (**IVIG**). When given within 10 days of disease onset, IVIG reduces symptom duration and risk of aneurysm formation.
- Consider **high-dose-aspirin** therapy after consultation with rheumatologist.

TABLE 5.24. Diagnostic Criteria for Kawasaki Disease

Fever = 5 d, **and** 4 of 5 of the following criteria:
1. Bilateral conjunctival injection
2. Oropharyngeal changes (fissuring or erythema of lips, strawberry tongue, erythema of pharynx)
3. Changes to skin on hands/feet (edema or erythema → desquamation)
4. Rash on torso (nonvesicular)
5. Cervical lymphadenopathy (at least 1 lymph node greater in size than 1.5 cm)
And no other diagnosis to explain symptoms

COMPLICATIONS

- **Aneurysms of coronary arteries** develop in 20% of patients who are untreated. Patients at highest risk are male, < 1 year old, and those with delayed diagnosis. Aneurysms can lead to myocardial infarction (MI), sudden cardiac death, or chronic ischemia.
- Cardiovascular (CV): CHF, myocarditis, pericarditis, valvular disease.
- CNS: Sensorineural hearing loss.
- GI: Hydrops of gallbladder.
- GU: Urethritis.
- Eye: Anterior uveitis.
- Mortality is < 1% for children in the United States.
- Recurs in 1%-2% of children within 12 months.

RHEUMATIC FEVER

- Mediated by the host immune response to a preceding GAS infection.
- Affected patients are typically school age.
- Rare in the United States.
- Symptoms develop 2-3 weeks after a strep infection, with target organs including heart, joints, CNS, and skin.

SYMPTOMS/EXAMINATION

- Variable, depending on which organ systems are affected. Fever is usually low grade.
- Polyarthritis, typically affecting > 5 large joints of limbs—must have true signs of joint inflammation not just pain.
- Carditis causing damage to mitral or aortic valves, resulting in valvular insufficiency, CHF, or pericarditis.
- Subcutaneous nodules (pea-sized bumps on the extensor surfaces of extremities): Often only develop with recurrent rheumatic fever.
- Erythema marginatum (serpiginous, evanescent, nonpruritic rash that typically spares the face).
- Sydenham chorea (involuntary nonsensical movements) due to CNS involvement.

DIFFERENTIAL

- JIA
- Septic arthritis
- Kawasaki syndrome
- Myocarditis/pericarditis
- SLE
- Serum sickness
- HSP

DIAGNOSIS

- The JONES criteria (Table 5.25) are used to confirm the diagnosis.
- Routine laboratory tests should include CBC, ESR, CRP, strep throat cultures, ASO titers, ECG, CXR, cardiac echocardiography.

TREATMENT

- Primary prevention of rheumatic fever: Treat streptococcal pharyngitis with antibiotics within 9 days of symptom onset.
- Secondary treatment once rheumatic fever is diagnosed requires admission to the hospital and penicillin.

MNEMONIC

JONES criteria for diagnosis of rheumatic fever:

Joints
Oh, no—carditis!
Nodules
Erythema marginatum
Sydenham chorea

KEY FACT

Reliance on the minor criteria for diagnosis of rheumatic fever can lead to false-positive diagnoses, because the minor criteria are all nonspecific.

TABLE 5.25. 1992 JONES Criteria for Diagnosing Rheumatic Fever

1. Evidence of preceding group A *Streptococcus* infection: ■ Elevated or rising ASO titer, or ■ + Throat culture, or ■ + Rapid antigen test
and
2. Either two major manifestations, or one major and two minor manifestations: **Major manifestations:** ■ Carditis ■ Polyarthritis ■ Sydenham chorea ■ Erythema marginatum ■ Subcutaneous nodules **Minor manifestations:** ■ Arthralgia ■ Fever ■ Elevated ESR or CRP ■ Prolonged PR interval on ECG

ASO, antistreptolysin O, CRP, C-reactive protein; ECG, electrocardiogram; ESR, erythrocyte sedimentation rate.

- High-dose aspirin.
- Steroids for carditis or chorea.

Complications

- Damage to heart valves
- Recurrent episodes of acute rheumatic fever (can be reduced with antibiotic prophylaxis)

Neurology

SEIZURES

Seizures are dramatic and panic provoking events for caregivers and often precipitate ED visits. Seizures are **the most common neurologic disorder** in childhood. Peak incidence is in the first year of life and then declines as children get older. **Fever is the most common cause of seizures in children**. However, the differential diagnosis, evaluation and management depend on the age of the patient and the type of seizure present (Table 5.26).

KEY FACT

While both seizures and syncope can lead to abnormal movements, altered consciousness, and loss of bowel/bladder, syncope is not associated with a postictal period.

Symptoms

- Careful history should be taken to determine the type and length of seizure as well as the presence or absence of postictal phase, loss of bowel/bladder control, and/or neurologic deficit.
- Many disorders can mimic seizures (Table 5.27). Careful history can usually differentiate mimics from true seizures.

TABLE 5.26. Classification of Pediatric Seizures

Seizure Type	Characteristics
Febrile	**Seizure in presence of fever, no CNS infection or other cause**
Simple	Generalized, < 15 min, age 6 mo-5 y, ≤ 1 in 24-h period
Complex	Focal, > 15 min or multiple in number
Generalized	**Convulsive or nonconvulsive, LOC**
Tonic–clonic	Alternating increased tone with spasms
Tonic	Increased tone
Clonic	Rhythmic spasms
Absence	Nonconvulsive, < 10-15 s LOC, no postictal phase
Myoclonic	Minor symmetric motor spasms
Atonic	Loss of muscle tone
Partial (focal)	**Focal seizures without LOC**
Simple	Focal seizure without change in mentation
Complex	Focal seizure **with** impaired consciousness or change in behavior
Neonatal	**Clinically subtle: Apnea, eye movements, chewing, "bicycling"**

CNS, central nervous system; LOC, loss of consciousness.

Examination

- The most important examination finding is to determine if the seizure is ongoing.
- A thorough neurologic examination should be completed to determine if any neurologic deficit is present. Such a finding suggests a structural cause for seizure.
- Signs of meningitis and elevated ICP (bulging fontanelle and papilledema) should be sought.
- Certain skin findings may suggest an underlying neurologic disease.
  - Café-au-lait spots: Neurofibromatosis
  - Ash leaf spot: Tuberous sclerosis
  - Port-wine stain on face: Sturge-Weber syndrome
- Unexplained ecchymoses may suggest intracranial hemorrhage secondary to bleeding disorder or child abuse.
- Pregnancy and hypertension may suggest eclampsia.

MNEMONIC

Causes of seizures in children:

TIMED IT

Trauma
Infection (meningitis)
Metabolic (hypoglycemia, hyponatremia, hypernatremia, hypocalcemia)
Epilepsy (medication noncompliance common)
Drugs (lead, cocaine, aspirin, carbon monoxide)
Inborn errors of metabolism
Tumor

TABLE 5.27. Seizure Mimics

Characteristics	Seizure Mimics
Loss of consciousness, no postictal phase	Syncope Complex migraine Breath-holding spells
No loss of consciousness	Tics Shuddering attacks Benign sleep myoclonus Night terrors Pseudoseizures

TABLE 5.28. Differential Diagnosis of Seizure by Age

Age	Differential
Neonatal	Hypoxic-ischemic encephalopathy: Most common (> 50%) Intracranial hemorrhage (~15%) Inborn errors of metabolism (~10%) CNS infection Congenital CNS disorders Drug withdrawal (intrauterine exposure) Metabolic disorders (hypoglycemia, hypo/hypernatremia, hypocalcemia, hypomagnesemia, pyridoxine deficiency) Benign familial neonatal convulsions ■ Present first 3 d with strong family history Benign idiopathic neonatal convulsions ("fifth day fits") ■ Present on day 5
Infant/young child (< 6)	Febrile seizure Seizure disorder Tumor Meningitis/encephalitis Head trauma (intracranial hemorrhage) Metabolic disorder Neurocutaneous disorders Toxins
Older child/ adolescent	Seizure disorder Meningitis/encephalitis Head trauma Tumor Toxins

CNS, central nervous system.

DIFFERENTIAL

The differential diagnosis of seizure depends on the age of the patient (Table 5.28).

DIAGNOSIS

The diagnosis of seizure is clinical. History from an eyewitness should help determine if the event in question was in fact a seizure or something else. If the event described was a seizure, the age of the patient, associated symptoms, and findings on examination will direct further evaluation.

Neonatal Seizures

- The differential for neonatal seizures is different from that of older children. While benign etiologies of neonatal seizures exist, the more common causes of neonatal seizures are concerning etiologies that necessitate an aggressive workup. The diagnostics below should be obtained on all neonates with seizures to rule in or rule out the following causes:
- Metabolic abnormalities: Glucose, electrolytes (Na, Ca, Mg)

- IEM: Ammonia, pH (+ anion gap), urine ketones, lactate
- Sepsis: CBC with differential, UA/UCx, Blood Cx, LP
- Meningitis/encephalitis: LP with CSF analysis and culture (include HSV)
- Structural abnormalities: Cranial ultrasound, CT, or MRI
- Drug withdrawal: Urine toxicology screen (if suspected)

Febrile Seizures

- Simple febrile seizures are defined as generalized seizures lasting < 15 minutes, that do not recur within 24-hours in a child between 3 months and 6 years of age, with a temperature > 38°C (100.4°F) in the absence of signs of CNS infection, the absence of metabolic derangements that could cause seizure activity, and with no prior history of afebrile seizures. Complex febrile seizures are those that have focal activity at onset, continue for longer than 15 minutes, or that recur within 24 hours.
- The main consideration for a child with a febrile seizure is whether or not the child has underlying meningitis or encephalitis. The **AAP** guidelines for febrile seizures state that an LP should be performed in a child with symptoms that suggest meningitis, considered for an infant aged 6-12 months who has not received the recommended *H influenzae* type b (Hib) or *S pneumoniae* immunization, and considered for children who have been pretreated with antibiotics. Recent studies suggest LP is not needed following a simple febrile seizure in a well-appearing, vaccinated child > 6 months without other clinical signs of meningitis. Additional diagnostics including electrolytes and imaging are also not necessary in a child with a simple febrile seizure.

Generalized and Partial Seizures

- History and physical examination should guide the need for further evaluation. If on examination the patient is asymptomatic (normal mental status and neurologic examination), it is unlikely that a metabolic or structural defect is present.
- Asymptomatic patient: Diagnostics beyond blood glucose and checking antiepileptic drug levels (when appropriate) are low yield.
- Symptomatic patient (altered mental status or abnormal neurologic examination).
  - Bedside glucose and electrolytes: Evaluate for metabolic abnormalities.
  - If toxins suspected: Urine tox, ethyl alcohol (EtOH), salicylate level, ECG, lithium, cardiac output, theophylline.
  - If meningitis/encephalitis is suspected: LP.
  - If stroke, hemorrhage, or tumor is suspected: CNS imaging (CT/MRI).

TREATMENT

- Treatment of ongoing seizures of all types should begin in the same manner.
- Maintain airway and give oxygen (airway, breathing, and circulation [ABCs]); intubate if necessary (check glucose first).
- Protect cervical spine if trauma suspected.
- Correct hypoglycemia if present.
- First-line anticonvulsant should be a benzodiazepine.
  - Lorazepam 0.05-0.1 mg/kg IV/IM/IO
  - Diazepam 0.2-0.3 mg/kg IV/IM/IO or 0.5 mg/kg PR
- If seizure stops, evaluate and treat suspected underlying pathology. See the following text for further treatment options for cases of status epilepticus.

KEY FACT

Phenobarbital is the preferred long-acting anticonvulsant in neonates and in seizures induced by toxins.

KEY FACT

Fosphenytoin has essentially replaced phenytoin. Phenytoin use was associated with arrhythmias and hypotension if given at a fast rate because of the propylene glycol it contains.

Children with seizure lasting > 15 minutes or multiple seizures without return to baseline between seizures should be considered to be in status epilepticus.

SPECIAL CONSIDERATIONS

Neonatal Seizures

- **Phenobarbital** (20-mg/kg IV load, 1-mg/kg/min IV gtt) is the preferred long-acting anticonvulsant in neonates.
- Underlying pathology should aggressively be sought.
- Antibiotics should be started after cultures obtained.
- Pyridoxine **can be given for refractory seizures because pyridoxine deficiency is a rare but potential cause of neonatal seizures that will be resistant to standard anticonvulsants.**

Status Epilepticus

- Status epilepticus is a true medical emergency with significant associated complications that necessitate aggressive treatment.
- Intubation and EEG monitoring can be required if seizures do not respond to medications or if respiratory depression develops.
- First-line anticonvulsant is a benzodiazepine (as discussed previously).
- Second-line treatment is loading of fosphenytoin (20 mg/kg IV) or Keppra (20- to 30-mg/kg IV).
- Third-line treatment is phenobarbital (20-mg/kg IV load at 1 mg/kg/min).
- Fourth-line treatments to be considered include propofol, pentobarbital, or valproic acid.

HEADACHE

Headache is common complaint among children. While the vast majority of children do not have a life-threatening or serious etiology for their headache, the EM physician must be able to identify those children that need further workup.

Symptoms

- Concerning headache features include:
- Sudden onset
- Visual changes
- Altered mental status or behavior changes
- Fever and/or neck pain
- Focal neurologic changes
- Associated trauma
- Nocturnal awakening
- Morning headache and vomiting
- Persistent unrelenting headaches
- Chronic progressive headaches

Examination

- Concerning examination findings include:
- Presence of a ventriculoperitoneal (VP) shunt
- Altered mental status or behavior changes
- Meningismus
- Hypertension
- Signs of head injury (hemotympanum, Battle sign, raccoon eyes, hematoma)
- Signs of increased ICP (papilledema, bulging fontanelle, vomiting)
- Focal neurologic deficits
- Abnormal eye movements
- Ataxia or gait disturbances
- Petechiae/purpura
- Signs of neurocutaneous disorders

TABLE 5.29. Differential Diagnosis of Pediatric Headache

LIFE-THREATENING/SERIOUS ETIOLOGIES	BENIGN ETIOLOGIES
Intracranial hemorrhage/hematoma	Migraine
Tumor	Tension headache
Infection: Meningitis/encephalitis/abscess	Cluster headache
Aneurysm/AV malformation	Viral syndrome
Pseudotumor cerebri	Frontal sinusitis (> 6 y old)
Congenital malformation	Dental pain or abscess
Hydrocephalus	Strep throat
Toxins: CO and heavy metals	Otitis media
Cavernous venus thrombosis	Stress

AV, arteriovenous.

Differential

See Table 5.29.

Diagnosis

- History and physical examination should dictate the need for further evaluation.
- While most children do not require emergent imaging, CT scan should be obtained if concern for intracranial bleeding, tumor, increased ICP, or abscess.
- Chronic progressive headaches necessitate CT or MRI scan.
- LP should be performed if concern for meningitis/encephalitis or suspected subarachnoid hemorrhage and negative CT. However, subarachnoid hemorrhage is much less common in children than adults.
- Sinus radiographs or CT is typically **not indicated** for cases of suspected sinusitis.
- Toxicology studies if indicated.
- Rapid strep testing if indicated.
- Patients with VP shunt need a shunt series and CT scan if history and physical examination are concerning for shunt malfunction. A shunt tap should be performed (by neurosurgery) if there is concern for meningitis or shunt infection.

SPECIAL CONSIDERATIONS

Migraine

Migraine headaches in children are different than in adults:

- May last 1-72 hours (vs 4-72 hours in adults)
- Pain more often bilateral (vs usually unilateral in adults)

Migraine with aura (classic migraine): ≥ 2 headaches meeting the below criteria:

- Fully reversible neurologic disturbances or deficits (auras)
  - Ophthalmic (most common)
  - Hemiparesthetic (second most common)
  - Hemiplegia
  - Hemiparetic
  - Aphasia
- At least 2 of the following:

KEY FACT

The diagnosis of new migraines should not be made in the ED.

- Gradual development of aura over > 4 minutes
- Each aura lasts 5-60 minutes
- Occurrence of headache before, during, or within 60 minutes of aura
- ≥ 1 aura is unilateral

TREATMENT

- Primary headaches and migraines can be treated similarly to adults.
- Tylenol and PO NSAIDs should be used first line.
- Preferred V medications for status migrainosus, in order based on evidence: Prochlorperazine, metoclopramide with or without diphenhydramine (to prevent dystonic reactions), IV fluids, ketorolac, valproic acid, sumatriptan in older children with preferred route intranasally.
- IV opiates may be used if headache is refractory, but often produce rebound headaches.

Orthopedics

LIMP

Evaluating a child with a limp can be difficult because the differential is large and the examination is often limited when the child is in pain or will not cooperate.

SYMPTOMS

- A thorough history from the parents can help narrow down the affected area.
- History should elicit the duration of symptoms, associated trauma, fever, abdominal pain or nausea/vomiting, bowel or bladder dysfunction, back pain, decreased strength or sensation, recent URI, morning stiffness, headache, rash or skin changes, and exposure to ticks, possible toxins, or drugs.
- Past medical history should also elicit whether the patient has known inflammatory diseases, hemoglobinopathies, or immunocompromised states.

EXAMINATION

- Physical examination should first focus on inspection of how the child is holding the affected limb and looking for skin changes, evidence of trauma, and joint effusions.
- Next, the long bones and joints should be palpated assessing for warmth, tenderness, skin lesions, rash, and induration. Once palpated, the joints should be ranged bilaterally looking for restricted range of motion.
- An abdominal examination should be done looking for signs of appendicitis or testicular pain.
- A thorough neurologic examination should also be done looking for weakness, sensory deficits, and abnormal reflexes. The spine and paraspinous areas should also be palpated for tenderness.
- If a spinal cord tumor is suspect, a rectal examination should be performed.
- Last, the child should be observed walking. A child too young to walk should be assessed for ability to bear weight on all extremities by holding the child up and allowing them to put weight on lower legs and then allowing them while prone to push up using upper extremities or crawl.

KEY FACT

Knee pain in a child is often referred pain from the hip.

DIFFERENTIAL

See Table 5.30.

TABLE 5.30. Differential Diagnosis of Limp by Location of Disease

Location of Disease	Etiologies
Joint	Trauma: Fracture, dislocation Septic arthritis Inflammatory arthritis: Transient synovitis, JRA Sickle cell (vaso-occlusive) Avascular necrosis (Legg-Calvé-Perthes) SCFE
Long bones	Trauma: Fracture Osteomyelitis Tumor
Soft tissues	Cellulitis Myositis Fasciitis
Abdomen	Appendicitis
Spine/back	Cord tumor Epidural abscess Psoas abscess
CNS	Cerebellar tumor/abscess Meningitis/encephalitis Guillain-Barré syndrome Tick paralysis Toxin exposure (heavy metals, alcohol)

CNS, central nervous system; JRA, juvenile rheumatoid arthritis; SCFE, slipped capital femoral epiphysis.

Q

A 13-year-old obese African American male has had a limp for 3 days. He has no fever and there is no associated trauma. What is a likely diagnosis?

Diagnosis

- A thorough history and physical examination should be able to narrow down the possible etiologies and guide further evaluation.
- Laboratory evaluation: CBC with differential, ESR, and CRP may be helpful if inflammatory or infectious process is suspected.
- Imaging:
  - X-rays should be taken if there is localized pain or history of possible trauma.
  - Ultrasound should be used to evaluate for joint effusions if there is concern for septic arthritis.
  - MRI can be used to further evaluate for musculoskeletal tumors, fractures not seen on x-ray, and inflammatory/infectious states.
- **Septic arthritis** has been associated with the following factors:
  - Fever > 38.5°C (101.3°F).
  - Inability to bear weight.
  - WBC > 12,000/mm^3.
  - ESR > 40 mm/h.
  - CRP > 2 mg/dL.
  - The absence of all these features makes septic arthritis unlikely, while the probability is quite high if ≥ 3 features are present.

A

Slipped capital femoral epiphysis (SCFE).

TREATMENT/COMPLICATIONS

Treatment and complications depend on the etiology identified. See the next section "Special Considerations" for further discussion of particular etiologies.

SPECIAL CONSIDERATIONS

Legg-CalvÉ-Perthes

Idiopathic avascular necrosis of the proximal femoral epiphysis. Occurs primarily in boys between the age of 2 and 12 years.

SYMPTOMS/EXAMINATION

- Insidious onset pain localized to groin and anteromedial thigh; worsened by activity and improved with rest
- Bilateral in approximately 10%

DIAGNOSIS/TREATMENT

- Anteroposterior (AP) and frog-leg lateral view of **both** hips should be obtained.
  - While multiple radiographic stages exist, in the early stages, the femoral head appears small with subchondral lucency and collapse ("crescent sign").
  - If normal radiograph but high index of suspicion—obtain MRI or bone scan.
- Treatment depends on the stage of deformity. Patients should be placed in non–weight bearing status and referred urgently to an orthopedist.

Without proper treatment, early degenerative joint disease occurs with approximately 17% needing total hip replacement. With proper treatment 70%-90% are pain free with good range of motion.

Slipped Capital Femoral Epiphysis

Slipped capital femoral epiphysis (SCFE) refers to posterior and inferior displacement of the proximal femoral epiphysis on the metaphysis. Typical patient is an obese, adolescent boy.

SYMPTOMS/EXAMINATION

- When ambulation is possible (stable SCFE), symptoms are usually insidious.
- When ambulation is NOT possible (unstable SCFE), symptoms are usually acute and associated with a traumatic event.
- Bilateral in 25%-50% of cases.

> **KEY FACT**
>
> Think of the femoral head as an ice cream cone (the epiphyseal portion is the "ice cream"; metaphyseal is the "cone"). The "ice cream" usually stays within the socket (acetabulum) and the "cone" usually slips laterally and anteriorly.

DIAGNOSIS/TREATMENT

- Diagnosis is made with AP and frog-leg lateral radiographs of the hip/pelvis (Figure 5.20).
- **Klein line** (line drawn along the superior border of the femoral neck) should intersect the femoral head; if not, suspect a SCFE.
- Once diagnosed, it is critical that the patient stay non–weight bearing. Stable SCFE requires urgent fixation. Unstable SCFE requires emergent fixation.

COMPLICATIONS

Complications include chondrolysis (~5%), avascular necrosis (10%-15%), nonunion, premature closure of the epiphyseal plate, and degenerative changes.

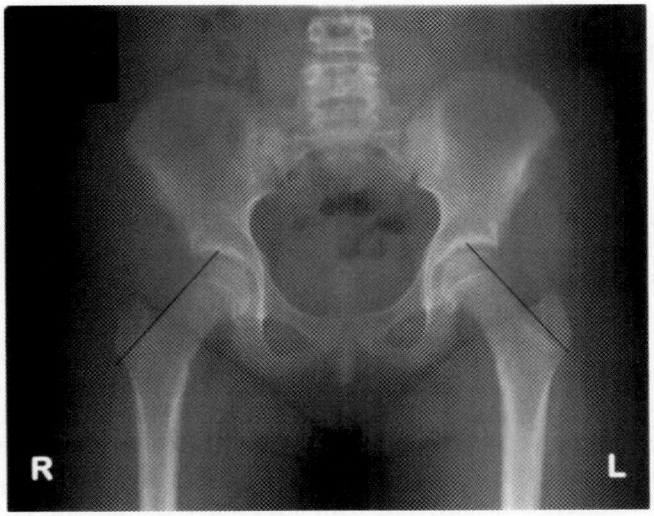

FIGURE 5.20. Klein line. (Reproduced, with permission, from Stead LG, Stead SM, Kaufman MS. *First Aid for the Pediatric Clerkship*. New York, NY: McGraw-Hill; 2004:336.)

Transient Synovitis

Self-limiting, noninfectious, inflammatory reaction in the synovium. **Most common cause of hip pain** in young children. Peak incidence 3-6 years.

SYMPTOMS/EXAMINATION

- Unclear etiology. Preceding URI (~50%) and trauma are often associated.
- Usually well appearing and complaining of hip and/or groin pain, but pain may also be referred to the knee.
- Unilateral (< 5% bilateral).

DIAGNOSIS/TREATMENT

- Diagnosis of exclusion. Radiographs and laboratory evaluations are needed to rule out other etiologies, most notably septic arthritis (see Chapter 4, Orthopedics).
- Treatment consists of joint rest (non–weight bearing) and NSAIDs.
- Prognosis is very good. More than 75% have resolution of pain by 2 weeks.

COMPLICATIONS

Long-term complications are rare but include coxa magna, degenerative changes, and progression to Legg-Calvé-Perthes.

Nursemaid's Elbow (Radial Head Subluxation)

Most common elbow injury in children < 5 years. The proximal radial head is help in place by the overlying annular ligament. It is fairly straight and does not become flared or nodular until approximately 5-6 years of age.

PATHOPHYSIOLOGY

Longitudinal traction on arm with elbow extended → partial slippage of radial head under annular ligament → displacement of annular ligament into radio-capitellar joint.

SYMPTOMS/EXAMINATION

- The child usually cries immediately after the injury and refuses to use the arm.

- Injured arm is held in a characteristic position—held at the side, slightly flexed at the elbow and pronated ("**thumb rotated in toward the body**").
- Usually well appearing, other than refusal to use the arm.
- No visible deformity or swelling of the arm.

Diagnosis

Clinical history and examination are usually sufficient. Radiographs are indicated if there is a history of direct trauma or history inconsistent with nursemaid's elbow, focal tenderness, any swelling, or deformity.

Treatment

- Supination technique: Stabilize the elbow with one hand; while applying pressure to radial head, firmly supinate the forearm, then flex the elbow.
- Hyperpronation technique (**reportedly more successful and less painful**): While holding elbow in extension, firmly pronate the forearm.
- A palpable click is usually felt with successful reduction. The child will typically begin to use the affected arm within several minutes, but may require prompting to do so. If they continue to refuse to use the arm, x-rays should be obtained. If x-rays do not demonstrate a fracture and the child still refusing to use arm, splinting and orthopedic follow-up are appropriate.

> **KEY FACT**
>
> Hyperpronation or supination/flexion can be utilized to reduce a nursemaid's elbow. If there is concern for a fracture, then x-rays should be obtained prior to attempting these maneuvers.

> **KEY FACT**
>
> Salter-Harris type II is the **most common form** of a physeal fracture (75%).

> **KEY FACT**
>
> Children with normal initial radiographs may still have a Salter I fracture; the presence of pain and tenderness over a growth plate should prompt splinting and orthopedic follow-up.

> **MNEMONIC**
>
> ***Salter-Harris fractures:***
>
> **SALTR**
>
> **S** (I) = Slipped epiphysis
> **A** (II) = fracture **A**bove physis
> **L** (III) = fracture be**L**ow physis
> **T** (IV) = fracture **T**hrough physis
> **R** (V) = **R**uined physis

> **KEY FACT**
>
> Children bend and bow, adults snap and break!

Fractures

FRACTURE PATTERNS UNIQUE TO CHILDREN

Physeal Fractures—Salter-Harris Classification System

The Salter-Harris classification is used for physeal injuries only (Figure 5.21). Types I and II have a lower risk of growth arrest.

Plastic Deformation, Greenstick, and Buckle Fractures

These fracture patterns occur almost exclusively in children due to the pliability of bone (Figure 5.22).

Plastic Deformation

- Also known as a **bowing** deformity.
- Mechanism is usually from **longitudinal compression**.
- Clinically, the patient will have a deformity suggesting a fracture. X-rays show a bowing deformity without an obvious break in the bony cortex. Comparison films of the other side may be useful to assess for deformity.
- Patients with plastic deformities should be discussed with and referred to an orthopedic surgeon for evaluation because remodeling is minimal, and these fractures are commonly associated with long-term cosmetic and functional deficits.

Greenstick Fractures

- Mechanism is usually **axial compression with twisting**, such as occurs with falling backward on a supinated or pronated forearm.
- X-rays show an intact bony cortex on one side with a fracture through the cortex on the opposite side (Figure 5.23).
- **Greenstick fractures** may require reduction of the rotational or angular deformity in addition to casting.

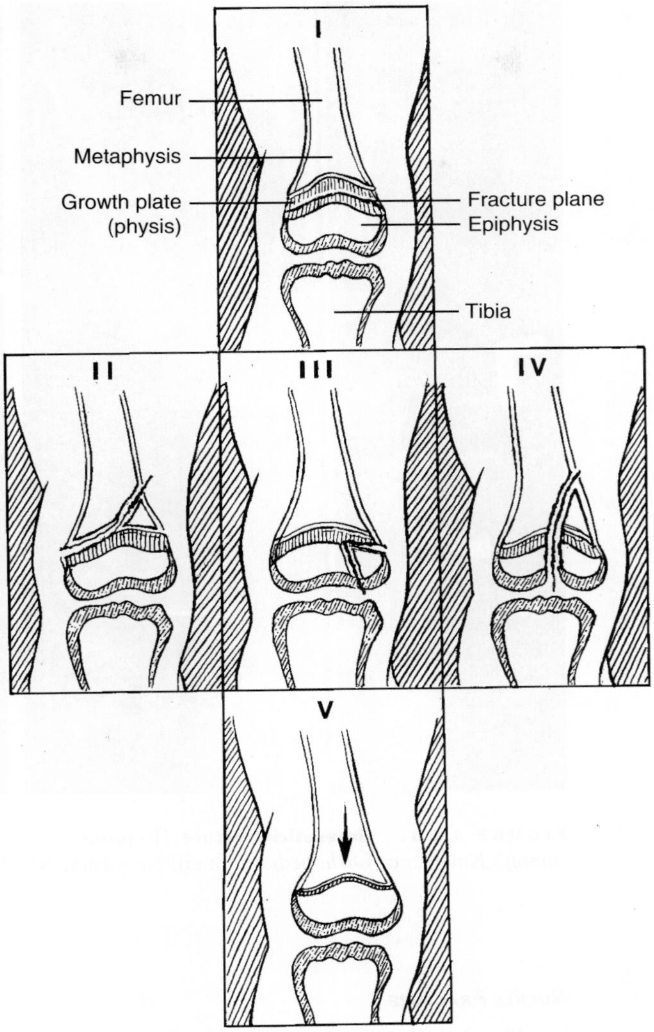

FIGURE 5.21. Salter-Harris classification of fractures. (Reproduced, with permission, from Knoop KJ, Stack LB, Storrow AB, Thurman RJ. *Atlas of Emergency Medicine*. 3rd ed. New York, NY: McGraw-Hill; 2010.)

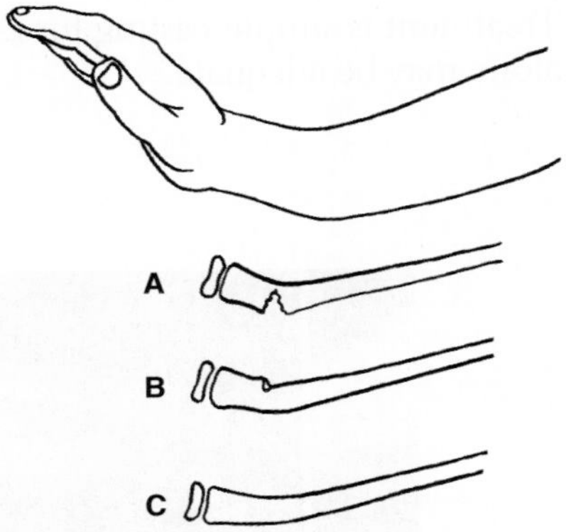

FIGURE 5.22. Pediatric fractures. (**A**) Greenstick fracture. (**B**) Torus fracture. (**C**) Plastic deformation (bowing fracture). (Reproduced, with permission, from Skinner HB. *Current Orthopedics*, 4th ed. New York, NY: McGraw-Hill; 2006:636.)

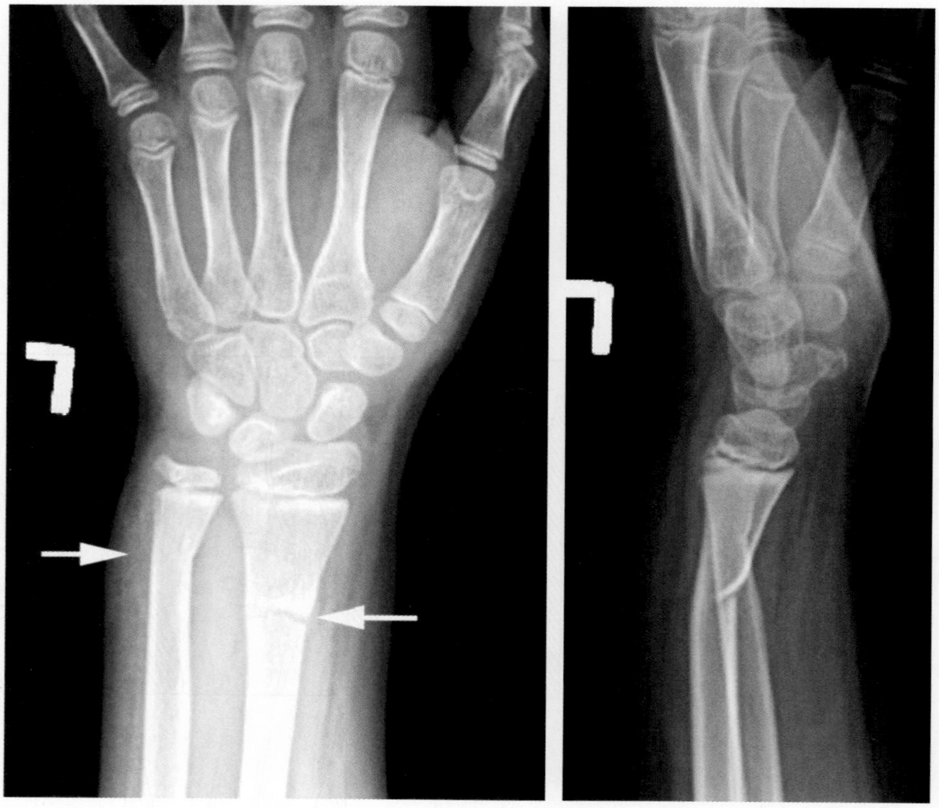

FIGURE 5.23. Greenstick fracture. (Reproduced, with permission, from Sherman S: *Simon's Emergency Orthopedics*. 7th ed. New York, NY: McGraw-Hill Education, 2015.)

BUCKLE FRACTURE

- Also known as a **torus** fracture.
- Mechanism is usually **axial compression**, such as occurs with a fall on an outstretched arm.
- **Most common site is the distal radius**.
- X-rays show a bulging or "buckling" of the bone on the side of the compressive force (Figure 5.24).
- Treatment is simple casting for 2-4 weeks. Recent studies suggest splinting alone may be adequate.

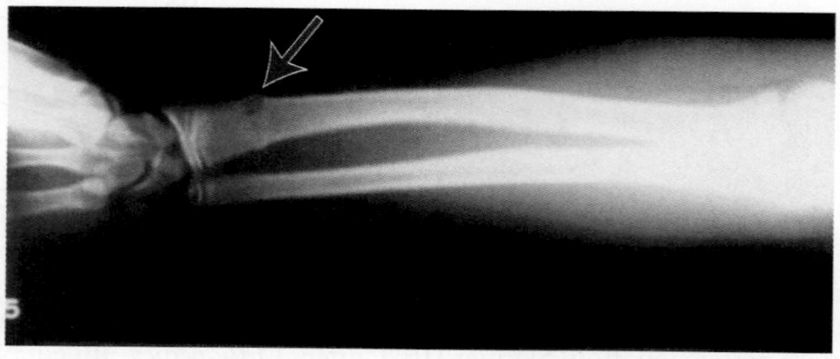

FIGURE 5.24. Torus fracture of the distal radius. (Reproduced, with permission, from Schafermeyer R, Tenenbein M, Macias CG, et al: Strange and Schafermeyer's. *Pediatric Emergency Medicine*. 4th ed. New York, NY: McGraw-Hill Education; 2015.)

Supracondylar Fracture of the Humerus

Symptoms/Examination

- **Most common elbow fracture** in children.
- Most fractures occur in children < 8 because the ligaments are stronger than the bones up to this point.
- Supracondylar fractures occur either by an extension or flexion mechanism.
- **Extension**: Most common (~95%). Hyperextension forces olecranon anteriorly causing displacement of the proximal humerus anteriorly.
- **Flexion**: Elbow is flexed when the distal ulna hits the ground causing energy to be transferred to the distal humerus resulting in anterior displacement of the distal humerus.
- Associated forearm fractures can occur, and it is important to also x-ray distal forearm in child with significant elbow injury.

Diagnosis

AP, lateral, and oblique x-rays of the elbow should be obtained. Most important view is the lateral view with the elbow flexed at 90°.

- Ossification of the elbow is not complete until approximately age 11 (Table 5.31).
- A normal lateral view should show a "figure-eight" or "hour-glass" appearance to the distal humerus with the anterior humeral line bisecting the middle third of the capitellum. A line drawn through the midshaft of the radius should also go through the center of the capitellum (Figure 5.25).
- Abnormal findings in the lateral view that suggest a supracondylar fracture include:
  - Posterior fat pad: Always pathologic.
  - Large anterior fat pad: "Sail sign." Small anterior fat pads can be normal. A normal anterior fat pad should tightly adhere to the distal humerus like a drop of water.
  - Posterior displacement of the capitellum in relation to the anterior humeral line (Figure 5.26).
  - Abnormal Baumann angle: Angle formed between the anterior humeral line and the radiocapitellar line. This should be approximately 75°.
- Classification of supracondylar fractures:
  - Type I: Nondisplaced fracture with anterior and posterior periostea intact).

MNEMONIC

Ossification centers of the pediatric elbow:

"CRITOE"—age of appearance of ossification center

Capitellum: 1 year
Radial head: 3 years
Internal (**m**edial) epicondyle: 5 years
Trochlea: 7 years
Olecranon: 9 years
External (**l**ateral) epicondyle: 11 years

TABLE 5.31. Sequence of Appearance of Ossification Centers of the Elbow

Ossification Center	Approximate Age of Appearance (add 1 y for boys)
Capitellum (*C*)	1 y old
Radial head (*R*)	3 y old
Medial epicondyle (*I*)	5 y old
Trochlea (*T*)	7 y old
Olecranon (*O*)	9 y old
Lateral epicondyle (*E*)	11 y old

(Reproduced, with permission, from Tintinalli JE, Stapczynski JS, Ma OJ, et al. *Tintinalli's Emergency Medicine*. 7th ed. New York, NY: McGraw-Hill; 2011:898.)

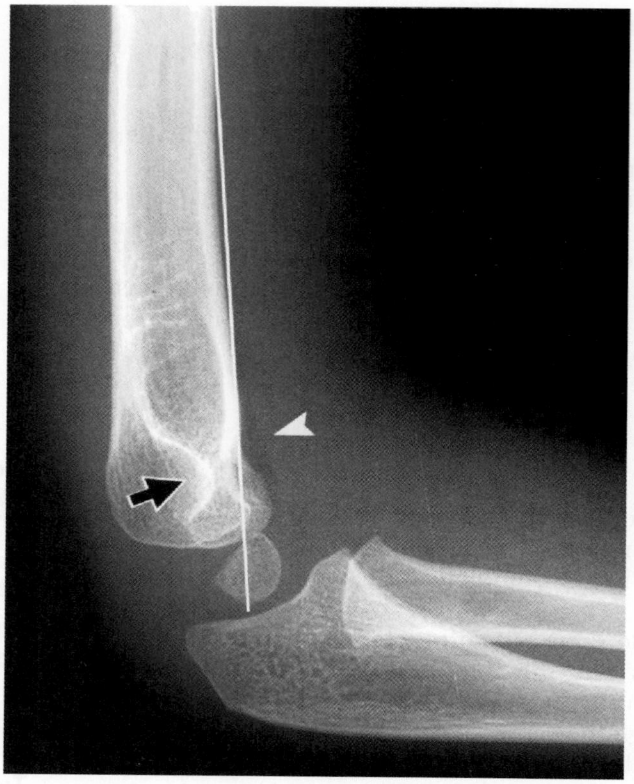

FIGURE 5.25. Anterior humeral line. A line drawn along the anterior cortex of the humeral shaft normally intersects the middle third of the capitellum. A normal radiographic teardrop is seen where the cortices of the olecranon and coronoid fossae come together (black arrow). A small normal anterior fat pad is visible (arrowhead). (Reproduced, with permission, from Schwartz D. *Emergency Radiology Case Studies*. New York, NY: McGraw-Hill; 2008.)

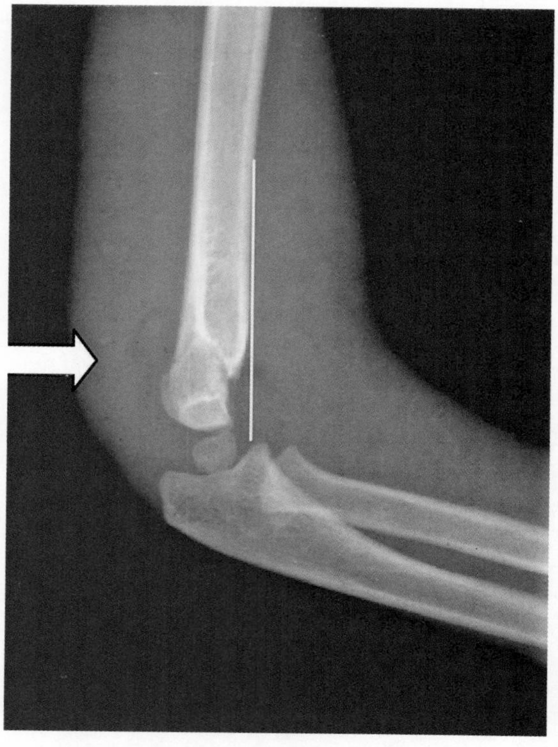

FIGURE 5.26. Supracondylar fracture of the humerus. Note displaced fat pads (arrow) signifying joint effusion. A line along the anterior cortex of the humerus should pass through the middle third of the capitellum on a true lateral view for a normal elbow.

- Type II: Displaced fracture with posterior periosteum intact. The anterior humeral line is displaced toward the anterior portion of the capitellum.
- Type III: Displaced fracture with disruption of the humerul periosteum anteriorly and posteriorly, a "through and through" fracture.

TREATMENT

- Treatment depends on the type of supracondylar fracture.
- Nondisplaced fractures: Posterior long arm splint with elbow at 90° and forearm in neutral (pronation) position followed by urgent follow-up with orthopedic surgeon. Repeat films after splinting should be obtained to assess for any new displacement prior to discharge.
- Displaced fractures require orthopedic consult for immediate reduction and/or operative repair.

COMPLICATIONS

- Complications are seen with high frequency in displaced fractures and include median nerve injury (anterior interosseus branch), radial nerve injury, and brachial artery injury.
- Compartment syndrome: Mostly seen with associated brachial artery injuries.
- Volkmann's ischemic contracture: The result of muscle necrosis in untreated forearm compartment syndrome.

KEY FACT

The anterior interosseous nerve is the most commonly injured nerve with a supracondylar fracture. Function of this nerve can be assessed by asking children to make the "OK" sign with their fingers.

Clavicle Fracture

The clavicle is one of the most frequently fractured bones in children and young adults because the physis doesn't close until early 20s. Most result from direct falls onto the shoulder/clavicle region.

- Midshaft (~80%) fractures are the most common.
- Medial third fractures are rare but can cause vascular injuries especially if displaced posteriorly.
- Treatment is usually rest, ice, simple sling and pain control. There is no benefit to figure-eight splinting.
- Distal fractures may require surgery if the coracoclavicular ligament is ruptured.
- Neonatal clavicular fractures are treated by swathing the arm.

KEY FACT

Only with significant tenting of the skin or displacement clavicle fractures require reduction or treatment beyond a sling. Younger children can tolerate much more displacement before operative repair than older, school-aged children and adolescents.

Monteggia Fracture

A Monteggia fracture is a fracture of the proximal ulna with dislocation of the radial head (see Figure 4.13).

- Isolated ulna fractures are rare in children. If found, imaging of the elbow is necessary to rule out a Monteggia fracture.
- The radial head should align with the capitellum in all elbow radiographs (see Figure 4.6). If it does not, a radial head dislocation should be suspected.
- Treatment involves immediate reduction and splinting. Surgery may be needed for repair of the ulna fracture, but closed reduction is often satisfactory in children.

Galeazzi Fracture

A Galeazzi fracture is a fracture of the radial shaft with an associated distal radioulnar joint dislocation (see Figure 4.12).

- Galeazzi fracture requires orthopedic intervention with open reduction and surgical pinning.

KEY FACT

Young children with lower leg pain but no fracture on standard x-rays, should have oblique x-rays obtained, because these will often demonstrate a toddler's fracture.

Toddler's Fracture

A toddler's fracture, now called a "childhood accidental spiral tibial" (CAST) fracture, is an oblique nondisplaced fracture caused by low-energy torsion, most commonly on the distal tibia.

- Child often presents with a limp often after seemingly minor or unrecognized trauma (going down slide, running and falling).
- AP, lateral, and oblique views are often needed to isolate the fracture.
- If CAST fracture suspected but no fracture seen, the child should be splinted and radiographs repeated in 1 week.
- Treatment of a toddler's fracture requires casting.
- Midshaft fractures, tibial fractures in nonambulating children, and fractures with a suspicious history of mechanism should prompt consideration for nonaccidental trauma.

MNEMONIC

Causes of apnea and bradycardia in infants:

HAS CRASH

Hypoglycemia
Aspiration
Sepsis (infections: respiratory syncytial virus [RSV], pertussis)
Cardiac arrhythmias
Reflux
Anemia
Seizures
Hydrocephalus

Pulmonary Disorders

ACUTE LIFE-THREATENING EVENT

An acute life-threatening event (ALTE) is defined as an acute, otherwise unexplained change in an infant's breathing, behavior, or appearance that causes the caretaker to be frightened. It may involve apnea or decreased respiratory rate, a change in color such as pallor or cyanosis, a change in muscular tone such as limpness or rigidity, or an episode of choking or gagging. ALTEs encompass a heterogeneous range of presentations, with causes that range from the benign to the life threatening. Clinically, the history is crucial for determining the severity of an event and the degree of evaluation required.

Symptoms/Examination

In the ED, all symptoms usually have resolved and the infant often has an unremarkable physical examination.

Diagnosis

- An accurate history is essential. It is important to know the length of the event, preceding symptoms or feedings, prior similar episodes, color change, associated movements or changes in tone, and resuscitative efforts.
- Supporting data including serum glucose, electrolytes, and an ECG may be helpful.
- CBC, blood and urine cultures only if signs of infection.
- Imaging should only be performed as dictated by the history and physical examination (eg, brain CT only if concern for ICH).

Treatment

- Supportive, with specific therapy directed toward the cause of the event.
- Disposition is dictated by the patient's history and appearance. Inpatient monitoring is recommended for the following patients:
  - Those who appear unwell, toxic, have poor tone, respiratory distress, or recurrent vomiting.
  - Patients who have signs of trauma, failure to thrive, or any suspicion for abuse.
  - Those with a history of prior ALTE, particularly within the preceding 24 hours.
  - A family history of a significant ALTE or death in a sibling.
  - Patients with congenital abnormalities.
  - Patients who had a severe ALTE (sustained loss of consciousness, apnea, or cyanosis), or who required resuscitation efforts such as rescue breaths or CPR.

BREATH-HOLDING SPELLS

These involuntary periods of apnea are often associated with color change, loss of consciousness, or postural tone in children usually between 6 months and 5 years of age. First event typically occurs before the age of 2 years. They typically develop in response to frightening or painful event and are often preceded by intense crying that suddenly stops as the patient becomes apneic. Breath-holding spells can run in families.

Symptoms

- Loss of consciousness
- Pallor or cyanosis
- May become limp or have associated clonic jerks
- No postictal period
- Inciting stimulus–anger, frustration, fear, or pain
- Last < 1 minute

Examination

Normal examination.

Differential

- Seizures: Unlike seizures, with breath holding the color change precedes the motor activity
- Syncope
- Arrhythmia
- Apnea

Diagnosis

- Clinical diagnosis
- Hemoglobin, may be associated with anemia
- ECG if any concern for arrhythmia

Treatment

- Reassure parents, and educate them that spells often recur, only terminating as children reach 5 years of age. During repeat episodes, parents should lay the patient in the lateral decubitus position and ensure their airway is clear.
- A study suggests iron supplementation may reduce recurrence, but this therapy should not be initiated in the ED.

> **Q**
>
> A 2-year-old boy becomes upset after his parents take away a favorite toy. He cries vigorously, then becomes limp, cyanotic, and his parents describe seizure-like activity. Upon arrival in the ED, he is alert with normal vital signs and a normal physical examination. What is the appropriate ED workup?

BRONCHOPULMONARY DYSPLASIA

Infants with bronchopulmonary dysplasia (BPD) received supplemental O_2 for the first 28 days of life and have characteristic radiographic findings. The condition arises from repeated episodes of injury and inflammation. Risk factors for BPD include prematurity, positive pressure ventilation, and genetic predisposition. BPD is becoming more common because more infants survive after being born prematurely. Infants with BPD usually present to the ED with acute deterioration of their chronic lung disease, often arising from viral respiratory infections such as respiratory syncytial virus (RSV).

Symptoms/Examination

- Respiratory distress.
- Tachypnea.
- Hypoxia is common.
- Crackles, rhonchi, wheezes, or decreased breath sounds.

A

Reassurance and education for breath-holding spell.

Diagnosis

- Clinical diagnosis.
- Baseline chest x-ray often shows hyperinflation, cystic areas, and signs of fibrosis—look for changes from prior radiographs to suggest pneumonia.

Treatment

- Supportive care with supplemental oxygen and suctioning.
- Trial of inhaled bronchodilators/corticosteroids and diuretics.
- IV fluids for patients who are dehydrated.
- Admit unless only extremely small degree of hypoxia or change from baseline.

Complications

- Apnea, hypercarbia, or hypoxemia
- Dehydration
- Cor pulmonale

ASPIRATION PNEUMONIA

When foreign material enters the lung, it causes inflammation and chemical injury. Aspiration can also lead to development of a bacterial pneumonia or an abscess from anaerobic organisms. It can be difficult to distinguish pneumonitis from pneumonia based on the clinical presentation. Children with impaired swallowing mechanisms from altered consciousness or chronic medical conditions are particularly prone to aspiration.

Symptoms/Examination

- Asymptomatic for approximately 30 minutes after aspiration event
- Fever
- Cough
- Tachypnea, respiratory distress
- Focal findings on auscultation

Diagnosis

X-ray may be normal initially and later show infiltrate either from pneumonitis or infection.

Treatment

- Supportive care with suctioning, oxygen, and positive pressure ventilation as needed.
- A reasonable initial approach is to defer antibiotic treatment in favor of careful observation and empirically treat only those with a tenuous respiratory status or compelling evidence of infection.
- Admission—including asymptomatic patients because they will often worsen within 24 hours.

PLEURAL EFFUSION

Excess fluid may accumulate in the pleural space leading to pleuritic chest pain, shortness of breath, and abnormalities on x-ray. Exudative effusions arise from increased capillary permeability or lymphatic obstruction from infections or neoplasms. Transudative effusions arise from increased capillary hydrostatic pressure from CHF, cirrhosis, nephritic syndrome, or hypoproteinemia.

Symptoms

- Pleuritic chest pain
- Shortness of breath
- Cough

Examination

- Decreased breath sounds
- Dullness to percussion

Diagnosis

- X-ray showing blunting of costophrenic angle can identify effusions as small as 50 mL.
- Decubitus x-ray will show layering of free-flowing fluid.
- Ultrasound helps determine effusion size, location, and presence of loculations.
- Thoracentesis: Protein, glucose, cell counts, LDH, pH, Gram stain, culture.

Treatment

- If pleural fluid is grossly purulent, has + Gram stain, glucose < 60 mg/dL, or pH < 7.2, surgical management with thoracostomy tube should be considered.
- Ultrasound can aid in diagnosis, thoracentesis, and chest tube placement.

> **KEY FACT**
>
> Pigtail chest tubes are replacing thoracentesis because they allow ongoing drainage if needed.

CYSTIC FIBROSIS

Cystic fibrosis (CF) is the **most common lethal congenital condition** in the United States, occurring in roughly 1 in 2500 Caucasians. It is extremely rare in other ethnic groups. The most common cause is the F508 deletion that causes impaired chloride and water transport, resulting in thick, dry secretions. These dry secretions produce chronic inflammation and infection in the respiratory tract, GI tract, and sweat glands.

Symptoms

- Frequent lung and sinus infections.
- Chest pain due to pleurisy, pneumonia, spontaneous pneumothorax, or gastroesophageal reflux disease (GERD).
- Shortness of breath related to respiratory tract infection or allergic bronchopulmonary aspergillosis.
- Hemoptysis due to infection or erosion into pulmonary vessel.
- Abdominal pain from constipation, obstruction, pancreatitis, cholecystitis GERD, malabsorption. There is an increased incidence of rectal prolapse.
- Failure to thrive and fatty stools due to malabsorption of fats.

Examination

- Increased AP diameter of the chest
- Small size for age
- Wheezing or focal findings on auscultation

Diagnosis

- Meconium ileus of newborn is virtually diagnostic. Most other cases are identified on newborn screening.
- Diagnosis is confirmed with sweat chloride testing.
- Children typically present to the ED with exacerbations of known CF.
- X-ray compared to prior imaging to look for pneumonia.
- Chemistries to assess for hyperglycemia or dehydration (often hyponatremic, hypochloremia).

TREATMENT

- Antibiotics: Inhaled and oral antibiotics tailored to particular pathogens of patient, typically require coverage of *Pseudomonas* sp
- Aggressive pulmonary hygiene
- Steroids for bronchospasm or allergic bronchopulmonary aspergillosis
- Consultation with pulmonology

COMPLICATIONS

- Respiratory failure
- Hemoptysis and/or massive pulmonary hemorrhage
- Dehydration
- Electrolyte abnormalities
- GI obstruction, specifically distal intestinal obstruction syndrome (DIOS)
- GI bleeding

ASTHMA

(See also Chapter 10, Thoracic and Respiratory Disorders.)

Asthma is the **most common chronic medical condition in children**. Often patients present to the ED with only mild exacerbations, but asthma can be life threatening. A history of ICU admission, intubation, multiple admissions in the past year, low socioeconomic status, and comorbidities place patients at risk for potentially deadly complications from asthma.

Asthma arises from chronic inflammation of the lower airways. Acute exacerbations result from the **triad** of airway inflammation (often with mucus plugging), bronchial hyperresponsiveness, and intermittent reversible airway obstruction. **Triggers** of asthma flares include viral URIs, cold weather, exercise, cigarette smoking, and other allergens (eg, dust mites, cockroaches). Younger children are particularly prone to status asthmaticus due to smaller airway diameters, lower respiratory reserves, and decreased elastic recoil.

SYMPTOMS/EXAMINATION

- Patients typically present with wheezing and respiratory distress, although there may be absence of wheezing in severe exacerbations due to limited air movement.
- Patients with cough-variant asthma may present with persistent cough that is worse at night.

DIFFERENTIAL

Wheezing does not always mean asthma! Other causes of wheezing are listed in the Table 5.32.

TABLE 5.32. Differential Diagnosis of Wheezing

Infection	Pneumonia Bronchiolitis
Allergy	Asthma Anaphylaxis
Cardiac	Pulmonary edema
Other	Foreign body aspiration BPD Bronchiectasis Vocal cord dysfunction

BPD, bronchopulmonary dysplasia.

DIAGNOSIS

- Mainly a clinical diagnosis
- Peak expiratory flow rate (PEFR) before and after treatment
- CXR if focal findings after therapy, failure to respond to therapy, or concern for foreign body or pneumothorax

TREATMENT

- O_2 as needed, to achieve $Spo_2 > 94\%$
- Mild exacerbation (FEV_1 or PEFR < 70% predicted):
  - Inhaled β-agonists (albuterol) and anticholinergic agents (ipratropium) by metered dose inhaler (MDI) or nebulizer
  - Oral corticosteroids

- Moderate exacerbation (FEV_1 or PEFR 40%-69% predicted):
  - Inhaled β-agonists (albuterol) and anticholinergics (ipratropium) by MDI or nebulizer with progression to possible continuous neb
  - Inhaled anticholinergics (ipratropium)
  - Oral or IV corticosteroids
  - IV magnesium (infuse over 20 minutes)
- Severe exacerbation (FEV_1 or PEFR < 40% predicted):
  - Inhaled β-agonists (albuterol) and anticholinergics (ipratropium) by nebulizer with progression to possible continuous neb
  - IV corticosteroids
  - IV magnesium
  - IV ketamine drip with or without loading dose (doses may vary 0.3-1mg/kg/h)
  - Consider heliox as temporizing measure
  - Consider IV terbutaline and noninvasive positive pressure ventilation adjuncts
  - Consider intubation: Use ketamine as induction agent (bronchodilates), tidal volumes of 6-10 mL/kg and long expiratory times (4-8 seconds); continue bronchodilation with short-acting β-agonists
- If well appearing 60-120 minutes after last treatment (Sao_2 > 91%, PEFR > 50% predicted, no distress), consider discharge on 5-day course of steroids with close follow-up.

COMPLICATIONS

- Pneumothorax
- Pneumomediastinum
- Hypokalemia from prolonged albuterol

INFECTIOUS DISORDERS

Epiglottitis

Epiglottitis is a life-threatening bacterial infection of the supraglottic space that can lead to significant inflammation and obstruction of the airway. Classically caused by Hib but since implementation of Hib vaccine, most cases are now due to streptococcal and staphylococcal species. Epiglottitis is most common in children between the ages of three and eight and in adults.

SYMPTOMS

Abrupt onset and rapid progression of fever, drooling, sore throat, and irritability often with hoarse, "hot potato" voice.

EXAMINATION

- Patient is anxious appearing, sitting upright with head in sniffing position.
- Soft inspiratory or biphasic stridor may be present.

DIAGNOSIS

- Do not attempt to visualize the pharynx unless can be done with minimal agitation and without a tongue blade.
- Lateral neck x-ray will show a swollen epiglottis (thumbprint sign); x-ray should not delay definitive management.
- Laboratory tests should be deferred until the airway is secure.

TREATMENT

- If impending airway occlusion, consult anesthesia/ENT stat, prepare for difficult intubation, and have surgical airway equipment at bedside.

Q

A 6-year-old boy with a history of asthma presents to the ED in severe respiratory distress. In the ED, he has already received inhaled bronchodilators, steroids, and magnesium, without any significant improvement. His RR is 45 breaths/min and O_2 saturation is 89% on a 100% Fio_2 albuterol neb. What additional medication should he receive?

A

Epinephrine 1:1000, intramuscularly, at a dose of 0.01 mg/kg (maximum single dose of 0.3 mg).

KEY FACT

Most stridor is due to croup but in the anxious, ill-appearing, or older child, consider epiglottitis, bacterial tracheitis, or foreign body aspiration and prepare for a potential airway emergency.

- Place patient in position of comfort and administer O_2.
- Place IV and administer ceftriaxone **only** if patient is cooperative.
- Transfer to operating room (OR) for definitive diagnosis with direct visualization and intubation.

Croup

Laryngotracheobronchitis is a viral infection of the upper airway most commonly caused by parainfluenza, but other viruses (influenza, RSV, rhinovirus) have also been implicated. It is most common during the winter in children < 3 years.

Symptoms/Examination

- Gradual onset of illness with barky cough, coryza, fever.
- Symptoms typically peak on days 3-4 of illness.
- Severe croup is characterized by prominent inspiratory stridor, marked sternal retractions, respiratory distress, and agitation.
- Lower lungs are clear with no wheezing.

Differential

- Other causes of stridor: Foreign body aspiration, hemangiomas, papillomas, subglottic stenosis
- Bacterial tracheitis
- Epiglottitis

Diagnosis

- Clinical diagnosis.
- Soft tissue neck x-ray may reveal classical "**steeple sign**" due to symmetric narrow of the supraglottic airway (Figure 5.27) but more often is normal.

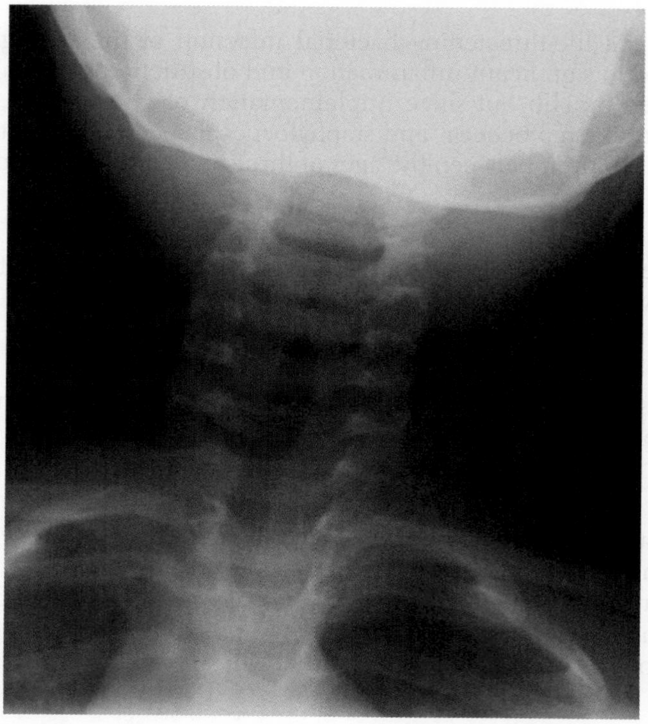

FIGURE 5.27. Steeple sign of croup. (Reproduced, with permission, from Shah BR, Lucchesi M. *Atlas of Pediatric Emergency Medicine*. New York, NY: McGraw-Hill; 2006:241.)

- Routine radiography is not necessary in patients of appropriate age for croup with history and examination consistent with croup.

TREATMENT

- Supplemental humidified O_2 and cool mist may be used in hospitalized patients but have not been shown to improve outcomes.
- A single dose of **oral dexamethasone** has 0.6 mg/kg been shown to be as effective as IM dexamethasone and should be given to all patients.
- **Epinephrine nebs** should be given to patients with stridor at rest or significant respiratory distress. Patients given an epinephrine neb should be observed for 2-4 hours to monitor for return of stridor. β-Agonists should not be used in the treatment of croup because they may worsen the airway edema.
- If impending respiratory compromise, consider trial of heliox.
- If intubation is necessary, use an endotracheal tube at least half a size smaller than calculated.
- Admit for ongoing stridor at rest or increased work of breathing despite initial treatments.

COMPLICATIONS

- Upper airway obstruction
- Dehydration

Bacterial Tracheitis

Bacterial tracheitis is a severe form of laryngotracheobronchitis caused by bacterial superinfection of the trachea with copious purulent tracheal secretions and membranes. *S aureus* (including MRSA) is the most commonly isolated organism, but many others have been identified (Hib, nontypeable *H influenzae*, *Moraxella*, *Peptostreptococcus*, *Fusobacterium*, anaerobes).

SYMPTOMS/EXAMINATION

- Typically preceded by a viral illness for a few days
- May be seen after infection with influenza
- Fever, often > 39°C (102.2°F)
- Rapid and severe biphasic stridor with toxic appearance
- Typically little response to therapy
- Often have foreign body sensation in lower throat/neck or sore throat
- Cough or raspy, hoarse voice

DIFFERENTIAL

Includes epiglottitis, croup, retropharyngeal abscess, viral URI, and foreign body in airway. See also Table 5.33.

DIAGNOSIS

- High index of suspicion based on clinical grounds.
- Soft-tissue neck x-ray showing subglottic tracheal narrowing with a shaggy rough-appearing tracheal lining.
- Bronchoscopy confirms diagnosis.

TREATMENT

- Similar to epiglottitis: Place patient in position of comfort, administer supplemental oxygen, pursue direct visualization and intubation only in OR.

KEY FACT

Neck radiographs in croup may show the classical "**steeple sign**" due to symmetric narrowing of the trachea.

KEY FACT

Stridor in a child > 4 years or who does not respond to standard therapy should raise concern for foreign body aspiration or bacterial tracheitis in an ill-appearing child with fevers.

KEY FACT

Inspiratory stridor = obstruction above larynx

Expiratory stridor = bronchial or tracheal obstruction

Wheezing = obstruction in bronchi

TABLE 5.33. Most Common Infectious Causes of Stridor in Children

	Epiglottitis	Bacterial Tracheitis	Croup
Anatomy	Supraglottic	Subglottic	Subglottic
Pathology	*Staphylococcus* sp *Streptococcus* sp	*S aureus* Other aerobes and anerobes	Parainfluenza
Age	3-8 y	< 3 y	< 3 y
Onset	Sudden	Sudden after URI	Gradual
Stridor	Inspiratory	Biphasic	Inspiratory
Drooling	+	–	–
Cough	–	+	+ (barky)
X-ray	Thumbprint	Tracheal narrowing with rough lining	Steeple sign
Treatment	OR for visualization	OR for visualization	Dexamethasone ± neb epinephrine

OR, operating room; URI, upper respiratory infection.

- If impending airway occlusion, consult anesthesia/ENT stat, prepare for intubation, and have surgical airway equipment at bedside.
- Administer antibiotics including coverage for MRSA (ceftriaxone ± vancomycin) **only** if patient is cooperative with IV placement.

KEY FACT

Recent croup in a toxic-appearing patient = bacterial tracheitis

Complication

Airway obstruction.

Retropharyngeal abscess

Children < 4 years can develop infection in the potential space between the esophagus and cervical spine. Most commonly caused by GAS, *S aureus*, and anaerobes.

Symptoms/Examination

- Fever, often > 39°C (102.2°F) and sore throat.
- Hoarseness, drooling, neck pain may develop.
- Can progress to toxic appearance.
- Swelling of posterior pharynx is difficult to visualize on examination and oropharynx often appears normal.

Diagnosis

- Lateral neck x-ray showing soft tissue widening anterior to cervical vertebrae (more than one-third width of adjacent vertebral body). Ensure that x-ray is obtained **during inspiration with neck in extension** to prevent false positives.
- CT of neck with contrast if high suspicion or neck x-ray abnormal.

TREATMENT

- Monitor airway closely.
- Antibiotics with MRSA coverage (IV clindamycin).
- Consult ENT for potential surgical drainage.

Peritonsillar Abscess

Children and adolescents with sore throat should be assessed for peritonsillar abscess. This occurs typically because of streptococcal pharyngitis, though the abscess itself is often polymicrobial.

SYMPTOMS/EXAMINATION

- Unilateral tonsillar swelling, sometimes with uvular deviation toward the contralateral side.
- Patients may develop trismus, drooling, pain with swallowing, and unilateral neck/ear pain.

DIAGNOSIS

- Diagnosis is typically made based on clinical history and examination.
- In uncertain cases, the presence or absence of purulent material on needle aspiration can confirm the diagnosis and differentiate peritonsillar abscess from cellulitis.

TREATMENT

- Supportive care with analgesics.
- IV fluids if there has been poor PO intake.
- Single dose of dexamethasone PO/IV/IM to reduce swelling.
- Antibiotics, usually clindamycin to cover MRSA.
- Needle aspiration or incision and drainage.
- Rapid ENT consultation should be obtained if there is any concern for airway occlusion.

Pertussis

Bordetella pertussis causes an infection of the lower airways leading to whooping cough. It is most common in unimmunized younger children but also is found in adolescents.

SYMPTOMS

- Catarrhal stage: Initial stage of cough, conjunctivitis, coryza for 1-2 weeks.
- Paroxysmal stage: Classic spasms of cough followed by "whoop" sound from sudden inspiration of air, lasting for 2-4 weeks. Young children cannot generate sufficient force to produce the whoop. Post-tussive emesis is common.
- Convalescent stage: Chronic cough.

EXAMINATION

Normal except during coughing spells.

DIAGNOSIS

- Clinical.
- Chest x-ray: Classically shows shaggy right heart border but more often unremarkable.
- Nasopharyngeal culture or PCR of nasopharyngeal secretions is confirmative.

KEY FACT

Lateral neck x-rays often result in false positives for retropharyngeal abscess, if they are taken during expiration or with the patient's neck in flexion.

KEY FACT

Young children with pertussis will have spasms of cough but do not generate the classic "whoop."

Treatment

- Antibiotics (azithromycin)
- Chemoprophylaxis with azithromycin for close contacts
- Admit if < 6 months
- Report to local health authorities

Complications

- Apnea
- Airway obstruction
- Pneumonia

Bronchiolitis

Bronchiolitis is an infection of the lower airways that leads to sloughing of the respiratory epithelium and obstruction in the lower airways. It is **most commonly caused by RSV** but also other viruses including adenovirus, parainfluenza, rhinovirus, influenza, and metapneumovirus. Affected children are usually < 2 years old, with the most severely affected being premature infants and infants < 6 months old. The peak incidence is winter to spring. Symptoms may last 2-4 weeks.

Symptoms/Examination

- 1-2 days of URI symptoms with fever, rhinorrhea, and cough, followed by wheezing, tachypnea (retractions, nasal flaring that can progress to grunting), and respiratory distress.
- Tachypnea often leads to decreased oral intake and dehydration.
- Hypoxia can be present.
- Apnea may occur in infants particularly premature infants.

KEY FACT

Bronchiolitis lasts for a median duration of 2 weeks but 25% of patients have symptoms for > 3 weeks.

Differential

- Pneumonia
- Asthma exacerbation
- Aspirated foreign body

Diagnosis

- Clinical diagnosis based on symptoms/examination
- Rapid antigen testing of nasopharyngeal sample as needed for cohorting in the hospital or risk stratification in the evaluation of infantile fever
- CXR not routinely required unless diagnosis uncertain or child ill enough for ICU—hyperinflation, peribronchial cuffing, and atelectasis

KEY FACT

Unlike URIs, patients with bronchiolitis will have lower respiratory tract findings: crackles and coarse or high pitched wheezing on auscultation.

Treatment

- Supplemental O_2 and suctioning.
- The latest guidelines do not recommend the routine use of nebulized β-agonists, epinephrine, or hypertonic saline in the ED.
- Consider hypertonic saline if patient requires admission to the hospital.
- Admission for supportive therapy if hypoxia, respiratory distress, comorbidities, or apnea present.

KEY FACT

Risk factors for apnea and therefore need for admission with bronchiolitis include age < 1 month, preterm birth and corrected age < 2 months, low birth weight, high or low respiratory rate, and report of any apneic episode.

Complications

- Apnea or respiratory failure
- Dehydration

Pneumonia

Pneumonia is a lower respiratory tract infection caused **most commonly by viruses** but also bacteria. *S pneumoniae* is common in younger children and *M pneumoniae* in children > 5 years (Table 5.34).

TABLE 5.34. Etiology of Pneumonia in Children

< 1 mo	Bacteria: Group B streptococci, *E coli, S aureus, C trachomatis* Viruses: CMV, rubella, HSV, RSV
1 mo-5 y	Viruses: RSV, influenza, parainfluenza, adenovirus Bacteria: *S pneumoniae, S aureus, H influenzae*
> 5 y	Viruses: Adenovirus, influenza Bacteria: *S pneumoniae, M pneumoniae*

CMV, cytomegalovirus; HSV, herpes simplex virus; RSV, respiratory syncytial virus.

SYMPTOMS/EXAMINATION

- Symptoms are variable and depend on the age of the child and severity of illness. Young infants may present only with fever, dehydration, and/or tachypnea.
- Cough: The cough of *C trachomatis* is classically described as "staccato" and may cause paroxysms similar to pertussis.
- Rales or decreased breath sounds.

DIAGNOSIS

- CXR: Lobar consolidation suggests bacterial pneumonia, while diffuse interstitial infiltrate or peribronchial cuffing suggests viral or *M pneumoniae* infection.
- WBC count may be elevated but nonspecific and not needed routinely.

TREATMENT

- Antibiotics: For young children, who are at risk for *S pneumoniae*, high-dose amoxicillin. For older children with concern for *M pneumoniae*, azithromycin.
- Any child discharged with the diagnosis of pneumonia should be reevaluated in 24-48 hours to ensure appropriate response to therapy.
- Admission should be considered for young infants, those with comorbidities, pleural effusion, dehydration, respiratory distress, or failure of outpatient therapy.

COMPLICATIONS

- High risk of dehydration.
- Bacteremia, with risk of developing second-degree infections, such as meningitis or septic arthritis, particularly in infants.
- Empyema or pleural effusion.
- Respiratory failure is possible but less common than with other lower respiratory tract infections.

KEY FACT

Children with lower lobe pneumonias may present with abdominal pain.

KEY FACT

Mycoplasma pneumoniae pneumonia is often associated with pharyngitis, otitis media, and rashes.

KEY FACT

Pleural effusions should raise concern for *S aureus* or MRSA. These patients should receive clindamycin and/or vancomycin.

Sudden Infant Death Syndrome

Sudden infant death syndrome (SIDS) is the unexplained death of an infant < 1 year. Peak incidence is ages 2-5 months. Ninety percent of all cases occur in infants before the age of 6 months.

PATHOPHYSIOLOGY

The etiology of SIDS is unclear. Some evidence suggests SIDS may be related to apnea, accidental suffocation, or an immature ability to respond to noxious stimuli (such as rising serum CO_2 and falling serum O_2). Fewer than 5% of cases are thought to be due to child abuse.

RISK FACTORS

- Sleeping in prone position
- Young maternal age
- Mother who smokes (during pregnancy or postnatally)
- Cosleeping
- Infants sleeping on excessively soft surface or with objects that may accidentally occlude airway (such as pillows, toys, loose bedding)
- Excessive ambient heat
- Prematurity
- Male sex
- Possibly a family history of SIDS (such as sibling who died from SIDS) may increase risk; consider child abuse if > 2 siblings with SIDS

SYMPTOMS/EXAMINATION

Infant is typically found lifeless in crib.

TREATMENT

- Support for family.
- No known treatment other than prevention.
- **"Back to sleep"** is the recommendation that infants sleep on their backs. Since the introduction of this campaign, the incidence of SIDS has decreased by > 40%.
- Encourage maternal smoking cessation.

Trauma

Trauma is the leading cause of death in children > 1 year.

HEAD TRAUMA

> **KEY FACT**
>
> Growing skull fractures present weeks to months after the initial injury with swelling over the fracture site. They result from a tear in the dura during the initial injury that allows brain parenchyma to herniate through the fracture site and prevent healing. They require surgical repair.

Most commonly due to falls in younger children and **MVAs or sporting accidents** in older children.

PATHOPHYSIOLOGY

Primary brain injury occurs from direct neuronal injury following the trauma. Secondary injury results from cerebral ischemia due to reduced cerebral blood flow. Blood flow is determined by the cerebral perfusion pressure (CPP), which in turn is determined by the mean arterial pressure (MAP) and ICP (CPP = MAP – ICP). In normal children, CPP is 50 mm Hg (MAP of 70 and ICP < 20 mm Hg). Following head injury, the volume in the skull often increases due to bleeding or edema leading to elevations in ICP that reduce CPP.

SYMPTOMS/EXAMINATION

- In minor head injury, patients often show only minimal symptoms. Less than 50% of infants with intracranial injury manifest the usual signs and symptoms such as decreased consciousness, vomiting, or lethargy.

- Nonfrontal scalp hematomas in children < 2 years increase risk of brain injury.
- Signs of elevated ICP include bradycardia, hypertension, and bradypnea.

DIAGNOSIS

In children, CT of the brain has more adverse side effects than in adults due to potentially harmful radiation exposure. Multiple clinical decisions rules have been proposed to reduce CT utilization in children following minor head injury. In 2009, Kuppermann et al published the Pediatric Emergency Care Applied Research Network. (PECARN) criteria based on > 40,000 patients that describe patients who likely do not need to undergo CT (Table 5.35).

> **KEY FACT**
>
> Skull radiographs should not be routinely obtained.

TREATMENT

- If there is concern for elevated ICP, the following measures should be implemented immediately while awaiting CT acquisition and/or neurosurgical consultation:
  - Avoid hypotension and hypoxia, both of which increase mortality.
  - Elevate the head of bed to 30°.
  - Very mild hyperventilation to $EtCO_2$ of 30-35 mm Hg if intubated.
  - Fluid resuscitation to maintain MAP > 60 mm Hg.
  - IV mannitol (1 g/kg): Use caution in polytrauma patients as mannitol will lead to an osmotic diuresis and may reduce MAP.
  - Hypertonic saline IV (2-6 mL/kg initial bolus of 3% saline and continuous infusion of 0.1-1 mL/kg/h to maintain ICP < 20 mm Hg). Unlike mannitol, it does not cause hypotension.

TABLE 5.35. Children at Low Risk for Clinically Important Brain Injury—PECARN Criteria

Children < 2 y do not need to undergo CT if they meet the following criteria following minor head injury (Kuppermann, 2009):
▪ Mild or moderate injury mechanism
▪ No LOC (or LOC < 5 s)
▪ Acting normally to parents
▪ Normal mental status
▪ No scalp hematoma (or frontal hematoma only)
▪ No skull fracture
Children > 2 y do not need to undergo CT if they meet the following criteria following minor head injury (Kuppermann, 2009):
▪ Mild or moderate injury mechanism
▪ No LOC
▪ No severe headache
▪ No vomiting
▪ Normal mental status
▪ No basilar skull fracture

Reproduced with permission from Kuppermann N, Holmes JF, Dayan PS, et al. Identification of children at very low risk of clinically important brain injuries after head trauma: *A prospective cohort study. Lancet.* 2009; 374:1160-70.

CT, computed tomography; LOC, loss of consciousness; PECARN, Pediatric Emergency Care Applied Research Network.

Note: The presence of one of these criteria (except altered mental status or basilar skull fracture) does not mandate the acquisition of brain CT but should raise suspicion for a potential brain injury. Concerns about radiation exposure should not delay CT acquisition in patients with signs of severe brain injury.

- None of these measures reduce ICP in the long term. They serve as temporizing measures, while awaiting definitive neurosurgical management.
- Many children with subdural hematomas can be managed conservatively following consultation with a neurosurgeon. Children with altered mental status, neurologic deficits, or large hematomas are more likely to require surgery.
- Children with simple skull fractures (linear, nondepressed without associated intracranial injuries) and no other concerning findings or concerns for nonaccidental trauma can be discharged from the ED with head injury precautions and neurosurgical follow-up after a period of observation.

CERVICAL SPINE TRAUMA

Unlike adults, trauma rarely produces fractures of the cervical spine in children < 8 years. With high mechanism trauma, these children can suffer devastating injuries to their spinal cord, but if they survive to the ED, they rarely have cervical fractures. In older children, fractures are more common and typically occur in the lower cervical spine.

SYMPTOMS/EXAMINATION

- Cervical injuries can be particularly difficult to detect in children, because they often cannot provide history or localize their symptoms.
- 50% of children with injury to their spinal cord will have a neurologic deficit on examination.

> **KEY FACT**
>
> Rarely, children can have atlantoaxial rotary fixation, in which the anterior facet of C1 becomes locked on the anterior facet of C2, preventing rotation around the joint. These children cannot turn their head past midline. Reduction should be performed by neurosurgery followed by immobilization in a cervical collar.

DIAGNOSIS

- Because of the difficulty in identifying injuries on examination, children are often subjected to radiation from imaging of their cervical spines. When employed universally to all trauma patients, imaging studies have extremely low yield.
- Clinical decision rules designed to identify adults at high risk for cervical injury have not been validated in young children.
- Children should only undergo imaging of their cervical spine, if they demonstrate the following:
  - Altered mental status
  - Neck pain
  - Focal neurologic deficit
  - Torticollis with history of trauma
  - High-risk injury, eg, high speed MVA, diving
  - Concomitant major injury to torso
- In children < 8 years, plain films can be obtained as an initial study. CT should be ordered if there are concerning findings on examination, history of significant trauma, neurologic deficit, alteration in mental status, or an abnormality on the plain films.
- In children > 8 years, National Emergency X-Radiography Utilization Study (NEXUS) criteria can be applied to rule out C spine injury without imaging. CT may be employed if there is significant concern for cervical injury or the patient cannot be cleared by NEXUS criteria.
- MRI is needed to evaluate for spinal cord injuries if the C spine cannot be cleared within 24-72 hours (such as in patients who are unconscious/intubated) or if there are focal neurologic deficits such as arm or hand weakness or any other deficit.

> **KEY FACT**
>
> Children < 8 years will often have pseudosubluxation of C_2 on C_3 on imaging with approximately 2-3 mm of anterior–posterior displacement of C_2 on C_3.

TREATMENT

- All children with potential cervical injury should be immobilized. Children < 8 years require elevation of their torso with a towel when placed on a back board to prevent flexion of their neck.

- Spinal surgeons should be consulted for any injuries identified on examination or imaging.
- No studies have shown a reliable benefit from steroid administration in children with cervical spine injury.

THORACIC TRAUMA

Unlike adults, thoracic trauma is uncommon in children and almost always occurs in the setting of multisystem injury. Rib fractures are less common in children due to increased compliance of the thoracic cavity. However, this increased compliance can lead to internal injuries such as pulmonary contusions without evidence of thoracic injury externally. Traumatic aortic tears are also much less common in children but should be considered in patients with hypotension or hard signs of vascular injury.

SYMPTOMS/EXAMINATION

Children often cannot localize their symptoms following chest trauma. Tachypnea, tachycardia, hypotension, abnormal auscultatory examination, and evidence of external trauma to the chest should raise suspicion of internal thoracic injury.

DIAGNOSIS

- CXR should be obtained in any child with evidence of trauma to the chest, significant mechanism or injury, or requiring intubation.
- Chest CT should only be obtained in patients with abnormal vital signs or plain film abnormalities. Great vessel injuries are extremely rare in children.

TREATMENT

- Pneumothoraces < 15% in size can be managed with oxygen and observation. Typically observation should be performed in the hospital because children are prone to rapid decompensation.
- Larger or symptomatic pneumothoraces should be managed with tube thoracostomy.

ABDOMINAL TRAUMA

Children are more prone to intra-abdominal injuries following trauma than adults because their overlying musculature is not as developed. Intra-abdominal injuries can often be managed without operative intervention in children.

SYMPTOMS/EXAMINATION

- The physical examination is difficult to interpret in children, because tenderness on palpation may arise from intra-abdominal injuries or from abdominal wall contusions.
- Serial abdominal examinations significantly improve the sensitivity and specificity of the examination for detection of intra-abdominal injury.
- The rectal examination is usually unnecessary. It can be particularly psychologically traumatic for children and adds little to their evaluation.

DIAGNOSIS

- Elevated transaminases or lipase levels can be the only sign of liver or pancreatic injuries.
- Gross hematuria should raise suspicion for renal or bladder injuries. The relevance of microscopic hematuria is unclear.

KEY FACT

Consider MRI to evaluate for SCIWORA (spinal cord injury without obvious radiologic abnormality) in children with neurologic signs or symptoms but normal x-rays/CT.

KEY FACT

Continued air leak following placement of a chest tube should raise suspicion of a tracheal rupture.

- Pelvic x-ray should not be routinely acquired in children < 8 years, because pelvic fractures are uncommon.
- Abdominal CT is the primary diagnostic modality for pediatric trauma although there is an emerging roll for focused assessment with sonography for trauma (FAST) ultrasound. Imaging should be obtained in hemodynamically stable children with abdominal tenderness, lower rib or femur fractures, elevated LFTs, hematuria, or anemia.
- Plain films, ultrasound, and even CT may miss pancreatic or hollow viscus injuries particularly in early stages of presentation.

KEY FACT

The presence of a handle bar sign from a bicycle injury should raise concern for a duodenal hematoma, an injury which is often missed on abdominal CT. Children with evidence of handle bar injuries should be admitted for observation.

Treatment

- Nonoperative management of isolated hepatic or splenic injuries is successful in 95% of injuries. Patients still require admission to monitor for deterioration and for serial hemoglobin checks.
- Pancreatic injury can lead to pseudocyst formation, but this can typically be managed nonoperatively.

KEY FACT

A compression or flexion-distraction of the lumbar spine (Chance fracture) is associated with duodenal perforation, mesenteric injuries, and bladder rupture. Patients with Chance fractures should undergo laparotomy or admission for serial abdominal examinations.

Free fluid on abdominal CT after abdominal trauma should raise concern for hollow viscus injury and prompt at laparotomy or admission for observation.

Airway Management

- 50% of a child's ventilation is through their nose. Therefore, suctioning of the nose can significantly improve a child's work of breathing.
- The pediatric epiglottis is larger and floppier than an adult's, often obscuring the underlying vocal cords.
- Children's vocal cords are located much more anterior and superior than in adults.

Symptoms/Examination

- Normal pediatric respiratory rates vary from 10 to 60 based on age.
- Low respiratory rates are ominous. A respiratory rate < 20 in children < 6 years should raise concern the patient is tiring and may require aggressive airway intervention.

Auscultatory Finding	Etiology
Stridor	Croup, RPA, foreign body
Wheezing	Asthma, foreign body
Grunting	Contusion, pneumonia, hemothorax
Crackles	Pneumonia, hemothorax, pulmonary edema, contusion
Decreased breath sounds	Foreign body, pneumothorax, hemothorax, contusion, asthma

Treatment

- Children have much large tongues that can obstruct the oropharynx and prevent adequate ventilation. An oropharyngeal airway should be employed to stent the tongue from the posterior pharynx.
- If there is any concern that intubation will be difficult, then bag valve mask ventilate the patient and consult a more experienced laryngoscopist or anesthesiologist.

- Endotracheal tube size can be determined by the formula: (age/4) + 4 (subtract 0.5 when using a cuffed tube). Cuffed tubes are now recommended for pediatric patients.
- Endotracheal tube depth can be determined by the formula: tube size × 3.

Gastric decompression is crucial following any attempt at intubation or bag-valve-mask ventilation. A distended stomach can reduce ventilation and venous return.

REVIEW QUESTIONS

QUESTIONS

1. In which of the following patients is outpatient management most appropriate?
   A. A 2-week-old previously healthy boy who presents with a temperature of 38.8°C (101.8°F) rectally, who has no other symptoms.
   B. A 1-month-old boy who presents with dyspnea and an O_2 sat of 88% not improved with supplemental oxygen.
   C. An otherwise healthy 3 month old who presents with a temperature of 39°C with rhinorrhea and cough, but who is otherwise well appearing, with normal RR and O_2 sat.
   D. A 3 week old otherwise asymptomatic boy who had a temperature of 38.5°C rectally at home, but who is afebrile in the emergency department after receiving Tylenol at home.

2. What is the most common cause of serious bacterial infections in newborns age 0-28 days?
   A. Urinary tract infections
   B. Necrotizing enterocolitis
   C. Maternal vaginal flora
   D. Meningitis
   E. Gastrointestinal pathogens

3. Which of the following most likely represents a benign murmur in a young child?
   A. A continuous murmur
   B. A 2/6 diastolic murmur
   C. A 2/6 systolic murmur with associated cyanosis
   D. A 3/6 systolic murmur
   E. A systolic murmur that increases in intensity with a Valsalva maneuver

4. Which of the following is the most common elbow fracture in children?
   A. Supracondylar humeral fracture
   B. "Nursemaid's elbow"
   C. Coronoid process fracture
   D. Radial head fracture
   E. Olecranon fracture

ANSWERS

1. **C.** Patients 28 days and younger who are febrile require a full workup, empiric antibiotics, and hospital admission, even if they are well appearing. At 3 months of age, a well-appearing infant with symptoms of an upper respiratory infection, who is not hypoxic, and has no symptoms of serious bacterial illness can be safely discharged.

2. **C.** In neonates, the most common source of serious bacterial illnesses is maternal vaginal flora, particularly Group B Streptococci.

3. **D.** Systolic murmurs are common in young children. They are typically benign and usually resolve with age. Diastolic murmurs and continuous murmurs are considered pathologic. A murmur that increases in intensity with Valsalva can be due to hypertrophic cardiomyopathy.

4. **A.** Supracondylar fractures are the most common elbow fractures in children. Nursmaid's elbow is the most common elbow injury in children, but is not a fracture. It is a subluxation of the annular ligament around the radial head.

CHAPTER 6

Toxicology

James Dazhe Cao, MD, Janetta L. Iwanicki, MD, Howard Kim, MD, and Java Tunson, MD

Differential Diagnosis by Chief Complaint

Although the poisoned patient may present with varied symptoms and complaints, the chief presenting complaint or symptom may suggest a diagnosis (Table 6.1).

Toxidromes

Recognition of grouped symptoms and findings consistent with a toxidrome (Table 6.2) can guide diagnosis and treatment in the poisoned patient.

Principles of Gastrointestinal Decontamination

Gastrointestinal (GI) decontamination refers to therapies that may decrease the amount of poison absorbed from the GI tract. Methods include induced emesis, gastric lavage (GL), activated charcoal (AC), or whole-bowel irrigation (WBI).

INDUCED EMESIS

Induced emesis utilizes syrup of ipecac to induce vomiting, theoretically emptying the stomach, and reducing absorption of an ingested agent. Syrup of ipecac induces vomiting by activation of both local and central emetic receptors.

- Induced emesis has largely been abandoned in clinical practice.
- Policy statements released by both the American Academy of Pediatrics and the American Association of Poison Control Centers **discourage the use of syrup of ipecac**.

GASTRIC LAVAGE

Gastric lavage (GL) attempts to directly remove stomach contents by using an orogastric tube.

Indications

- Ingestion of a substance with high-toxic potential **and:**
  - Within 1 hour of ingestion.
  - Ingested substance is not bound by AC or has no effective antidote.
  - Potential benefits outweigh risks.

Contraindications

- Spontaneous emesis.
- Diminished level of consciousness/unprotected airway reflexes (intubate first).
- Ingestion of hydrocarbons, caustic agents, or foreign body.
- Patient is at high risk for esophageal or gastric injury (GI hemorrhage, recent surgery, abnormal anatomy, etc).

Technique

- Recommended tube size is 36F-40F for adults, 22F-28F for children.
- Secure airway via intubation, if necessary.

TABLE 6.1. Primary Considerations for Presenting Chief Complaint in the Poisoned Patient

Chief Complaint	Common Causes
Coma	Alcohols Antipsychotics Antiseizure medications Carbon monoxide Cyanide Muscle relaxants Opioids Sedative/hypnotics
Delirium	Anticholinergics/cholinergics Muscle relaxants Neuroleptic malignant syndrome Serotonin syndrome Sympathomimetics Withdrawal syndromes
Seizure	Antidepressants (tricyclics, bupropion) Anticholinergics/cholinergics Isoniazid Local anesthetics Methylxanthines (caffeine, theophylline) Mushrooms (*Gyromitra* sp.) Sympathomimetics Toxic alcohols Withdrawal syndromes
Hepatic injury	Acetaminophen Carbon tetrachloride Ethanol Iron Mushrooms (*Amanita phalloides*)
Renal injury	Ethylene glycol Heavy metal salts (mercury) Mushrooms (*Cortinarius orellanus*) Rhabdomyolysis (cocaine, amphetamines)

- Position patient in left-lateral decubitus position, with head lowered below level of feet.
- Confirm tube placement following insertion.
- Aspirate any available stomach contents.
- Lavage with 250 mL (10-15 mL/kg in children) aliquots of warm water or saline.
- Continue until fluid is clear and a minimum of 2 L has been used.
- Instill AC through same tube, if indicated.

Complication

Primary risks are vomiting, aspiration, and esophageal injury or perforation.

TABLE 6.2. Toxidromes

Toxidrome	Common Agents	Presentation	Treatment
Anticholinergic (see also Table 6.7)	Antihistamines Jimsonweed (scopolamine) Deadly nightshade (atropine)	Altered mentation Dry, flushed skin Mydriasis Hyperthermia Seizures Tachycardia Urinary retention	Benzodiazepines Physostigmine
Cholinergic (see also Table 6.8)	Organophosphates Carbamates Sarin	Altered mentation Bradycardia Bronchospasm ↑ Secretions Miosis nausea/vomiting, defecation Seizures Urination	Atropine 2-PAM (for organophosphates)
Sympathomimetic (see also p. 431)	Ephedrine Ma Huang (Ephedra) Cocaine Amphetamines	Agitation Diaphoresis Hallucinations HTN Hyperthermia Mydriasis Muscular rigidity Tachycardia	Benzodiazepines Sodium bicarbonate (for wide complex dysrhythmias)
Opioid (see also p. 414)	Morphine Heroin	CNS depression Bradycardia Hypothermia Miosis Respiratory depression	Naloxone

CNS, central nervous depression; HTN, hypertension.

ACTIVATED CHARCOAL

Activated charcoal (AC) is ingested by the patient in order to adsorb poison within the GI tract lumen.

Dose

- AC should be given in a 10:1 ratio (ie, ingestion of 1 g of poison requires 10 g of AC), so larger or repeated doses may be required in cases of massive overdose.
- Empiric dosing typically starts with 50-100 g (1 g/kg in children).

Indications

- Patient presents within 1 hour after ingestion.
- Patient has ingested a potentially dangerous amount of a poison adsorbed by charcoal.
- Multiple-dose activated charcoal (MDAC) maybe appropriate after 2 hours for some agents (eg, carbamazepine, dapsone, phenobarbital, quinine, theophylline) that undergo enterohepatic or enteroenteric recirculation or form concretions.

Contraindications

- Ingested substance is poorly adsorbed by AC (eg, metals or alcohols) or presents greater danger if AC induces vomiting (eg, caustics or hydrocarbons).
- Diminished level of consciousness/unprotected airway reflexes (AC can be given by naso- or orogastric tube following intubation).
- Patient presentation over 2 hours after ingestion unlikely to benefit from AC unless ingestion of massive quantities, sustained-release products, or part of MDAC strategy.
- Cases where endoscopy will be required or patient may be at risk for hemorrhage or perforation (ie, caustic agents).

KEY FACT

Substances for which AC is **contraindicated:** Metals (eg, iron, lead, lithium), caustics, hydrocarbons, alcohols.

Risks

- Primary risk of single-dose AC is vomiting resulting in aspiration.
- Repeated doses of cathartics given with charcoal may cause diarrhea, dehydration, and/or electrolyte abnormalities.

WHOLE-BOWEL IRRIGATION

Whole-bowel irrigation (WBI) flushes the GI tract to decrease the transit time of luminal contents, thereby limiting absorption.

Dose

- Polyethylene glycol (PEG) solution is administered at a rate of 1-2 L/h (usually requires a naso- or orogastric tube) with endpoints of clear rectal effluent or a total irrigation volume of 10 L

Indications

- Removal of ingested drug packets (eg, body packers) without suspicion of packet rupture, large ingestion of a sustained-release drug, or potentially toxic ingestion that cannot be treated with AC (eg, metals)

KEY FACT

Common indications for WBI: Body packers, sustained-release formula medications, and metals.

Contraindication

- Diminished level of consciousness/unprotected airway reflexes (intubate first), decreased GI motility, bowel obstruction, significant GI hemorrhage, or persistent emesis

Complications

- Primary risks associated with WBI are vomiting and aspiration.
- Patient discomfort: Bloating, cramping, and flatulence.
- WBI with balanced PEG solutions does not generally cause electrolyte abnormalities.

KEY FACT

Endpoints for WBI: Clear rectal effluent or total irrigation volume of 10 L.

Principles of Enhanced Elimination

The goal of enhanced elimination is to increase the clearance of a poison from the body after it has been systemically absorbed. The following methods of enhanced elimination are available (Table 6.3):

- MDAC
- Urinary alkalinization
- Hemodialysis (HD)

MULTIPLE-DOSE ACTIVATED CHARCOAL

Uses repeated doses of AC (every 2-4 hours) to increase poison clearance. MDAC exerts its effects through disruption of enterohepatic circulation or direct adsorption across the GI mucosal surface ("gut dialysis").

Indications

- Drugs that have enterohepatic or enteroenteric circulation, sustained-release agents, and agents that form concretions or bezoars can possibly be treated with MDAC include the following: Carbamazepine, dapsone, phenobarbital, quinine, and theophylline.

Contraindications

- Unprotected airway, GI obstruction or ileus, or GI tract not anatomically intact

Risks

- Risks associated with MDAC are similar to those with AC; however, there is a greater risk of bowel obstruction with MDAC

KEY FACT

Single-dose AC is used to decrease poison absorption. MDAC is used to increase poison elimination.

KEY FACT

Urinary alkalinization will not occur unless hypokalemia is corrected because the renal tubules will reabsorb potassium ions in exchange for hydrogen ions preventing alkalinization.

TABLE 6.3. Enhanced Elimination: Drug Characteristics and Examples

Technique	Drug Characteristics	Examples
Multiple-dose activated charcoal	Enterohepatic or enteroenteric circulation, or known to form bezoars or concretions	Carbamazepine Dapsone Phenobarbital Quinine Theophylline
Urinary alkalinization	Weak organic acid with renal excretion	Aspirin Methotrexate Phenobarbital
Hemodialysis	Low molecular weight, low plasma protein binding, small volume of distribution, poor endogenous clearance *OR* Acidosis caused by toxin	Alcohols Aspirin Lithium Metformin

URINARY ALKALINIZATION

Urinary alkalinization increases renal elimination of a drug by ion trapping. Urinary acidification to increase the clearance of weak bases is not recommended due to the risk of renal injury.

Dose

Alkalinization is accomplished via a sodium bicarbonate ($NaHCO_3$) infusion. The most common method uses 150 mEq of $NaHCO_3$ (3 amps) in 1 L D_5W, infused at 1.5 to 2 × the normal intravenous (IV) fluid maintenance rate. If indicated, potassium can also be given with fluids.

Indications

- Urinary alkalinization only affects the clearance of drugs that are weak organic acids.
  - Aspirin (most common use for alkalinization)
  - Methotrexate
  - Phenobarbital

KEY FACT

Urinary alkalinization is used for weak organic acids: Aspirin, methotrexate, and phenobarbital.

Contraindications

- Poisoning with agents that are not weak organic acids or are not primarily cleared by the kidneys
- Patients who cannot tolerate excess sodium/water loading (eg, congestive heart failure [CHF], renal failure)

Risks

Fluid overload

HEMODIALYSIS

Hemodialysis (HD) directly removes toxins from plasma, using the same technology applied to renal failure

Indications

- The ingested poison should have low molecular weight, low plasma protein binding, small volume of distribution, and poor endogenous clearance.
- HD can also treat severe acidosis caused by a toxin, even if the toxin itself is not readily dialyzable (eg, metformin toxicity).

Contraindication

- Toxins that do not satisfy the conditions are listed previously.

Risks

- HD requires central venous access, with all the usual accompanying risks (bleeding, pneumothorax, etc).
- HD must be used cautiously in patients who are hemodynamically unstable due to large volume shifts, but continuous renal replacement therapy (CRRT) may be considered in these patients.

ECG Principles in Toxicology

The electrocardiogram (ECG) is used as a screening tool in the evaluation of the patient with a suspected ingestion/overdose. Specific ECG findings may be associated with ingestion of certain classes of drugs (Table 6.4).

TABLE 6.4. ECG Findings and Associated Classes of Drugs

ECG Findings	Classes of Drugs
Bradydysrhythmias Sinus bradycardia AV block	β-Blockers Ca^{++} channel blockers Cardiac glycosides Clonidine Other antidysrhythmic agents
Tachydysrhythmias Sinus tachycardia SVT VT	Anticholinergics Stimulants Sympathomimetics
QRS widening	Na^{+} channel blocking drugs: Quinidine Sedating antihistamines Cocaine Tricyclic antidepressants
QTc prolongation Screening tool for conduction abnormality that could degenerate into torsade de points	Antidepressants Antidysrhythmic agents Antipsychotic medications Hydrofluoric acid Many others
Ischemic changes	Stimulants Sympathomimetics
Classic toxicology-related ECG findings	**Digoxin** Digitalis effect—seen in both therapeutic use and overdose Bidirectional VT (rare) Atrial fibrillation with slow ventricular response **Tricyclic antidepressants** Rightward deviation of the QRS axis Terminal R wave in aVR QRS prolongation

AV, atrioventricular; SVT, supraventricular; VT, ventricular tachycardia.

Q

A 35-year-old man presents to the emergency department (ED) with a complaint of abdominal pain, nausea, and blurry vision. He has a history of ethyl alcohol (EtOH) abuse and reports running out of alcohol today. On examination, he appears inebriated and tachypneic. His laboratory test results reveal an osmole gap and a wide anion gap metabolic acidosis. What is the most appropriate initial treatment?

Alcohols

The alcohol ingestions most commonly seen in the ED include ethanol, methanol, ethylene glycol, and isopropyl alcohol. However, there are many other "toxic alcohols" like diethylene glycol that may cause severe morbidity and mortality. If the ingested product's name sounds like a toxic alcohol, call your poison center for clarification.

Alcohols are primarily metabolized in the liver via alcohol dehydrogenase (ADH) using NAD+ as a cofactor. In the case of methanol and ethylene

A

This patient has likely ingested methanol, based on his presentation of inebriation with visual changes and wide anion gap acidosis. Initial therapies include administration of fomepizole or ethanol to decreased formation of formic acid (the toxic metabolite) and urinary alkalinization to increase its clearance. Visual changes are an indication for treatment with HD.

glycol, the metabolites (**not** the parent compound) cause severe toxicity, making ADH blockade a key factor in treatment.

ETHANOL

Ethanol is the most common poison seen in the ED. In addition to typical preparations, it can be found in products such as aftershave, vanilla extract, cold/allergy medications, glass cleaners, mouthwash, and perfumes.

Symptoms/Examination

Symptoms and examination findings include behavioral changes (eg, increased sociability, irritability, aggressiveness, etc), ataxia/ gait instability, and CNS depression ranging from mild sedation to coma and respiratory failure.

Differential

- Consider other etiologies of CNS depression, especially with relatively low serum ethanol levels.
- Common conditions associated with ethanol use include hypoglycemia, electrolyte disturbances, vitamin depletion (folate, thiamine, B12), withdrawal, head trauma, hypothermia, and other toxin/drug overdose.

Diagnosis

Diagnosis is usually clinical or based on serum ethanol concentrations; however, correlation between serum concentrations and patient symptoms varies widely due to individual tolerance.

Treatment

- Supportive care
- Be careful not to overlook concomitant injuries or medical illness

Complications

Chronic alcohol use is associated with a wide variety of illnesses, including hypoglycemia, alcoholic ketoacidosis, cirrhosis, pancreatitis, GI bleeding, malnutrition, neurologic disease, and trauma.

METHANOL (CH_3OH)

Methanol is found in windshield wiper fluid, antifreeze, photocopier fluid, and solid fuels (eg, Sterno). Patients may ingest methanol by accident, as a suicide attempt, or as an ethanol substitute.

Mechanism/Toxicity

- Methanol itself has minimal toxicity, causing mild intoxication.
- Metabolized by ADH to a toxic metabolite, **formaldehyde and then by aldehyde dehydrogenase (ALDH) to formic acid.**
- Formic acid accumulation → anion gap metabolic acidosis.

Symptoms/Examination

- **Neurologic:** Intoxication similar to ethanol, headache, CNS depression, basal ganglia injury resulting in Parkinsonism.
- **Visual changes:** Classic description is "looking through a snow field," hyperemic optic discs, retinal edema (sluggish fixed pupils), blindness.
- **Cardiovascular/Pulmonary:** Tachycardia, tachypnea.
- **GI:** Abdominal pain, nausea/vomiting, pancreatitis.

Differential

- Consider other causes of acute metabolic acidosis.
- Combination of acute onset visual changes with acidosis is highly suggestive of methanol toxicity.

Diagnosis

- Gold standard is direct serum methanol measurement, but serial bicarbonate measurements may be used if levels are not available.
- Suspect methanol ingestion if patient has a high osmole gap, anion gap metabolic acidosis, and visual symptoms.
- An osmole gap > 10 mOsm/kg may be abnormal and may suggest the presence of a toxic alcohol. Osmole gap = measure osmolality − calculated osmolarity, where calculated serum osmolarity = $2(Na^+) + (BUN/2.8) + (glucose/18) + (ethanol/4.6)$.
- Late presenting cases may have no osmole gap due to metabolism of the ingested alcohol (early = high osmole gap/no anion gap and late = high anion gap/no osmole gap).
- Metabolism, and therefore toxicity, may be **delayed** with coingestion of ethanol.

Treatment

- **Antidote = fomepizole or ethanol**
  - Fomepizole blocks ADH, preventing production of formic acid.
  - Ethanol is preferentially metabolized by ADH over methanol.
  - Evaluate response to treatment using serial bicarbonate measurements.
- **Folate:** Improves the metabolism of formic acid to carbon dioxide and water.
- Consider **HD** in cases of severe acidosis, renal failure, visual changes, or a serum level ≥ 50 mg/dL; effectively removes both the parent compound and formic acid.

Complication

Permanent visual losses and parkinsonian motor dysfunction may occur.

KEY FACT

Osmole gap may also be elevated by ethanol, mannitol, sorbitol, or recent contrast administration. Don't forget to check a serum ethanol level.

KEY FACT

"Blind drunk," osmole gap, and anion gap metabolic acidosis = methanol toxicity.

ETHYLENE GLYCOL ($OHCH_2CH_2OH$)

Ethylene glycol is most commonly found in engine coolants (antifreeze). It is also found in aircraft deicing fluid, water-based latex paints (low concentrations), hydraulic brake fluids, and some cleaning products. It is ingested under similar circumstances as methanol.

Mechanism/Toxicity

- Ethylene glycol itself has minimal toxicity, causing mild intoxication.
- Metabolized by ADH and ALDH to toxic metabolites: **Oxalic acid causes direct renal toxicity, and glycolate causes anion gap metabolic acidosis.**

Symptoms/Examination

- There are four stages of toxicity: (1) acute neurologic stage (30 minutes to 12 hours); (2) cardiopulmonary stage (12- 24 hours); (3) renal stage (24-72 hours); and (4) delayed neurologic sequelae (6-12 days).
- **Neurologic:** Intoxication similar to ethanol, headache, CNS depression. Delayed findings include cranial neuropathy, petechial brain hemorrhage, and cerebral edema with papilledema.
- **Cardiopulmonary:** Hypertension, tachycardia, tachypnea, pulmonary edema, ARDS. Delayed findings include myocardial depression and cardiogenic shock.

- **GI:** Abdominal pain, nausea/vomiting
- **Renal:** Acute renal failure, hematuria
- **Electrolytes:** Symptoms of hypocalcemia (carpal pedal spasm)

Diagnosis

- Gold standard is direct serum measurement of ethylene glycol, or serial bicarbonate measurements if levels are not available.
- Suspect ethylene glycol ingestion if patient has an osmole gap, anion gap metabolic acidosis, and acute renal failure. Oxalic acid may also falsely increase the serum lactate with some assays.
- Presence of **oxalate crystals in the urine** (suggestive of diagnosis, but is not sensitive or specific).
- Some brands of antifreeze contain fluorescent dyes to aid in the identification of coolant leaks and will fluoresce under Woods lamp (UV [ultraviolet] light); however, the practice of examining a patient's urine under UV light is highly unreliable and should not be used to confirm or rule out ingestion.

Treatment

- **Antidote = fomepizole or ethanol**
  - Fomepizole blocks ADH, preventing production of toxic metabolites.
  - Ethanol is preferentially metabolized by ADH over ethylene glycol.
  - Evaluate response to treatment using serial bicarbonate measurements.
- **Thiamine** (vitamin B_1) and **pyridoxine** (vitamin B_6) may help convert glyoxylic acid to nontoxic metabolites.
- Consider **HD** in cases of severe acidosis (pH < 7.25), renal failure, or electrolyte disturbances.

Complication

- Renal damage is generally reversible, but may be irreversible in severe poisonings.

ISOPROPANOL (ISOPROPYL ALCOHOL—$CH_3CHOHCH_3$)

Isopropanol is found in rubbing alcohol, perfumes, and some hand sanitizers. It is most often ingested as an ethanol substitute. Intoxication due to isopropanol is more severe than that due to an equivalent amount of ethanol.

Unlike methanol and ethylene glycol, isopropanol is **not** metabolized to an organic acid. It is converted directly to **acetone** by ADH.

Mechanism/Toxicity

CNS toxicity effects are mediated through γ-aminobutyric acid (GABA) receptors, and isopropanol is directly toxic to GI mucosa.

Symptoms/Examination

- Neurologic: Intoxication, CNS depression, coma
- GI: Abdominal pain, nausea/vomiting, hemorrhagic gastritis

Diagnosis

- Isopropanol can be directly measured in serum.
- Ingestion should be suspected in patients who appear intoxicated but have low or undetectable ethanol levels.
- Other clues include an increased osmolal gap and detectable serum acetone.
- Isopropanol does **not** directly cause a metabolic acidosis.

KEY FACT

Intoxicated patient with osmole gap, anion gap metabolic acidosis, and acute renal failure = ethylene glycol.

KEY FACT

Antidote to methanol and ethylene glycol poisoning = fomepizole or ethanol.

In pediatric patients, use fomepizole to avoid complications from ethanol: sedation and (theoretically) hypoglycemia.

KEY FACT

Isopropanol intoxication (as compared to ethanol) = "twice as drunk for twice as long."

KEY FACT

Ketosis without acidosis.

KEY FACT

All alcohols will cause an elevated osmole gap. Methanol and ethylene glycol metabolism cause an anion gap metabolic acidosis because they are primary alcohols and metabolized to acids.

TREATMENT

Supportive care only

Antidepressants

The broad classes of antidepressants are:

- TCAs
- Selective serotonin reuptake inhibitors (SSRIs)
- Monoamine oxidase inhibitors (MAOIs)
- Newer drugs that act at multiple CNS receptors

TRICYCLIC ANTIDEPRESSANTS

Tricyclic antidepressants (TCAs) are associated with life-threatening CNS and cardiovascular toxicity. Safer medications, such as SSRIs, have decreased the use of TCAs for depression, and they are now more commonly used at lower doses for treatment of chronic pain syndromes, migraine prophylaxis, and enuresis. Examples include amitriptyline (Elavil), nortriptyline (Aventyl), and imipramine (Tofranil).

MECHANISM/TOXICITY

TCAs have several pharmacologic effects that contribute to toxicity, including:

- Histamine receptor blockade → antihistamine effects.
- Muscarinic receptor inhibition → anticholinergic effects.
- α-Adrenergic receptor blockade → hypotension.
- GABA receptor antagonism → seizures.
- Na^+ channel blockade prolongs phase 0 (rapid depolarization) of the cardiac action potential → quinidine-like QRS prolongation.
- K^+-channel antagonism → QTc prolongation → dysrhythmia.

SYMPTOMS/EXAMINATION

Table 6.5 summarizes the clinical findings in TCA poisonings.

- Early: Tachycardia, hypertension, rapid mumbled speech, urinary retention, alteration of consciousness.
- Late: Myocardial depression, hypotension, ECG with wide QRS >100 milliseconds → seizures, wide complex cardiac dysrhythmia.
- **Seizures** are typically self-limited but are associated with acidosis, which worsens the cardiovascular effects.
- Rapid deterioration can occur.

DIFFERENTIAL DIAGNOSIS

- Sedating antihistamine overdoses may present similarly to early TCA toxicity.
- Na^+ channel blockade can also be seen with quinidine, flecainide, propafenone, amantadine, carbamazepine, cocaine, and diphenhydramine.

DIAGNOSIS

- Suspect based on history and presentation
- ECG findings of Na^+ channel blockade:
  - QRS widening
    - QRS > 100 milliseconds is associated with increased risk of seizures.
    - QRS > 160 milliseconds is associated with increased risk of wide complex dysrhythmias.

Q

A 33-year-old woman with a history of depression and chronic pain is brought to the ED via emergency medical services (EMS) for a suspected overdose. On arrival, her BP is 80/40 mm Hg with an HR in the 120s. She is lethargic but responds to tactile stimuli. Her ECG shows sinus tachycardia with a QRS duration of 160 milliseconds. What is the best treatment for this patient?

KEY FACT

Life-threatening cardiac toxicity results from Na^+ channel blockade.

KEY FACT

Acidosis worsens Na^+ channel blockade.

KEY FACT

ECG findings consistent with sodium channel blockade: QRS > 100 milliseconds, terminal R in aVr > 3 mm, rightward deviation of the terminal 40 milliseconds of the QRS, and QTc prolongation.

A

Any patient with a suspected ingestion who presents with CNS depression and QRS widening > 100 milliseconds should be presumed to have tricyclic antidepressant (TCA) toxicity. TCA-mediated Na^+ channel blockade may result in life-threatening cardiovascular toxicity, manifesting as hypotension with QRS widening > 100 milliseconds. The drug of choice is sodium bicarbonate, given initially in boluses. IV fluids and pressors can be used for hypotension.

TABLE 6.5. Clinical Findings in TCA Toxicity

Pharmacologic Effect	Symptoms/Examination
Antihistamine	CNS depression ↔ coma
Anticholinergic	Dry, flushed skin Mydriasis Hyperthermia Tachycardia Urinary retention CNS excitation Hallucinations
α-Adrenergic receptor blockade	Reflex tachycardia Orthostatic hypotension Miosis
GABA receptor blockade	Seizures
Na^+ channel blockade	QRS widening Decreased contractility Hypotension Seizures
K^+ channel antagonism	QT prolongation
Inhibition of amine uptake	Initial hypertension CNS excitation ↔ coma

CNS, central nervous depression; GABA, γ-aminobutyric acid; TCA, tricyclic antidepressant.

    - Rightward deviation of the terminal 40 milliseconds of the QRS.
    - Terminal R in lead aVr > 3 mm (Figure 6.1).
- Prolongation of QTc interval.
- Plasma TCA concentrations are not highly correlated with clinical effects and of no use in management.
- Urine drug screen for TCAs are fraught with false positives, including diphenhydramine, carbamazepine, cyclobenzaprine, and phenothiazines.

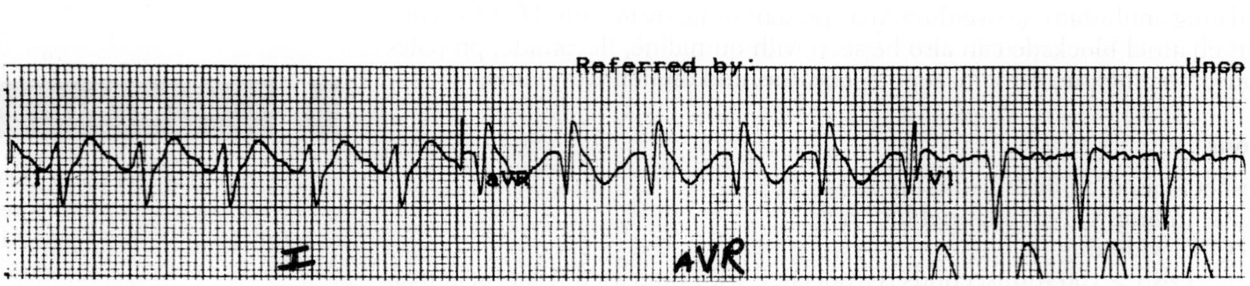

FIGURE 6.1. Sodium channel blockade in TCA toxicity. (Reproduced, with permission, from Tintinalli JE, Kelen GD, Stapczynski JS. *Emergency Medicine: A Comprehensive Study Guide*. 6th ed. New York, NY: McGraw-Hill; 2004:1031.)

TREATMENT

- Supportive care
  - Early intubation to avoid respiratory acidosis
- Charcoal if within 1 hour of ingestion, but intubate sedated patients prior to administering charcoal.
- **Sodium bicarbonate,** indications:
  - QRS > 120 milliseconds or longer
  - Ventricular dysrhythmias
  - Hypotension unresponsive to fluids
  - Administer boluses of 1-2 mEq/kg until narrowing of QRS

Sodium bicarbonate is the treatment of choice for TCA-induced dysrhythmias.

- **Benzodiazepines** for seizures.
- IV fluids and sodium bicarbonate boluses for hypotension, but may require **norepinephrine** or epinephrine if unresponsive to initial interventions.
- **Magnesium sulfate** if torsade de pointes.
- **Avoid:**
  - Physostigmine has no treatment benefit and may cause adverse events.
  - Respiratory and/or metabolic acidosis (worsens Na^+ channel blockade): Hyperventilate intubated patients to induce mild respiratory alkalosis (target pH 7.45-7.5).
  - Class IA and IC antidysrhythmics (fast Na^+ channel blockers) will worsen cardiotoxicity.
  - Class III antidysrhythmics (K^+ channel blockers).
  - Phenytoin (no treatment benefit).

COMPLICATIONS

- Aspiration
- Hypoxic brain injury
- Cardiovascular collapse

SELECTIVE SEROTONIN REUPTAKE INHIBITORS

Selective serotonin reuptake inhibitors (SSRIs) are widely used for depression because of their large therapeutic window. Fatal overdoses are rare. Examples include fluoxetine (Prozac), citalopram (Celexa), and paroxetine (Paxil).

> **KEY FACT**
>
> Serotonin syndrome may occur with overdose or routine use.

MECHANISM/TOXICITY

Inhibition of presynaptic serotonin reuptake → increased CNS serotonin

SYMPTOMS/EXAMINATION

- Most common signs and symptoms include nausea, vomiting, abdominal pain, sinus tachycardia, CNS sedation, and tremors, but seizures and more serious cardiovascular toxicity can occur
- **Serotonin syndrome** may occur with overdose or routine use:
  - Autonomic dysfunction → hyperthermia (> 38°C), diaphoresis
  - CNS dysfunction → agitation and/or altered mental status (AMS)
  - Neuromuscular dysfunction → nystagmus, myoclonus, ocular clonus, hyperreflexia, muscular rigidity (lower extremities predominantly), tremors

> **KEY FACT**
>
> Serotonin syndrome is characterized by a triad of altered mentation, autonomic instability, and increased neuromuscular activity in the setting use of a serotonergic medication.

DIAGNOSIS

- Clinical diagnosis is based on history of ingestion, constellation of signs, and symptoms.

- Typical history includes increasing the dose of an SSRI or more commonly, adding a second serotonergic agent (eg, MAOIs, TCAs, some opioids, CNS stimulants).
- SSRIs are not typically detected on standard toxicology screens.

Treatment

- Supportive care
- Benzodiazepines for agitation, neuromuscular hyperactivity, and seizures
- **Antidote = cyproheptadine** (serotonin antagonist)
  - Indicated for serotonin syndrome in the patient able to take oral medication (oral formulation only)

> **KEY FACT**
>
> Antidote to SSRIs, used in serotonin syndrome = cyproheptadine.

MONOAMINE OXIDASE INHIBITORS

Rarely used today as first-line agent for depression due to narrow therapeutic window and drug interactions. Examples include phenelzine (Nardil), tranylcypromine (Parnate), and St. John's wort (an herbal preparation for depression thought to have some monoamine oxidase inhibitor action). MAOI-B inhibitors (selegiline, rasagiline) are used to treat Parkinson disease and are much less toxic in overdose.

Mechanism/Toxicity

- MAOI reactions can be due to toxicity or interactions with other medications or food products.
- Inhibition of monoamine oxidase → decreased inactivation of biogenic amines, including epinephrine, norepinephrine, serotonin → excessive circulating catecholamines.
- Monoamine oxidase may take weeks to regenerate after discontinuation of MAOIs! Remember to ask about recent discontinuation if you suspect toxicity.

> **KEY FACT**
>
> Symptom onset following MAOI overdose is frequently delayed 6-12 hours.

Symptoms/Examination

- Characterized by **excessive sympathetic activity**
- Symptoms are usually **delayed 6-12 hours** following overdose:
  - Cardiovascular: Tachycardia, hyperthermia, hypertension
  - Musculoskeletal: Muscle rigidity, hyperreflexia, myoclonus
  - CNS: Seizures, coma, agitation, mydriasis
- **Tyramine reaction (occurs with therapeutic use)**—after ingestion of tyramine-containing foods (red wine, cheese, etc)
  - Headache, hypertension, diaphoresis, palpitations, and neuromuscular excitation lasting for several hours

Differential

Cocaine, sympathomimetics, phencyclidine, serotonin syndrome

> **KEY FACT**
>
> MAOI overdose symptoms are those of life-threatening excessive sympathetic activity.

Diagnosis

- Clinical diagnosis based on history and patient presentation.
- MAOIs are usually not detected on standard toxicology screens.

Treatment

- Supportive care including aggressive treatment of agitation, rigidity, seizures, tachycardia, and hyperthermia with benzodiazepines
- Sodium nitroprusside or phentolamine, if severely hypertensive
- Avoid:
  - β-Blockers → unopposed α-adrenergic stimulation, theoretical
  - All indirect sympathomimetics (eg, dopamine)

TABLE 6.6. Toxicity Related to Newer Antidepressants

MEDICATION	MAJOR TOXICITY
Bupropion (Wellbutrin)	Seizures (hallmark of toxicity)
Mirtazapine (Remeron)	Hypotension Serotonin syndrome
Trazodone (Desyrel)	Similar to SSRIs Serotonin syndrome Hypotension Priapism
Venlafaxine (Effexor)	CNS sedation Serotonin syndrome Dysrhythmias Seizures

CNS, central nervous depression; SSRIs, selective serotonin reuptake inhibitors.

COMPLICATIONS

- Serotonin syndrome
- Sequelae of hypertensive emergency
- Rhabdomyolysis

NEWER ANTIDEPRESSANTS

Heterogeneous group of newer medications that block dopamine, norepinephrine, and serotonin CNS reuptake to varying degrees. Common examples and toxicities are listed in Table 6.6.

Antibiotics and Antiretrovirals

Most antibiotics and antivirals are associated with adverse drug effects (eg, allergic reactions) or complications from chronic therapy.
This section is limited to medications that are associated with severe toxicity in overdose.

ISONIAZID

Isoniazid is one of the first-line agents used to treat tuberculosis (TB).Chronic use is associated with peripheral neuropathy, hepatitis, drug-induced systemic lupus erythematosus (SLE). Acute toxicity can cause seizures refractory to treatment with benzodiazepines.

MECHANISM/TOXICITY

- Reduction of vitamin B_6 in brain → ↓ GABA production (the inhibitory neurotransmitter in the brain) but ↑glutamate (the excitatory neurotransmitter in the brain) → seizures

KEY FACT

Seizing patient refractory to treatment with benzodiazepines? Consider isonicotinic acid hydrazide (INH) toxicity or hyponatremia.

Q

A 23-year-old man with a history of depression presents to the ED via EMS for altered mentation. On presentation, he is agitated and delirious. Physical examination reveals tachycardia, dilated pupils, mild hypertension, hyperthermia, dry mucous membranes, and flushed, dry skin. Ingestion of which groups of drugs is suggested by this patient's symptoms?

SYMPTOMS/EXAMINATION

- Mild: Nausea, vomiting
- Severe: Slurred speech, ataxia, depressed mental status, seizures, status epilepticus, metabolic acidosis

DIAGNOSIS

Consider in any patient with seizures who is undergoing treatment for TB or is refractory to standard treatment.

TREATMENT

- Supportive care.
- AC if early and no CNS depression.
- Barbiturates and benzodiazepines for status epilepticus until antidote available.
- **Antidote: Pyridoxine (vitamin B_6)** replenishes vitamin B_6 stores to help replete GABA.

KEY FACT

INH is listed as a cause of an anion gap metabolic acidosis because it causes a profound lactic acidosis from seizure activity.

COMPLICATION

Chronic large doses of pyridoxine = peripheral neuropathy

REVERSE TRANSCRIPTASE INHIBITORS

Reverse transcriptase inhibitors are antiretroviral agents used in the treatment of human immunodeficiency virus (HIV). Highly active antiretroviral therapy (HAART) refers to a drug regimen combining reverse transcriptase inhibitors with agents from 2 other antiretroviral classes—protease inhibitors and fusion inhibitors. Reverse transcriptase inhibitors include didanosine (ddI), stavudine (d4T), lamivudine (3TC), and others.

MECHANISM/TOXICITY

Mitochondrial toxicity → lactic acidosis, hepatotoxicity, pancreatitis

KEY FACT

Reverse transcriptase inhibitors may cause a profound lactic acidosis due to mitochondrial toxicity.

SYMPTOMS/EXAMINATION

- Malaise
- Tachypnea, hyperpnea
- Nausea/vomiting, abdominal pain

DIAGNOSIS

- Suspect based on history and clinical presentation.
- Confirmed with laboratory findings (elevated lactate, etc).
- Muscle or liver biopsy is definitive for diagnosis of mitochondrial toxicity but rarely required.

A

This patient is presenting with an anticholinergic toxidrome, which may be caused by over-the-counter antihistamines, certain plants, or a variety of prescription medications.

TREATMENT

- Discontinue implicated drug and provide supportive care
- If severe lactic acidosis → sodium bicarbonate, HD, or CRRT for correction of acidosis

Anticholinergics/Cholinergics

ANTICHOLINERGICS

The anticholinergic toxidrome may result from exposure to medications or plants (Table 6.7).

MECHANISM/TOXICITY

Competitive antagonism of acetylcholine at muscarinic receptors in the central nervous system (CNS), parasympathetic nervous system, and sweat glands

TABLE 6.7. Common Anticholinergic Agents

Pupillary dilators
Atropine
Homatropine
Cyclopentolate
Antispasmodic medication
Dicyclomine
Motion sickness medication
Scopolamine
Asthma medications (rarely cause systemic symptoms)
Ipratropium
Tiotropium
Airway secretion medication
Glycopyrrolate
Antiparkinsonian medications
Benztropine
Trihexyphenidyl
Amantadine
Urinary incontinence and bladder spasms medications
Tolterodine
Oxybutynin
Medications with anticholinergic side effects
Antihistamines
Tricyclic antidepressants
Carbamazepine
Cyclobenzaprine
Phenothiazines
Plants
Jimsonweed (*Datura stramonium*)
Deadly nightshade (*Atropa belladonna*)

KEY FACT

Anticholinergic toxidrome: Mad as a hatter, red as a beet, dry as a bone, blind as a bat, hot as a hare, full as a flask, seizing like a squirrel, tachy as a pink flamingo.

MNEMONIC

Cholinergic toxidrome:

SLUDGE

Salivation/Sweating
Lacrimation
Urination
Defecation
Gastrointestinal distress
Emesis
plus

"The Killer Bs"
Bradycardia
Bronchorrhea
Bronchospasm

Symptoms/Examination

- Anticholinergic toxidrome: Agitation, delirium, hallucinations, hyperthermia, dry/flushed skin, mydriasis, tachycardia, hypertension, decreased bowel sounds, decreased defecation, and urinary retention.
- Cardiac sodium channel blockade may be seen with diphenhydramine overdose.

Differential

Sympathomimetic toxicity (will have diaphoretic skin), neuroleptic malignant syndrome, serotonin syndrome, hallucinogen intoxication, phencyclidine intoxication, withdrawal syndromes (alcohol, benzodiazepines), primary psychosis, sepsis, encephalitis

Diagnosis

- Clinical diagnosis is based on exposure history and physical examination.
- Laboratory tests and imaging as needed to exclude nontoxicologic causes.
- ECG used to screen for sodium channel blockade.

Treatment

- Supportive care with IV fluids and benzodiazepines (for seizures, agitation, hyperthermia).
  - Intubation, passive and active cooling measures may be needed for severe hyperthermia.
- **Antidote = physostigmine**
  - Indication include agitation and delirium uncontrolled with sedatives.
  - Contraindicated with QRS > 100 milliseconds or history of TCA overdose.
  - Monitor for bradycardia and seizures during administration.
- **Avoid**
  - β-Blockers and sedatives with anticholinergic effects such as diphenhydramine or antipsychotic agents

Complications

- Rhabdomyolysis may be a result of agitation, coma, or hyperthermia.
- Sedate with benzodiazepines to control psychomotor agitation and hyperthermia, treat with IV fluids, and follow serial creatinine kinase (CK) and creatinine, as indicated.
- QRS prolongation and wide complex dysrhythmias may be seen with certain agents (TCAs, diphenhydramine) due to sodium channel blockade.
  - Treat with sodium bicarbonate.

CHOLINERGICS

The cholinergic toxidrome is uncommon, but may result from exposure to cholinergic agents (Table 6.8).

Mechanism/Toxicity

Inhibition of the enzyme acetylcholinesterase → excess acetylcholine at muscarinic and nicotinic receptors

Symptoms/Examination

AMS (delirium to coma), seizures, lacrimation, salvation, sweating, bronchorrhea, bronchospasm, bradycardia, miotic (constricted) pupils, urinary/bowel incontinence, hyperactive bowel sounds, and muscle fasciculations

TABLE 6.8. Cholinergic Agents

Alzheimer medication Donepezil
Myasthenia gravis medications Pyridostigmine Edrophonium
Insecticides Organophosphate compounds Carbamate compounds
Chemical weapons Nerve agents (Sarin, Soman, Tabun, VX)
Glaucoma medication Pilocarpine
Nicotine
Mushrooms ***Clytocybe* and *inocybe* species**

Diagnosis

- Clinical diagnosis is based on exposure history and physical examination.
- Red blood cell (RBC) cholinesterase levels may be indicated in chronic exposures.
- ECG used to screen for atrioventricular (AV) block, dysrhythmias.

Treatment

Supportive care: **Atropine to dry up airway secretions and treat unstable bradycardia** (very high doses often needed), benzodiazepines for seizures and agitation, and pralidoxime (2-PAM) to regenerate acetylcholinesterase in organophosphate poisoning

KEY FACT

Warfarin blocks the activation of vitamin K–dependent clotting factors II, VII, IX, X.

Anticoagulants

WARFARIN

Warfarin is an oral anticoagulant used for the management of atrial fibrillation.

Mechanism/Toxicity

- Blocks conversion of vitamin K to its active form, thereby preventing activation of vitamin K–dependent clotting factors (II, VII, IX, X).
- Effect is delayed until preformed stores of clotting factors are depleted (typically ≥ 15 hours).
- Duration of action may be up to 6 days.
- Blocks the synthesis of antithrombotic proteins C and S → prothrombotic period before vitamin K–dependent factors are depleted.

Symptoms/Examination

Bleeding—may be spontaneous or related to trauma. This can range from bruising and joint effusions to major GI bleeding or intracranial hemorrhage.

Differential

Other "warfarin-like" anticoagulants (brodifacoum—rat poison), heparin/Low-molecular-weight heparin (LMWH), direct thrombin inhibitors, factor Xa inhibitors

Diagnosis

- Usually clear from patient's history and examination.
- Prothrombin time (PT) and international normalized ratio (INR) should be monitored for 3-4 days.

Treatment

- Supportive therapy, including packed red blood cell (PRBC) transfusion as needed.
- AC—if within 1 hour (with airway control as needed).
- Approach depends on INR level and presence of bleeding (Table 6.9).
- **Vitamin K1:**
  - Will reverse the blockade, but will not activate enough factors to reverse coagulopathy for several hours.
  - Do NOT administer prophylactically in an acute overdose.

KEY FACT

Onset of effect in overdose is delayed and PT and INR should be monitored for 3-4 days.

KEY FACT

PCCs and recombinant factor VIIa are used when immediate and complete reversal of warfarin anticoagulation is desired in life-threatening bleeding.

TABLE 6.9. Guidelines for Treatment of Overanticoagulation with Warfarin

Condition	Treatment
INR < 5, no clinically significant bleeding	Lower or skip dose Resume when INR therapeutic
INR 5-9, no clinically significant bleeding	Omit next one or two doses *Or* Skip dose and give vitamin K1 (1-2 mg PO) Resume at lower dose when INR therapeutic
INR > 9, no clinically significant bleeding	Hold warfarin Give higher dose of vitamin K1 (5-10 mg PO) Resume at lower doses when INR therapeutic
Serious bleeding at any elevation of INR	Hold warfarin Give vitamin K1 (10 mg slow IV) Give FFP or PCC Recombinant factor VIIa is an alternative therapy
Life-threatening bleeding	Hold warfarin Give vitamin K1 (10 mg slow IV) Give FFP, PCC, or recombinant factor VIIa Repeat as necessary

FFP, fresh frozen plasma; INR, international normalized ratio; IV, intravenous;PCC, prothrombin complex concentrate; PO, by mouth.

- **Fresh frozen plasma (FFP):**
  - 10-15 mg/kg will restore factor levels to ≥ 30% of normal.
- **Prothrombin complex concentrate (PCC), recombinant factor VIIa, or others.**
  - Allow for factor replacement and immediate complete reversal of anticoagulation.

COMPLICATIONS

- IV vitamin K1 therapy can rarely cause anaphylactoid reactions.
- Warfarin-induced skin necrosis:
  - Occurs 3-8 days after initiating warfarin therapy in patients with protein C deficiency (transient hypercoagulable state leading to thrombosis of cutaneous vessels)
  - Prevented by coadministration of heparin during initiation of warfarin therapy
  - Treated with discontinuation of warfarin and initiation of heparin therapy

HEPARIN

MECHANISM/TOXICITY

- Binds antithrombin III → heparin-antithrombin III complex → inhibits multiple steps (IXa, Xa, XIa, XIIa, and thrombin) in intrinsic and extrinsic pathways.
- LMWHs are obtained from heparin, but have a longer half-life, greater bioavailability, and greater activity against factor Xa.

SYMPTOM/EXAMINATION

Bleeding may be spontaneous or related to trauma

DIFFERENTIAL

Warfarin, "warfarin-like" anticoagulants (brodifacoum—rat poison), fondaparinux, direct thrombin inhibitors, factor Xa inhibitors

DIAGNOSIS

- Usually clear from patient's history and examination.
- Elevation of aPTT and anti-Xa levels, but levels may not correlate with bleeding in LMWH use.

TREATMENT

- Stop heparin/LMWH
- **Antidote = Protamine sulfate**
  - Indicated for severe bleeding complications only (risk of serious anaphylaxis with administration) and reverses the effect of heparin (only partially inactivates LMWH)
  - 1 mg of protamine neutralizes 100 units of unfractionated heparin

> **KEY FACT**
>
> HIT is associated with systemic venous and arterial thrombotic events.

COMPLICATIONS

Heparin-induced thrombocytopenia (HIT): May occur 5-10 days after initiating therapy or as late as 3 weeks after stopping therapy. Antibodies cause significant drop in platelets (> 50%) and skin changes at injection sites. Systemic **venous and arterial thrombotic events** can cause a wide variety of end organ damage. This is more common with heparin than LMWH.

NEWER ANTICOAGULANTS

- Pentasaccharides (fondaparinux): Bind antithrombin-like heparin but unlikely to cause HIT.
- Direct Xa inhibitors (rivaroxaban, apixaban): Currently there is no reliable diagnostic assay to predict bleeding risk, but PCC may be of benefit for acute hemorrhage.
- Direct thrombin inhibitors (hirudins, dabigatran, ximelagatran, melagatran): Currently there is no reversal agent but may consider the use of FFP or PCC for active hemorrhage.

Anticonvulsants

Anticonvulsant medications were developed for treatment of seizures, but they are also used for treatment of pain (carbamazepine, gabapentin), mood disorders (carbamazepine, valproic acid, lamotrigine), and migraines (valproic acid, topiramate).

KEY FACT

Cardiac toxicity with IV phenytoin administration is due to its propylene glycol diluent.

KEY FACT

Carbamazepine is structurally similar to TCAs. At high levels, it can cause similar CNS and rarely cardiac toxicity.

MECHANISM/TOXICITY

- Na^+ channel blockade: Phenytoin, carbamazepine, topiramate, valproic acid
- GABA agonism: Phenobarbital
- Calcium channel blockade: Gabapentin, pregabalin, valproic acid
- Rapid IV infusion of phenytoin → myocardial depression and cardiac arrest from **propylene glycol diluent** (not present in fosphenytoin)

DIAGNOSIS

- Clinical laboratories can measure serum concentrations for many antiepileptics; however, concentrations may not accurately predict toxicity.
- Valproic acid may induce hyperammonemia from depletion of carnitine and interference with the urea cycle.
- Free phenytoin concentration depends on serum albumin and may be estimated after measuring total phenytoin concentration and albumin concentration.

SYMPTOMS/EXAMINATION

- All → CNS depression in overdose
- Carbamazepine
  - Mild/moderate toxicity: Ataxia and nystagmus
  - Severe toxicity (concentrations > 40 mg/L): Seizures, respiratory and CNS depression, and dysrhythmias (AV block, QRS/QTc prolongation)
- Phenytoin
  - Mild to moderate toxicity: Nystagmus, ataxia, and dysarthria
  - Severe toxicity (concentrations > 50 mg/L): Stupor, coma, and respiratory arrest
  - Rapid IV injection → hypotension, bradycardia, and cardiac arrest due to diluent (propylene glycol)
  - Serious soft tissue reaction → "**purple glove syndrome**": Edema, pain, ischemia, tissue necrosis, compartment syndrome
- Valproic acid
  - Mild to moderate toxicity: Nausea, vomiting, CNS depression
  - Severe toxicity (levels > 850 mg/L): Coma, respiratory depression, seizures, metabolic disturbances, cardiac arrest

TREATMENT

- Supportive therapy.
- Observe asymptomatic patients for at least 6 hours—peak serum concentrations may be delayed with ingestion of modified-release products.
- AC in patients presenting early without CNS depression.
- HD is **not** effective in most overdoses; may be considered in massive valproic acid ingestions.
- MDAC increases the clearance of phenytoin, carbamazepine, and phenobarbital.
- L-carnitine can be used to treat valproic acid induced hyperammonemia.

COMPLICATIONS

- **Drug reaction with eosinophilia and systemic symptoms (DRESS) syndrome:** Hypersensitivity reaction associated with aromatic antiepileptics such as phenytoin, carbamazepine, phenobarbital, and lamotrigine.
  - Initial symptoms include fever, malaise, pharyngitis with progression to drug rash, lymphadenopathy, and multiorgan involvement with fatality rates as high as 10%.
- **Gingival hyperplasia** can be seen with chronic phenytoin therapy.

NEWER ANTICONVULSANTS

Gabapentin

- Adjunctive treatment for seizure, postherpetic neuralgia, posttraumatic stress disorder, behavioral disorder, mood disorders, bruxism, migraine prophylaxis, trigeminal neuralgia, neuropathic pain
- Adjust doses with **renal failure**
- Clinical effects: Sedation, ataxia, movement disorder, nausea, vomiting, psychosis with pregabalin, and **coma rare**
- Treatment: Supportive, AC

Lacosamide (Vimpat)

- Functionalized amino acid approved as an adjunct antiepileptic
- Clinical effects: AV blockade, ataxia, diplopia, sedation
- Treatment: Supportive, AC

Lamotrigine (Lamictal)

- Broad spectrum; used for bipolar disorder
- Clinical effects: Nausea, vomiting, lethargy, ataxia, nystagmus, **seizures, coma QRS widening/ventricular dysrhythmias**
- Chronic use: Rash, rhabdomyolysis, and increased liver function tests (LFTs)
- Treatment: Supportive, AC, benzodiazepines for seizures, sodium bicarbonate for QRS prolongation

Levetiracetam (Keppra)

- Also neuroprotective and anti-inflammatory
- Wide margin of safety with no CYP effects
- Clinical effects: Lethargy, coma, and respiratory depression, and rarely psychosis
- Treatment: Supportive, AC

Q

A 45-year-old woman is brought in by family due to nonsensical speech and strange behavior over the last day. They report a medical history of seizure disorder on an unknown antiepileptic drug. Laboratory workup is remarkable for an elevated ammonia level. What medication is responsible for this presentation?

KEY FACT

Severe valproic acid toxicity (as compared to phenytoin and carbamazepine) can be treated with HD. Valproic acid-induced hyperammonemia is treated with L-carnitine.

A

Valproic Acid.

Oxcarbazepine (Trileptal)
- Clinical effects: Somnolence, tinnitus, bradycardia, and ↓ BP
- Treatment: Supportive, AC

Tiagabine (Gabitril)
- Adjunctive treatment of seizures and psychiatric disorders
- Clinical effects: Lethargy, **facial myoclonus** (grimacing), nystagmus, **posturing**, coma, and seizures (stimulation of $GABA_B$ receptors on thalamus)
- Treatment: Supportive, AC; seizures, posturing, or grimacing with benzodiazepines as first line

Topiramate (Topamax)
- Long duration of action
- **Inhibits carbonic anhydrase** causing a nongap acidosis, renal tubular acidosis (renal tubular acidosis [RTA]—↑ urine pH), hypokalemia, and hyperchloremia
- Clinical effects: **Nephrolithiasis**, lethargy, ataxia, nystagmus, echolalia, **psychosis,** hallucinations, myoclonus, waxing and waning lucid intervals, myopia, acute angle **glaucoma,** coma, seizures, and status epilepticus
- Treatment: Supportive, AC, sodium bicarbonate (1-2 mEq/kg) for severe RTA, and rarely **HD**

Vigabatrin (Sabril)
- Long duration of action
- Clinical effects: **Agitation, psychosis** (more common in kids), coma
- Chronic effects: Depression, psychosis, dizziness, peripheral **vision defects, vision loss**, and tremor
- Treatment: Supportive, agitation benzodiazepines, psychosis resolves with removal of drug

Zonisamide (Zonegran)
- Sulfonamide derivative
- **Weak carbonic anhydrase inhibitor**
- Clinical effects: Nephrolithiasis, psychosis, bradycardia, hypotension, RTA, ↑ BUN/Cr (blood urea nitrogen/creatinine), coma, and seizure
- Treatment: Supportive, AC

Antiparkinsonism Drugs

KEY FACT

Acute overdose of antiparkinsonism drugs is rare.

Parkinson disease is a neurodegenerative disorder affecting the substantia nigra resulting in reduced production of dopamine, an essential neurotransmitter for the control of movement and coordination.

The drugs used in the treatment of Parkinson disease can be divided into six main groups: Levodopa, dopamine agonists, catechol-O-methyltransferase (COMT) inhibitors, monoamine oxidase B inhibitor, amantidine, and anticholinergics (Table 6.10).

Mechanism/ Toxicity

- Levodopa and dopamine agonists: Excessive activation of dopaminergic neurons and activation of serotonergic systems
- COMT inhibitor and monoamine oxidase B inhibitor: Excessive circulating catecholamines
- Amantidine and anticholinergics: Inhibition of central and peripheral muscarinic receptors

TABLE 6.10. Drugs Used in the Treatment of Parkinson Disease and Mechanisms of Action

Drug	Mechanism of Action
Levodopa	Converts to dopamine
Dopamine Agonists Bromocriptine Pergolide Pramipexole Ropinirole	Dopamine receptor agonist
COMT inhibitors Tolcapone Entacapone	Extend the duration of effect of levodopa
Monoamine oxidase B inhibitor Selegiline	Blocks reuptake of dopamine
Amantidine	Inhibits excessive glutamate neurotransmission in the basal ganglia, increased dopamine release, decreased dopamine reuptake, and anticholinergic
Anticholinergics Benztropine Trihexyphenidyl	Inhibit the excess central muscarinic activity caused by dopamine deficiency

COMT, catechol-*O*-methyltransferase.

Symptoms/Examination

- Levodopa and dopamine agonists:
  - Acute toxicity: Anxiety, confusion, agitation, tachycardia, orthostatic hypotension, nausea/vomiting, dyskinesias
  - Chronic toxicity: Dystonia, hallucinations, hypersexuality, delusions, fibrotic changes (dopamine agonists only)
- Amantidine and anticholinergics: **Agitation/confusion, hallucinations, hyperthermia, tachycardia, dry mucous membranes, decreased bowel sounds, and urinary retention**
- COMT inhibitor and monoamine oxidase B inhibitor: Limited information; may see classic MAOI and serotonin toxicity

Diagnosis

- Clinical diagnosis is based on history and examination.
- Selegiline is metabolized to L-methamphetamine, which can be detected on urine toxicology screening.

Treatment

- Supportive care and cessation of medication
- Sedation with benzodiazepines as needed

KEY FACT

Remember removal of dopaminergic agents may precipitate neuroleptic malignant syndrome.

Antipsychotics

Antipsychotics were developed for the treatment of psychoses, but are also commonly used in the treatment of intractable vomiting, migraines, and in the chemical restraint of severely agitated patients. Therapeutic effects are due to antagonism of mesolimbic dopamine receptors, but variable affinity for other receptors causes a variety of side effects and toxicity. They are divided into two major groups (Table 6.11).

TYPICAL ANTIPSYCHOTICS

Originally introduced in the 1950s, characterized by nonspecific receptor affinity → greater incidence of side effects than newer agents

ATYPICAL ANTIPSYCHOTICS

Acute overdose of newer generation antipsychotics (introduced in the 1970s) is common, but toxicity resulting in severe morbidity or mortality is rare.

Mechanism/Toxicity

- Nonspecific dopamine receptor antagonism → extrapyramidal symptoms and neuroleptic malignant syndrome (NMS)
- $\alpha 1$-Adrenergic antagonism → hypotension and reflex tachycardia
- Muscarinic receptor antagonism → anticholinergic symptoms
- Histamine receptor antagonism → sedation
- Cardiac fast sodium channel blockade → QRS widening
- Cardiac K^+ channel blockade → prolonged QTc

Symptoms/Examination

- Adverse effects related to nonspecific receptor blockade are common (Table 6.12), and typical agents are more likely to have adverse effects than atypical agents.
- Findings in acute overdose are an extension of adverse effects:
  - Highest incidence of NMS with typical antipsychotics (haloperidol)
  - Highest rate of QTc prolongation with ziprasidone
  - Quetiapine most sedating with notable hypotension

TABLE 6.11. Common Antipsychotic Agents

Typical Antipsychotics	Atypical Antipsychotics
Haloperidol (Haldol)/Droperidol	Risperidone (Risperdal)
Chlorpromazine (Thorazine)	Quetiapine (Seroquel)
Fluphenazine	Olanzapine (Zyprexa)
	Aripiprazole (Abilify)

TABLE 6.12. Adverse Effects of Antipsychotics

Adverse Effect	Mechanism/Toxicity	Symptoms/Examination	Treatment
Extrapyramidal symptoms	Basal ganglia dopamine receptor antagonism	See Table 6.13	Diphenhydramine, benztropine, or benzodiazepines
NMS	Anterior hypothalamus and basal ganglia dopamine receptor antagonism	Altered mental status Hyperthermia Muscular rigidity	Stop medication Benzodiazepines Intubate and paralyze as needed
Altered mental status	Histamine and muscarinic receptor antagonism	Agitated delirium Somnolence Coma	Benzodiazepines for agitation Support airway as needed
Hypotension	α_1-Adrenergic receptor antagonism	Mild to moderate hypotension	Intravenous fluids Pressors may be needed
Tachycardia	α_1-Adrenergic (reflex tachycardia) and muscarinic receptor antagonism	Mild to moderate sinus tachycardia	Benzodiazepines and supportive care
Prolonged QTc	K^+ channel blockade	Theoretical concern for torsade de pointes	Cardiac monitoring Check electrolytes Treat torsade (Mg^{++}, overdrive pacing)
Blood dyscrasias	Adverse drug effect associated with clozapine	Agranulocytosis, leukopenia, neutropenia	Stop medication

NMS, Neuroleptic malignant syndrome.

Diagnosis

- Clinical diagnosis is based on history of exposure and physical examination findings.
- ECG is used to monitor prolonged QRS and QTc.

Treatment

- Supportive therapy and continuous monitoring
- AC for large ingestions within 1-2 hours (with airway protection as needed)
- Norepinephrine for hypotension unresponsive to IV fluids
- IV magnesium sulfate, overdrive pacing, isoproterenol for torsade de pointes
- Benzodiazepines to control agitation and seizures
- Aggressive sedation and cooling measures for NMS

Q

A 65-year-old man presents to the ED via EMS with weakness and dizziness. He has a history of depression, CHF, and hypertension (HTN), and is on multiple "heart" medications. Physical examination reveals sinus bradycardia, hypotension, mild temperature depression, and normal mentation. Overdose of which groups of cardiac drugs is suggested by this patient's presentation?

KEY FACT

Class IA and IC antidysrhythmic agents are notorious for prolonging the QRS and/or QTc, causing ventricular tachycardia (VT) or torsade de pointes.

A

Overdose of β-blockers, calcium channel blockers, clonidine, digoxin, and central-acting agents should be suspected in any patient presenting with hypotension and bradycardia.

TABLE 6.13. Extrapyramidal Symptoms

Name	Onset/Reversibility	Symptoms/Examination	Treatment
Akathisia	Hours to days Reversible	Anxiety Acute motor restlessness	Stop medication Benzodiazepines Diphenhydramine Benztropine
Acute dystonia	Hours to days after exposure Reversible	Sustained muscle contractions → facial grimacing Torticollis Trismus Laryngospasm Opisthotonos	Stop medication Benzodiazepines Diphenhydramine Benztropine
Parkinsonism	Days to months of exposure Usually reversible	Akinesia or bradykinesia Masked facies Muscular rigidity Tremor Gait instability Cognitive impairment	↓ Dose or stop medication Benztropine
Tardive dyskinesia	Months to years of exposure Usually irreversible	Involuntary, repetitive orofacial, trunk, and extremity movements	No specific treatment available

Cardiovascular Medications

ANTIDYSRHYTHMIC AGENTS

KEY FACT

Propranolol, due to its lipophilicity, can cause delirium in the absence of cardiovascular effects.

Antidysrhythmic agents are classified into groups based on electrophysiology properties (Table 6.14). Toxicity is unique to each class.

β-Blockers

Normal function of β-adrenergic receptors:

- β_1: Heart (increases rate, contractility, conduction), kidney (increased secretion of renin), eye (increased production of aqueous humor)
- β_2: Smooth muscle relaxation
- β_3: Adipose tissue (lipolysis)

Mechanism/Toxicity

β-Adrenergic receptors blockade

Symptoms/Examination

- Cardiovascular: Varying degrees of hypotension, bradycardic, cardiogenic shock, QRS, and QTc prolongation
- Pulmonary: Respiratory depression, apnea, and bronchospasm (β_2-blockade)
- Neurologic: AMS, coma, seizures with lipophilic agents (eg, propranolol)
- Endocrine/Electrolytes: Hyperkalemia, hypoglycemia (potentially, in children)

TABLE 6.14. Overview of Antidysrhythmic Agents

Vaughn-Williams Classification	Mechanism of Action	Examples	Symptoms of Toxicity	Treatment
Class I	Na^+ channel blockers → cardiac conduction delay	**IA:** Procainamide, Quinidine, Disopyramide **IB:** Lidocaine, Phenytoin **IC:** Flecainide, Propafenone	Vary with agent Agitation, confusion Hypotension Ventricular or bradydysrhythmias	Supportive care Activated charcoal (if early) Sodium bicarbonate for QRS widening (1A and 1C only)
Class II	β-Blockers	See text	See text	See text
Class III	K^+ channel blockers → prolongation of repolarization Sotalol also has β-blocking activity	Amiodarone Sotalol	Vary with agent Hypotension and bradycardia QTc prolongation → VT, VF, torsade Chronic amiodarone therapy: interstitial pneumonitis, grey or bluish skin changes, corneal microdeposits	Supportive care GI decontamination (if early) Sodium bicarbonate for QRS widening Magnesium/pacing for torsade de pointes
Class IV	Calcium channel blockers	See text	See text	See text

GI, gastrointestinal.

Differential

Calcium channel blocker, clonidine, and digoxin toxicity

Diagnosis

Should be considered in the differential of any patient with bradycardia and hypotension

Treatment

- Supportive therapy
- GI decontamination
  - GL: Consider only if presenting within 1 hour of ingestion of a large quantity of potentially lethal agents that lack effective antidotes (eg, verapamil, diltiazem, or propranolol).
  - AC: Consider administration in patients presenting within 1 hour of ingestion of potentially lethal medication with protected airway.
  - WBI: If large overdose of modified-release preparation in patients with a patent airway.
- Bradycardia and hypotension
  - Treat initially with **IVF, atropine,** and β-adrenergic **vasopressors** (norepinephrine, epinephrine, dopamine).
  - **Calcium** supplementation for increased intracellular calcium and contractility.

- **Glucagon** bypasses β-adrenergic receptors to increase cyclic AMP, resulting in increased calcium influx into the cell.
  - Requires high doses (5-10 mg).
- **High-dose insulin** increases cardiac output.
  - Start at 1 unit/kg of regular insulin bolus and then a drip at 1 unit/kg/h and titrate
  - Consider bolus of 0.5 g/kg of dextrose and start an infusion to maintain blood glucose between 100 and 200 mg/dL
- Cardiac pacing, intra-aortic balloon pump, and bypass should be considered if pharmacologic measures fail.
- Sodium bicarbonate for prolonged QRS in propranolol toxicity.
- HD may be considered for atenolol toxicity.

Calcium Channel Blockers

Prescribed for the treatment of hypertension, arrhythmias, and migraines.

Mechanism/Toxicity

- Blockade of L-type voltage-gated Ca^{++} channels → decreased Ca^{++} influx into cells
- In cardiac cells → decreased SA node activity, decreased contractility, slowed AV conduction
- In smooth muscle cells (peripheral vascular system) → relaxation and vasodilatation
- In pancreatic β-islet cells → decrease insulin release
- Agent specificity:
  - Verapamil: Major effect at sinoatrial and AV nodes
  - Diltiazem: Intermediate activity at both cardiac and peripheral vasculature
  - Dihydropyridines (eg, nifedipine): Major effect on peripheral vasculature

KEY FACT

Specificity between peripheral and central cardiovascular effect may be lost in overdose.

Symptoms/Examination

- Cardiovascular: Varying degrees of hypotension, including cardiogenic shock, bradycardia, QRS widening, and QTc prolongation
- Neurological: AMS, seizures, and coma, and respiratory depression
- Endocrine: Hyperglycemia

KEY FACT

Hyperglycemia is suggestive of calcium channel blocker overdose in the undifferentiated hypotensive and bradycardic patient.

Differential

β-Blockers, clonidine, and digoxin

Diagnosis

Should be considered in the differential of any patient with bradycardia, hypotension, and hyperglycemia

KEY FACT

Hyperglycemia may help differentiate between calcium channel blocker overdose (where hyperglycemia is common) and β-blocker overdose (where patients are typically euglycemic).

Treatment

- GI decontamination:
  - GL: Consider only if presenting within 1 hour of ingestion of a large quantity of potentially lethal agents that lack effective antidotes (eg, verapamil, diltiazem, or propranolol) or sustained-release products
  - AC: Best if administered in patients presenting within 1 hour of ingestion with protected airway
  - WBI: If large overdose of sustained-release preparation with patent airway
- Bradycardia and hypotension:
  - Treat initially with IVF, **atropine**, and **vasopressors** (norepinephrine, epinephrine, dopamine).

- **Calcium** supplementation for increased intracellular calcium and contractility.
- Glucagon may be less successful than with β-blocker toxicity, but consider in undifferentiated patients.
- **High-dose insulin** increases cardiac output.
  - Start at 1 unit/kg of regular insulin bolus and then a drip at 1 unit/kg/h and titrate.
  - Consider bolus of 0.5 g/kg of dextrose and start an infusion to maintain blood glucose between 100 and 200 mg/dL.
- Cardiac pacing, intra-aortic balloon pump, and bypass should be considered if pharmacologic measures fail.

Digoxin

Digoxin is a cardiac glycoside derived from the foxglove plant. It is used to increase the force of myocardial contraction in systolic heart failure and to decrease AV conduction in atrial fibrillation. Digoxin has a narrow therapeutic-toxic window and is eliminated primarily via renal excretion.

Mechanism/Toxicity

- Inactivation of the Na^+/K^+ ATPase pump on the cardiac cell membrane → increased intracellular Ca^{++} and extracellular K^+
- Increased automaticity
- Decreases conduction through the AV node via increased vagal tone

Toxicity may be either acute or chronic:

- Acute toxicity:
  - Results from an acute ingestion.
  - Severe Na^+/K^+ ATPase pump inhibition → hyperkalemia.
  - Hyperkalemia in acute toxicity is a predictor of poor outcome without treatment.
- Chronic toxicity:
  - Caused by increase in dose or decrease in renal excretion of digoxin in a patient on chronic therapy.
  - Hypokalemia may enhance chronic toxicity → toxicity at lower digoxin levels.
  - Higher overall mortality (sicker patient population at baseline).

KEY FACT

Hyperkalemia in acute digoxin toxicity is a predictor of poor outcome.

Symptoms/Examination

- Onset of symptoms is often insidious in chronic toxicity
- Cardiovascular: Acute toxicity → more bradycardia and blocks, chronic toxicity → ventricular dysrhythmias more common
  - Bidirectional VT, slow atrial fibrillation, and almost any dysrhythmia except supraventricular tachydysrhythmias or torsade de pointes
- GI: Nausea/vomiting, anorexia
- Neurological: Visual disturbances (eg, scotomata, yellow halos around lights), headaches, generalized weakness, mental status changes

KEY FACT

Hypokalemia in a patient on chronic digoxin therapy may lead to toxicity at lower digoxin levels.

KEY FACT

Bidirectional VT is fairly specific for cardiac glycoside toxicity.

Diagnosis

- Serum digoxin concentration: May not correlate with symptoms and may take 4-6 hours to reach steady state in acute ingestion.
- Potassium and renal function monitoring are essential.

Treatment

- Supportive therapy.
- Hyperkalemia: Treat in the normal manner. Until recently, it was often recommended to avoid calcium in the setting of digoxin toxicity. However, IV Ca^{++} is reasonable and not dangerous.

TABLE 6.15. Indications for Digoxin-Specific Antibodies

Ventricular dysrhythmias
Bradycardia unresponsive to therapy
$K^+ > 5.0$ mEq/dL in acute ingestion
Potentially massive overdose Adults: > 10 mg Pediatrics: > 4 mg (or 0.1 mg/kg)

- Hypokalemia in chronic toxicity: Replete if < 4.0 mEq/L
- Consider magnesium repletion
- Bradycardia: Treat with atropine and/or pacing
- Tachydysrhythmias:
  - Cardioversion and defibrillation may induce VT/VF (ventricular fibrillation).
  - Phenytoin and lidocaine are felt to be safest drugs.
    - Phenytoin can increase AV nodal conduction.
- **Antidote = digoxin-specific antibodies** (see Table 6.15 for indications)
  - Acute empiric dosing = 10-20 vials.
  - Chronic adult = 2-4 vials.
  - Chronic children = 1-2 vials.
  - Known concentration: # vials = [weight (kg) × concentration (ng/mL)/100], round up to next vial.
  - Give over 30 minutes; IV bolus is acceptable in cardiac arrest.
  - Do NOT follow total digoxin concentrations after antidote is given, assay cannot differentiate between free digoxin and bound digoxin.

Angiotensin-Converting Enzyme Inhibitors and Angiotensin Receptor Blockers

Both are prescribed for the treatment of hypertension (HTN) and CHF. Angiotensin-converting enzyme inhibitors (ACEI) are also used post-MI and for diabetic nephropathy.

> **KEY FACT**
>
> Serious toxicity is not expected in ACEI or ARB overdose as a single agent.

Complications of chronic use include angioedema, nonproductive cough, and renal insufficiency (with renal artery stenosis).

Mechanism/Toxicity

- ACEI: Decreases angiotensin II formation.
- Angiotensin receptor blockers (ARB): Blocks the receptor for angiotensin II on the blood vessels, heart, and adrenal cortex.
- Blockage of angiotensin II results in decreased aldosterone release (→ decreased sodium and water retention) and vasodilation.

Symptoms/Examination

- Mild hypotension
- Hyperkalemia

Diagnosis

Clinical based on patient history, physical examination, and laboratory analysis

TREATMENT

- Supportive care with IVF and vasopressors (rarely needed)
- Unlikely to cause significant toxicity

Clonidine

An imidazoline compound prescribed for the treatment of hypertension and pediatric behavioral disorders. Other imidazoline compounds include oxymetazoline and tetrahydrozoline (ophthalmologic topical vasoconstrictors and nasal decongestants), tizanidine (centrally acting muscle relaxant), guanfacine (used to treat pediatric behavioral disorder), and dexmedetomidine (ICU IV sedation).

MECHANISM/TOXICITY

- Central presynaptic α_2-adrenergic agonist → decreased sympathetic (norepinephrine) outflow → hypotension and bradycardia.
- Peripherally, presynaptic α_2-agonism may result in vasoconstriction and paradoxical transient hypertension.

SYMPTOMS/EXAMINATION

- Cardiovascular: Initial, short-lived hypertension progresses to hypotension and bradycardia
- Respiratory: Hypoventilation
- Neurologic: Mental status depression, coma, and miosis

DIFFERENTIAL

β-Blockers, calcium channel blockers, digoxin, and opioids

DIAGNOSIS

- Clinical diagnosis based on patient history and physical examination
- Consider in the differential of any patient with bradycardia and hypotension

TREATMENT

- Supportive care.
- Bradycardia and hypotension typically respond to IV fluids, but may require atropine or vasopressors.
- Naloxone has been reported to reverse some of the sedation.

KEY FACT

Clonidine overdose may resemble opioid overdose with miosis, but hypotension will be more notable with clonidine.

OTHER ANTIHYPERTENSIVE AGENTS

Table 6.16 lists other hypertensive agents that may present with acute toxicity in overdose.

These drugs will usually cause symptoms, but are rarely life threatening as a single drug ingestion.

DIAGNOSIS

Clinical based on patient history and physical examination

TREATMENT

Supportive care with IV fluids and vasopressors (if needed) is usually sufficient.

Q

A 72-year-old man presents to the ED via EMS for weakness and AMS. He has a history of dementia and diabetes. EMS found bottles of metformin and acarbose in the bathroom. Physical examination reveals a finger stick of 48, sinus tachycardia, and sweaty skin. The patient is awake, but confused. Which of the drugs found in his house is likely responsible for his hypoglycemia?

TABLE 6.16. Toxicity From Other Hypertensive Agents

Antihypertensive Agent	Mechanism/Toxicity	Symptoms/Examination
Furosemide **Hydrochlorothiazide**	Diuretics	Hypotension Electrolyte disturbances
Hydralazine	Direct-acting vasodilator	Hypotension Tachycardia Hypokalemia
Minoxidil	Inhibits Ca^{++} uptake into cells → vasodilation	Hypotension Tachycardia
Nitroprusside **Nitroglycerin**	Direct-acting venodilator	Hypotension Tachycardia Cyanide toxicity (nitroprusside)
Methyldopa	Metabolite stimulates central α_2-receptors → ↓ sympathetic output	Hypotension Miosis Sedation Respiratory depression
Doxazosin **Prazosin** **Terazosin**	Selective α_1-receptor blocker → ↓ PVR	Hypotension Tachycardia Dizziness/syncope

Diabetes Medications

SULFONYLUREAS

Agents include glipizide, glyburide, and glimepiride.

Mechanism/Toxicity

- ↑ Secretion of preformed insulin from pancreatic β-islet cells → hypoglycemia.
- Hepatic or renal impairment and drug interactions may be inciting event.

Symptoms/Examination

- Most agents require hours to reach peak effect, but hypoglycemia may be delayed as long as 24 hours after ingestion.
- Symptoms of hypoglycemia:
  - Cardiac: Tachycardia, hypertension.
  - Dermatologic: Diaphoresis.
  - GI: Nausea.
  - Neurologic: Mental status changes, agitation, headache, focal neurologic deficits, or seizures.
  - Symptoms may be masked by the concurrent use of β-adrenergic antagonists.

Differential

Other causes of hypoglycemia, including insulin excess, sepsis, hepatic dysfunction, endocrine disorders, or ethanol intoxication

KEY FACT

Ingestion of a single sulfonylurea tablet can produce severe hypoglycemia in young children.

KEY FACT

Octreotide inhibits the release of insulin from the pancreas and therefore can be used in sulfonylurea-induced hypoglycemia.

A

Neither biguanides (metformin) nor α-glucosidase inhibitors (acarbose) typically cause hypoglycemia. Consider insulin, sulfonylureas, or other nontoxicologic causes of hypoglycemia.

Diagnosis

Clinical based on patient history, physical examination, and evidence of hypoglycemia by rapid glucose measurement

Treatment

- AC if recent ingestion and protected airway
- Correct hypoglycemia with dextrose boluses as needed to maintain normal serum glucose
- **Antidote = octreotide**
  - Long-acting synthetic analog of somatostatin, inhibits release of insulin from pancreas
  - Use for recurrent hypoglycemia
  - Decreases dextrose requirements and further episodes of recurrent hypoglycemia
  - Monitor for recurrent hypoglycemia after termination of octreotide therapy
- All patients who become symptomatic should be admitted for 24 hours of observation regardless of response to treatment.
- All children ingesting one or more sulfonylurea tablets should be observed for at least 12 hours and possibly longer if there is any hypoglycemia or glucose administration.

Complication

Disulfiram reactions (headache, flushing, nausea/vomiting) are possible with all sulfonylureas following exposure to alcohol

KEY FACT

Nonspecific symptoms in patient on metformin? Suspect lactic acidosis.

OTHER ANTIHYPERGLYCEMIC AGENTS

Table 6.17 lists other diabetic agents that may present with acute toxicity in overdose.

Hormonal Agents

THYROID HORMONES

Thyroid hormones are used as replacement therapy in hypothyroidism. Levothyroxine (T_4, Synthroid) is the most commonly used agent, though triiodothyronine (T_3), liotrix (both T_3 and T_4), and natural desiccated animal thyroid (both T_3 and T_4) are also available.

Onset of symptoms from levothyroxine (T_4) overdose may be delayed by 2-5 days as T_4 requires in vivo conversion to the active hormone, T_3. In contrast, T_3 ingestions will usually produce symptoms within 6 hours after ingestion.

Mechanism/Toxicity

Increases sympathetic activity

Symptoms/Examination

- Tremor, confusion, agitation, hyperreflexia
- Tachycardia, hypertension, palpitations, flushing, diaphoresis, diarrhea, mydriasis
- Fever, weight loss, and heat intolerance with chronic overdose

Q

A 32-year-old woman presents 5 days after ingesting #50 Levothyroxine 112 μg (tetraiodothyronine [T_4] tablets). Patient was asymptomatic until day of presentation when she presented with palpitations and agitation. Upon ED arrival, her vital signs showed: HR 160 bpm, BP 130/90 mm Hg, RR 16 breaths/min, temperature of 37.5°C 99.5°F. On physical examination, patient was found to be restless, tachycardic, with brisk reflexes. ECG showed sinus tachycardia. Laboratory results were as follows: Total T_4 30 μg/dL (normal 5-12 μg/dL), total T_3 220 ng/dL (normal 40-132 ng/dL), and undetectable thyroid-stimulating hormone level (TSH). How would you manage this patient?

TABLE 6.17. Toxicity from other Hypoglycemic Agents

Antihyperglycemic Class	Mechanism of Action	Symptoms/Exam
Biguanides (Metformin)	↑ Peripheral glucose use ↓ Hepatic production and intestinal absorption of glucose	Lactic acidosis → nausea/vomiting, malaise, tachypnea Does NOT cause hypoglycemia Treatment: hemodialysis if severe lactic acidosis (more likely to occur in underlying renal failure)
Meglitinides (Nateglinide, Repaglinide)	↑ Release of insulin	Hypoglycemia (rare and less severe than sulfonylureas)
α-Glucosidase inhibitors (Acarbose, Miglitol)	Delays breakdown of complex carbohydrates in small intestines	Abdominal cramping, diarrhea
Thiazolidinediones (Rosiglitazone, Pioglitazone)	↑ Insulin sensitivity Inhibits gluconeogenesis	Hepatotoxicity, CHF
Gliptins (Sitagliptin, Saxagliptin)	Inhibits enzyme responsible for inactivation of incretin	Nasopharyngitis, skin lesions
Incretin mimetic (Exenatide)	Enhances insulin release	Hypoglycemia rare, GI distress, pancreatitis

CHF, congestive heart failure; GI, gastrointestinal.

KEY FACT

Acute ingestions of levothyroxine will not produce symptoms for several days.

Differential

- Primary hyperthyroid states (Graves disease)
- Sympathomimetic toxicity (cocaine, amphetamines)
- Methylxanthine toxicity (theophylline, caffeine)

Diagnosis

- Clinical diagnosis based on history and physical examination
- Elevated T_4:T_3 ratio is suggestive of chronic, excess levothyroxine intake though concentrations do not correlate well with clinical symptoms

Treatment

- AC if presenting within 1-2 hours of large acute ingestion may prevent later toxicity.
- Benzodiazepines for agitation.
- β-Antagonists, such as propranolol or esmolol, to control severe tachydysrhythmias.
- Agents that block endogenous thyroid hormone production (PTU, methimazole) have limited utility.

A

Use β-antagonists, such as propranolol or esmolol, to control severe tachyarrhythmias, benzodiazepines for agitation.

Household Chemicals

CAUSTICS

Many household products are caustic or corrosive, causing direct tissue damage by burns and necrosis. Examples include cleaning products. Most severe injuries are caused by intentional ingestion or industrial-strength products.

Mechanism/Toxicity

- Produce damage by direct cellular injury
- Acids: Low pH, cause coagulation necrosis, may cause very deep injury but form eschar, most injury occurs rapidly
- Alkali/bases: High pH, cause liquefactive necrosis, ongoing slower injury causes deep tissue penetration
- Factors affecting toxicity include pH, concentration, quantity ingested, titratable acid reserve, and viscosity

Symptoms/Examination

- Acute GI: Pain, burning sensation, vomiting, drooling, GI bleed, perforated viscus
- Acute Pulmonary: Airway burns if aspiration event, upper airway edema, stridor, airway obstruction
- Dermal exposure: Pain, chemical burns
- Ocular exposure: Pain, lacrimation, hyperemia, chemosis, vision changes, globe rupture
- Delayed symptoms: GI tract scarring, strictures, obstruction

Diagnosis

- Clinical diagnosis based on history of exposure.
- In pediatric unintentional ingestions, higher likelihood of significant injury if vomiting, drooling, or stridor is present.

Treatment

- ABCs and supportive care
- Avoid vomiting, charcoal, and gastric emptying (only consider nasogastric [NG] aspiration if large volume of caustic present in stomach)
- Early intubation if airway involvement suspected
- Urgent GI consult for endoscopy if significant ingestion or symptoms (scope within 24 hours or delay for 2 weeks), useful for evaluation of grade of injury and prognosis for risk of strictures
- Emergent surgical consult if suspected perforation
- Dermal exposure: Decontaminate thoroughly with large volume irrigation, pain control, treat like any other burn, consider burn surgery evaluation if severe
- Ocular exposure: Decontaminate thoroughly with large volume irrigation via Morgan lens if available until pH normal, consult ophthalmology if any symptoms remain after irrigation

HYDROCARBONS

Hydrocarbons include any compound containing both hydrogen and carbon, and include subcategories such as aliphatic (butane, octane, hexane), cyclic (cyclohexane), aromatic (benzene, toluene, naphthalene), and halogenated (chloroform, carbon tetrachloride). Hydrocarbons are extremely common in household products, including in solvents, degreasers, fuels, and oils.

Mechanism/Toxicity

- Systemic toxicity may include CNS depression, similar to general anesthetics.
- Specific hydrocarbons may be associated with unique toxicities, such as RTA and non-gap acidosis with toluene exposure.
- Hydrocarbon aspiration causes chemical pneumonitis and acute lung injury/acute respiratory distress syndrome (ALI/ARDS) due to direct injury and disruption of pulmonary surfactant.

Symptoms/Examination

- CNS: CNS depression, intoxication, obtundation, coma, seizures
- GI: Nausea, vomiting
- Pulmonary: Aspiration pneumonitis, ALI/ARDS
- Cyclic variation: Myocardial sensitization to catecholamines leading to cardiac dysrhythmias after a patient is startled (sudden sniffing death syndrome)
- Chronic exposure: Most common with abuse by huffing or inhalation, leukoencephalopathy, slowed mentation

Diagnosis

Clinical diagnosis based on history of exposure

Treatment

- ABCs and supportive care
- Avoid vomiting, charcoal, and gastric emptying (only consider NG aspiration if large volume of hydrocarbon present in stomach, or substance with severe systemic toxicity)
- Monitor for signs/symptoms of aspiration pneumonitis (persistent cough, dyspnea, tachypnea, hypoxia, wheezing), consider chest x-ray (CXR) if any symptoms at 6 hours after exposure
- Admit any patient with persistent symptoms or evidence of aspiration on CXR

CHLORINE AND CHLORAMINE

Chlorine gas is yellow-green in color with an irritating odor, and may be released from bleach (hypochlorite) especially when used in closed rooms or high concentrations. Chloramine gas is a similarly irritating gas that is released from the mixing of ammonia and bleach.

Mechanism/Toxicity

Chlorine and chloramine are irritants that cause direct mucous membrane irritation and inflammation

Symptoms/Examination

Pulmonary: Mucous membrane irritation, wheezing, upper airway edema, stridor, pneumonitis, pulmonary edema (more common with chlorine gas)

Diagnosis

Clinical diagnosis based on history of exposure

Treatment

- Remove from exposure to fresh air, consider warmed humidified air if available
- ABCs and supportive care
- Bronchodilators as needed for significant wheezing, especially if history of asthma
- Observe patients (up to 24 hours) exposed to high concentrations of chlorine gas for upper airway and pulmonary edema

TABLE 6.18. Common Nontoxic Household Chemicals

Cyanoacrylate glues	Ballpoint-pen ink
Soap	Ink (w/out aniline dyes, EG)
Lipstick	Watercolors
Hand lotion	Crayons
Suntan lotion	Chalk
Perfume (except alcohol)	Candles
Air fresheners	Fire extinguishers
Toothpaste	Plaster
Deodorant	Indelible markers
Shampoo	Silica gel packets
Eye makeup	Fabric softener
Shoe polish	Fertilizers
Hydrogen peroxide (unless food-grade)	Household bleach (< 5% sodium hypochlorite)

COMMON NONTOXIC HOUSEHOLD CHEMICALS

See (Table 6.18).

Industrial Toxins

HYDROGEN FLUORIDE

Hydrogen fluoride (HF, hydrofluoric acid) is a water soluble weak acid that is most commonly encountered as a solution. HF is found in rust removers, oven cleaners, and automotive wheel cleaners. Commercial uses include glass etching, graffiti removal, and manufacture of semiconductors and certain fuels.

Mechanism/Toxicity

- Absorbed through skin and mucous membranes → penetrates deeply and causes cellular destruction → pain
- Highly reactive free fluoride ion avidly binds extracellular Ca^{++} and Mg^{++} → hypocalcemia and hypomagnesemia
- Systemic hypocalcemia and hypomagnesemia may occur with ingestion or heavy dermal exposure
- Hyperkalemia may be delayed in onset and occurs due to cellular breakdown, acidosis and direct fluoride effects on K^+ efflux

Symptoms/Examination

- Direct relationship between solution concentration and time to symptom onset.
  - Concentrated solutions > 10% produce symptoms earlier.
  - Onset can be delayed up to 24 hours after exposure to dilute solution.
- Dermal exposure to low concentrations cause local pain, erythema, swelling, and a white-blue discoloration (especially subungual).
  - Pain "out of proportion" to skin findings
  - Local pain due to direct tissue injury
- Systemic hypocalcemia from oral ingestions and large dermal exposures → tetany, weakness, Chvostek sign, life-threatening dysrhythmias, and sudden death

KEY FACT

Onset of symptoms from dermal exposure to low concentrations of HF may be delayed up to 24 hours.

DIAGNOSIS

- Usually determined from history and examination.
- ECG findings with severe hypocalcemia include prolonged QTc and peaked T waves.
- Direct measurement of total or ionized Ca^{++} confirms severe toxicity.

TREATMENT

- HF ingestions should be considered life threatening-> obtain central access, provide aggressive empiric calcium repletion, and monitor closely.
- **Give calcium chloride via central access** if possible to avoid vascular injury, can also use calcium gluconate (requires 3× as much for same effect) IV for systemic toxicity.
- **Copious water irrigation** for surface decontamination.
- **Calcium gluconate** administration for local pain:
  - Topical paste
  - Subcutaneous and intradermal injections (caution in digits)
  - Bier block
  - Regional intra-arterial infusion
  - Nebulized (for inhalation exposure)

> **KEY FACT**
>
> Calcium gluconate paste, injection, and arterial infusions are key to treating ongoing pain and toxicity from dermal HF exposure.

LEAD

Lead is a heavy metal used extensively in commercial products and manufacturing processes. Adult lead exposure is primarily occupational (construction, mining, welding, smelting, manufacture of batteries, plastic and rubber, "moonshine"). Pediatric exposure usually results from accidental ingestion of lead-containing material, especially paint chips, imported toys and jewelry.

> **KEY FACT**
>
> Most lead toxicity is due to chronic, low-level exposure. Acute toxicity from single exposures is rare.

MECHANISM/TOXICITY

Inhibits a wide variety of cellular enzymes, decreases ability to synthesize heme, directly damages peripheral nerves

SYMPTOMS/EXAMINATION

- **Chronic lead toxicity:** Subtle, insidious, and nonspecific symptoms, including headache, peripheral motor neuropathy (wrist drop), HTN, anemia, gout, and cognitive impairment
- Acute lead toxicity
  - Nausea/vomiting, constipation, abdominal pain (lead colic)
  - Anemia
  - **Encephalopathy**, ataxia, and seizures

> **KEY FACT**
>
> Most lead toxicity is chronic and causes subtle neurologic changes, anemia, and hypertension.

DIAGNOSIS

- Lead can be directly measured in whole blood, consider in cases of anemia with basophilic stippling.
- Lead-containing material is usually visible on x-ray if ingested.

TREATMENT

- Remove the patient from the source of exposure
- AC does **not** bind metals
- WBI is indicated in cases of lead ingestion with visible material on x-ray
- **Chelators = BAL (British anti-lewisite, dimercaprol) and Ca-EDTA (calcium disodium ethylenediaminetetraacetic acid)**
  - Use for the severely poisoned patient (symptomatic with encephalopathy or level >100 μg/dL)
  - Treat with BAL first then follow with Ca-EDTA for encephalopathy

- **Chelator = DMSA** (2,3-dimercaptosuccinic acid, succimer) oral chelation therapy if no acute symptoms and child with level > 45 μg/dL or level > 80 μg/dL in asymptomatic adults

ARSENIC

Arsenic-containing compounds are used in a wide variety of applications:
- Pesticides, wood preservatives, metal alloys, chemical synthesis, and glass manufacturing, folk remedies.
- Arsenic trioxide is used as a chemotherapeutic agent for acute promyelocytic leukemia.

Mechanism/Toxicity

- Inhibits multiple key enzymes in cellular oxidative metabolism
- Arsine gas causes acute hemolysis

Symptoms/Examination

- Chronic poisoning
  - Peripheral neuropathy, headache, ataxia, confusion, malaise
  - Hyperpigmentation, **Mees lines** (transverse white lines on nails), alopecia
  - Skin lesions: Hyperkeratotic lesions palms and soles
  - Cancer: Skin, lung, bladder
- Acute poisoning
  - GI symptoms predominate: **Violent gastroenteritis**
  - Confusion, coma, seizures
  - Hypotension, tachycardia, **prolonged QTc interval**, torsade de pointes
  - ARDS
- Arsine gas poisoning
  - Findings consistent with acute hemolysis: Hematuria, jaundice, renal failure
  - Abdominal pain, nausea/vomiting
  - Hypotension, tachycardia, pulmonary edema
  - Symptoms may be delayed 2-24 hours

KEY FACT

Mees lines appear weeks to months after arsenic exposure.

Diagnosis

- Suspect based on clinical presentation and possible exposure
- 24-hour urine arsenic levels
  - Blood levels not typically useful.
  - Urine levels may be elevated following consumption of seafood because of the presence of nontoxic, organic arsenic compounds, check levels after seafood holiday or determine concentration of specific organic/inorganic species.

KEY FACT

Acute arsenic exposure is characterized by violent gastroenteritis.

Treatment

- Identify and remove the source of arsenic exposure
- WBI: If radiopaque objects visible on x-ray
- **Antidote = BAL** (British anti-lewisite, dimercaprol) for chelation in patients with severe GI symptoms
- DMSA (2,3-dimercaptosuccinic acid, succimer) in chronic poisoning and in acute poisonings once hemodynamically stable and GI symptoms resolved

MERCURY

Mercury is pervasive in industrial processes and commercial products. It is encountered in three forms:
- Elemental mercury (quicksilver): Mercury-containing devices in workplace or home

- Inorganic mercury salts: Calomel (mercurous chloride) in skin-lightening creams
- Organic mercury: Occupational/agricultural exposure

Elemental mercury primarily causes toxicity when inhaled and has negligent oral absorption. The principal route of exposure for mercury salts and organic mercury is through GI absorption.

Mechanism/Toxicity

- Reacts with sulfhydryl groups causing inhibition of multiple cellular enzyme systems.
- Inhalation of elemental mercury may lead to severe pneumonitis and noncardiogenic pulmonary edema.

Symptoms/Examination

- Elemental mercury (quicksilver) inhalation
  - Acute: Rapid onset shortness of breath, cough, chills, fever, respiratory distress
  - Chronic: Tremor, neuropsychiatric disturbances (erethism = shyness, withdrawal, depression), gingivostomatitis, acrodynia (pain in extremities, HTN, sweating, anorexia, irritability, pink discoloration, and desquamation in extremities = "pink disease")
- Acute ingestion of inorganic mercury salts: Corrosive gastroenteritis with shock (from massive fluid loss), renal failure, grayish discoloration of mucous membranes, metallic taste
- Acute ingestion of organic mercury: Delayed permanent neurotoxicity—ataxia, dysarthria, constricted visual fields

> **KEY FACT**
>
> Elemental mercury (inhaled) → respiratory distress. Inorganic mercury (ingested) → severe corrosive gastroenteritis. Organic mercury (ingested) → delayed neurotoxicity.

Diagnosis

- Based on presenting symptoms and history of exposure
- Mercury can be measured in whole blood or urine
- Ingested mercury-containing material is usually visible on x-ray

Treatment

- Remove source of exposure, supportive care and aggressive fluid resuscitation if severe GI symptoms
- WBI: If radiopaque objects visible on x-ray
- **Antidote = BAL** (British anti-lewisite, dimercaprol) if severe GI symptoms or **DMSA** (2,3-dimercaptosuccinic acid, succimer) if able to tolerate PO

Inhaled Toxins

SIMPLE ASPHYXIANTS

Simple asphyxiants include carbon dioxide, methane gas, and helium. Methane gas is present in high concentrations in bogs of decaying organic matter and in natural gas.

Mechanism/Toxicity

Produce toxicity by displacing oxygen from the lungs → hypoxia

Symptoms/Examination

- Pulmonary: Rapid onset with hypoxia, tachypnea, and shortness of breath
- Neurological: Dizziness and confusion progressing to coma
- Cardiovascular: Tachycardia, may lead to cardiac arrest

DIAGNOSIS

Clinical diagnosis based on history of exposure

TREATMENT

- Remove patient from source of exposure
- Supportive care with administration of oxygen

CARBON MONOXIDE

Carbon monoxide (CO) is an odorless and colorless gas produced by incomplete combustion of fuels or organic material.

Common sources of CO include vehicle exhaust, ovens, house fires, furnaces, and portable generators.

Methylene chloride, a solvent found in paint removers, degreasers, and similar products, is metabolized in vivo to CO following absorption.

MECHANISM/TOXICITY

- Binds to hemoglobin → carboxyhemoglobin (COHb) incapable of carrying O_2 → impaired O_2 delivery, cellular hypoxia, lactic acidosis
- Shifts the oxyhemoglobin dissociation curve to left → ↓ release of O_2 to tissues from normal hemoglobin
- Binds to heme groups in mitochondria and triggers oxidative injury
- CO has even greater affinity for fetal hemoglobin → higher fetal levels and toxicity for any given maternal exposure

SYMPTOMS/EXAMINATION

The symptoms and signs of CO toxicity are vague and nonspecific, and, if not severe, will resolve shortly after removal from CO source.

- Cardiopulmonary: Tachycardia, syncope, chest pain, myocardial ischemia, dyspnea, cardiac arrest
- GI: Nausea/vomiting
- Musculoskeletal: Rhabdomyolysis
- Neurologic: Headache, dizziness, weakness, confusion, delayed neurologic sequelae (memory loss, parkinsonism, chorea), ataxia, cerebellar symptoms, seizure, coma

DIAGNOSIS

- Carbon monoxide is a common and serious poisoning, for which the diagnosis is often missed.
- Consider in any case with headache, nausea/vomiting, especially if multiple patients affected.
- Direct measurement of COHb in either arterial or venous blood via co-oximetry.
  - Normal nonsmoker = 2%-3%
  - Smokers = < 10%
- Pulse oximetry **cannot** distinguish COHb from oxyhemoglobin.
- Expected arterial blood gas (ABG) findings:
  - Normal PaO_2 (measuring dissolved O_2)
  - Metabolic acidosis (from **lactate** accumulation)
  - Normal **calculated** O_2 saturation (calculated from PaO_2)
- Consider ECG, troponin, lactate, and CK.

Q

A 40-year-old woman presents to the ED with complaints of headache, nausea, and dizziness. Other family members have recently reported similar symptoms. She reports recent problems with her water heater at home. What diagnostic test can most easily aid in the diagnosis?

KEY FACT

The solvent methylene chloride is metabolized to carbon monoxide in the liver after absorption.

KEY FACT

CO poisoning: Normal pulse oximetry, ABG with metabolic acidosis, and normal PaO_2.

KEY FACT

Elimination half-life of CO:

Room air: 4-5 hours
100% O_2: 1-1.5 hour
Hyperbaric O_2: 20-30 minutes

Carbon monoxide poisoning should always be suspected when several members of the same household have headache or mild flulike symptoms. A venous or arterial carboxyhemoglobin level > 5% (10% in a smoker) confirms the diagnosis.

TABLE 6.19. Suggested Indications for HBO Treatment of CO Poisoning

Any history of loss of consciousness
COHb level > 25%
Coma
Fetal distress in pregnancy
Persistent neurologic symptoms/cerebellar dysfunction
Prolonged CO exposure (> 24 hours)
Seizure

CO, carbon monoxide COHb, carboxyhemoglobin HBO, hyperbaric O_2.

Treatment

- Remove the patient from CO source
- Acute stabilization as required
- Administration of **100%** O_2 by non-rebreather:
  - Reduces the elimination half-life of CO from approximately 4-5 hours (room air) to 1-1.5 hours
- **Hyperbaric O_2 (HBO)**
  - Further reduces the elimination half-life of CO to 20-30 minutes.
  - HBO therapy may prevent the development of delayed or persistent neurologic sequelae, but studies are not conclusive.
  - Use of hyperbaric oxygen is controversial but some proposed indications are listed in Table 6.19.
  - Lower threshold for HBO in pregnant patients.

Complication

Delayed or persistent neurocognitive deficits on neuropsychiatric testing

CYANIDE

Cyanide (CN) is a rapid-acting, highly toxic poison found in a wide variety of chemicals. Poisoning is rare in the United States, but can be life threatening.

Sources of CN include:

- Combustion of plastics, synthetic fibers, or wool; house fires (smoke inhalation) represent the most likely source of exposure.
- Prolonged infusion of nitroprusside.
- Industry including mining, plastics manufacturing, welding, fumigation, chemical synthesis, and research.
- Pits and seeds of certain fruits (apricots, bitter almonds) contain amygdalin, which releases CN in vivo during its metabolism.

Mechanism/Toxicity

Inhibits cytochrome oxidase, disrupting oxidative phosphorylation → cellular hypoxia and lactic acidosis

SYMPTOMS/EXAMINATION

- Effects are within seconds following hydrogen cyanide gas (HCN) inhalation, and within minutes of cyanide salt ingestion.
- Toxicity due to amygdalin seeds is rare unless they are pulverized and eaten in large quantities, but if toxicity occurs, it may be delayed by hours as CN is released by metabolism of amygdalin.
- Early symptoms of nausea/vomiting, headache, and confusion are followed rapidly by seizures and coma.
- Cardiopulmonary: Early hypertension and tachypnea, followed by pulmonary edema, dysrhythmias, hemodynamic collapse, and cardiac arrest.

DIFFERENTIAL

Hydrogen sulfide, seizure, postcardiac arrest state

DIAGNOSIS

- CN poisoning should be considered in any patient presenting with rapid onset of coma, shock, and marked lactic acidosis.
- Clues to the diagnosis include:
  - History of smoke inhalation or occupational access to CN.
  - ABG evidence of decreased tissue extraction of O_2: Metabolic acidosis, arterial appearance of venous blood, and elevated venous oxygen saturation (> 90%).
  - Marked lactic acidosis (> 8 mmol/L).
  - Patient has a distinctive bitter almond-like odor, although many individuals are genetically incapable of detecting this odor.
- Blood CN levels can be measured but usually not available in a timely manner.

TREATMENT

- Removed from exposure
- Acute stabilization as required
- Surface decontamination, if indicated
- **Antidote = cyanide antidote kit**; three components:
  - **Amyl nitrite pearls (for inhalation, prior to IV access)**
    - Induces methemoglobinemia, which strongly binds CN and pulls it away from cellular enzymes
  - **Sodium nitrite (IV)**
    - Induces methemoglobinemia
    - Use with caution in smoke inhalation victims who may have concurrent carboxyhemoglobinemia and nitrate-induced methemoglobinemia may worsen tissue oxygenation
  - **Sodium thiosulfate (IV)**
    - Binds to CN to form thiocyanate, a much less toxic compound that is renally excreted
- **Antidote = hydroxocobalamin**
  - Reacts with CN to form cyanocobalamin (vitamin B_{12}), a nontoxic compound which is readily excreted in urine
  - May replace the cyanide antidote kit in the future due to its ease of use and improved risk profile
  - Causes body fluids to become red and causes transient hypertension
  - Typically used as a single agent

HYDROGEN SULFIDE

Hydrogen sulfide (H_2S) is a gas formed as a byproduct of organic decomposition as well as many industrial processes. It has a very strong, distinctive "rotten egg" odor. Sources of H_2S include:

Q

A 25-year-old man is brought to the ED after being found unresponsive inside a burning house. He was intubated by EMS en route. On arrival he is hypotensive, comatose, and markedly tachypneic. There is no evidence of trauma or skin/airway burns. ABG reveals a severe metabolic acidosis and a normal measured Pao_2. What is the most appropriate next step?

KEY FACT

Suspect CN poisoning if a patient presents with rapid onset of coma, shock, and severe metabolic acidosis.

KEY FACT

Laboratory clues to CN poisoning: Marked lactic acidosis, arterial appearance of venous blood, elevated measured venous O_2 saturation, and bitter almond-like odor.

KEY FACT

Antidote should be administered empirically if CN poisoning is considered.

KEY FACT

Avoid using nitrites in smoke inhalation victims with suspected CO poisoning. Use sodium thiosulfate alone or hydroxocobalamin.

- **Sewer or manure gas**
- Chemical or industrial processes, such as tanning, rubber vulcanizing, mining, and manufacture of paper, silk, rayon, refrigerants, soap, and petroleum products
- Natural sources include hot springs and volcanic eruptions

A

This patient should be presumed to have a combined CO and cyanide (CN) poisoning based on his hemodynamic instability and coma. Initial treatment of CO poisoning consists of O_2 therapy, which has already been initiated. The next most appropriate step, therefore, is administration of either hydroxocobalamin or sodium thiosulfate for treatment of CN poisoning. In the smoke inhalation victim, administration of nitrites is not recommended, as a nitrite-induced methemoglobinemia will further decrease tissue O_2 delivery in the CO-poisoned patient. If the COHb level is low on co-oximetry, nitrites may be initiated.

Mechanism/Toxicity

- H_2S is a stronger inhibitor of cytochrome oxidase than CN → disruption of oxidative phosphorylation → cellular hypoxia and lactic acidosis.
- Spontaneously dissociates from cytochrome oxidase.
- Direct mucous membrane irritant.
- High concentrations of H_2S may overwhelm the olfactory system and extinguish the odor.

Symptoms/Examination

- Severity of symptoms depends on the concentration and duration of exposure. Low-concentration exposure may only produce mild mucous membrane irritation. Brief exposures to very high concentrations → immediate loss of consciousness
- Cardiovascular: Hypotension, bradycardia, dysrhythmias, cardiac arrest
- GI: Nausea/vomiting
- Mucous membrane irritation: Conjunctivitis, rhinitis, bronchorrhea, pulmonary edema
- Neurologic: Headache, seizures, rapid loss of consciousness, coma

KEY FACT

Sewer or manure gas exposure? Rotten egg odor? Think hydrogen sulfide toxicity.

Diagnosis

- H_2S poisoning should be considered in any patient presenting with rapid onset of coma, shock, and marked lactic acidosis.
- Clues to the diagnosis include:
  - Relevant occupational setting
  - Rapid loss of consciousness
  - Odor of rotten eggs at scene
  - Silver jewelry on scene may be darkened
  - ABG evidence of decreased tissue extraction of O_2: Metabolic acidosis, arterial appearance of venous blood, and elevated venous oxygen saturation (> 90%)
  - Marked lactic acidosis
- Blood levels of sulfide and thiosulfate can serve as markers of H_2S exposure but are not readily available in most clinical laboratories.

KEY FACT

Hydrogen sulfide toxicity: Rapid coma, shock, and lactic acidosis (as with CN); spontaneous improvement after exposure is ended.

Treatment

- Removed from exposure (first responders require self-contained breathing apparatus)
- Acute stabilization as required
- Administer 100% O_2
- Observe several hours for delayed-onset pulmonary edema
- Most patients will not require further therapy
- **Antidote = sodium nitrite** (if prolonged symptoms; limited evidence for effectiveness)
  - Induces methemoglobinemia, which binds H_2S to produce sulfmethemoglobin

Lithium

Lithium is a mood stabilizer used to treat bipolar disorder. It has a narrow therapeutic window.

Mechanism/Toxicity

- Lithium is a cation and behaves like Na^+ or K^+.
- Exact mechanism of action is unclear, but thought to affect catecholamine and serotonin neurotransmission.
- Though lithium is completely absorbed in approximately 6 hours, CNS uptake and elimination are slow; therefore, serum lithium levels do NOT correlate with CNS effects.
- Lithium elimination is glomerular filtration rate (GFR) dependent.
- Precursors to chronic toxicity:
  - ↑ Therapeutic dose
  - ↑ Renal reabsorption in dehydration
  - ↓ GFR (renal insufficiency, use of NSAIDs, ACEI, diuretics)
  - Drug–drug interactions with SSRIs and antipsychotic agents

Symptoms/Examination

The expected effects from lithium intoxication depend on whether the ingestion is acute or chronic.

Severe toxicity is more common secondary to chronic ingestion versus acute overdose.

Acute ingestion:

- Occurs in patients who do not normally take lithium but acutely ingest a large quantity
- GI toxicity > > CNS toxicity (no time for CNS uptake)
- GI toxicity = nausea/vomiting/diarrhea
- CNS findings are typically mild, but can develop over hours and include hyperreflexia, tongue fasciculations, clonus, agitation, AMS, seizures

Chronic ingestion:

- Acute-on-chronic or chronic toxicity:
  - CNS toxicity > > GI toxicity.
  - CNS effects may range from lethargy and confusion to coma and seizures.
  - ECG changes include T-wave inversions, T-wave flattening, depressed ST segments, and less commonly bradycardia and sinus node arrest.

Diagnosis

- Clinical diagnosis based on history and examination
- Lithium levels:
  - Measure 4-6 hours postingestion, follow levels until clear peak and decline
  - Peak serum level with large ingestion, especially sustained-release preparations, may occur > 12 hours postingestion
  - Falsely elevated if placed in a green-top tube (lithium heparin)

Treatment

- Lithium does **not** adsorb well to charcoal.
- **WBI may be useful in acute ingestion of sustained-release preparations** although likely to be limited by vomiting.

Q

A 30-year-old man on chronic lithium therapy for bipolar disorder is brought to the ED by his mother for mental status changes. She reports he has had a flulike illness over the past few days with vomiting and diarrhea. On examination the patient appears dehydrated, lethargic, and confused but has normal vital signs. His lithium level returns at 2.5 mmol/L (upper level of normal). What is the single most important therapeutic intervention for this patient with presumed lithium toxicity?

KEY FACT

A decrease in GFR (↓ drug clearance) is a common precursor to chronic lithium toxicity.

KEY FACT

Acute lithium ingestion → high serum levels, minimal CNS effects. Chronic lithium toxicity → lower serum levels, significant CNS effects.

A

This patient likely has chronic lithium toxicity related to a decreased GFR from dehydration. In chronic toxicity, CNS effects predominate. The single most important therapy for this patient is to reestablish GFR with IV hydration.

TABLE 6.20. Suggested Indications for Hemodialysis in Lithium Toxicity

Renal failure/anuria
Inability to handle aggressive hydration (history of CHF or pulmonary edema)
Severe CNS toxicity/seizures

CHF, congestive heart failure; CNS, central nervous depression.

- **Hydration** is essential to correct dehydration and increase GFR
- **HD**
  - Lithium is effectively removed by HD (Table 6.20).
  - Because HD removes lithium only from the plasma, a "rebound lithium level" may occur from peripheral tissue redistribution; a lithium concentration should be checked after HD and 6 hours later.
- Benzodiazepines for seizures and agitation
- Avoid:
  - Phenytoin: Decreases renal excretion of lithium
  - Forced diuresis or diuretics (not effective)

Complications

- Hypothyroidism (Lithium concentrates in thyroid gland)
- Nephrogenic diabetes insipidus (via blockage of antidiuretic hormone) with chronic therapy
- Increased risk of serotonin syndrome when taken with other serotonergic agents
- Syndrome of irreversible lithium-effectuated neurotoxicity (SILENT): Irreversible neurologic and neuropsychiatric sequelae

Local Anesthetics

KEY FACT

All amide local anesthetics have 2 "i"s in their name.

Local anesthetics are typically divided into two classes:
- **Esters:** Procaine, tetracaine, benzocaine
- **Amides:** Lidocaine, bupivacaine, mepivacaine

Effect is usually local, but may become systemic with in inadvertent injection into a blood vessel, use of large volumes, or premature release of cuff with IV regional anesthetics (Bier block).

Mechanism/Toxicity

- Inhibition of Na^+ channels → reversible blockade of the initiation and propagation of action potentials along affected nerve.
- Systemic toxicity occurs with accumulation of local anesthetics in the brain and cardiac tissue where the drugs exert sodium channel blocking affects.

KEY FACT

Toxicity is characterized primarily by neurologic symptoms, but may include cardiovascular symptoms in large overdoses.

Symptoms/Examination

- Local toxicity may lead to prolonged anesthetic effects, permanent sensory and motor deficits, and respiratory arrest secondary to blocking nerves to respiratory muscles.
- Systemic toxicity progresses from mild neurologic symptoms (confusion, anxiety, and sense of impending doom, headache, drowsiness, dizziness/lightheadedness, tremors, tinnitus, or numbness of the mouth) to seizures to hemodynamic collapse.

- Cardiac toxicity may progress from widening of PR interval and QRS complex to bradycardia, VT, VF, hypotension, asystole.
- Methemoglobinemia is possible with exposure to benzocaine and prilocaine.
- Bupivacaine is more cardiotoxic than other local anesthetics and is not indicated for IV regional anesthesia.

KEY FACT

Pregnant women are disproportionately affected by bupivacaine, and it is no longer indicated for obstetric spinal anesthesia.

DIAGNOSIS

- Usually clear from history and examination
- ECG and cardiac monitoring, as needed
- Co-oximetry if methemoglobinemia is suspected

TREATMENT

- Supportive care including benzodiazepines for seizures, methylene blue for methemoglobinemia, and advanced cardiovascular life support (ACLS) for cardiac dysrhythmias
- **Antidote = IV fat emulsions (Intralipid),** acts as a lipid sink pulling local anesthetics away from site of toxicity, given as a 20% solution 1.5-mL/kg bolus followed by 0.25 mL/kg/min over 30-60 minutes
- Discontinue use of agent
- No role for decontamination or enhanced elimination

COMPLICATIONS

- Allergic reactions:
  - Ester anesthetics are responsible for most, due to metabolite **para-aminobenzoic acid (PABA)**.
  - Preservative **methylparaben** is found in multidose vials of amide anesthetics and is chemically related to PABA.
  - Hypersensitivity reaction to either an ester or amide class local anesthetic should not cross-react with the other.
- Inadvertent IV injection of epinephrine (in "with epi" preparations)

Methylxanthines

Agents in this class include:

- **Caffeine:** Most commonly used drug in the world; marketed for increased alertness, weight loss, migraine therapy, and neonatal apnea and bradycardia
- **Theophylline:** Still occasionally used for asthma and chronic obstructive pulmonary disease (COPD) (although largely replaced by newer safer agents)
- **Theobromine:** Found in chocolate and various teas

MECHANISM/TOXICITY

- Triggers release of preformed epinephrine and norepinephrine → adrenergic receptor stimulation, stimulates β-adrenergic receptors and hypokalemia
- Phosphodiesterase inhibition
- Adenosine receptor antagonism

SYMPTOMS/EXAMINATION

- **Severe nausea/vomiting** in majority of patients
- CNS stimulation ranging from elevated mood to nervousness, agitation, and seizures
- Cardiovascular stimulation with tachycardia, hypertension, and dysrhythmias
- At high concentrations: Peripheral vasodilation and hypotension

Q

A 32-year-old woman presents to the ED via EMS after ingesting #50 theophylline 600 mg extended release that belong to her grandfather approximately 2 hours prior. She arrived complaining of nausea, vomiting, palpitations. On arrival her vital signs were: HR 160 bpm, BP 90/60 mm Hg, RR 18 breaths/min, and temperature 37.7°C (99.9°F). On physical examination, patient was diaphoretic, tremulous with mydriasis and tachycardia. ECG showed sinus tachycardia. While in the ED, the patient had a seizure that resolved with benzodiazepines. Her theophylline level returned at 110 mg/L (therapeutic: 10-20 mg/L). What is the optimal management for this patient?

DIAGNOSIS

- Usually clear from history and examination.
- Serum theophylline levels, repeated every 2-4 hours until peak and decline.
- In chronic ingestions, severe symptoms occur at significantly lower levels.

TREATMENT

- Symptomatic and supportive care, IV hydration.
- Hypotension caused by increased β-adrenergic stimulation can be treated with low-dose β-blocker.
- Most patients autodecontaminate with profuse vomiting.
- **MDAC** enhances elimination but use typically limited by vomiting.
- **WBI** for large ingestion of sustained-release preparations but use typically limited by vomiting.
- Charcoal hemoperfusion or HD for severe toxicity.
- Benzodiazepines and barbiturates for seizures and status epilepticus.
- Hypokalemia caused by intracellular movement of potassium usually self-resolves.

Opioids

Opioid toxidrome may result from exposure to:

- Prescription medications (eg, fentanyl, methadone, hydrocodone, oxycodone, hydromorphone)
- Illicit drugs (eg, heroin)

MECHANISM/TOXICITY

Stimulate opioid receptors (μ, κ, and δ) in the CNS, spinal cord, and GI tract

SYMPTOMS/EXAMINATION

- Classic triad includes CNS depression, respiratory depression, and pinpoint pupils.
- Cardiovascular: Bradycardia, orthostatic hypotension, peripheral vasodilatation.
  - Wide complex dysrhythmias may be associated with Na^+ channel blockade in propoxyphene overdose (propoxyphene is no longer available in the United Kingdom and United States).
- GI: Reduced motility, reduced gastric acid secretion, increased anal sphincter tone.
- Otologic: Sensorineural hearing loss (generally with prolonged use).
- Metabolic: Hypoglycemia, hypothermia.
- Neurologic: Miosis (may not be seen with propoxyphene, pentazocine, meperidine), seizures may be associated with propoxyphene or meperidine.
- Pulmonary: Noncardiogenic pulmonary edema.

DIAGNOSIS

- Clinical diagnosis based on history and examination
- Reversal of symptoms by naloxone

TREATMENT

- Support ventilation/oxygenation as needed.
- **Antidote = naloxone (Narcan).**
  - Pure opiate receptor antagonist
- Sodium bicarbonate for wide complex dysrhythmias (propoxyphene).
- Seizures are typically self-limited but can be treated with benzodiazepines.

KEY FACT

Opiate toxidrome = CNS depression, respiratory depression, and pinpoint pupils.

KEY FACT

Naloxone is only indicated for reversal of hypoventilation and is not useful in the intubated patient.

A

Treat hypotension with IVF and low-dose β-blockers. Immediate arrangements should be made for HD.

COMPLICATIONS

- Aspiration and global hypoxic/anoxic injury.
- Rhabdomyolysis and compartment syndrome can occur from prolonged immobilization.
- Withdrawal syndrome can lead to significant distress but is not life threatening.

Nutritional Supplements

In 1994, Congress passed the Dietary Supplement Health and Education Act (DSHEA)—reducing FDA oversight of dietary supplements. The FDA can warn the public, suggest changes, recall the product, or ban the product if the product is proved to be unsafe. Manufacturers only have to demonstrate good manufacturing practices under sanitary conditions without guarantee of safety, efficacy, or the quality of the product.

VITAMINS

Largely nutritional deficiencies are uncommon in developed countries, but supplementation remains commonplace. Fat-soluble vitamins (A, D, E) can lead to toxicity in overdose. Water-soluble vitamins are excreted efficiently in the urine and do not cause toxicity (Table 6.21).

MECHANISM/TOXICITY

- Vitamin A maintains growth and differentiation of epithelial cells.
- Vitamin D regulates calcium homeostasis.
- Vitamin E functions as an antioxidant but may be pro-oxidant and antagonizes vitamin K in overdose.

SYMPTOMS/EXAMINATION

In overdose:

- Vitamin A: Headache, papilledema, photophobia, seizures, psychosis, nausea/vomiting, abdominal pain, liver injury, and desquamation

TABLE 6.21. Vitamins

VITAMIN	NATURAL SOURCES	DEFICIENCY	TOXICITY
Vitamin A	Liver, fish, cheese, and whole milk	Dry skin/hair, broken fingernails, blindness, susceptible to respiratory infections, diarrhea, urinary calculi	Headache, papilledema, photophobia, seizures, psychosis, nausea/vomiting, abdominal pain, liver injury, desquamation. Hypercarotenemia causes yellow-orange discoloration of skin
Vitamin D	Cod liver oil, butter, cheese, cream, eggs, and fatty fish	Rickets	Hypercalcemia
Vitamin E	Nuts, wheat germ, whole-grain, and vegetable/seed oils	Peripheral neuropathy and spinocellular syndrome	Nausea/vomiting, diarrhea, abdominal cramps, coagulopathy

- Vitamin D: Hypercalcemia
- Vitamin E: Nausea/vomiting, diarrhea, abdominal cramps, coagulopathy

Diagnosis

- Vitamin A: Diagnosis is largely clinical but maybe supported by evaluation of serum electrolytes, hepatic enzymes, and vitamin A concentration.
- Vitamin D: Elevated serum calcium concentration and hyperphosphatemia.
- Vitamin E: Clinical diagnosis based on history and physical examination.

Treatment

- Vitamin A: Discontinuation of vitamin A supplementation and supportive care
- Vitamin D: Discontinuation of vitamin D and calcium supplementation with fluid hydration
- Vitamin E: Discontinuation of vitamin E and reversal of coagulopathy, if present

Complications

- Vitamin A: Blindness can be a complication due to both overdose and deficiency.
- Vitamin D: Hypercalcemia can result in water depletion and metastatic calcification of skin and organs.

Herbal Preparations

Herbal preparations are considered a subset "alternative therapies" with variety of mechanisms and toxicities (Table 6.22).

Athletic performance enhancers

Performance-enhancing xenobiotics can be categorized as anabolic steroids, peptide hormones/growth factors, hormone agonists/metabolic modulators, or stimulants.

Mechanism/Toxicity

- Anabolic steroids: Agents related to testosterone that increase muscle mass and lean body weight
- Peptide hormones/growth factors:
  - Creatine: Resynthesized as adenosine triphosphate (ATP) for use as short-term energy burst during exercise
  - Human growth hormone/insulin-like growth factor: Stimulants protein synthesis
- Stimulants: Caffeine and amphetamines are both used as performance enhancement agents (see previous sections on methylxanthine and sympathomimetics)

Symptoms/Examination

- Anabolic steroids can lead to multisystem dysfunction:
  - Oncologic: Increase cancer risk
  - Cardiac: Acute myocardial infarction, venous thromboembolism, and sudden cardiac death
  - Dermatologic: Acne, stray, and gynecomastia
  - Endocrine: Gynecomastia in men and menstrual irregularities/breast atrophy in women
  - Hepatic: Peliosis hepatis—blood-filled sinuses in the liver
  - Infectious: Immunosuppression

TABLE 6.22. Herbal preparations

Herbal preparation	Purported Usage	Active/Toxic Ingredient(s)	Adverse Effects
Aconite (monkshood, wolfsbane)	Topical analgesic, asthma, heart disease	Aconite alkaloid	GI upset and dysrhythmias
Aristolochia	Human stimulant, cancer treatment, antibacterial	Aristolochic acid	Nephrotoxicity, renal cancer, retroperitoneal fibrosis
Comfrey	Ulcers, hemorrhoids, bronchitis, burns, sprains, swelling, bruises	Pyrrolizidine alkaloids	Haptic veno-occlusive disease
Ephedra (ma huang)	Stimulant, bronchospasm	Ephedrine, pseudoephedrine	Headache, dizziness, seizure, sympathomimetic effects
Evening Primrose	Premenstrual syndrome, diabetes, eczema, rheumatoid arthritis	Cis-γ-linoleic acid (prostaglandin precursor)	Lowers seizure threshold
Foxglove	Asthma, sedative, diuretic/cardiotonic	Cardioactive steroids	Blurred vision, GI upset, weakness, dysrhythmias
Ginkgo	Asthma, chilblain, digestive aid, cerebral dysfunction	Ginkgolides and bilobalide	Extracts: GI upset, headache, skin reaction; leaf: antiplatelet, allergic reactions
Ginseng	Increase metabolism and regulate blood pressure/glucose, aphrodisiac, respiratory illnesses, antiinflammatory	Ginsenosides (panax, ginseng)	Stimulant effect, hypertension, hypoglycemia
Saw palmetto	Benign prostatic hypertrophy	5-α-reductase inhibitor	Diarrhea
St. John's wort	Anxiety, depression, gastritis, insomnia, promote healing, AIDS	Hyperforin, hypericin	MAOI properties and drug–drug interaction (CYP3A4 inducer)
Valerian root	Anxiety, insomnia, antispasmodic	Valepotriates, valerenic acid	Sedation
Yohimbe	Body building, aphrodisiac, stimulant	Yohimbine	Hypertension, tachycardia, abdominal pain, weakness

GI, gastrointestinal; MAOI, monoamine oxidase inhibitor.

  - Musculoskeletal: Tendon and ligament rupture
  - Neuropsychiatric: Mood lability, aggression, psychosis, insomnia
- Peptide hormones/growth factors:
  - Creatine: Water retention and diarrhea
  - Human growth hormone/insulin-like growth factor: Myalgia, arthralgia, carpal tunnel syndrome, and edema

Diagnosis

- Clinical diagnosis based on history and physical examination
- Comprehensive urinary and blood testing available for athletic performance enhancers but unlikely to influence clinical medical decision making

Treatment

Supportive care with discontinuation of inciting agent

Complications

Anabolic steroids: Avascular necrosis in osteoporosis from prolonged use

Dieting Xenobiotics and Regimens

Weight loss supplements are commonly encountered. Many agents are inherently dangerous and some have been banned by the FDA. Supplements can be classified into sympathomimetics, GI agents, serotonergic agents, or uncouplers (Table 6.23).

Mechanism/Toxicity

- Sympathomimetics: As a dieting agent, sympathomimetics may decrease appetite and increase basal metabolic rates.
- GI agents: Decreased intestinal absorption of macronutrients.
- Serotonergic agents: Increased metabolic demands.
- Uncouplers: Increase heat generation and metabolic demand.

TABLE 6.23. Dietary weight-loss supplements

Dietary Supplement	Mechanism of Action	Adverse Effects
	Sympathomimetics	
Bitter orange extract	Contains synephrine and octopamine	Sympathomimetic effects
Clenbuterol	β_2-Adrenergic agonist	Sympathomimetic effects
Guarana	Contains caffeine	Nausea, vomiting, insomnia, anxiety, palpitations, tachycardia, seizures
Ma huang	Contains ephedrine	Sympathomimetic effects
	GI Agents	
Chitosan	Insoluble marine fiber that binds dietary fat	Decreased absorption of fats soluble vitamins, diarrhea
	Serotoninergic Agent	
Fenfluramine	Increases release and decreases uptake of serotonin	Valvular heart disease, primary pulmonary hypertension
	Uncouplers	
Dinitrophenol	Uncouples oxidative phosphorylation	Hyperthermia, hepatotoxicity

GI, gastrointestinal.

SYMPTOMS/EXAMINATION

- Sympathomimetics: Tachycardia, hypertension, palpitations, hyperthermia (sympathomimetic toxidrome)
- GI agents: GI distress, risk for nutritional deficiencies
- Serotonergic agents: Serotonin toxicity
- Uncouplers: Increase heat generation and metabolic demand

DIAGNOSIS

Clinical diagnosis based on history and physical examination

TREATMENT

Supportive care with benzodiazepines, IV fluids, cardiac monitoring, and discontinuation of inciting drug

COMPLICATION

Life-threatening hyperthermia may be associated with sympathomimetics, serotonergic agents, and uncouplers, may need aggressive cooling measures, including intubation and paralysis.

Over-the-Counter Medications

ACETAMINOPHEN

Acetaminophen (APAP) ingestions are typically divided into acute overdoses **(single ingestion)** and **repeated supratherapeutic ingestions**. An ingestion of > 150 mg/kg (children) or 7.5 g (adults) in less than an 8-hour period should be considered potentially toxic.

MECHANISM/TOXICITY

- APAP is primarily metabolized by the liver, where in therapeutic doses, 90% of APAP is conjugated with glucuronide or sulfate to nontoxic metabolites, while 5% is oxidized by cytochrome P450 2E1 (CYP2E1) to a **toxic metabolite, N-acetyl-p-benzoquinone imine (NAPQI).**
- Hepatic stores of **glutathione** rapidly combine with NAPQI to form nontoxic metabolites.
- In APAP overdose, normal glucuronide and sulfate conjugation are overwhelmed, and a large amount of NAPQI is produced.
- When NAPQI formation exceeds glutathione stores, free NAPQI binds to cellular proteins causing hepatotoxicity (centrilobular or zone III).
- High-risk patients: Patients with decreased glutathione stores (alcoholics, malnourished) and those on cytochrome P450–inducing medications (INH, anticonvulsants) may have increased risk of hepatotoxicity.

> **KEY FACT**
>
> In acetaminophen toxicity, glutathione stores become depleted, allowing NAPQI (toxic metabolite) to accumulate.

SYMPTOMS/EXAMINATION

- **Acute overdose:**
  - Potential toxic dose: ≥ 10 g or 200 mg/kg (whichever is less) in patients > 6 years and ≥ 200 mg/kg in patients < 6 years.
  - The most severe cases will develop delayed fulminate hepatic failure with hepatic encephalopathy, severe coagulopathy, renal failure, cerebral edema, and acidosis; liver transplantation may be indicated.
- **Repeated supratherapeutic ingestion potential toxic doses:**
  - Patients > 6 years:
    - ≥ 10 g/d or 200 mg/kg/d for a single 24-hour period
    - ≥ 6 g/d or 150 mg/kg/d (whichever is less) for > 48 hours

- Children < 6 years:
  - ≥ 200 mg/kg over 8-24 hours
  - ≥ 150 mg/kg/d for 2 days
  - ≥ 100 mg/kg/d for 3 days or longer
- Patients may present with normal transaminase, asymptomatic elevation of enzymes or even hepatic failure.

KEY FACT

Unknown time of acetaminophen ingestion? If the APAP level is > 20 μg/mL or the AST/ALT is elevated → treat with NAC.

DIAGNOSIS

- **Acute ingestion (time of ingestion known)** of both immediate and extended-release formulations:
  - Obtain a 4-hour (up to 24 hours) postingestion serum acetaminophen concentration and plot the concentration on the Rumack-Matthew nomogram (Figure 6.2).

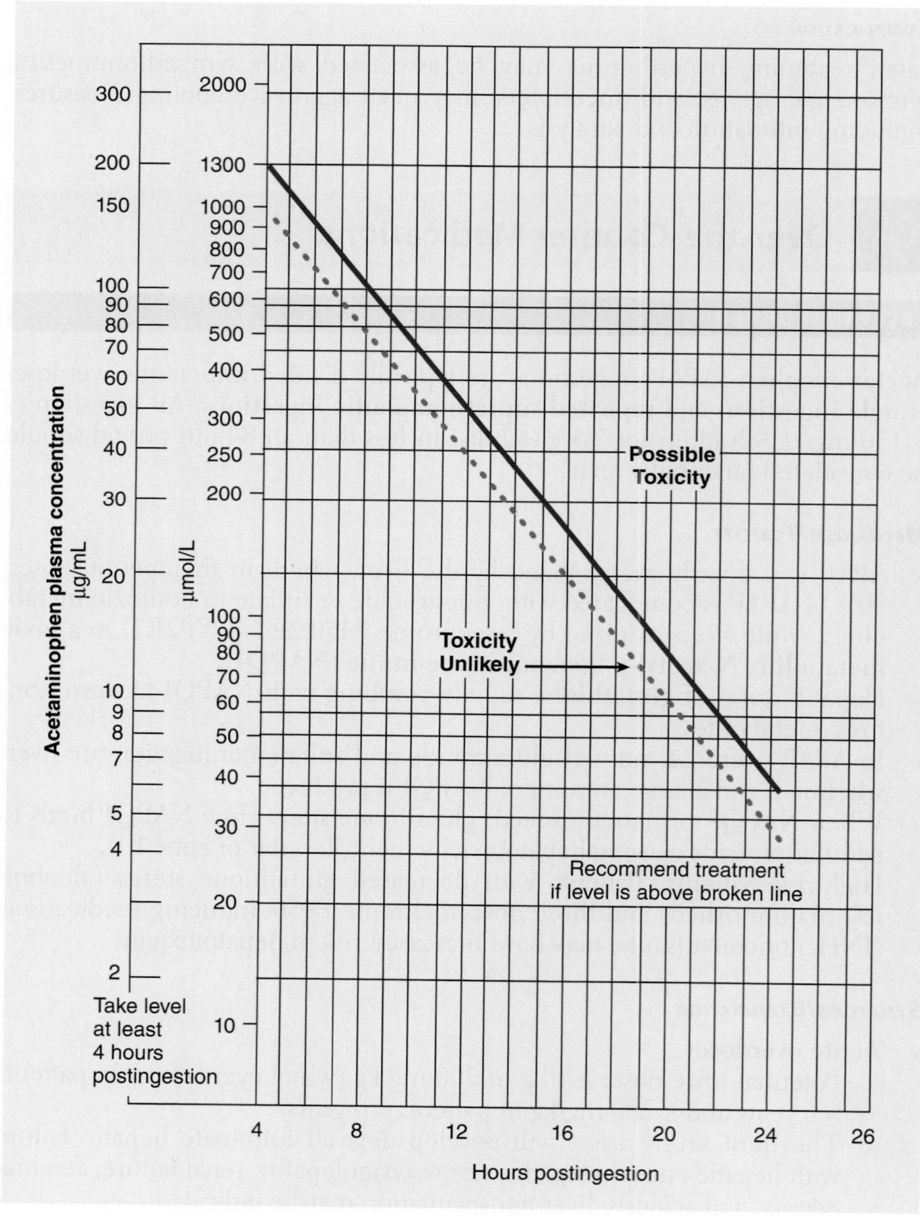

FIGURE 6.2. Rumack-Matthew nomogram. Serum acetaminophen concentration vs time after acute ingestion. (Reproduced, with permission, from Tintinalli JE, Stapczynski JS, Ma OJ, et al. *Tintinalli's Emergency Medicine: A Comprehensive Study Guide*. 7th ed. New York, NY: McGraw-Hill Education, 2011. Figure 184.2.)

- The solid line (Rumack-Matthew line) is the original line developed from the study, above which hepatotoxicity was observed.
- The dotted line (treatment line) is the line accepted as the standard of care in the United States and is 25% lower as a safety margin.
- If the patient's serum APAP concentration is above the treatment line (150 μg/mL at 4 hours postingestion), start treatment with N-acetylcysteine (NAC)
- **Repeated supratherapeutic ingestion**
  - Do not plot an acetaminophen concentration on the Rumack-Matthew nomogram.
  - Obtain an APAP concentration and alanine transaminase/aspartate transaminase (AST/ALT) at time of presentation.
  - If APAP is > 20 μg/mL **OR** the AST/ALT are elevated, treatment with NAC is recommended.

TREATMENT

- Supportive therapy as indicated.
- AC may be considered if < 2 hours from time of an acute ingestion and without airway compromise.
- **Antidote = N-acetylcysteine (NAC)**
  - Very effective if given within 8-10 hours of acute ingestion, but even late administration is beneficial (ie, **always** give NAC).
  - If no APAP concentration available and patient approaching (or exceeding) 8 hours from ingestion → give NAC while awaiting APAP level.
  - Oral (Mucomyst): 140 mg/kg load, then 70 mg/kg every 4 hours for 72 hours.
  - IV (Acetadote): 150 mg/kg load, then 12.5 mg/kg/h × 4 hours, then 6.25 mg/kg/h × 16 hours.
    - May cause dose-, rate-, and concentration-dependent anaphylactoid reactions.
  - Patients with repeated supratherapeutic ingestions may be treated with NAC for 12 hours with repeat APAP level and LFTs performed nearing the end of treatment: If patient is clinically well, APAP is nondetectable, and LFTs are trending down, the patient may be cleared.

COMPLICATIONS

- Patients with severe toxicity may develop fulminant hepatic failure, metabolic acidosis, hyperglycemia, hepatorenal syndrome, hepatic encephalopathy, coagulopathy, infection, and cerebral edema
- **Indications for liver transplantation (King's College Criteria)** include pH < 7.3 after resuscitation, or all 3 of INR > 6.5, creatinine > 3.4 mg/dL, grade 3 or 4 encephalopathy

SALICYLATES

Salicylates are found in a variety of over-the-counter preparations such as analgesics (eg, Bayer aspirin), cold medicines, antidiarrheal agents (bismuth subsalicylate in Pepto-Bismol), topical products (methylsalicylate), aminosalicylates in treatment of inflammatory bowel disease, and as combination products in decongestants, antihistamines, and narcotic medications.

Salicylic acid is a weak acid that at normal serum pH is mostly ionized and therefore will not cross the blood–brain barrier or the renal tubules (for reabsorption). Acidemia promotes the nonionized form, allowing salicylate to enter the brain and be reabsorbed by the kidneys (decreasing renal excretion). Chronic excessive use of salicylates is associated with toxicity at a lower serum salicylate concentration.

Q

A 33-year-old woman presents to the ED with complaint of nausea/vomiting and back pain. The back pain has been ongoing since she lifted some heavy boxes 2 days earlier and was severe enough that she took a "handful" of aspirin 4 hours earlier to treat the symptoms. On examination she is tachypneic, but otherwise alert and hemodynamically stable. ABG reveals a pH of 7.51, P_{CO_2} of 13.9, P_{O_2} of 110 mm Hg. Serum HCO_3^- is 12 mEq/L. What is the goal of initial therapy in this patient?

KEY FACT

NAC is most effective if given within 8-10 hours of acute ingestion and before the transaminase is elevated.

KEY FACT

Even late administration of NAC can be beneficial.

KEY FACT

Acetaminophen toxicity: Toxic level at 4 hours = 150 μg/mL; Oral NAC loading dose = 140 mg/kg; IV NAC loading dose = 150 mg/kg.

KEY FACT

At a given salicylate concentration, chronic salicylate ingestion results in greater toxicity than acute ingestion.

A

Therapy with sodium bicarbonate boluses, and then drip should be initiated with a goal of urinary alkalinization to a pH of 7.5-8.0. Alkalinization traps salicylate in the nonionized form, which increases renal clearance and decreases CNS uptake of salicylate.

KEY FACT

Patient with respiratory alkalosis and anion-gap metabolic acidosis? Think salicylate toxicity.

KEY FACT

Suspect chronic salicylate intoxication in elderly patients with AMS or hearing complaints.

MECHANISM/TOXICITY

- **Direct stimulation of respiratory center** → hyperventilation, respiratory alkalosis
- **Stimulation of chemoreceptor trigger zone** → vomiting
- **Uncoupling of oxidative phosphorylation** → anaerobic metabolism, anion-gap metabolic acidosis, hyperthermia
- Permanent inhibition of platelet aggregation
- **Ototoxicity** → tinnitus and hearing loss correlate with salicylate level
- Alterations in capillary integrity → cerebral and pulmonary edema

SYMPTOMS/EXAMINATION

- **Acute ingestion**
  - Early: Nausea/vomiting, tinnitus, hearing loss, lethargy, hyperventilation, diaphoresis, and hyperthermia
  - Mixed acid-base picture with a respiratory alkalosis and anion-gap metabolic acidosis
    - Blood gases early in toxicity often show a respiratory alkalosis with pH > 7.5
  - Severe toxicity: Metabolic acidosis, marked hyperthermia, cerebral edema, seizure, coma hypoglycemia, pulmonary edema, cardiovascular collapse
- **Chronic ingestion**
  - Symptoms similar to acute ingestion but slower in onset and often nonspecific.
  - Patients often present with confusion, dehydration, and metabolic acidosis.
  - Neurologic symptoms are common, including confusion, hallucinations, agitation, and coma.
  - Pulmonary edema, cerebral edema, seizures, and renal failure occur more frequently compared to acute ingestions.

DIAGNOSIS

- Based on history, physical examination, and acid-base findings
- Maintain high level of suspicion in patients with:
  - Unexplained respiratory alkalosis
  - Metabolic acidosis or mixed acid-base disorders
  - Elderly with AMS
  - Patients with hearing complaints
- Key laboratory tests: Salicylate concentration, ABG, electrolytes

TREATMENT

- Goal of treatment is to keep salicylate ionized, thereby inhibiting its movement into the brain and enhancing its urinary excretion.
- Supportive and symptomatic care:
  - Avoid CNS/respiratory depressants, which may inhibit respiratory alkalosis and worsen overall acidemia
  - If intubated, hyperventilate to match the preintubation P_{CO_2}
- AC if no significant CNS depression or vomiting, or protected airway.
- IV hydration (**not** forced diuresis) to maintain renal perfusion.
- **Sodium bicarbonate therapy:**
  - 1- to 2-mEq/kg IV bolus, followed by drip
  - Goal is **urinary alkalinization** to pH 7.5-8.0
- **Correct hypokalemia:**
  - Results from intracellular shifts and body losses
  - Urinary alkalinization will not occur unless hypokalemia is corrected

TABLE 6.24. The Five Phases of Iron Toxicity

Phase 1: GI phase
Phase 2: Latent phase
Phase 3: "Shock" phase
Phase 4: Fulminant hepatic failure
Phase 5: Delayed sequelae

GI, gastrointestinal.

- Obtain basic metabolic panel and salicylate levels every 1-2 hours
  - Monitor salicylate levels until levels have declined below therapeutic concentrations
- **HD:** Indications listed in Table 6.24

NONSTEROIDAL ANTI-INFLAMMATORY DRUGS

Nonsteroidal anti-inflammatory drugs (NSAIDs) inhibit the enzyme cyclo-oxygenase, causing decreased prostaglandin formation. Prostaglandins have a variety of functions, including mediating pain and inflammation, maintaining the gastric mucosa, and regulating blood flow in the kidneys. Ibuprofen is the most common NSAID seen in overdose.

Mechanism/Toxicity

- Symptomatic overdose occurs with ibuprofen ingestion > 200 mg/kg
- GI: Nausea, vomiting, gastritis, upper GI bleed
- Renal: Renal insufficiency due to decreased renal blood flow; more common in chronic than acute exposure
- Metabolic: NSAIDs or metabolites may be organic acids that contribute to an anion gap metabolic acidosis
- Systemic: May be seen with massive ibuprofen overdose; symptoms include cerebral and pulmonary edema, seizures, coma

Symptoms/Examination

- Abdominal pain, nausea/vomiting, and renal insufficiency
- AMS, seizure, and metabolic acidosis in severe ingestions
- Agents with specific toxicities:
  - Ibuprofen (massive ingestions): Seizures, coma, cerebral and pulmonary edema
  - Mefenamic acid: Seizures
  - Phenylbutazone (discontinued in the United States): Aplastic anemia and agranulocytosis

Diagnosis

- Based primarily on history and examination
- Follow basic metabolic panel

Treatment

Supportive and symptomatic therapy

Q

A 2-year-old boy presents after ingestion of an unknown amount of his mother's iron supplements. Upon arrival to the ED approximately six episodes of vomiting and hematemesis in the first hour. His vitals are as follows: HR 140 bpm, BP 85/60 mm Hg, RR 35 breaths/min, temperature 37°C. The child receives an IV fluid bolus (20 mL/kg), and an abdominal x-ray showed a large number of tablet fragments in the stomach. The child is intubated, undergoes orogastric lavage, and WBI. His ABG show pH 7.1, Pco_2 35 mm Hg, Po_2 450 mm Hg. What should be your next step in management?

A

The child should be chelated with deferoxamine given the severe acidosis and shock.

KEY FACT

A key feature of iron toxicity is the uncoupling of oxidative phosphorylation → anaerobic metabolism.

IRON

For any given iron compound, determine the amount of elemental iron to determine potential toxicity of ingestion—toxic dose > 20 mg/kg of elemental iron

MECHANISM/TOXICITY

- **Direct corrosive effect** on GI tract
- **Toxicity from free circulating iron** → cellular uncoupling of oxidative phosphorylation and production of free radicals → anaerobic metabolism and multiorgan failure

SYMPTOMS/EXAMINATION

Classically described as five phases of toxicity (Table 6.25):

- **Phase 1: GI phase**
  - Nausea, vomiting, diarrhea, GI bleeding from corrosive effect
  - No vomiting within 6 hours = no toxicity
- **Phase 2: Latent phase (6-24 hours postingestion)**
  - Clinical improvement after resuscitation.
  - Patients with mild toxicity will not progress beyond this stage.
- **Phase 3: "Shock" phase**
  - Recurrence of GI symptoms
  - Anaerobic metabolism → shock, lactate production, anion gap metabolic acidosis
  - Multiorgan involvement with cardiac dysfunction, bleeding, renal failure
- **Phase 4: Fulminant hepatic failure (2-3 days postingestion)** from cellular oxidative injury
- **Phase 5: Delayed sequelae** from GI scarring, including strictures

DIFFERENTIAL

Most metals (eg, mercuric salts, lead, arsenic) cause GI effects in overdose.

DIAGNOSIS

KEY FACT

Asymptomatic patients 6 hours after iron exposure will not have significant systemic toxicity.

- History of ingestion and presence of GI (phase 1) symptoms indicate toxicity.
- Presence of anion gap metabolic acidosis (primarily lactate) indicate cellular toxicity.
- Total serum iron concentration at 4-6 and 6-8 (for sustained-release or enteric-coated preparations, respectively) hours postingestion.
- Iron concentration > 500 µg/dL = severe toxicity.
- Measurement of TIBC is not clinically useful.
- Abdominal radiograph: A negative radiograph for radiopaque pills does not rule out ingestion.

KEY FACT

Not all iron pills are visible on abdominal x-ray.

TREATMENT

- Supportive and symptomatic care
- Decontamination:
  - AC does **not** adsorb iron.
  - WBI if large burden of pills visualized on abdominal x-ray, but may be limited by vomiting.
- **Antidote = Deferoxamine** (chelating agent)
  - Indications:
    - Systemic illness (severe acidosis, shock)
    - Serum iron levels > 500 µg/dL (with clinical symptoms)
  - Renally excreted deferoxamine-iron complexes may cause urine color to pink-red ("vin-rose").

KEY FACT

Iron antidote = deferoxamine.

TABLE 6.25. Antidotes for Specific Toxicologic Agents

Antidote	Ingestion/Exposure	Indications for Treatment
Atropine	Cholinergic poisoning	Symptomatic bradycardia Excessive secretions
Black widow spider antivenom	Black widow spider (*Latrodectus*)	Persistent symptoms despite analgesia Pregnancy Very young or elderly
Calcium	HF acid exposure	Local symptoms or burns (dermal application) Hypocalcemia or high-concentration exposure (IV dosing)
CroFab	Family Viperidae: Rattlesnakes Copperheads Water moccasins	Progressive swelling Increased pain Coagulopathy Systemic symptoms
Cyanide antidote kit	Cyanide	Suspicion for exposure in patients with acidosis, coma, seizures, and hypotension
Deferoxamine	Acute iron intoxication	Systemic symptoms Iron level > 500 μg/dL
Digoxin-specific Fab	Digoxin toxicity	Ventricular dysrhythmias Bradycardia unresponsive to therapy K > 5.0 mEq/dL in acute ingestion Potentially massive overdose
Flumazenil	Benzodiazepine overdose	Severe respiratory depression; not routinely used in acute overdose; used more with procedural sedation Contraindicated in: chronic use; if coingestion of seizure-inducing medication; elevated ICP
Fomepizole	Ethylene glycol Methanol	Metabolic acidosis or known significant ingestion of a toxic alcohol
Glucagon	Ca^{++} channel blocker toxicity β-Blocker toxicity	Symptomatic bradycardia Hypotension
Hydroxocobalamin	Cyanide	Suspicion of exposure in patients with acidosis, coma, seizures, and hypotension
Insulin/glucose	Ca^{++} channel blocker toxicity β-Blocker toxicity	Symptomatic bradycardia Hypotension
Methylene blue	Methemoglobinemia	Levels > 30% Mental status changes Chest pain, Shortness of breath

(Continued)

TABLE 6.25. Antidotes for Specific Toxicologic Agents (*Continued*)

Antidote	Ingestion/Exposure	Indications for Treatment
NAC	Acetaminophen	Acute single ingestion: Use Rumack-Matthew nomogram Unknown time or repeated supratherapeutic ingestion: Elevated AST/ALT APAP level > 10 μg/mL
Naloxone	Opioid toxicity	Respiratory depression
Octreotide	Sulfonylurea overdose	Recurrent hypoglycemia
Physostigmine	Anticholinergic toxidrome (rarely indicated)	Delirium Seizures Dysrhythmias
Pralidoxime (2-PAM)	Organophosphates	Symptomatic poisonings
Vitamin K	Warfarin	Increased INR (escalating dosing) Bleeding

AST/ALT, alanine transaminase/aspartate transaminase; APAP, acetaminophen ICP, intracranial pressure; INR, international normalized ratio; IV, intravenous; NAC, *N*-acetylcysteine.

Complications

- *Yersinia enterocolitica* GI infection or sepsis may occur from chronic iron overload or deferoxamine therapy (both foster the growth of the organism).
- Deferoxamine is associated with duration-related risk for ALI/ARDS in children and rate-related hypotension.

DEXTROMETHORPHAN

- Found in many over-the-counter cough preparations
- Frequently used recreationally by adolescents
- Structurally related to levorphanol, a synthetic opioid agonist

Mechanism/Toxicity

- Antagonizes N-methyl-D-aspartate (NMDA) receptors (similar to ketamine or phencyclidine [PCP]), inhibits serotonin reuptake, and at high doses, acts as an agonist at opioid receptors

Symptom/Examination

- Mild to moderate overdose: Agitation, ataxia, nystagmus, visual and auditory hallucinations.
- Severe overdose: Coma and respiratory depression.
- Serotonin syndrome is rare but may occur when ingested with other serotonergic agents.

Treatment

Supportive and symptomatic therapy

Complication

May be ingested as combination products including acetaminophen (hepatotoxicity)

DIPHENHYDRAMINE

Diphenhydramine is a sedating antihistamine with anticholinergic, antitussive, antiemetic, and local anesthetic properties.

Mechanism/Toxicity

- H_1-receptor antagonism → smooth muscle relaxation, sedation
- Muscarinic receptor antagonism → anticholinergic toxidrome
- Na^+ channel blockade (at high doses) → QRS prolongation, seizure

Symptoms/Examination

- CNS depression.
- Anticholinergic toxidrome.
- Extremely large doses may cause seizures and dysrhythmias.

Diagnosis

- Based on history and clinical presentation
- ECG to evaluate for QRS widening/dysrhythmias

Treatment

- Supportive and symptomatic therapy
- Benzodiazepines for agitation or seizures
- Sodium bicarbonate if QRS prolongation or wide complex dysrhythmias

Pesticides/Insecticides/Rodenticides

ORGANOPHOSPHATES AND CARBAMATES

Organophosphates and carbamates are insecticides used extensively in agricultural and commercial applications.

Mechanism/Toxicity

- Inhibition of cholinesterase → increases synaptic acetylcholine → increased activity at all nicotinic and muscarinic receptors.
- Carbamates bind cholinesterase transiently (minutes to hours).
- Organophosphates can undergo "aging" → irreversible binding of the insecticide to cholinesterase.

Symptoms/Examination

- Cholinergic (muscarinic) toxidrome (see mnemonic "Sludge + Killer Bs" and Table 6.2)
- Sympathomimetic excess from pregangilionic nicotinic receptor stimulation
- Muscle weakness, fasciculation, and paralysis from nicotinic excess at the neuromuscular junction
- AMS (delirium to coma), seizures

Differential

Toxicity from nerve agents (VX, Sarin, Soman, Tabun), nicotine, donepezil, pilocarpine, or *Clitocybe* species mushrooms (see Table 6.8)

Diagnosis

- Usually apparent from clinical symptoms and history of exposure.
- Measured RBC cholinesterase or pseudocholinesterase (plasma cholinesterase) levels are reduced in toxicity but are not available in a timely manner and often not clinically useful.

KEY FACT

Unlike carbamates, the organophosphate bond to cholinesterase will "age" and become irreversible over time.

Q

A 54-year-old man farm worker called EMS after ingesting an insecticide in a self-harm attempt. On ED arrival, he is confused and smells of garlic. Further examination reveals pinpoint pupils, excessive salivation, lacrimation, and muscle fasciculations. What is the most appropriate initial medication to give in the treatment of this patient?

Treatment

- Immediate surface decontamination to prevent secondary contamination of rescuers and health care providers
- Supportive therapy with close airway monitoring and benzodiazepines for seizures
- **Antidote = atropine,** used for hemodynamically unstable bradycardia and excessive secretions (endpoint is drying of airway secretions)
  - Very high doses often needed; 0.5-2 mg IV initially with doubling of dose every 5 minutes until drying of airway secretions
- **Antidote = pralidoxime (2-PAM), used to reactivate inhibited cholinesterase in organophosphate poisoning prior to "aging"**

KEY FACT

Antidotes to organophosphate poisoning: Atropine and pralidoxime.

SUPERWARFARINS

Most home rodenticide products contain a superwarfarin such as brodifacoum. Laboratory abnormalities occur 1-2 days following ingestion.

Mechanism/Toxicity

Superwarfarins act similarly to warfarin by inhibiting activation of vitamin K–dependent clotting factors (II, VII, IX, X); however, the duration of anticoagulation may extend for weeks.

KEY FACT

Duration of anticoagulation following superwarfarin ingestion may extend for weeks.

Symptoms/Examination

- Symptoms are due to bleeding (brain, GI, vaginal, etc).
- Onset of anticoagulation is 1-2 days following ingestion and may last for months.

Diagnosis

- PT/INR measurement at 24 and 48 hours can determine the extent of anticoagulation from superwarfarins.
- Normal PT/INR at 48 hours in the absence of vitamin K or FFP treatment excludes toxicity.

Treatment

- Vitamin K supplementation for elevated INR. Large ingestions may require high doses for prolonged periods of time.
- Prophylactic vitamin K (prior to elevation of INR) is **not** indicated because it may mask impending INR elevation and not allow it to be an accurate future marker of anticoagulation (duration of action of superwarfarin is much longer than that of vitamin K).
- Acute bleeding requires FFP, cryoprecipitate, or PCC to reverse anticoagulation.

STRYCHNINE

A rodenticide with significant human toxicity, its use in home products has largely been supplanted by the superwarfarins. Has also been found as an adulterant in illicit drugs.

Mechanism/Toxicity

Inhibits glycine receptors within the spinal cord → uncontrolled muscular contraction

A

This patient is presenting with cholinergic excess consistent with organophosphate poisoning. Atropine is the initial medication and should be used to control airway secretions and symptomatic bradycardia. Large doses are often needed.

Symptoms/Examination

- Strychnine poisoning produces rapid onset involuntary muscle contractions, opisthotonus, hyperreflexia, clonus, and trismus usually within 15-30 minutes of ingestion.
- Mental status is not affected.

Diagnosis

Based on history and examination, specific testing for strychnine is not available.

Treatment

- Benzodiazepines or barbiturates are administered to relieve excessive muscular activity.
- More severe cases may require intubation and neuromuscular blockade.

Sedative Hypnotics

Sedative-hypnotic agents are medications used to treat anxiety, panic disorders, and insomnia. Medications in this class include barbiturates, benzodiazepines, antihistamines, antidepressants, and other agents with sedating side effects. This section is limited to a discussion of barbiturates and benzodiazepines.

BARBITURATES

Barbiturates are used as sedatives, to induce anesthesia, and to treat epilepsy, including status epilepticus.

They are categorized by their duration of action:

- Ultrashort-acting (eg, methohexital, thiopental)
- Short-acting (eg, pentobarbital)
- Intermediate-acting (eg, amobarbital, butalbital)
- Long-acting (eg, phenobarbital)

The magnitude and duration of effect depends on the agent and dose. Chronic exposure often leads to tolerance.

Mechanism/Toxicity

- Binds to $GABA_A$ chloride channel → increased duration of channel opening, depression of neuronal firing
- Depresses medullary respiratory centers
- Inhibits myocardial contractility and conduction

Symptoms/Examination

- Mild to moderate intoxication: Lethargy, nystagmus, ataxia, slurred speech (similar to alcohol intoxication)
- Severe intoxication: Small/midsized pupils, hypothermia, coma, respiratory depression, hypotension, bradycardia

Diagnosis

- Usually based on history of exposure and clinical examination.
- Serum levels may be available for agents used to treat epilepsy (eg, phenobarbital).
- In overdose, clinically correlate levels and monitor for peak and decline.

Q

A 2-year-old girl is brought in to the ED by her parents following suspected ingestion of rat poison containing difenacoum 1 hour earlier. She has no past medical history, is acting normally, and the physical examination is unremarkable. What workup and intervention should be considered at this time?

KEY FACT

Generalized, uncontrolled muscular activity with normal mental status ("awake seizures") is suggestive of strychnine poisoning.

KEY FACT

Severe barbiturate intoxication depressed/decreased:

HR
BP
RR
Temperature
CNS

Q

A 21-year-old man is brought in by the police after being found running naked in the park on a hot summer night. Physical examination reveals an agitated patient chewing on the restraints and fighting to get loose. His airway and breathing are intact and the nurse states that his pulse is "fast." What are the first actions to take in treating this patient?

A

Nothing at this time. It is very unlikely that the laboratory test results will be abnormal and very rare to have clinically significant bleeding after a 1-time unintentional ingestion. A conservative approach is to have follow-up coagulation studies done daily for 2-3 days.

KEY FACT

Flumazenil contraindications: (1) Chronic benzodiazepine use (2) Coingestion of seizure-inducing meds (3) Suspected ↑ ICP; Not used routinely in acute benzodiazepine overdose.

A

Sedation with benzodiazepines and temperature control are essential with the undifferentiated sympathomimetic patient. Although it would be ideal to know what he took, determining the temperature and reversing the psychomotor agitation are of paramount importance.

TREATMENT

- Supportive therapy.
- **MDAC** may be beneficial in phenobarbital overdose only if airway is protected.
- **WBI** if large ingestion of long-acting agents only if conditions are appropriate.
- HD for severely intoxicated patients refractory to above therapy.

COMPLICATION

- Barbiturate withdrawal is similar to alcohol/benzodiazepine withdrawal and may be life threatening.

BENZODIAZEPINES

Benzodiazepines are used as sedatives, to induce anesthesia, and to treat seizures including status epilepticus.

They are categorized by their duration of action.

- Short-acting (eg, midazolam)
- Intermediate-acting (eg, lorazepam)
- Long-acting (eg, diazepam)

The shorter-acting agents are more lipophilic, and therefore cross the blood–brain barrier more rapidly (rapid on, rapid off). Half-life is **not** a good indicator of duration of effect.

Severe toxicity from benzodiazepine exposure is rare unless combined with other agents that have synergistic effects.

MECHANISM/TOXICITY

- Enhanced binding of GABA to $GABA_A$ channels → depression of neuronal firing
  - Toxicity limited by availability of GABA and hence safer in overdose then barbiturates.
- Peripheral vasodilatation

SYMPTOMS/EXAMINATION

- Mild to moderate intoxication: Lethargy, slurred speech, ataxia
- Severe intoxication: Coma, respiratory depression

DIAGNOSIS

- Usually based on history of exposure.
- Most urine toxicology tests screen for older benzodiazepines (diazepam, oxazepam, temazepam, chlordiazepoxide).

TREATMENT

- Supportive therapy
- **Antidote = Flumazenil**
  - Benzodiazepine receptor antagonist.
  - Duration of effect = 1 hour (recurrent sedation possible, similar to naloxone).
  - Limited utility in the ED: Mostly for reversal of procedural sedation, whereas routine use in acute overdose is not recommended because benzodiazepine overdose alone is rarely fatal, may have significant side effects especially in benzodiazepine-dependent patients.
  - Contraindications:
    - Chronic benzodiazepine use (may induce withdrawal)
    - Coingestion of seizure-inducing medication (eg, TCAs)
    - Suspected increased intracranial pressure (ICP)

Sympathomimetics

The sympathomimetic toxidrome may result from exposure to any of the following:

- Prescription medications: Attention deficit disorder/attention deficit hyperactivity disorder (ADD/ADHD) medications (Ritalin, Adderall)
- Over-the-counter medications and herbal preparations: Ephedrine, pseudoephedrine, Ma Huang
- Illicit drugs: Cocaine, methamphetamines (see the section "Drugs of Abuse")

Mechanism/Toxicity

Excessive epinephrine/norepinephrine due to:

- Increased release from α- and β-adrenergic receptors
- Decreased enzymatic breakdown
- Decreased reuptake
- Cocaine → Na^+ channel blockade causing wide complex dysrhythmias

Symptoms/Examination

Fight or flight response

- Agitation, hallucinations
- Tachycardia, hypertension
- Hyperthermia, diaphoresis
- Mydriasis
- Muscular rigidity

Diagnosis

- Clinical diagnosis based on exposure history and physical examination
- ECG to evaluate rhythm, rule out cardiac sodium channel blockade (especially for cocaine), evaluate for ischemia

Treatment

- Supportive care
  - Passive and active cooling measures; may need aggressive sedation, and occasionally intubation and paralytics, to maintain normothermia
  - IV hydration
- **Benzodiazepines:** For agitation, hyperthermia, tachycardia, seizures, muscular rigidity
- **Sodium bicarbonate:** For wide complex dysrhythmias
- **Avoid**
  - β-Blockers due to concern for unopposed α-receptor stimulation.
  - Consider WBI for body packers. These patients may need surgical removal of packets if any concern for packet rupture or obstruction.

Complications

- Cardiac ischemia
- Aortic dissection
- Ruptured abdominal aortic aneurysm
- Ischemic bowel
- Intracranial hemorrhage
- Rhabdomyolysis

> **KEY FACT**
>
> **Sympathomimetic toxidrome:**
> Agitation, anxiety
> Tachycardia
> Hypertension
> Mydriasis
> Diaphoresis

> **KEY FACT**
>
> Diaphoretic, not dry, skin and hyperactive, not hypoactive, bowel sounds are the key to differentiating the sympathomimetic toxidrome from the anticholinergic toxidrome.

REVIEW QUESTIONS

QUESTIONS

1. A 42-year-old man presents with a chief complaint of abdominal pain and nausea. Vital signs are temperature 36.6°C, HR 108 bpm, BP 132/86 mm Hg, RR 18 breaths/min, O_2 sat 92% room air. On further interview, he reports ingesting a "handful of Tylenol PM" 2 hours prior to arrival in an effort to harm himself. What is the next step in this patient's management?
   A. Urine drug screen
   B. Acetaminophen concentration
   C. Electrocardiogram
   D. Intravenous *N*-acetylcysteine

2. A 22-year-old woman is brought in by ambulance shortly after ingesting an entire bottle of unknown medication. The patient complains of abdominal pain, but refuses to disclose the name of the medication. Vital signs are temperature 36.4°C, HR 89 bpm, BP 118/79 mm Hg, RR 23 breaths/min, O_2 sat 100% room air. Several minutes later, a roommate arrives with an empty bottle of aspirin that she found in the patient's room. A point of care ABG is obtained and shows pH 7.42, Pco_2 33, HCO_3 21. Aside from obtaining a salicylate level, what is the next step in this patient's management?
   A. Activated charcoal
   B. Intubation
   C. Hemodialysis
   D. Recheck ABG in 30 minutes

3. A 42-year-old woman with history of depression presents with headache, sweating, and flushing after a wine tasting tour. She denies any current medications. Vital signs are temperature 37.1°C, HR 104 bpm, BP 180/93 mm Hg, RR 18 breaths/min, O_2 sat 98% room air. What class of antidepressant medication did she most likely recently discontinue?
   A. SSRI
   B. MAOI
   C. Tricyclic antidepressant
   D. SNRI

4. A 63-year-old man with history of diabetes is brought in by ambulance after being found by a family member with altered mental status, nausea, vomiting, and abdominal pain. Blood glucose in the field is 123. On arrival you find the patient to be tachypneic and difficult to arouse. Your laboratory test results return with Cr of 2.1 mg/dL, lactate 10 mmol/L, ABG pH 6.98, Pco_2 30, HCO_3 11. What is the best next step in management?
   A. Call nephrology to initiate dialysis
   B. Start empiric antibiotics
   C. Administer charcoal and initiate whole-bowel irrigation
   D. Initiate a bicarbonate drip

5. A 54-year-old male farmer presents to the emergency department with diaphoresis, miosis, wheezing, frothy secretions, and bradycardia after a chemical exposure. Current vital signs are temperature 36.8°C, HR 45 bpm, BP 104/68 mm Hg, RR 32 breaths/min, O_2 sat 90% room air. Endpoint of treatment with the antidote should be:
   A. Dried airway secretions
   B. Resolution of bradycardia
   C. Mydriasis
   D. Improvement of mental status

6. A 6-year-old child was found crying and arching his back uncontrollably after playing in the garage. Upon EMS arrival, paramedics described the child as having seizure-like activity but conscious. Parents are worried that he may have gotten into some gopher bait. The implicated toxin affects which of the following area of the nervous system?
   A. Basal ganglia
   B. Neuromuscular junction
   C. Parasympathetic ganglion
   D. Spinal cord

ANSWERS

1. **C.** The most appropriate answer here is an electrocardiogram to evaluate for evidence of QRS widening and/or terminal R wave in aVR from sodium channel blockade from the diphenhydramine portion of the ingestion. Urine drug screen is unlikely to change clinical management because of the high likelihood for false positives and false negatives. For acute ingestions of acetaminophen, an acetaminophen concentration < 4 hours postingestion can only help if the concentration is 0 μg/mL. The Rumack-Matthew nomogram cannot be applied to an acetaminophen concentration < 4 hours. The most prudent course of action is to send an acetaminophen concentration 4 hours postingestion. Empirically initiating intravenous *N*-acetylcysteine is not needed if an acetaminophen concentration can be obtained < 8 hours postingestion.

2. **A.** The most appropriate next step should be administration of activated charcoal in the setting that the patient has ingested acetylsalicylate (aspirin) without

alteration a mental status or significant nausea/vomiting. Activated charcoal may be beneficial for salicylate overdose given the propensity for salicylates to cause delayed absorption secondary to bezoar formation and pyloric spasm. Patient is mentating appropriately without evidence of hypoventilation. Intubation is not warranted at this point. Patient has no significant metabolic acidosis with a mild respiratory alkalosis. Without clinical evidence of severe toxicity, renal insufficiency, cerebral edema, pulmonary edema, or intolerance of fluids, hemodialysis is not warranted at this point. Repeat laboratory evaluation will likely be necessary starting with intervals of every 1-2 hours.

3. **B.** Fermented foods such as cheese and wine may contain high concentrations of biologic amines including tyramine. Coadministration of foods high in tyramine and MAOIs may lead to a hypertensive crisis or the so-called "cheese effect." This interaction is unlikely to be associated with SSRIs, tricyclic antidepressants, or SSRIs.

4. **A.** In a diabetic patient with normal glucose, nausea/vomiting, elevated lactate, and severe metabolic acidosis, metformin toxicity should be high on the differential. For this patient, metformin toxicity may have been exacerbated or triggered by his renal insufficiency. After initial attention to airway, breathing, and circulation, nephrology should be consulted to initiate dialysis to correct patient's severe acid-base disturbance with the added benefit of enhanced elimination of metformin in the patient's system. Bicarbonate drip may only be a temporizing measure and should be initiated after nephrology has been consulted. Activated charcoal and whole-bowel irrigation are unlikely to be beneficial in this setting without known chronicity and degree of altered mentation. The risk of aspiration is high in the setting of altered mentation without a protected airway. One should keep a broad differential for this presentation, including sepsis and ischemic bowel, but antibiotics may not be the definitive treatment here.

5. **A.** Patient presents with a cholinergic toxidrome (bradycardia, bronchospasm, bronchorrhea, salivation, lacrimation, urination, defecation/mydriasis, GI distress, emesis) likely secondary to an organophosphate pesticide. The correct first-line antidote here is atropine. Large doses of atropine may be needed to resuscitate the patient with an end point of dried airway secretions. Remember the ABCs of resuscitation. Patient's bradycardia is not causing malperfusion with a blood pressure of 104/68 mm Hg. Pupillary size is a poor marker of cholinergic toxicity and should not be used to guide treatment. Mental status improvement is likely secondary to improvement in airway and perfusion. Pralidoxime may be needed as a second-line antidote for organophosphate poisoning to regenerate acetylcholinesterase and prevent permanent aging of the toxin to the enzyme.

6. **D.** The poison in this scenario is likely to be strychnine which can be found in gopher bait or other forms of rodenticide. Strychnine can be highly lethal and acts by inhibiting glycine receptors within the spinal cord leading to this inhibition of muscular contraction. Larger muscle groups will contract more strongly leading to the clinical picture of opisthotonus. Mental status for these patients is unaffected leading to the appearance of "awake seizures." Treatment is sedation with benzodiazepines or barbiturates. Intubation and/or neuromuscular blockade may be necessary in severe cases. Generalized tetanus can present similarly but acts by irreversibly inhibiting the release of inhibitory neurotransmitter release (GABA and glycine) in the autonomic and somatic nervous systems. Some common basal ganglia toxins include carbon monoxide, cyanide, and methanol. Botulism- and curare-like agents act to decrease transmission across the neuromuscular junction and lead to flaccid paralysis.

CHAPTER 7

Endocrine, Metabolic, Fluid, and Electrolyte Disorders

Lauren M. Abbate, MD, PhD

Fluid and Hydration

BASIC DEFINITIONS

- Solute: Particles dissolved in a solvent (ie, electrolytes, glucose, urea, proteins)
- Solvent: Liquid that dissolves the solute creating a solution, usually H_2O
- Osmolality: Number of dissolved particles in a solution, expressed as osmoles per kilogram of solvent (Osm/kg)

TOTAL BODY WATER AND DISTRIBUTION

KEY FACT

Total blood volume in adults is 70 mL/kg or about 5 L in a 70-kg person. Total blood volume is 80-90 mL/kg in children.

- Total body water (TBW) = about 60% of total body weight.
- Two-thirds of TBW is intracellular = 40% of TBW (Table 7.1).
- Cell membranes are semipermeable and allow free passage of solvent, allowing water to move freely down concentration gradients between intracellular, interstitial, and plasma compartments to maintain equilibrium.
- In contrast, solutes require energy to be actively pumped across membranes or need ion gradients to flow through opened channels within a membrane.

Hyper- and Hypo-Osmolar States

- Serum osmolality can be measured in the laboratory using an osmometer. Normal circulating solutes include sodium salts, glucose, and urea. **The normal *measured* serum osmolality is around 285 mOsm/kg**. A rise in the measured serum osmolality can be due to an increase in a normal circulating solute (eg, hypernatremia, uremia) or the presence of additional particles (eg, alcohols, mannitol).
- Osmolality can also be **calculated** using the following formula:

$$2\,[Na^+] + \frac{\text{Glucose}}{18} + \frac{\text{BUN}}{2.6} = \text{calculated osmolality (mOsm/kg)}$$

KEY FACT

In patients with altered mental status and an unexplained increased anion gap, use the osmolal gap as a screening test for unmeasured osmoles, such as methanol or ethylene glycol.

- If additional particles are present, the measured osmolality will be much larger than the calculated osmolality = **osmolal gap**. A normal osmolal gap should be **< 10 mOsm/kg**. High osmolal gaps are caused by increases in measured (but not calculated) serum particles. Causes include:
  - Acetone
  - Glycerol
  - Ethylene glycol
  - Mannitol
  - Isopropyl alcohol
  - Sorbitol
  - Methanol
  - Ethanol
  - Formaldehyde
  - Paraldehyde
  - Severe hyperlipidemia
  - Severe hyperproteinemia

TABLE 7.1. Comparison of Intracellular and Interstitial Fluid Electrolyte Concentrations

	% TBW	% Weight	Na^+	Cl^-	HCO_3^-	K^+	Ca^{2+}	Mg^{2+}	Includes
Intracellular	2/3	40%	14	4	10	150	< 1	30	Proteins
Interstitial	1/3	20%	140	113	27	5	9	3	Plasma

Electrolytes measured in mEq/L

- Account for ethanol's contribution to the osmolal gap by dividing the blood ethanol in mg/dL by 4.6:

$$2\,[Na^+] + \frac{\text{Glucose}}{18} + \frac{\text{BUN}}{2.6} + \frac{\textit{serum}\ \text{EtOH}}{4.6}$$
$$= \text{calculated osmolality (mOsm/kg)}$$

- Hypo-osmolar states are usually caused by hyponatremia.

> **Q**
>
> An 86-year-old man with urosepsis presents dehydrated. How much intravascular fluid does 1 L of 0.9 normal saline (NS) provide? How about 1 L of 0.45 NS or D_5W?

FLUID BALANCE

Water

- Adults need 2000-3000 mL of water a day on average.
- Water loss can be categorized as sensible or insensible.
  - Sensible water loss = urinary output = approximately 1500 mL/d
  - Minimum normal urine output of a hydrated adult without renal compromise is approximately 0.5 mL/kg/h.
- Insensible water loss includes:
  - Respiratory losses of approximately 600 mL/d
  - Integumentary/evaporative skin losses of about 300 mL/d
  - Gastrointestinal (GI)/feces losses of about 100 mL/d
- The body handles water regulation with three major mechanisms:
  - Antidiuretic hormone (ADH)
    - Dehydration → decreased free water → increased serum osmolality → ADH release from the posterior hypopituitary → retention of free water in the kidney
  - Renin-angiotensin-aldosterone
    - Hypovolemia → release of renin by kidneys → conversion of circulating angiotensinogen to angiotensin → release of aldosterone by adrenals → retention of sodium and water in renal tubules
  - Hypothalamic osmoreceptors
    - Increased thirst driven by increases in serum osmolality, renin-angiotensin-aldosterone, β-adrenergic stimulation, and drugs such as lithium, as well as by drops in intracellular and extracellular volume.

Diabetes Insipidus

Decreased release of ADH (central diabetes insipidus [DI]) or resistance to ADH action in the kidney (nephrogenic DI) leads to inability to concentrate urine and loss of free water.

- Patients present with polyuria, nocturia, and polydipsia.
- An elevated plasma sodium level > 142 mEq/L in the setting of dilute urine suggest diagnosis.
- A water restriction test (evaluating urine and plasma osmolality) with administration of exogenous ADH (DDAVP) is diagnostic and differentiates central from nephrogenic DI.
- Treatment for central DI is DDAVP. Nephrogenic DI treatment focuses on decreasing the polyuria and restricting salt intake.

SIADH

Inappropriate production of ADH centrally, from ADH secreting tumors, or by enhanced release or effect from drugs or illness leading to renal water retention. Other natriuretic mechanisms (listed previously) are activated resulting in sodium and water loss and euvolemia

- Patients present with hyponatremia with euvolemia.

A

After redistribution with the extravascular space, 1 L of NS provides 250 mL of intravascular fluid, while 0.45 NS provides only 125 mL of intravascular fluid. D_5W initially provides 333 mL of intravascular fluid, but this volume decreases to 83 mL once the sugar is metabolized.

KEY FACT

Lithium is a common cause of nephrogenic diabetes insipidus.

KEY FACT

Digoxin directly inhibits the Na^+/K^+ pump. Thus, acute digoxin toxicity is associated with hyperkalemia. However, severe hypokalemic states increase digoxin's inotropic effect on myocardium because digoxin and K^+ bind to the same site on the Na^+/K^+ pump.

- Laboratory test results show a low serum osmolarity (due to hyponatremia), high urine osmolarity, and high urine sodium.
- Treatment is via water restriction, salt administration, and vasopressin receptor antagonists.

Psychogenic Polydipsia

Excessive free water intake from psychiatric cause.

- These patients present with hyponatremia.
- Laboratory test results show a low serum osmolarity, low urine osmolarity and low urine sodium.

RESUSCITATIVE FLUIDS

- Fluid tonicity:
  - 0.9% NS and Ringer's lactate solution are approximately isotonic to plasma.
  - D_5W is approximately isotonic, but glucose is then metabolized leaving hypotonic free water.
- Fluid distribution:
  - 1 L of 0.9 NS will distribute 250 mL intravascularly and 750 mL in the interstitial space.
  - 1 L of 0.45 NS places only 125 mL in the intravascular space.
  - 1 L of D_5W places 333 mL initially in the intravascular spaces, but after the sugar is metabolized only one-quarter (83 mL) remains.

Electrolyte Pump Physiology

While water freely moves between cells, it follows the gradient set up by electrolyte cell pumps. These pumps can be active (requiring ATP) or passive. The most important ones to be familiar with are:

- **Na^+/K^+ ion pump:** The major active pump in the human body exchanges 3 Na^+ out of cells for 2 K^+ into cells. This creates Na^+ and K^+ gradients across the cell membrane and also an electrical gradient that is used for many processes from neurotransmission to muscle contraction.
- **H^+/K^+ ion pump:**
  - In acidosis, H^+ is pumped intracellularly in place of K^+ to act as a cell buffer.
  - This is why patients with diabetic ketoacidosis (DKA) are initially hyperkalemic despite a total body potassium deficit from renal and GI losses. When the acidosis is corrected, this hypokalemia is unmasked. This only occurs with organic acids such as ketones that do not freely cross the cell membrane.

Sodium

Sodium is the major extracellular cation and key component of serum osmolality as opposed to K^+ and Mg^{2+}, which are the major intracellular cations. Strict sodium homeostasis is maintained by ADH, thirst, and renal absorption/excretion. Sodium regulation is followed passively by water regulation through osmosis; hence, problems with sodium usually represent problems with water balance.

HYPONATREMIA ($Na^+ < 135$ mEq/L)

Most cases of hyponatremia are associated with a hypo-osmolar or hypotonic state, but there are exceptions. Severe hyponatremia is defined as a serum $Na^+ < 120$ mEq/L.

Causes

- **Hypervolemic hypotonic hyponatremia** is due to heart failure, cirrhosis, or renal failure with salt and water retention.
- **Euvolemic hypotonic hyponatremia** has a varied etiology:
  - Endocrine: Hypothyroidism, glucocorticoid deficiency
  - Psychogenic polydipsia
  - SIADH (caused by central nervous system [CNS] disease, pulmonary disease, drugs, neoplasms)
- **Hypovolemic hypotonic hyponatremia** is caused by dehydrated states where the kidney is actively trying to reabsorb water.
- **Pseudohyponatremia** or isotonic hyponatremia is a falsely low sodium measurement in patients with high levels of lipid or protein in their plasma (hyperlipidemia, multiple myeloma, or intravenous [IV] immunoglobulin).
- **Hypertonic hyponatremia** is a state of increased serum osmolality due to hyperglycemia, radiocontrast, glycerol, or mannitol administration resulting in extracellular free water accumulation.
  - Hyperglycemia is by far the most common cause. The correction factor is an expected decrease in sodium by 1.6 mEq/L for every 100 mg/dL rise in glucose for glucose levels > 100 mg/dL. For glucose levels > 400 mg/dL, some authors advocate a correction factor of 2.4 mEq/L.

Symptoms

Symptom severity is associated with the level and rate of development of hyponatremia.

- Headache, nausea, and vomiting
- Confusion
- Seizures

Examination

Besides altered mental status, patients may have findings consistent with the underlying cause of their hyponatremia including CHF, cirrhosis, vomiting/diarrhea, excessive thirst, or water intake.

Differential

A wide differential for altered mental status should include vital sign abnormalities (hypoxia, hypotension), head injury, toxic/metabolic abnormality, infection, or psychiatric illness.

Diagnosis

- Evaluation depends on suspected underlying volume status based on HPI. Useful laboratory tests include serum electrolytes, serum osmolality, urine osmolality, and urine sodium.
- Figure 7.1 charts the basic algorithm for evaluation of hyponatremia.
- **Hypervolemic hypotonic hyponatremia**
  - If urine sodium is low (< 10 mEq/L) = cirrhosis, CHF, or nephrotic syndrome (perceived low intravascular volume causing kidneys to actively retain sodium and reabsorb water)
  - If urine sodium is high (> 20 mEq/L) = acute or chronic renal failure (inability to appropriately excrete sodium)

KEY FACT

Hypervolemic hyponatremia may be caused by **liver, heart,** or **renal** failure.

KEY FACT

The serum sodium will decrease by 1.6 mEq/L for every 100 mg/dL rise in glucose above normal.

KEY FACT

Rapid sodium decreases are more likely to produce symptoms and severe sequelae.

MNEMONIC

Differential for altered mental status:

AEIOU TIPS

Acidosis/Alcohol
Epilepsy
Infection
Overdose
Uremia
Trauma to head
Insulin
Psychosis
Stroke

Q

A 59-year-old man with a history of CHF presents to the emergency department altered with pitting edema and crackles in his lungs. His mentation is normal. His sodium is 115 mEq/L. What therapies should you initiate?

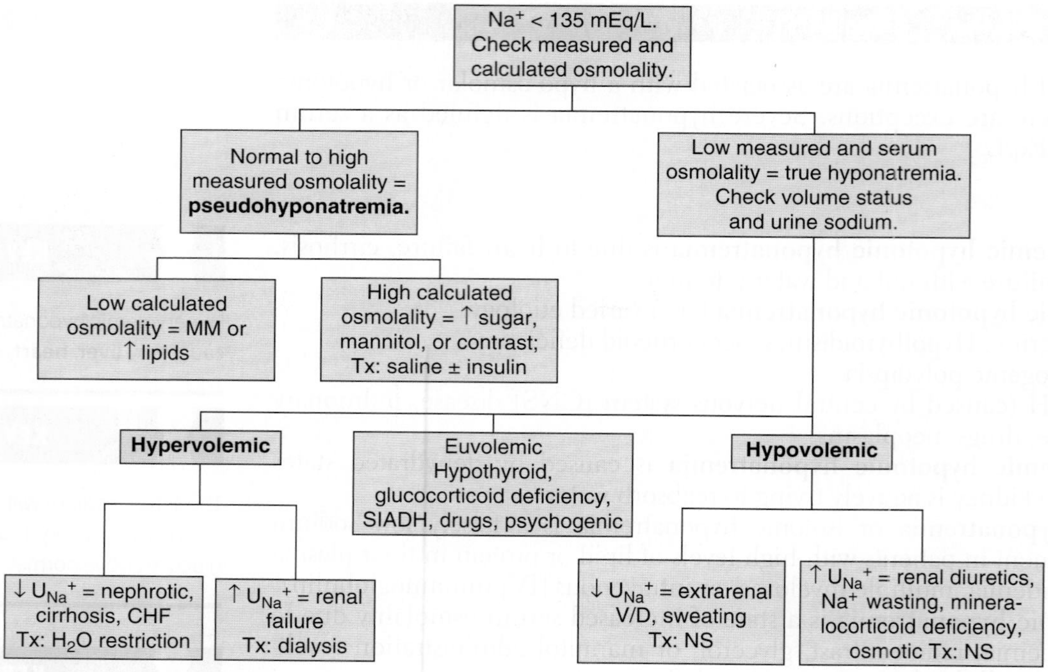

FIGURE 7.1. Evaluation of hyponatremia.

- **Euvolemic hypotonic hyponatremia**
  - Urine sodium is usually high (> 20 mEq/L). SIADH is associated with high urine osmolality and low BUN.
- **Hypovolemic hypotonic hyponatremia (dehydrated)**
  - Signs of dehydration likely present including poor skin turgor and tachycardia
  - Low urine sodium (< 10 mEq/L) = extrarenal sodium loss (eg, vomiting, diarrhea, GI suction, fistula)
  - High urine sodium (> 20 mEq/L) = renal sodium loss (eg, diuretics, nephropathy, mineralocorticoid deficiency)

TREATMENT

- Identify and correct the underlying cause.
- Dehydrated patients need to be volume resuscitated with isotonic fluid first.
- Patients with symptomatic **severe hyponatremia** (eg, altered level of consciousness or seizures) emergently require **hypertonic 3% saline** (513 mEq of Na^+/L) (initially, 100-mL bolus over 10 minutes, may repeat) until these severe symptoms have resolved with a goal of **raising the serum sodium by 4-6 mEq/L** (NOT to a predetermined sodium level).
- Have a lower threshold for giving hypertonic saline in patients who have rapid onset hyponatremia (water intoxication, marathon runners, use of ecstasy) as they are more likely to develop fatal brain herniation without aggressive treatment.
- Check laboratory test results frequently. **Do not increase sodium more rapidly than 0.5 mEq/L/h or 8 mEq/L in the first 24 hours.**
- Pseudohyponatremia does not require treatment.
- Hypertonic hyponatremia secondary to mannitol or contrast requires saline; due to hyperglycemia requires insulin and saline.
- **Hypervolemic hypotonic hyponatremia** secondary to renal failure may require dialysis; due to CHF, cirrhosis, or renal failure requires fluid restriction diuresis with loop diuretic, and treating the underlying disorder.

KEY FACT

Sodium should not be corrected more rapidly than 0.5 mEq/L/h (12 mEq/L /d).

A

This patient likely has hypervolemic hyponatremia and needs water restriction, diuresis with a loop diuretic and additional pharmacologic therapy for his underlying CHF. He will need admission for close monitoring, but given the normal mentation and likely chronic nature of his hyponatremia does not need hypertonic saline.

- **Euvolemic hypotonic hyponatremia** requires free water restriction and treating the underlying disorder.
- **Hypovolemic hypotonic hyponatremia** requires aggressive hydration with saline.

Complications

- **Fatal brain herniation** is seen in patients with acute postoperative hyponatremia, rapidly developing hyponatremia and those with underlying intracranial pathology.
- **Seizures** are more likely to occur in those with rapid onset severe hyponatremia.
- Rapid correction of **chronic** hyponatremia has been associated with neurologic deterioration known as *osmotic demyelination syndrome (ODS)*, formerly known as *central pontine myelinolysis (CPM)*. No such risk has been seen in patients with acute (< 24 hours) development of hyponatremia.
  - ODS presents with flaccid paralysis, dysarthria, dysphagia, and hypotension.
  - Alcoholics, malnourished, liver disease patients and those with Na < 105 mEq/L or hypokalemia are at increased risk.

KEY FACT

Reserve use of hypertonic saline for severe hyponatremia with seizures or decreased mental status, typically in patients with Na < 115 mEq/L.

KEY FACT

ODS occurs with rapid correction of chronic hyponatremia.

HYPERNATREMIA ($Na^+ > 145$ mEq/L)

Hypernatremia results from either a dehydrated state or iatrogenic Na^+ gain. In general, this state develops only in those who are unable to experience thirst or access water: elderly, infants, disabled, comatose, or intubated patients. Hypernatremia that has been present for > 48 hours is considered to be chronic. There are three major types: hypovolemic, euvolemic, and hypervolemic.

Causes

- **Hypovolemic:** Sweating, GI losses, diuretic medication, hyperglycemic osmotic diuresis, mannitol osmotic diuresis
- **Euvolemic**
  - Inadequate water intake due to physical or neurologic disability (infants, intubated patients)
  - Diabetes insipidus either central or nephrogenic
- **Hypervolemic:** Iatrogenic (hypertonic saline, saline enemas, sodium bicarbonate administration), seawater ingestion, acute renal failure

Symptoms

- Symptoms correlate with severity and chronicity of condition.
- Lethargy, weakness, irritability, and symptoms of the underlying disease process

Examination

- Altered mental status or seizures
- Increased tone and reflexes
- Poor skin turgor, tachycardia, low urine output

Treatment

- Identify and treat the underlying cause.
- Rehydrate hypovolemic patients with 0.9% NS (to euvolemia).
- Correct sodium by free water repletion with D_5W or oral tap water using the following formula to calculate the patient's free water deficit (replace 0.6 with 0.5 for adult women and elderly men and 0.45 for elderly women):

$$\text{Free water deficit} = \text{Total body weight (kg)} \times 0.6 \times \left(\frac{\text{Serum Na}}{140} - 1\right)$$

- For **acute hypernatremia,** aim to lower the sodium to near normal in < 24 hours.
- For **chronic hypernatremia,** the goal is to lower the serum sodium by 10 mEq/L over 24 hours using the following formula:

$$\text{Free water replacement over 24 h} = \text{Free water deficit} \times \left(\frac{10 \text{ mEq/L}}{\text{Serum Na} - 140}\right)$$

- Add a loop diuretic, such as furosemide to free water regimen in hypervolemic patients.

Complications

Chronic hypernatremia is associated with the gradual accumulation of intracellular osmolytes in the brain to maintain cell volume. The loss of these osmolytes is also gradual; therefore, rapid correction of chronic hypernatremia can lead to cerebral edema and cell death.

Potassium

Potassium is the body's major intracellular cation (98% of K^+ is intracellular) and determinant of cell membrane potential. It must be actively pumped into cell to maintain gradient. K^+ is freely filtered through the glomerulus, absorbed in the proximal and ascending tubules, and secreted in the distal tubules through an Na^+/K^+ gate.

HYPOKALEMIA ($K^+ < 3.5$ mEq/L)

Causes

- Renal losses:
  - Common: Renal tubular acidosis, postobstructive diuresis, diuretic therapy.
  - Uncommon: Cushing syndrome, licorice ingestion, Bartter syndrome (rare inherited defect in the ascending limb of the loop of Henle), Gitelman syndrome (closely related to Bartter syndrome but milder)
- Nonrenal losses: Vomiting, diarrhea, excessive sweating or suctioning, colon cancer, or villous adenoma.
- Decreased intake: Either low dietary content or pica
- Intracellular shifts:
  - **Hypokalemic periodic paralysis:** Rare familial channelopathy characterized by episodes of muscle weakness; typical setting includes recent heavy exercise, high-carbohydrate, high-salt meal, or alcohol intake.
  - **Thyrotoxic hypokalemic period paralysis:** Similar to familial periodic paralysis in presentation, but due to hyperthyroid state.
  - Insulin or albuterol administration.

> **KEY FACT**
>
> A familial channelopathy with perioidic **hyperkalemia** can also cause periodic paralysis. Symptoms are often less severe but more frequent than hypokalemic periodic paralysis.

Symptoms

- Typically requires a $K^+ < 3$ mEq/L to be symptomatic. Severity is proportional to degree of hypokalemia and its duration.
- Include malaise, muscle weakness, paresthesias, and symptoms of underlying cause

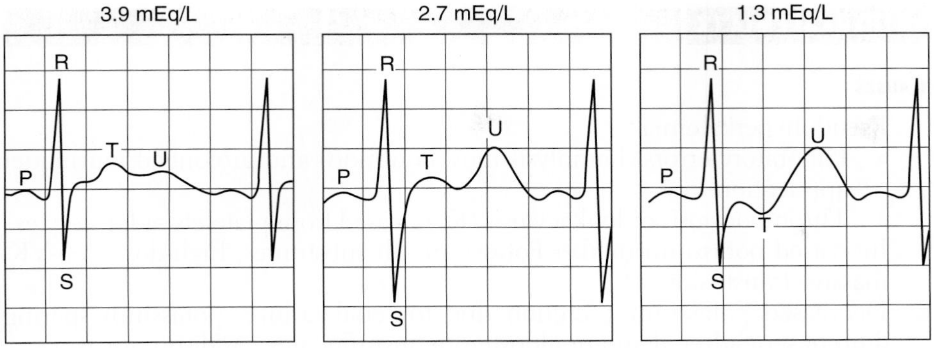

FIGURE 7.2. ECGs of hypokalemia with characteristic U waves and ST depression.

Q

A patient with a history of renal failure missed her last few dialysis sessions and presents with weakness. When attached to the cardiac monitor, you notice a very wide QRS complex resembling a sine wave. What treatments should be initiated? Which of these treatments is definitive?

Examination

- Muscle weakness which can progress to respiratory failure, paralysis, ileus
- Hyporeflexia in severe cases but DTRs usually preserved
- Electrocardiogram (ECG) findings are not sensitive, but see Figure 7.2.
- Bradycardia and AV block
- Ventricular fibrillation (Vfib) or ventricular tachycardia (VTach)
- U waves and flat T waves
- ST depression or QT prolongation

Diagnosis

History and physical are usually sufficient in diagnosing the cause of potassium loss.

A low urine potassium-to-creatinine ratio suggests hypokalemia due to intracellular shifts, poor intake, or nonrenal losses.

Treatment

- Severe hypokalemia (K < 2.5 mEq/L)
  - Considered life threatening
  - Replete with KCl 10 mEq/h by peripheral IV or 20 mEq/h if central venous access is available.
  - As a guideline, 10 mEq of KCl will increase serum K by ~0.1 mEq/L.
  - Goal is to correct K^+ to at least 3.5 mEq/L.
  - ECG and cardiac monitoring for ectopy or arrhythmia
  - Aggressive fluid administration if hypovolemic. Dehydrated patients continue to secrete the hormone aldosterone which causes the kidney to excrete potassium in exchange for sodium. This will make it difficult to replenish potassium stores until volume is restored.
  - Remember to check for hypomagnesemia which can inhibit potassium repletion unless corrected. In patients with hypokalemia and malnutrition, it is appropriate to presumptively **give magnesium along with potassium** replacement.
- Mild-moderate hypokalemia (K = 2.5-3.5 mEq/L)
  - Not usually life threatening
  - K^+ replacement should be done orally if there is no contraindication.

KEY FACT

Do not forget to replace K^+ in DKA patients, even if they have normal serum K^+ initially. Correction of acidosis can lead to a precipitous and dangerous drop in the K^+.

Complications

- **Rhabdomyolysis** due to muscle ischemia
- **Rebound hyperkalemia** is a real concern in patients with distributive hyperkalemia, especially period paralysis. The maximum dose of K^+ replacement for these patients should be 90 mEq in 24 hours.

A

Initiate treatment with calcium, insulin with glucose, and Kayexalate and prepare for dialysis. Consider sodium bicarbonate and albuterol as adjuncts. Ultimately, only Kayexalate, dialysis, and diuretics are definitive treatments as they remove potassium from the body.

HYPERKALEMIA ($K^+ > 5.5$ mEq/L)

Causes

- Pseudohyperkalemia
  - Laboratory errors (hemolysis most common) and prolonged tourniquet application
  - Thrombocytosis or leukocytosis (K^+ released from platelets or leukocytes)
- Increased potassium intake: Potassium salt substitutes, high-dose Pen-VK, massive transfusion
- Decreased potassium excretion due to renal failure, potassium sparing diuretics, or adrenal and/or aldosterone insufficiency (Addison disease)
- Cellular release
  - DKA or other states of acidosis
  - Cell breakdown (eg, burns, crush injuries, tumor lysis syndrome)
  - Medications (succinylcholine and digoxin)

Symptoms

Similar to hypokalemia

Examination

- Weakness and areflexia
- Hypotension
- ECG findings: Symmetric peaked T waves → P wave flattening → widened QRS → sine waves (Figure 7.3)

KEY FACT

Hyperkalemia due to digoxin toxicity needs digibind, not calcium.

Treatment

- Three categories of treatment (Table 7.2)
- Without ECG findings, treatment can be limited to decreased intake and potassium excreting drugs.
- ECG findings prompt emergent use of the rapid-onset protective agents such as calcium and insulin until definitive excretory methods can take effect or dialysis can be arranged. Generally, **give calcium if there is QRS widening**.
- Sodium bicarbonate has no effect on nonacidotic patients.

KEY FACT

Do not use succinylcholine for RSI on patients who have known or suspected hyperkalemia or in patients with neurologic conditions (Guillain-Barré, muscular dystrophy, old stroke, burn, crush, or spinal cord injury) that may predispose them to a large increase in serum K^+ with succinylcholine.

Complications

- Inadequate treatment of hyperkalemia can lead to life-threatening cardiac dysrhythmias.
- Only Kayexalate, dialysis, and diuretics remove potassium, but they are time dependent. The other measures are more rapid but only temporarily shift potassium intracellularly without changing total body potassium.

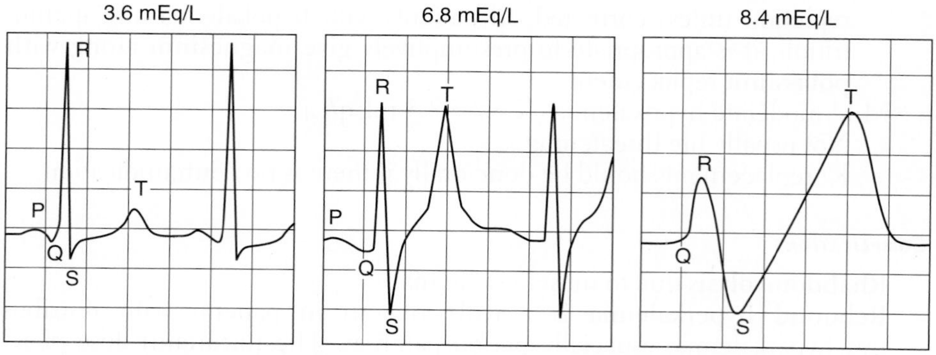

FIGURE 7.3. **ECGs of hyperkalemia with peaked T waves progressing to sine waves.**

TABLE 7.2. Treatments for Hyperkalemia

Intervention	Mechanism Category	Usual Dose	Onset of Action	Duration of Effect on K^+
Kayexalate	Excretory	15 g PO or 30 g PR	1-2 h	4-6 h
Furosemide	Excretory	40 mg IV	< 1 h	6 h
Dialysis	Excretory	—	Immediate	Continuous
Insulin and glucose	Redistribution	10 U regular insulin and 50 g of D_{50}	30 min	4-6 h
Sodium bicarbonate	Redistribution	1 mEq/kg IV	5 min	2 h
Albuterol	Redistribution	10 mg inhaled	30 min	2-4 h
Calcium gluconate/ chloride	Membrane stabilization	10-20 mL IV of 10%	1-3 min	30-60 min

IV, intravenous; PO, by mouth; PR, per rectum.

Q

A 54-year-old woman undergoing treatment for breast cancer presents to your ED with abdominal pain, nausea, and vomiting. Her electrolytes show a creatinine of 3.1 mg/dL and a Ca^{2+} of 13.6 mg/dL. What treatments should you initiate?

Calcium

Almost all calcium (99%) is in bone as the calcium phosphate salt hydroxyapatite. The rest is in plasma with half bound to proteins and half as free ionized ions. Normal plasma calcium levels are maintained at approximately 8.8-10.3 mg/dL by vitamin D and parathyroid hormone (PTH). Decreased serum Ca^{2+} results in release of PTH from parathyroid glands, which increases calcium resorption from bones and kidneys. PTH also increases vitamin D to augment intestinal absorption of calcium.

Calcium plays a key role in neuromuscular transmission and is an important cofactor for many physiologic processes:

- Control of cell membrane depolarization
- Coagulation and platelet aggregation
- Hormone secretion
- Contractile protein function
- Intracellular enzyme regulation

HYPOCALCEMIA ($Ca^{2+} < 8.5$ mg/dL)

Ionized calcium (free calcium not bound to protein) is the metabolically active serum calcium but *total calcium*, which takes into account both ionized calcium and calcium bound to albumin, is reported by most laboratory tests.

Causes

- Pseudohypocalcemia = Low total Ca^{2+}, but normal metabolically active ionized Ca^{2+} due to hypoalbuminemia. To correct for low albumin levels, add 0.8 mg/dL to the measured Ca^{2+} for every 1 mg/dL the albumin is below normal. Acid-base disturbances can alter albumin binding and the correction factor. In this setting, measure ionized Ca^{2+} instead.

A

Treat this patient with saline hydration and either calcitonin or a bisphosphonate. Furosemide should be added if there is evidence of volume overload.

KEY FACT

Causes of Hypocalcemia

- Hypoparathyroidism
- Vitamin D deficiency/resistance
- Malabsorption states
- Chelation or binding
- Sepsis/severe illness
- Phosphate overload
- Hypomagnesemia
- Renal failure
- Drugs

- Hypoparathyroidism (most common) from surgery or infiltrative processes such as sarcoidosis or malignancy
- Vitamin D deficiency/resistance or malabsorption causing decreased Ca^{2+} uptake from gut
- Increased chelation and protein binding
  - Rapid and massive blood transfusions (high citrate levels complex with calcium)
  - Acute pancreatitis (the free fatty acids produced saponify calcium)
  - Rhabdomyolysis (chelation with phosphate from damaged muscle cells)
- Sepsis or severe illness (multifactorial)
- Hyperphosphatemia
- Hypomagnesemia causes end organ resistance to PTH.
- Renal failure: Due to phosphate overload and vitamin D deficiency
- Numerous drugs

Symptoms

- Neuromuscular irritability: Paresthesias (particularly perioral and distal extremities), muscle spasms, and/or tetany. Bronchospasm and laryngospasm can occur.
- Neuropsychiatric: Altered mental status, irritability, extrapyramidal symptoms.

Examination

- Hyperreflexia
  - **Chvostek sign** (spasm when percussing facial nerve)
  - **Trousseau sign** (carpal spasm when brachial blood pressure cuff is inflated)
- Cardiovascular findings:
  - QT prolongation (rarely progressing to torsade or heart block)
  - Hypotension due to loss of vascular tone
  - CHF

Diagnosis

Evaluation should be based on suspected underlying cause. Serum magnesium levels should be measured if the cause is not immediately apparent.

Treatment

- Emergent treatment of acutely symptomatic patients = IV 10% calcium
  - **Calcium gluconate** is the preferred agent over calcium chloride in most cases (exception being cardiac arrest). Calcium gluconate has one-third of the available elemental calcium per 10 mL, but has a much lower risk of tissue necrosis with extravasation than calcium chloride.
- Massive transfusion-associated hypocalcemia: Higher incidence in patients with liver disease (liver metabolizes citrate). Replete only if symptomatic.

KEY FACT

Calcium chloride: Three times the available elemental calcium than calcium gluconate. Much higher risk of tissue necrosis with extravasation.

HYPERCALCEMIA ($Ca^{2+} > 10.5$ mg/dL)

Hypercalcemia is generally a product of another underlying disorder and not a primary process in itself. Primary hyperparathyroidism and malignancy account for 90% of cases. The total calcium level should be corrected in the presence of hypoalbuminemia.

CAUSES

- Excessive bone resorption
  - **Hyperparathyroidism** due to parathyroid adenoma (primary) or severe chronic kidney disease (secondary and tertiary hyperparathyroidism)
  - Also occurs with thyrotoxicosis, immobilization, Paget disease
- Malignancy
  - Primary hematologic or metastatic to bone
  - Parathyroid hormone-related peptide producing tumor (small cell lung cancer, kidney and ovarian cancers)
- Increased calcium absorption in small bowel
  - **Milk-alkali syndrome:** High intake of milk or calcium carbonate that leads to metabolic acidosis, hypercalcemia, and renal insufficiency. The alkalosis stimulates calcium resorption in the distal tubule, perpetuating the problem.
  - Vitamin D toxicity.
  - Granulomatous disease (via calcitriol): Sarcoidosis, TB, Croh'n, granulomatosis with polyangiitis (Wegener's), etc.
- Medications: **Lithium, thiazide diuretics,** vitamin A

Q

You respond to a code on the floor to find an elderly man seizing. After treating the seizures, you review the chart to see the patient has been admitted for CHF and has been receiving IV diuretics for the last few days. With a basic metabolic panel that shows a normal sodium and potassium, what electrolyte abnormality could cause the seizure?

SYMPTOMS

- Lethargy and weakness
- Constipation and anorexia
- Bone and muscle pain
- Altered mentation

EXAMINATION

- Neuromuscular
  - Confusion → lethargy → stupor → coma with increasing Ca^{2+}
  - Weakness, hypotonia, and hyporeflexia
  - Apathy or depression
- Cardiovascular
  - Hypertension
  - Arrhythmias
  - Shortened QT interval
  - PR and QRS widening
  - ST and T wave coving or T wave widening
- Renal
  - Renal failure
  - Nephrolithiasis
  - Polyuria

MNEMONIC

Symptoms of hypercalcemia:

Stones: Kidney stones
Bones: Pain, fractures, metastases
Groans: Anorexia, constipation
Moans: Fatigue, myalgias, weakness
Psychic Overtones: Depression, apathy, confusion

TREATMENT

- Treatment is necessary for symptomatic patients and those with levels > 14 mg/dL.
- Increase calcium excretion from the kidney:
  - **Hydration with 0.9% NS** adjusted to urine output of 200-300 mL/h.
  - Furosemide 20 mg IV once rehydrated can enhance calcium excretion. Controversial due to side effects (hypokalemia especially) and availability of bisphosphonates and calcitonin that inhibit calcium release from bone
- **Bisphosphanates (eg, pamidronate) or calcitonin** to block bone resorption
- Hydrocortisone for hematologic cancers, vitamin D deficiency, or granulomatous diseases.
- Treat underlying cause.

A

This patient likely has iatrogenic hypomagnesemia.

Magnesium

Approximately 60% of total body magnesium is contained in bone, linking its regulation closely to calcium and phosphate. Of the remaining magnesium, 39% is intracellular, and just 1% is extracellular and detectable by laboratory testing. Magnesium plays crucial roles in skeletal growth, calcium and potassium metabolism, energy production, neuromuscular activity, and the function of the Na-/K-ATPase pump in the myocardium.

HYPOMAGNESEMIA (Mg^{2+} < 1.4 mEq/L)

Causes

- Decreased GI absorption:
  - Diarrhea > vomiting
  - Malnutrition
  - Malabsorption states (ie, small bowel bypass surgery)
  - Pancreatitis
- Renal losses:
  - Diuresis (alcohol, loop diuretics, hyperglycemia)
  - Nephrotoxic drugs (ie, aminoglycosides)
  - Hypercalcemia
  - Other acquired or congenital renal defects

Symptoms/Examination

- Lethargy, altered mental status, seizures
- Neuromuscular irritability with hyperreflexia, tremor, tetany, or carpopedal spasms
- Cardiovascular effects
  - Hypotension
  - Dysrhythmias
  - QT and PR prolongation
  - Widened QRS
  - ST depression
  - T wave flattening and inversion

Treatment

- For emergent management of life-threatening dysrhythmias or seizures, give 2 g of $MgSO_4$ IV over 2 minutes followed by infusion of 4-8 g over 12-24 hours.
- For the stable patient with significant symptoms, start with 1-2 g over 15-60 minutes, followed by infusion of 4-8 g over 12-24 hours.
- Lower dose by at least 50% in patients with chronic kidney disease.
- Check and correct for associated **hypokalemia** and **hypocalcemia**.
- $MgSO_4$ administration is also indicated for preeclampsia/eclampsia, is possibly efficacious in severe asthma, but has no clear role in acute MI.

Complications

- $MgSO_4$ administration can result in flushing, hypotension, or dysrhythmias.
- Monitor for signs of magnesium toxicity (loss of **deep tendon reflexes**).

HYPERMAGNESEMIA (Mg^{2+} > 2.2 mEq/L)

The primary clinical effects of hypermagnesemia are from **neuromuscular toxicity** due to decreased impulse transmission across the neuromuscular junction and **cardiovascular toxicity** due to its calcium and potassium channel-blocking effects.

Causes

- Excessive administration
  - Most commonly from administration to preeclamptic patients
  - Mg^{2+} containing antacids, laxative, or enemas
- Decreased renal clearance (renal failure)
- Other causes include DKA, adrenal insufficiency, lithium therapy, rhabdomyolysis, tumor lysis syndrome, and accidental ingestion of Epsom salts (nearly100% $MgSO_4$)

Symptoms

- Early: Flushing, nausea/vomiting, lightheadedness
- Generalized weakness and slurred speech
- Drowsiness → lethargy → coma and respiratory failure

Examination

- Hyporeflexia is early finding and progresses to somnolence, areflexia and finally, muscle paralysis
- Cardiovascular effects:
  - Hypotension
  - Prolonged PR and QT
  - ST and T wave elevation
  - Bradycardia → AV block → asystole

KEY FACT

Loss of DTRs is an early finding of hypermagnesemia.

Magnesium Level	Finding
4-6 mEq/L	Hyporeflexia
6-10 mEq/L	Hypotension Somnolence Bradycardia
> 10 mEq/L	Muscle paralysis Respiratory failure
> 15 mEq/L	Complete heart block Cardiac arrest

Treatment

- Discontinue exogenous magnesium
- NS 0.9% IV + diuretics to increase renal excretion
- IV calcium (Mg antagonist) 100-200 mg over 5-10 minutes if life-threatening
- Dialysis for severe cases or in setting of renal failure

Phosphorus

The majority of body's phosphorous is stored in bone as hydroxyapatite. Of the circulating phosphate, most is intracellular. Phosphate is essential to energy storage and production (ATP). Isolated PO_4^{3-} abnormalities requiring treatment are rare, but abnormal levels are frequently encountered in conjunction with chronic disease states.

HYPOPHOSPHATEMIA ($PO_4^{3-} < 2.5$ mg/dL)

Symptoms are primarily due to cellular dysfunction from decreased intracellular ATP levels. Chronic hypophosphatemia also leads to decreased calcium resorption in the kidney and subsequent demineralization of bone.

Causes

- Decreased GI absorption (malnutrition, inflammatory bowel disease, phosphate-binding antacids)
- Renal losses (diuresis, hyperparathyroidism)
- Transcellular shifts:
  - Acute respiratory alkalosis
  - Insulin (intrinsic or extrinsic)
  - Postoperative parathyroidectomy (hungry bone syndrome)

Symptoms/Examination

Occur if deficit is severe (typically $PO_4^{3-} < 1$ mg/dL)
- Generalized weakness with muscle dysfunction
- Encephalopathy/coma

Treatment

- Treat underlying cause
- IV replacement for severe symptoms with PO_4^{3-} level < 1 mg/dL
  - Monitor for tetany.
- Oral phosphorus replacement for mild to moderate symptoms

Complication

Do not infuse IV phosphorous with lactated Ringer solution or PO_4^{3-} will precipitate out of solution with Ca^{2+}.

HYPERPHOSPHATEMIA ($PO_4^{3-} > 5$ mg/dL)

Causes

- Increased intake, most commonly phosphate containing laxatives
- Decreased excretion (commonly chronic renal failure, also hyperparathyroidism)
- Extracellular shift or release
  - Rhabdomyolysis
  - Hemolysis
  - Tumor lysis syndrome

Symptoms/Examination

Follows symptomatology and examination of associated hypocalcemia if severe.

Treatment

- **Calculate calcium-phosphate product (CPP) = serum Ca^{2+} × serum PO_4^{3-}.**
- CPP > 70 correlates with accelerated myocardial, vascular, and soft tissue calcification.
- Treat by diuresis with 0.9% NS (when possible).
- Oral phosphate binders and diet adjustment for outpatient treatment with mild-moderate cases
- Dialysis is temporary, but indicated for severe symptoms or $PO_4^{3-} > 14$ mg/L.

Chloride

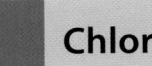

Extracellular anion that follows changes of other anions. Disorders in chloride are rarely the primary problem but a reflection of another process. Chloride functions in water, osmotic, and acid-base balance.

HYPOCHLOREMIA ($Cl^- < 95$ mEq/L)

Causes

- Vomiting or diarrhea
- Excessive sweating or heat exhaustion
- Hypokalemic alkalosis
- Acute infections

Treatment

- Replace chloride with normal saline.
- Check and correct for other associated electrolyte abnormalities.

HYPERCHLOREMIA ($CL^- > 105$ mEq/L)

Causes

- Dehydration
- GI or renal losses of bicarbonate
- Hyperparathyroidism

Treatment

- For GI loss administer normal saline.
- For renal loss administer oral bicarbonate.

Acid-Base Disorders

INTERPRETING BLOOD GASES

Basic Definitions

- Acidosis/alkalosis: A process that leads to acidemia/alkalemia.
- A metabolic disorder results in change in HCO_3^-.
- A respiratory disorder results in change in Pco_2.
- Buffering capacity: Body's immediate response to change in serum pH by protein release or capture of free H^+.
  - Extracellular proteins (one-third of buffering capacity)
  - Intracellular proteins (two-thirds of buffering capacity)
- Respiratory compensation: Body's attempt to correct metabolic acidosis or alkalosis by changes in ventilation with retention or exhalation of CO_2.
- Renal (metabolic) compensation: Body's attempt to correct respiratory acidosis or alkalosis by net excretion or regeneration of hydrogen ions through the urine.

Q

A 70-year-old woman presents with fever, tachypnea, and altered mental status. Her arterial blood gas shows pH = 7.44, $Po_2 = 90$, $Pco_2 = 20$, $HCO_3^- = 12$. The chemistry panel shows an increased anion gap. What acid-base disorders are present?

KEY FACT

Hypochloremic hypokalemic metabolic alkalosis is the classic electrolyte disorder seen with pyloric stenosis.

KEY FACT

Acidemia: pH < 7.38

Alkalemia: pH > 7.42

KEY FACT

Respiratory compensation is rapid.

Metabolic compensation is relatively slow.

A mixed respiratory alkalosis and metabolic acidosis, consider salicylate toxicity. Initially, salicylates directly stimulate the respiratory center causing hyperventilation and a respiratory alkalosis. Then, salicylates uncouple the oxidative phosphorylation in the mitochondria resulting in a metabolic acidosis.

KEY FACT

Peripheral VBG has:

pH 0.02-0.04 units lower

HCO_3^- 1-2 mEq/L higher

Pco_2 3-8 mm Hg higher than ABG

MNEMONIC

Causes of a high anion gap metabolic acidosis:

MUDPILES

Methanol, **M**etformin
Uremia
Diabetic or alcoholic ketoacidosis (AKA)
Paraldehyde
INH/iron/inhalant (ie, CO) poisoning
Lactic acidosis (sepsis, shock, hypoxia, seizures, cyanide)
Ethylene glycol
Salicylates, Solvents

Diagnosis

Use the history and examination for clues to the disorder.

- Respiratory status (increased RR suggests respiratory alkalosis; decreased RR or respiratory failure suggests respiratory acidosis)
- Dehydration/vomiting = metabolic alkalosis; diarrhea = metabolic acidosis
- Past medical history, medication, and toxin exposures

Step 1: Evaluate the blood gas and chemistry.

- Look at the pH to determine if there is an acidemia or alkalemia.
- Check the Pco_2 to determine if there is a respiratory acidosis or alkalosis.
- Examine the HCO_3^- to determine if there is a metabolic acidosis or alkalosis.

Step 2: Classify the disturbance.

- Respiratory alkalosis ($Pco_2 < 40$); causes include anxiety, CHF, hypoxia, ↑ ICP, toxic salicylates, and sympathomimetics.
- Respiratory acidosis ($Pco_2 > 40$); causes include respiratory failure, sedatives, and opiates; common and often chronic in patients with COPD; considered a sign of respiratory failure in asthmatics
- Metabolic alkalosis (↑ HCO_3^-); causes include hypovolemia, hyperaldosteronism, and Bartter syndrome
- Metabolic acidosis (↓ HCO_3^-); causes are subdivided by the presence or absence of an elevated anion gap.

Step 3: Calculate the anion gap = $Na^+ - (Cl^- + CO_2)$.

- Low anion gap metabolic acidosis (anion gap < 1); causes include increases in unmeasured serum cations (seen in multiple myeloma), lithium toxicity, decreased serum albumin, or bromide/iodine poisoning (mistaken for chloride in many laboratory tests)
- Normal anion gap metabolic acidosis; causes include diarrhea, renal tubular acidosis, ketone wasting, toluene
- High anion gap acidosis (anion gap > 15, depending on analyzer); caused by increased concentrations of anions other than K^+ and Cl^- (MUDPILES mnemonic)

Step 4: Assess compensation for acute or chronic disturbances.

If the primary disturbance is:

Respiratory:

- Acute respiratory acidosis, the HCO_3^- should increase by 1 for each 10 mm Hg of Pco_2
- Chronic respiratory acidosis, the HCO_3^- should increase by 4 for each 10 mm Hg of Pco_2
- Acute respiratory alkalosis, the HCO_3^- should decrease by 2 for each 10 mm Hg of Pco_2
- Chronic respiratory alkalosis, the HCO_3^- should decrease by 5 for each 10 mm Hg of Pco_2

Metabolic:

- Metabolic acidosis, the $Pco_2 = 1.5\ (HCO_3^-) + 8 \pm 2$ = **Winter's formula**
- Metabolic alkalosis, the Pco_2 increases 0.75 for every 1 mEq/L increase in HCO_3^-

Step 5: Consider mixed disorders.

Three rules assist in identifying a mixed disorder:

1. Neither respiratory nor renal compensation completely normalizes the pH, so if pH is normal, look for a mixed disorder.
2. Inadequate compensation suggests:
   - Measured Pco_2 < predicted = respiratory alkalosis

- Measured P_{CO_2} > predicted = respiratory acidosis
- Measured HCO_3^- < predicted = metabolic acidosis
- Measured HCO_3^- > predicted = metabolic alkalosis

3. If the AG is high, calculate the delta-delta. ΔΔ = [(calculated AG – expected AG)/(normal HCO_3^- – measured HCO_3^-)], where expected AG = [albumin] × 2.5 and normal HCO_3^- = 24.
   - ΔΔ < 1 = AG metabolic acidosis + non-AG metabolic acidosis
   - ΔΔ of 1-2 = AG metabolic acidosis only
   - ΔΔ > 2 AG = metabolic acidosis + metabolic alkalosis

KEY FACT

There are only three endogenous causes of an anion gap acidosis: Lactate, ketones, and uremia. All other causes are exogenous.

METABOLIC ACIDOSIS (↓pH + ↓ HCO_3^-)

An extremely common presentation, both in the ED and on the examination. These patients are often ill- or septic-appearing on presentation.

Causes

See *Step 3: Calculate the Anion Gap.*

Symptoms/Examination

- Tachypnea is a compensatory response in any patient with a metabolic acidosis, but may be greatest (ie, Kussmaul) in DKA or salicylate poisoning.
- Look for symptoms or findings of underlying cause (eg, visual disturbance with methanol poisoning).

Diagnosis

A metabolic acidosis is present in any patient with a pH < 7.38 and HCO_3^- < 20 mEq/L. In patients with mixed disorders, the pH may be normal or elevated. Use the anion gap and the serum K^+ to help narrow the differential.

- Normal anion gap [Na^+ – (Cl^- + HCO_3^-)] ≈ 12
  - Look for chloride losses.
- Hypokalemic normal gap acidosis:
  - Renal losses: Renal tubular acidosis or carbonic anhydrase inhibitors, such as acetazolamide
  - GI losses: Diarrhea or malabsorption
- Hyperkalemic normal gap acidosis:
  - Adrenal insufficiency
  - Renal insufficiency
  - Posthypocapnia
- Increased anion gap [Na^+ – (Cl^- + HCO_3^-)] > 15 indicates presence of excess organic acids.

KEY FACT

Measure the serum osmolar gap to screen for toxic alcohol ingestion in patients with AMS and an increased anion gap. Normal osmolar gap is < 10 mOsm/L.

TABLE 7.3. Commonly Tested Acid-Base Disorders

pH	P_{CO_2}	HCO_3^-	Anion Gap	Causes
↓ or ↑	↓↓	↓	↑	Salicylates
↓	↓	↓	↑	DKA, toxic alcohol, sepsis
↓	↑↑	—	—	Narcotic OD, COPD (pure respiratory acidosis)

COPD, chronic obstructive pulmonary disease; DKA, diabetic ketoacidosis; OD, overdose.

- Causes of a high anion gap acidosis can be remembered with the MUDPILES mnemonic.
- For patients with a high anion gap without obvious identifiable cause, calculate a serum osmolar gap to screen for the presence of toxic alcohols. See the section "Fluid and Hydration" for a more detailed explanation.

TREATMENT

Treating the underlying cause is the most important action.

- Sodium bicarbonate administration is controversial and potentially dangerous because of the risk of electrolyte disturbances and paradoxical cerebral acidosis. The cerebral acidosis occurs 2° to the inability of HCO_3^- to quickly cross the blood–brain barrier. Bicarbonate for the treatment of acidosis should only be considered for extremely ill patients with severe acidosis.
- Treatments for specific underlying causes of toxin-mediated metabolic acidosis include:
  - Ethylene glycol and methanol: Ethanol or fomepizole and dialysis
  - Salicylate toxicity: Sodium bicarbonate to keep serum pH between 7.5 and 7.8 with resultant **urine alkalinization**; dialysis
  - Iron overdose: Deferoxamine
  - Isoniazid: Pyridoxine (vitamin B_6)

METABOLIC ALKALOSIS (↑ pH + ↑ HCO_3^-)

CAUSES

Increased bicarbonate usually occurs in the setting of:

- Gastric acid loss from vomiting or NG suctioning
- Diuretic use
- Adrenocortical hormone excess

DIAGNOSIS

Categorized as:

- *Chloride (saline) sensitive* (most common): Diuretic or GI losses of K^+ and Cl^- responds to replacement
- *Chloride (saline) resistant*: Mineralocorticoid excess → renal absorption of Na^+ and HCO_3^- and excretion of K^+, H^+, and Cl^- → large K^+ replacement required.

RESPIRATORY ACIDOSIS (↓ pH + ↑ HCO_3^-)

CAUSES

Primarily caused by inadequate ventilation or increased dead space. Causes include:

- Head or chest trauma
- Oversedation, obtundation, or coma
- Neuromuscular disorders
- Pickwickian syndrome (obesity-hypoventilation syndrome)
- COPD

Renal compensation occurs after 48 hours of steady state.

> **KEY FACT**
>
> Compensation, whether renal or respiratory, should never completely correct the pH by itself. Complete or overcorrection is an indicator of another process occurring.

TREATMENT

- Ventilatory support.
- O_2 may be necessary to treat hypoxia, but may worsen hypercapnia in patients with COPD or in heavily sedated patients.

RESPIRATORY ALKALOSIS (↑ pH + ↓ HCO_3^-)

CO_2 ventilation is greater than CO_2 production.

Causes

- The most common cause in ill patients is a **secondary** compensatory respiratory alkalosis in response to a metabolic acidosis (seen in sepsis, DKA).
- **Primary** causes of respiratory alkalosis include:
  - Hyperventilation secondary to anxiety
  - CNS disorder
  - Hypermetabolic states
  - Hypoxia
  - Hepatic insufficiency
  - Aspirin toxicity

Treatment

Treatment focuses on identifying and addressing the underlying cause of tachypnea.

ALCOHOLIC KETOACIDOSIS

Alcoholic ketoacidosis (AKA) is a high anion gap metabolic acidosis that occurs in alcohol-dependent patients who do not consume their usual liquid calories.

Pathophysiology

- Ethanol is normally metabolized to acetaldehyde by alcohol dehydrogenase and aldehyde dehydrogenase with NAD^+ as a coenzyme. Chronic ethanol use shifts the NAD^+/NADH ratio toward the reduced NADH.
- Concurrent illness (pancreatitis, gastritis) with nausea and vomiting → depletion of glycogen stores and suppression of insulin secretion → suppression of aerobic metabolism and stimulation of lipolysis → increased ketone (acetoacetate, β-hydroxybutyrate, acetone) production
- Due to depletion of NAD^+, β-hydroxybutyrate is the predominate ketone produced, and lactate levels are elevated (conversion of pyruvate to lactate).

Symptoms

- Nausea and vomiting
- Lethargy or altered mental status
- History of alcohol abuse but not usually intoxicated at time of evaluation

Examination

- Tachypnea, tachycardia, dehydration
- "Fruity" breath

Differential

DKA, sepsis, GI bleed, uremia, toxic ingestion (methanol, ethylene glycol salicylates)

Diagnosis

- Key findings in diagnosing alcoholic ketoacidosis (AKA):
  - A low bicarbonate level (< 18) indicating acidosis
  - The high anion gap (> 15) is primarily from β-hydroxybutyrate. **The nitroprusside (ketone) test is often *negative* or weakly positive because it tests for acetoacetate.** The test often becomes positive as the patient improves due to the presence of NAD^+ and a shift from β-hydroxybutyrate to acetoacetate
  - **A low or negative blood alcohol level**

Q

A 50-year-old homeless man is brought in altered and dehydrated with a history of chronic alcohol use. His laboratory test results are negative for alcohol or ketones, but he has an HCO_3^- of 15 with an anion gap of 22 mEq/L and a glucose of 150 mg/dL. What is his diagnosis?

KEY FACT

Be careful administering O_2 to COPD patients. Chronic hypercapnia in COPD patients lowers the CO_2 respiratory drive, leaving hypoxia as the only respiratory trigger.

KEY FACT

Nondistilled alcohol (beer, wine) contains lots of carbohydrates, which is why AKA doesn't usually occur while a patient is still intoxicated.

A

Likely AKA. Check an osmolal gap to exclude the possibility of methanol or ethylene glycol poisoning. The nitroprusside test can be negative due to redox shift of ketones. Lactate levels are often elevated due to conversion from pyruvate.

KEY FACT

If IV dextrose is administered to a chronic alcoholic prior to giving thiamine, it may precipitate acute Wernicke encephalopathy by stimulating further consumption of thiamine by the TCA cycle.

- Blood glucose levels can be low, normal or elevated.
- Concomitant hypokalemia, hyponatremia, hypomagnesemia and hypophosphatemia may be present.

Treatment

- Thiamine 50-100 mg IV prior to dextrose.
- IV hydration with D5NS: The combination of fluid and carbohydrate corrects the ketoacidosis quicker than fluid alone. Cerebral edema is not a concern.
- Insulin is not required.
- Correct electrolyte losses.
- Bicarbonate only if the patient is severely acidotic.

LACTIC ACIDOSIS

Lactate is a byproduct of anaerobic metabolism. Both acute and chronic conditions can cause elevated lactate levels. A normal lactate level is typically given as < 2 mEq/L. Levels > 4-5 mEq/L are considered significantly elevated. Typically, such patients will have an anion gap acidosis.

Acute conditions:

- **Inadequate tissue perfusion** due to either hypotension or hypoxia
- Toxic causes of disruption in cellular metabolism such as cyanide
- Exercise
- Insulin or epinephrine injections

Chronic conditions:

- Alcoholism
- Diabetes mellitus
- Liver disease
- Renal Failure
- Acquired immunodeficiency syndrome

Differential

Other causes of high anion gap acidosis must be considered

Diagnosis and Causes

History should lead to one of the four categories of lactic acidosis

- Type A: Inadequate tissue perfusion → cellular hypoxia
- Type B1: Disorders
  - Diabetes
  - Renal or hepatic failure
  - Leukemia or cancer
  - Seizures
  - Infectious etiology
- Type B2: Toxins
  - Ethanol or methanol
  - Fructose and sorbitol
  - Epinephrine
  - Metformin
- Type B3: Inborn errors of metabolism and hepatic fructose-bisphosphatase deficiency

Treatment

- Hydration as indicated
- Support oxygenation and blood pressure as needed.
- Treat infection or underlying cause.
- Sodium bicarbonate administration is controversial and should be reserved for extremely acidotic and deteriorating patients.

Glucose Disorders

Plasma glucose is the primary metabolic fuel used by the CNS and under normal circumstances is derived from the diet, hepatic gluconeogenesis, and breakdown of glycogen stores in the liver.

INSULIN PHYSIOLOGY

- Functions in glucose uptake and storage in liver as glycogen
- Increases lipogenesis and inhibits lipolysis leading to increased triglycerides

KETONES

Production is increased during states of cellular starvation with absence of available glucose resulting in lipolysis to provide free fatty acids and ketone bodies used for energy. Three types are produced:

- β-Hydroxybutyrate: Not detected by serum or urine ketone (nitroprusside) tests
- Acetoacetate
- Acetone: A ketone, but not an acid

HYPOGLYCEMIA (BLOOD SUGAR < 70 mg/dL)

One of the most common causes of altered mental status in the ED.

Causes

- Critical illness: Sepsis, liver failure
- Drugs:
  - Most commonly insulin or oral hypoglycemic (Table 7.4)

TABLE 7.4. Sulfonylureas

Drug	Common Medication Interactions	Duration of Effect
Tolbutamide	Warfarin SMX chloramphenicol rifampin digoxin	6-12 h
Glipizide	TMP/SMX miconazole ASA	12-24 h
Glyburide	TMP/SMX ciprofloxacin H_2-blockers rifampin	12-24 h
Chlorpropamide	Warfarin chloramphenicol probenicid allopurinol rifampin	4-5 d

SMX, Sulfamethoxazole; TMP, Trimethoprim.

Q

A lethargic 5-year-old boy is brought in with an empty bottle of his father's glipizide. His accucheck is 30 mg/dL, and upon administration of glucose the boy returns to baseline. When can he be discharged home?

A

This patient needs to be observed for a minimum of 24 hours with normal sugars before discharge, usually prompting admission.

- Alcohol: Inhibition of gluconeogenesis and depletion of glycogen stores
- Salicylate: Primary hypoglycemia and seizures in children
- Haloperidol
- Phenothiazines
- Monoamine oxidase (MAO) inhibitors
- Cimetidine

- Malnourishment
- Cortisol deficiency
- Nonislet cell tumor
- Endogenous hyperinsulinism: eg, islet cell tumor
- Hypoglycemia of infancy
  - Seen in 4 in 1000 births, usually with diabetic or narcotic-abuse mothers or premature or small for gestational age infants
- Disorders that cause hypoglycemia in the postprandial (vs fasting) state include endogenous hyperinsulinism, factitious disorder, and unripened ackee fruit ingestion.

SYMPTOMS

Patients usually become symptomatic < 50 mg/dL. They can present with complaints of:

- Tremors and agitation/ anxiety
- Diaphoresis
- Seizures

EXAMINATION

Patient examinations are usually consistent with their symptoms but you may also find:

- Altered mental status or focal neurologic signs (including hemiparesis)
- Tachycardia

KEY FACT

Sepsis should be considered in all patients with a low blood sugar.

DIAGNOSIS

- All patients with seizures or altered mental status should have an immediate bedside glucose measurement.
- Administering glucose to a hypoglycemic patient should quickly resolve their symptoms. If not, further investigation is required.
- If the glucose is < 55 mg/dL and the patient is not a diabetic, send glucose, insulin, and C-peptide levels (produced during insulin cleavage from endogenous proinsulin).
  - Factitious (exogenous) hypoglycemia: High insulin level, low C-peptide level
  - Insulinoma: High insulin and high-C-peptide levels

KEY FACT

Sulfonylureas (glipizide, glyburide) increase insulin release. Octreotide inhibits insulin release.

TREATMENT

- IV glucose is the mainstay of treatment.
- IV dextrose is fast and effective but not a large or long-lasting source of carbohydrate. An ampule of D_{50} provides only 25 g or 100 calories.
- IM glucagon can also be used when IV access is not available but may not be effective in elderly or alcoholic patients who do not have adequate glycogen stores.
- **Octreotide** inhibits insulin release. Consider using for recurrent hypoglycemia following sulfonylurea overdose
- As soon as the patient is able, he/she should be encouraged to eat. A complex meal consisting of protein, fat, and complex carbohydrates is preferable to simple sugars such as fruit juice or candy bars.

KEY FACT

Do not discharge patients with an overdose of a long-acting hypoglycemic agent until they have been observed beyond the duration of the drug.

HYPERGLYCEMIA

Diabetes mellitus, the most common endocrine disorder, is characterized by an absolute (type 1) or relative (type 2) insulin deficiency. It can also occur during pregnancy (gestational diabetes) and from a secondary disease process or drug. A hemoglobin A_{1C} of ≥ 6.5% confirms the diagnosis. A random glucose of ≥ 200 mg/dL also suggests the diagnosis.

Hyperglycemia occurs when enough insulin is not produced or administered to maintain a normal glucose. ED presentations range from uncomplicated hyperglycemia requiring medication adjustment or initiation (low-dose sulfonylurea or metformin) to DKA and hyperglycemic hyperosmolar states (HHS) requiring aggressive therapy.

DIABETIC KETOACIDOSIS (DKA)

DKA is the presenting illness in 15%-25% of newly diagnosed diabetics. There is a 5% mortality (often due to concurrent illness).

Pathophysiology

- Insulin insufficiency → inability of glucose to enter cells → cellular starvation despite hyperglycemia, stress hormone upregulation → increased gluconeogenesis, glycogenolysis, and lipolysis → further elevation of glucose and free fatty acid production → ketone formation (β-hydroxybutyrate predominates; also acetoacetate, acetone).
- High extracellular sugar levels create an osmotic diuresis. Patients with DKA are usually severely dehydrated, acidotic, and electrolyte depleted.

Cause

A precipitating factor usually initiates this cascade of events:

- Lack of insulin/medication noncompliance
- Infection (commonly a urinary tract infection or pneumonia)
- Acute myocardial infarction or stroke
- Trauma or surgery
- Pregnancy
- Hyperthyroidism
- Pancreatitis
- Alcohol or illicit drug use
- Steroids

Symptoms

- Patients usually present with a history of one of the precipitating factors, but may also complain of:
  - Thirst, nausea/vomiting, abdominal pain, polyuria, agitation, or altered mental status

Examination

- Dehydration
- Tachycardia
- Deep and rapid breathing (Kussmaul respirations)
- Hypotension and altered mentation if critically ill

Differential

- Hyperosmolar nonketotic coma
- Other acidosis (eg, AKA, lactic acidosis, toxic alcohols, salicylates)

MNEMONIC

Common causes of DKA:

Insulin (lack of)
Infection
Ischemia (MI, CVA)
Illicit drug use (cocaine)

KEY FACT

Hyperglycemia lowers measured serum sodium by dilution. To correctly interpret the sodium level, add 1.6 mEq/L for each 100 mg/dL of glucose above 100 mg/dL.

KEY FACT

In DKA, insulin should start late and end late. Start insulin late because you need to wait for the serum potassium. End insulin late because you need to close the anion gap (not just bring down the glucose).

Diagnosis

- The diagnosis of DKA requires the presence of **hyperglycemia** (may be mild), **ketosis,** and an **anion gap metabolic acidosis**. Serum HCO_3^- may be normal due to the presence of both an anion gap acidosis and metabolic alkalosis with concurrent vomiting and dehydration.
  - Bedside glucose will indicate level of hyperglycemia. Glucose is usually > 250 mg/dL.
  - Serum ketones (acetoacetate, β-hydroxybutyrate, and acetone). A positive nitroprusside test for ketones is consistent with DKA but only tests for acetoacetate. **β-hydroxybutyrate is not measured with the nitroprusside test** and ketone tests may therefore be normal in patients with DKA. Some centers have β-hydroxybutyrate assays.
  - Anion gap metabolic acidosis based on ABG and/or chemistry panel showing (2 of 3) pH < 7.30, serum bicarbonate < 18 mmol/L, and anion gap > 15mEq/L.
- Electrolytes, including potassium, magnesium, calcium, and phosphorus (repeat q2h)
- BUN/creatinine: Indicator of renal function and dehydration
- Chest x-ray and urinalysis (UA) to look for evidence of infection
- ECG and cardiac enzymes if appropriate for patient
- Other studies depending on clinical suspicion

Treatment

- DKA treatment encompasses a multisystem approach, including hydration, electrolyte replacement, and insulin administration under careful monitoring. The goal is to correct deficits over 24 hours to avoid cerebral edema.
- **Rehydration:**
  - Patients are usually significantly dehydrated. Most patients will benefit from an initial 2-L isotonic NS (10-20 mL/kg in peds).
  - Continue isotonic saline until hyponatremia is corrected, then consider switch to 0.45% NS.
  - Once glucose falls < 250 mg/dL, switch to a glucose solution to avoid hypoglycemia and cerebral edema.
  - In pediatric patients, **do not** exceed 40 mL/kg in the first 4 hours (higher risk of cerebral edema).
- **Potassium replacement:**
  - DKA may cause significant total body K^+ depletion that is sometimes only unmasked once the acidosis is reversed and the remaining extracellular K^+ shifts back into the cell.
  - Patients with serum K^+ < 3.5 mEq/L should receive 20-40 mEq/L in infusion fluids.
  - Patients with serum K^+ 3.5-5 mEq/L should receive 20-30 mEq/L in infusion fluids.
- **Insulin:**
  - **IV insulin drip at 0.1 units/kg/h;** titrate rate as needed
  - Large bolus doses of insulin may cause hypoglycemia and hypokalemia and has fallen out of practice.
  - **Do not** initiate insulin therapy until serum potassium is > 3.5 mEq/L as insulin promotes transport of K^+ into cells leading to fatal arrhythmias (See the section "Hypokalemia").
  - **Do note** start insulin until hydration of patient is established and at lease 500-1000 mL of fluid is given.
- Sodium bicarbonate has not been shown to be beneficial in DKA patients and carries a risk of causing paradoxical cerebrospinal fluid acidosis and worsening hypokalemia. It should be reserved for critically ill patients with a pH ≤ 6.9 and evidence of shock with impending cardiovascular collapse or life-threatening hyperkalemia.

COMPLICATIONS

- **Cerebral edema** is responsible for the majority of death with DKA in children.
  - Seen mostly in children < 5 years with severe acidosis or dehydration 6-10 hours after initiation of therapy
  - Early and frequent monitoring for headache, recurrent vomiting, and altered mental status is essential. Findings on head computed tomography (CT) occur late.
  - Treatment includes reducing rate of IVF and administering mannitol.
- Other morbidity is typically related to therapy: **Hypokalemia,** hypoglycemia, and other electrolytes disturbances.

Q

An elderly nursing home resident with a history of DM presents with altered mental status. She appears ill and dehydrated. Her bedside blood glucose is 950. What is her most likely diagnosis?

KEY FACT

The most common cause of death in children with DKA is cerebral edema, which is associated with age < 5 and severe acidosis or dehydration.

HYPEROSMOLAR HYPERGLYCEMIC STATE (HHS)

Formerly known as HHNK (hyperglycemic hyperosmolar nonketotic coma). Less common than DKA and generally a slower process, frequently occurring in the elderly diabetic patient with limited access to water. 33% have no prior history of diabetes. The degree of volume contraction is generally greater in HHS than DKA. Mortality ranges from 20% to 60% (increased if patients are comatose).

PATHOPHYSIOLOGY

Hyperglycemia and stress → increased glucagon secretion (along with catecholamines, cortisol, and growth hormone) coupled with insulin resistance/deficiency → gluconeogenesis and glycogenolysis → hyperglycemia without ketosis → elevated osmolality → diuresis and dehydration without ketoacidosis

SYMPTOMS/EXAMINATION

- Weakness, fatigue, thirst, and altered mental status are common symptoms.
- Most patients have some altered mental status but are not comatose.
- Focal neurologic signs.
- Dehydration.

DIAGNOSIS

- Extremely elevated blood glucose (> 400 mg/dL but often > 800 mg/dL)
- Negative ketones
- No acidosis on ABG

TREATMENT

- Identify and treat precipitating event.
- Treatment is similar to DKA, although patients with HHS have incredibly large water deficits averaging 8-12 L.
- **Fluid resuscitation:** Administer 2 L of NS over the first 1-2 hours, continue until patient is hemodynamically stable. Replace half the fluid deficit with NS over 12 hours, then switch to 0.45% NS.
- **Potassium replacement:** as with DKA above
- **Insulin:** Start drip at 0.1 U/kg/h once K^+ is > 3.5 mEq/L and continue until the patient's glucose reaches approximately 300 mg/dL.
- Correct hypomagnesemia and hypophosphatemia.
- Thiamine administration (malnutrition common in these patients).

COMPLICATIONS

Cerebral edema in children (see the section "Diabetic Ketoacidosis")

A

This patient has a hyperglycemic hyperosmolar state.

Pituitary Disorders

The pituitary gland is composed of two parts: the anterior pituitary (adenohypophysis) and the posterior pituitary (neurohypophysis) and is connected to the hypothalamus by the pituitary stalk (infundibulum).

The pituitary gland releases hormones based on regulatory input from the hypothalamus.

Anterior Pituitary Hormones	Posterior Pituitary Hormones
Growth hormone	ADH (vasopressin)
Prolactin	Oxytocin
Follicle-stimulating hormone and luteinizing hormone	
Thyroid-stimulating hormone (TSH)	
Adrenocorticotropic hormone (ACTH)	

HYPOPITUITARISM

Decreased production of hormones from the pituitary due to loss of stimulation from hypothalamus or a dysfunctioning pituitary gland. Destruction of 90% of the pituitary is necessary before hypopituitarism becomes apparent.

Causes

- Pituitary tumor (primary or metastatic) = most common cause.
- **Pituitary apoplexy** (pituitary hemorrhage).
- Sheehan syndrome—postpartum pituitary hypoperfusion and infarction secondary to volume depletion resulting in eventual necrosis
- Additional causes include infection, trauma, vascular event, infiltrative disease, radiation, or surgery.

Symptoms/Examination

The clinical picture depends on the underlying cause and which pituitary hormones have been affected but may include signs and symptoms of:

- Headache, AMS, meningismus
- Visual field deficits, CN palsy
- Signs and symptoms of:
  - Hypothyroidism
  - Hypogonadism
  - Adrenal insufficiency
  - Failure to lactate postpartum
  - Diabetes insipidus

KEY FACT

Always give steroids to patients with suspected hypopituitarism before you administer levothyroxine to prevent precipitation of an adrenal crisis because thyroid hormone will increase metabolism of cortisol.

Diagnosis

- Magnetic resonance imaging (MRI)
- Multiple coinciding hormone deficiencies: Measure TSH, free T4, cortisol, prolactin, testosterone/follicle-stimulating hormone (men), estradiol/luteinizing hormone (women), and insulin-like growth factor 1.
- Endocrine referral

TREATMENT

- Supportive care
- Glucocorticoid replacement (dexamethasone or hydrocortisone); must occur prior to thyroid hormone replacement to prevent worsening cortisol deficiency
- Thyroid hormone replacement (levothyroxine)

PITUITARY ADENOMAS

Pituitary adenomas are uncommon benign neoplasms of the **anterior** pituitary. They are characterized by size (microadenoma < 1 cm, macroadenoma > 1 cm) and the type of pituitary hormone secreted.

SYMPTOMS/EXAMINATION

Patients can present with symptoms related to mass effect, apoplexy (hemorrhage), and/or secreted hormone excess *or* deficiency.

- Headache, AMS, meningismus
- Visual field deficits, classically **bitemporal hemianopsia** from mass effect on optic chiasm; diplopia can occur.
- CSF rhinorrhea
- Gigantism (peds) or acromegaly (adults) with growth hormone excess; short stature (peds) or decreased lean body mass/increased fat mass (adults) with deficiency
- Hypogonadism with gonadotropin deficiency; symptoms from excess are uncommon
- Hyperthyroidism if excessive TSH; hypothyroidism if deficiency
- Galactorrhea if excess prolactin; failure of lactation with deficiency
- Cushing syndrome if excessive ACTH; adrenal insufficiency with deficiency

DIFFERENTIAL

Other causes of suprasellar mass includes pituitary hyperplasia, other benign tumors (eg, meningioma), malignant tumors (eg, lymphoma), metastatic disease, cysts, abscess, AV malformation.

DIAGNOSIS

- Neuroimaging (MRI)
- Hormone levels upon consultation with endocrinology

TREATMENT

- Supportive therapies as indicated
- Hormone replacement or suppression in consultation with endocrinology
- Definitive treatment with radiation or surgery

Parathyroid Disorders

The parathyroid glands produces parathyroid hormone which functions in calcium homeostasis and acts on:

- Kidneys to increase renal calcium resorption and phosphate excretion and to facilitate conversion of vitamin D to its more active metabolite in the renal tubules
- Bone to activate osteoclasts to digest bone and increase osteoclast production
- GI system to increase calcium absorption

HYPOPARATHYROIDISM

A state of parathyroid hormone deficiency

Causes

- Iatrogenic—accidental excision (often during thyroid surgery)
- Congenital—DiGeorge syndrome
- Pseudohypoparathyroidism—kidney unresponsiveness to PTH, autosomal recessive inheritance associated with short stature and shortened fourth/fifth digits

Symptoms/Examination

Similar to hypocalcemia

Diagnosis

Low serum calcium, low PTH (may be high in pseudohypoparathyroidism)

Treatment

- Calcium repletion
  - IV calcium for severe symptoms
  - PO calcium if stable

HYPERPARATHYROIDISM

A state of parathyroid hormone excess.

Causes

- Primary hyperparathyroidism:
  - 81% parathyroid adenomas (usually in inferior glands)
  - 18% parathyroid hyperplasia
  - < 1% parathyroid carcinoma
- Secondary hyperparathyroidism:
  - Hyperplasia of parathyroid glands in response to chronic renal disease causing decreased production of vitamin D
  - Elevated PTH levels

Symptoms/Examination

- Similar to hypercalcemia
- Rarely palpable parathyroid nodules

Diagnosis

- Elevated calcium—extremely high calcium levels should raise suspicion of parathyroid carcinoma
- Elevated PTH levels with secondary hyperparathyroidism
- Check other electrolytes (especially potassium).
- Imaging as indicated

Treatment

- Hydrate with 0.9% NS.
- Furosemide 40 mg IV to increase calcium excretion
- Calcitonin or bisphosphonates to block bone resorption
- Electrolyte repletion as indicated
- Refer to appropriate specialist.

Thyroid Disorders

Thyroid hormones (T_3 and T_4) stimulate cellular protein production triggering increases in bone growth, CNS activity, basal metabolic rate, oxygen consumption, respiratory and heart rate.

Physiology

Thyrotropin-releasing hormone (TRH) is produced by the hypothalamus and regulates anterior pituitary production of thyroid-stimulating hormone (TSH). TSH in turn activates the production and release of iodine-containing T_3 and T_4 by the thyroid. Once released, T_4 is converted to T_3 (which is more biologically active) in peripheral tissues. The hormones feedback to the hypothalamus to decrease TRH production. Measurements of TSH and free T_4 can indicate the type of underlying disorder (see Table 7.5).

HYPOTHYROIDISM AND MYXEDEMA COMA

Hypothyroidism is a state of insufficient production of thyroid hormones by the thyroid gland. It is more common in women than men. Iodine deficiency is the most common cause worldwide, but Hashimoto thyroiditis (a chronic autoimmune condition) is the predominate cause in developed countries. Myxedema coma is a severe form of hypothyroidism that has a high mortality rate.

Causes

- Primary hypothyroidism
  - Hashimoto thyroiditis (most common in the United States)
  - Iodine deficiency (most common worldwide)
  - Treatment of hyperthyroidism
  - Medications: Lithium, amiodarone
  - Radiation therapy or thyroidectomy
  - Less common: Congenital, pituitary failure, pregnancy, infiltrative disorders
- Secondary and tertiary hypothyroidism due to TSH or TRH deficiency, respectively
  - Pituitary tumors
  - Sheehan syndrome: Postpartum hemorrhage of pituitary gland
  - Hypothalamic damage or dysfunction

TABLE 7.5. TSH and Thyroid Hormone Levels

TSH Level	Free T_4 Level	Disorder
Normal	Normal	None
Low	Low	2° hypothyroidism
Low	High	Thyrotoxicosis
High	Low	1° hypothyroidism
High	High	TSH-mediated hyperthyroidism

Q

A 75-year-old woman presents to the ED with the chief complaint of anorexia, weakness, and weight loss. On examination, she has sleepy-looking eyes, rales on lung exam, and atrial fibrillation (AFib) on the cardiac monitor. Her TSH is markedly decreased. What is the most appropriate treatment for her Afib?

KEY FACT

Lithium causes hypothyroidism by Inhibiting T_3 and T_4 formation and release.

A

This patient has apathetic hyperthyroidism, which is common in the elderly. The Afib should be treated with B-blocker therapy.

Symptoms

- Fatigue, lethargy, depression, weight gain, cold intolerance
- Menstrual irregularity, constipation
- Coarse hair, dry skin
- Hoarseness, dyspnea, peripheral edema

Examination

- Mild disease can be hard to detect on examination.
- Goiter is common in Hashimoto thyroiditis and iodine deficiency.
- **Myxedema coma** is characterized by **hypothermia and altered mental status.**
- Other findings that may be present, depending on severity of disease:
  - Bradycardia, hypertension
  - Respiratory failure (decreased respiratory rate, CO_2 narcosis)
  - Edema, loss of eyebrows, enlargement of tongue
  - Woltman sign (brisk DTRs but delayed relaxation)
  - Low voltage on ECG 2° to pericardial effusion
  - Hypoglycemia and hyponatremia

Diagnosis

- Primary hypothyroidism: Elevated TSH with a low free T_4
- Secondary/tertiary hypothyroidism is harder to diagnosis, but free T_4 levels are typically low.

Treatment

- **Thyroid hormone:**
  - Myxedema coma, administer 300-500 μg IV thyroxine
  - If uncomplicated hypothyroidism, PO levothyroxine, start 50 μg daily
- Supportive care and rewarming
- Correct electrolytes, blood glucose.
- Identify and treat inciting event (antibiotics if underlying infection).
- Administer **hydrocortisone** empirically for possible coexisting adrenal insufficiency (send cortisol level).

HYPERTHYROIDISM AND THYROID STORM

Hyperthyroidism is a state of overproduction of thyroid hormones, leading to an increase in metabolic drive. Hyperthyroidism most commonly presents in patients with Graves disease (80%) due to the production of an IgG antibody that mimics TSH. Thyroid storm is the severe form of hyperthyroidism that has a nearly 100% mortality due to severe CNS dysfunction or cardiovascular collapse if left untreated.

KEY FACT

Precipitants of thyroid storm

Infection
DKA or hypoglycemia
Iodine load
CVA
Acute coronary syndrome (ACS)
Pulmonary embolism
Trauma
Surgery
Emotional stress

Causes

- Graves disease
- Thyroid nodule (single/adenoma or multinodular): Autonomously functioning thyroid nodule(s)
- Thyroiditis
  - Hashimoto thyroiditis: **Painless**, hyperthyroid early in the course of disease (then hypothyroid)
  - Subacute (de Quervain) thyroiditis: **Painful**, self-limited, often follows viral illness
  - Postpartum thyroiditis: **Painless**, 1-6 months post delivery, typically self-limited
  - Drug-induced: Amiodarone

- Pituitary adenoma
- Thyroid cancer: Can present with hyperthyroidism (sometimes hypothyroidism).
  - Papillary, follicular, medullary, anaplastic (in order of increasing mortality and decreasing prevalence)
  - Palpable nodule may be present

SYMPTOMS

- Symptoms and examination depend on severity of disease.
- Weight loss, heat intolerance, sweating
- Thinning of hair
- Anxiety, agitation, psychosis
- Palpitations, shortness of breath
- Increased frequency of bowel movements
- **Apathetic hyperthyroidism** seen in elderly patients: Lethargy, weakness, weight loss, blepharoptosis (eye drooping), and atrial fibrillation with CHF

EXAMINATION

- Goiter
- Lid lag (sclera seen above iris when looking down) and lid retraction
- Exophthalmos (Graves only)
- Hyperdynamic precordium with tachycardia and hypertension, possibly AFib
- Proximal muscle weakness
- **Thyroid storm** is the severe form of hyperthyroidism characterized by varying degrees of:
  - **Hyperthermia**
  - **Tachycardia**
  - **Heart failure**
  - **CNS effects** (agitation, delirium, seizures, coma)
  - **GI-hepatic dysfunction** (abdominal pain, nausea\vomiting\diarrhea, jaundice)

DIAGNOSIS

- Hyperthyroidism: Decreased TSH with elevated free T_4.
- Thyroid storm: Based on clinical findings. The Burch-Wartofky scoring system that rates the 5 findings listed above is fairly sensitive (but not specific) in identifying thyroid storm.

TREATMENT

- Treat underlying cause.
- Supportive care, cooling, hydration, electrolyte replacement.
  - **Avoid** aspirin because it displaces thyroid hormone from thyroglobulin, increasing the availability of active hormone.
- **β-Blockers** to decrease hyperadrenergic state. Propranolol is preferred because it also decreases T_4 to T_3 peripheral conversion. Consider esmolol in patients with CHF.
- **Propylthiouracil** to inhibit stored thyroid hormone release; preferred over methimazole 2° to conversion inhibition and rapid onset
- **Inorganic iodine** to inhibit stored thyroid hormone release
- **Dexamethasone *or* hydrocortisone** to decrease T_4 to T_3 peripheral conversion and treat relative adrenal insufficiency
- Pharmacotherapy and disposition depends on degree of illness:
  - Mild symptoms: Oral β-blocker therapy alone with outpatient follow up and for endocrine referral

KEY FACT

Thyroid Storm
Hyperthermia
Tachycardia
Heart failure
CNS effects
GI-hepatic dysfunction

KEY FACT

Levothyroxine is a synthetic T_4. Levothyroxine overdose is usually asymptomatic because the breakdown of T_4 occurs more rapidly than the conversion to T_3.

KEY FACT

Do not give iodine contrast to a thyrotoxic patient; it can cause increased thyroid hormone synthesis.

MNEMONIC

Thyroid Storm Treatment:

***P**roptotic **P**olly **(W**ait**) I**s **D**ying*

Propranolol
Propylthiouracil (PTU)
Wait 1 hour
Iodine
Dexamethasone

- Moderate symptoms: β-Blocker therapy, supportive care, treat CHF, admit, endocrine consult
- Thyroid storm: All of the above therapy, admit ICU, endocrine consult
- Definitive treatment is radioactive therapy or thyroidectomy.

KEY FACT

Always administer PTU at least 1 hour before iodine to prevent increased thyroid hormone synthesis.

Adrenal Insufficiency and Crisis

The adrenal glands are paired organs that sit in the retroperitoneum superior to each kidney. They are made up of an outer cortex and inner medulla. The cortex secretes aldosterone while the medulla secretes cortisol, catecholamines, and androgens or sex steroids.

Physiology

- Cortisol production: Corticotropin-releasing factor from hypothalamus → pituitary secretion of ACTH → adrenal cortex secretion of cortisol. Regulates carbohydrate, protein, and lipid metabolism.
- Aldosterone is the major mineralocorticoid and is controlled by the renin-angiotensin system and K^+ concentrations. Regulates fluid and electrolyte balance.
- Epinephrine and norepinephrine are released from the medulla in response to sympathetic stimulation by the CNS.

ADRENAL INSUFFICIENCY

Primary adrenal insufficiency (**Addison disease**) is a failure of the adrenal gland to produce cortisol, aldosterone, or both due to destruction of the gland itself. Secondary adrenal insufficiency results from pituitary or hypothalamic dysfunction and lack of ACTH secretion. Only cortisol levels are affected in secondary adrenal insufficiency.

Causes

- Primary adrenal insufficiency
  - **Autoimmune** (70%): Associated with DM, Hashimoto disease, and Graves disease
  - Infectious/infiltrative: Tuberculosis (TB), fungal, acquired immune deficiency syndrome (AIDS), sarcoid, malignancy
  - Drugs: Methadone, rifampin, and ketoconazole
  - Adrenal apoplexy (bilateral adrenal hemorrhage), associated with anticoagulation
  - **Waterhouse-Friderichsen syndrome,** bilateral adrenal hemorrhage due to infection (often meningococcus)
- Secondary adrenal insufficiency
  - **Suppression after prolonged steroid use,** etomidate, fluconazole
  - Pituitary tumors or infarction (eg, Sheehan syndrome)
  - Basilar skull fracture
  - Infiltrative disease (eg, sarcoidosis)
  - Infection
  - Internal carotid artery aneurysm

Symptoms

- Weakness, malaise, lassitude
- Depression, impaired memory
- Nausea, anorexia, and weight loss
- Orthostasis

EXAMINATION

- **Brownish hyperpigmentation of the skin,** particularly on pressure points and hand creases. Seen with 1° adrenal insufficiency (due to elevation of ACTH and related peptides) but not with 2° adrenal insufficiency.
- Hypotension or orthostatic hypotension
- Hypoglycemia
- Electrolyte abnormalities: ↓Na^+, ↑K^+ (1° adrenal insufficiency)

DIAGNOSIS/TREATMENT

- Low AM cortisol and poor response to stimulation test establishes diagnosis of adrenal insufficiency; high ACTH confirms a primary process
- Glucocorticoid replacement: Hydrocortisone PO
- Mineralocorticoid replacement (1° disease): Fludrocortisone acetate PO

ACUTE ADRENAL CRISIS

Acute adrenal crisis presents with more extreme findings of adrenal insufficiency in the setting of an acute physiologic stress, pituitary apoplexy, or acute withdrawal of chronic steroids. This life-threatening crisis is more commonly seen with primary adrenal insufficiency due to the combined lack of cortisol and aldosterone.

DIAGNOSIS

- Patients are usually altered and near cardiovascular collapse.
- Refractory hypotension and hypoglycemia are common.
- Hyponatremia and hyperkalemia (with primary adrenal insufficiency)
- A single cortisol level < 15 mcg/dL or an abnormal ACTH stimulation test with associated clinical findings suggests the diagnosis. **Do not** delay treatment while tests are performed.

TREATMENT

- IV fluid resuscitation and glucose as indicated; treat hyperkalemia > 6 mEq/L with standard therapy.
- Hydrocortisone 100 mg IV will provide both glucocorticoid and mineralocorticoid replacement and is preferred in the setting of adrenal crisis with hyperkalemia for this reason.
- Dexamethasone 4-6 mg IV does not interfere with the ACTH stimulation diagnostic test and is therefore preferred, when possible, in patients **without** a known diagnosis of adrenal insufficiency and $K^+ < 6$ mEq/L
- Identify and treat the underlying condition.

CUSHING SYNDROME

Cushing syndrome is a state of hypercortisolism resulting in **symptomatic glucocorticoid** excess. It may predispose to disseminated infections. Fevers and other signs of systemic infection may be masked.

CAUSES

- Exogenous steroid administration (iatrogenic disease) = most common cause
- Adrenal tumors—50% become malignant
- Cushing disease: Excessive ACTH secretion from pituitary tumor or hyperplasia
- Ectopic ACTH producing tumor (small cell lung cancer, pancreatic cancer)

Q

An elderly patient presents with pneumonia and sepsis. After treatment with antibiotics and fluid, the patient remains hypotensive. Laboratory test results reveal a blood glucose of 50 and a sodium of 124. Her potassium is 4.5 mEq/L. What other diagnosis might this patient have and how do you treat it?

KEY FACT

Patients with adrenal insufficiency will need 2-3 times their daily glucocorticoid replacement in setting of physiology stress.

KEY FACT

Hydrocortisone interferes with the cosyntropin stimulation test, but dexamethasone does not.

KEY FACT

Dexamethasone has no mineralocorticoid effect.

A

Adrenal insufficiency. Give dexamethasone and check a serum cortisol level. An ACTH stimulation test is definitive, but should not delay initiation of treatment.

SIGNS AND SYMPTOMS

- Truncal obesity, "buffalo hump," moon facies, striae
- Proximal muscle weakness
- Osteoporosis
- Hypertension

DIAGNOSIS

- Salivary cortisol along with low-dose dexamethasone suppression testing
- Usually can be done as outpatient

TREATMENT

- Depends of cause of excess
- Gradual withdrawal and taper of exogenous steroids.
- Surgical removal for ACTH-producing tumors. Drugs that target the corticotroph tumor or antagonize glucocorticoids can be used in patients who are not surgical candidates.

PHEOCHROMOCYTOMA

KEY FACT

The 10% rule of pheochromocytomas:

10% bilateral
10% extra-adrenal
10% malignant
10% calcify
10% kids
10% familial

Pheochromocytoma is a chromaffin cell tumor of the adrenal glands that results in paroxysmal release of catecholamines. It is difficult to diagnose (75% are identified postmortem) and is associated with multiple endocrine neoplasia (MEN) Types II and III. It most commonly occurs in the fourth to fifth decade.

SIGNS AND SYMPTOMS

- Episodic headache, sweating, and tachycardia are the classic triad, but all 3 are reported in a minority of patients.
- Weight loss.

DIFFERENTIAL

- Consider other causes of hypertension/hypertensive crisis (< 1% of hypertensive patients are found to have a pheochromocytoma).
- Catecholamine-secreting paragangliomas ("extra-adrenal pheochromocytomas") have similar clinical effects, but are not associated with MEN.

DIAGNOSIS

- Evaluate for end-organ damage (ECG, creatinine).
- 24-hour urine collection to demonstrate elevated catecholamine levels.
- Plasma metanephrine level: Less well studied, but has reports of high sensitivity

TREATMENT

- Lower blood pressure in controlled manner.
- Combined α- and β-adrenergic blockade:
  - α-Blockade with phentolamine: 1- to 4-mg bolus followed by continuous infusion
  - β-Blockers **after** α-blockade (to avoid unopposed α-stimulation and further elevation in BP)
- Tumor resection is definitive treatment.

Nutritional Disorders

Vitamins are organic substances needed to sustain normal metabolic functions.

- Fat-soluble vitamins include vitamins A, D, E, and K. These vitamins typically regulate specific metabolic activities. Vitamin K therapy is discussed further in chapter 9, Hematology and Oncology.
- Water soluble vitamins include the B vitamins, vitamin C, biotin, and folic acid. These vitamins generally provide a coenzyme function in the body.

VITAMIN DEFICIENCY AND EXCESS

- Deficiencies are less common in the developed world due to largely adequate nutrition. Patients at risk include those with various malabsorption syndromes.
- Excess: 23% of Americans regularly use vitamin supplements, which leads to a large number of acute poisonings. 92% are unintentional and 79% involve children < 6 years. Most adverse reactions are related to the overdose of multivitamins containing iron, discussed in more depth in chapter 6, Toxicology.

Vitamin A

Vitamin A is a subclass of retinoic acid. Two main types are found in diet: Preformed retinols (from animal products) and provitamin A (β-carotenes from fruits and vegetables). It plays a major role in vision. It also facilitates bone growth and the maintenance of healthy skin, mucous membranes, and immune system. Deficiency is rare in the United States but may occur in patients with fat malabsorption, cystic fibrosis, inflammatory bowel disease, chronic alcoholism, impoverishment, or in recent refugees from developing countries.

SYMPTOMS/EXAMINATION

- Deficiency: Includes abnormal night vision, dry skin and hair, broken fingernails, poor bone growth, and decreased resistance to infection.
- Toxicity:
  - Acute toxicity is typically due to excessive vitamin supplementation or accidental ingestions by children. Symptoms include nausea/vomiting, vertigo, and blurry vision.
  - Chronic ingestion of higher-than-recommended doses can lead to hepatotoxicity and cirrhosis, but common symptoms include dry skin, hair loss, fatigue, irritability, and nausea.
  - Vitamin A in excess is teratogenic in the first trimester.

DIAGNOSIS

- Vitamin A levels to confirm
- Calcium levels and liver function panel recommend in suspected toxicity

TREATMENT

- For deficiency, encourage vitamin A rich foods and supplement as indicated.
- For toxicity, supportive treatment, IV hydration, treat associated electrolyte abnormalities. Rarely in acute ingestion will GI decontamination be recommended.

KEY FACT

Vitamin D deficiency has been implicated in predisposition to infections, immune disorders, cardiovascular disease and worse prognosis in sepsis.

Vitamin D

Vitamin D has a structure similar to steroids and is formed from 7-dehydroxycholesterol through several steps to 1,25-hydroxycholecalciferol, a more potent metabolite. In this form, vitamin D regulates calcium and phosphorus absorption from the gut and resorption from bone. Acute toxicity is rare. Deficiency (often found in elderly and hospitalized patients) can be due to inadequate sunlight exposure, malabsorption, or medication effects.

Symptoms/Examination

- Deficiency in children manifests as **rickets** which presents as bowing of the legs.
- Deficiency in adults manifests as **osteomalacia**.
- In acute overdose, symptomatology correlates with hypercalcemia.
- Chronic overuse can also exhibit hypercalcemia and may have osteoporosis from increased bone resorption.

Diagnosis

- Serum levels of vitamin D
- PTH levels
- Calcium levels and liver function panel recommended in suspected toxicity

Treatment

- Treat underlying cause.
- Vitamin D supplementation for deficiency.

Vitamin B_1 (Thiamine)

Vitamin B_1 (thiamine) functions in the body as a cofactor for enzymes in carbohydrate metabolism. Thiamine is not toxic in patients with normal renal function, even in high concentrations. Patients at risk for deficiency include chronic alcoholics, those on fad diets, or peritoneal dialysis. Deficiency results in **beriberi**.

Symptoms/Examination

- Dry beriberi: Symmetric motor and sensory peripheral neuropathy and Wernicke encephalopathy (see also Chapter 16, Psychobehavioral Disorders)
- Wet beriberi: Dry beriberi plus cardiovascular manifestations culminating in high-output heart failure, tachycardia, and peripheral edema.

Diagnosis/Treatment

- Blood thiamine concentrations are diagnostic.
- Treat with thiamine replacement, but use with caution if heart failure is present, may precipitate low-output heart failure.

KEY FACT

Niacin flushing can occur at even low doses in some patients

Vitamin B_3 (Niacin)

Vitamin B_3 (niacin) is found in the body as the functional component of NAD^+ and $NADP^+$, which are important cofactors in cellular respiration. It is also used as a medication to treat hyperlipidemia, and has the known side effect of **flushing reaction** caused by direct vasodilation of small blood vessels and histamine release. Deficiency, which is caused by a diet lacking in plant and animal foods (mostly developing countries) results in **pellagra**.

Symptoms/Examination

- Pellagra: Photosensitivity dermatitis, diarrhea, dementia are classic; glossitis and neuropsychiatric problems are also common

Diagnosis/Treatment

- Testing levels of urinary metabolites can aid diagnosis.
- Balanced diet and supplementation as needed are treatments of choice.

MNEMONIC

The 3 Ds of pellagra:

Dermatitis
Diarrhea
Dementia

Vitamin B_6 (Pyridoxine)

Vitamin B_6 (pyridoxine) is a necessary coenzyme for biotransformations of amino acids and is the **treatment for isoniazid toxicity,** covered in chapter 6, Toxicology. Malnutrition and peritoneal dialysis may predispose to deficiency.

Symptoms/Examination

Symptoms of deficiency include stomatitis, glossitis, cheilosis along with depression, irritability, and confusion.

Diagnosis/Treatment

- Plasma levels are diagnostic.
- Balanced diet and supplementation as needed are treatments of choice.

Vitamin B_{12} (Cyanocobalamin)

Vitamin B_{12} (cyanocobalamin) plays an active role in DNA synthesis of cells undergoing rapid turnover (such as red blood cells [RBCs]). Folate has a similar role. Deficiency of either results in megaloblastic anemia. B_{12} deficiency is also associated with neuropathy. The most common cause of deficiency is a **lack of gastric intrinsic factor** (necessary for absorption of B_{12}) resulting in **pernicious anemia**. This is seen in the setting of chronic atrophic gastritis or gastrectomy. Malabsorption of B_{12} is another cause seen in the setting of chronic alcohol abuse, *Helicobacter pylori* infection, long-term antacid use, gastric atrophy, gastric surgery, and pancreatic exocrine failure.

Symptoms/Examination

- Patients typically present with symptoms of anemia along with easy bruising or bleeding and peripheral neuropathy with ataxia.
- Other symptoms include cognitive difficulties and hallucinations.

KEY FACT

Pernicious anemia = lack of intrinsic factor causing B_{12} deficiency and megaloblastic anemia.

Diagnosis/Treatment

- Suspected by finding a macrocytic anemia.
- Serum levels of Vitamin B_{12} confirms diagnosis. Folate levels should also be checked as folate has similar function in RBCs.
- Treatment consists of cobalamin injections until the cause of deficiency can be eliminated. High-dose oral supplementation can work in some patients.

Vitamin C (Ascorbic Acid)

Vitamin C (ascorbic acid) is involved in a number of reactions responsible for the growth and repair of tissues. It is a strong antioxidant. It also enhances absorption of iron from the intestine. It is obtained from consumption of fresh fruits and vegetables. Deficiency occurs in the severely malnourished or those existing on diets devoid of fruits and vegetables. The end result is **scurvy.** Excess with toxicity is often due to over-supplementation and fad diets.

Symptoms/Examination

- Toxicity may result in nausea, diarrhea, abdominal cramps. Large overdoses with IV ascorbic acid may result in renal oxalate crystal formation that can lead to renal failure.
- **Scurvy** manifests as bruising, bleeding gums, petechiae, poor wound healing, fatigue, and muscle and joint pain.

DIAGNOSIS

- Serum levels of vitamin C
- UA and creatinine levels

TREATMENT

- Treat underlying cause.
- Vitamin C supplementation and diet rich in fresh fruits and vegetables for deficiency.

Folate

As with vitamin B_{12} (cyanocobalamin) folate plays an active role in DNA synthesis of cells undergoing rapid turnover (such as RBCs). Deficiency results in megaloblastic anemia. Causes include malnutrition, alcoholism, drugs that interfere with folate metabolism (methotrexate, phenytoin), and increased folate requirements (pregnancy, hemolytic anemia, exfoliative skin conditions). It is found in leafy vegetables and fortified flour.

SYMPTOMS/EXAMINATION

- Patients typically present with symptoms of anemia along with easy bruising or bleeding.
- Other symptoms include cognitive difficulties and hallucinations.

DIAGNOSIS/TREATMENT

- Suspected by finding a macrocytic anemia.
- Serum levels of folate confirm diagnosis. Vitamin B_{12} levels should also be checked as B_{12} has similar function in RBCs.
- Treatment is with oral folate supplementation.

REVIEW QUESTIONS

QUESTIONS

1. A 29-year-old man with a history of alcohol dependence and depression is brought in by family for altered mental status. The family is concerned that he may have ingested antifreeze about 12 hours ago in an attempt to kill himself as he has done this in the past. The patient has a temperature of 37.4°C (99°F), HR 85 bpm, BP 130/88 mm Hg, RR 16 breaths/min with an oxygen saturation of 98% on room air. He is somnolent but arousable to voice and oriented to person only with slurred speech. Laboratory test results show Na^+ 135 mEq/L, K^+ 4.5 mEq/L, Cl^- 105 mEq/L, CO_2 18 mEq/L, BUN 10 mg/dL, Cr 0.9 mg/dL, blood glucose 180 mg/dL. Serum Osm are 369 mOsm/kg with a serum ethyl alcohol (EtOH) of 395 mg/dL and a venous blood gas pH of 7.40. You send a toxic alcohols panel and consult your local toxicologist. You tell your consultant that the patient has a(n):
   A. AG metabolic acidosis and osmolal gap of 89, which is explained by his EtOH intoxication
   B. Non-AG metabolic acidosis and osmolal gap of 69, which is not explained by his EtOH intoxication
   C. No evidence of a metabolic acidosis and an osmolal gap of 86, which is explained by his EtOH intoxication
   D. No evidence of a metabolic acidosis and an osmolal gap of 69, which is not explained by his metabolic acidosis.

2. A 68-year-old woman with a history of small cell lung cancer is brought in by ambulance from her care facility for altered mental status and concern for seizure activity. The patient is unresponsive on arrival with a temperature of 37.3°C, HR 98 bpm, BP 134/78 mm Hg, RR 14 breaths/min, O_2 saturation is 95% on her baseline 3 L home O_2. You order a bedside glucose which is 90. Her laboratory test results return with a Na^+ 108 mEq/L, K^+ 4.5 mEq/L, Cl^- 100 mEq/L, CO_2 22 mEq/L, BUN 10 mg/dL, Cr 0.9 mg/dL. You order:
   A. 100-mL hypertonic 3% saline
   B. 100-g mannitol
   C. 1000-mL normal saline
   D. 1000-mg levetiracetam

3. A 65-year-old man with end-stage renal disease on dialysis presents with shortness of breath and chest pain. Initial electrocardiogram (ECG) shows flat P waves and QRS widening, and a bedside potassium is 7.4. You order calcium to stabilize the cardiomyocyte membranes. You also order insulin and glucose to:
   A. Decrease the total body stores of potassium
   B. Further stabilize the cardiac membrane
   C. Optimize glycemic control prior to dialysis
   D. Redistribute the potassium intracellularly

4. A 39-year-old woman with a history of Graves disease presents with fever, cough, and shortness of breath for 4 days with increased confusion and lethargy as well as vomiting today per family. On arrival, temperature of 40.2°C, HR 171 bpm, BP 110/74 mm Hg, O_2 sat 95% RA. Laboratory test results return and are significant for a decreased TSH and elevated free T_4. The correct order for the treatment of her condition is:
   A. Propranolol, propylthiouracil (PTU), iodine, steroids
   B. Steroids, propranolol, iodine, PTU
   C. Propranolol, steroids, iodine, PTU
   D. Propranolol, steroids, iodine, PTU

5. A 58-year-old man with alcohol dependence presents with confusion, abdominal pain and diarrhea. On examination, he has an erythematous, blistering rash on his forearms and on the back of his neck over areas that are not covered by his shirt. In addition to thiamine, he is likely deficient in which other vitamin:
   A. Vitamin A
   B. Vitamin B_1 (thiamine)
   C. Vitamin B_3 (niacin)
   D. Vitamin B_6 (pyridoxine)

6. A 71-year-old female with history of hypertension and coronary artery disease is brought in by EMS with altered mental status after being found by her neighbor on a welfare check. Blood glucose was 50 mg/dL and IV D50 was given. On arrival, temperature 34°C (93°F), HR 50 bpm, BP 150/90 mm Hg. She is confused and agitated with puffy eyelids and bilateral lower extremity pitting edema. She has no focal neurologic deficits, but slow reflexes throughout. Her repeat blood glucose is 150 mg/dL. Lab tests return and are significant for an elevated TSH and low free T_4 and low normal cortisol. What is the most appropriate next treatment?
   A. Hydrocortisone 100 mg IV
   B. Thyroxine (T_4) 400 ug IV plus hydrocortisone 100 mg IV
   C. Active core rewarming
   D. Glucose infusion and broad-spectrum antibiotics

ANSWERS

1. **C.** The patient has a decreased bicarbonate consistent with a metabolic acidosis. His AG [Na^+ – (Cl^- + HCO_3^-)] is 12 indicated that he has a non-anion gap acidosis. His calculated osmolality [2(Na^+) + Glucose/18 + BUN/2.6] is 284 leaving an osmolal gap of 85, which is equal to the contribution of alcohol to the gap (EtOH/4.6 = 86).

2. **A.** This patient has symptomatic severe hypernatremia and should be treated with hypertonic 3% saline, initial 100-mL bolus over 10 minutes, repeated until these severe symptoms resolve. The goal is an increase in serum sodium by 4-6mEq/L.

3. **D.** Medications used in the treatment of hyperkalemia have different actions. Medications that shift potassium intracellularly include bicarbonate, nebulized albuterol, and insulin. Kayexalate and furosemide decrease the total body stores of potassium.

4. **A.** The order of medications for thyroid storm treatment can be remembered by using the mnemonic "**P**roptotic **P**olly (**W**ait) is **D**ying": **P**ropranolol, **P**ropylthiouracil, **W**ait 1 hour, **I**odine, **D**examethasone. Propranolol is used first to treat the hyperadrenergic state, followed by PTU to inhibit thyroid hormone synthesis. The administration of iodine is delayed until hormone synthesis is fully blocked, as iodine increased thyroid hormone synthesis, at which time it will inhibit release of stored hormone. Dexamethasone is used empirically to treat relative adrenal insufficiency. It also decreases T_4 to T_3 peripheral conversion.

5. **C.** Niacin deficiency results in pellagra which is characterized by the 3 Ds: dermatitis, diarrhea, and dementia.

6. **B.** This patient has myxedema coma, which caries a high mortality rate. She should be treated with thyroid hormone replacement along with hydrocortisone, which treats possible coexisting adrenal insufficiency. Broad-spectrum antibiotic therapy is also reasonable along with close glucose monitoring. Glucose infusion is not necessary unless there are repeat episodes of hypoglycemia.

CHAPTER 8

Infectious Disease

Joseph Hemerka, MD and Christopher Davis, MD, DTMH

Sepsis

Sepsis is a systemic disorder characterized by an inflammatory and immune-mediated response to infection. Aggressive and early fluid resuscitation, early antibiotic therapy, and source control are the cornerstones of sepsis management. See also Chapter 1, Resuscitation.

Selected Bacteria

> **KEY FACT**
>
> **MRSA**
> Gram + cocci
> *mecA* gene: β-Lactam resistance
> PVL toxin gene: Necrotizing cytokines

METHICILLIN-RESISTANT *STAPHYLOCOCCUS AUREUS*

Methicillin-resistant *Staphylococcus aureus* (MRSA) was first recognized in the early 1960s shortly after the introduction of semisynthetic penicillins, such as methicillin. The *mec*A gene confers resistance to all β-lactam antibiotics such as methicillin, dicloxacillin, and many cephalosporins. MRSA infections are classified as either health care–associated MRSA (HA-MRSA) or community-associated MRSA (CA-MRSA). CA-MRSA strains have an additional Panton-Valentine leukocidin (PVL) toxin gene that allows production of necrotizing cytokines, increasing its invasiveness and virulence.

- HA-MRSA:
  - Hospital prevalence rates are as high as 60%.
  - Most common mode of transmission is patient-to-patient spread by health care workers with contaminated hands/gloves.
  - Risks for HA-MRSA include hospitalization, indwelling catheter, recent antibiotic therapy, and residence in a long-term care facility.
- CA-MRSA:
  - Occurs primarily in the absence of health care exposure and often in otherwise healthy individuals.
  - Most common mode of transmission is skin-to-skin contact.
  - High-risk populations include day care attendees, athletes participating in contact sports, those living in close quarters (eg, military, prisoners), injection drug users and men having sex with men.

Symptoms/Examination

- HA-MRSA: Most commonly presents as bacteremia or a device-associated infection.
- CA-MRSA: Most common presentation is **purulent (pus forming) skin/soft tissue infection.**
- Other presentations include necrotizing pneumonia, endocarditis, osteomyelitis (Figure 8.1).

Diagnosis

- Suspect (and initiate treatment) based on risk factors and clinical presentation.
- Gold standard is culture.
- Polymerase chain reaction (PCR) is most accurate.

Treatment

- HA-MRSA:
  - Treat empirically with vancomycin; consider linezolid/daptomycin.
- CA-MRSA:
  - Abscess: Incision and drainage (I&D) is the mainstay of therapy. Consider antibiotics for:

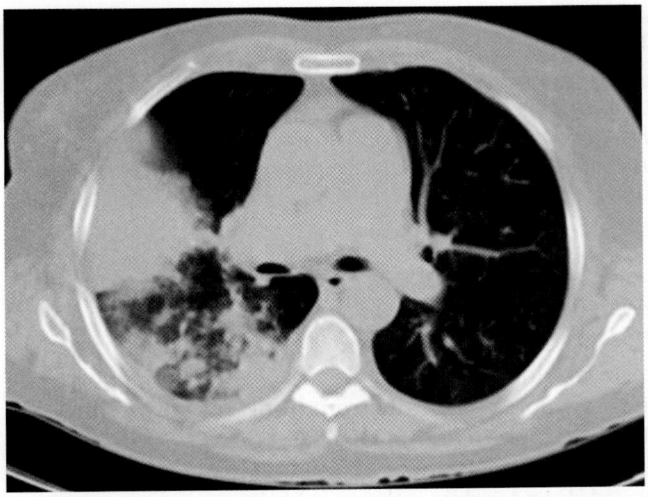

FIGURE 8.1. CT illustrating necrotizing pneumonia due to community-acquired methicillin-resistant *Staphylococcus aureus* (MRSA). (Reproduced, with permission, from Longo DL, Fauci AS, Kasper DL, et al. *Harrison's Principles of Internal Medicine*. 18th ed. New York, NY: McGraw-Hill Education; 2012. Figure 135.4.)

- Abscess > 5 cm per or multiple lesions
- Evidence of surrounding cellulitis
- Associated comorbidities or immunosuppression such as diabetes or transplant patients
- Systemic signs of infection
- Lack of response to initial I&D

- Trimethoprim-sulfamethoxazole, clindamycin, and doxycycline are typically safe in adults though each has its own side-effect profile.
- Antibiotic choice should be guided whenever possible by a regional antibiogram.
- Eradication of colonization:
  - Consider for recurrent MRSA infections or recurrent close contact transmission despite appropriate cleaning and hygiene.
  - Done with mupirocin 2% ointment 0.5 g in each nostril twice a day for 5 days in conjunction with a skin cleansing antiseptic.

BOTULISM

Botulism is caused by the spore-forming bacterium *Clostridium botulinum*. It is prevalent in soil and marine sediment worldwide. The spores are heat and acid resistant and under anaerobic conditions, germinate and produce the **heat-labile botulinum** neurotoxin. The toxin is remarkably potent—estimates suggest that 1 g evenly dispersed and inhaled would be enough to kill 1 million people. Unfortunately, such potency makes botulism a potential bioterrorism agent.

Pathogenesis

Ingestion of preformed botulinum toxin or spore germination and production of toxin in gastrointestinal tract (infants) or wound → blockage of presynaptic release of acetylcholine at the neuromuscular junction → **flaccid descending paralysis**, mydriasis, ptosis, and eventual respiratory paralysis, which is the primary cause of death.

Q

A 4-month-old infant presents with 4 days of constipation and poor feeding. He is afebrile, appears lethargic, and has decreased muscle tone with depressed deep tendon reflexes (DTRs). What food product did the child likely consume?

KEY FACT

Clostridium botulinum
- Gram + anaerobic rod
- Spore forming
- Blocks release of acetylcholine at neuromuscular junction
- Causes neuromuscular blockade

A

Honey

Infectious History!

Botulism was first described in the early 1800s by Dr Justinus Kerner. He studied an epidemic of "sausage poisoning" affecting > 70 victims in rural Germany who experienced weakness and dilated pupils after eating contaminated blood sausage. Botulism gets its name from the Latin "botulus," which means sausage!

Symptoms/Examination

- **Infant** (72%)
  - Age < 1 year old
  - Ingestion of spores (typically from honey or corn syrup)
  - Constipation, poor feeding, weak cry
  - Decreased muscle tone/loss of head control
  - Depressed deep tendon reflexes (DTRs)
  - Respiratory failure (50%)
  - Fever is absent.
- **Foodborne** (25%)
  - Direct toxin ingestion (classically, home-canned foods)
  - Incubation: Approximately 1 day (range: 6 hours-10 days)
  - Cranial nerve palsies (eg, diplopia, dysphagia, dysarthria)
  - Descending paralysis and respiratory failure
- **Wound** (rare)
  - From open wounds, injection drug use (eg, "black tar" heroin)
  - Incubation period approximately 1 week
  - Lower mortality than foodborne

KEY FACT

Adults don't get botulism from eating honey because the presence of normal intestinal flora prevents colonization of the GI tract.

Diagnosis

- Presumptive diagnosis is based on clinical presentation.
- Confirmed by presence of **toxin** in blood, stool, or food, **or growth of bacteria** from wound

Treatment

- Supportive care, may require early intubation
- Immediate administration of botulinum antitoxin
  - Trivalent antibodies to toxin (derived from horse serum), neutralizes only circulating toxin.
  - Not recommended in infant type (low efficacy/high risk of anaphylaxis); use human-derived botulinum immune globulin intravenous (BIG-IV) instead.
- Consider decontamination/bowel irrigation for foodborne or infant botulism.
- For wound botulism, irrigate wound and administer antibiotics **after** antitoxin; early antibiotics → increased cell lysis and toxin release.

KEY FACT

In cases of clear-cut wound botulism, withhold antibiotics until antitoxin administered.

KEY FACT

Clostridium tetani
- Gram + rod
- Obligates anaerobe
- Spore forming → "drumstick appearance"
- Blocks release of inhibitory neurotransmitters

TETANUS

Tetanus is caused by the **exotoxin tetanospasmin** produced by the spore-forming bacteria *Clostridium tetani*. Spores of *C. tetani* are found in soil and animal feces and can persist for years. Tetanus typically occurs after a break in the skin from a wound, a rusty nail, or even a dirty needle used for injection drug use. Tetanus presents in 1 of 4 clinical patterns: local, generalized (most common), neonatal, or cephalic.

RISK FACTORS

- Temperate climates (Texas, Florida, California)
- Diabetes, elderly (> 60 years old)
- Injection drug use (15%)
- Puncture wounds or crushed/devitalized tissue
- Inadequate immunization

Infectious History!

Tetanus is an ancient disease first described by Hippocrates. An effective immunization program was not available until World War II. During the Civil War, the rate of tetanus was nearly 2000 cases per 1 million wounds. After the introduction of tetanus immunization to army recruits, only 12 cases of tetanus were reported in US troops in World War II.

Q

An 80-year-old man presents with pain and stiffness in his masseter muscles 1 week after stepping on a rusty nail. Muscle rigidity has progressed to his neck, torso, and upper extremities. What treatment needs to be initiated before wound debridement?

KEY FACT

Many patients with tetanus cannot recollect any injury or trauma.

PATHOGENESIS

- Germination of *C. tetani* from spores present in damaged or devitalized tissue → production of tetanospasmin exotoxin → blockage of release of inhibitory neurotransmitters glycine and γ-aminobutyric acid (GABA) at the motor endplates of skeletal muscle, spinal cord, brain, and sympathetic nervous system → spastic paralysis and tetany

SYMPTOMS/EXAMINATION

- Traumatic injury (no apparent injury in ~30%)
- Incubation period: 1 day to > 1 month (shorter = more severe)
- **Local tetanus**
  - Muscle spasms near site of injury that spontaneously resolve in weeks to months
  - Normally no permanent sequelae but may progress to generalized form
- **Generalized tetanus (80% of cases)**
  - Characterized by diffuse muscle rigidity and periodic spasms, resulting in:
    - Trismus due to masseter spasm ("lockjaw")
    - Risus sardonicus (sardonic smile)
    - Opisthotonus: Severe muscle spasms causing arching of the back
    - Respiratory failure
- **Neonatal tetanus**
  - Common in developing countries due to lack of passive immunity from nonimmunized mother and use of nonsterile instruments to cut umbilical stump
  - Characterized by irritability and poor feeding in first week of life
  - Case fatality rate is approximately 15%-30%.
- **Cephalic tetanus (rare)**
  - Occurs after facial trauma or otitis media
  - Cranial nerve dysfunction, most commonly CN VII, (mimics Bell's palsy)
  - Variable clinical course, 15%-30% mortality

DIFFERENTIAL

- **Strychnine poisoning** can have similar appearance.
  - Found in some pesticides, homeopathic medications, and adulterated street drugs
  - Waxing and waning intense muscle contractions, back arching, grimacing
  - Treatment is with benzodiazepines.

KEY FACT

Strychnine acts by blocking an inhibitory glycine receptor, rapidly causing convulsions and death.

A

Tetanus immunoglobulin (TIG).

KEY FACT

In addition to tetanus, diphtheria and pertussis (Tdap) vaccination, give TIG for high-risk wounds with uncertain or < 3 prior immunizations.

DIAGNOSIS

- Clinical
- The spatula test, in which a tongue depressor is used to touch the posterior oropharynx, will cause a patient with tetanus to uncontrollably bite down on the depressor with a reported sensitivity and specificity of > 90% for tetanus infection.

TREATMENT

- Aggressive supportive care
- Immediate treatment with human tetanus immunoglobulin (TIG)
  - 3000-5000 units IM
  - Neutralizes circulating tetanospasmin
  - Does not affect toxin already absorbed by central nervous system (CNS)
- Wound debridement **after** TIG as additional toxin may be released during procedure!
- Tetanus immunization (give opposite site of TIG)
- Benzodiazepines muscle relaxation
- Magnesium and labetalol for sympathetic hyperactivity (avoid isolated β-blockade)
- Antibiotics are of questionable utility, but commonly given after TIG and immunization.
  - **Metronidazole** is drug of choice.
  - Penicillin is theoretically contraindicated (may potentate neurotoxin effects).
- Long-term neuromuscular blockade with vecuronium may be necessary.

WOUND PROPHYLAXIS

For prophylaxis in the absence of clinical tetanus, see Table 8.1.

KEY FACT

Neisseria gonorrhoeae
Gram-negative diplococcus
Intracellular
Mucosal surfaces
Thayer-Martin media

GONORRHEA

Gonorrhea is caused by the gram-negative diplococcus *Neisseria gonorrhoeae*. Because *N gonorrhoeae* invades columnar or transitional epithelium, infections can involve a multitude of locations including the cervix, urethra, epididymis, rectum, prostate, pharynx, and conjunctiva. An uncomplicated infection is one that has no associated bacteremia or ascending spread of infection. Unfortunately, increasing antibiotics resistance is common.

SYMPTOMS/EXAMINATION

- Incubation period: 1-14 days
- Asymptomatic infection is common.

TABLE 8.1. Tetanus Prophylaxis

PRIOR IMMUNIZATION	LOW-RISK WOUND (CLEAN/MINOR)	HIGH-RISK WOUND[a]
≥ 3	Tdap or Td if > 10 y since last dose	Tdap or Td if > 5 y since last dose
Uncertain or < 3	Tdap	Tdap and TIG (250 U IM)

Tdap, tetanus, diphtheria and pertussis; Td, tetanus, diphtheria; IM, intramuscular; TIG, tetanus immunoglobulin.

[a]High risk is defined as > 6 h old; contaminated (eg, dirt, saliva, feces); puncture, crush wounds, or avulsions; foreign bodies, burns, frostbite.

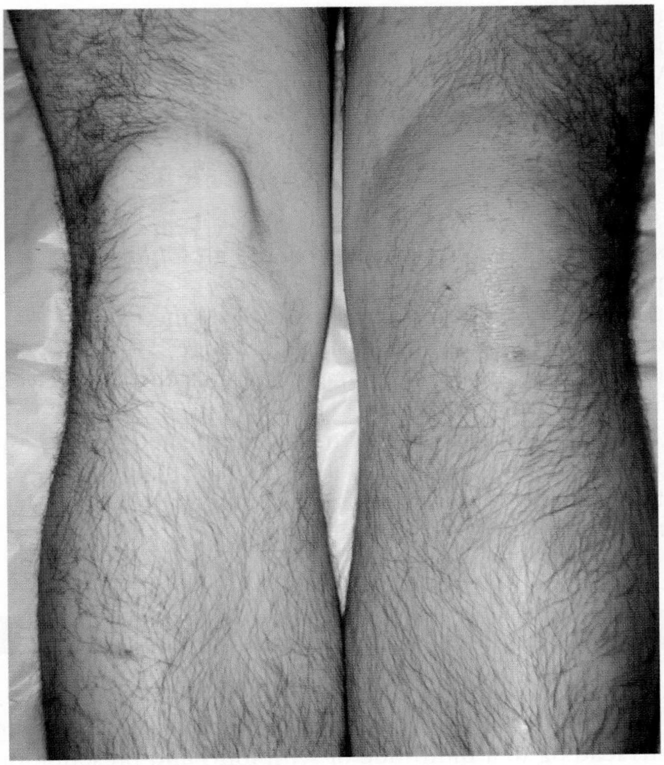

FIGURE 8.2. Septic arthritis of knee. (Reproduced with permission from *the clinical slide collection on Rheumatic Diseases*, 1991, 1995. American College of Rheumatology.)

Q

A 24-year-old woman presents with several days of fever and tenderness over the dorsum of one wrist and one ankle, with decreased range of motion of both. She also notes hemorrhagic pustules on her distal extremities. What is the most likely diagnosis and treatment?

- Symptoms depend on location of infection—typically pain and purulent discharge are present.
- **Disseminated gonococcal (GC) infection** (~2% of patients with GC infection, usually women) presents with fevers/chills, malaise followed by 1 of 2 distinct syndromes:
  - **Purulent (septic) arthritis** of wrist, knee, or ankle without skin lesions (Figure 8.2)
  - **Tenosynovitis, dermatitis, polyarthralgia syndrome**
    - Tenosynovitis, often of distal extremities
    - Skin lesions: Most often vesiculopustular or pustular; few in number; peripherally located
    - Asymmetric polyarthralgia that may progress to a purulent septic arthritis

KEY FACT

Septic arthritis in young adult? Think disseminated GC infection!

KEY FACT

Empirically treat all patients with suspected gonorrhea for *Chlamydia*, because estimates suggest a 40%-50% coinfection rate.

Infectious History!

Gonorrhea is known colloquially as "the clap." One theory for this is that historical French brothels were known as "les clapiers." Thus, if you visited one les clapiers you were likely to get "the clap."

DIAGNOSIS

- Uncomplicated/localized:
  - Nucleic acid amplification test (NAAT) of urethral/first-catch urine, cervical, pharyngeal, or rectal specimen; sensitivity approximately 95%

A

Disseminated gonococcal (GC) infections. Admit for ceftriaxone 1 g daily and possible surgical drainage, along with empiric coverage for chlamydia.

- Disseminated:
  - Blood cultures
  - NAAT of synovial, skin, urethral/cervical, rectal and pharyngeal specimens; Thayer-Martin media culture as alternative if NAAT not available

Treatment

- All cases should also be empirically covered for *Chlamydia*.
- Uncomplicated infection:
  - Ceftriaxone 250 mg IM × 1 or cefixime 400 mg PO.
  - Avoid fluoroquinolones (increasing resistance).
- Pelvic inflammatory disease: See Chapter 12, Obstetrics and Gynecology.
- Disseminated:
  - Joint drainage for purulent arthritis via repeated needle aspirations or in operating room.
  - Treat empirically if high suspicion as test sensitivity is low.
  - Ceftriaxone 1 g IV daily is initial therapy.

KEY FACT

Treponema pallidum
- Gram-negative bacterium
- Obligate intracellular
- Spirochete (corkscrew shaped)
- Visible with darkfield microscopy

SYPHILIS

Syphilis is caused by the bacterial spirochete *Treponema pallidum*. It is often called the "**great imitator**" because it is able to infect nearly every organ in the body, thus leading to a multitude of symptoms and presentations. Syphilis was very common prior to the antibiotic era. Currently an estimated 10,000 cases occur each year in the United States. However, the incidence is rising, especially in those with human immunodeficiency virus (HIV).

Symptoms/Examination

- Incubation period: 2-4 weeks
- **Primary syphilis (Figure 8.3)**
  - **Painless** genital ulcer with indurated border (chancre) that heals spontaneously over 2-6 weeks
- **Secondary syphilis**
  - 4-8 weeks after healing of chancre
  - Maculopapular **rash** that is nonpruritic and spreads from trunk → extremities (often involves **palms and/or soles**) (Figure 8.4)
  - **Condyloma lata**: Wartlike anogenital lesions (Figure 8.5)
  - Flulike illness with sore throat, low-grade fevers, malaise, and generalized lymphadenopathy
  - Symptoms resolve spontaneously.
- **Latent syphilis**
  - Asymptomatic period (serologies positive)
  - Normally lasts 3-4 years
- **Tertiary syphilis**
  - Tabes dorsalis (myelopathy involving the dorsal columns of the spinal cord)
  - Dementia
  - Gummatous lesions of mucous membranes
  - Thoracic aortic aneurysms
- **Neurosyphilis**
  - Can occur during any stage of infection
  - Acute neurosyphilis may be asymptomatic but typically presents with meningitis or a CNS vasculitis (stroke, headaches, etc).
  - Chronic neurosyphilis presents with tertiary symptoms above.

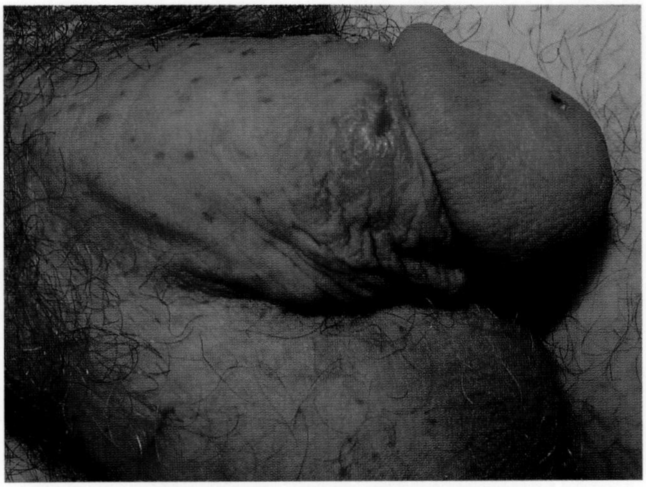

FIGURE 8.3. Chancre of primary syphilis. (Reproduced, with permission, from Wolff K, Johnson RA, Saaredra AP. *Fitzpatrick's Color Atlas & Synopsis of Clinical Dermatology*, 7th ed. New York, NY: McGraw-Hill Education; 2013. Figure 30.25.)

Diagnosis

- Screening test = serum rapid plasma reagin (RPR) or VDRL
  - Tests for nontreponemal antibodies, therefore nonspecific and false positives occur; cheap to perform
  - Positive > 2 weeks **after** 1° chancre (4-6 weeks after infection)
- Confirmatory test = serum florescent treponemal antibody absorption test (FTA-ABS)
- Tests for treponemal specific antibodies; stays positive for life
- Dark-field microscopy of chancre or oral/genital lesions has a high sensitivity of detecting the organism.
- Cerebrospinal fluid-VDRL is used to diagnose neurosyphilis in patients with positive serum FTA-ABS.

KEY FACT

RPR and VDRL false positives occur frequently in patients with HIV, malaria, pneumonia, and lupus.

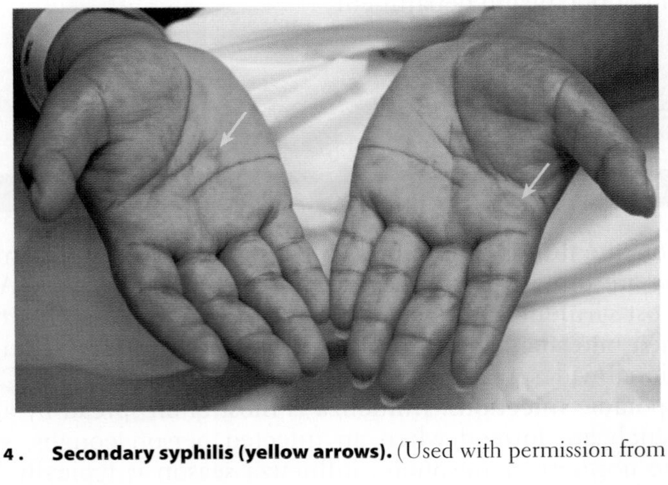

FIGURE 8.4. Secondary syphilis (yellow arrows). (Used with permission from Dr. William Griffith.)

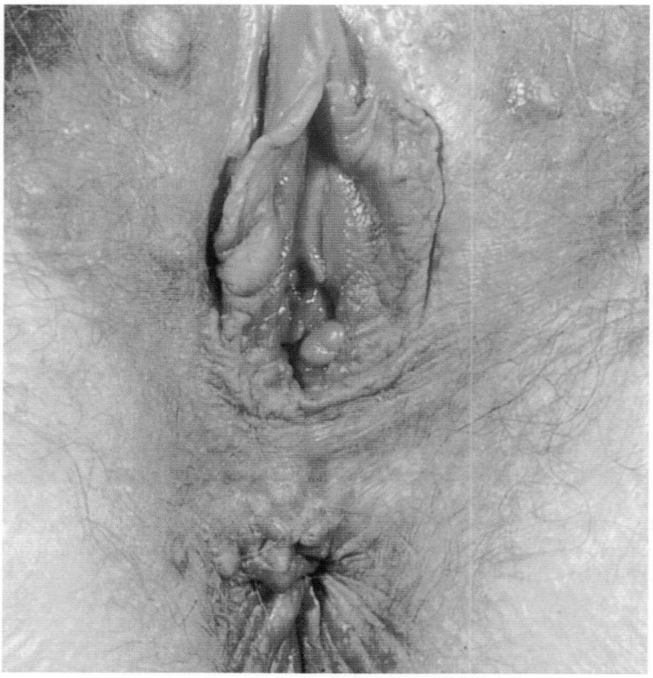

FIGURE 8.5. Condyloma lata. (Reproduced, with permission, from Handsfield HH. *Atlas of Sexually Transmitted Diseases*. New York, NY: McGraw-Hill; 1992.)

TREATMENT

- Primary or secondary:
  - Benzathine penicillin 2.4 million U IM (alternative = doxycycline × 14 days)
- Latent or tertiary:
  - Benzathine penicillin 2.4 million U IM weekly × 3 (alternative = doxycycline PO × 28 days)
- Neurosyphilis:
  - Aqueous penicillin G 3-4 million units IV q4h × 10-14 days or benzathine penicillin 2.4 million units IM qd plus probenecid PO qid × 10-14 days
- **Jarisch-Herxheimer reaction:** Acute fevers, headaches, myalgias, sweating within 24 hours of initial treatment of **spirochete** infections; self-limited (12-14 hours); worse with HIV
- Partners should be tested; treat empirically if sexual contact within 90 days.
- Report to public health department

> **KEY FACT**
>
> Consider 2° syphilis in any patient with a rash involving the palms and/or soles.

Selected Viruses

INFLUENZA

> **KEY FACT**
>
> **Influenza A**
> - Etiology of most flu epidemics and pandemics
> - Most virulent
> - Various strains based on surface proteins

Influenza, or "the flu," is caused by a single-stranded RNA Orthomyxoviridae virus. There are three types that cause illness in humans: Type A is considered the most virulent and is associated with pandemics. This type is further classified into strains based on two surface proteins (H1N1, etc). Type B causes regional/widespread epidemics every 2-3 years. Type C is associated with sporadic infections. Influenza is most often spread by **aerosolized droplets** which are formed when an infected person coughs, sneezes, or talks. In the northern hemisphere, influenza season is typically November through April.

SYMPTOMS/EXAMINATION

- Incubation period: 1-4 days
- Characterized by:
  - Sudden onset, high fever (2-4 days)
  - Headache, myalgias, fatigue/malaise
  - Coryza, sore throat, nonproductive cough
  - GI symptoms (more common in children)

Infectious History!

The Spanish flu occurred between 1918 and 1920 and infected an estimated 500 million people. More than 50 million people died because of this H1N1 strain, making it one of the deadliest pandemics ever recorded. The rapid spread of flu during this period is believed to be facilitated by troop movements at the end of World War I.

DIAGNOSIS

- Clinical suspicion (~85% accurate during known outbreak)
- Rapid antigen test has low sensitivity of approximately 40%-70% but high specificity.
- Reverse transcriptase-polymerase chain reaction (RT-PCR) is highly sensitive and specific but takes 4-6 hours to perform.
- Viral culture is still the laboratory gold standard and should be considered for hospitalized patients or surveillance purposes.
  - Less sensitive but more specific than RT-PCR
  - Results take 48-72 hours

KEY FACT

All antivirals for influenza are only efficacious if started within 48 hours of symptom onset.

TREATMENT

- Supportive measures
- Antivirals agents:
  - Zanamivir or oseltamivir (neuraminidase inhibitors)
  - Amantadine and rimantadine are no longer recommended due to high resistance.
- Indications for treatment:
  - Symptom duration < 48 hours
  - Severe illness requiring hospitalization
  - **High risk for complications** (age < 2 or > 65 years, hospitalized, children with long-term aspirin use, pregnant, immunosuppressed, chronic organ dysfunction, resident of long-term care facility, morbid obesity)

COMPLICATIONS

- 1° (influenza) or 2° (bacterial) pneumonia
  - Occurs most frequently in the elderly and those with comorbidities
- Reye syndrome (with aspirin in pediatric patients)
- Rare: Aseptic meningitis, pericarditis, Guillain-Barré syndrome

PANDEMIC INFLUENZA

A flu pandemic occurs when a novel influenza strain appears and causes widespread worldwide infection. All past flu pandemics have been caused by influenza A, with H1N1 subtypes responsible for the 1919 Spanish flu pandemic and the more recent 2009 pandemic.

- Reasons for pandemic potential:
  - Rapid mutation
  - Airborne transmission
  - Migratory animal hosts worldwide
  - High morbidity and mortality
- Current influenza viruses with pandemic potential; Avian influenza A (H5N1 and H7N9)
- Vaccination and exposure prevention keys to disease control

MONONUCLEOSIS

KEY FACT

If patients with mono are falsely diagnosed with strep pharyngitis and given antibiotics, they can develop a diffuse maculopapular rash and be incorrectly told they have a drug allergy.

Infectious mononucleosis is the clinical infection caused by the Epstein-Barr virus (EBV). Although > 90% of adults have antibodies to EBV, only approximately 10% have a symptomatic primary infection. EBV is typically **transmitted via bodily secretions**, leading to the nickname "kissing disease." Most pediatric infections are asymptomatic.

Symptoms/Examination

- Incubation period: 1-2 months
- Patients typically complain of fever, fatigue, and sore throat.
  - Examination findings include exudative pharyngitis (often severe), cervical lymphadenopathy (particularly posterior cervical lymphadenopathy), and hepatosplenomegaly (> 50%).
- Rash is common following antibiotics.
  - Classically amoxicillin; also Levaquin and azithromycin

Diagnosis

- Transaminitis (95%)
- Atypical lymphocytes in peripheral blood smear
- Definitive: Heterophil antibody tests, eg, Monospot (viral capsid immunoglobulin M [IgM])
  - May have false negatives early in disease

Treatment

Primarily supportive. Avoid contact sports for 4 weeks.

Complications

- Airway obstruction from tonsillar hypertrophy; treat with steroids
- **Splenic rupture**; can be spontaneous or after minor trauma
- Hemolytic anemia or thrombocytopenia; treat with steroids
- Guillain-Barré syndrome
- Bilateral Bell palsy
- Implicated in Burkitt and Hodgkin lymphoma as well as nasopharyngeal carcinoma

RABIES

A *Lyssavirus* (specifically genotype 1) transmitted by the bite, scratch, or open skin contact with saliva or secretions of an infected animal. Aerosol transmission from caves filled with bats is also a likely source. Rabies reservoirs in the United States include raccoons, foxes, skunks, and bats.

No human transmission from rodents or lagomorphs has been known to occur. Stray cats and dogs are important reservoirs for infection in developing countries, including Mexico.

PATHOGENESIS

Virus enters motor and sensory nerves at wound or injection site → travels centrally via peripheral nerves to spinal cord and CNS → widely disseminates in CNS → passes centrifugally via somatic and autonomic nerves to wide variety of tissues, including salivary glands, and skin of head and neck (sites used for identification of the virus).

Infectious History!

Rabies is an ancient disease with reports stretching back to 2300 BC. Around 100 AD the Roman writer Cardanus describes the saliva of a rabid dog as "virus," the Latin word for poison.

SYMPTOMS/EXAMINATION

- Incubation period: 2-12 weeks before onset of generalized symptoms in most cases
- Bites to head and neck have a shorter incubation period
- Pain, paresthesia, and **itching** may occur at site of bite
- Initial symptoms are otherwise nonspecific and flu-like.
- **Encephalitic form** of the disease:
  - Periodic episodes of hyperactivity, restlessness, or agitation.
  - Hypersalivation is common.
  - Periodic spasms in response to stimuli, including inspiratory (aerophobia) and (pharyngeal) hydrophobia
- **Paralytic form** of disease is less common and presents with a Guillain-Barré–like progressive paralysis associated with urinary incontinence.

DIAGNOSIS

- In the United States, wildlife reservoirs for rabies include bats, skunks, raccoons, foxes and coyotes.
- Diagnosis of active infection is confirmed by identification of virus in saliva (most reliable), punch biopsy of hair-bearing skin from nape of neck, serum, or CSF (if obtained).

TREATMENT

- Postexposure management (Table 8.2).
- Clean wound ASAP, preferably with a virucidal agent such as povidone-iodine.

TABLE 8.2. Postexposure Rabies Prophylaxis

ANIMAL	ANIMAL DISPOSITION	RECOMMENDATION[a]
Dog, cat, ferret	Healthy/captured	Observe animal for 10 d, no treatment unless clinical signs develop
	Escaped	Consult public health
	Sick	HRIG + vaccination
Skunks, raccoons, foxes, bats	Captured	HRIG + vaccination (stop series if euthanized animal tests negative)
	Escaped	HRIG + vaccination
Squirrels, hamsters, guinea pigs, gerbils, chipmunks, rats, mice, rabbits	N/A	Almost never requires treatment (consult public health for specific recommendations)

HRIG, human rabies immunoglobulin.

[a]If treated with pre-exposure vaccine → finish vaccine course, but do not give H-RIG.

Q

A 30-year-old otherwise healthy man gardener presents with ulcerating lesions progressing up his arm 3 weeks after planting a new rose bush. What is the diagnosis and treatment?

KEY FACT

Symptomatic rabies infections are almost invariably fatal. Postexposure management with both rabies immunoglobulin and vaccine is critical.

A

Sporotrichosis from the fungus *Sporothrix schenckii*. Treatment is with itraconazole.

- Administer rabies immune globulin—as much as possible around site, the rest IM.
- Administer rabies vaccine in five doses: 0, 3, 7, 14, and 28 days after exposure.
- Postexposure prophylaxis of closed-room bat exposure without clear bite is controversial, but still recommended in the United States.

Selected Fungal Infections

Also see Chapter 10, Thoracic and Respiratory Disorders for agents typically presenting with fungal pneumonia (aspergillosis, blastomycosis, coccidiomycosis, and histoplasmosis).

SPOROTRICHOSIS

Sporotrichosis is caused by the fungal agent S. *schenckii* and is found on plants and in the soil. Dubbed "rose gardener's disease," it most commonly causes a subacute infection in individuals with outdoor occupations such as gardeners and landscapers who experience a traumatic inoculation.

Symptoms/Examination

- Incubation period: 1-10 weeks (average 3 weeks)
- $\geq$ 1 suppurating subcutaneous nodules
- Progresses proximally along lymphatic channels

Diagnosis

- Treat based on clinical suspicion
- Definitive: Biopsy/fungal culture

Complications

- Osteomyelitis, septic arthritis, bursitis, tenosynovitis
- Systemic forms: Pulmonary and meningeal (rare)

Treatment

Itraconazole for 3-6 months

MUCORMYCOSIS

Rare infection caused by organism belonging to the group of fungi called Mucoromycotina. These fungi are found in soil and in decaying organic matter. Human infection nearly always occurs in the setting of diabetes or immunocompromise.

Symptoms/Examination

- **Rhino-orbital-cerebral:** Acute sinusitis (fevers, facial pain, purulent nasal drainage) that rapidly spreads to contiguous structures of the orbit and brain. Symptoms depend on structures involved.
- **Pulmonary:** Rapidly progressive pneumonia often with hemoptysis due to necrosis of structures; may spread to adjacent structures or disseminate
- GI, skin, and renal mucormycosis can also occur.

DIAGNOSIS/TREATMENT

- Emergency department (ED): Begin treatment with amphotericin B based on clinical suspicion.
- Definitive: Biopsy/fungal culture

> **Q**
>
> A 3-year-old boy presents with nightly perianal itching and a normal physical examination. What is the most likely diagnosis?

Common Parasitic Helminths

While rare in the United States and Europe, it is estimated that nearly one-fourth of the population of Sub-Saharan Africa is infected with one or more helminths. These parasites thrive in warm and humid environments with poor sanitation and a lack of clean drinking water. There are three basic types of helminths: nematodes (roundworms), trematodes (flukes), and cestodes (flatworms). Consider in travelers, immigrants or patients with unexplained fever, abdominal pain, diarrhea, or **eosinophilia**.

INTESTINAL NEMATODES (ROUND WORMS)

Round worms (Table 8.3) are cylindrical, unsegmented, elongated white worms that enter the human host through ingestion of eggs, penetration of skin, or insect bite.

Pinworm (*Enterobius vermicularis*)

- The most common helminth infection in the United States. Adult females migrate to anal verge to lay eggs in perianal folds, causing intense **perinanal itching**. Scratching leads to spread of eggs via fecal-oral route.
- Perianal itching, worse at night
- Diagnosed via scotch-tape swab of anal verge and direct visualization of worms (Figure 8.6)
- Treat with albendazole or mebendazole.

TABLE 8.3. Intestinal Nematodes (Roundworms)

NAME	NEMATODE	ROUTE	SYMPTOMS/EXAMINATION	DIAGNOSIS
Pinworm	*Enterobius vermicularis*	Fecal–oral (mostly children)	Nocturnal perianal itching	Scotch-tape swab
Common roundworm	*Ascaris lumbricoides*	Ingestion of contaminated food/soil	Pneumonitis, abdominal cramps, worm passage obstruction	O&P
Hookworm	*Ancylostoma duodenale, Necator americanus*	Penetration of skin via soil	Localized dermatitis (normally feet), pneumonitis, abdominal pain, anemia	O&P
Whipworm	*Trichuris trichiura*	Ingestion of contaminated food/soil	Dysentery, tenesmus, rectal prolapse	O&P
Strongyloides	*Strongyloides stercoralis*	Ingestion of contaminated food/soil	Eosinophilia, perianal rash, abdominal pain, overwhelming infection in immunosuppressed	Serology, O&P
Trichinella	*Trichinella spiralis*	Ingestion of raw or undercooked wild game	Fever, periorbital edema, myalgias, CNS abnormalities	Serology, muscle biopsy

CNS, central nervous system; O&P, ova and parasite exam.

A

Pinworm (Enterobius vermicularis).

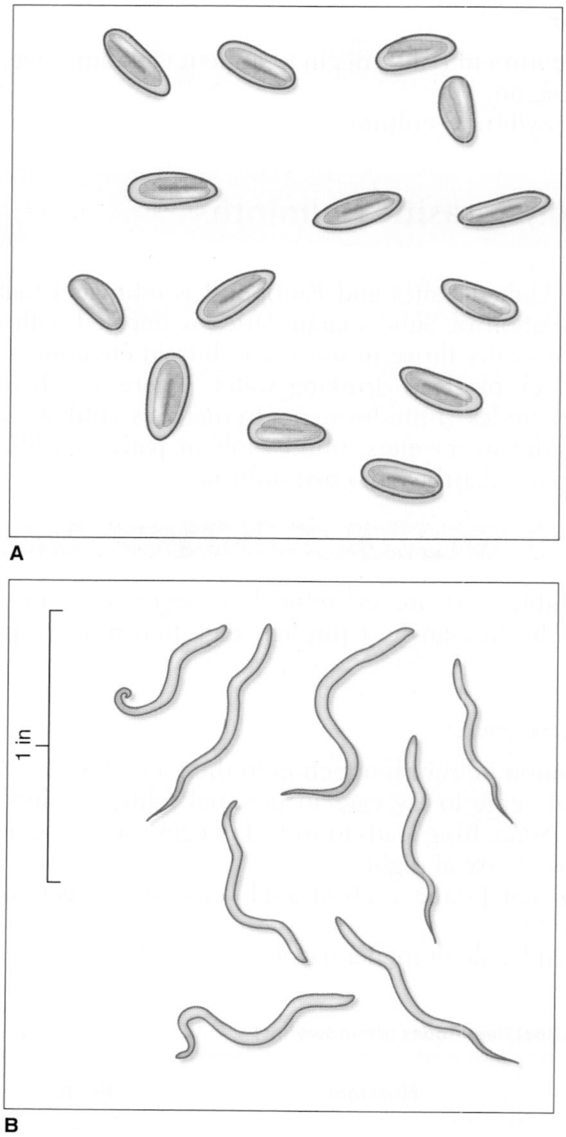

FIGURE 8.6. Pinworm tape test. Microscopic examination of tape applied to both sides of the anus first thing in the AM may show pinworm eggs (**A**) or less commonly the adult worm (**B**). (Reproduced, with permission, from Nicoll D, Lu CM, Pignone M, et al. *Pocket Guide to Diagnostic Tests*. 6th ed. New York, NY: McGraw-Hill Education; 2012. Figure 2.6.)

Common Roundworm (*Ascaris lumbricoides*)

A soil-transmitted helminth, caused by ingestion of fertilized eggs. Eggs hatch in the small intestine and larvae migrate via blood to lungs where they mature, ascend the bronchial tree, and are swallowed.

- Often asymptomatic, but large burdens may cause **bowel obstruction or nutritional deficiencies.**
- **Löeffler syndrome:** Dry cough, chest pain, and low-grade fever due to eosinophilic pneumonitis during migration through lung.
- Worms can also migrate into biliary or pancreatic ducts causing obstruction and symptoms.
- Diagnosed via stool microscopy (O&P)
- Treat with albendazole or mebendazole.

Hookworm (*Ancylostoma duodenale, Necator americanus*)

Hookworm eggs hatch into larvae in soil. Once mature, the larvae penetrate human skin and migrate via blood to lungs (usually without symptoms) where they ascend the bronchial tree and are swallowed. In the intestines, they attach to intestinal mucosa causing chronic blood loss.

- Nonspecific GI symptoms are common initially, but chronic infection leads to **iron-deficiency anemia and nutritional deficiencies.**
- Diagnosed via microscopic examination (O&P) of stool (Figure 8.7)
- Treat with albendazole or mebendazole

Whipworm (*Trichuris trichiura*)

A soil-transmitted helminth caused by ingestion of *T. trichiura* eggs. The mature worm burrows into the colon.

- Infection may be asymptomatic, but heavy worm burden often causes **bloody diarrhea**.
- **Rectal prolapse** can also occur.
- Diagnosed via microscopic identification (O&P) of stool
- Treat with albendazole or mebendazole.

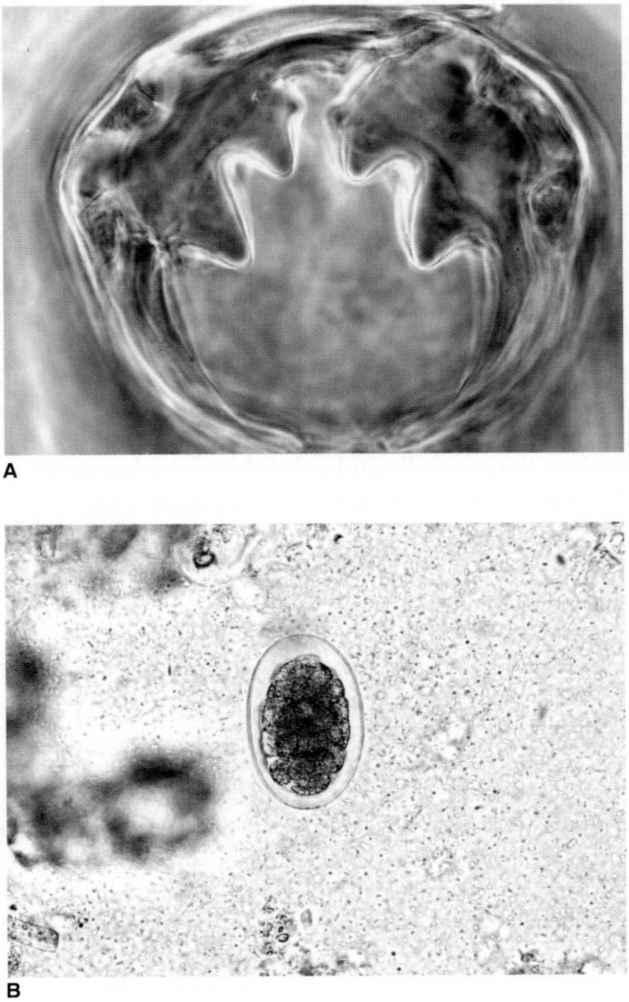

FIGURE 8.7. ***Ancylostoma duodenale.*** Microscopic images showing two pairs of teeth in anterior end of an adult worm (**A**) and an egg from a fecal saline preparation (**B**) (Reproduced, with permission, from Sullivan JT. A *Color Atlas of Parasitology*. 8th ed. San Francisco, CA: University of San Francisco; 2009).

Strongyloides (*Strongyloides stercoralis*)

Mature larvae are passed in human feces to soil or other materials. Upon contact with humans these larvae penetrate the skin and migrate via blood to the lungs where they ascend the bronchial tree and are swallowed. The adult worms burrow into the mucosa of the small intestines. After infection is established, the mature larvae are able to penetrate the colon or anal mucosa of the host and travel to the lungs to repeat the lifecycle (a process called **autoinfection**; seen mostly with immunocompromise).

- Nonspecific GI, skin, or pulmonary symptoms (Löeffler syndrome) that wax and wane
- Diagnosed by microscopy of concentrated stool or serologic testing for IgG antibodies
- Treat with ivermectin or albendazole.

Trichinella (*Trichinella spiralis*)

Caused by the ingestion of encysted *Trichinella* larvae in raw or undercooked meat of wild game or pigs. They mature into adults worms in the intestines. The female worm then releases larvae that migrate via blood to host striated muscle where they encyst.

- Initial intestinal stage: Nonspecific gastroenteritis symptoms for first week
- Muscle stage: **Muscle pain and tenderness**, fever, and **periorbital swelling**
- Diagnosed by serologic testing (a variety exist) or muscle biopsy (definitive).
- Treat with albendazole plus steroids.

KEY FACT

Löeffler syndrome: Eosinophilic pneumonitis with pulmonary symptoms such as cough and wheezing due to worm migration through the lungs.

BLOOD AND TISSUE NEMATODES (FLUKES)

Nematodes (Table 8.4) are leaflike, symmetrical flatworms with ventral sucker and no body cavity. They live in intermediate hosts, such as snails, crabs, fish, and their larvae infect humans.

Lymphatic Filariasis/Elephantiasis (*Wuchereria bancrofti* and *Brugia malayi*)

Larvae migrates through mosquito bite wound and enter lymphatic vessels where they mature into adult worms. New larvae are eventually produced and enter blood stream allowing mosquito-borne transmission to another host.

- Acute infection: Fevers/chills and painful lymphadenopathy
- Pneumonitis can occur as larvae migrate through lung.

TABLE 8.4 Blood and Tissue Nematodes

Name	Distribution	Vector	Symptoms/Examination	Treatment
Lymphatic filariasis (elephantiasis)	Southeast Asia, equatorial regions	Mosquito	Lymphangitis and lymphedema, pneumonitis	Ivermectin or DEC
Onchocerca volvulus (river blindness)	Africa, Central or South America	Blackfly (*Simulium*)	Blindness (sclerosing keratitis), subcutaneous nodules	Ivermectin
Loa loa (eye worm)	Africa	Deerfly (*Chrysops*)	Larvae migrating across conjunctiva	DEC
Dracunculus medinensis (guinea worm)	Africa	Ingestion of infected water (copepods)	Painful worm extruding from lower extremity	Wrap worm around stick, metronidazole

DEC, diethylcarbamazine.

- Chronic disease: **Chronic lymphedema (elephantiasis)**
- Treat with diethylcarbamazine (DEC) or ivermectin.

Onchocerciasis/River Blindness (*Onchocerca volvulus*)

Larvae are deposited into human skin by the bite of the black fly (found near fast-flowing rivers and streams). The larvae mature into adults worms (called microfilariae) and mate in the subcutaneous tissue. Offspring microfilariae migrate to the ocular tissues, lymphatics, and skin causing intense inflammatory responses.

- Eye findings include keratitis, uveitis, and chorioretinitis.
- Subcutaneous nodules and other skin findings may be present.
- Treat with ivermectin.

Loiasis (*Loa Loa*)

Larvae are deposited into human skin by the bite of the African horse or deer fly. The larvae mature into adults worms (called microfilariae) which live in the subcutaneous tissue and migrate throughout body including the subconjunctival tissue of eye,

- Worm can be visible on conjunctival examination of eye.
- Subcutaneous swelling from migration of worm in tissue may be seen.
- Treat with DEC.

CESTODES (TAPEWORMS)

Tapeworms (Table 8.5) are structurally characterized by a scolex (head) with hooks/suckers and segmented bodies. Each segment has a complete set of reproductive organs.

Taeniasis (*Taenia saginata* or *Taenia solium*)

Humans become infected with *Taenia* by ingestion of raw or undercooked beef (*T. saginata*) or pork (*T. solium*) containing larval cysts (cysticerci). These cysts then mature in the small intestine and attach to the wall. Matured segments of the worm (proglottids) and eggs are released into stool.

TABLE 8.5. Cestodes (Tapeworms)

Parasite	Ingestion	Clinical Findings
T. saginata	Raw beef	Nausea, anorexia, abdominal pain
Cysticercosis (*T. solium*)	Raw pork	New onset seizures, CNS or muscle cysts
Diphyllobothrium latum	Undercooked fish	Megaloblastic anemia due to B_{12} deficiency
Hymenolepis nana, Hymenolepis diminuta	Rodent feces or fleas	Abdominal cramps, diarrhea
Dipylidium caninum	Dog fleas	Abdominal cramps, diarrhea
Echinococcus sp	Feces of sheepdogs, cattle, wolves, foxes	Hydatid disease (liver, lung, and/or CNS abscesses)

CNS, central nervous system.

Larval spread in humans can occur with *T. solium* but not *T. sagitum* as follows: Human ingestion of *T. solium* eggs from food or water contaminated with infected human feces → eggs hatch into larvae in small intestines → larvae disseminate via blood with formation of **larval cysticerci in brain, striated muscle and liver** (= **cysticercosis**).

- Most adults are asymptomatic and diagnosis is suspected after passage of segments in feces.
- Symptoms due to cysticercosis depend on location of cysts but may include **headaches, seizures**, elevated intracranial pressure, and focal neurologic signs.
- Diagnosis is based on clinical presentation and imaging.
- Treat with praziquantel.

KEY FACT

In endemic areas, cysticercosis (*T. solium*) is responsible for more than one-third of the cases of adult-onset epilepsy.

Fish Tapeworm (*Diphyllobothrium latum*)

Humans become infected with *D. latum*, the largest human tapeworm, by ingestion of raw or undercooked freshwater fish. *D. latum* prevents host vitamin B_{12} absorption.

- Most adults are asymptomatic but symptomatic vitamin B_{12} deficiency (glossitis, anemia, peripheral neuropathy) may develop.
- Treat with praziquantel.

HIV/AIDS

The human immunodeficiency virus (HIV) is a RNA retrovirus responsible for causing the acquired immunodeficiency syndrome (AIDS). HIV namely targets CD4 helper T cells and causes direct (cell lysis) and indirect (immune-mediated) cellular destruction leading to immunosuppression. As the CD4 counts drop, the host becomes more susceptible to opportunistic infections. Antiretroviral treatment decreases rate of opportunistic infection and decreases spread of disease, but needs strict compliance given the virus' ability to rapidly mutate and create resistance.

- Agent: RNA retrovirus, HIV
- Incidence: Approximately 40,000 new cases per year in the United States (stable)
- Increasing incidence in women, minorities, and children

Risk Factors

- Men who have sex with men
- Injection drug use
- Unprotected intercourse
- Blood transfusion prior to 1985
- Maternal transmission (rare in the United States)

Symptoms/Examination

See Table 8.6.

KEY FACT

Suspect acute HIV?

Send HIV viral load as HIV antibody tests will be negative for 3-12 weeks after exposure.

Diagnosis

- Acute HIV: High titers of viral RNA with negative antibody screen
- Seroconversion occurs 3-12 weeks after exposure at which time standard HIV testing can be used.
- Enzyme-linked immunosorbent assay (ELISA) assay: Testing of oral fluids, whole blood, or urine for HIV-specific antibodies
- Rapid HIV test: Technology similar to ELISA using blood or oral fluids
- Positive result must be confirmed by Western blot (99% sensitive/specific).

TABLE 8.6. HIV Time Course

Stage	CD4 Count	Time Course	Clinical Findings
Exposure	Normal	N/A	Via blood/blood products, semen, vaginal secretions, breast milk, or transplacentally
Acute HIV syndrome	Normal	2-4 wk after exposure	Flulike illness for 1-3 wk Very high viral loads can be detected
Seroconversion	Normal	3-12 wk after exposure	HIV antibody tests become positive
Asymptomatic period	> 500	Mean: Adults = 8 y Children = 2 y	Asymptomatic, generalized lymphadenopathy
Early symptomatic	200-500	Variable	Thrush, bacterial pneumonia, herpes zoster, hairy leukoplakia, B-cell lymphoma, Hodgkin disease, ITP, Kaposi sarcoma, tuberculosis
Late symptomatic	< 200 < 100	Variable	Esophageal candidiasis, PCP, HIV encephalopathy, *Salmonella septicemia*, disseminated coccidiomycosis or histoplasmosis, PML CMV retinitis, cryptococcal meningoencephalitis, cerebral toxoplasmosis
End-stage AIDS	< 50	Variable	Disseminated CMV, MAC, primary CNS lymphoma

AIDS, acquired immune deficiency syndrome; CMV, cytomegalovirus; CNS, central nervous system; HIV, human immunodeficiency virus; ITP, idiopathic thrombocytopenic purpura; MAC, mycobacterium avium complex; PCP, *Pneumocystis* pneumonia; PML, progressive multifocal leukoencephalopathy.

Definition of AIDS

- CD4 count < 200 cells/mm^3 (or CD4 < 14% of total T lymphocytes)
- HIV positive plus AIDS-defining illness

PULMONARY COMPLICATIONS

For *Mycobacterium tuberculosis*, please see Chapter 10, Thoracic and Respiratory Disorders.

See Table 8.7 for chest x-ray (CXR) differential diagnosis.

Bacterial Pneumonia

Bacterial pneumonia is the primary cause of pulmonary infection in HIV-positive patients. Common organisms include *Streptococcus pneumoniae*, *Haemophilus influenzae*, and atypical bacterial pathogens. This presents similarly to other community-acquired pneumonias (see Chapter 10, Thoracic and Respiratory Disorders).

Histoplasmosis

Histoplasma capsulatum is a fungus endemic in the moist soil of the Mississippi and Ohio River valleys. The infection is often clinically silent in healthy patients. Severe or disseminated disease can occur in HIV with CD4 counts < 200 cells/mm^3 and is considered an AIDS-defining illness.

KEY FACT

Histoplasma capsulatum

Fungus
Moist soil with bird/bat droppings
Mississippi and Ohio River valleys
Inhalation of spores

Q

A 25-year-old man with known HIV/AIDS (last CD4 count < 200 cells/mm^3) presents with hypoxia, a chronic cough, and a chest x-ray (CXR) showing diffuse interstitial infiltrates. In addition to normal bacterial pneumonia treatment, what other organism should be emergently covered and what test should be done before initiating treatment?

TABLE 8.7. Differential Diagnosis for AIDS-Associated CXR Findings

CXR	Differential Diagnosis
Normal	Histoplasmosis (40%) PCP (20%) TB Cryptococcosis
Focal consolidation	Bacterial pneumonia *M. pneumoniae* PCP TB *M. avium*
Nodular lesions	Kaposi sarcoma TB *M. avium* Fungal lesions Toxoplasmosis
Cavitary lesions	PCP TB Bacterial abscess Fungal abscess
Diffuse interstitial infiltrates	PCP CMV TB *M. avium* Histoplasmosis Coccidioidomycosis Lymphoid interstitial pneumonitis *M. pneumoniae*

AIDS, acquired immune deficiency syndrome; CMV, cytomegalovirus; CXR, chest x-ray; PCP, *Pneumocystis* pneumonia; TB, tuberculosis.

Symptoms/Examination

- Fevers, chills, night sweats, fatigue
- Shortness of breath
- Nausea/vomiting

Diagnosis

- Pancytopenia is common.
- CXR: Diffuse interstitial infiltrates, hilar adenopathy, effusions; normal radiograph does not rule out disease (Figure 8.8)
- Diagnosis: Combination of culture and direct microscopy of peripheral blood

Treatment

- Admit for IV amphotericin for severe disease.
- Itraconazole for mild disease.

A

When considering *Pneumocystis* pneumonia (PCP), obtain an arterial blood gas (ABG) to determine the need for prednisone. Steroids should be given if the A-a gradient is > 35 or Pao_2 is < 70 mmHg.

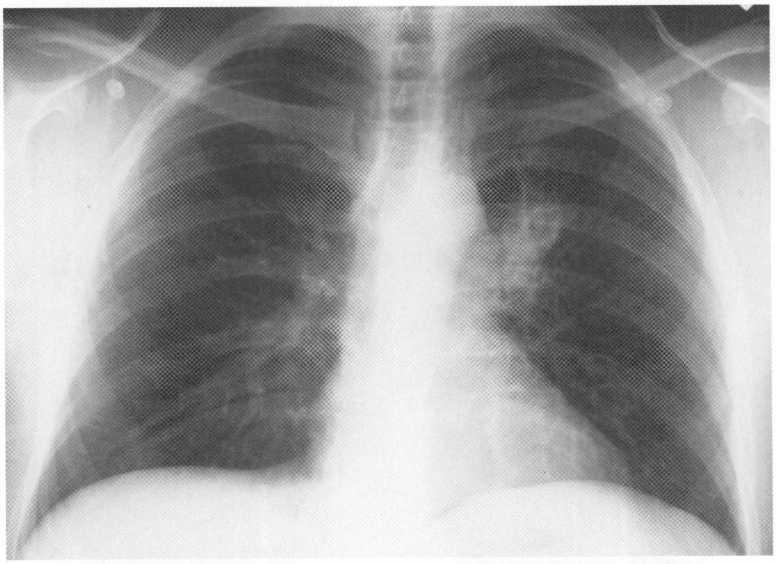

FIGURE 8.8. Histoplasmosis in a 33-year-old man with 6-month history of fatigue. (Used with permission from Lacey Washington, MD.)

Coccidiomycosis

Coccidioides immitis is a fungus endemic to the arid soils of the Southwestern United States and Northern Mexico. Infection results from inhalation of dust from disturbed soil. The infection is often clinically silent in healthy patients. Severe or disseminated disease can occur in HIV with CD4 count < 200 cells/mm^3 and is considered an AIDS-defining illness.

Symptoms/Examination

- Fevers, chills, night sweats, fatigue
- Shortness of breath, cough
- Disseminated disease: Meningitis and skin or subcutaneous tissue lesions most common

Diagnosis

- Pancytopenia is common.
- CXR: Diffuse interstitial infiltrates, hilar adenopathy, effusions; normal radiograph does not rule out disease.
- Diagnosis: Combination of serologic testing, histopathology, and culture.

Treatment

- Depends on severity of disease with amphotericin B (severe disease) vs oral itraconazole and fluconazole.

Pneumocystis Pneumonia (PCP)

Caused by the yeast-like fungus ***P. jirovecii*** **(previously *Pneumocystis carinii*)**. It is an opportunistic infection and the leading cause of AIDS-associated mortality.

Symptoms/Examination

- Gradual onset of dyspnea, nonproductive cough, fever
- Ambulatory desaturation < 90% may be the only finding if early.

KEY FACT

Coccidioides immitis
Fungus
Arid soils
Southwestern United States and Northern Mexico
Inhalation of spores

KEY FACT

The Patient Pneumonia Outcome Research Team (PORT) criteria did not included HIV-positive patients in their derivation and should not be applied to this population.

KEY FACT

Pneumocystis jirovecii
Fungus
World-wide distribution
Aerosolized transmission

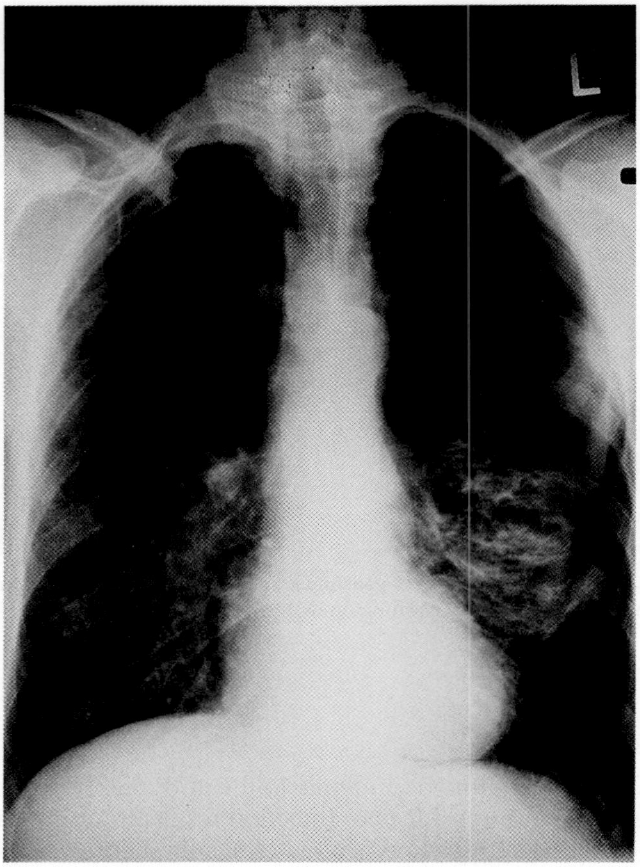

FIGURE 8.9. Posteroanterior chest x-ray of a patient with *Pneumocystis* pneumonia (PCP) who presented with a left-sided pneumothorax. (Reproduced, with permission, from Hall JB, Schmidt GA, Kress JP. *Principles of Critical Care*. 4th ed. New York, NY: McGraw-Hill Education; 2015. Figure 69.4.)

KEY FACT

A normal CXR is common in early PCP, but a normal chest CT makes the diagnosis unlikely.

Diagnosis

- CXR (Figure 8.9):
  - Classic: Diffuse interstitial infiltrates
  - Negative CXR reported in 15%-20% of patients
- Chest computed tomography (CT) has a high sensitivity for diagnosis, but is not required in most cases.
- Lactate dehydrogenase (LDH) and A-a gradient are frequently elevated.
- Definitive: Isolation of the organism from lower respiratory tract secretions (induced sputum, bronchoscopy).

Treatment

- TMP-SMX (in sulfa allergy, treat with clindamycin + primaquine)
- Prednisone if A-a gradient > 35 or Pao_2 < 70 mm Hg
- Prophylaxis with TMP-SMX, 1 DS tab daily is indicated for CD4 < 200 cells/mm^3 and greatly decreases the incidence of PCP.

NEUROLOGIC COMPLICATIONS

CNS disease occurs in 75%-90% of AIDS patients, and it is the AIDS-presenting illness in 10%-20% of HIV-positive patients (Table 8.8).

TABLE 8.8. Head CT and CSF Findings in HIV

Disease	Head CT	CSF	Definitive Diagnosis
HIV encephalopathy	Atrophy	Normal	Diagnosis of exclusion
Cryptococcus neoformans	Normal	↑ Opening pressure (66%), ↑ monos, + India ink (70%)	+ Cryptococcal antigen
Toxoplasma gondii	Multiple ring-enhancing lesions (subcortex or basal ganglia)	↑ Opening pressure, ↑ monos	Brain biopsy
CNS lymphoma	Solitary ring-enhancing lesion (periventricular)	↑ Protein	Monoclonal malignant lymphocytes on CSF cytology
Progressive multifocal leukoencephalopathy	Nonenhancing white matter lesion(s)	Normal or ↑ protein	PCR of JC virus

CNS, central nervous system; CSF, cerebrospinal fluid; CT, computed tomography; HIV, human immunodeficiency virus; PCR, polymerase chain reaction.

Cryptococcal Meningitis

CNS infection caused by the fungus *Cryptococcus neoformans*. The portal of entry for the fungus is the lung, and a focal or diffuse pneumonia can result. The CNS is the most common site of disseminated infection leading to focal cerebral lesions or diffuse meningoencephalitis. It is most common in patients with CD4 < 100 cells/mm^3.

> **KEY FACT**
>
> ***Cryptococcus neoformans***
> Encapsulated yeast
> Round-oval
> Found in soil
> Entrance via respiratory tract

Symptoms/Examination

- Subacute onset of fever, headache, and malaise
- Meningismus is uncommon (25%).
- Altered mental status may occur.
- Focal neurologic deficits are uncommon.

Diagnosis

- CT brain: Typically normal; a mass lesion suggests an alternative diagnosis.
- Lumbar puncture (LP) CSF studies:
  - Mononuclear pleocytosis with low numbers (< 50 cells/mm^3) is typical, but CSF is normal in up to one-third of cases.
  - Elevated opening pressure = high fungal burden. CSF removal to lower pressures is recommended.
- India ink stain of CSF is positive in 75% of cases.
- CSF cryptococcal antigen is highly sensitive and specific.
- Fungal culture is definitive.
- Serum cryptococcal antigen is highly sensitive and can be used in patients in whom LP is not possible.

Treatment

- Admit for IV amphotericin and PO flucytosine.
- Lifelong therapy with fluconazole
- Predictors of bad outcome include significantly elevated opening pressure, altered mental status, high CSF cryptococcal antigen titers, low CSF white blood cell count.

> **KEY FACT**
>
> HIV is an indication for a head CT before performing an LP.

KEY FACT

Toxoplasma gondii
- Protozoan parasite
- Obligates intracellular
- Found worldwide
- Felines are host

Toxoplasmosis

An encephalitis caused by reactivation of a chronic *Toxoplasma gondii* infection in HIV patients with CD4 counts < 100 cells/mm^3. It is the #1 cause of intracranial mass in AIDS.

Symptoms/Examination

- Fever, headache, AMS
- Focal neurological deficits (80%) or seizures

Diagnosis

- CT: **Multiple bilateral subcortical contrast-enhancing lesions** (Figure 8.10)
  - Most common in **basal ganglia** (often multiple)
- Presumptive diagnosis is based on clinical presentation, consistent CT findings, and presence of toxoplasma IgG indicating prior exposure.
- Definitive diagnosis: Identification of organism in biopsy specimen

Treatment

- Pyrimethamine + sulfadiazine (+ folinic acid)
- Steroids are indicated for significant edema/mass effect.
- Routine seizure prophylaxis is not recommended.

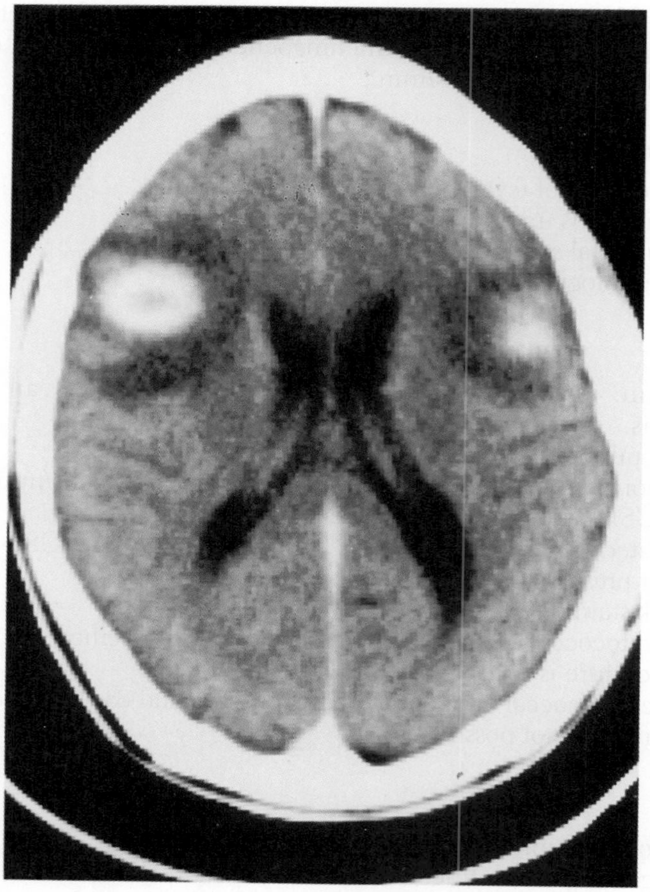

FIGURE 8.10. CT scan of the head demonstrating 2 lesions of cerebral toxoplasmosis. (Reproduced, with permission, from Hall JB, Schmidt GA, Kress JP. *Principles of Critical Care*. 4th ed. New York, NY: McGraw-Hill Education; 2015. Figure 69.10.)

Differential

The presence of a single contrast-enhancing lesions is more consistent with primary CNS lymphoma (see below).

Primary CNS Lymphoma

A non-Hodgkin B-cell lymphoma. The Esptein-Barr virus (EBV) is identified in 100% of cases and plays a pathogenetic role. Occurs most frequently with CD4 < 50 cells/mm^3.

Symptoms/Examination

- Headache, confusion, lethargy, memory loss
- Focal neurologic deficits and seizures may occur.

Diagnosis

- CT: **Focal lesion (usually solitary) that enhances with contrast**. Hyperdense/isodense periventricular enhancement is often seen.
- May appear similar to toxoplasmosis
- Magnetic resonance imaging (MRI) has higher diagnostic yield and is the preferred imaging modality to determine extent of disease.

Treatment

- Chemotherapy + radiation
- Median survival < 1 month

Progressive Multifocal Leukoencephalopathy (PML)

Severe demyelinating CNS disease caused by reactivation of polyomavirus JC (JC virus). PML is seen with CD4 counts < 200 cells/mm^3 as well as in other immunosuppressed states.

Symptoms/Examination

- Most commonly presents with subacute neurologic deficits including AMS, motor deficits, and ataxia
- Seizures can occur.

Diagnosis

- CT: **Single or multiple nonenhancing** white-matter lesions
- PCR of the JC virus (80% sensitive)

Treatment

- Highly active antiretroviral therapy (HAART)
- Prognosis is poor.

HIV Encephalopathy (AIDS Dementia)

Characterized by a progressive impairment of memory/cognitive processes caused directly by HIV. It is a diagnosis of exclusion.

HIV Peripheral Neuropathy

- May be due to HIV virus itself or its treatment. Most commonly a distal symmetric polyneuropathy but numerous other types are possible
- Rarely emergent
- Diagnoses is based on clinical presentation along with EMG and nerve conduction studies.

Q

35-year-old female with HIV and unknown CD4 count presents with headache, confusion and subtle right arm weakness. CT brain shows multiple ring-enhancing lesions. What is the likely cause? What is the approximate CD4 count?

KEY FACT

Any new alteration of mental status must be fully worked up in a patient with HIV including head CT and LP.

A

Given the presence of multiple contrast-enhancing lesions, the likely cause is toxoplasmosis and the CD4 count is likely to be below 100 cells/mm³. If a single lesion was present the likely cause would be primary CNS lymphoma with a CD4 count of < 50 cells/mm³. Non-enhancing lesions indicate PML.

KEY FACT

Hairy leukoplakia (unlike thrush) is normally located on the lateral portions of the tongue. Lesions do not scrape off easily.

GASTROINTESTINAL COMPLICATIONS

Thrush (Oral Candidiasis)

Thrush is caused by the unicellular diploid fungus or "yeast" *Candida albicans*. It affects > 80% of patients with AIDS.

SYMPTOMS/EXAMINATION

- Whitish plaques to tongue and buccal mucosa that easily scrape off to leave an erythematous base
- Often asymptomatic; may cause soreness, burning, dysphagia

DIFFERENTIAL

Hairy Leukoplakia: An EBV-induced lesion seen almost exclusively in HIV patients characterized by white plaques that do not easily scrape off, located on the **lateral portions** of the tongue.

TREATMENT

- Mild disease: Nystatin or clotrimazole topical therapy
- Recurrent/refractory or severe disease: Fluconazole

Esophagitis

An infectious etiology should be the primary concern in the HIV-positive patient with symptoms of esophagitis. The presence of thrush raises the likelihood of *C albicans* esophagitis, where its absence is associated with an ulcerative etiology such as herpes simplex virus or cytomegalovirus.

SYMPTOMS/EXAMINATION

Odynophagia and/or dysphagia

DIAGNOSIS/TREATMENT

- Presence of thrush: Empiric trial of fluconazole
- Absence of thrush or no response to fluconazole: Endoscopy and biopsy to guide treatment

Diarrhea

Diarrhea is the most common GI symptom in HIV.

CAUSES

- Routine enteric pathogens, with more severe disease as immunity wanes
- *Cryptosporidium*, *Cyclospora*, and *Cystoisospora* (previously called *Isospora*) are intestinal parasites that can cause self-limited diarrhea in the healthy host, but intractable diarrhea in advance HIV.
- Opportunistic infections such as CMV, *Mycobacterium avium-intracellulare*, (see below) and microsporidium are seen with CD4 < 50 cells/mm³.
- Noninfectious causes include medications and infiltrative diseases.

DIAGNOSIS

- Evaluation varies with CD4 count and clinical suspicion for pathogen
- Stool culture for enteric bacteria
- Stool for *Clostridium difficile* toxin
- Three stool specimens for ova and parasites
- Acid-fast smear of stool (*Cryptococcus*, *Cystoisospora*, *Cyclospora*)
- If these are unrevealing, consider upper and lower endoscopy

Mycobacterium Avium Complex (MAC)

Also known as *Mycobacterium avium-intracellulare* (MAI) infection, MAC is infection with 1 of 2 non-TB mycobacterial species *M. avium* or *Mycobacterium intracellulare*. These organisms are common in water and soil. A TB-like pulmonary infection is occasionally seen in the elderly or those with underlying lung disease. Disease in HIV is most common with CD4 < 50 cells/mm^3.

Symptoms/Examination

- Localized disease: Focal lymphadenitis
- Disseminated disease: Fever, weight loss, night sweats, **diarrhea**, abdominal pain

Diagnosis/Treatment

- Definitive diagnosis is by isolation of organism in blood or lymph node.
- Treatment: Clarithromycin or azithromycin + ethambutol

CUTANEOUS COMPLICATIONS

Kaposi Sarcoma

An angioproliferative disease occurring in HIV patients with prior human herpesvirus-8 (HHV-8) infection. It is more common in men who have sex with men and is an AIDS-defining illness.

Symptoms/Examination

- Papules or nodules that are pink, red, or purple in color
- Painless/nonblanching
- Commonly on lower limbs, face, mouth, and genitals
- Respiratory and GI involvement can occur

Treatment

- Antiretroviral therapy; disease may regress as CD4 count rises
- Palliation: Cryotherapy, radiotherapy, and systemic chemotherapy

Varicella-Zoster Virus Reactivation

There is a 27 × higher incidence of varicella-zoster virus (VZV) in HIV-positive patients. It may occur at any stage of HIV illness and is associated with an increased risk of neurologic (eg, aseptic meningitis) and ophthalmologic (eg, retinal necrosis) complications.

Treatment

- Oral acyclovir, famciclovir, or valacyclovir
- Admit for IV antiviral therapy if severe, disseminated, or ophthalmologic involvement.

> **KEY FACT**
>
> Shingles in a multidermatomal pattern is suspicious for HIV coinfection or other immunocompromised state.

OPHTHALMOLOGIC COMPLICATIONS

Cytomegalovirus Retinitis

Cytomegalovirus (CMV) retinitis is reactivation of latent CMV infection, typically with CD4 < 100 cells/mm^3. It causes a severe necrotic vasculitis and retinitis and is the #1 cause of AIDS-associated blindness.

Symptoms/Examination

- Visual acuity changes, photophobia, floaters, scotoma, redness, and/or pain
- Retina: Fluffy white perivascular lesions ("**cotton-wool spots**") (Figure 8.11)

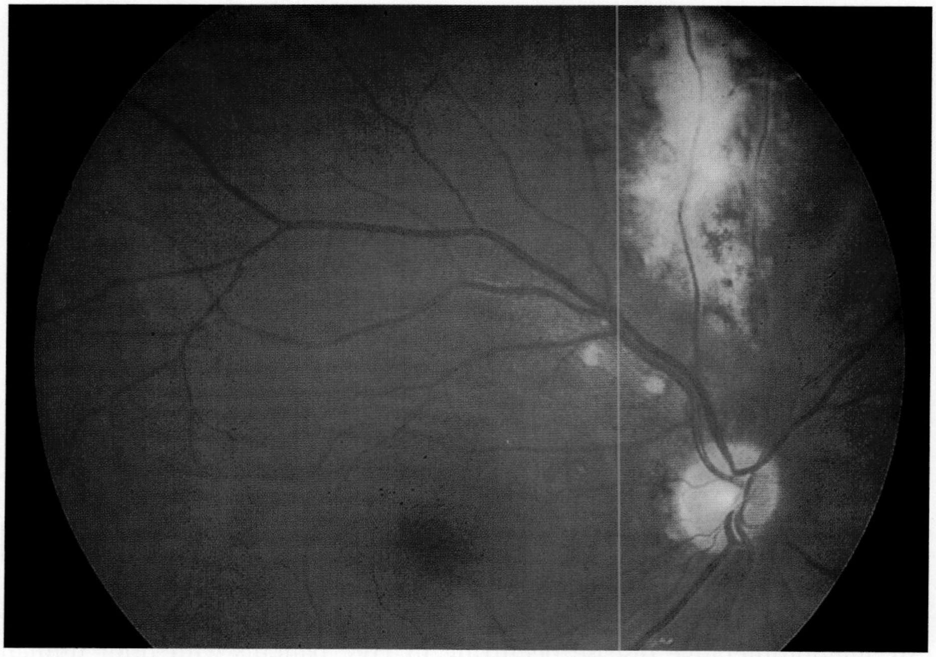

FIGURE 8.11. Cytomegalovirus retinitis. (Reproduced, with permission, from Knoop KJ, Stack LB, Storrow AB, et al. *The Atlas of Emergency Medicine*. 3rd ed. New York, NY: McGraw-Hill Education; 2010. Figure 20.18. Photographer: Edward C. Oldfield III, MD.)

Treatment

Ganciclovir

ADVERSE MEDICATION REACTIONS IN HIV TREATMENT

> **KEY FACT**
>
> NRTIs can cause a life-threatening lactic acidosis.

- Drug fever, rash, nausea, diarrhea, headache, neuropathy, and liver disease are common.
- Lactic acidosis associated with nucleotide reverse transcriptase inhibitors (NRTIs), eg, stavudine, zidovudine, didanosine, and lamivudine has untreated mortality rate up to 50%.
- For specific HIV medication side effects, see Table 8.9.

Infection in Transplant Recipients

While new powerful immunosuppressants have decreased rejection rates, they predispose to infection and mask the typical signs and symptoms of inflammation. Infection in transplant recipients is typically related to the level of immunosuppression a patient requires and their infectious exposures.

INFECTION IN THE FIRST MONTH

In the first month after transplant, heavy immunosuppression predisposes to acquired donor-related disease, reactivation of latent host diseases, and standard perioperative/hospitalization infections.

- Hospital-associated pathogens including methicillin-resistant *Staphyloccocus aureus*, vancomycin-resistant enterococcus, Candida, *C. difficile*

TABLE 8.9. Specific Side Effects for HIV-Associated Medications

Drug	Side Effect
Nucleoside/nucleotide reverse transcriptase inhibitors	**Class effects:** Lactic acidosis, hepatic steatosis (mitochondrial toxicity)
Specific medications	
Didanosine	Pancreatitis, neuropathy
Zidovudine	Bone marrow suppression
Zalcitabine	Neuropathy
Stavudine	Pancreatitis, neuropathy
Non-nucleoside reverse transcriptase inhibitors	**Class effects:** Rash and hepatotoxicity
Specific medications	
Efavirenz	Rash, sleep disturbance, teratogenic
Nevirapine	Rash, hepatitis
Delavirdine	Rash, hepatitis
Protease inhibitors	**Class effects:** Gastrointestinal symptoms, hyperlipidemia, glucose intolerance
Specific medications	
Atazanavir	Hyperbilirubinemia, prolonged QT
Darunavir	Headaches, rash
Ritonavir	Paresthesias, hepatotoxicity
Tipranavir	Hepatotoxicity
Fusion inhibitors	
Enfuvirtide	Nausea, eosinophilia

HIV, human immunodeficiency virus.

- Donor-associated infections are uncommon with prescreening but include HSV, rabies, West Nile virus and HIV.
- Recipient-derived infections via expansion of colonized patients include *Aspergillus* and *Pseudomonas*.

INFECTION FROM THE FIRST TO SIXTH MONTH

In the 1- to 6-month period post-transplant, patients are at risk for reactivation of latent disease as well as opportunistic infections.

- CMV
  - Presentation includes pneumonitis, GI symptoms, renal injury, CNS infection and skin manifestations
  - Can trigger or exacerbate organ rejection
  - Treat with IV ganciclovir.
- EBV
  - Clinical effects are similar to CMV, but also causes a mononucleosis-like syndrome.
- VZV
  - Primacy varicella infection can result in disseminated disease.
  - Seronegative patients should receive varicella-zoster immune globulin after exposure to chickenpox or zoster.
  - Consider inpatient treatment/IV acyclovir with cutaneous zoster.
- Also consider viral hepatitis, *Listeria*, PCP, endemic fungal infections.

Q

55-year-old male six months s/p renal transplant who presents to the ED after exposure to nephew with chicken pox. He has a documented inadequate response to prior varicella immunization. What is the most appropriate therapy?

KEY FACT

Symptomatic infection with CMV begins a median of 40 days after transplantation.

A

Because live vaccines are contraindicated in the transplant recipient, he should receive varicella-zoster immune globulin.

INFECTION AFTER SIX MONTHS

After six months, the level of immunosuppression decreases in healthy transplant patients. The risk of opportunistic infection is much less, leaving patients with a slightly increased risk for typical community-acquired infections, especially pneumonia. Exceptions include:

- Patients who require higher levels of immunosuppression are at high-risk for both opportunistic infections and severe community-acquired infections.
- Patient may develop reactivated or chronic viral infections including CMV, EBV, hepatitis B or C, HSV, and JC virus.

Zoonotic Infections

HANTAVIRUS

Viruses of the Bunyaviridae family with a worldwide distribution. This includes the Sin Nombre virus. Their primary natural reservoir is wild rodents. Although suspected as the cause of at least one medieval outbreak, the first confirmed hantavirus outbreak occurred during the Korean War and affected roughly 2000 patients. Today, the majority of cases occur in the **southwestern United States** and occur via **inhalation of feces/urine or direct bite from rodents** (primarily deer mouse). It causes two major clinical syndromes: Hantavirus pulmonary syndrome and hantavirus hemorrhagic fever with renal syndrome.

SYMPTOMS/EXAMINATION

- **Hantavirus pulmonary syndrome** is characterized by a flulike prodrome for 3-4 days, followed by noncardiogenic pulmonary edema and hypotension.
- Hantavirus hemorrhagic fever with renal syndrome is characterized by fever, hemorrhage, hypotension, and renal failure.
- Mortality rate of 10%-50%

DIAGNOSIS

- Suspect based on history of exposure and clinical presentation.
- **Thrombocytopenia** and marked leukocytosis are often keys to the diagnosis.
- Definitive: Immunofluorescent or immunoblot assays

TREATMENT

Supportive care

WEST NILE VIRUS

A Flavivirus transmitted by several species of mosquito. Birds are an important reservoir. West Nile Virus is endemic to most of North America and is responsible for seasonal epidemics (peaking July-October) of infections ranging from simple viral illness to encephalitis. Older patients are primarily at risk for encephalitis and death.

SYMPTOMS/EXAMINATION

- Incubation: 3-14 days
- Most infections are asymptomatic.

- West Nile fever (20% of infections):
  - Fever and flulike illness with upper respiratory infection (URI) symptoms and maculopapular central rash (50%)
  - Symptoms usually last for 3-6 days.
- Meningoencephalitis (1 in 150 infections):
  - Fever, headache, AMS
  - Motor disturbances including CN palsies, myelitis, movement disorders (eg, myoclonus)
  - Sensory abnormalities are not seen.

DIAGNOSIS

- Suspect based on clinical presentation during summer/fall months
- CSF findings with meningoencephalitis: ↑lymphocytes, ↑protein, normal glucose
- Definitive diagnosis is by identification of IgM antibody in CSF or serum.

TREATMENT

Supportive

COMPLICATIONS

- Mortality rate in admitted patients is 4%-18%.
- Prolonged neurologic complaints are common.

LYME DISEASE

Lyme disease is a syndrome caused by the spirochete *Borrelia burgdorferi*. The ticks *Ixodes scapularis* (deer tick) and *Ixodes pacificus* are responsible for disease transfer, with peak transmission in summer months. Lyme disease is endemic to the Northeast Coast (Connecticut, New York, New Jersey, Pennsylvania, Rhode Island), the Midwest (Wisconsin, Minnesota), and the West Coast (California, Oregon). The majority of people with Lyme disease do not recall a tick bite.

> **KEY FACT**
>
> ***Borrelia burgdorferi***
> Gram-negative bacterium
> Spirochete (helical shape)
> Extracellular
> Tick transmitted

PATHOGENESIS

Immature tick (nymph) or adult tick attaches for 24-48 hours → transmission of spirochete and early localized stage → dissemination of spirochete via blood or lymphatics → early disseminated stage → if persistent infection, late disseminated stage develops

SYMPTOMS/EXAMINATION

- **Early localized**/Stage 1 (1 week after exposure)
  - Flulike symptoms (80%)
  - Rash (90%): Localized **erythema migrans**
    - "Target lesion" at site of bite (Figure 8.12)
    - Average 10 cm diameter
    - May have additional smaller secondary lesions
- **Early disseminated**/Stage 2 (weeks to months after exposure)
  - Disseminated erythema migrans
  - Large joint arthritis
  - Neurological symptoms (15%)
    - Cranial neuropathies (may mimic Bell palsy)
    - Meningitis
    - Radiculopathy (motor or sensory)
  - Carditis, AV blocks (4%-10%)

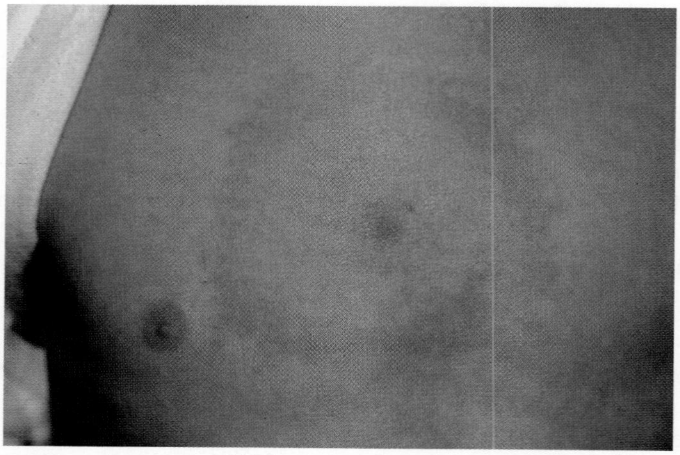

FIGURE 8.12. Erythema migrans. Spreading redness with central clearing in patient with Lyme disease. (Reproduced, with permission, from Rudolph CD, Rudolph AM, Hostetter MK, Lister G, Siegel NJ. *Rudolph's Pediatrics*. 21st ed. New York, NY: McGraw-Hill; 2003:Color Plate 22.)

KEY FACT

Suspect Lyme disease in the patient presenting with bilateral seventh nerve palsy.

- **Late disseminated**/Stage 3 (> 1 year after exposure)
  - Chronic encephalopathy
  - Chronic arthritis
  - Peripheral neuropathy

DIAGNOSIS

- Summer visit to endemic area + suggestive clinical symptoms (eg, rash, meningitis)
- Screening test: ELISA (89% sensitive, 72% specific, false positives common)
- Confirmatory test: Western blot assay
- Lyme meningitis: CSF with ↑lymphs, ↑protein, normal glucose; positive CSF ELISA confirms diagnosis

TREATMENT

- Symptomatic support, antibiotics
- For treatment regimens, see Table 8.10.

TABLE 8.10. Lyme Disease Treatment Regimens

STAGING	TREATMENT[a]
Early localized	Doxycycline PO × 21 d
Early disseminated (arthritis)	Doxycycline PO × 30 d
Early disseminated (neurologic)	Doxycycline PO × 21 d (if isolated CN palsy) or Ceftriaxone IV at meningitic doses (all others)
Early disseminated (cardiac)	Doxycycline PO × 21 d (if first-degree AV block) or Ceftriaxone IV at meningitic doses (all others)

AV, atrioventricular; CN, cranial nerve; IV, intravenous; PO, by mouth.

[a]Substitute amoxicillin for doxycycline in children < 8 y old and pregnant or lactating women.

PROPHYLAXIS

- Only indicated for *Ixodes* tick bite and only if tick is attached > **36 hours**
- Single 200-mg dose doxycycline within 72 hours of tick removal

ROCKY MOUNTAIN SPOTTED FEVER

Rocky Mountain spotted fever (RMSF) is caused by *Rickettsia rickettsii*. The ticks *Dermacentor variabilis* (dog tick) and *Dermacentor andersoni* (wood tick) are responsible for the bacteria's spread, with peak transmission occurring between April and September (95% of cases). The majority of cases occur in the South Atlantic States (eg, North Carolina), and it is actually rare in the Rocky Mountain States.

PATHOGENESIS

Tick bite and transmission → invasion and proliferation of organism within capillary and precapillary endothelial cells → perivascular inflammation → platelet and fibrin occlusion of vessels and multisystem disease

SYMPTOMS/EXAMINATION

- Incubation period: 2-14 days
- Clinical illness is characteristic of a vasculitis.
- Sudden onset of flulike or meningitis-like symptoms; headache is often a prominent feature.
- Fever (~75%).
- Rash (~50%).
  - Maculopapular → **petechial/purpuric**
  - Starts on **wrists/ankles**
  - Spreads **centripetally** (extremities → trunk)
  - Classically involves palms and soles (50%)
- Multisystem involvement is common including lethargy, confusion, myocarditis, acute lung injury, interstitial nephritis and GI symptoms.

DIAGNOSIS

- Based on clinical suspicion
- Hyponatremia and thrombocytopenia are common with advanced disease.
- Serology with fourfold increase in Ab titers (positive 6-10 days after onset, 94% sensitive/specific)
- Skin rash biopsy (3-mm punch biopsy, results in ~ 4 hours, 70% sensitive)

TREATMENT

- Treat empirically for clinical suspicion due to high mortality rates (roughly 3%-5% despite treatment, 25% if untreated).
- Supportive therapy, low threshold for admission
- Antibiotics: Doxycycline, tetracycline, or chloramphenicol

COMPLICATIONS

- Interstitial pneumonitis leading to adult respiratory distress syndrome (ARDS)
- Myocarditis, congestive heart failure
- Disseminated intravascular coagulation
- Seizures, encephalitis

Q

A 17-year-old man presents with fever and flulike symptoms a few days after a hiking trip in North Carolina. He has recently developed a maculopapular rash, which started on his wrists/ankles and progressed to involve his palms/soles and trunk. What treatment should be initiated?

KEY FACT

In Lyme endemic regions, give a single dose of doxycycline for the prophylaxis of high-risk tick bites.

KEY FACT

Rickettsia rickettsii

Gram-negative coccobacillus
South Atlantic states
Tick transmitted
Perivascular inflammation

KEY FACT

The classic triad of tick exposure, fever, and rash is present initially in only a minority of RSMF cases.

A

Doxycycline, tetracycline, or chloramphenicol

EHRLICHIOSIS

Ehrlichiosis is divided into **human monocyte ehrlichiosis** caused by *Ehrlichia chaffeensis* and **human granulocytic ehrlichiosis** caused by *Anaplasma phagocytophilum*. These bacteria are spread via bites from the *Ixodes*, *Dermacentor*, or *Amblyomma* ticks, whose reservoirs include deer, elk, and mice and are endemic to regions similar to those of Lyme disease.

KEY FACT

Ehrlichia chaffeensis

Anaplasma phagocytophilum

- Gram-negative coccobacilli
- Obligates intracellular (monocyte or granulocyte)
- Tick transmitted

Pathogenesis

Tick bite with transmission of organism → invasion of either monocyte or granulocyte → symptoms via poorly defined mechanisms

Symptoms/Examination

- Incubation period: 1-21 days (median = 7 days).
- Typically presents with flulike symptoms.
- Maculopapular rash that **may** involve palms/soles is seen in a minority of patient; more common in peds.

Diagnosis

- **Leukopenia, thrombocytopenia, transaminitis** (50%-90%)
- Peripheral blood smear may show mulberry-like clusters within monocyte or granulocyte in first week of illness.
- IgG antibody titers or culture/biopsy
- Definitive: PCR

Treatment

Doxycycline, tetracycline, or rifampin

KEY FACT

If suspected, both RMSF and ehrlichiosis must be treated immediately, because the illnesses can be rapidly fatal.

Complications

- Multisystem involvement with renal failure, respiratory failure, encephalitis, or DIC
- Opportunistic infections can occur due to leukopenia.

BABESIOSIS

KEY FACT

***Babesia* sp**

- Parasitic protozoan
- Pleomorphic
- Intraerythrocytic
- Transmitted by ticks

Babesiosis is caused by protozoan parasites of the genus *Babesia*. Similar to malaria, they infect red blood cells (RBCs) and cause a hemolytic anemia. *Babesia* is spread via the *Ixodes* ticks with a reservoir in deer and mice and similar geographic/temporal distributions to Lyme disease.

Pathogenesis

Nymph and adult state *Ixodes* ticks feed on human → organism enters erythrocyte and differentiate into merozoite → multiplication occurs and infected erythrocyte ruptures → organisms invades other erythrocytes → hemolytic anemia

Symptoms/Examination

- Incubation: 1-4 weeks
- Mild cases present as flulike illness with possible splenomegaly.
- Severe cases:
  - Hemolytic anemia, jaundice
  - Renal insufficiency
  - ARDS

Diagnosis

- Thick and thin Giemsa-stained smears
  - Erythrocytes show budding tetrad in "Maltese cross" formation.
- Also: PCR, serology (requires Centers for Disease Control and Prevention involvement)

Treatment

- Mild disease → no treatment
- Severe disease or postsplenectomy → quinine + clindamycin
- Exchange transfusion if fulminant

Complications

- Mortality approximately 6.5%
- 20%-50% of patients are coinfected with Lyme disease.

> **KEY FACT**
>
> Babesiosis is of greatest concern in the splenectomized patient.

Q FEVER

Q Fever is caused by *Coxiella burnetii*, and can be transmitted by the *Dermacentor* tick or via the ingestion of raw milk, inhalation of dried byproducts of cattle, sheep, or goats, or blood transfusions. It should be considered in patients who have significant exposure to animal byproducts (eg, slaughterhouse workers).

> **KEY FACT**
>
> ***Coxiella burnetii***
> Gram-negative bacterium
> Obligates intracellular
> Transmitted by ticks, exposure to animal products or raw milk
> Highly infectious

Symptoms/Examination

- Incubation: 2-6 weeks
- Flulike symptoms, pneumonia, hepatitis

Diagnosis

- Often clinical
- Definitive: PCR, serologies (positive 2-3 weeks after infection)

Treatment

Doxycycline, tetracycline, or chloramphenicol

Complications

Endocarditis (up to 68%), granulomatous hepatitis, osteomyelitis (peds)

COLORADO TICK FEVER

Caused by the Colorado tick fever virus and transmitted by *D. andersoni* (wood tick). Found in the Western United States or Canada in mountainous areas between 4000 and 10,000 ft.

Symptoms/Examination

- Incubation: 1-14 days
- Classic biphasic fever and flulike symptoms, each lasting for a few days
- Rare meningoencephalitis

Diagnosis/Treatment

- Clinical; most recall a tick bite
- PCR is available.
- Treatment is supportive.

TICK PARALYSIS

Caused by a tick-produced neurotoxin. Most commonly reported in the Western United States. Several species of tick have been implicated with *D. variabilis* (dog tick) and *D. andersoni* (wood tick) being most common. The tick attaches and feeds, releasing salivary toxins for several days before the onset of symptoms.

SYMPTOMS/EXAMINATION

Classic presentation is generalized weakness and ataxia followed by ascending paralysis with loss of DTRs.

DIAGNOSIS/TREATMENT

- Diagnosed by finding feeding tick
- Treatment is supportive.
- Improvement starts with removal of tick.

KEY FACT

Malaria symptoms are often nonspecific; consider the diagnosis in any febrile person with a history of travel to the tropics.

KEY FACT

***Plasmodium* sp**

- Parasitic protozoan
- Transmitted by mosquitoes
- RBC lysis
- Severe disease: *Falciparum*
- Recurrent disease: *Ovale* and *vivax*

The Febrile Traveler

MALARIA

Malaria is a devastating disease caused by a protozoan genus *Plasmodium*. Several species cause disease in humans including *Plasmodium falciparum*, *Plasmodium vivax*, *Plasmodium ovale*, *Plasmodium malariae* and *Plasmodium knowlesi*. Malaria is spread by the *Anopheles* mosquito which most commonly bites at dusk or at night. Globally there are > 200 million infections annually with an estimated 700,000 deaths. Most of the deaths are in children and occur in sub-Saharan Africa with *P. falciparum* being responsible for most fatalities.

PATHOGENESIS

Mosquito transmits asexual haploid form of *Plasmodium* → migrates to liver and matures to produce merozoites → released from liver and invade RBCs → mature in 48-72 hours causing RBC lysis and release of additional merozoites → invade more RBCs → hemolytic anemia

Infectious History!

Prior to the discovery of the plasmodium parasite, it was believed that malaria was caused by "miasma" or toxic air. The word malaria in fact comes from the Italian for "bad air!"

SYMPTOMS/EXAMINATION

- Incubation period: 1-4 weeks
- Longer with partial immunity or antimalarial use
- Classic febrile cycles (from RBC lysis) are frequently absent, especially in *P. falciparum*.
- **Uncomplicated malaria**
- Flulike illness; mild jaundice and splenomegaly may be present after several days of illness.
- **Severe or complicated malaria** (higher burden of parasites):
  - Toxic/septic appearance
  - Acute lung injury

TABLE 8.11. Malaria Treatment Regimens for the United States

Setting	Adult Drug Regimen[a]	Pediatric Drug Regimen[a]
Uncomplicated, chloroquine sensitive (Central America and Caribbean)	Chloroquine phosphate	Chloroquine phosphate
Uncomplicated, chloroquine resistant (South America, South Asia, Africa)	Quinine sulfate (PO) + doxycycline or Atovaquone/proguanil or Mefloquine	Quinine sulfate (PO) + pyrimethamine sulfadoxine[b] or Atovaquone/proguanil or Mefloquine
Complicated (possible *P. falciparum*, unable to tolerate PO)	Quinidine gluconate (IV) + doxycycline	Quinidine gluconate (IV)

IV, intravenous; PO, by mouth.

[a]For *P. vivax, P. ovale*, which have a dormant hepatic phase, add primaquine phosphate to prevent relapse (test first for G6PD deficiency).

[b]Contraindicated in infants < 2 mo old.

- **Cerebral malaria (*P. falciparum*, mortality ~20%):**
  - Progressive delirium
  - Seizures
  - Coma → death
- **"Blackwater fever" (massive intravascular hemolysis, *P. falciparum*):**
  - Characteristic jaundice
  - Hemoglobinuria (causes "black" urine)

Diagnosis

- Suspect in febrile traveler from endemic region.
- Laboratory findings in uncomplicated disease: Mild anemia with mild liver function test (LFT) abnormalities.
- Laboratory findings in severe disease: Lactic acidosis, hypoglycemia, DIC, multisystem organ dysfunction.
- Definitive diagnosis: Plasmodial parasites on **Giemsa-stained thick and thin smears**.
- Speciation is important as *P falciparum* infections are more severe; *P vivax* and *P ovale* require additional treatment (see the following text).

KEY FACT

If unsure about chloroquine sensitivity in the region, treat as if resistant.

KEY FACT

Patients must be first tested for G6PD deficiency before taking primaquine due to a potentially fatal hemolysis reaction.

Treatment

- DEET-containing insect repellent and mosquito nets for prevention
- Supportive care including antipyretics, and fluid resuscitation as needed
- Consider exchange transfusion for severe disease/signs of end-organ damage.
- See Table 8.11 for treatment regimens.

Complications

Relapse can occur months-years after initial infection with *P vivax* and *P ovale* due to their **dormant hepatic phase**.

Q

A 60-year-old ill-appearing woman presents with headache, high fevers, and drenching sweats a week after returning from visiting relatives in West Africa. What diagnostic test should be sent and (if positive) what treatment should be initiated?

EBOLA

The Ebola virus causes a viral hemorrhagic fever similar to other viruses such as Marbug, Lassa, and Crimean-Congo hemorrhagic fever. It is spread via bodily fluids, and although bats have been speculated as a reservoir this is still unclear. Ebola was typically limited to Central Africa until the 2014 epidemic when it appeared in West Africa. The 2014 epidemic was the largest Ebola outbreak to date, infecting natives, travelers and health care workers caring for the ill and spurned health care organizations nationwide to revamp their safety protocols.

Symptoms/Examination

- Fever, headaches, myalgias
- Nausea, vomiting, or diarrhea
- Rash
- Unexplained easy bruising/bleeding

Diagnosis

- Suspect in a patient with recent travel to an endemic area.
- Contact local health authorities for further diagnostic guidance.

Treatment

- Isolation precautions
- Supportive care

DENGUE

KEY FACT

Dengue presents with fever and dramatic bone pain in the traveler.

Flavivirus transmitted to humans by the *Aedes* mosquito. In contrast to the mosquito vector for malaria, the *Aedes* mosquito typically bites during the day. The disease is endemic in many tropical regions worldwide and has been found with increasing frequency in nontravelers in Southern Florida. The World Health Organization definitions of dengue syndromes include undifferentiated fever, classic dengue fever, and dengue hemorrhagic fever. The risk for severe disease includes prior exposure, age, malnutrition, DEN-2 serotype, and genetic factors.

Symptoms/Examination

- Incubation: 5-10 days
- High fever, nausea, vomiting
- Nicknamed "break-bone fever" for severe bone pain/myalgias/arthralgias
- "Dengue facies": Classic facial edema
- Pale morbilliform rash develops following defervescence; starts on trunk, spreads to extremities/face

Diagnosis

- Clinical diagnosis based on travel history
- Rule out malaria if from malaria endemic region.
- Definitive diagnosis is via ELISA.

Treatment

Supportive

Complications

- **Dengue hemorrhagic fever:**
  - Most often occurs following **exposure to a second serotype**
  - Initial clinical course is similar to classic dengue.
  - Second phase of illness begins as initial symptoms are resolving
  - Manifestations include:
    - Fatigue
    - Shock

A

Thick and thin smears; quinidine gluconate and doxycycline.

- Bleeding diathesis with hemorrhagic pleural effusions
- Thrombocytopenia
- Mortality is 50% without care, < 5% with care.

LEPTOSPIROSIS

Leptospirosis is caused by the bacterial spirochete *Leptospira interrogans*. It is the #1 zoonosis affecting humans worldwide and is common in tropical climates. Transmission occurs with percutaneous or mucus membrane contact with freshwater contaminated by the urine of infected rodents, livestock, or domestic animals. Outbreaks are often after periods of heavy rainfall or flooding. The illness has a biphasic course with an acute febrile illness followed by the more severe "Weil disease."

SYMPTOMS/EXAMINATION

- Incubation: 2-30 days
- **Secondary immune phase**
  - Aseptic meningitis is a common finding.
- **Acute bacteremic phase (4-7 days duration)**
  - Symptoms range from mild illness to abrupt high fever/chills, intense headache (often worst of life) and severe myalgias.
  - **Conjunctival suffusion** (redness without exudates) is pathognomonic.
- **Weil syndrome (up to 1 month duration)**
  - Characterized by severe icterus, renal failure, hemorrhage and acute lung injury/ARDS

DIAGNOSIS

- Clinical in acute phase
- ↑ WBC, ↑ bilirubin (relatively mild increase in alk phos and transaminases)
- CSF consistent with aseptic meningitis
- Definitive: Isolation of leptospires in urine or CSF

TREATMENT

- Treatment is most effective in first 4 days and may prevent Weil syndrome. Treat empirically if clinical suspicion is high.
- Mild disease: Treat with doxycycline/amoxicillin.
- Severe disease: Treat with penicillin/ampicillin/ceftriaxone.

Q

A 35-year-old man presents with fever and the worst headache of his life 2 weeks after returning from a white-water rafting trip to Peru. Physical examination reveals bilateral conjunctivitis. An LP shows aseptic meningitis. If untreated, what life-threatening syndrome may develop?

KEY FACT

Leptospirosis interrogans
Gram-negative spirochete
Obligates anaerobe
"Weil syndrome"

KEY FACT

Leptospirosis: Contaminated freshwater, fever, headache, conjunctival suffusion.

CHAGAS DISEASE

Chagas disease is caused by the protozoan parasite *Trypanosoma cruzi* and is endemic to South and Central America as well as Mexico. The disease is transmitted by contact with feces of the blood-sucking triatomine type of reduviid bugs ("kissing" bugs). Transmission occurs during/after their nocturnal feeding on a human host. These bugs have been identified in the Southern United States where increased numbers of infections are being reported. It is diagnosed most often in children. After initial circulation in the blood, the parasite invades tissues including the muscles of the heart, esophagus, and colon.

SYMPTOMS/EXAMINATION

- Incubation: 2-30 days
- **Acute phase (weeks-months duration)**
  - Edema at the inoculation site (often the eyelid)
  - Malaise, fever, anorexia, myalgias
  - Hepatosplenomegaly, lymphadenopathy

KEY FACT

Trypanosoma cruzi
Protozoan parasite
American trypanosomiasis
Latin America
Triatomine (reduviid/kissing) bug

Weil syndrome.

- **Chronic phase (10-20 years postinfection)**
  - Cardiomyopathy
  - Megaesophagus
  - Megacolon

DIAGNOSIS

- Observation of the parasite on thick and thin blood smears in acute phase
- Serologic testing for chronic disease

TREATMENT

Nifurtimox

OTHERS

- For additional geographically limited causes of acute fever in the return traveler, see Table 8.12.

TABLE 8.12. Geographically Limited Causes of Acute Fever

NAME	VECTOR	ORGANISM/DISTRIBUTION	SYMPTOMS/EXAMINATION	DIAGNOSIS/TREATMENT
Schistosomiasis	Penetration of skin by fresh water cercariae (eg, while swimming)	*Schistosoma* sp, a parasitic blood fluke Africa, Asia, Middle East, South America, Caribbean	Acute: Severe fever, headache, cough, urticaria, hypereosinophilia Chronic: Dermatitis, hematochezia, hepatic cirrhosis	O&P, serology Praziquantel
Chagas disease (American trypanosomiasis)	Triatomines (reduviid or kissing) bugs	*T. cruzi,* a protozoan parasite South and Central America, Mexico	Acute: Swelling at site of inoculation, fever, malaise, anorexia Chronic: Cardiomyopathy megaesophagus, megacolon	Blood smear or xenodiagnosis Nifurtimox
Human African trypanosomiasis (sleeping sickness)	Glossina (tsetse) fly	*T. brucei gambiense*, a protozoan parasite West and Central Africa	Early: Headache, fever, arthralgias, LAD, hepatosplenomegaly, pruritus Late: Personality changes, with slow progression to coma	Increased serum IgM Pentamidine or eflornithine
East African Trypanosomiasis (sleeping sickness)	Glossina (tsetse) fly	*T. brucei rhodesiense,* a protozoan parasite East and Southeast Africa	High fever, rash, leading rapidly to encephalitis and coma	Increased serum IgM Suramin or melarsoprol
Epidemic typhus	Body lice	*Rickettsia prowazekii*, a gram-negative obligate intracellular aerobacterium East Africa, Himalayas, Central/ South America	High fever, severe HA, rash	Serology Doxycycline or chloramphenicol
Leishmaniasis	Sandflies (*Phlebotomus* sp)	*Leishmania* sp, a protozoan parasite Asia, Middle East, Africa, Mexico, Central and South America	Cutaneous form: Papules or nodules that ulcerate Visceral form: Hepatosplenomegaly, pancytopenia	Serology, histology Sodium stibogluconate

IgM, immunoglobulin M; LAD, lymphadenopathy; O&P, ova and parasite exam.

Postexposure Prophylaxis

OCCUPATIONAL EXPOSURE

Health care provider contact with potentially infectious blood, tissue or body fluids via needle stick, mucus membrane, or nonintact skin.

HIV Transmission Risk

HIV transmission has been greatly reduced by universal precautions (Table 8.13). The majority of occupational seroconversions are percutaneous via needle stick or other sharp injury. There has been no confirmed seroconversion with a suture needle. The risk of HIV transmission depends on both types of exposure and patient factors (Table 8.14).

Hepatitis B Transmission Risk

Hepatitis B is highly infectious, but transmission to health care workers has been dramatically decreased by mandatory hepatitis B immunizations for all health care workers.

Hepatitis C Transmission Risk

The rate of seroconversion to hepatitis C is approximately 1.8% after a needle stick or sharps exposure.

Diagnosis

- **Source patient testing** (unless source patient is known to be positive) should be performed.
  - Varies based on patient agreement and state law
  - Includes hepatitis B surface antigen, hepatitis C antibody, and rapid HIV
  - Skip hepatitis B testing if provider has received vaccine series and has proven immune response.

TABLE 8.13. Risk for HIV Transmission by Route (Per Episode)

Type	Exposure	Estimated Risk (%)
Occupational	Percutaneous	0.3
	Mucocutaneous	0.09
Nonoccupational (assumes no condom use)	Needle-sharing injection drug	0.7
	Receptive anal intercourse	0.5
	Receptive penile-vaginal intercourse	0.1
	Insertive anal intercourse	0.07
	Insertive penile-vaginal intercourse	0.05
	Receptive oral (male) intercourse	0.01
	Insertive oral (male) intercourse	0.005

HIV, human immunodeficiency virus.

Q

A 28-year-old surgical intern presents after being stuck with a bloody 18G needle while placing a femoral line. The patient has known AIDS with a high viral load. What is the HIV transmission risk and what treatment should be initiated?

KEY FACT

Needlestick injuries are associated with risk for bacterial infections, hepatitis B, hepatitis C, and HIV.

KEY FACT

Exposure of bodily fluids onto intact skin is not a risk for HIV transmission.

A

High-risk source; high-risk exposure. Although the transmission rate is probably < 1% for this exposure, you should recommend expanded HIV postexposure prophylaxis regimen with first dose given as soon as possible. Also, don't forget to confirm prior hepatitis B vaccination with immune response.

TABLE 8.14. Risk Stratification for HIV Transmission

Type	Low Risk	High Risk
Source	Asymptomatic HIV Viral load < 1500 copies/mL	Symptomatic HIV/AIDS Acute seroconversion High viral load
Exposure (Occupational)	Superficial Solid needle Contact with intact skin = no risk	Deep injuries Visible blood on device Injuries sustained placing a catheter in a vein/artery
Exposure (nonoccupational)	Urine, nasal secretions, saliva, sweat, or tears not visibly contaminated with blood	Blood, semen, vaginal secretions, rectal secretions, breast milk, or any body fluid visibly contaminated with blood Exposure of vagina, rectum, eye, mouth or other mucous membrane, nonintact skin, or percutaneous contact

AIDS, acquired immune deficiency syndrome; HIV, human immunodeficiency virus.

- **Health care provider testing**
  - Hepatitis B surface antibody level (immune response) if not previously documented
  - Rapid HIV

TREATMENT

- Wound care: Skin cleaning with soap and water; irrigation of mucus membranes
- Tetanus immunization as indicated
- **HIV postexposure prophylaxis (PEP)**:
  - **Tenofovir-emtricitabine (Truvada) + raltegravir (Isentress)** unless known resistant strain
  - Associated with 79% reduction in transmission
  - Initiate ASAP (goal = 1-2 hours).
  - After 36 hours, HIV PEP is usually not indicated, unless particularly high risk.
  - Common side effects = constitutional, GI
- **Hepatitis B PEP** for those who have not completed vaccine series or known nonresponders.
  - Hepatitis B immunoglobulin (HBIG)
  - Hepatitis B vaccination: Usually given as three doses over 4-6 months with first dose given with HBIG in different site
- No current PEP is available for hepatitis.

NONOCCUPATIONAL POSTEXPOSURE PROPHYLAXIS

Experts recommend HIV PEP for persons exposed to a source known to be HIV positive or at high risk of HIV. High-risk exposure include unprotected vaginal/anal intercourse, needle/syringe sharing, or mucus membrane exposure to blood. Hepatitis B PEP is recommended for any blood or body fluid exposure. See Tables 8.13 and 8.14.

Diagnosis

- Source testing (unless source is known to be positive) should be performed when available.
  - Varies based on source agreement and state law
  - Includes hepatitis B surface antigen, hepatitis C antibody, and rapid HIV
  - May skip hepatitis B testing if patient has received vaccine series and has proven immune response
- Patient testing
  - Hepatitis B surface antibody level (immune response) if not previously documented
  - Rapid HIV

Treatment

- **HIV PEP.**
- **Tenofovir-emtricitabine (Truvada) + raltegravir (Isentress)** unless known resistant strain.
- Initiate ASAP (goal = 1-2 hours).
- After 36 hours, HIV PEP is usually not indicated, unless particularly high risk.
- **Hepatitis B PEP** for those who have not completed vaccine series or known nonresponders.
  - HBIG
  - Hepatitis B vaccination: Usually given as three doses over 4-6 months with first dose given with HBIG in different site

Vaccinations

- See Figure 8.13 for standard immunization schedule.
- For vaccine contraindications, see Table 8.15.

LIVE VACCINES

- Give multiple live vaccines either together or > 30 days apart.
- Contraindications:
  - 1° immunodeficiency
  - 2° immunodeficiency (eg, HIV, immune-modulating agents, high dose corticosteroids > 14 days)
  - Pregnant patients
  - Significant contacts of the previous

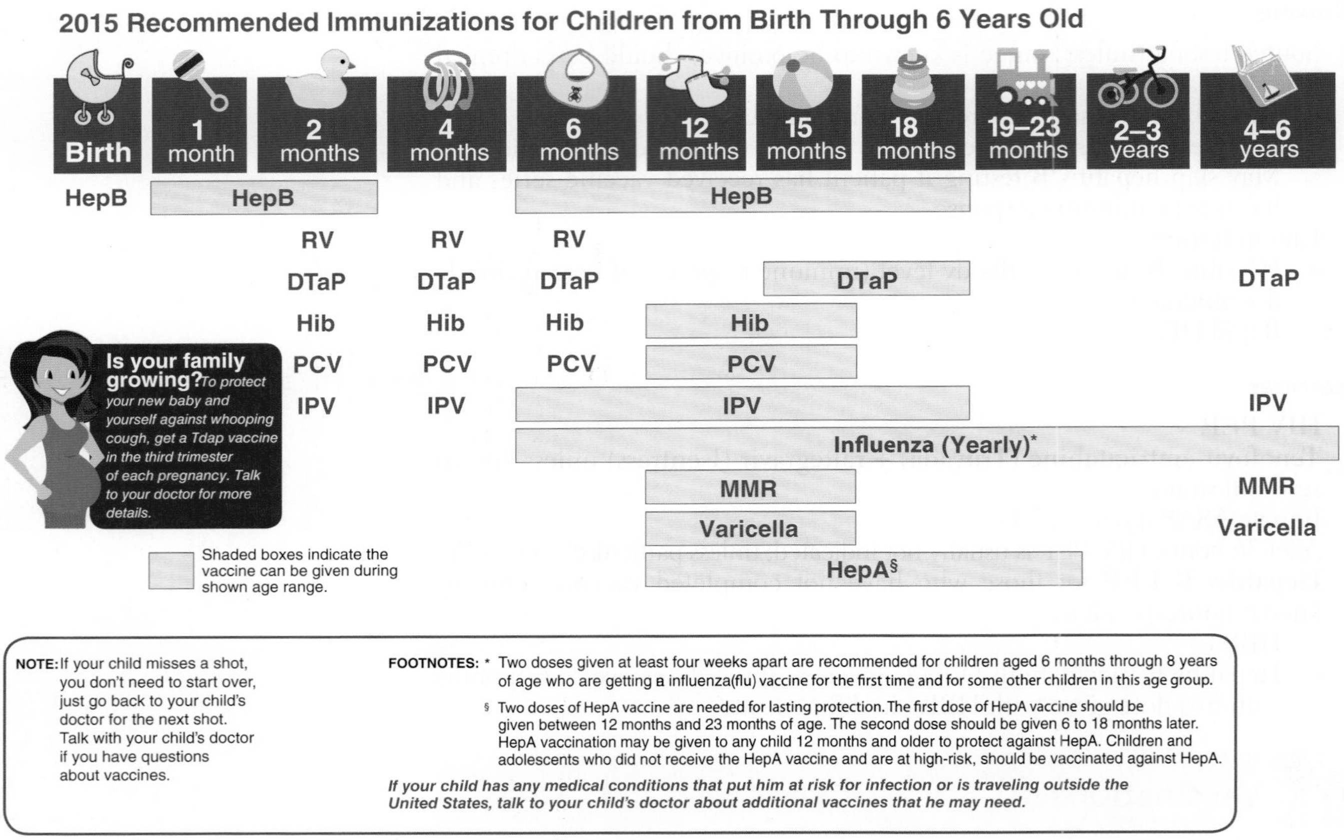

2015 Recommended Immunizations for Children from Birth Through 6 Years Old
Birth
1 month
2 months
4 months
6 months
12 months
15 months
18 months
19–23 months
2–3 years
4–6 years
HepB
HepB
HepB
RV
RV
RV
DTaP
DTaP
DTaP
DTaP
DTaP
Hib
Hib
Hib
Hib
PCV
PCV
PCV
PCV
IPV
IPV
IPV
IPV
Influenza (Yearly)*
MMR
MMR
Varicella
Varicella
HepA§
Is your family growing? To protect your new baby and yourself against whooping cough, get a Tdap vaccine in the third trimester of each pregnancy. Talk to your doctor for more details.
Shaded boxes indicate the vaccine can be given during shown age range.
NOTE: If your child misses a shot, you don't need to start over, just go back to your child's doctor for the next shot. Talk with your child's doctor if you have questions about vaccines.
FOOTNOTES: * Two doses given at least four weeks apart are recommended for children aged 6 months through 8 years of age who are getting a influenza(flu) vaccine for the first time and for some other children in this age group.
§ Two doses of HepA vaccine are needed for lasting protection. The first dose of HepA vaccine should be given between 12 months and 23 months of age. The second dose should be given 6 to 18 months later. HepA vaccination may be given to any child 12 months and older to protect against HepA. Children and adolescents who did not receive the HepA vaccine and are at high-risk, should be vaccinated against HepA.
If your child has any medical conditions that put him at risk for infection or is traveling outside the United States, talk to your child's doctor about additional vaccines that he may need.

FIGURE 8.13. **HepB:** HepB vaccine protects against hepatitis B. **RV:** RV vaccine protects against rotavirus. **DTaP:** DTaP vaccine protects against diphtheria, tetanus, and pertussis (whooping cough). **Hib:** Hib protects against *H. influenzae* type b. **PCV:** PCV vaccine protects against pneumococcus. **IPV:** IPV protects against polio. **Influenza:** Influenza protects against flu. **MMR:** MMR protects against measles, mumps, and rubella. **Varicella:** Varicella protects against chickenpox. **HepA:** HepA vaccine protects against hepatitis A. (Reproduced from the Centers for Disease Control and Prevention (CDC).

TABLE 8.15. Common Vaccines and Their Contraindications

Vaccine	Contraindications
All	Previous anaphylactic reaction to specific vaccine or vaccine constituent
Live vaccines MMR Varicella OPV Influenza (live) Oral yellow fever typhoid Smallpox (vaccinia)	1° or 2° immunodeficiency Pregnancy Significant contacts of previous[a]
Influenza (inactivated)	Anaphylactic reaction to eggs
HBV	Anaphylactic reaction to baker's yeast
HAV	Anaphylactic reaction to 2-phenoxyethanol or alum
DTaP	History of encephalopathy < 7 d from prior DTaP

DTaP, diphtheria, tetanus, acellular pertussis vaccine; HAV, hepatitis A virus; HBV, hepatitis B virus; MMR, measles, mumps, rubella vaccine; OPV, oral polio vaccine.

[a]For live flu and vaccinia vaccines.

REVIEW QUESTIONS

QUESTIONS

1. Which of the following is an appropriate antibiotic for the treatment of community-associated methicillin-resistant S. *aureus* (CA-MRSA)?
   A. Cephalexin
   B. Azithromycin
   C. Trimethoprim-sulfamethoxazole (TMP)
   D. Levofloxacin

2. An otherwise health 35-year-old man steps on a rusty nail. He states he received all his routine childhood vaccinations. His believes his last booster was 6 years ago. You should:
   A. Administer a tetanus booster and tetanus immunoglobulin because this is a tetanus prone wound.
   B. Administer a tetanus booster.
   C. Do not administer a booster. He is covered for 10 years.
   D. Do not administer a booster. He is covered for 10 years. However, prescribe antibiotics for cellulitis prophylaxis.

3. Patients with suspected gonorrhea often are coinfected with *Chlamydia*. Coinfection rates are estimated to be as high as:
   A. 40%
   B. 50%
   C. 60%
   D. 70%

4. The classic lesion of primary syphilis is the:
   A. Chancroid
   B. Condyloma lata
   C. Rash on the palms and soles of the feet
   D. Chancre

5. Which of the following is not a treatment indication for influenza?
   A. Hospitalized patient
   B. 70-year-old woman with chronic obstructive pulmonary disorder (COPD)
   C. 12 month old who tests positive for flu by polymerase chain reaction (PCR)
   D. 48 year old with 3 days of symptoms

6. A patient with a previous history of human immunodeficiency virus (HIV) presents to your emergency room complaining of eye pain and vision loss. He has not taken highly active antiretroviral therapy (HAART) therapy "for months." On funduscopic examination you note "cotton wool" spots. You estimate his CD4 count to be:
   A. 75 cells/mm^3
   B. 150 cells/mm^3
   C. 250 cells/mm^3
   D. 350 cells/mm^3

7. Which of the following statements regarding hantavirus is FALSE?
   A. Leukocytosis, hemoconcentration, and thrombocytopenia are common laboratory findings.
   B. Hypoalbuminemia and acidosis are predictors of disease severity.
   C. Antiviral therapy has been shown to provide improvement in mortality in confirmed infections.
   D. Has had an expanding geographic distribution in the United States, starting in the southwest and now with > 30 states reporting confirmed cases.

8. A patient presents to the emergency department with a fever and malaise 1 year after having a solid organ transplant. What is the most likely etiology of their underlying infection?
   A. Wound infection
   B. Nosocomial infection
   C. Opportunistic infection
   D. Community-acquired infection

9. A patient presents having just pulled off a tick they believe was attached for < 12 hours. They currently have no symptoms and wonder what they should do. What is the correct course of action?
   A. Reassurance
   B. Provide prophylactic antibiotics to prevent superficial skin tract infection.
   C. Provide prophylactic antibiotics to prevent Lyme disease.
   D. Check Lyme serologies.

ANSWERS

1. **C.** The remaining antibiotics have little to no effect on CA-MRSA. Health care–associated MRSA (HA-MRSA) is often treated with vancomycin.

2. **B.** A "tetanus prone" wound should receive a tetanus booster if the last vaccination was > 5 years ago. Because this individual had his routine vaccinations, there is no indication for tetanus immunoglobulin.

3. **A.** Empiric treatment for sexually transmitted diseases should cover both gonorrhea and *Chlamydia*.

4. **D.** The chancroid lesion is painful rather than painless and is associated with *Haemophilus ducreyi*. Condyloma lata and a palmar rash are associated with the later stages of syphilis.

5. **D.** Those hospitalized with influenza should be treated regardless of symptom onset. Those with underlying lung or heart disease should also be treated. However, health individuals > 2 years old and < 65 years old should not receive treatment if symptoms have been present for > 2 days.

6. **A.** This patient has cytomegalovirus (CMV) retinitis which is typically found in patients with a CD4 count of < 100 cells/mm^3.

7. **C.** Supportive care remains the standard of care; however, current studies are underway to evaluate the utility of antivirals in confirmed infections.

8. **D.** Although the immunosuppression transplant patients receive predisposes them to a multitude of infections, once a patient is approximately 6 months status post transplant, their most likely source of infection is community-acquired pathogens.

9. **A.** The current recommendations for asymptomatic tick bites are to only provide prophylaxis for Lyme disease if the patient is in a Lyme endemic region, bitten by *Ixodes scapularis* tick that was attached > 36 hours (or engorged) and is < 72 hours since removal of tick. There are no recommendations to check serologies or provide other prophylaxis.

CHAPTER 9

Hematology, Oncology, Allergy, and Immunology

Jesse W. Loar, MD

RBC Disorders

ANEMIA

Various standards. However, the World Health Organization (WHO) definition: Hemoglobin < **12** g/dL (hematocrit [Hct] < 36%) **in women** and < 13 g/dL **in men** (Hct < 39%).

Causes

Generally caused by decreased production or increased destruction/loss of new erythrocytes. In the emergent setting, the most common cause of acute anemia is rapid erythrocyte loss from bleeding. Chronic anemia is frequently caused by abnormal erythrocyte formation and can be further categorized by MCV values (Table 9.1).

Symptoms/Examination Findings

Signs and symptoms are variable and depend on chronicity and severity of anemia. Clinically severe anemia is indicated by hypotension, tachycardia, tachypnea, altered mental status (AMS), chest pain, syncope, AMS, and severe dyspnea.

Patients with chronic anemia generally present with a more insidious onset of dyspnea, decreased exercise tolerance, fatigue, generalized weakness, and orthostatic dizziness. They tend to have more normal vital signs and less pronounced examination abnormalities.

KEY FACT

Ancillary testing for anemia is affected by blood transfusion, so extra blood should be drawn and saved prior to transfusion.

Diagnosis

- Initial laboratory tests include complete blood count (CBC) with differential, reticulocyte count, and peripheral smear.
- Other testing based on clinical suspicion for underlying cause (eg, iron studies, B_{12} and folate levels, Coombs testing, serum protein electrophoresis [SPEP], etc).

TABLE 9.1. Classification of Anemia

Type	Pathophysiology	Causes
Microcytic anemia (MCV < 80 fL)	Decreased hemoglobin production	Fe deficiency Thalassemia Lead poisoning Sideroblastic anemia Chronic disease
Macrocytic anemia (MCV > 100 fL)	Decreased DNA synthesis	Vitamin B_{12} deficiency Folate deficiency Sulfa drugs Alcohol abuse
Normocytic anemia	Decreased marrow production of RBCs **or** increased loss or destruction of RBCs	Hemorrhage Hemolysis Aplastic anemia Sickle cell disease Anemia of chronic disease/renal disease

RBC, red blood cell.

Treatment

- Transfuse packed red blood cell (PRBC) as indicated.
  - Symptomatic patients with hemoglobin < 10 g/dL, including patients with acute coronary syndromes.
  - Recent clinical trial evidence proposes a more restrictive policy of transfusing a hemodynamically stable patient to a hemoglobin > 7 g/dL.
  - However, transfuse emergently for any hemodynamically unstable patient.
- Treat underlying causes.

MICROCYTIC ANEMIA

Defined by an MCV < 80 fL. Causes of microcytic anemia can be remembered by the mnemonic FALTS.

Iron Deficiency

One of the most common causes of microcytic anemia. It may be related to poor intake but should prompt evaluation for occult gastrointestinal (GI) bleed. Evaluation of iron studies can help in differentiating the etiology of patient's anemia; see Table 9.2.

Anemia of Chronic Disease

Although typically normocytic and normochromic, it can also be microcytic. Can be differentiated from iron-deficiency anemia by iron studies; see Table 9.2.

MNEMONIC

FALTS

Fe deficiency
Anemia of chronic disease (may also be normocytic)
Lead poisoning
Thalassemia
Sideroblastic anemia

TABLE 9.2. Interpretation of Iron Studies

Test	Normal Result	Iron-Deficiency Level	Notes
Fasting serum iron	60-180 µg/dL	< 60 µg/dL	May be decreased by infection May be increased by hepatitis, hemochromatosis, hemolytic anemia, and aplastic anemia
Total iron-binding capacity	250-400 µg/dL	> 400 µg/dL	May be decreased by infection May be increased by late pregnancy or hepatitis
Percentage saturation of total iron-binding capacity	15%-45%	< 15%	
Serum ferritin	10-10,000 mg/mL	< 10 mg/mL	Reflects iron stores May increase as an acute phase reactant
Bone marrow stainable iron	Presence of hemosiderin granules in reticuloendothelial cells	Absence of hemosiderin granules	Gold standard for assessment of iron stores

Lead Poisoning

Typically associated with construction or manufacturing, though may also be related to paint removal related to paints made prior to 1977. In children typical exposure is ingestion; in adults typical exposure is via inhalation.

Thalassemia

See the following section.

Sideroblastic Anemia

Caused by acquired or congenital defect in porphyrin synthesis. Can be preleukemic state in elderly. Often related to toxins (like chloramphenicol, isoniazid, cycloserine, lead); infections; malignancy; rheumatologic disease; or hemolytic anemia.

MACROCYTIC/MEGALOBLASTIC ANEMIA

Defined by MCV > 100 fL. Megaloblastic anemia (ie, bone marrow) is the most frequent cause of macrocytic anemia (ie, peripheral blood) and occurs with abnormal DNA synthesis, usually related to deficiencies in folic acid or vitamin B_{12} levels. Other causes of macrocytic anemia include liver dysfunction, alcohol abuse, and thyroid disease.

KEY FACT

Vitamin B_{12} deficiency is also associated neurologic findings: typically paresthesias of the hands and feet with decreased proprioception and decreased vibratory sense.

APLASTIC ANEMIA

May be acquired or congenital, although most cases are congenital. Most cases of acquired aplastic anemia are idiopathic; other common causes are listed in Table 9.3.

Therapy involves a combination of removing any clear causative agent, providing supportive care via transfusions and antibiotics (in cases of neutropenia), and some combination of bone marrow transplant and/or immunosuppressive therapy.

TABLE 9.3. Causes of Aplastic Anemia

Congenital disorders	Fanconi anemia is most common.
Drug reaction	Multiple drugs are implicated, though this is uncommon. ▪ NSAIDs ▪ Chloramphenicol ▪ Sulfonamides ▪ Antiepileptic drugs ▪ Nifedipine
Toxin related	Solvents, pesticides/insecticides, radiation.
Viral	Most common is parvovirus B19. HIV and hepatitis have also been implicated.

HIV, human immunodeficiency virus; NSAID, nonsteroidal anti-inflammatory drug.

TABLE 9.4. Classification of Hemolytic Anemia

Hereditary Disorders	Acquired Disorders
Abnormal membrane - Hereditary spherocytosis - Hereditary elliptocytosis - Hereditary pyropoikilocytosis	Immune related - Warm antibody (related to autoimmune disorders, medications, lymphoproliferative disorders) - Cold antibody (usually related to infection like mycoplasma or EBV)
Abnormal enzymes - G6PD	Microangiopathic anemia - DIC, TTP, Preeclampsia
Hemoglobinopathies - Sickle cell disease, thalassemia	Mechanical shear from cardiac valves
	Sequestration from splenomegaly
	Membrane abnormality - Paroxysmal nocturnal hemoglobinuria

DIC, disseminated intravascular coagulation; EBV, Epstein-Barr virus; TTP, thrombotic thrombocytopenic purpura.

HEMOLYTIC ANEMIAS

Hemolytic anemia results from the destruction of red blood cells (RBCs) due to an **inherited** or **acquired** disorder (Table 9.4). Destruction may occur within the blood vessels (intravascular hemolysis) or because of sequestration elsewhere in the body (extravascular hemolysis). A component of both intra- and extravascular hemolysis is often present.

Pathophysiology

- **Intravascular hemolysis:** Intravascular RBC lysis leads to release of hemoglobin and lactate dehydrogenase (LDH) with associated reduction in haptoglobin (binds free hemoglobin), hemoglobinuria; presence of schistocytes (Figure 9.1).
- **Extravascular hemolysis:** RBCs with membrane alterations or antibody/complement bound membranes are phagocytized by macrophages in spleen and liver leading to increased levels of unconjugated bilirubin and LDH and partially ingested RBCs present (spherocytes).

KEY FACT

Patients with hemolysis may present with signs and symptoms of cholelithiasis or cholecystitis because of bilirubin gallstone formation.

Symptoms/Examination

- Signs and symptoms are typically attributed to the resultant anemia and include shortness of breath, fatigue, and pale or yellow skin. Dark urine related to hemoglobinuria usually indicates intravascular hemolysis. Splenomegaly is more common in extravascular hemolysis.
- Intravascular hemolysis tends to produce a more severe and more acute anemia so tends to have more dramatic presentation.

KEY FACT

Red cell production, measured by a reticulocyte count, should be increased in patients with hemolytic anemia.

Diagnosis

- In intravascular hemolysis, look for increased LDH, decreased haptoglobin, hemoglobinuria, and schistocytes.
- In extravascular hemolysis, look for indirect hyperbilirubinemia, increased LDH, and spherocytes.

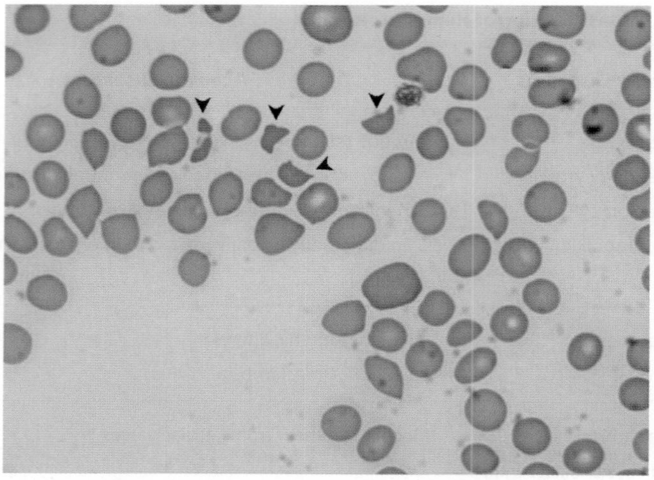

FIGURE 9.1. Schistocytes. Multiple fragmented red blood cells (black arrowheads) seen on this peripheral smear at 100X in a patient with microangiopathic hemolytic anemia. (Reproduced, with permission, from Knoop KJ, Stack LB, Storrow AB, et al. *The Atlas of Emergency Medicine*. 3rd ed. New York, NY: McGraw-Hill Education; 2010. Figure 25.25. (Photographer: James P. Elrod, MD, PhD.)

- Reticulocyte count should be elevated (> 4%-5%).
- **Positive direct or indirect Coombs** test (if due to membrane antibodies).

Hereditary Spherocytosis

Autosomal dominate disease caused by a defect in red cell membrane protein. More common among persons of Northern European decent. Severity of hemolysis ranges from mild to severe.

Pathophysiology

RBCs take on a microspherocytic shape that is unable to pass through the spleen leading to RBC destruction.

Symptoms/Examination

- Anemia, jaundice, splenomegaly.
- Symptoms/findings consistent with cholelithiasis are common.

Diagnosis

- Peripheral smear with **spherocytes**.
- Negative Coombs test (to rule out autoimmune hemolytic anemia).
- **Osmotic fragility test** is confirmative.

> **KEY FACT**
>
> Spherocytes may also be seen in microangiopathic hemolytic anemia.

Treatment

Folic acid supplementation in mild-moderate disease; splenectomy is curative and indicated for severe anemia.

G6PD Deficiency

This X-linked recessive disorder results in RBCs that are more susceptible to oxidant stress. Level of G6PD deficiency ranges from mild to severe. The disease is common in people of African, Asian, and Mediterranean descent.

Pathophysiology

Oxidant stress (Table 9.5) leads to hemoglobin precipitation within the RBC and subsequently both intravascular cell lysis and removal of cell from circulation via spleen.

TABLE 9.5. Common Precipitants of Hemolysis in G6PD Deficiency

Drugs (oxidizing agents) Dapsone, methylene blue, **nitrofurantoin, phenazopyridine (Pyridium)**, primaquine sulfonamides, antimalarials
Infection
Fava beans

Symptoms/Examination

- Asymptomatic unless exposed to precipitant.
- Hemolytic crisis = severe hemolysis with dark urine (hemoglobinuria), jaundice, pallor, splenomegaly, dyspnea, and possible vascular collapse.
- Symptoms/findings consistent with cholelithiasis are common.

Diagnosis

- Laboratory findings of both intravascular and extravascular hemolysis.
- Peripheral smear showing **Heinz bodies** (RBCs with precipitated hemoglobin) and degmacytes (aka *"bite cell"* which is an abnormally shaped RBC with ≥ 1 semicircular portions removed from the cell margin).
- Confirm diagnosis with G6PD enzyme activity; should delay testing by 3 weeks after acute event because reticulocytes have more normal levels of G6PD enzyme.

KEY FACT

The classic story for hemolysis due to G6PD deficiency is the **African American male** soldier in Vietnam receiving **treatment for malaria.**

Treatment

Prevention by avoiding precipitants is key; supportive care if hemolysis occurs.

Immune-Mediated Hemolytic Anemia

RBC destruction caused by autoimmune, alloimmune, or drug-induced immunologic reactions targeting RBC cell membranes (Table 9.6).

- **Autoimmune (warm and cold antibody) hemolytic anemia** caused by antibodies formed against native RBC antigens

TABLE 9.6. Classification of Immune-Mediated Hemolytic Anemia

Type	Pathophysiology	Common Triggers
Autoimmune: Warm antibody	IgG antibodies form against native RBC antigens Bind at body temperature	Lymphoproliferative disorder
Autoimmune: Cold antibody	IgM antibodies form against native RBC antigens Bind at cool temperatures	Acute: *Mycoplasma pneumonia* or Epstein-Barr infection Chronic: Lymphoma or Waldenström macroglobulinemia
Alloimmune	Antibodies form in response to foreign RBC antigens	Transfusion reaction Hemolytic disease of newborn
Drug induced	Three possible mechanisms: IgG autoantibody Hapten formation Immune complex formation	Cephalosporins, levodopa, methyldopa, penicillin, sulfa, quinidine, oral hypoglycemic agents, some NSAIDs

IgG, immunoglobulin G; IgM, immunoglobulin M; NSAID, nonsteroidal anti-inflammatory drug; RBC, red blood cell.

- **Alloimmune (transfusion reaction) hemolytic anemia** where RBC antibodies form in response to foreign RBC antigens (ie, transfused blood products)
- **Drug-induced hemolytic anemia** where medication results in antibody, hapten or immune complex formation, and subsequent RBC destruction

PATHOPHYSIOLOGY

Antibody, hapten, or immune complex binding to RBCs leads to rapid cell destruction via complement fixation and/or sequestration by the spleen where affected portions of the RBC membrane are digested by macrophages leading to development of microspherocytes.

SYMPTOMS/EXAMINATION

Degree of symptoms depends on the type and severity of the immune response. Symptoms can include dark urine (hemoglobinuria), jaundice, pallor, splenomegaly, dyspnea, and possible vascular collapse.

DIAGNOSIS

- Microspherocytes on peripheral smear suggest splenic sequestration.
- Positive Coombs test in the case of autoimmune reactions (direct Coombs test measures immunoglobulin G [IgG]-mediated reactions like warm antibody hemolytic anemia; indirect Coombs test measures immunoglobulin M [IgM] or complement mediated reactions like cold antibody hemolytic anemia).

TREATMENT

- Treat underlying cause or stop implicated medication/transfusion.
- Warm antibody hemolytic anemias may respond to high-dose corticosteroids, intravenous (IV) gamma globulin, cytotoxic agents, or splenectomy.
- Cold antibody hemolytic anemia is generally mild and self-limited; therefore, primary treatment is supportive and includes avoidance of cold.

Fragmentation Hemolytic Anemia

Caused by mechanical destruction of RBCs in circulation. Frequently related to mechanical shear from abnormal or artificial heart valves, breakdown of cell wall integrity from repetitive pounding motion related to marching or long distance running, or cellular destruction during passage through small, damaged, fibrin-containing vessels (termed *microangiopathic hemolytic anemia*) (Table 9.7).

SYMPTOMS/EXAMINATION

General signs and symptoms of intravascular hemolysis. May also see signs and symptoms of underlying disease process.

DIAGNOSIS

Evidence of intravascular hemolysis; schistocytes on peripheral smear.

TABLE 9.7. Causes of Microangiopathic Hemolytic Anemia

DIC
TTP
HUS
Pregnancy
Malignant HTN
Malignancies

DIC, disseminated intravascular coagulation; HTN, hypertension; HUS, hemolytic uremic syndrome; TTP, thrombotic thrombocytopenic purpura.

TREATMENT

Treat underlying cause. Supportive care.

Thrombotic Thrombocytopenic Purpura—Hemolytic Uremic Syndrome

A spectrum of disease marked by **microangiopathic hemolytic anemia and thrombocytopenia** with varying degrees of renal or neurologic involvement.

- Typical or classic hemolytic uremic syndrome (HUS) occurs in children and is recognized as microangiopathic anemia, thrombocytopenia, and renal dysfunction following a diarrheal illness (classically caused by Shiga toxin–producing bacteria-like *Escherichia coli*, *Shigella*, *Salmonella*).
- Classic thrombotic thrombocytopenic purpura (TTP) is caused by congenital or acquired deficiency in ADAMTS13 protein activity.
- Other risk factors for development of TTP-HUS in adults include Shiga toxin–producing bacteria; drugs (quinine, antiplatelet agents, chemotherapeutic agents); malignancy; and pregnancy.

PATHOPHYSIOLOGY

Fibrin deposition and **platelet aggregation** in capillaries and arterioles lead to intravascular hemolysis (microangiopathic hemolytic anemia) and thrombocytopenia.

- Microthrombi in renal vasculature > renal failure
- Microthrombi in central nervous system (CNS) vasculature > neurologic symptoms

SYMPTOMS/EXAMINATION

- Patients often present with nonspecific symptoms. In adults, may see symptoms of anemia and thrombocytopenia primarily. In children, frequent prodrome of diarrheal illness.
- Low-grade fever (90%), jaundice, and purpura are commonly seen.
- Neurologic symptoms may include headache, **AMS**, seizures, and focal neurologic deficits.
- The classic pentad of TTP (fever, anemia, thrombocytopenia, renal failure, and neurology problems) is rarely seen on presentation.

DIAGNOSIS

- Initially based on clinical suspicion such as anemia, jaundice, and low platelet count.
- Confirmed by laboratory findings of microangiopathic hemolytic anemia (ie, anemia with decreased haptoglobin, elevated LDH, and presence of schistocytes on peripheral smear) and thrombocytopenia is adequate to start therapy.
- Need to rule out other causes of microangiopathic anemia like immune hemolytic anemia (rule out with Coombs testing) and disseminated intravascular coagulation (DIC) (rule out with fibrinogen, coagulants, D-dimer). If diarrheal illness is present should collect sample to test for the presence of Shiga toxin–producing bacteria.

TREATMENT

- The mainstay of treatment for TTP-HUS (except children with typical HUS) is **plasma exchange therapy**. Other treatment options that have been suggested, though appear to be less effective, include plasma transfusion, aspirin, and high-dose steroids alone (there may be a role for adjuvant glucocorticoid therapy in certain populations).
- In children with typical HUS, supportive care is usually sufficient for recovery; however, in more severe cases plasma exchange is indicated.

KEY FACT

In children with bloody diarrhea, test for **HUS**: thrombocytopenia, microangiopathic anemia, and renal failure.

Low-grade fevers are common in TTP-HUS; however, high fevers should prompt evaluate for sepsis with DIC as the cause for microangiopathic anemia and thrombocytopenia.

Hemoglobinopathies

THALASSEMIA

Normal hemoglobin is made of paired globin chains ($\alpha_2\beta_2$, $\alpha_2\delta_2$, $\alpha_2\gamma_2$). Thalassemia is an autosomal recessive disorder characterized by deficient synthesis of these globin chains. The most common forms are α- and β-thalassemia, which occurs in people of Mediterranean, African, Middle Eastern, Indian, and Asian descent.

PATHOPHYSIOLOGY

Globin chain gene deletion or mutation leads to deficient α- or β-globin chain synthesis and premature cell death and/or hemolysis.

> **KEY FACT**
>
> Patients with severe forms of thalassemia are at risk of anemia-related heart failure and transfusion-induced iron toxicity.

α-Thalassemia

Occurs when ≥ 1 of the 4 α-globin chain genes fail to function. Severity of disease depends on number of mutated genes.

- Carrier state: one mutated gene; asymptomatic, normal CBC
- α-Thalassemia minor: two mutated genes; usually asymptomatic, mild microcytic anemia
- **Hemoglobin H disease:** three mutated genes; splenomegaly, jaundice, chronic microcytic anemia
- α-Thalassemia major/hydrops fetalis: four mutated genes; fetal demise

β-Thalassemia

Occurs when one or both β-globin chain genes fail to function normally.

- **β-Thalassemia minor:** one mutated gene; asymptomatic, hypochromic, microcytic anemia.
- **β-Thalassemia major/Cooley anemia:** two mutated genes; severe anemia, splenomegaly, frontal bossing. Patients require transfusions to sustain life and iron chelation therapy to prevent complications from chronic transfusions. Splenectomy may reduce transfusion requirements.

SICKLE CELL DISEASE

This autosomal recessive disease is caused by an abnormal structure to both β-globin chains of hemoglobin, resulting in sickling of deoxygenated RBC. Sickle cell trait is caused by defect in only one β-globin chain and produces a less severe form of the disease with sickling only under conditions of **severe** hypoxia.

PATHOPHYSIOLOGY

Deoxygenated RBCs take on sickle shape, which leads to obstruction of RBCs in microcirculation causing vaso-occlusive ischemic tissue injury. Sickled cells are ultimately sequestered and destroyed by liver and spleen.

> **KEY FACT**
>
> Hypoxia, dehydration, and acute infections commonly precipitate or exacerbate sickling.

Vaso-Occlusive Pain Crisis

Most common manifestation of sickle cell crisis.

SYMPTOMS/EXAMINATION

- Usually pain in ribs, back, limbs.
- Pattern of pain is usually consistent from crisis to crisis and may last 5-7 days.

DIAGNOSIS

- A clinical diagnosis and diagnosis of exclusion
- CBC ± reticulocyte count (if hemoglobin levels are below baseline) to evaluate for acute hemolysis or aplastic crisis
- Urinalysis (UA), chest x-ray (CXR), and cultures to evaluate for infection

TREATMENT

- Mainstay of treatment is analgesia. Hydration via IV or PO fluid replacement is indicated for dehydrated patients. Antibiotics should be considered in all patients and should be started empirically in children < 2 years old with a temperature ≥ 39.5°C/103.1°F or white blood cells (WBCs) > 20,000/μL.
- Exchange transfusions are indicated for sickle cell patients with cardiopulmonary collapse, acute CNS event, acute chest syndrome, and priapism.
- Other therapies include hydroxyurea to reduce the frequency of pain crisis, and folic acid supplementation may help reduce degree of chronic anemia.

Acute Chest Syndrome

This disease is caused by a combination of pulmonary vascular **infarction** and/or **infection,** most often by *Chlamydia*, *Mycoplasma*, respiratory syncytial virus (RSV), *Staphylococcus aureus*, and *Streptococcus pneumoniae*.

SYMPTOMS/EXAMINATION

Chest pain, fever, cough, hypoxia.

DIAGNOSIS

CXR showing new pulmonary infiltrate.

TREATMENT

- Supportive care with supplemental O_2, IV hydration, and adequate analgesia. Antibiotics should be started empirically and typically include azithromycin and/or cephalosporins.
- **Exchange transfusion** is indicated for multiple lobe involvement, severe hypoxia, and disease refractory to antibiotics and supportive care.

Splenic Sequestration Crisis

Rapid sequestration of RBCs in spleen causing splenomegaly and severe anemia; occurs in **children 6 months-6 years old**. Usually occur in the setting of a viral illness.

SYMPTOMS/EXAMINATION

Abdominal pain, pallor, splenomegaly, possible shock.

DIAGNOSIS

Very low hemoglobin with evidence for reticulocytosis and palpable splenomegaly.

TREATMENT

- Hemodynamic support
- PRBC transfusion as needed
- Splenectomy for recurrent events

Aplastic Crisis

Sudden decrease in hemoglobin production by bone marrow resulting in severe anemia; usually precipitated by infection (**parvovirus B19**).

TABLE 9.8. Other Presentations of Sickle Cell Disease

Disease	Symptoms	Treatment
Stroke	Aphasia, hemiparesis, visual changes	Exchange transfusions to HbS < 25%.
Ulceration	Most commonly on the medial malleoli of the ankle	Rest, elevate leg, local wound care.
Priapism	Sustained erection, caused by vaso-occlusive crisis	Aspiration of corpus cavernosum with saline irrigation and injection of phenylephrine, surgical intervention if no response after 12 h. Exchange transfusion often used (uncertain efficacy).
Infections	Signs of sepsis, meningitis, pneumonia, osteomyelitis	Increased susceptibility to encapsulated organisms from function asplenism. Low threshold for broad-spectrum antibiotics.
Cholelithiasis	Intermittent RUQ pain	Elective cholecystectomy.
Osteonecrosis	Pain at affected joint (most commonly humeral and femoral heads)	Analgesia, avoid weight bearing, arthroplasty.
Osteomyelitis	Bone pain, fever	Antibiotics for *Streptococcus aureus* and *Salmonella*.

RUQ, right upper quadrant.

Symptoms/Examination

Pallor, lethargy, shock.

Diagnosis

Hemoglobin fall > 2 g/dL from baseline without reticulocytosis (< 2%).

Treatment

- Hemodynamic support
- PRBC transfusion

Other complications of sickle cell disease.

- See Table 9.8.

POLYCYTHEMIA (ERYTHROCYTOSIS)

Polycythemia is defined as an increase in RBC count to a hemoglobin > 16.5 g/dL (Hct > 48%) **in women** and > 18.5 g/dL (Hct > 52%) **in men**. **Primary** polycythemia, called polycythemia vera, is on the spectrum of myeloproliferative disorders and generally affects RBCs, WBCs, and platelets. Causes of **secondary** polycythemia include conditions that increase erythropoietin levels such as lung disease, heart disease, high altitude, and erythropoietin-secreting tumors.

Pathophysiology

Increased RBC production leads to increased blood viscosity with sluggish flow, as well as general venous engorgement.

SIGNS/SYMPTOMS

Usually presents with nonspecific complaints of pruritus, headache, dizziness, blurry, vision changes, and plethora. Other symptoms include:

- Cerebrovascular accident, myocardial infarction (MI), and deep venous thrombosis related to hyperviscosity
- Vertigo, dizziness, blurred vision, and headache related to hypervolemia syndrome
- Epistaxis, easy bruising, and GI bleeding related to platelet dysfunction

DIAGNOSIS

CBC and serum erythropoietin level; a low erythropoietin level and elevated hemoglobin level indicate polycythemia vera; a high erythropoietin level suggests a secondary cause.

TREATMENT

Phlebotomy is primary therapy for both primary and secondary polycythemia with goal Hct of 55%; in secondary polycythemia, treat underlying causes as well.

> **KEY FACT**
>
> Polycythemia vera can lead to both thrombosis (hyperviscosity) and bleeding (platelet dysfunction). Deaths are usually the result of one or both these mechanisms.

DYSHEMOGLOBINEMIAS

Methemoglobinemia

In the presence of oxidizing agents, ferrous iron (Fe^{2+}) changes to ferric iron (Fe^{3+}). Hemoglobin-containing ferric iron does not bind O_2 and is referred to as methemoglobin.

COMMON CAUSES

- Nitrates (in well water or vegetables)
- Medications: Lidocaine, benzocaine, nitrates, nitroglycerin, nitroprusside, sulfonamides, dapsone, phenazopyridine (Pyridium), inhaled nitric oxide

SYMPTOMS/EXAMINATION

- Symptoms range on a spectrum from tachypnea and tachycardia to myocardial ischemia, seizures, or coma. May also see bluish skin discoloration (cyanosis), anxiety, headache, and light-headedness.
- Classically see pulse oximetry of 80%-85% without response to supplemental O_2. However, pulse oximetry is an unreliable test in the presence of methemoglobinemia. Actual tissue O_2 availability may be much lower than suggested by pulse oximetry.
- Chocolate brown blood on venipuncture.

DIAGNOSIS

- Diagnosis should be considered in patients with low SaO_2 and normal PaO_2 on arterial blood gas (ABG). It can be confirmed via co-oximetry, which utilizes varying wavelengths of light to differentiate between oxy-, deoxy-, carboxy-, and methemoglobinemia.
- Symptoms of methemoglobinemia usually occur with methemoglobin levels > 20%; and significant mortality exists for levels > 40%.

TREATMENT

Methylene blue (1-2 mg/kg IV) facilitates the reduction of Fe^{3+} to Fe^{2+} and is indicated for use in any patient that is symptomatic. Methylene blue is contraindicated for use in patients with G6PD deficiency because it may cause hemolysis and worsen symptoms.

> **KEY FACT**
>
> Treat methemoglobinemia with methylene blue (treat blue with blue).

> **KEY FACT**
>
> The amyl nitrite and sodium nitrite in the Cyanide Antidote Kit or "Lilly Kit" work by inducing a methemoglobinemia, which scavenges cyanide. Use the "Lilly Kit" to treat cyanide toxicity, not methemoglobinemia.

> **KEY FACT**
>
> Paradoxical methemoglobinemia—excess methylene blue can cause methemoglobinemia.

Sulfhemoglobinemia

Pathophysiology and causes are similar to methemoglobinemia, but toxicity is usually less severe because sulfhemoglobinemia causes a rightward shift of the O_2 dissociation curve, favoring the release of O_2 (whereas methemoglobinemia causes a leftward shift).

KEY FACT

Inhaled **hydrogen sulfide** (H_2S) acts as a mitochondrial toxin similar to cyanide and is treated with **nitrates** in order to induce a methemoglobinemia. The primary described mechanism of toxicity is not via sulfhemoglobinemia.

CAUSES

Nitrates, sulfonamides, trinitrotoluene.

DIAGNOSIS

Co-oximetry will identify the presence of an abnormal hemoglobin but cannot differentiate between met- and sulfhemoglobin. Adding cyanide to the blood sample changes the absorption pattern of methemoglobin and allows for the identification of sulfhemoglobin.

TREATMENT

- Supportive care. Transfusions may be necessary for severe toxicity.
- Methylene blue does not reduce sulfhemoglobin.

Disorders of White Blood Cells

LEUKOCYTOSIS

This is defined by an elevation in the total WBC count on CBC. Typically, one cell line predominates resulting in a neutrophilia (absolute neutrophil count [ANC] > 7500 cells/μL) or lymphocytosis (defined by > 9000 cells/μL in patients aged 1-6 years; > 7000 cells/μL in patients aged 7-16 years; and > 4000 cells/μL in patients aged > 16 years).

KEY FACT

Neutrophilia without "left shift" is seen when demargination occurs in response to stress, exercise, or drugs (most commonly steroids).

- Neutrophilia usually occurs in response to inflammatory condition or bacterial infection, but can also occur in the setting of physiologic stress (ie, seizures, trauma, ketoacidosis, pain). Presence of a "left shift" (increase in circulation of immature neutrophils) suggests neutrophil destruction as occurs with infection or inflammation. Total WBC counts > 50,000 cells/μL should prompt consideration for a malignancy, but can occur in response to certain infection or metastasis of nonhematologic malignancies and is termed a *leukemoid reaction*.
- Lymphocytosis suggest viral infection or immunologic response, although can be elevated in certain bacterial infections (pertussis and tuberculosis). Sustained lymphocytosis should prompt an evaluation for malignancy.

Leukemoid Reaction

- Nonleukemic leukocytosis of granulocytes: Difficult to differentiate clinically from chronic myeloid leukemia (CML). Usually associated with a normal to elevated leukocyte alkaline phosphatase (LAP) level, compared with CML where LAP is low
- Seen in sepsis, tuberculosis, Hodgkin disease, and metastatic nonhematologic cancers

LEUKEMIAS

Chronic Myeloid Leukemia

- **Least common** of the four major leukemias; primarily an adult disease with median age at diagnosis being 50 years.

- Increased polymorphonuclear neutrophils and myelocytes, anemia seen in 50% of cases.
- **Philadelphia chromosome** is almost uniformly present (translocation between chromosomes 9 and 22).
- Typically asymptomatic. However, symptoms may include fatigue, malaise, weight loss, excessive sweating, abdominal fullness (usually related to splenomegaly), sternal pain (from bone marrow expansion), and bleeding (from platelet dysfunction).

Acute Myeloid Leukemia

- **Most common *acute* leukemia in adults,** median age of onset is 65 years.
- Typically presents with nonspecific symptoms including generalized weakness, fatigue, petechiae or epistaxis and potentially with infection.
- Laboratory findings include anemia, thrombocytopenia, and leukocyte count that is highly variable and can range from < 1000 cells/μL to > 100,000 cells/μL; with blast forms present. Ultimate diagnosis requires bone marrow biopsy.

Chronic Lymphocytic Leukemia

- **Most common leukemia in adults** with diagnosis usually after 65 years of age. Clinically synonymous with small lymphocytic lymphoma (SLL).
- Patients are frequently asymptomatic, although up to 10% have classic "B" symptoms of lymphoma (ie, weight loss, fever, night sweats, extreme fatigue). On examination, the most common finding is nontender lymphadenopathy (usually cervical, supraclavicular, or axillary) with varying degrees of hepatosplenomegaly.
- Laboratory evaluation demonstrates significant lymphocytosis (> 5000 lymphocytes/μL) with neutropenia, anemia, and thrombocytopenia (all of which are typically mild). Diagnosis is made via flow cytometry.

Acute Lymphocytic Leukemia

- Malignancy of childhood with most cases occurring in children from 2-5 years of age.
- Frequently presents with nonspecific symptoms of fever, malaise, bleeding, long bone pain, and painless lymphadenopathy.
- Laboratory test results typically show some degree of anemia, thrombocytopenia, and neutropenia with lymphocytosis and lymphoblasts present on peripheral smear. Final diagnosis requires bone marrow biopsy.

MULTIPLE MYELOMA

Malignant proliferation of a single plasma cell clone with subsequent uncontrolled production of a single immunoglobulin.

Symptoms/Examination

Most patients present with nondescript back pain or other bony pain related to lytic lesions. About one-quarter to one-third of patients also complain of weight loss and generalized fatigue.

Diagnosis

- Diagnosis should be suspected in the setting of new onset, unexplained anemia with renal failure. Elevated protein:albumin ratio can provide some hint to presence of disease.
- Confirmation of disease requires serum/urine electrophoresis. Bone survey should follow confirmation of disease given extensive bony involvement.

Complications

Concern for hypercalcemia, pathologic fracture, hyperviscosity syndrome, and spinal cord compression syndrome.

Treatment

- Only patients with evidence of end-organ disease need treatment. Findings of end-organ damage include anemia, hypercalcemia, renal insufficiency, lytic bone lesions, severe osteopenia, and extramedullary plasmacytoma.
- Mainstay of therapy is **hematopoietic cell transplant**.
- Adjunctive therapy includes bisphosphonates for patients with bony lesions.

Patient should also be advised to stay active to maintain good bone density.

LYMPHOMAS

Hodgkin Lymphoma

A group of lymphoid malignancies characterized by the presence of Reed-Sternberg cells (owl eye cells) contained within a reactive cellular background (Figure 9.2). Typically a disease of young adults (20s-30s) although there is a bimodal distribution with second peak over the age of 50 years.

KEY FACT

Pain at the site of Hodgkin lymphoma disease shortly after drinking alcohol is uncommon, but is specific to the diagnosis of Hodgkin lymphoma.

Symptoms/Examination

- Less than 20% of patients with early disease and > 50% of patients with advanced disease have "B" symptoms (fever > 38.0°C/100.4°F without evidence of an infection, unintentional loss of 10% of body weight in last 6 months, and drenching night sweats).
- Most common clinical findings are painless lymphadenopathy, most commonly in the cervical or supraclavicular nodes.
- Mediastinal adenopathy or mass may be incidentally found on x-ray.

Diagnosis

- Lymph node biopsy

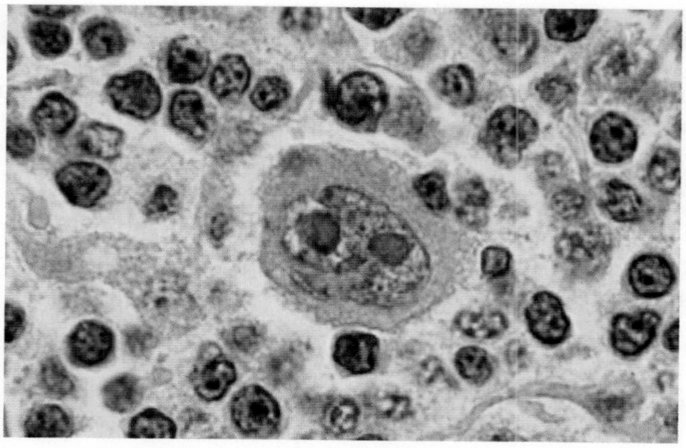

FIGURE 9.2. Diagnostic Reed-Sternberg cell in Hodgkin lymphoma. (Reproduced, with permission, from Lichtman MA, Kipps TJ, Seligsohn U, et al. *Williams Hematology*. 8th ed. New York, NY: McGraw-Hill Education; 2010. Figure 98.34.)

TREATMENT

This is a highly curable disease. Traditionally radiation therapy is the mainstay of therapy for early stage disease; however, given increasing understanding of the risk for development of solid organ tumors (specifically in patient's receiving chest radiation therapy), a combination of radiation and chemotherapy has become more common.

Non-Hodgkin Lymphoma

Heterogeneous group of B-cell and T-cell malignancies that range from indolent to highly aggressive and rapidly fatal. This is generally a disease of the elderly.

Indolent non-Hodgkin lymphomas

- Include follicular lymphomas and small lymphocytic lymphoma (SLL) (synonymous with chronic lymphocytic leukemia).
- Usually present with painless lymphadenopathy. May also have insidious hepatomegaly, splenomegaly, and cytopenias. Extranodal disease (most commonly of the GI tract, but also including skin, testis, bone, and kidney) is less common.
- "B" symptoms are less common.
- Poorly curable and most people present with late stage disease. Treatment can include radiation and chemotherapy but is generally reserved for patients with symptoms.

Aggressive non-Hodgkin lymphoma

- Include diffuse large B-cell lymphoma, anaplastic large cell lymphoma, peripheral T-cell lymphoma, Burkitt lymphoma, and lymphoblastic lymphoma.
- Presentation is often much more dramatic with high prevalence of "B" symptoms, and elevated levels of LDH and uric acid related to rapid cell turnover.
- Extra nodal disease (especially GI and skin disease) is much more common.
- Lymph node biopsy is diagnostic.
- Highly curable so generally treated aggressively, may include admission for urgent biopsy and initiation of therapy. Most common chemotherapy regimen is CHOP (cyclophosphamide, doxorubicin, vincristine, and prednisone) with or without rituximab (an anti-CD20 monoclonal antibody).

> **KEY FACT**
>
> While less commonly seen in the United States, Burkitt lymphoma in Africa is usually associated with Epstein-Barr virus (EBV) infection.
>
> When assessing lymphadenopathy in patients with concern for lymphoma, make sure to evaluate Waldeyer ring (tonsils, base of the tongue, nasopharynx).

LEUKOPENIA

Defined by an absolute WBC count < 4000 cells/μL. Typically one cell line accounts for the drop in total WBC count. Leukopenia is associated with increased susceptibility to infections.

Neutropenia

- Common causes: Aplastic anemia, leukemias, chemotherapy agents
- Mild: ANC 1000-1500 cells/μL—minimal increased risk of infection
- Moderate: ANC 500-1000 cells/μL—moderate increased risk of infection
- Severe: ANC < 500 cells/μL—high risk of overwhelming infections

> **KEY FACT**
>
> ANC = WBC count × (segmented neutrophils + bands)%

Lymphopenia

Common causes: Human immunodeficiency virus (HIV), corticosteroids, leukemias, radiation, chemotherapy agents.

Disorders of Hemostasis

Hemostasis is a balance between clot formation and breakdown.

PRIMARY HEMOSTASIS

Immediate response to vessel injury. Localized vasoconstriction is followed by formation of a primary plug via platelets and von Willebrand factor (vWF).

SECONDARY HEMOSTASIS

Slower process, with activation of the coagulation cascade leading to formation of a fibrin clot. (See Figure 9.3.)

- **Intrinsic** pathway
  - Measure with activated partial thromboplastin time (**aPTT**).
  - Foreign substance (eg, atherosclerotic plaque) leads to factor XII activation that causes a cascade of reactions leading to sequential activation of factors XI, IX, VIII, and ultimately X.
- **Extrinsic** pathway
  - Measure with prothrombin time (**PT**).
  - Tissue damage exposes tissue factor, leading to activation of factor VII activation and subsequently factor X.
- Intrinsic and extrinsic coagulation pathways share a **common final pathway**: Activated factor X leads to activation of factor V that activates thrombin and causes conversion of fibrinogen to fibrin.

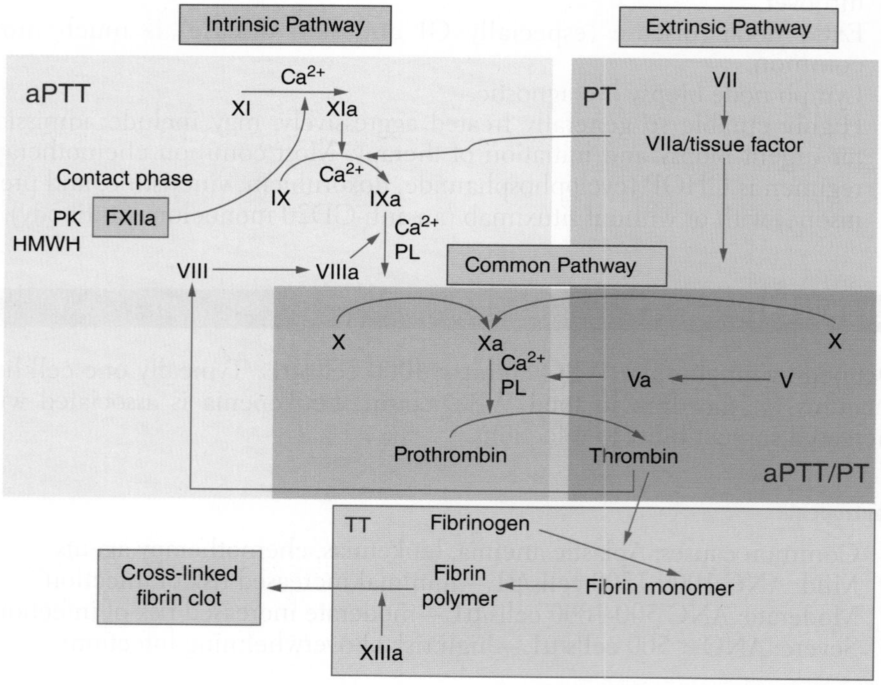

FIGURE 9.3. The coagulation cascade. The intrinsic pathway is measured by the activated partial thromboplastin time (PTT). The extrinsic pathway is measured by the prothrombin time (PT). (Reproduced, with permission, from Longo DL, Kasper DL, Jameson JL, et al. *Harrison's Principles of Medicine*. 18th ed. New York, NY: McGraw-Hill; 2012.)

TABLE 9.9. Use of Laboratory Values to Identify Cause of Increased Bleeding

Laboratory Finding	Causes
Low platelets	See Table 9.10.
Prolonged bleeding time	Platelet dysfunction von Willebrand disease, DIC, antiplatelet medications, uremia, liver disease
Prolonged PT	Abnormality of extrinsic or common pathway Vitamin K deficiency, warfarin, DIC, factor deficiency, liver disease
Prolonged PTT	Abnormality of intrinsic or common pathway Hemophilia A and B, von Willebrand disease, heparin, factor deficiency, liver disease
Low fibrinogen level	Hypoproduction or overconsumption Disseminated intravascular coagulation, large volume transfusion, liver disease, severe malnutrition

DIC, disseminated intravascular coagulation.

FIBRINOLYTIC SYSTEM

Limits size of fibrin clot that forms

- Tissue plasminogen activator (tPA), released from endothelial cells, activates plasminogen to plasmin leading to breakdown of fibrinogen and cross-linked fibrin (creating the degradation product D-dimer).

Evaluation

- Common coagulation studies include CBC with peripheral smear, platelet count, bleeding time, PT, partial thromboplastin time (PTT), fibrinogen level (Table 9.9).
- Other studies may include thrombin time, clot solubility, factor levels, and inhibitor screens.

THROMBOCYTOPENIA

Defined as a platelet count < 100,000/μL. Thrombocytopenia may result from decreased platelet production, increased platelet destruction, or splenic sequestration (Table 9.10).

Symptoms/Examination

Usually presents with petechiae or ecchymosis; bleeding from mucus membranes (including epistaxis and gum bleeding), menorrhagia, or GI bleeding.

Diagnosis

- Diagnosis is based on CBC values.
- Increased bleeding (usually with procedures) may occur when platelets are < 50,000/μL. Risk of life-threatening spontaneous hemorrhage occurs with counts < 20,000/μL and substantially increases with counts < 10,000/μL.

KEY FACT

Prolonged bleeding after injury/surgery or bleeding into joints? Think clotting-factor problems and not low platelets.

KEY FACT

Petechiae, epistaxis, gum bleeding, or vaginal bleeding? Think platelet problems and not coagulation factor disorders.

TABLE 9.10. Common Causes of Thrombocytopenia

Decreased bone marrow production	Marrow infiltration Drugs Toxins Infection/sepsis
Increased platelet destruction	Immunologic ITP Collagen vascular disease (eg, SLE) Leukemia, lymphoma Drug induced (eg, heparin) Infection (typically viral) Mechanical TTP HUS Disseminated intravascular coagulation HELLP syndrome Vasculitis
Splenic sequestration	Hypersplenism

HUS, hemolytic uremic syndrome; ITP, idiopathic thrombocytopenic purpura; SLE, systemic lupus erythematosus; TTP, thrombotic thrombocytopenic purpura.

KEY FACT

Thrombocytopenia in patients with alcoholism results from direct toxicity to the bone marrow from alcohol, folic acid deficiency, and increased sequestration from splenomegaly.

Treatment

- Treat underlying cause if possible.
- Platelet transfusion if:
  - Life-threatening hemorrhage and abnormal platelet level or function
  - Significant hemorrhage or major procedure with platelets < 50,000/μL
  - Platelets < 10,000/μL regardless of bleeding status, exception is in idiopathic thrombocytopenic purpura (ITP), TTP, heparin-induced thrombocytopenia (HIT), HUS

Idiopathic Thrombocytopenic Purpura

Idiopathic thrombocytopenic purpura (ITP) is likely due to immune-mediated removal of platelets by the reticuloendothelial system. It may be an acute (mostly children) or chronic (mostly adults) process. Peak incidence occurs in children (2-6 years old) and adults (20-50 years old). Platelet counts of < 20,000/μL may cause life-threatening hemorrhage.

Symptoms/Examination

- In children, often occurs within 3 weeks of a viral infection.
- Petechiae, gingival bleeding, epistaxis, menorrhagia, and GI bleeding are most common.

KEY FACT

ITP is the most common hemorrhagic disease in children. It is usually self-limited, resolving in weeks to months.

Diagnosis

- Isolated thrombocytopenia on CBC, and peripheral smear with a small number of well-granulated platelets.
- This is a diagnosis of exclusion so must rule out other myelodysplastic disorders, malignancies, and consumptive disorders.

TREATMENT

- Treatment is reserved for severe bleeding with platelets < 50,000/μL or platelet count < 10,000/μL without bleeding.
- For children, the majority have spontaneous remission within 2 months; children should avoid physical activity and nonsteroidal anti-inflammatory drugs (NSAIDs).
- In adults, the mainstays of treatments are prednisone 1-1.5 mg/kg/d and intravenous immunoglobulin (IVIG) or anti-D immunoglobulin. Those unresponsive to steroids and IVIG may need splenectomy or immune modulation therapy. Platelet transfusion is not normally indicated and should be limited to patients with life-threatening hemorrhage.

> **KEY FACT**
>
> ITP: IVIG, steroids
>
> TTP: Exchange transfusions

DISSEMINATED INTRAVASCULAR COAGULATION

Disseminated intravascular coagulation (DIC) is widespread activation of the coagulation and fibrinolytic cascade leading to a life-threatening bleeding disorder. Common causes are listed in Table 9.11.

SYMPTOMS/EXAMINATION

- **Bleeding (most common manifestation)**, involving skin (ie, petechiae and purpura), mucus membranes, venipuncture sites, surgical wounds, GI tract, genitourinary (GU) tract, CNS
- **Thrombosis (uncommonly seen)**, causing focal ischemia in areas of end circulation (extremities, nose, genitalia) and mental status changes

> **KEY FACT**
>
> Infection is the most common cause of DIC. Specific causes include gram-positive and gram-negative sepsis, meningococcemia, typhoid fever, and Rocky Mountain spotted fever.

DIAGNOSIS

- Evidence of:
  - Coagulation product consumption: Prolonged PT and aPTT, low platelet count, low fibrinogen level, increased thrombin time
  - Active clot formation and remodeling: Elevated fibrin degradation product, elevated D-dimer
  - Microangiopathic hemolytic anemia (ie, schistocytes on peripheral smear)

TREATMENT

- Treat underlying disease.
- Other treatment is essentially supportive. Can use fresh frozen plasma (FFP) and cryoprecipitate to replace consumed coagulation factors with significant bleeding. Platelet transfusion should be considered for levels < 50,000/μL

TABLE 9.11. Common Causes of disseminated intravascular coagulation (DIC)

Infection (bacterial, viral, fungal)
Carcinoma (adenocarcinoma, lymphoma, acute leukemia)
Trauma (burns, crush, head injuries)
Shock
Liver disease
Complications of pregnancy (placental abruption, amniotic fluid emboli, fetal death in utero)
Envenomation
ARDS
Transfusion and drug reactions
Surgical procedures
Heat stroke

DIC, disseminated intravascular coagulation; ARDS, acute respiratory distress syndrome.

if serious bleeding persists or patient will need invasive procedures; should consider transfusion prophylactically if levels are < 10,000/μL.
- Use of heparin should be considered if thrombosis predominates.
- Purpura fulminans (protein C deficiency, often seen with meningococcemia) should be treated with protein C concentrate.

VON WILLEBRAND DISEASE

Defined by decreased production or function of vWF; this is the most common hereditary bleeding disorder. The vWF functions to facilitate adherence of platelets to injured blood vessels and also stabilizes factor VIII in plasma.

There are three forms of vWF characterized by their quantitative or qualitative defects:

1. **Type I**, the most common form, has a partial decrease in quantity of vWF; generally mild symptoms only.
2. **Type II (four types)** has dysfunctional vWF, including abnormal binding of factor VIII in some cases.
3. **Type III** has almost no vWF and low-factor VIII levels; this is a rare disorder.

Symptoms/Examination

Usually presents with epistaxis, gingival bleeding, menorrhagia, and GI bleeding. Hemarthrosis and deep tissue bleeding may be present in forms with low-factor VIII levels or activity.

Diagnosis

- aPTT may be prolonged but is usually normal, normal platelet count, normal PT, and **increased bleeding time**.
- Abnormal assay of vWF activity, vWF antigen, or factor VIII coagulant (C) activity.

> **KEY FACT**
>
> Bleeding disorder with normal platelet count, PT, and PTT suggests von Willebrand disease.

Treatment

- **Desmopressin (DDAVP)**
  - Stimulates release of vWF (and factor VIII) stored in vascular endothelial cells
  - Indicted for type I disease and most types of type II disease
- vWF concentrate (either purified or present in intermediate purity factor VIII concentrates)
  - Primary therapy for types II and III disease
  - Should be used in all cases of serious bleeding
- Cryoprecipitate
  - Contains vWF, but carries risk of infectious disease transmission; therefore, it is only recommended when factor VIII concentrates with vWF are not available.

Topical thrombin and antifibrinolytic agents (aminocaproic acid and tranexamic acid) have been used for treatment or prophylaxis of bleeding in select cases (ie, related to dental extraction, tonsillar surgery, epistaxis).

HEMOPHILIA

Hemophilia A (classic hemophilia) and hemophilia B (Christmas disease) are X-linked coagulation disorders characterized by a deficiency in factor VIII and factor IX, respectively. Patients may have mild, moderate, or severe disease depending on their factor activity (5%-10% activity = mild disease, 1%-5% activity = moderate disease, < 1% activity = severe disease).

SYMPTOMS/EXAMINATION

Easy bruising, hemarthrosis, hematuria, and muscle hematoma are most common. May also see excessive bleeding after procedures, severe and/or delayed bleeding after apparent minor trauma (including intracranial hemorrhage and retroperitoneal hematoma formation).

DIAGNOSIS

Prolonged PTT, normal PT, abnormal factor specific assay.

TREATMENT

Treatment is guided by the type of hemophilia, bleeding site, bleeding severity, and presence or absence of inhibitors (see later). In general, factor replacement is required after trauma and prior to any invasive procedure, including central line, lumbar puncture, and arterial puncture. Adjunctive tranexamic acid and aminocaproic acid can be used to help prevent clot dissolution in patients with hemophilia. Disease specific treatment recommendations are as follows:

Hemophilia A

- **DDAVP**
  - Triggers release of preformed vWF and factor VIII from endothelial cells and leads to an increase in plasma factor VIII levels by 3- to 5-fold within 30 minutes. Indicated for mild-to-moderate bleeding in patients with mild hemophilia (ie, > 10% factor activity).
- **Factor VIII replacement**
  - See Table 9.12 for factor replacement guidelines.
  - Each U/kg of factor VIII raises factor VIII levels by 2%.
  - Units of factor VIII required = weight (kg) × 0.5 × (% activity desired – % intrinsic activity).
  - For those with low concentrations of inhibitors, an increased factor dose can be given in attempt to overwhelm existing antibodies.

Hemophilia B

Congenital, X-linked deficiency in factor IX. See Table 9.12 for factor replacement guidelines.

- **Factor IX replacement**
  - Each U/kg of factor IX raises factor IX levels by 1%.
- Units of factor IX required = weight (kg) × 1 × (% activity desired – % intrinsic activity).

TABLE 9.12. Factor Replacement Guidelines

Bleeding Site	Desired Factor Level (%)
Deep muscle	40-50
Joint	30-50
Epistaxis	80-100
Oral mucosa	50
GI tract	100
CNS	100

CNS, central nervous system; GI, gastrointestinal.

Q

A 25-year-old hemophiliac weighing 70 kg presents with a head injury and decreased mental status after a high-speed MVC. What is the level of factor (in %) that is desired in this patient? How much replacement should be given?

KEY FACT

Assume the present level of factor VIII is zero unless it is previously known.

A

This patient must be presumed to have intracranial hemorrhage and requires 100% factor replacement. Based on a starting factor level of 0% and with each unit/kg of factor VIII raising the plasma level by 2%, the number of units of factor required is 3500 (0.5 U/kg × 70 kg × 100% increase needed).

Inhibitors in Hemophilia

Patients may develop inhibitors (antibodies against replacement factors) limiting effectiveness of factor replacement and leading to risk of anaphylaxis during factor replacement in patients with hemophilia B.

- Presence of inhibitors is determined via the clotting factor mixing test. The clotting factor mixing test mixes normal plasma with a patient's serum. Under normal circumstances, the PTT should normalize. If the PTT remains prolonged, then the patient's serum contains an inhibitor.
- Patients with low levels of inhibitors may be treated with increased factor VIII replacement to attempt to overwhelm the inhibitor; because of the risk for anaphylaxis, factor XI replacement should be used with extreme caution in patients with hemophilia B and known inhibitors. Hemophiliacs with serious bleeding and high inhibitor levels, or a history of anaphylaxis to factor replacement should be treated with alternative therapy such as activated prothrombin complex concentrates (PCCs) or factor VIIa.

KEY FACT

Inhibitors are present in all patients with acquired hemophilia and also develop in about 20% of patients with inherited hemophilia.

Anticoagulation and Antiplatelet Agents

Anticoagulant and antiplatelet therapy are used to treat and prevent thrombosis.

UNFRACTIONATED HEPARIN

Primarily works through antithrombin III to inhibit thrombin and factor Xa to prevent clot propagation.

Contraindications

Hypersensitivity, active GI bleeding, intracranial hemorrhage, current bacterial endocarditis, HIT.

Monitoring

Follow aPTT and titrate based on therapeutic range (usually 1.5-2.5 × the normal value).

Complications

- Major bleeding
  - Treatment: Stop heparin, administer **protamine sulfate** (1 mg for every 100 unit of heparin over the previous 4 hours, max 50 mg). There is a risk of severe anaphylaxis with protamine, so administer slowly.
- **HIT syndrome**
  - Autoimmune response to heparin with typical onset within 5-7 days of heparin therapy; delayed onset is possible.
  - **Diagnosis**: Suspect if > 50% reduction in platelets or thrombosis; confirmed with HIT-specific assays.
  - **Treatment**: Anticoagulation with direct thrombin inhibitor (eg, bivalirudin) or heparinoids.

KEY FACT

HIT syndrome is less common with low-molecular-weight heparin (LMWH) than with heparin. In patients with HIT, stop the heparin or LMWH and start a direct thrombin inhibitor.

LOW-MOLECULAR-WEIGHT HEPARIN

Works by primarily inhibiting factor Xa activity; includes enoxaparin, dalteparin, and ardeparin. Cleared by kidneys, therefore needs dose adjustment in renal failure.

CONTRAINDICATIONS

Allergy to low-molecular-weight heparin (LMWH), active bleeding.

MONITORING

Generally no monitoring is necessary; if it is, monitoring is via factor Xa activity. Recommend monitoring in third trimester of pregnancy, in morbid obesity, and for patient with renal failure (ie, glomerular filtration rate [GFR] < 50 mL/min).

> **KEY FACT**
>
> The dosing of LMWF must be reduced in patients with severe renal impairment.

COMPLICATIONS

- Major bleeding: Protamine sulfate has some benefit, but will not completely reverse factor Xa inhibition.
- HIT occurs, but less frequently than with unfractionated heparin; treat with direct thrombin inhibitors or heparinoids.

FONDAPARINUX

Synthetic heparin derivative; inhibits activated factor X. Used primarily as prophylaxis in hip or knee replacements, but can be used for treatment of deep vein thrombosis (DVT)/pulmonary embolism (PE). Cleared by kidneys so contraindicated if GFR < 30 mL/min and must be used with caution if GFR < 50 mL/min.

COMPLICATIONS

- Bleeding can occur; if severe treat with recombinant factor VIIa (can partially reverse effects).
- Does **not** cause HIT, however has not been approved for treatment of patients with HIT.

PARENTERAL DIRECT THROMBIN INHIBITORS

Medications in this class include lepirudin, desirudin, argatroban, and bivalirudin. They function via direct inhibition of thrombin (compared with indirect inhibition produced by heparin and LMWH). They are primarily indicated for use in patients with HIT.

- Lepirudin and desirudin are renally cleared so should be used with caution in patients with renal failure.
- Argatroban is hepatically metabolized so should be used with caution in patients with liver failure.

COMPLICATIONS

Bleeding can occur; no specific antidote for these medications, but has a relatively short half-life so care is supportive.

WARFARIN

Oral anticoagulant that inhibits formation and activation of vitamin **K–dependent** coagulation factors. Vitamin K–dependent factors include II, VII, IX, X; also the anticoagulant factors protein C and protein S.

CONTRAINDICATIONS

Medication allergy, active bleeding, pregnancy, liver failure.

TABLE 9.13. Common Medications Affecting International Normalized Ratio (INR)

Increases INR	Decreases INR
Acetaminophen, amiodarone, amoxicillin, antifungals, cimetidine, doxycycline, fluoroquinolones, macrolides, metronidazole, sulfonamides, SSRIs, garlic, ginger, ginkgo biloba	Carbamazepine, phenytoin, phenobarbital, cholestyramine, dicloxacillin, griseofulvin, haloperidol, nafcillin, ranitidine, rifampin

INR, international normalized ratio; SSRI, selective serotonin reuptake inhibitor.

KEY FACT

IV Vitamin K administration may cause anaphylaxis; use IV form only if major bleeding.

Oral route is the overall preferred route; subcutaneous (sub Q) route is the preferred parenteral route; intramuscular (IM) route should be avoided due to the risk of hematoma formation.

Monitoring

- For most indications, therapeutic international normalized ratio (INR) is 2.0-3.0. For mechanical valves, therapeutic INR is 2.5-3.5.
- Warfarin has a large number of drug-drug interactions, so INR is commonly affected by interaction with concomitant medications. Table 9.13 shows a list of medications that can interfere with INR.

Complications

- Over- or under-anticoagulation. See Table 9.14 for guidelines on treatment of supra-therapeutic INR (ie, over-anticoagulation). Subtherapeutic INR (ie, under-coagulation) is treated with increased dose of warfarin with or without bridge.
- Major bleeding occurs in about 3% of patients. See Table 9.14 for guidelines on warfarin reversal.

Paradoxical thrombosis and **warfarin-induced skin necrosis** can occur between the second and tenth day after initiating therapy. Risk is greatly reduced by concurrent use of heparin or LMWH.

THE "NEW ORAL ANTICOAGULANTS"

- **Dabigatran**: Direct thrombin inhibitor. FDA approved for prevention of stroke in nonvalvular atrial fibrillation; treatment of DVT/PE after LMWH bridge; and secondary prevention of PE/DVT. Dose adjustments in renal failure.

TABLE 9.14. Warfarin Reversal

INR	Bleeding	Treatment
< 5	No/minor	Hold or lower dose, recheck INR in 24 h
5-9	No/minor	Hold dose, consider oral vitamin K 1-2.5 mg PO, recheck INR in 24 h
> 9	No/minor	Hold dose, vitamin K 2.5-5 mg PO, recheck INR in 24 h
Any elevation	Major bleeding	Hold dose, vitamin K 10 mg slow IV or sub Q, administer FFP, PCC, or recombinant factor VIIa

FFP, fresh frozen plasma; INR, international normalized ratio; IV, intravenous; PO, by mouth; PCC, prothrombin complex concentrate.

- **Rivaroxaban**: Factor Xa inhibitor. FDA approved for prevention of stroke in nonvalvular atrial fibrillation; treatment of PE/DVT (without LMWH bridge); primary prevention of PE/DVT related to hip or knee surgery; secondary prevention of PE/DVT. Dose adjustments for renal failure.
- **Apixaban**: Factor Xa inhibitor. Same FDA indications as rivaroxaban. May use in renal failure but caution with liver failure.
- **Bleeding risk**: There is no direct reversal agent for bleeding with any of the "new oral anticoagulants." Some studies suggest that minor bleeding can be managed supportively and major bleeding can be treated with PCCs, FFP, and antifibrinolytic agents like tranexamic acid. Charcoal has been suggested for overdoses of these agents given risk for bleeding and general inability to reverse supratherapeutic medication levels. Hemodialysis may be helped in dabigatran overdoses.

KEY FACT

Rivaro**Xa**ban and Api**Xa**ban inhibit factor **Xa**.

ASPIRIN

Aspirin irreversibly inhibits cyclooxygenase (COX-1), which prevents synthesis of thromboxane A_2 and associated platelet aggregation. Onset of action is delayed in enteric-coated formulations.

CONTRAINDICATIONS

Hypersensitivity reaction, severe hepatic disease, bleeding disorder, major GI bleed.

COMPLICATIONS

- Bleeding, related to platelet dysfunction and not thrombocytopenia. Some controversy about platelet transfusion in this population.
- Allergic reactions (usually manifested by bronchospasm), more common in patients with other atopic disease (ie, frequent urticaria or asthma).

THIENOPYRIDINES

Irreversibly inhibit platelet aggregation via adenosine diphosphate receptor antagonism; includes clopidogrel, ticlopidine.

CONTRAINDICATIONS

Active severe bleeding, hypersensitivity.

COMPLICATIONS

- Bleeding. Theoretically this is related primarily to platelet dysfunction, and transfusion of unaffected platelets should help: This practice is still controversial.
- Hypersensitivity reaction.
- Rarely, may see TTP or thrombocytopenia and neutropenia (more common with ticlopidine).

GLYCOPROTEIN IIb/IIIa INHIBITORS

Glycoprotein (GP) IIb/IIIa inhibitors transiently prevent binding of fibrinogen on the IIb/IIIa receptor which inhibits platelet activation. Most sources recommend addition of GP IIb/IIIa inhibitors to conventional anticoagulation for patient receiving percutaneous coronary intervention. GP IIb/IIIa inhibitors include abciximab, tirofiban, and eptifibatide.

Contraindications

Hypersensitivity, bleeding disorder, severe hypertension (systolic blood pressure [SBP] > 200 mm Hg), severe renal insufficiency, major surgery in the preceding 6 weeks, history of hemorrhagic stroke, ischemic stroke within past 30 days.

Complications

- Bleeding; treat with platelet transfusion (somewhat variable response).
- Hypersensitivity reaction.
- Thrombocytopenia has been seen but is rare.

Blood Products

PACKED RED BLOOD CELLS

RBCs that are separated from plasma and packaged into uniform units with an Hct of 55%-80% (depending on additives used). All products are packaged with anticoagulant preservatives of citrate, phosphate, dextrose, and adenine. RBC storage results in the following RBC changes:

- Reduced levels of 2,3-DPG—leads to reduced dissociation of oxygen (so less efficient oxygen delivery), generally reversible within 24 hours of transfusion
- Leakage of potassium in serum
- Spherical and rigid shape of cells—leads to increased small vessel hemolysis

Available Products

Use the most type-specific blood available, depending on urgency of transfusion. Full type and cross-match takes 45-60 minutes, longer (several hours to days) if antibodies are present. Type specific blood can typically be available in 15 minutes if cross-match is not completed. Type O blood is used for immediate, life-threatening hemorrhage. Women of childbearing age or younger should receive O-negative blood.

- Adult unit = 350 mL, Hct 55%-80%; pediatric units = 60 mL, Hct 72%.
- Leukoreduced PRBCs will decrease febrile nonhemolytic reactions; prevent sensitization in patients eligible for bone marrow transplant; prevent platelet alloimmunization in some cases; and minimize risk of virus (cytomegalovirus [CMV], HIV) transmission.

Clinical Indications and Usage

Primary indication for transfusion is end-organ damage related to anemia (ie, MI, stroke, etc). Some other indications include:

- Active or recent bleeding with a hemoglobin level of < 7 g/dL (most literature now supports this hemoglobin level as a transfusion trigger in all patients; however, some sources still debate a trigger of 8-10 g/dL in patients with known cardiac disease).
- Typically, begin by administering two units in adults or 15 mL/kg in children. One unit of PRBCs is sufficient to raise hemoglobin by 1 g/dL.

Complications

In massive transfusion, (> 10 units of PRBCs in 24 hours for the adult patient) coagulopathy, hypothermia, and hypocalcemia (from binding to citrate preservative) may occur. Current clinical trials are evaluating the optimal ratio of empiric PRBC:platelet:FFP transfusion in massive transfusion; however, these ratios have not yet been clearly established. Currently, transfusion of platelets, FFP, and cryoprecipitate should be based on clinical evidence of bleeding and abnormal laboratory values.

- Transfuse 2-4 units of FFP if INR > 1.5.
- Transfuse 1 unit of platelets if count < 50,000/μL.
- Transfuse 10 units of cryoprecipitate if fibrinogen < 100 mg/dL.
- Treat symptomatic hypocalcemia with calcium gluconate.

Febrile transfusion reaction

Most common transfusion reaction; characterized by fevers/chills, malaise. Treatment is symptomatic, usually with Tylenol.

Acute hemolytic transfusion reaction

- Most serious transfusion reaction, typically due to clerical error. ABO incompatibility leads to lysis of transfused RBCs with associated hemoglobinemia and hemoglobinuria.
- Characterized by immediate fevers/chills, headache, back pain, nausea/vomiting, dark urine, hypotension.
- Treatment includes stopping the transfusion, immediate vigorous crystalloid infusion, and diuretic therapy to maintain urine output at 1-2 mL/kg/h.

Allergic reaction

Usually urticaria or hives only (rarely anaphylaxis). Treatment is symptomatic, usually with Benadryl.

Transfusion-related acute lung injury (TRALI)

- Can occur with any plasma-containing blood transfusion, however is most common with FFP or platelets. Usually occurs within 6 hours of transfusion. Signs and symptoms are indistinguishable from acute respiratory distress syndrome.
- Stop transfusion. Treatment is otherwise primarily supportive, no evidence for use of steroids, antihistamines, or diuretics.

Delayed transfusion reaction

- Characterized by delayed extravascular hemolysis due to presence of small amounts of RBC antibodies (not detected on blood-type screening) directed against transfused RBC antigens. Treatment is supportive.

Transfusion-associated graft-versus-host disease

- Occurs when immunocompromised patients are transfused with PRBC containing immunocompetent T lymphocytes, effectively resulting in an unintentional bone marrow transplant. Carries 80% mortality.
- Characterized by rash, elevated liver function tests (LFTs), pancytopenia.
- Prevention is key—use irradiated blood products in immunocompromised patients.

Risk of transfusion-related infection

- **Viral:** Hepatitis B (1:1 million) > hepatitis C (1:1.2 million) > HIV (1:1.5 million). CMV, EBV, and parvovirus are not screened for and can affect immunocompromised patients.
- **Bacterial:** Contaminated samples can lead to bacteremia and sepsis and should be considered in post-transfusion fevers.

PLATELETS

One unit of platelets is sufficient to raise platelet count by 30,000/μL. ABO cross-matching is **not** necessary, though Rh matching is recommended.

Clinical Indications

- Significant hemorrhage or major procedure with platelet count < 50,000/μL.
- Life-threatening hemorrhage with abnormal platelet level or function (as with aspirin or thienopyridine [eg, Plavix] usage).
- As bleeding prophylaxis with platelet level < 10,000/μL. Generally want to avoid empiric/prophylactic platelet transfusion in ITP, TTP, and HIT.

KEY FACT

The most common transfusion reaction = febrile transfusion reaction.

KEY FACT

The most serious transfusion reaction = hemolytic transfusion reaction.

KEY FACT

Patient receiving blood transfusion may develop urticaria or hives, but anaphylaxis is rare.

KEY FACT

Graft-versus-host disease is an extremely rare but usually fatal complication of a transfusion. Give irradiated blood products to immunocompromised patients.

KEY FACT

One unit of platelets will raise the platelet count by 30,000/μL.

FRESH FROZEN PLASMA

One unit of fresh frozen plasma (FFP) contains 1 U/mL of each clotting factors in addition to 1-2 mg/mL of fibrinogen. It **must be ABO compatible** and is typically dosed as 4-6 units (200-250 mL volume per unit) in adults or 15 mL/kg in children.

KEY FACT

FFP contains fibrinogen and all clotting factors.

CLINICAL INDICATIONS

- Significant hemorrhage secondary to coagulopathy; NOT indicated as primary intravascular volume expander.

CRYOPRECIPITATE

Cryoprecipitate contains concentrated factors VIII and XIII, **fibrinogen**, and vWF. Standard dosage is 6-10 units (10-40 mL volume per unit). Does not require ABO matching.

CLINICAL INDICATIONS

- Significant hemorrhage in the setting of low fibrinogen states
- May be used to treat bleeding in hemophilia or von Willebrand disease, although specific factor replacement is preferred over cryoprecipitate

KEY FACT

Cryoprecipitate contains factors VIII and XIII, fibrinogen, and vWF.

PROTHROMBIN COMPLEX CONCENTRATE

Prothrombin complex concentrate (PCC) is a pooled plasma product that **replaces vitamin K–dependent factors II, VII, IX, and X**. There are three factor formulations with only low levels of factor VII, and four factor formulations containing larger amounts of factor VII. It is beneficial in that it can be reconstituted quickly, delivers much lower volume, and therefore can be given faster than FFP.

CLINICAL INDICATIONS

Reversal of warfarin anticoagulation in setting of life-threatening hemorrhage. Reversal occurs within about 10 minutes but is transient so vitamin K should still be given.

RECOMBINANT FACTOR VIIa

Harvested from hamster cells expressing the human factor VII gene. Currently FDA approved only for the control of bleeding in hemophiliacs with inhibitors. It has been used off label for treatment of massive hemorrhage that is not responsive to other therapy or when blood product transfusion has been declined by patients or is not available. There is little data and no standardization of doses for off label uses.

Oncologic Emergencies

HYPERCALCEMIA OF MALIGNANCY

There are a number of neoplastic and non-neoplastic etiologies for hypercalcemia (see the following text). In the setting of cancer, hypercalcemia results from bone destruction (metastasis, multiple myeloma), paraneoplastic syndrome (parathyroid hormone [PTH]-like substance), or osteoclast activation (lymphoma, leukemia).

SIGNS/SYMPTOMS

- Generally present when levels exceed 12 mg/dL, though symptoms vary with acuity and degree of elevation.
- Primary symptoms include anorexia, abdominal pain, nausea and vomiting, constipation, polyuria/polydipsia, hypertension, weakness, confusion, and generalized itching.

> **KEY FACT**
>
> Symptoms of hypercalcemia: Stones, bones, abdominal groans, and psychiatric overtones.

DIAGNOSIS

Serum calcium levels confirm hypercalcemia. In addition, should get a serum PTH level. At high levels, look for electrocardiogram (ECG) with shortened QT interval.

TREATMENT

- **Aggressive saline rehydration** is mainstay of therapy.
- **Bisphosphonates** (pamidronate, zoledronate) inhibit bone resorption and have become the pharmacologic treatment of choice for cancer-associated hypercalcemia.
- **Calcitonin** inhibits bone resorption and increases calcium excretion and can be used until bisphosphonates reach therapeutic effect (in 48-72 hours).
- Phosphate administration can help to bind calcium but cause calcium-phosphate depositions in soft tissue and renal parenchyma; **not** part of emergency department (ED) treatment.
- Loop diuretics are no longer considered first-line therapy but should be considered for use in controlling hypervolemia related to extensive IV hydration.
- Avoidance of medications like thiazide diuretics or lithium to avoid worsening disease.

HYPERVISCOSITY SYNDROME

This syndrome is characterized by microvascular sludging related to increased quantity of cells (ie, lymphocytosis, neutrophilia, polycythemia, thrombocytosis) or paraproteins. Common causes include Waldenström macroglobulinemia (increased IgM), multiple myeloma (increased IgG or immunoglobulin A [IgA]), leukemias with blast transformation, or polycythemia vera.

SIGNS/SYMPTOMS

- Classic presentation: Blurred vision, mucosal bleeding, and neurologic symptoms (headache, dizziness, AMS, dyspnea).
- These may be the first symptoms associated with previously undiagnosed hematologic malignancy.

DIAGNOSIS

- CBC with peripheral smear and serum/urine electrophoresis form the basis of diagnosing underlying illness. Leukocytosis range is generally >100,000/μL but hyperviscosity may occur with lower cell counts during blast crisis.
- Peripheral smear may show rouleaux formation, stacks of RBCs that form in the presence of increased serum proteins, particularly fibrinogen and globulins.
- May see lymphocytosis, neutrophilia, polycythemia on CBC.

> **KEY FACT**
>
> The tendency of RBCs to stack in the presence of fibrinogen causes them to settle faster and provides the basis for the erythrocyte sedimentation rate (ESR) test.

- Serum and urine electrophoresis will show abnormal spikes with Waldenström's macroglobulinemia and multiple myeloma.

TREATMENT

- Two units of phlebotomy with IV fluids hydration can be temporizing measure (and is definitive therapy for polycythemia).
- **Emergent plasmapheresis** for dysproteinemias.
- **Emergency leukapheresis** for blast transformations.
- Chemotherapy.

NEUTROPENIC FEVER

Neutropenic fever is defined as sustained temperatures > 38.0°C/100.4°F or single temperature > 38.3°C/101.0°F in the presence of neutropenia (ANC < 500 cells/μL). Fever may be the only presenting sign. Risk of death increases as the ANC decreases.

> **KEY FACT**
>
> Typhlitis is inflammation or necrosis of the ileum and cecum in neutropenic patients. It is similar to necrotizing enterocolitis in newborns. The mortality rate is 40%-50%.

CAUSES

Most likely sources include respiratory, urinary, GI, and line infection:

- Common bacterial organisms:
  - Gram-negative (*Pseudomonas, E coli, Proteus, Klebsiella*)
  - Gram-positive (*Staphylococcus, Streptococcus*)
- Viral infection (CMV, herpes)
- Opportunistic infections (*Candida* spp; *Pneumocystis jiroveci*, etc)

SIGNS/SYMPTOMS

Range from minimal symptoms to septic shock

DIAGNOSIS

- Signs of inflammation may be diminished by degree of neutropenia; therefore, thorough examination is necessary. Digital rectal examination may increase risk of infection and should **not** be performed.
- Empiric studies should include CBC, chemistries, LFTs, coagulation panel, urinalysis; cultures from indwelling catheter, blood, urine; and CXR.

TREATMENT

- Hemodynamic support.
- Initiate empiric broad-spectrum antibiotic: Monotherapy with cefepime (or equivalent). Add vancomycin if methicillin-resistant *Staphylococcus aureus* (MRSA) suspected or in presence of vascular catheter or soft tissue infection. Add other agents depending on clinical suspicion regarding source of infection.
- Control source of infection with debridement if appropriate or surgical consultation for intra-abdominal infections.

SPINAL CORD COMPRESSION

Presents with back pain at the level of compression with motor, sensory, and autonomic dysfunction below the level of compression.

CAUSES

Common etiologies include multiple myeloma, lymphoma, and metastatic cancer (lung, breast, prostate). The most common site is the thoracic spine followed by lumbar and cervical spine.

Signs/Symptoms

- Back pain is initial symptom in most, although neurologic symptoms are often present by time of diagnosis.
- Vertebral tenderness, sensory abnormality, motor weakness, and cauda equina syndrome may be present.

Diagnosis

Magnetic resonance imaging (MRI) is the gold standard for identifying compressive lesions. Plain films can help to evaluate for bony abnormality (ie, lytic lesions or pathologic fractures). Myelography can be used if MRI is unavailable.

Treatment

- Initial therapy involves pain control and steroids to reduce localized inflammation.
- Spinal cord compression syndrome is an indication for emergent radiation therapy for radiosensitive tumors.
- Neurosurgery may be needed to perform decompressive laminectomy.

SUPERIOR VENA CAVA SYNDROME

Superior vena cava (SVC) syndrome is obstruction of the SVC from underlying malignancy. Obstruction may be due to external pressure on the SVC or invasion of the SVC by tumor and resultant thrombosis.

Causes

Lung cancers and lymphoma are the most common cause of SVC syndrome. Nonmalignant causes include thrombosis around intravascular catheters or devices and compression from large goiter.

Signs/Symptoms

- Earliest signs are periorbital edema, conjunctival suffusion, and facial swelling. Early in the disease course signs are typically present only in the morning with generalized resolution as the day progresses.
- The most common overall presentation is dyspnea (related to tracheal edema), and edema of the face, trunk, and upper extremities.
- Neurologic symptoms, such as severe headache, AMS, and coma may represent cerebral edema or ischemia and represents one of the only true emergencies with SVC syndrome.

Diagnosis

- CXR to evaluate for widened mediastinum
- Computed tomography (CT) of chest with IV contrast
- MRI if cervical or thoracic pain is present—to rule out tumor compressing spinal cord (Rubin syndrome)

Treatment

Primary therapy is supportive and can include supplemental O_2 and elevation of the head of bed to promote venous drainage. Vascular stents with or without radiation is generally indicated for evidence of CNS involvement and may be useful for nonemergent treatment. Steroids and diuretics have been used but have unclear long-term benefit.

Q

A 60-year-old man presents with complaints of fever. His temperatures at home have been running 38.5°C. He has an indwelling catheter in place that is red and tender. Otherwise, he denies other symptoms and does not appear toxic. His CBC shows an ANC of 400/μL. What are your next steps in management?

KEY FACT

Cauda equina syndrome is a form of spinal cord compression involving the terminal portion of the cord. Patients present with some combination of low back pain, saddle anesthesia, bowel and bladder dysfunction, and lower extremity motor and sensory loss.

A

Obtain cultures and start broad-spectrum antibiotics (eg, cefepime or piperacillin/tazobactam, and vancomycin). Remove indwelling catheter. Also do a careful skin examination and check CXR and urine for alternative source of infection.

TUMOR LYSIS SYNDROME

Rapid destruction of large numbers of neoplastic cells associated with rapidly growing malignancies or with initiation of chemotherapy leads to the release of intracellular contents with subsequent metabolic derangements potentially leading to life-threating cardiac arrhythmias and renal failure. Of note, preexisting renal failure greatly increases the risk of developing tumor lysis syndrome.

SIGNS/SYMPTOMS

Constellation of symptoms related to metabolic derangements including fatigue, lethargy, nausea, vomiting, cloudy urine, muscle spasm, AMS, palpitations, and syncope.

DIAGNOSIS

- Hallmarks: Hyperuricemia, hyperkalemia, hyperphosphatemia, and associated hypocalcemia.
- Oliguric renal failure results from uric acid precipitation in the renal tubules.

TREATMENT

- Hyperuricemia should be treated with **vigorous IV hydration and allopurinol** (to reduce production of uric acid). Many sources recommend alkalization of urine to pH > 7, but this should be done with caution because it can exacerbate other metabolic abnormalities.
- Mild-to-moderate hypocalcemia and hyperkalemia should be treated in the standard fashion.
- Hemodialysis can be used for refractory hyperkalemia > 6 mEq/L or hyperuricemia > 10 mg/dL, phosphate levels > 10 mg/dL, creatinine > 10 mg/dL, symptomatic hypocalcemia, or volume overload.

KEY FACT

To make a bicarbonate drip for alkalization of the urine, add three ampules of bicarbonate to 1 L of D_5W.

Dermatologic Manifestations Of Malignancy

Skin manifestations of malignant disease are related to direct tumor spread or via hematogenous or lymphatic metastasis. Table 9.15 lists common skin manifestation of malignancy. Many of these skin findings can also be seen in nonmalignant conditions (eg, acanthosis nigricans in diabetes mellitus [DM], or erythema multiforme in herpes simplex or *Mycoplasma pneumoniae* infection).

Hypersensitivity Reactions

There are four classes of immune-mediated (hypersensitivity) reactions (Table 9.16).

ANAPHYLAXIS

Anaphylaxis is an almost immediate, rapidly progressive, multisystem allergic reaction. Common causes are listed in Table 9.17.

TABLE 9.15. Dermatologic Manifestations of Malignancy

MANIFESTATION	APPEARANCE	ASSOCIATION
Acanthosis nigricans	Hyperpigmentation, velvet-like hyperplasia and hypertrophy of the skin with accentuated skin markings	Gastrointestinal (GI) malignancies primarily, lung and breast cancer
Dermatomyositis	Violaceous rash of eyelids and periorbital region; erythema of face, neck, and upper trunk; progressive muscle weakness	Breast, ovarian, stomach, colon, and lung cancer
Erythema multiforme	Erythematous plaques with pale centers and bright red borders on extremities and oral mucosa	Leukemias and Hodgkin lymphoma
Erythema nodosum	Painful, erythematous nodules on extensor surfaces of lower extremities	Leukemia, Hodgkin lymphoma, and metastatic cancer
Erythroderma	Diffuse erythema of the skin. Associated with intractable pruritus	Hodgkin lymphoma, leukemia, and mycosis fungoides
Acquired ichthyosis	Diffuse, dry scaling lesions; hyperkeratosis of palms and soles	Hodgkin lymphoma; breast, cervical, lung, and colon cancer
Pruritus	Itching and burning sensation of the skin	Hodgkin lymphoma, leukemia, multiple myeloma, polycythemia vera, adenocarcinoma, carcinoid syndrome
Sister Mary Joseph node	Periumbilical nodule	Advanced adenocarcinoma (gastric or ovarian)
Urticaria	Transient areas of raised, red wheels	Hodgkin lymphoma, leukemia, internal malignancy, multiple myeloma
Purpura	Red or purple discoloration of the skin	Hodgkin lymphoma, leukemias, lymphoma, multiple myeloma, polycythemia vera

PATHOPHYSIOLOGY

- **Immune-mediated anaphylaxis**: Allergen exposure in a sensitized individual or immune complex binding leads to immune-mediated mast cell and/or basophil degranulation and release of histamine, serotonin, leukotrienes, and prostaglandins.
- Nonimmune-mediated (previously termed "anaphylactoid reaction") results from direct release of mediators listed earlier (not immunoglobulin E [IgE] mediated).

SYMPTOMS/EXAMINATION

- Flushing, urticaria, pruritus, angioedema, wheezing, stridor, hypotension, abdominal cramps, nausea/vomiting, diarrhea.
- Hypotension during anaphylaxis is a form of distributive shock (like sepsis) in which systemic vascular resistance is decreased. The skin should be warm.

DIAGNOSIS

According to expert consensus, the diagnosis of anaphylaxis can be made if 1 of the following three clinical criteria is met:

1. Acute onset reaction with involvement of skin and/or mucosal tissue along with either respiratory compromise **or** reduced blood pressure **or** symptoms of end-organ dysfunction.

KEY FACT

Most serious reactions occur within minutes of exposure. Some patients, however, may experience a recurrence of symptoms in 4-8 hours.

Q

An 18-year-old patient with Burkitt lymphoma presents 3 days after his last chemotherapy with fatigue, muscle spasms, and palpitations. Laboratory test results obtained show elevated potassium, uric acid, and phosphate levels, and decreased calcium level. The patient's monitor shows a widened QRS complex. What is your suspected diagnosis and next step in management?

TABLE 9.16. Hypersensitivity Reaction

Type of Reaction	Mechanism	Example
Type I: Anaphylactic	IgE-mediated degranulation of mast cells with release of mediators	Anaphylaxis Urticaria Angioedema
Type II: Cytotoxic	IgG or IgM antibodies react with cell antigens with resultant complement activation	Autoimmune hemolytic anemia Goodpasture syndrome
Type III: Immune complex	Immune complex deposition and subsequent complement activation	Serum sickness SLE RA
Type IV: Cell-mediated	Activated T cells against cell surface bound antigens	Contact dermatitis

IgE, immunoglobulin E; IgG, immunoglobulin G; IgM, immunoglobulin M; RA, rheumatoid arthritis; SLE, systemic lupus erythematosus.

KEY FACT

Penicillins and cephalosporins cause > 100 anaphylaxis deaths each year in the United States and are among the most common causes of fatal anaphylaxis.

2. Occurrence of ≥ 2 of the following signs rapidly after exposure to a **likely** allergen: involvement of the skin/mucosal tissue, respiratory compromise, reduced blood pressure (or associated symptoms), or persistent GI symptoms.
3. Reduced blood pressure after exposure to **known** allergen (usually minutes to hours).

Treatment

- Stop offending agent.
- Ensure adequate airway, supplemental O_2, and IV fluids.
- **Epinephrine**: 0.3-0.5 mg (1:1000) IM (pediatric, 0.01 mg/kg, max 0.5 mg). Patients with cardiovascular collapse should receive IV epinephrine (0.1-0.5 mg IV over 5 minutes). Glucagon can be used for patients on β-blockers with symptoms refractory to fluids and epinephrine.
- Antihistamines: H_1 blocker (diphenhydramine) and H_2 blocker (ranitidine, famotidine).

TABLE 9.17. Common Causes of Anaphylaxis

Immune Mediated	Nonimmune Mediated
Medications (any prescription or OTC medications)	Radiographic IV dye
Food (shellfish, nuts, milk, eggs)	Opioids (morphine)
Insect stings (hymenoptera)	Protamine
Blood products	
Latex	

IV, intravenous; OTC, over the counter.

A

Tumor lysis syndrome and severe hyperkalemia. Administer calcium gluconate, insulin IV, one ampule D_{50}, one ampule bicarbonate, albuterol nebulizer, and Kayexalate.

- **Steroids** (prednisone, methylprednisolone).
- Albuterol for bronchospasm.
- Observe patients who receive epinephrine for at least 4 hours prior to discharge. Admit patients with recurrent symptoms.

ANGIOEDEMA

Edema of the deeper dermal and subcutaneous layers of the skin.

CAUSES

- Hereditary angioedema (HAE), an autosomal dominant hereditary disorder associated with C1-inhibitor deficiency
- Medication related:
  - Angiotensin-converting enzyme inhibitor (ACEI) or angiotensin II receptor blockers (ARBs). Accounts for 20%-30% of angioedema seen in the ED. Mediated through bradykinin and substance P. Not associated with features of anaphylaxis or urticarial.
  - NSAIDs have also been implicated in causing angioedema.
- Mast cell mediated: Associated with IgE-mediated hypersensitivity (ie, anaphylaxis, urticarial, etc) or direct mast cell stimulation.

SYMPTOMS/EXAMINATION

Edema may occur anywhere in the body but most concerning is its involvement with tongue, face, and neck. Other common locations involve hands, feet, eyelids, and genitalia. In congenital angioedema, GI tract involvement with associated abdominal pain is not uncommon. Upper airway involvement may lead to dyspnea, cough, hoarseness, and stridor.

DIAGNOSIS

Clinical diagnosis but may obtain a C1 level to screen for HAE; the C1 level is usually low in affected individuals. Nasopharyngoscopy can be used to evaluate for laryngeal edema.

TREATMENT

- Care is primarily supportive after stopping offending medication.
- Epinephrine can be used for severe cases. Antihistamines, epinephrine, and steroids are of limited benefit in HAE and uncertain benefit in ACEI and ARB angioedema.
- For severe, acute attacks of HAE, first-line therapy includes administration of purified human C1 inhibitor, icatibant (a bradykinin B_2-receptor agonist), or ecallantide (a kallikrein inhibitor). FFP contains C1 inhibitor and is an alternative when these medications are not available.

URTICARIA (HIVES)

Pruritic, raised, erythematous, well-demarcated skin lesions; causes listed in Table 9.18.

TREATMENT

Mainstay of treatment is antihistamines. Steroids and/or epinephrine can be used for severe cases. Patients should be counseled to identify and avoid causative agents.

Q

A 40-year-old man with hypertension presents with angioedema involving his tongue. He was prescribed an angiotensin-converting enzyme (ACE) inhibitor last month. After treatment with steroids, H_1/H_2 blockers, and epinephrine, he reports feeling better but continues to have swelling on examination. Nasopharyngoscopy shows laryngeal edema. What is the patient's disposition?

KEY FACT

Sixty percent of cases of ACEI-induced angioedema occur within 1 week of starting the medication. It may, however, occur years after starting the medication.

A

Admit to ICU to closely monitor his airway.

TABLE 9.18. Common Causes of Urticaria

Drugs	PCN, sulfa, ASA, local anesthetics, diuretics, NSAIDs, morphine, codeine, progesterone
Infection	EBV, HBV, Coxsackie, parasitic infections
Environmental	Heat, cold, exercise, metals, animal saliva
Food	Fish, eggs, nuts, shellfish, fruits
Other	Latex, pregnancy, malignancy

ASA, Aspirin; EBV, Epstein-Barr virus; HBV, hepatitis B virus; NSAID, nonsteroidal anti-inflammatory drug; PCN, penicillin.

SERUM SICKNESS

A **type III (immune complex) hypersensitivity reaction,** serum sickness results when injection of an offending agent (Table 9.19) results in antigen-antibody complex formation. These complexes deposit in vessel walls and result in activation of the complement cascade.

KEY FACT

Serum sickness occurs 6-21 days after exposure to foreign antigen or 1-4 days after a reexposure. Symptoms that occur during the initial treatment of a Crotalidae envenomation are not due to serum sickness.

Symptoms/Examination

Onset of symptoms is typically 7-10 days after exposure to causative agent. This may occur much earlier (12-36 hours) in recurrent exposures. Usually presents with a pruritic rash and flulike symptoms (fever, malaise, arthralgia, myalgia).

Diagnosis

This is a clinical diagnosis based on signs/symptoms and history of inciting agent. Serum complement (C3, C4) levels will be decreased.

Treatment

Generally a self-limited illness that stops within 1-2 weeks of stopping offending agent. Initial symptomatic treatment includes antihistamines, NSAIDs, and steroids. Plasmapheresis has been used for severe cases with symptoms that are not responsive to other treatments or when causative agent cannot be withdrawn.

TABLE 9.19. Common Causes of Serum Sickness

Medications	Envenomation
Antibiotics (eg, PCN, sulfonamides)	Hymenoptera
Phenytoin	
Thiazide diuretics	
Barbiturates	
Horse serum antivenom	

PCN, penicillin.

DRUG ALLERGIES

Reactions can range from widespread rash to anaphylaxis to Stevens-Johnson syndrome (SJS).

Hypersensitivity

- Generally characterized by widespread, symmetrical maculopapular rash that erupts shortly after staring medications. Treatment consists of withdrawing offending agent and treating symptomatically with antihistamines and/or steroids.
- Anaphylaxis can occur and needs to be recognized and treated rapidly.

Drug rash with eosinophilia and systemic symptoms (DRESS)

- Widespread rash that usually occurs within 14 days of exposure to offending medication. Mucous membranes are spared. Associated with fever, malaise, lymphadenopathy, and end-organ damage (80% of cases include liver).
- Diagnosis is clinical based on the rash and presence of eosinophilia and end-organ damage on laboratory test results.
- Treatment involves withdrawing offending agent and is otherwise generally supportive including histamines and glucocorticoids. IVIG has not shown clear benefit and perhaps some harm so is not recommended for treatment of DRESS.
- Medications frequently associated with DRESS include allopurinol, antiepileptic medications (carbamazepine, lamotrigine, phenytoin), sulfasalazine, vancomycin, minocycline, dapsone, and sulfamethoxazole.

Stevens-Johnson syndrome—toxic epidermal necrolysis (SJS-TENS)

- Severe, acute, widespread blistering rash that often includes mucous membrane lesions. SJS is defined by sloughing of $< 10\%$ total body surface area, and TENS is defined by sloughing of $> 10\%$ of total body surface area. Typically associated with systemic symptoms including fever, malaise, and symptoms of mucous membrane involvement (sore throat, eye pain, dysuria, dysphagia).
- Commonly associated with allopurinol, antiepileptic medications, sulfa medications.
- Treatment involves withdrawal of culprit agent and transfer to ICU (preferably burn unit). Supportive care is similar to burn care involving wound management, fluid and electrolyte management, and infection prevention.
- Use of steroids, IVIG, and immunomodulators has been suggested but benefit is unclear so their usage is still considered controversial.

Inflammatory Disorders

RAYNAUD PHENOMENON

Disease marked by abnormal vascular response to cold temperatures. May be primary and idiopathic or may be secondary. Secondary causes of Raynaud phenomenon include associated rheumatic diseases (scleroderma, systemic lupus erythematous, Sjögren syndrome, dermatomyositis), toxin related (amphetamines or chemotherapeutic agents), or related to environmental exposures (hypothenar hammer syndrome, frostbite, usage of vibrating tools or frostbite).

Symptoms/Examination

Typical episode involves sharply demarcated color changes of skin to fingers (or toes) related to cold exposure (Figure 9.4). Usually go from white

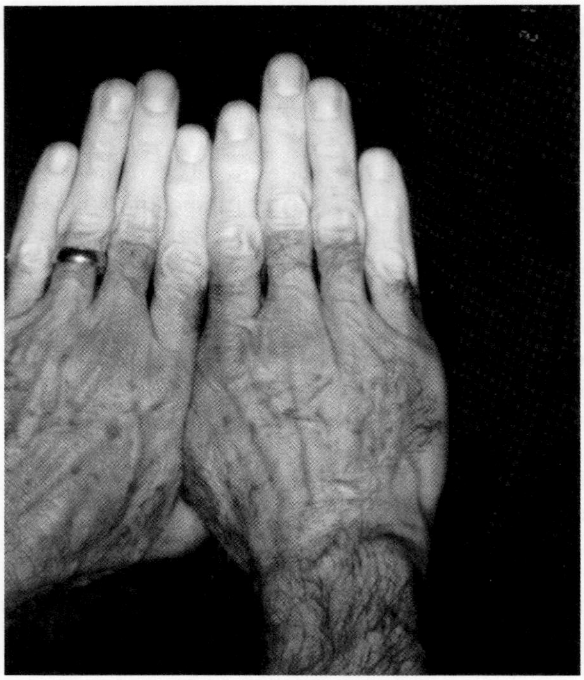

FIGURE 9.4. A typical Raynaud phenomenon attack characterized by a sharp demarcation of skin pallor. (Reproduced, with permission, from Imboden JB, Hellmann DB, Stone JH. *Current Diagnosis & Treatment: Rheumatology*. 3rd ed. New York, NY: McGraw-Hill Education; 2013. Figure 24.1.)

(vasoconstriction) to blue (cyanosis) to red and flushed after rewarming. This is associated with symptoms ranging from paresthesias or burning up to severe pain from tissue ischemia.

Treatment

- Acute attacks should be treated with rewarming.
- After resolution of the initial episode, patients should be educated about cold avoidance, smoking cessation, maintaining whole body warmth, and avoiding sympathomimetic medications.
- Some studies suggest the use of low-dose calcium channel blockers to help prevent or mitigate further attacks.

> **KEY FACT**
>
> **Reactive arthritis symptoms:**
> **Can't see** (conjunctivitis)
> **Can't pee** (urethritis)
> **Can't climb a tree** (arthritis)

REACTIVE ARTHRITIS (FORMERLY KNOWN AS REITER SYNDROME)

Seronegative spondyloarthropathy that is predominantly seen in young males and usually preceded by an GI or GU infections caused by *Chlamydia*, *Yersinia*, *Shigella*, *Salmonella*, *Campylobacter*, or *Clostridium difficile*. The syndrome lasts from one to several months and may recur.

Symptoms/Examination

- Typically 1-4 weeks after acute infection.
- Asymmetric oligoarthritis, predominantly of weight bearing joints of lower extremities, including hips, knees, and heels ("lover's heels").

Extra-articular manifestations may include urethritis, conjunctivitis and/or uveitis, mucocutaneous lesions, and nonspecific systemic symptoms like fevers and malaise.

TREATMENT

- If urethritis—treat for *Chlamydia* and gonorrhea because of frequency of coexisting infection.
- Patients with recurrent ocular inflammation may require immunosuppressant therapy.
- NSAIDs for arthritis. Patients with arthritis who are not responsive to NSAIDs may require intra-articular or systemic glucocorticoids or immune-modulating therapies.

RHEUMATOID ARTHRITIS

Rheumatoid arthritis is a chronic inflammatory autoimmune disease, involving not only the joints but also other organs, including the lung and heart.

SYMPTOMS/EXAMINATION

- Frequent prodrome of generalized fatigue, weakness, and musculoskeletal pain.
- Joints become visibly inflamed during active disease—typically joint involvement is symmetric and starts with small joints, characteristically involving the metacarpophalangeal (MP) and proximal interphalangeal (PIP) joints of hands. Overtime see characteristic and chronic deformities of the hand including ulnar deviation, **swan-neck deformity, and Boutonnière deformity** (Figure 9.5).
- Extra-articular manifestations: Pleural effusion, pericarditis, splenomegaly, vasculitis, subcutaneous nodules (over bony prominences or bursa/tendon sheaths).

> **KEY FACT**
>
> Degeneration of transverse ligaments of C1-C2 can cause instability of the cervical spine so caution during intubation.

DIAGNOSIS

- Inflammatory arthritis involving ≥ **3 joints**.
- Elevated levels of C-reactive protein (CRP) or erythrocyte sedimentation rate (ESR).
- Rheumatoid factor and anti-cyclic citrullinated peptide (anti-CCP) antibodies are present in most.

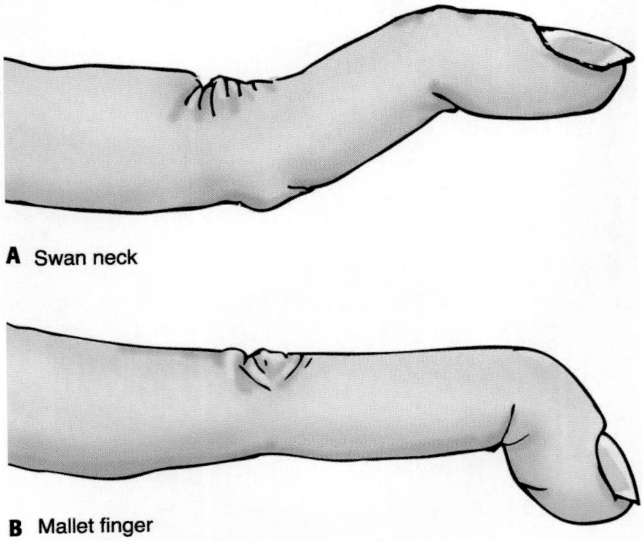

FIGURE 9.5. (A) Swan finger. (B) Boutonnière deformity. (Reproduced, with permission, from Tintinalli JE, Stapczynski S, Ma OJ, et al. *Tintinalli's Emergency Medicine: A Comprehensive Guide*. 7th ed. New York, NY: McGraw-Hill Education; 2011. Figure 41.5.)

Treatment

- NSAIDs or low-dose oral prednisone for arthritis, arthralgias, serositis.
- Additional disease-modifying antirheumatic drugs (DMARDs) include methotrexate, tumor necrosis factor (TNF)-blockers, and monoclonal antibodies.

SYSTEMIC LUPUS ERYTHEMATOSUS

This is an autoimmune disorder affecting multiple organ systems. Systemic lupus erythematosus (SLE) is usually first diagnosed in women of childbearing age. Disease course is highly variable and patients may have acute flares. Drug-induced SLE is often reversible. Disease may be a primary autoimmune disease or may be related to exposure.

KEY FACT

SLE is associated with accelerated ischemic coronary artery disease, and has earned, along with diabetes, the status of "CAD-risk equivalent."

Symptoms/Examination

Symptoms are highly variable and generally include some combination of constitution symptoms, including fatigue, malaise, weight loss, fever; malar rash (Figure 9.6), arthritis, neuro/psychiatric disease, renal disease, pleuritis, and hematologic abnormality (see the following text).

MNEMONIC

Drugs that induce SLE:

HIPPS

Hydralazine
Isoniazid
Phenytoin
Procainamide
Sulfonamides

Diagnosis

The presence of 4 of 11 criteria outlined in mnemonic "DOPAMINE RASH" is diagnostic.

- Hematologic findings can include hemolytic anemia, thrombocytopenia, and leukopenia.

MNEMONIC

SLE criteria:

DOPAMINE RASH

Discoid rash
Oral ulcers
Photosensitive rash
Arthritis
Malar rash (Figure 9.6)
Immunologic criteria (+anti-dsDNA test or +anti-Sm test)
NEeurologic or psychiatric symptoms
Renal disease
Antinuclear antibody+
Serositis (pleural, pericardial, peritoneal)
Hematologic disorders

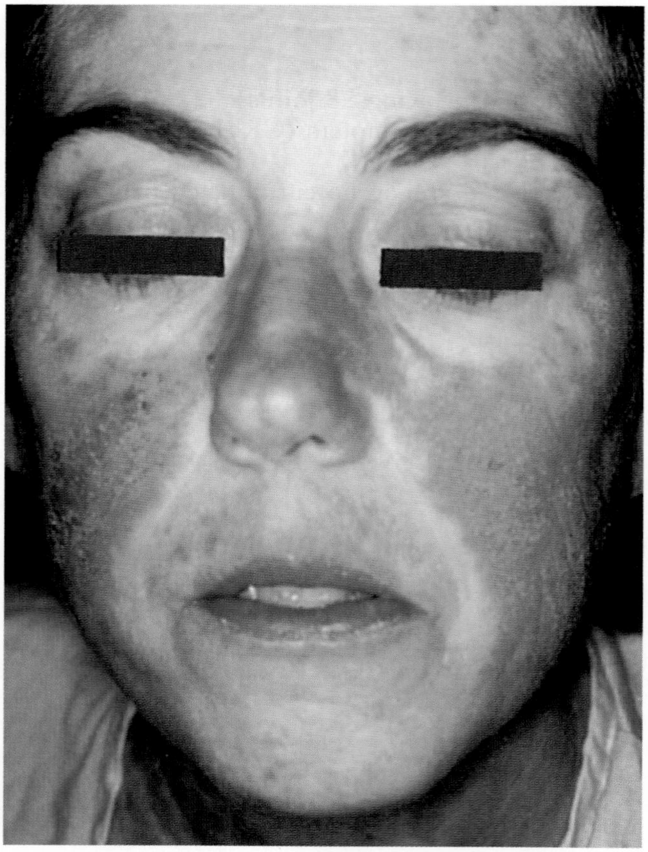

FIGURE 9.6. Malar rash. (Reproduced, with permission, from Kasper D, Fauci A, Hauser S, et al. *Harrison's Principles of Internal Medicine*. 19th ed. New York, NY: McGraw-Hill Education; 2015. Figure 73.5A.)

- Persistent proteinuria (nephritis) is common.
- During acute flares, there is a decrease in C3, C4 levels but an increase in ESR and CRP levels.

TREATMENT

- Highly individualized and based on severity.
- NSAIDs are primary therapy and used to treat arthritis, arthralgias, and serositis. Hydroxychloroquine or chloroquine for rash, malaise, arthralgias. Steroids for life-threatening manifestations, acute flares, and symptoms refractory to conservative therapy. A steroid-sparing immunosuppressive agent such as azathioprine or methotrexate may be required for moderate cases.
- Severe cases may require immunosuppressive agents such as mycophenolate, cyclophosphamide, or rituximab.

COMPLICATIONS

- Nephrotic syndrome or renal failure
- Purulent pericarditis (caused by superinfection with S *aureus*)
- Pleural effusion/tamponade
- Interstitial lung disease, pulmonary hypertension
- Coronary artery vasculitis with acute MI
- Libman-Sacks endocarditis: A noninfectious endocarditis
- Mesenteric vasculitis

SCLERODERMA

A heterogeneous group of disorders characterized by thickening and hardening of skin with varying degrees of associated systemic or other organ system involvement. Broadly scleroderma can be divided into systemic sclerosis or limited cutaneous systemic sclerosis.

SYMPTOMS/EXAMINATION

- Skin findings generally including hardening and thickening of the skin. This may be limited to fingers (sclerodactyly) or more widespread. Other skin findings include edema and pruritus at early stages of the disease; skin ulceration and pitting of fingernails.
- Vasculitic changes typical of Raynaud phenomenon are commonly present.
- Extracutaneous involvement include the GI tract (esophageal dysmotility and incompetence of the lower esophageal sphincter); lung (primary pulmonary hypertension, interstitial lung disease, lung cancer); renal dysfunction; cardiac abnormality (pericarditis, pericardial effusion, myocardial fibrosis, heart failure, myocarditis, MI, arrhythmia/conduction abnormality); and neuropathies.

CREST

A subgroup of limited cutaneous systemic sclerosis that is defined by **C**alcinosis cutis, **R**aynaud phenomenon, **E**sophageal dysmotility, **S**clerodactyly, and **T**elangiectasia.

TREATMENT

- Most treatment is target organ specific (ie, ACE inhibitors for hypertensive renal crisis; calcium channel blockers for Raynaud phenomenon).
- Immunosuppressive therapies are reserved for patients with severe disease (like interstitial lung disease, myocarditis, severe arthritis) or diffuse skin involvement.

Q

A 70-year-old woman presents with new-onset severe, throbbing, unilateral headache. She has also noted proximal muscle weakness and blurry vision. Physical examination shows tender, pulseless temporal artery, and vision loss. What is the suspected diagnosis and next step?

TABLE 9.20. Predominantly Large Vessel Vasculitis

SYNDROME	SIGNS/SYMPTOMS	DIAGNOSIS	TREATMENT
Giant cell arteritis	Involvement of branches of carotid artery → headache, jaw claudication, scalp tenderness, vision changes Polymyalgia rheumatic symptoms are often present	Temporal artery biopsy, ESR > 50 mm/h	Prednisone Low-dose ASA
Behçet disease	Recurrent painful oral and genital ulcers	Biopsy of affected tissue	Prednisone
Takayasu arteritis	Uveitis, iritis, or optic neuritis	Aortic arch arteriogram	Immunosuppressants

ASA, Aspirin; ESR, erythrocyte sedimentation rate.

KEY FACT

The ESR is elevated > 50 mm/h in most patients with giant cell arteritis. Start prednisone 1-2 mg/kg/d immediately to prevent irreversible blindness.

VASCULITIS

Vasculitis is a group of disorders characterized by inflammation and necrosis of blood vessels leading to tissue damage. These disorders are commonly classified according to the size of predominant blood vessels involved, though frequent overlap exists. See Tables 9.20 through 9.22.

SYMPTOMS/EXAMINATION

- Constitutional symptoms include fever, weight loss, malaise, and arthralgias/arthritis.
- Mononeuritis multiplex—defined as nerve damage to at least two named nerves in separate parts of the body.

TABLE 9.21. Predominantly Medium Vessel Vasculitis

SYNDROME	SIGNS/SYMPTOMS	DIAGNOSIS	TREATMENT
Polyarteritis nodosa	Skin ulcers Nephritis Mesenteric ischemia	Biopsy (skin, kidney) Mesenteric angiogram HBV/HCV testing	Prednisone Cyclophosphamide
Wegener granulomatosis	Sinusitis Pulmonary infiltrates Nephritis	*c*-ANCA Lung biopsy	Prednisone Cyclophosphamide
Buerger disease (thromboangiitis obliterans)	Young male smoker with necrotic digits and superficial thrombophlebitis	MRA or angiography	Smoking cessation
Microscopic polyangiitis	Pulmonary infiltrates Nephritis	*p*-ANCA Renal biopsy	Cyclophosphamide

HBV, hepatitis B virus; HCV, hepatitis C virus; MRA, magnetic resonance angiography.

A

Temporal arteritis (giant cell arteritis). The patient will require immediate high-dose oral steroids and temporal artery biopsy within 1-2 days.

TABLE 9.22. Predominantly Small Vessel Vasculitis

Syndrome	Signs/Symptoms	Diagnosis	Treatment
Hypersensitivity vasculitis	Palpable purpura	Skin biopsy	Prednisone
Henoch-Schönlein purpura	Palpable purpura (buttocks, lower extremities) Abdominal pain, nausea/vomiting/diarrhea Hematuria	Skin biopsy Rectal biopsy	Supportive Prednisone
Goodpasture syndrome	Cough and dyspnea Hemoptysis glomerulonephritis	Renal or lung biopsy showing basement membrane antibodies	Supportive Prednisone cyclophosphamide plasmapheresis

- Large vessel involvement: Limb claudication, aortic dilation.
- Medium vessel involvement: Cutaneous nodules, ulcers, digital gangrene, livedo reticularis.
- Small vessel involvement: Purpura, urticaria, splinter hemorrhages, uveitis, episcleritis/scleritis.

KEY FACT

The classic case of Henoch-Schönlein purpura is a boy between 2 and 11 years old who presents with palpable purpura on his legs, edema, and abdominal pain with a history of recent upper respiratory infection (URI).

Diagnosis

Based on combination of clinical, laboratory, biopsy, and radiographic findings.

Treatment

Generally involve glucocorticoid therapy with additional supportive measures as needed.

Transplant-Related Problems

TRANSPLANT-RELATED INFECTIONS

Transplant-related infection may be related to infection of the host with latent, chronic infectious agents from donor tissue (ie, CMV, hepatitis C virus [HCV]); infection of the host with more acute infectious agents from donor tissue (ie, occult bacteremia, influenza), reactivation of latent host infections related to immunosuppression (ie, *Mycobacterium tuberculosis*), or infection of the immunocompromised host by community-acquired (ie, *S pneumoniae*) or opportunistic infections (ie, *P jiroveci*).

Infection risk related to time since transplant

Infectious risk changes during the first year after a transplant as the degree of immunosuppression changes.

- **First month after transplant:** Two common infectious etiologies include latent acute infections (ie, bacteremia, candida species, antimicrobial resistant bacteria, West Nile virus, HIV), that are in donor tissue infect the host; and postsurgical infection (cellulitis, abscess, pneumonia, etc).

- **1-6 months:** CMV, EBV, *P jiroveci*, Chagas disease, endemic fungal disease, and tuberculosis (TB) all become common.
- **More than 6 months:** Usually the lowest levels of immunosuppression so most infections are related to community-acquired agents.

Of note, when patients have graft failure they are typically treated with increasing doses of immunosuppressant therapy that lead to increased risk for opportunistic infections.

Cytomegalovirus (CMV)

- In immunocompetent hosts, CMV infection is generally asymptomatic or causes a mononucleosis type syndrome.
- In immunocompromised hosts, can see a systemic disease that includes nonspecific fever, weakness, and myalgia/arthralgia with some degree of end-organ damage such as nephritis, hepatitis, carditis, pneumonitis, retinitis, or encephalitis.
- Most donor recipients receive prophylaxis with an antiviral like valacyclovir, at least during the early phases of immunosuppression. Acute infections or flairs are typically treated with ganciclovir.

Epstein-Barr virus (EBV)

- Has been associated with post-transplantation lymphoproliferative disorder (PTLD)—a heterogeneous group of conditions potentially leading to malignant lymphoma type disease.
- PTLD carries a 40%-60% mortality rate.
- There is no good therapy for EBV. PTLD is treated supportively with frequent adjunct chemotherapy.

Other viral infections

- Polyomavirus BK has been associated with nephropathy and hemorrhagic cystitis. Treatment involves reduction in immunosuppression. There are no antivirals with good activity against polyomavirus BK.
- John Cunningham (JC) virus is associated with progressive multifocal leukoencephalopathy (marked by rapidly progressive focal neurologic deficits and alteration in mental status).

Central Nervous System Infections

Differential diagnosis includes listeria, herpes simplex virus (HSV), JC virus and *Cryptococcus neoformans*; in addition to more traditional organisms causing bacterial or viral meningitis.

Pneumocystis jiroveci

KEY FACT

Immunocompromised patients cannot receive live vaccines including measles, mumps, and rubella (MMR), varicella, or rotavirus.

- Usually associated with more aggressive immunosuppression during the first 6 months post-transplant, or related to graft failure.
- Presents with cough, dyspnea, and hypoxia out of proportion to radiographic findings.
- Treated with Bactrim. Adjuvant therapy with glucocorticoids has been shown to be beneficial for patients with a $PaO_2 < 70$ mm Hg on room air or A-a gradient of ≥ 35 mm Hg.

Disease prevention

- Patients should have all their vaccines updated prior to starting on immunosuppressive therapies.

- Most patients are maintained on Bactrim prophylaxis and antiviral prophylaxis during the period immediately following transplantation or after increase in immunosuppression. These help to prevent *P jiroveci*, CMV, HSV, etc.

TRANSPLANT REJECTION

Common immunosuppressants for transplant recipients:

- Cyclosporine (Sandimmune, Neoral): Acute toxicity causes reversible vasoconstriction and renal ischemia. Calcium channel blockers and antibiotics (doxycycline, erythromycin) can increase cyclosporine levels.
- Mycophenolate (Cellcept): Side effects include diarrhea, nausea/vomiting, and leukopenia.
- Tacrolimus (Prograf): Side effects include diabetes, nephrotoxicity, seizures, and neuropathy.
- Corticosteroids.

There are three categories of transplant rejection: Hyperacute, acute, and chronic.

- **Hyperacute**: Occurs from a few minutes to hours after surgery and results in irreversible graft destruction.
- **Acute**: Generally occurs 1-12 weeks after transplant and may be reversed.
- **Chronic**: Progressive, insidious decline results in tissue fibrosis, ischemia, and death; no effective therapy.

KEY FACT

A transplant patient's failure to take immunosuppressant medications should be considered an emergency.

Renal Transplant Rejection

SYMPTOMS/EXAMINATION

- Tenderness over allograft (in the left or right iliac fossa)
- Decreased urine output, increased edema, and weight gain
- Elevated serum creatinine
- Worsening hypertension

DIFFERENTIAL DIAGNOSIS

Volume contraction, urinary leak or obstruction, cyclosporine nephrotoxicity, infection.

DIAGNOSIS

UA, serum creatinine, urine protein to creatinine ratio, cyclosporine level (to rule out toxicity), renal ultrasound (to exclude urinary leak or obstruction), and biopsy, if necessary.

KEY FACT

A subtle rise in creatinine may be the only indication of acute rejection of a transplanted kidney.

TREATMENT

- Methylprednisolone, 500 mg IV × 3 days.
- May wait for results of biopsy before initiating steroids.

Lung Transplant Rejection

SYMPTOMS/EXAMINATION

- Cough, dyspnea
- Chest tightness
- Fever (> 0.5°C above baseline)

DIFFERENTIAL DIAGNOSIS

Infection.

KEY FACT

Findings on CXR for acute lung rejection are usually nonspecific and may include perihilar infiltrates, interstitial edema, and pleural effusions.

KEY FACT

An infant has had a cardiac transplant for myocarditis. How might acute cardiac rejection present? **Feeding intolerance, fever, or fussiness.**

KEY FACT

Atropine does not increase HR in patients with a heart transplant. Use isoproterenol, dopamine, or dobutamine.

Transplanted hearts are denervated. Myocardial ischemia will not present with angina but will present as heart failure or with sudden death.

Diagnosis

CXR, ABG, spirometry, drug levels, bronchoscopy.

Treatment

Methylprednisolone, 0.5-1 g IV × 3-5 days.

Heart Transplant Rejection

Symptoms/Examination

Patient may be asymptomatic or complain of generalized fatigue. Evidence of myocardial dysfunction includes signs and symptoms of heart failure (orthopnea, dyspnea, jugular venous distention, paroxysmal nocturnal dyspnea) or dysrhythmias.

Diagnosis

ECG, cardiac enzymes, echocardiogram, **biopsy**.

Treatment

- Methylprednisolone, 0.5-1 g IV × 3-5 days
- Isoproterenol for bradydysrhythmias
- Dopamine or dobutamine for hypotension

Liver Transplant Rejection

Symptoms/Examination

Fever, anorexia, abdominal pain, hepatosplenomegaly; rarely, ascites.

Differential Diagnosis

Vascular thrombosis, biliary anastomotic leak/obstruction, infection, drug toxicity.

Diagnosis

LFTs and biopsy.

Treatment

- Methylprednisolone, 500mg-1g IV
- Broad-spectrum antibiotics if biliary leak is present

Immunodeficiency/Immunosuppression

Immunodeficiency results in increased susceptibility to infection. Patients with defects in **antibody-mediated** immunity (also known as humoral or B cell–mediated immunity) are at particularly increased risk of infection by encapsulated bacteria. By contrast, **cellular** immunity (also known as T-cell–mediated immunity) is more important in protecting patients against viral, intracellular, bacterial, and fungal infections as well as malignancies. There are a wide variety of congenital and acquired immunodeficiencies. Initial evaluation for suspected immunodeficiency includes CBC with differential, quantitative immunoglobulin levels, complement levels, HIV test.

ANTIBODY-MEDIATED IMMUNE DYSFUNCTION

- **IgA deficiency (a selective immunoglobulin deficiency)**
  - Usually presents with recurrent sinus and pulmonary infections
  - At risk for developing severe transfusion reactions

- **Common variable immunodeficiency (CVID)**
  - Low or dysfunctional levels of IgG, IgA, and IgM antibodies.
  - Typically presents with recurrent sinus and pulmonary infections.
- **Hyper-IgE syndrome (Job syndrome)**
  - Presents with recurrent pyogenic infections of the skin and lower respiratory tract.
- **Multiple myeloma**
  - Pathophysiology and treatment discussed more thoroughly earlier.
  - Immunosuppression occurs because of defect in production of opsonizing antibodies.
- **Splenectomy patients**
  - Increased susceptibility to encapsulated bacteria and fungi (*Streptococcus* spp, *Haemophilus influenzae*, *N meningitides*, *Klebsiella pneumoniae*, *Salmonella*, *Pseudomonas*, *Cryptococcus*).
  - Administer pneumococcal, meningococcal, and *H influenzae* type b vaccines.

CELLULAR IMMUNE DYSFUNCTION

- **Bruton agammaglobulinemia**
  - See recurrent bacterial infections.
- **DiGeorge syndrome**
  - Thymic hypoplasia leads to reduced T-cell numbers.
  - Recurrent viral, fungal, and protozoan infections.
- **Chronic mucocutaneous candidiasis**
  - Recurrent candida infections.
- **Severe combined immunodeficiency syndrome**
  - Recurrent viral, bacterial, fungal, and protozoan infections.
- **Wiskott-Aldrich syndrome**
  - Decreased antibody production.
  - Recurrent pyogenic infections, eczema, thrombocytopenia.
- **Hodgkin disease**
  - Impaired delayed-type hypersensitivity recall to antigens.
- **Acquired immune deficiency syndrome (AIDS)**
  - Defined by CD4 counts < 200/μL or AIDS-defining opportunistic infection.
  - See opportunistic infections with *Pneumocystis jiroveci*, *Cryptococcus meningitis*, CNS toxoplasmosis, *Mycobacterium avium* complex, tuberculosis, candidiasis, and CMV.
  - Please see the section on "AIDS" for further discussion.

KEY FACT

Patients with cellular immune dysfunction are susceptible to intracellular infections including *Listeria*, mycobacterium, *Cryptococcus*, fungi, HSV, CMV, and *Pneumocystis jiroveci*.

REVIEW QUESTIONS

QUESTIONS

1. A 4-year-old boy is brought in by his mother for complaint of painless bloody diarrhea for the last several days. There has been no recent travel. Family has no pets although there is a turtle in his class at school. The child is potty trained so the mother is not sure how often he has been going to the bathroom. What should you tell the mother and child about the differential diagnosis and plan for evaluation?
   A. There is a "stomach bug" going around and this probably just represents a viral illness and should resolve in the next 3-5 days.
   B. You just read about how "Flamin' Hot Cheetos" can make stool appear red and you are sure that is probably all this is.
   C. You would like to do some blood work to check on his kidney function and blood counts and would like to collect a stool sample to check for bacteria.
   D. You would like to put in an intravenous (IV), collect a complete blood cell (CBC) count and chemistry, and order an ultrasound to look for "abnormal telescoping of the bowels."

2. A 25-year-old woman who is several hours postpartum from a C-section performed emergently for fetal bradycardia becomes tachycardiac and is noted to have recurrence of severe vaginal bleeding and oozing from IV sites. Which of the following blood tests would not be useful in evaluating this patient's condition?
   A. CBC with differential
   B. Bleeding time
   C. Coagulants (PT/INR, PTT)
   D. D-*dimer*

3. A middle-aged man comes rushing into the emergency department (ED) carrying his 9-year-old nephew. He reports his nephew is in town visiting and they decided to ride bicycles when his nephew collided with a parking block and struck his head on a building wall. When the uncle called the child's father, he was told the child had "Christmas disease" and needed to get to the ED right away. The child weighs 26 kg. How much reversal agent does he need to get?
   A. 1300 units of factor VIII
   B. 2600 units of factor VIII
   C. 1300 units of factor IX
   D. 2600 units of factor IX

4. A 65 year-old man is diagnosed with acute myeloid leukemia (AML) in blast crisis and admitted to hospital to start chemotherapy. He receives no premedications. On the second day of his hospitalization, the patient develops oliguria and widening of his QRS on electrocardiogram (ECG). What laboratory abnormality does NOT fit with this patient's condition?
   A. Hyperkalemia
   B. Hypercalcemia
   C. Hyperuricemia
   D. Elevated creatinine

5. A 30-year-old women presents with swelling of her face, lips, and hands. She has some associated cramping abdominal pain. She reports one similar episode several years ago and reports that her mother used to have similar episodes. She appears to be protecting her airway and you decide to try medical management. What medication is likely to help her the most?
   A. Epinephrine 0.3 mg IM
   B. Solumedrol
   C. Benadryl
   D. Icatibant

6. A 40-year-old woman is started on Bactrim therapy for treatment of a urinary tract infection (UTI). She returns several days later complaining about pain with breathing, pain in multiple joints, and a rash on her face. A CBC is obtained and notable for platelet count of 75,000/μL. What should you tell her?
   A. This is a drug reaction and should get better after she stops taking the antibiotic.
   B. You would like to collect another urine sample and treat her with ceftriaxone IM and doxycycline.
   C. You think it is probably viral and advise her to use Tylenol and ibuprofen for symptom control.
   D. You are not really sure what is going on and would like to ask another colleague.

7. A 55-year-old man with a history of renal transplant 5 years prior presents with cough, low-grade fever, and dyspnea. His vital signs are notable for a room air SaO_2 of 82%. Chest x-ray (CXR) shows mild peribronchial cuffing without focal consolidation. Review of the patient's records shows a recent elevation in his creatinine concerning for possible graft failure with subsequent changes in his immunosuppression. When asked about his graft function, the patient reports he has been working with his nephrology team and did get a couple of new prescriptions several weeks ago but didn't have the money to fill them. What is the next step?
   A. Start azithromycin and ceftriaxone and admit the patient to the hospital.
   B. Start Bactrim and admit the patient to the hospital.
   C. Discharge the patient home with a tank of oxygen a diagnosis of viral illness.
   D. Obtain a computed tomography (CT) angiogram of the chest to evaluate for pulmonary embolism (PE).

8. A 23-year-old man presents with complaints of painful, red, nodular lesions on his shins and several weeks of intermittent subjective fevers, night sweats, and generalized malaise. What are your next steps?
   A. Mark the areas of erythema and start the patient on IV antibiotics.
   B. Consult dermatology to get a punch biopsy before starting him on an empiric steroid.
   C. Ask the patient's about his substance usage and look for other evidence of trauma from falls.
   D. Do a head-to-toe examination including palpation of the cervical, axillary, and inguinal regions; and obtain a CBC with differential and peripheral smear.

ANSWERS

1. **C.** This is a case of hemolytic uremic syndrome (HUS). In childhood, HUS is related to Shiga toxin–producing bacteria such as *Salmonella* which his turtle school pet would put him at risk for. Stool sample should be collected to test for *Salmonella*. CBC to look for anemia and thrombocytopenia. Basic chemistries to look for elevated creatinine.

2. **B.** Patient here is in disseminated intravascular coagulation (DIC). While bleeding time gives insight into platelet function, the pathophysiology of DIC includes consumptive coagulopathy with abnormal fibrin clot formation and associated microangiopathic anemia. These abnormalities will manifest microangiopathic anemia, thrombocytopenia, elevated PT/INR and PTT, and elevated D-dimer.

3. **D.** Christmas disease is hemophilia B, a factor IX deficiency. Replacement is calculated at 1 U/kg × 26 kg (body weight) × 100% replacement (given head injury and unknown starting activity level) = 2600 units of factor IX.

4. **B.** Tumor lysis syndrome is marked by hyperkalemia, hyperuricemia (with subsequent renal failure and elevation of creatinine), and hyperphosphatemia (with associated hypocalcemia).

5. **D.** Patient has a good description for hereditary angioedema. In this case, the bradykinin receptor agonist (icatibant) is more likely to help her than epinephrine IM, Solumedrol, or Benadryl (all of which are used to treat angioedema related to anaphylaxis).

6. **A.** Patient meets criteria for diagnosis of systemic lupus erythematous (malar rash, thrombocytopenia, arthritis, and pleuritis). This is likely related to the sulfa medication she is using for her UTI (ie, Bactrim).

7. **B.** Patient likely has *Pneumocystis jiroveci* pneumonia related to his increasing immunosuppression in the setting of graft reduction. Likely the medications he did not fill are his prophylactic antibiotics.

8. **D.** Presentation is consistent with "B" symptoms and erythema nodosum. Both these are associated with a diagnosis of Hodgkin lymphoma, so a complete examination looking for adenopathy and a CBC looking for lymphocytosis should be done.

CHAPTER 10

Thoracic and Respiratory Disorders

Stephanie A. Crapo, MD

Signs and Symptoms

DYSPNEA

Dyspnea is the uncomfortable awareness of difficult, labored, or unpleasant breathing. Normal resting patients are unaware of the act of breathing. For most patients presenting with dyspnea, there is either a cardiac or pulmonary cause of their symptoms (Table 10.1). Other, less common, causes include psychogenic factors, gastroesophageal reflux disease (GERD), and deconditioning.

Symptoms/Examination

Look for signs of impending respiratory failure (severe tachypnea, tachycardia, stridor, agitation) and evidence for underlying etiology (eg, rash and hypotension with anaphylaxis).

Diagnosis/Treatment

- Conduct a systematic diagnostic and therapeutic evaluation for the cause of dyspnea.
- Obtain a chest x-ray (CXR) at minimum. Obtain other studies (CT-PE, echocardiogram) based on clinical suspicion.

Treatment

Treat underlying condition.

TABLE 10.1. Differential Diagnosis of Dyspnea

	Acute Dyspnea (Minutes to Hours)	Chronic Dyspnea (Days to Years)
Pulmonary disorders	Pneumonia/bronchitis Pulmonary embolism Pneumothorax Bronchospasm (asthma, COPD) Obstruction (angioedema, foreign body)	COPD Asthma Interstitial lung disease Pulmonary hypertension
Cardiovascular disorders	Ischemia CHF Cardiac tamponade	Cardiomyopathy CHF
Other disorders	Metabolic acidosis Anaphylaxis Panic attack/hyperventilation Upper airway obstruction (FB, angioedema, hemorrhage)	Severe anemia Anxiety Gastroesophageal reflux Obesity Neuromuscular disorders (MG, GBS, botulism)

CHF, congestive heart failure; COPD, chronic obstructive pulmonary disease; FB, foreign body; GBS, Guillain-Barré syndrome; MG, myasthenia gravis.

COUGH

Causes

Cough results from stimulation of irritant receptors in the larynx, trachea, and major bronchi. Triggers include mucus, allergens, chemical irritants, gastric acid, and others. Likely etiologies differ depending on whether the cough is acute (< 3 weeks) or more persistent.

Acute Cough

- Acute upper respiratory infection (pertussis, rhinitis, sinusitis)
- Lower respiratory infection
- Asthma/COPD (chronic obstructive pulmonary disease) exacerbation
- Environmental irritants, such as pets, dust, and other allergens
- Airway foreign body

Chronic Cough

- Smoking: Chemical irritant, chronic bronchitis
- Postinfectious postnasal drip
- GERD
- Chronic asthma/COPD
- Angiotensin-converting-enzyme (ACE) inhibitor
- *Bordetella pertussis*
- Other causes: Bronchiectasis, congestive heart failure (CHF), environmental irritants, and recurrent aspiration

Symptoms/Examination

- Inquire about postnasal drip symptoms, asthma, GERD, treatment with ACE inhibitors or angiotensin receptor blockers (ARBs), and smoking.
- Determine if cough is productive (infection, bronchiectasis) or bloody (malignancy, infection, Goodpasture syndrome, Wegener granulomatosis).
- The physical examination should focus on the nasal mucosa, lungs, heart, and extremities (for clubbing).

Diagnosis/Treatment

- Evaluation should be guided by history and examination findings.
- CXR should be obtained if etiology is unclear or if cough persists.
- Treatment should be geared to underlying cause.

> **KEY FACT**
>
> **DDx of Clubbing**
>
> Interstitial lung disease
> Chronic lung infections
> Lung malignancy
> Pulmonary arteriovenous malformation (AVM)
> Cyanotic congenital heart disease
> Infective endocarditis
> Cirrhosis
> Inflammatory bowel disease
> Hyperthyroidism
> Idiopathic
> Hereditary

WHEEZING

A wheeze is a continuous musical sound lasting > 100 milliseconds. It is caused by turbulent airflow through bronchioles narrowed by edema, compression, secretions, hypertrophy, or bronchospasm. Wheezes can be high or low pitched, consist of a single or multiple tones, and occur during inspiration or expiration. Wheezing is most likely to occur in obstructed airways (Table 10.2) but may occasionally be heard in a normal airway.

Symptoms/Examination

Look for symptoms/findings that suggest an underlying cause (eg, unilateral wheezing in toddler suggesting foreign body aspiration).

> **KEY FACT**
>
> All that wheezes is not asthma.

Differential

- **Stridor**: High-pitched and musical, but harsher and of constant pitch; results from narrowing of the upper airway.

TABLE 10.2. Differential Diagnosis of Consequence: Wheezing

Upper airway (more likely to be stridor, may have element of wheezing)
Angioedema: allergic, angiotensin-converting enzyme inhibitor, idiopathic
Foreign body
Infection: croup, epiglottis, tracheitis
Lower airway
Asthma
Transient airway hyperreactivity (usually caused by infection or irritation)
Bronchiolitis
Chronic obstructive pulmonary disease
Foreign body
Cardiovascular
Cardiogenic pulmonary edema ("cardiac asthma")
Noncardiogenic pulmonary edema (acute respiratory distress syndrome)
Pulmonary embolus (rare)
Psychogenic

(Reproduced, with permission, from Tintinalli JE, Stapczynski JS, Ma OJ, et al. *Tintinalli's Emergency Medicine*. 7th ed. New York, NY: McGraw-Hill; 2011:468.)

- **Rhonchi**: Lower in pitch and longer in duration; a "snoring" quality; associated with secretions in larger airways.
- **Crackles**: Intermittent, nonmusical, explosive sounds of very brief duration; due to forced opening of alveoli and small airways held closed due to airway secretions or interstitial diseases.

Diagnosis

- Conduct a systematic diagnostic and therapeutic evaluation for the cause of wheezing.
- If no prior history of wheezing, obtain a CXR at minimum. Obtain other studies based on clinical suspicion.

Treatment

Treat underlying disorder.

CYANOSIS

Cyanosis is a bluish discoloration of the skin or mucous membranes due to the presence of deoxygenated hemoglobin (deoxyhemoglobin or abnormal hemoglobin) in skin capillaries. It is generally detected when there is 5 g/dL (**absolute level**) of deoxygenated hemoglobin in the circulating capillary blood, although it can sometimes be detected at lower levels. The presence of cyanosis suggests (but does not diagnose) tissue hypoxia.

Central Cyanosis

- When abnormal or deoxygenated hemoglobin is circulated
- **Causes** include:
  - R-to-L cardiac shunt
  - Ventilation-perfusion (V/Q) mismatch (eg, PE, interstitial fibrosis)
  - Hypoventilation
  - Hemoglobinopathy (eg, methemoglobinemia)
  - Toxins (eg, cyanide)
  - High altitude

Peripheral Cyanosis

- This is due to slowing of flow of normally oxygenated hemoglobin to the extremity or extremities resulting in ↑ O_2 extraction.
- Causes include shock, arterial/venous obstruction (eg, thrombus, vasoconstriction), and cold.

Symptoms/Examination

- Central cyanosis is best seen on perioral skin, oral mucosa, or conjunctivae.
- Look for symptoms/findings that suggest an underlying cause (eg, lower extremity [LE] cyanosis, hypotension, and abdominal pain in ruptured abdominal aortic aneurysm [AAA]; murmur and central cyanosis in cardiac shunt).

Differential

Pseudocyanosis from heavy metals or drugs (amiodarone, phenothiazine); skin does not blanch with pressure.

Diagnosis

- Conduct a systematic diagnostic and therapeutic evaluation for the cause of cyanosis.
- If central cyanosis is present, the presence of an abnormal form of hemoglobin must be ruled out by arterial blood gas (ABG) with co-oximetry (gold standard). Peripheral cyanosis: ABG normal, central cyanosis: ↓ Sao_2.
- Other tests that may be helpful include a complete blood count (CBC) and CXR.

Treatment

- Administer supplemental O_2, although this will not improve cyanosis in hemoglobinopathy, cyanide poisoning, and anatomic shunt.
- Treat underlying cause.

HEMOPTYSIS

Defined as the coughing up of blood from the lower (below larynx) respiratory tract, hemoptysis can range from blood-streaked sputum to life-threatening bleeding. **Massive hemoptysis** carries a high mortality and is variably defined as the coughing up of > 100-600 mL of blood in a 24-hour period. Massive hemoptysis is almost always due to the bronchial vessels (rather than pulmonary vessels).

> **KEY FACT**
>
> Mild hemoptysis = blood-streaked sputum or tiny amounts of frank blood.

Bronchitis, bronchogenic carcinoma, and bronchiectasis are the most common causes of hemoptysis (Table 10.3), but up to 30% of patients have no identifiable cause even after extensive evaluation.

Symptoms/Examination

Historical clues that suggest a cause:

- A history of tuberculosis (TB) or sarcoidosis → aspergilloma
- Frequent/multiple episodes of pneumonia as a child → bronchiectasis
- A diastolic heart murmur → mitral stenosis
- A history of epistaxis, telangiectasias, and a bruit in the posterior aspect of the lungs → hereditary hemorrhagic telangiectasia with a ruptured pulmonary arteriovenous malformation (AVM)
- Renal insufficiency and hemoptysis → Wegener granulomatosis or Goodpasture syndrome
- Weight loss, tobacco abuse, and cachexia → malignancy

> **KEY FACT**
>
> Autoimmune etiologies of hemoptysis include Goodpasture syndrome and Wegener granulomatosis. Think of these syndromes when there is also hematuria and renal failure.

TABLE 10.3. Causes of Hemoptysis

Most Common Causes	Other Causes
Bronchiectasis[a]	Infection
Bronchitis	Pneumonia
Lung neoplasm	Aspergilloma
	Lung abscess
	TB
	Parasitic infection
	Autoimmune disorder
	Goodpasture syndrome
	Wegener granulomatosis
	Systemic lupus erythematosus
	Cardiovascular
	Pulmonary embolism
	Arteriovenous malformation
	Mitral stenosis
	CHF
	Arterial-tracheal/bronchial fistula
	Bleeding disorder or anticoagulant use
	Trauma
	Cystic fibrosis
	Crack cocaine

CHF, congestive heart failure; TB, Tuberculosis.

[a]Most common cause of massive hemoptysis

KEY FACT

CXR often localizes the site of bleeding in massive hemoptysis.

KEY FACT

Massive hemoptysis almost always originates from the high-pressure bronchial arteries.

Differential

Blood expectorated from the upper respiratory tract and the upper gastrointestinal (GI) tract.

Diagnosis

- Obtain a CXR in all patients with hemoptysis.
- Laboratory studies include CBC with differential, coagulation studies, urinalysis (UA), blood urea nitrogen (BUN), and creatinine.
- Further diagnostic options include high-resolution computed tomography (CT) scan with contrast (stable patients) and bronchoscopy.

Treatment

Nonmassive Hemoptysis

- Treatment is directed at the specific cause (eg, antifungals for aspergilloma).
- Healthy patients with blood-streaked sputum can usually be managed as outpatients. All others require chest CT and consideration for admission.

Massive Hemoptysis

- Treatment is directed toward bringing about abrupt cessation of bleeding.
- Correct coagulopathies if present.
- Place the patient with bleeding side down to theoretically maximize V/Q ratio.

- Intubate with a large bore single-lumen endotracheal tube (ET); selectively intubate the nonbleeding mainstem bronchus, when possible. Double-lumen ETs are **not** preferred (difficult to place, small lumens).
- Urgent bronchoscopy is usually first line: diagnostic and therapeutic (balloon tamponade, topical medications).
- Angiography of the bronchial arteries (a more common site of bleeding than the pulmonary arteries) has been shown to identify the bleeding site in > 90% of patients. Very effective when combined with bronchial artery embolization.
- Emergency surgery for massive hemoptysis is controversial and usually reserved for those with failed embolization.

PLEURAL EFFUSION

Defined as the abnormal accumulation of fluid in the pleural space. In the United States, the most common causes are CHF, pneumonia, and cancer. Pleural effusions are classified as **transudative** or **exudative**.

Transudative Effusion

- Occurs because of an imbalance between hydrostatic and oncotic pressures in the pleural space.
- The main causes are CHF, cirrhosis, and nephrotic syndrome.

Exudative Effusion

- Occurs when inflammation → altered vascular permeability and protein-rich pleural fluid.
- Common causes include malignancy, bacterial, and viral pneumonia, TB, PE, pancreatitis, esophageal rupture, collagen vascular disease, chylothorax, and hemothorax.
- Pleural effusions associated with pneumonia are termed *parapneumonic effusions*. These effusions become **complicated** when ongoing infection leads to formation of empyema with loculations and pleural thickening.

Symptoms/Examination

- Dyspnea, pleuritic chest pain
- Dullness to percussion, ↓ or absent fremitus, and ↓ breath sounds on the affected side
- Findings of underlying disease process (eg, productive cough, fever, and consolidation in parapneumonic effusion)

Diagnosis

- **CXR:** Upright CXR confirms diagnosis in most cases (Figure 10.1). Decubitus films help determine if fluid is free-flowing or loculated. The presence of > 1 cm of fluid on decubitus CXR suggests the presence of a significant amount of fluid.
- Ultrasound can rapidly identify pleural fluid and loculations.
- **Diagnostic thoracentesis:** Most new effusions require diagnostic thoracentesis. An exception would be a new effusion with a clear clinical diagnosis and no evidence for superimposed infection. Fluid is analyzed to distinguish transudate from exudate via Light's criteria (Table 10.4).
  - If exudative effusion is suspected or confirmed, additional pleural fluid analysis should occur (Table 10.5), guided by clinical suspicion for underlying disease process.
- **Chest CT**: Can confirm diagnosis and aid in differentiating underlying disease process (eg, PE, malignancy).

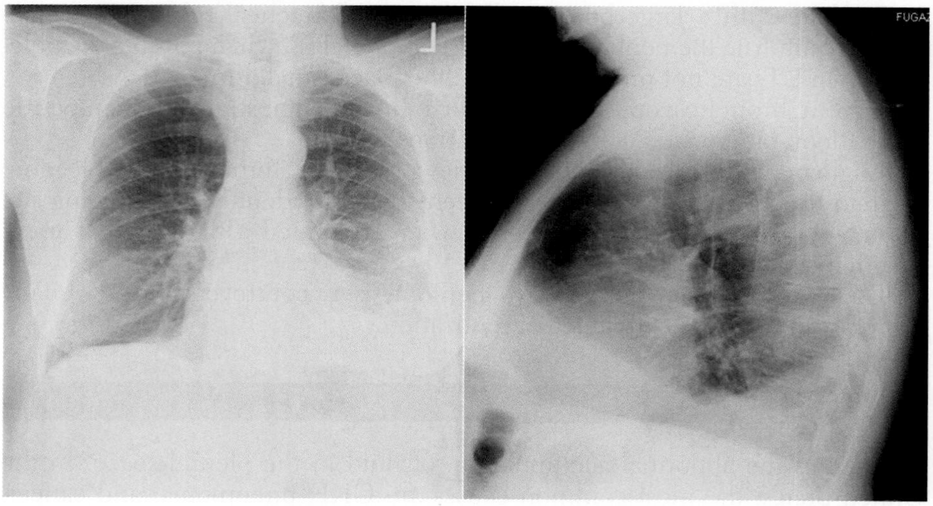

FIGURE 10.1. Left pleural effusion. (Reproduced, with permission, from Longo DL, Kasper DL, Jameson JL, et al. *Harrison's Principles of Internal Medicine*. 18th ed. New York: McGraw-Hill; 2011.)

TABLE 10.4. Light's Criteria for Distinguishing Transudative from Exudative Effusion

Pleural fluid/serum protein ratio > 0.5
Pleural fluid LDH > 2/3 upper limit of serum reference range
Pleural fluid/serum LDH ratio > 0.6
The fluid is an exudate if at least one of the above criteria is present.
The fluid is a transudate if none of the above criteria is present.

LDH, lactate dehydrogenase.

TABLE 10.5. Exudative Pleural Fluid Analysis and Interpretation

Pleural Fluid Test	Interpretation
RBC count	Grossly bloody or > 100,000 cells/mm^3 suggests trauma, malignancy, PE, pneumonia
Neutrophils	> 50% suggests acute pleural process (infection, PE)
Lymphocytes	> 50% suggests chronic pleural process (TB, malignancy)
Eosinophils	Presence suggests air or blood in pleural space
Glucose	< 60 mg/dL suggests a complicated parapneumonic effusion, malignancy, ruptured esophagus, TB, or rheumatoid arthritis
Triglycerides	> 110 mg/dL suggests chylothorax
pH	Pleural pH < 7.2 with parapneumonic effusion indicates the need for drainage

TB, tuberculosis.

TREATMENT

- **Transudative pleural effusion:** Treatment is aimed at the underlying cause with therapeutic thoracentesis if the patient is symptomatic.
- **Parapneumonic effusion:** Large effusions, or evidence of empyema (loculations, thickened parietal pleura, pH < 7.2, pus, glucose < 60 mg/dL, Gram stain+) are indications for further drainage or more aggressive intervention.
- **Hemothorax:** Drainage is required or fibrothorax will likely develop.

Abnormalities in Gas Exchange

HYPOXEMIA

Defined as a decrease in blood O_2 (in general, a Pao_2 of < 60 mm Hg). Hypoxemia may result in inadequate delivery of O_2 to tissues (tissue hypoxia). The five major etiologies of hypoxemia are listed in Table 10.6.

SYMPTOMS/EXAMINATION

Hypoxemia can lead to **tissue hypoxia** and cause impaired judgment, motor dysfunction, fatigue, drowsiness, respiratory distress, and respiratory failure.

TABLE 10.6. Etiologies of Hypoxemia

CAUSE	MECHANISM	DISEASE STATES	COMMENTS
Reduced inspired O_2	O_2 is replaced by other gases *or* low total O_2	Enclosed spaces, fire, high altitude, air travel	Normal A-a gradient
Diffusion abnormality	Reduction in diffusion capacity	Interstitial lung disease	↑ A-a gradient, improves with O_2. An uncommon cause of hypoxemic respiratory failure
Hypoventilation	↓ Minute ventilation results in ↑ $Paco_2$ and ↓ Pao_2	See Table 10.5	Normal A-a gradient
V/Q mismatch	Altered ratio of perfusion to ventilation	Pulmonary embolus, asthma, COPD, pneumonia, interstitial lung disease	↑ A-a gradient. Pao_2 corrects with supplemental O_2
R-to-L shunt	Physiologic shunt: Perfusion to nonventilated lung Anatomic shunt: Communication between the arterial and venous systems	ARDS, pneumonia Pulmonary AVM, congenital heart disease, patent foramen ovale with right-to-left flow	↑ A-a gradient. Pao_2 does not correct with supplemental O_2

A-a, alveolar-arterial; ARDS, acute respiratory distress syndrome; AVM, arteriovenous malformation; COPD, chronic obstructive pulmonary disease; V/Q, Ventilation-perfusion.

DIAGNOSIS

- Formal diagnosis of hypoxemia requires ABG analysis.
- Perform history, examination, and obtain studies (eg, CXR, CT-PE), as indicated, to search for the underlying cause.
- Calculate the alveolar-arterial (A-a) O_2 gradient to narrow the etiology:
  - Alveolar-arterial (A-a) gradient = [Fio_2 × (Atmospheric pressure − H_2O pressure)] − ($Paco_2$/0.8) − Pao_2.
  - Assuming sea level, a shortened formula is A-a gradient = 150 − ($Paco_2$ × 1.2 + Pao_2).
  - A conservative estimate of a normal A-a gradient is (age in years/4) + 4.

TREATMENT

- All patients with hypoxemia should be treated with supplemental O_2. Titrate Sao_2 > 90% in acute on chronic hypercapnia with hypoxia to avoid respiratory depression. No improvement with supplemental O_2? Suspect anatomic shunt.
- Treat underlying cause.

KEY FACT

Hypoxemia due to shunt does not correct with 100% O_2 therapy.

HYPERCAPNIA

Hypercapnia is elevated CO_2 in the blood ($Paco_2$ > 45 mm Hg). It is nearly always a result of alveolar hypoventilation from a variety of disease processes. In rare cases, it can be the result of exogenous CO_2 poisoning (dry ice, volcanic eruption).

ETIOLOGIES

See Table 10.7.

TABLE 10.7. Etiologies of Hypercapnia

Cause	Mechanism	Disease States
Depressed central respiratory drive	↓ Minute ventilation	Drug overdose Brainstem lesion/infarction Central sleep apnea Hypothyroidism
Peripheral nerve disorders	Same as above	Guillain-Barré syndrome ALS Poliomyelitis West Nile virus
Neuromuscular junction disorders	Same as above	Myasthenia gravis Botulism
Muscle disorders	Same as above	Muscular dystrophy Glycogen storage disease
Lung disorders	↓ Alveolar ventilation due to obstructive lung disease	COPD Asthma Cystic fibrosis
Chest wall disorders	Chest wall mechanics are altered, leading to ↓ alveolar ventilation	Kyphoscoliosis Massive obesity

ALS, Amyotrophic lateral sclerosis; COPD, chronic obstructive pulmonary disease.

SYMPTOMS/EXAMINATION

From mild to severe: Headache, confusion, lethargy, seizure, coma, cardiovascular collapse

DIAGNOSIS

- ABG
- Perform history, examination, and obtain studies (eg, CXR, CT-PE), as indicated, to search for the underlying cause.

TREATMENT

- Treatment depends on underlying cause (eg, Narcan in opiate-induced hypoventilation).
- In all cases, provide supplemental O_2 and support ventilation via bag-valve mask ventilation, noninvasive positive-pressure ventilation, or intubation (as appropriate).

Acute Respiratory Distress Syndrome

Acute respiratory distress syndrome (ARDS) is an acute, diffuse, inflammatory lung injury characterized by rapid onset dyspnea, hypoxemia, and bilateral pulmonary infiltrates. The root problem underlying the development of ARDS is acute lung injury (ALI), which arises for many different reasons. Not all ALI progresses to ARDS, but all cases of ARDS begin as ALI.

CAUSES

See Table 10.8.

TABLE 10.8. Causes of Acute Lung Injury and ARDS

Direct pulmonary injury
Pneumonia
Aspiration
Embolism (fat, air, thrombus)
Toxic inhalation
Ventilator associated
Drowning
Indirect pulmonary injury
Transfusion reaction (TRALI)
High-altitude exposure
Systemic infection, DIC
Pancreatitis
Drug reactions (heroin, ASA)
Trauma
Shock
Severe burns

ARDS, acute respiratory distress syndrome; ASA, aminosalicylic acid; DIC, disseminated intravascular coagulation; TRALI, Transfusion-related acute lung injury.

PATHOPHYSIOLOGY

- Triggering event → complex inflammatory response → both alveolar epithelial cell and vascular endothelial cell injury.
- Cell injury → capillary leak, cell death, and loss of surfactant resulting in diseased alveoli that do not participate in oxygenation (shunt).
- Diseased segments of the lung are interspersed with healthy segments.

SYMPTOMS/EXAMINATION

Presents with rapid onset of dyspnea, tachypnea, and diffuse crackles.

DIFFERENTIAL

Includes cardiogenic pulmonary edema, pneumonia, diffuse alveolar hemorrhage, acute idiopathic eosinophilic pneumonia, miliary TB, cancer (most often lymphoma or leukemia), idiopathic pulmonary fibrosis.

DIAGNOSIS

ALI and ARDS are diagnoses of exclusion and are characterized by acute onset of symptoms, bilateral infiltrates (similar appearance to pulmonary edema) and low/normal L atrial pressures (Figure 10.2). Only the $Pa{O_2}$ to $Fi{O_2}$ ratio distinguishes ALI from ARDS (Table 10.9). Additional findings are as follows:

- **CT chest:** May demonstrate alveolar filling and consolidation that is more apparent in dependent lung zones with sparing of other areas (Figure 10.3).
- **Bronchoalveolar lavage (BAL):** May help differentiate the etiology (eg, *Pneumocystis* in the immunocompromised patient).
- B-type natriuretic peptide (BNP), echocardiogram, right heart catheterization as indicated to exclude cardiac pulmonary edema.

KEY FACT

To improve mortality in patients with ARDS, target a tidal volume of 6 mL/kg **predicted** body weight.

TREATMENT

- Search for and treat the underlying cause of acute respiratory failure (ARF).

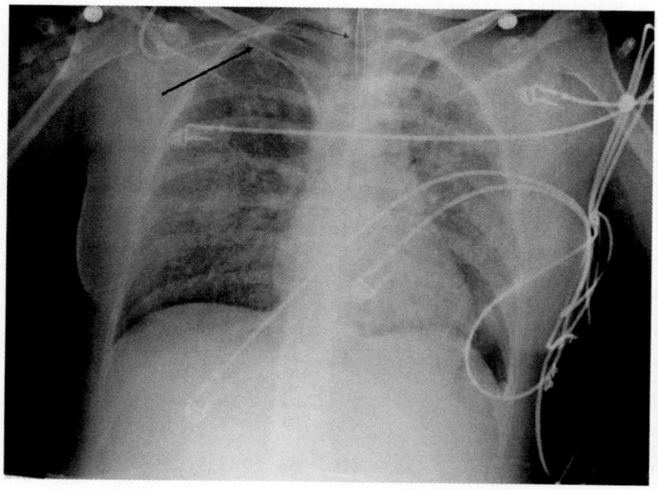

FIGURE 10.2. Acute respiratory distress syndrome (ARDS). Note diffuse, bilateral alveolar infiltrates with normal heart size. (Reproduced, with permission, from Longo DL, Kasper DL, Jameson JL, et al. *Harrison's Principles of Internal Medicine*. 18th ed. New York: McGraw-Hill; 2011.)

TABLE 10.9. Required Features for Diagnosis of ALI and ARDS

	Onset of Symptoms	Oxygenation	Hemodynamics	CXR
ALI	Acute	$Pao_2/Fio_2 \leq 300$	Low or normal left atrial pressure	Bilateral infiltrates
ARDS	Acute	$Pao_2/Fio_2 \leq 200$	Low or normal left atrial pressure	Bilateral infiltrates

ALI, acute lung injury; ARDS, acute respiratory distress syndrome; CXR, chest x-ray.

- Most patients with ARDS require mechanical ventilation during the course of the disease.
- **Use of tidal volumes ≤ 6 mL/kg of predicted body weight has been shown to ↓ mortality.**
- Add positive end-expiratory pressure (PEEP) as needed to maintain Fio_2 < 60%.
- Inverse ratio ventilation with permissive hypercarbia allows for more inspiratory time and may improve oxygenation.
- Plateau pressure must be kept at < 30 cm H_2O to prevent barotrauma.
- A conservative fluid management strategy (ie, one involving less volume) is preferred over a liberal fluid strategy.
- The use of corticosteroids, inhaled bronchodilators, exogenous surfactant, high-frequency ventilation, liquid ventilation, and antioxidant therapy has been studied with no proven benefit.
- Mortality is approximately 40%. Of the survivors, approximately 25% have no pulmonary impairment at 1 year, 50% have mild impairment, 25% moderate impairment, and a small fraction severe impairment.

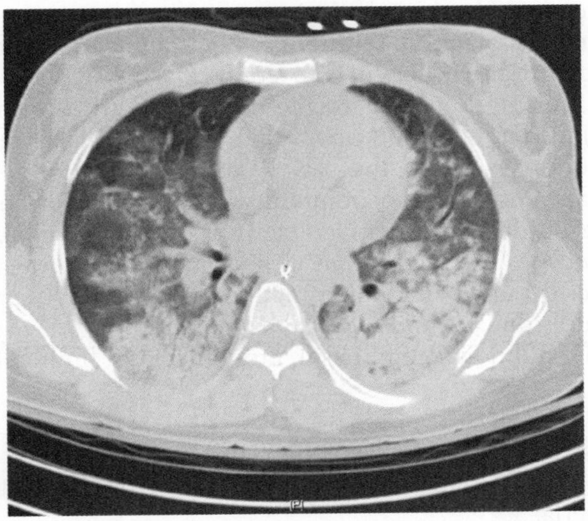

FIGURE 10.3. CT scan of ARDS demonstrates "ground-glass" opacities with more consolidated areas in the dependent lung zones. (Reproduced, with permission, from Longo DL, Kasper DL, Jameson JL, et al. *Harrison's Principles of Internal Medicine*. 18th ed. New York: McGraw-Hill; 2011.)

Q

An 80-year-old woman presents to the emergency department (ED) with 1 day of cough, fever, and weakness. She lives independently and has been healthy with the exception of a weeklong hospitalization 2 months prior for hip replacement (complicated by urosepsis). She has been to the clinic several times in follow-up and has done well since discharge. Vital signs are normal with exception of mild tachypnea and low-grade fever. CT shows R lower lobe infiltrate and no evidence for PE. Laboratory test results are unremarkable. Your intern would like to treat her with azithromycin. Do you agree?

A

No! This patient was hospitalized for > 2 days within the past 90 days and had several clinic visits, therefore, should be treated for a health care–associated pneumonia. Antibiotics coverage should be expanded to include *Pseudomonas* (and other gram-negatives) and methicillin-resistant *Staphylococcus aureus* MRSA.

KEY FACT

Streptococcus pneumoniae and *Staphylococcus aureus* are common causes of postinfluenza pneumonia.

KEY FACT

Pneumonia in alcoholics is most likely due to *S pneumoniae*, anaerobes, *Klebsiella pneumoniae*, and *Acinetobacter*.

Pneumonia and Complications

COMMUNITY-ACQUIRED PNEUMONIA

An infection of the lower respiratory tract in an individual who has not been recently hospitalized.

CAUSES

The single leading cause of community-acquired pneumonia (CAP) is *Streptococcus pneumoniae*. Common organisms are listed in Table 10.10. Less common pathogens will be discussed further.

PATHOPHYSIOLOGY

Both the virulence of the infecting organism and host factors contribute to the risk of CAP. Table 10.10 lists the epidemiologic conditions and/or risk factors related to specific pathogens.

- Decreased mucociliary clearance of airway (eg, cystic fibrosis [CF], smoking, COPD, elderly, mechanical obstruction) →↓ host defenses.
- Relative/absolute immunosuppression (eg, chronic disease, human immunodeficiency virus [HIV]) →↑ susceptibility to bacterial infection.
- Hematogenous spread of organism to lung is less common (eg, injection drug users [IDU]).

SYMPTOMS/EXAMINATION

- Fever, dyspnea, or cough productive of purulent/bloody sputum are most common.
- Pleuritic chest pain, tachypnea, and abnormal breath sounds.
- In the elderly, the presenting complaint may be vague and nonspecific, eg, altered mental status, poor appetite, or a fall.

DIFFERENTIAL

- **Hospital-acquired pneumonia:** Occurs 48 hours or more after admission.
- **Ventilator-associated pneumonia:** Pneumonia developing 48 hours or more after endotracheal intubation.
- **Health care–associated pneumonia:** Pneumonia in a nonhospitalized patient with extensive health care contact. This includes patients who reside in a nursing home or long-term care facility, have received intravenous (IV) therapy or wound care within the past 30 days, were hospitalized for 2 or more days within the past 90 days, dialysis patients, patients on chemotherapy, or immunocompromised patients. Common pathogens include aerobic gram-negative bacilli (eg, *Pseudomonas*, *Klebsiella*, *Escherichia coli*, *Acinetobacter*) as well as gram-positive organisms such as *Staphylococcus aureus* (including methicillin-resistant *S aureus* [MRSA]). They are rarely due to viral or fungal pathogens.
- Also consider pulmonary embolism, bronchiectasis, bronchitis, CHF.

DIAGNOSIS

- Suspect based on clinical presentation.
- It is not possible to differentiate atypical from typical infections based on clinical criteria.
- CXR
  - Radiographic findings cannot accurately predict the microbial cause, but lobar infiltrates are more likely due to typical bacterial pathogens (Figure 10.4) and interstitial infiltrates due to atypical pathogens.
  - The initial CXR may be negative in patients with significant dehydration.

KEY FACT

Health care–associated pneumonia is most likely due to aerobic gram-negative and gram-positive organisms (including MRSA).

TABLE 10.10. Common Community-Acquired Pneumonia Pathogens

Organism	Classic Patient	Classic Clinical Presentation
Typical Aerobic Organisms		
Streptococcus pneumoniae	Extremes of age and chronically ill Immunocompromised (eg, HIV, splenectomy)	Peak incidence in winter and early spring Abrupt onset of **single**-shaking chill **Rust-colored sputum** Sepsis or multisystem illness Lobar infiltrate
Haemophilus influenzae	Elderly Underlying lung disease (eg, **COPD**)	Peak incidence in winter and early spring Less abrupt in onset Patchy, bibasilar infiltrates
Klebsiella sp	Alcoholic or chronically debilitated patient	Abrupt onset rigors (multiple) and chills **Currant-jelly sputum** Right upper lobe infiltrate with **bulging fissure**
Staphylococcus aureus (MSSA, MRSA)	Elderly Hematogenous (**IDU**) Postinfluenza pneumonia	Insidious onset Low-grade fever Patchy, often multilobar necrotizing pneumonia (empyema, lung abscess)
Anaerobes		
Peptostreptococcus *Fusobacterium* *Bacteroides* *Prevotella*	Aspiration Alcoholic Poor dental hygiene	Subacute or chronic presentations Necrotizing pneumonia (empyema or lung abscess) Putrid sputum
Atypical Organisms		
Mycoplasma sp	Younger, healthy patient	Year round Subacute illness Interstitial infiltrates May see extrapulmonary manifestations (eg, rash, bullous myringitis, pericarditis)
Legionella sp	Immunosuppressed Smokers, chronic lung disease Outbreaks associated with aerosolized water (eg, showers) and hotel or cruise ship stay in previous 2 wk	Year round Mild to multisystem illness **GI symptoms** **Hepatic dysfunction** **Hyponatremia** Pleuritic CP and pleural effusions common
Chlamydophila (formerly *Chlamydia*) *pneumoniae*	Elderly	Year round Mild, subacute illness
Viral Pathogens		
RSV Parainfluenza Influenza	Infants and young children	Autumn and winter months

COPD, chronic obstructive pulmonary disease; CP, chest pain; GI, gastrointestinal; HIV, human immunodeficiency virus; IDU, injection drug users; RSV, respiratory syncytial virus.

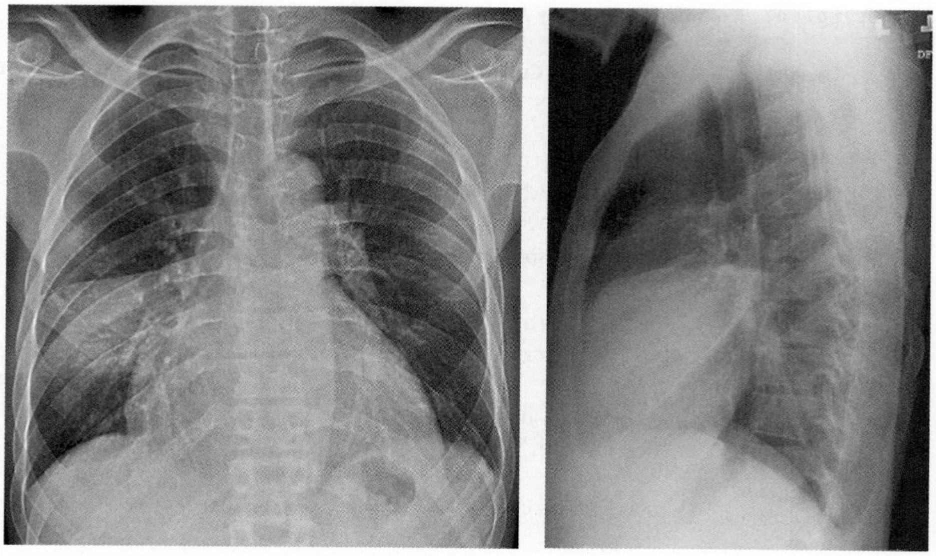

FIGURE 10.4. Right middle lobe infiltrate c/w pneumonia. (Reproduced, with permission, from Chen MY, Pope TL, Ott DJ, eds. *Basic Radiology*. 2nd ed. New York: McGraw-Hill; 2011.)

- Microbiological diagnosis is reserved for more seriously ill admitted patients:
  - Blood cultures: Low yield overall but accurately identifies organism when positive.
  - Sputum Gram stain is rarely helpful. Diagnostic sample must have **< 10 epithelial cells and > 25 WBC/hpf**. See Table 10.11 for Gram stains of common organisms that cause pneumonia.
  - Specific culture and urinary antigen testing if *Legionella* is suspected.
  - Pleural fluid aspiration and evaluation should be performed on effusions > 10 mm thick on lateral decubitus radiograph. Large or complicated parapneumonic effusions require further drainage (see sections on empyema and pleural effusion for further discussion).

TABLE 10.11. Gram Stains of Common Organisms That Cause Pneumonia

Organism	Gram Stain Findings
Streptococcus pneumoniae	Gram+ lancet-shaped cocci, usually in pairs, PMNs
Haemophilus influenza	Gram– coccobacillus, PMNs
Staphylococcus aureus	Gram+ cocci in clusters, PMNs
Klebsiella sp	Gram– rod, PMNs
Legionella sp	Few weakly Gram– rods, many PMNs
Oral flora (aspiration)	Mixed Gram+ and – cocci and rods, PMNs
Atypicals *Legionella* sp Viral	Few bacteria, many PMNs, or monos

PMN, polymorphonuclear neutrophil.

- **Findings associated with poor outcome** include pleural effusion, multilobar involvement, ARDS, septic shock, older or immunocompromised patient, failure to clear lactate by at least 15%-20% in the first 6 hours, cavitation, and WBC count > 30,000 or < 4000 cells/mm^3.

TREATMENT

- The **Pneumonia Patient Outcomes Research Team (PORT)** score can help guide decisions regarding the need for hospitalization in **immunocompetent adults** (Tables 10.12 and 10.13). In general, older people with comorbid disease who reside in a health care facility have systemic signs of illness and abnormal laboratory test results tend to have increased morbidity.
- **Outpatient empiric therapy:**
  - Healthy adults: Macrolide (azithromycin or clarithromycin) or doxycycline.
  - Adults with comorbidities or recent antibiotic use: Respiratory fluoroquinolone **or** β-lactam (eg, high-dose amoxicillin-clavulanate) plus either a macrolide or doxycycline.
- **Inpatient empiric therapy:**
  - Ceftriaxone + azithromycin or single-agent treatment with respiratory fluoroquinolone.
  - ICU care: ceftriaxone + azithromycin; ceftriaxone + fluoroquinolone.
  - Add vancomycin for HCAP or ICU care.
- Special considerations:
  - Suspected *Pseudomonas*: Treat with antipseudomonal β-lactam and an aminoglycoside. Another option is carbapenems with antipseudomonal quinolones plus an aminoglycoside.
  - Suspected *Legionella* sp: Add fluoroquinolone or azithromycin.
  - Suspected MRSA: Add vancomycin or linezolid.
  - Suspected aspiration pneumonia: Add piperacillin-tazobactam or clindamycin.

FUNGAL PNEUMONIA

Fungal pneumonia occurs when disruption of contaminated soil or other media results in inhalation of fungal spores.

Histoplasmosis

The fungus *Histoplasma capsulatum* is endemic in the moist soil of the **Mississippi** and **Ohio River valleys** (most of the area between the Rocky and the Appalachian Mountains). Spores are concentrated where there are bat and bird droppings—caves, chicken coops, old buildings, etc. Severe or disseminated infection is more common in immunocompromised patients.

SYMPTOMS/EXAMINATION

- Infection is often clinically silent in healthy patients.
- Symptomatic infection is characterized by fever, cough, and flulike symptoms.
- Chronic illness typically manifests as TB-like symptoms (weight loss, fevers, malaise, hemoptysis).

> **KEY FACT**
>
> Respiratory illness in a patient with exposure to bird or bat droppings? Think *Histoplasma capsulatum*.

DIFFERENTIAL

TB, sarcoidosis, other fungal infections.

TABLE 10.12. PORT Prediction Rule for CAP

Patient Characteristic	Points Assigned[a]
Demographic Factor	
Age: men	Number of years
Age: women	Number of years minus 10
Nursing home resident	10
Comorbid Illnesses	
Neoplastic disease[b]	30
Liver disease[c]	20
CHF[d]	10
Cerebrovascular disease[e]	10
Renal disease[f]	10
Physical Examination Finding	
Altered mental status[g]	20
Respiratory rate ≥ 30 breaths/min	20
Systolic BP < 90 mm Hg	20
Temperature ≤ 35°C or ≥ 40°C	15
Pulse ≥ 125 bpm	10
Laboratory or Radiographic Finding	
Arterial pH < 7.35	30
BUN ≥ 30 mg/dL	20
Sodium < 130 meq/L	20
Glucose > 250 mg/dL	10
Hematocrit < 30%	10
Arterial Po_2 < 60 mm Hg	10
Pleural effusion	10

BP, blood pressure; bpm, beats per minute; BUN, blood urea nitrogen; CAP, community-acquired pneumonia; CHF, congestive heart failure; PORT, Patient Outcomes Research Team.

[a]A total point score for a given patient is obtained by summing the patient's age in years (age minus 10 for women) and the points for each applicable characteristic.

[b]Any cancer except basal or squamous cell carcinoma of the skin that was active at the time of presentation or diagnosed within 1 year before presentation.

[c]Clinical or histologic diagnosis of cirrhosis or another form of chronic liver disease.

[d]Systolic or diastolic dysfunction documented by history, physical examination and CXR, echocardiogram, multiple uptake gated acquisition (MUGA) scan, or left ventriculogram.

[e]Clinical diagnosis of stroke or TIA or stroke documented by MRI or CT scan.

[f]History of chronic renal disease or abnormal BUN and creatinine concentration documented in the medical record.

[g]Disorientation (to person, place, or time, not known to be chronic), stupor, or coma.

(Adapted, with permission, from Fine MJ, Auble TE, Yealy DM, et al. A prediction rule to identify low-risk patients with community-acquired pneumonia. *NEJM* 1997 Jan 23;336(4):243-250.)

TABLE 10.13. Risk Stratification Based on PORT Score

Number of Points	Risk Class	Mortality at 30 Days (%)	Recommended Site of Care
Absence of predictors	I	0.1-0.4	Outpatient
≤ 70	II	0.6-0.7	Outpatient
71-90	III	0.9-2.8	Outpatient or brief inpatient
91-130	IV	8.2-9.3	Inpatient
≥ 130	V	27.0-31.1	Inpatient

PORT, Patient Outcomes Research Team.

(Data from Fine MJ, Auble TE, Yealy DM, et al. A prediction rule to identify low-risk patients with community-acquired pneumonia. *NEJM*. 1997[336]:243.)

Diagnosis

- **CXR:** Often normal or showing hilar adenopathy with focal infiltrates in primary infection (can look like **sarcoidosis**); scattered nodules (histoplasmomas) or upper lobe cavitary lesions may develop in chronic illness.
- Positive fungal stains, cultures, antigen detection, or serologic testing are confirmatory.

Treatment

Amphotericin B is reserved for severe disseminated illness; itraconazole is used for mild to moderate illness and for step-down from amphotericin B.

Complications

- Pericarditis
- Disseminated disease with multiorgan involvement
- Mediastinal granulomas
- **Fibrosing mediastinitis** (superior vena cava [SVC] syndrome, airway obstruction, dysphagia)
- Broncholithiasis: Calcified lymph nodes erode into adjacent bronchi causing wheezing, hemoptysis, cough, sputum production (that may contain small calcium stones)

Coccidiomycosis (Valley Fever)

The fungi *Coccidioides immitis* and *Coccidioides posadasii* are endemic to the arid soils of the **southwestern United States** and northern Mexico. Infection results from inhalation of dust from disturbed soil. Severe or disseminated infection is more common in immunocompromised patients.

> **KEY FACT**
>
> Flulike illness with pneumonia in resident or traveler to southwestern United States? Don't forget coccidiomycosis or hantavirus.

Symptoms/Examination

- Infection is clinically silent in most healthy individuals.
- Symptomatic infection is characterized by cough, fevers/chills, and flulike symptoms.
- Classic presentation is triad of pneumonitis, rash (erythema nodosum), and arthralgias.

Diagnosis

- **CXR:** In acute infection it may be normal or show hilar adenopathy, thin-walled cavities, or unilateral infiltrates.
- Positive fungal stains, cultures, or serologic testing is confirmatory.

Treatment

Subacute, mild infection often resolves without antifungals. Antifungals (fluconazole, itraconazole, ketoconazole) are reserved for patients with severe acute disease or those with chronic illness or immunosuppression.

Complication

Disseminated disease with multiorgan involvement (skin, bone, joints, central nervous system [CNS]).

Blastomycosis

The fungus *Blastomyces dermatides* is found in the **Midwest** and the **southeastern United States** (overlapping the distribution of histoplasmosis, but extending farther north into Canada). Disease is caused by inhalation of spores. Dissemination occurs frequently.

Symptoms/Examination

- Most common presentation is a chronic indolent pneumonia with weight loss, night sweats, and low-grade fevers.
- Acute pulmonary infection is characterized by cough, fever/chills, and flulike symptoms.
- Severe pulmonary infectious do occur and can cause ARDS.

Diagnosis

- CXR: Fibronodular, interstitial, or alveolar infiltrates
- Positive fungal stains, cultures, or serologic testing are confirmatory
- Disseminated disease can be mistaken for malignancy

Treatment

- Life-threatening illness, pregnancy, immunocompromise, CNS disease: Amphotericin B
- Mild to moderate illness: Itraconazole
- **Almost all cases require therapy**

Complications

Dissemination to skin (ulcerative or verrucous lesions), bones, joints, prostate.

Aspergillosis

The Aspergillus fungus is commonly found growing on decaying vegetation (eg, leaf or compost piles). Aspergillosis results from inhalation of fungal spores in patients with underlying lung disease or immunosuppression. It is the most common cause of noncandidal invasive fungal infection in transplant patients. Symptoms result from either an allergic reaction to presence of fungus or invasive infection.

Symptoms/Examination

- Allergic bronchopulmonary disease: Patient with underlying asthma or CF; fever, cough, hemoptysis, wheezing, malaise, rash.
- Invasive infection: Insidious onset fever, cough, malaise, dyspnea; chronic sinusitis if spread to sinuses; altered mental status, focal weakness, or seizures if spread to CNS.
- Aspergilloma (colonization of preexisting lung cavities): Pleuritic chest pain, cough, hemoptysis (severe in 25%).

Diagnosis

- Eosinophilia and high IgE levels should raise suspicion of allergic bronchopulmonary disease; IgG antibody levels can help confirm diagnosis.
- CXR is insensitive early in the disease; later it can show single or multiple nodules or patchy consolidation.
- Confirmation can be difficult; gold standard is identification of *Aspergillus* in tissue sample or culture.

Treatment

- Life-threatening invasive disease should be treated with voriconazole or amphotericin B.
- Less severe disease can be treated with itraconazole or voriconazole (depending on extent); add steroids if allergic disease.

Complications

Life-threatening hemoptysis, bronchiectasis, respiratory failure, stroke, endocarditis, and bone destruction.

ZOONOTIC PNEUMONIA

Anthrax—see Chapter 20, EMS and Disaster Medicine.

Brucellosis

Causes

Caused by organism *Brucella* species and is most often acquired through consumption of unpasteurized milk and dairy products or by slaughterhouse workers.

Symptoms/Examination

- Upper respiratory infection (URI) with hoarse voice, cough, wheezing
- Fever, joint and muscle pain, sweating

Diagnosis

- Paratracheal and hilar lymphadenopathy on CXR
- Confirmation (when necessary) is by serologic testing, histology, or culture

Treatment

Doxycycline + rifampin

Complications

Orchitis, spondylodiscitis, Sacroileitis

Psittacosis (Parrot Fever)

Causes

Caused by organism *Chlamydophila* (formerly *Chlamydia*) *psittaci*, which is transmitted from **birds** to humans. It is found worldwide.

Symptoms/Examination

- History of occupational or recreational exposure to birds.
- Abrupt onset of fever; severe headache and dry cough are common.
- Rales or other lung examination findings are common.
- Extrapulmonary manifestations are common.

DIAGNOSIS

- Primarily a clinical diagnosis
- Patchy infiltrates on CXR
- Confirmation (when necessary) is by serologic testing

TREATMENT

- Tetracyclines, eg, doxycycline and tetracycline
- Erythromycin as second-line agent
- Chloramphenicol and rifampin have also been used effectively

COMPLICATIONS

Renal failure, encephalitis, endocarditis, DIC

Pulmonic Plague—see Chapter 20, EMS and Disaster Medicine.

Q FEVER

> **KEY FACT**
>
> Consider Q fever in patients with pneumonia and exposure to farm animals or parturient cats.

CAUSES

Caused by the organism *Coxiella burnetii*, a gram-negative bacterium, similar to rickettsia, which is transmitted to humans from **farm animals or parturient (ie, about to give birth) cats. It is aerosolized from urine, birth products, or feces.**

SYMPTOMS/EXAMINATION

- History of occupational or recreational exposure to farm animals or parturient cats.
- Flulike illness along with dry cough and pleuritic chest pain.
- Confusion and GI symptoms are common.
- Hepatomegaly, rash.

DIAGNOSIS

- Patchy infiltrates on CXR
- Diagnosed by serologic testing

TREATMENT

- Doxycycline for those with moderate to severe symptoms
- Trimethoprim-sulfamethoxazole (TMP-SMX) for pregnant patients

COMPLICATIONS

- Pericarditis/myocarditis/endocarditis, vascular aneurysm/graft infection and hepatitis are seen with chronic infection. Mortality is high.
- Growth retardation, fetal demise. and other complication if acquired during pregnancy.

PNEUMOCYSTIS PNEUMONIA

Pneumocystis pneumonia (PCP) results from infection with the fungus *Pneumocystis jiroveci* (formerly *carinii*) in an immunocompromised host. The exact mode of transmission (reactivation of latent state or primary infection) is unclear.

Risk factors include HIV infection (CD4 count < 200), recent glucocorticoid use, other immunosuppressive therapy, malignancy, bone marrow or organ transplantation, and primary immunodeficiency. PCP is unlikely to occur in patients who are compliant with PCP prophylaxis.

SYMPTOMS/EXAMINATION

- Patients without HIV-infection: Fulminate respiratory failure with fever and dry cough.
- HIV-infected patients: Symptom progression over a 2- to 3-week period with dyspnea, dry cough, low-grade fever.
- Hypoxic, tachypneic, tachycardic.
- The patient may have normal lung sounds or rales.

DIAGNOSIS

- **CXR:** May be normal if early in the disease process or may have a classic bilateral interstitial infiltrate that projects out from the perihilar region (Figure 10.5).
- **Chest CT:** More sensitive than CXR in early disease (see Figure 10.5).
- **Ambulatory pulse oximetry:** If CXR is normal but diagnosis is suspected, O_2 desaturation to < 90% with ambulation is enough to initiate treatment.
- A lactate dehydrogenase (LDH) > 450 IU is common, and the degree of elevation is prognostic.
- **Immunofluorescent staining** of sputum or bronchoalveolar lavage sample (gold standard) is confirmative.

TREATMENT

- **TMP-SMX** is the preferred agent.
  - High-dose oral therapy (2 DS tabs TID) may be used for patients with mild or early disease. IV therapy should be given to all admitted patients.
  - Patients with HIV have a high-incidence of hypersensitivity reactions to TMP-SMX (fever, rash, hepatitis, etc); continued therapy should be based on confirmed diagnosis.
  - Second-line agents include pentamidine or dapsone.
- **Steroids** are also considered first-line adjuvant therapy in patients with Po_2 < 70 mm Hg and/or an A-a gradient > 35.

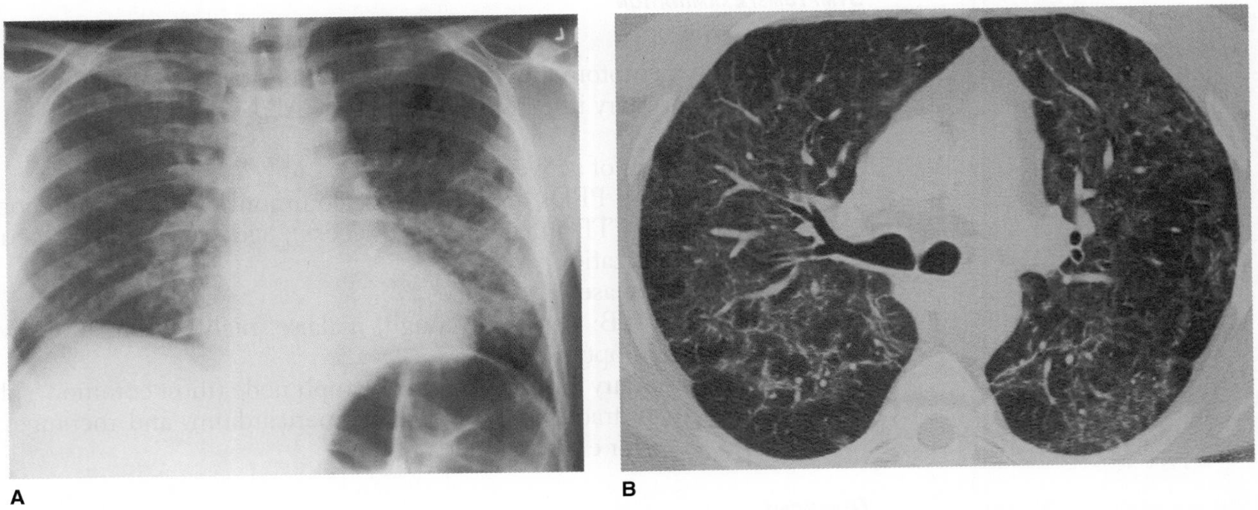

FIGURE 10.5. Pneumocystis pneumonia in an HIV-infected person. (**A**) Chest radiograph depicting diffuse infiltrates in an HIV-infected patient with PCP. (**B**) High-resolution CT of the lung showing ground-glass opacification in an HIV-infected patient with PCP. (Reproduced with permission from Longo DL, Fauci AS, Kasper DL, et al: *Harrison's Principles of Internal Medicine*. 18th ed. New York, NY: McGraw-Hill; 2011. Figure 207.1. A&B. Photo Contributor: Dr. Cristopher Meyer.)

TABLE 10.14. Tuberculosis Risk Factors

Immigration from high-prevalence country
Immunocompromise (eg, chronic steroids, HIV, transplant)
Older age
Substance abuse
Tobacco use
Malnutrition
Systemic diseases (eg, silicosis, DM, renal failure)
Close contact with infected person
Crowded living conditions
Travel to endemic areas
Health- or residential-care work

DM, diabetes mellitus; TB, tuberculosis.

TUBERCULOSIS

Infection with *Mycobacterium tuberculosis*, a slow-growing acid-fast aerobic rod, affects approximately one-third of the world's population.

- Transmitted human-to-human via respiratory droplets; the lungs are the major site of infection.
- Humans are the only natural reservoir and usually must be in confined environments over extended periods of time to transmit the disease.
- See Table 10.14 for TB risk factors.

Pathophysiology

- **Primary infection** in immunocompetent host → small number of organisms contained in granulomas in the lungs or spread through the body → **latent (dormant) infection** and +PPD (purified protein derivative).
- Host becomes immunocompromised (eg, HIV, malignancy, immunosuppressant medications) → **reactivation** of latent disease and symptoms.
- Hematogenous spread during primary or reactivation → **miliary TB.**

Symptoms/Examination

- **Primary TB**
  - Usually asymptomatic, but a small number of cases may develop progressive primary infection, resembling CAP.
- **Latent TB**
  - No symptoms of active disease, +PPD.
  - False-negative PPDs are seen most commonly with immunocompromised, recent TB infection (< 10 weeks), age < 6 months, recent live virus immunization.
- **Reactivation disease**
  - **Pulmonary TB**: Persistent cough, malaise, night sweats, fever, weight loss, and hemoptysis.
  - **Extrapulmonary TB:** Sites include lymph node (most common), pleura, genitourinary tract, bones and joints, pericardium, and meninges. See Table 10.15 for clinical clues.

Diagnosis

- CXR
  - **Primary TB:** May be completely normal or reveal nonspecific infiltrate in any region of the lung. This infiltrate in association with regional

TABLE 10.15. Clinical Clues with Extrapulmonary Tuberculosis

Extrapulmonary Location	Clinical Clue
Meninges	Meningitis Lumbar puncture: High opening pressure and protein Lymphocyte predominance ↓ Glucose
Pleura	Exudative pleural effusion with predominance of lymphocytes and pleural fluid glucose < 60 mg/dL
Genitourinary tract	Urinary tract complaints WBCs without bacteria on UA
Miliary (disseminated)	Abnormal CBC Hepatosplenomegaly Lymphadenopathy Hyponatremia CXR with millet seed-like densities
Bone	Pott disease (bony destruction, often in spine) Osteomyelitis Arthritis

CBC, complete blood count; CXR, chest x-ray; TB, tuberculosis; UA, WBC, white blood cell.

lymphadenopathy is termed the *Ghon complex*. PPD will be positive 1-2 months after exposure.
- **Reactivation TB: Upper lobe infiltrates** with or without cavitation is most common findings, though atypical patterns (eg, lower lobe, effusion only) may be seen.

- **Sputum smears** are stained for **acid-fast bacilli**.
- Cultures of sputum, blood, or tissue are the gold standard for diagnosing active infection but may take weeks to grow.
- Latent infection can be diagnosed via the **tuberculin skin test or the interferon-gamma release assay** (IGRA) that detects the host immune response to the organism. The IGRA has an advantage in that there is no cross reactivity with the tuberculin vaccine (BCG). The tuberculin skin test is interpreted as positive based on the degree of induration (not redness) in a given patient risk group:
  - Low-risk individuals (eg, aged > 4 years, without any risk factors): > 15 mm
  - Medium risk individuals (IDU, immigrant, diabetes): > 10 mm
  - High risk patients (HIV, TB close contact, concerning CXR, transplants, chronic steroids): > 5 mm
- Many foreign-born patients may have been immunized with BCG, the therapeutic effectiveness of which is unclear. Therefore, the CDC recommends that history of such is ignored when interpreting the PPD response.
- TB serologic test: Fewer false negatives, BCG vaccination does not affect result.

Treatment

- **Latent TB (newly +PPD)**: 6-9 months of isoniazid (INH) **or** 3 months of INH plus rifapentine.

- **Active TB: Initial therapy with 4 drugs is now recommended until a multidrug-resistant strain can be ruled out by culture**. There are 10 drugs to treat TB, but 4 are commonly employed: INH, rifampin, pyrazinamide, and ethambutol. The drugs are selected for treatment based on local practice, patterns of resistance, and patient tolerance. Baseline laboratory test results, particularly liver function tests, are indicated before use of these drugs.
- **Corticosteroids:** For TB meningitis and pericarditis.

Complications

- Hemoptysis, pneumothorax, bronchiectasis, or empyema may be seen with pulmonary disease
- Disseminated disease
- Adverse drug reactions (eg, hepatitis or peripheral neuropathy secondary to INH, optic neuritis from ethambutol)
- Inadequate therapeutic effect of warfarin, steroids, oral contraceptives (OCPs), oral hypoglycemics, digoxin, anticonvulsants, and methadone secondary to treatment with INH
- Immune reconstitution syndrome can be seen with initiation of therapy; it is more common in HIV+ patients, and it manifests with symptoms, including fever, respiratory distress, and meningitis

ASPIRATION PNEUMONITIS AND PNEUMONIA

This disease occurs when normal protective mechanisms of the airway are compromised and foreign material enters the tracheobronchial tree. The aspiration can occur either in community or hospital settings. The airway becomes inflamed and the parenchyma collapses.

Causes

Risk factors for aspiration include drug or alcohol intoxication, general anesthesia/sedation, seizures, stroke, brain injury and dementia, and esophageal dysmotility, reflux, obstruction, or nasogastric (NG) tube. Periodontal disease and poor oral hygiene increases the risk of infection once aspiration occurs.

Common pathogens include:

- **Oral anaerobes: *Peptostreptococcus*, *Fusobacterium*, *Bacteroides*, *Prevotella***
- ***Klebsiella pneumoniae*** and other gram-negative enteric pathogens
- *S aureus*
- *Streptococcus*

Pathophysiology

- Aspiration of gastric contents → immediate inflammatory response and **chemical pneumonitis** → breakdown of pulmonary defense mechanisms → risk of aspiration **pneumonia.**
- Severity of the insult depends on the volume of the aspirate, presence of particulate matter, and the pH of the material. High-risk aspirates include those with **volumes > 25 mL, particulate food matter, a low pH, and bacterial contamination**.

Symptoms/Examination

- Aspiration event may be immediately followed by coughing or choking in the awake patient.
- **Chemical pneumonitis** (Mendelson syndrome): Tachypnea, shortness of breath, and fever with minimal sputum production developing within

hours of aspiration event. Symptoms within the first 24-48 hours of the aspiration event are likely due to pneumonitis.
- **Aspiration pneumonia**: Low-grade fevers, malaise, cough with sputum production developing over several **days** after the aspiration event.
- Wheezing, rhonchi, or rales over involved lung fields may be present.

KEY FACT

Aspiration pneumonia develops over days (not hours) of the aspiration event.

Diagnosis

- Suspect based on clinical history and presentation.
- **CXR:** May be completely normal immediately after event; infiltrates may develop in dependent portion of lung (depends on position of patient at time of aspiration—eg, bilateral lower lungs if standing).

Treatment

- Supportive care.
- Prophylactic antibiotics are not recommended.
- Indications for antibiotic therapy (piperacillin-tazobactam or clindamycin) include expanding infiltrate, new fever, or progressive symptoms > **48 hours** after aspiration event.
- **Avoid**: Systemic corticosteroids, which are of no benefit and may be harmful.

Complications

- Respiratory failure and shock.
- Empyema/abscess development.
- Pulmonary fibrosis.
- If the pH of the aspirated material is < 2.5, the lungs have suffered a chemical burn in addition to the ensuing secondary bacterial infection, and the mortality rate may be as high as 70%.

LUNG ABSCESS

A lung abscess is defined as necrosis of the lung parenchyma by a microbial infection. It is most commonly due to aspiration (primary lung abscess), but may also result from a complication of another process such as hematogenous spread of bacteria, penetrating trauma, malignancy, or pulmonary infarction (secondary lung abscess). A primary lung abscess has a mortality of 2%-3%, and a secondary lung abscess has a mortality approximating 70%.

Causes

Common organisms include:
- **Oral anaerobes (most common)**
- *S aureus*
- *K pneumoniae*
- Other gram-negative bacilli
- *Streptococcus pyogenes*
- *Nocardia asteroids*
- *Actinomyces* sp

Symptoms/Examination

Indolent course of fever, chest pain, weight loss, and night sweats.

Differential

The differential diagnosis of the cavitary lung lesion includes fungal infections, TB, neoplasm, Wegener granulomatosis, sarcoidosis.

DIAGNOSIS

- CXR: Usually confirms the presence of cavitary lesion with air-fluid levels
- Chest CT: May be needed to confirm cavitation

TREATMENT

Piperacillin-tazobactam or clindamycin. Surgical intervention is sometimes required.

EMPYEMA

Defined as pus in the pleural space or pleura fluid with presence of organisms on Gram stain.

Risk factors for empyema include:
- Pneumonia with parapneumonic effusion (most common)
- Penetrating trauma
- Esophageal perforation/rupture
- Presence of hemothorax, hydrothorax, or chylothorax

PATHOPHYSIOLOGY

The infection generally progresses through three stages:
1. **Exudative stage:** Free-flowing fluid present
2. **Fibrinopurulent stage:** Fibrin strands develop → loculations
3. **Organizational stage:** Thick pleural peel present

Identification and treatment in the exudative stage is essential to ensure good patient outcome.

SYMPTOMS/EXAMINATION

- Presence of risk factor, eg, recent pneumonia.
- Persistent fevers, dyspnea, pleuritic chest pain, and cough.
- Dullness to percussion and ↓ breath sounds over the effusion.

DIAGNOSIS

- **CXR:** Can confirm the presence of pleural effusion.
- **Decubitus CXR:** To determine if fluid is free-flowing or loculated.
- **Pleural fluid evaluation**. Findings consistent with empyema include aspiration of frank pus, pleural fluid pH < 7.2, pleural fluid glucose < 60 mg/dL and positive Gram stain or culture.
- **Chest CT:** To further delineate underlying pathology and evaluate extent of loculations and/or pleural peel, as needed.

TREATMENT

- **Drainage of pleural space:** Required in all cases.
- If exudative stage: Tube thoracostomy and IV antibiotics.
- Fibrinopurulent and organizational stage empyemas often require more aggressive and/or surgical management (eg, intrapleural fibrinolytics, surgical removal of fibrous peel).

> **KEY FACT**
>
> **Commonly encountered pathogens in acute exacerbations of bronchiectasis:**
> *Pseudomonas aeruginosa*
> *Haemophilus influenza*
> *Burkholderia cepacia*
> *Staphylococcus aureus*

BRONCHIECTASIS

Defined as the irreversible dilatation and destruction of bronchi with inadequate clearance of mucus in the airways. Cycles of infection and inflammation → permanently dilated airways and focal constrictive areas.

Causes

Caused by recurrent inflammation or infection of the airway:

- Inability to clear secretions (ciliary abnormalities, CF, tracheobronchomalacia)
- Severe or repeated episodes of pneumonia
- Recurrent aspiration (eg, severe GERD, disordered swallow)
- Lower airway obstruction with tumor

Symptoms

Patients often have cough productive of yellow or green sputum together with dyspnea and hemoptysis.

Examination

- Lung examination reveals crackles and wheezes.
- Acute exacerbations typically include changes in sputum production, increase in dyspnea, cough and wheezing, fatigue, low-grade fever, ↓ pulmonary function, changes in chest sounds, and radiographic changes.

Differential

COPD, interstitial fibrosis, pneumonia, asthma.

Diagnosis

- Suspect based on history and patient risk factors.
- CXR shows dilated and thickened bronchi ± scattered irregular opacities, atelectasis, and focal consolidation.
- High-resolution CT is diagnostic study of choice.

Treatment

- **Antibiotics:** The standard of care for acute exacerbations, a reasonable first-line choice would include a fluoroquinolone.
- **Inhaled bronchodilators:** Helpful when there is acute airway inflammation.
- **Inhaled corticosteroids:** Not routinely used except for coincident asthma and/or wheezing. Can improve pulmonary function in severe cases.
- Other treatment aimed toward specific underlying cause (eg, percussive vests to aid in clearance of secretions in patients with CF, proton pump inhibitor for severe GERD).
- **Surgical resection** remains an option for patients with localized focal bronchiectasis.
- **Double-lung transplantation** has been performed in patients with severe bronchiectasis.

BIOTERRORISM AGENTS

Pulmonary infections related to biological weapons of mass destruction include anthrax, plague, and tularemia. These are discussed further in Chapter 20, EMS and Disaster Medicine.

Asthma

Reactive airway disease consists of three classic components: **Airway inflammation, bronchial hyperresponsiveness, and reversible airflow obstruction**. Asthma is more prevalent in blacks than whites, and in childhood, asthma is more prevalent in boys than girls.

Q

A 30-year-old man presents to the ED with a severe asthma exacerbation requiring intubation. The initial CXR shows good ET tube position without complication or infiltrate. After approximately 30 minutes on the ventilator, the patient becomes hypotensive. End-expiratory pressures are increased. What should you do?

A

Suspect decreased venous return and cardiac output due to breath stacking and resultant increased intrathoracic pressure. Disconnect the patient from the ventilator allowing for a long expiration while squeezing the lower chest walls. Remember to use a low tidal volume (6-8 mL/kg) and low respiratory rate (10-12 bpm) for intubated patients with severe asthma exacerbation. Hypotension with increasing peak airway pressures suggests pneumothorax.

KEY FACT

Previously rising, mortality due to asthma has been declining since the mid-1990s.

KEY FACT

Symptoms after exposure to aminosalicylic acid (ASA) in aspirin-sensitive asthma: Rhinorrhea, conjunctival injection, periorbital edema, facial flushing, and wheezing.

PATHOPHYSIOLOGY

- Inhalation of allergen → production of IgE. Further exposure to allergen causes IgE binding to airway mast cells → release of inflammatory mediators (histamine, leukotrienes, cytokines) → bronchospasm, airway edema and accumulation of eosinophils and other cells in airway.
- Permanent airway remodeling can occur with chronic asthma.
- Aspirin sensitive asthma: Occurs in 5%-20% of all asthmatics, most often with prior sensitization to NSAID + chronic rhinosinusitis + nasal polyps + asthma.

CAUSES

Common triggers include respiratory infections, environmental allergens/ irritants, weather changes, and exercise. Rarer causes include aspirin or nonsteroidal anti-inflammatory drug (NSAID) hypersensitivity, β-blocker use, and emotional stressors.

Risk factors for death include:

- Previous ICU admission/intubation
- More than two hospitalizations or three ED visits in the past year
- Use of systemic corticosteroids or > 2 canisters of β_2-agonist metered-dose inhalers (MDIs) per month
- Difficulty perceiving presence or severity of airflow obstruction
- Low socioeconomic status
- Illicit drug use
- Serious comorbidities

SYMPTOMS/EXAMINATION

- Dyspnea, wheezing, coughing, chest tightness.
- Fever and purulent sputum usually represent a complicating process such as pneumonia.
- Wheezes are usually present, but may be absent in either mild or severe cases (minimal airflow). Presence of inspiratory wheezing or stridor should prompt evaluation for upper airway obstruction.
- Prolonged expiratory phase.
- Findings suggestive of **severe airway obstruction** include poor air movement that can manifest itself as **absence of wheezing,** tachypnea (> 40 bpm), tachycardia (> 120 bpm), pulsus paradoxus (> 10 mm Hg), accessory respiratory muscle use, altered mental status, hypoxemia, peak expiratory flow rate (PEF) < 100 L/min before treatment or PEF < 300 L/min after aggressive treatment.

DIFFERENTIAL

- **"All that wheezes is not asthma."** Consider CHF, upper airway obstruction, foreign-body aspiration, vocal cord dysfunction
- Other causes include COPD, bronchiectasis, CF

DIAGNOSIS

- **PEF** is most predictive of the severity of exacerbation and should guide therapy. PEF < 100 L/min or < 40% predicted is considered severe exacerbation.
- **Pulse oximetry** is helpful to establish adequate oxygenation, but it is not a good indicator of ventilation. **Capnography** is the noninvasive method of choice for monitoring ventilation.
- **ABG analysis** does not predict clinical outcome and should not supersede clinical findings in determining need for intubation. However, stages of asthma have been described based on ABG findings (Table 10.16).

TABLE 10.16. ABG Findings in Asthma

SEVERITY	pH	P_{CO_2}	P_{O_2}
Mild	↑	↓	Normal
Moderate	Normal	Normal	↓
Severe	↓	↑	↓

ABG, arterial blood gas.

- **CXR** is usually normal or shows hyperinflation and is necessary only when a secondary process is suspected such as pneumonia, CHF, pneumothorax, or foreign body. Obtain CXR for all first episodes of wheezing.

TREATMENT

Treatment should proceed as follows (Table 10.17).

- **O_2 therapy** to keep the O_2 saturation > 90%.
- **Inhaled β_2-agonist (racemic albuterol or its R isomer levalbuterol).**
  - Amount and frequency depend on the degree of airflow obstruction. Patients with severe exacerbation should receive three treatments within the first hour or continuous therapy for at least 1 hour.
  - **Drug delivery is equivalent** with handheld MDIs and nebulizer therapy in multiple studies; however, the latter is clinically more effective in patients who are in acute distress.
- **Combination therapy** with ipratropium bromide (0.5 mg per 3-mL vial) may improve bronchodilation and decrease the need for hospitalization and should be used for the first three treatments in all patients with severe exacerbations.
  - **Systemic corticosteroids** decrease the need for hospitalization and subsequent relapse rate. Requires about 4 hours to take effect; so, **administer early**! Oral and intravenous delivery are equally effective. Discharged patients should continue oral therapy for 3-10 days.
- **Inhaled steroid therapy** is not useful for acute exacerbation but is the mainstay of outpatient treatment.
- **Antibiotics** are generally unnecessary. Reserve for patients with suspected underlying bacterial pneumonia.
- **Magnesium sulfate** is somewhat controversial but has been shown to improve airflow obstruction in patients with severe exacerbations (FEV_1 < 25% predicted).
- **Subcutaneous epinephrine or terbutaline** can be used for patients unable to adequately inhale due to severe bronchospasm. Give 0.2-0.5 mg of epinephrine (1:1000) or 0.25 mg terbutaline every 20 minutes as needed for 3 doses.

TABLE 10.17. Treatment of Acute Asthma Exacerbations

ALL PATIENTS	SELECTED PATIENTS	NOT USEFUL/HARMFUL
O_2 (maintain Sa_{O_2} > 90%)	Ipratropium therapy	Theophylline
Inhaled bronchodilators	Magnesium sulfate	Mucolytic agents
Corticosteroids	Assisted ventilation	Sedatives
	Antibiotics	

KEY FACT

Levalbuterol is the R isomer of albuterol.

KEY FACT

A normal Pa_{CO_2} in the patient with an acute asthma exacerbation indicates moderately severe airflow obstruction.

- **Heliox** may be helpful. Usually delivered in an 80% (helium)/20% (O_2) mixture. As the proportion of O_2 rises, this modality becomes less effective, so it should not be used in a patient with a significant oxygen requirement.
- **Assisted ventilation** in severe cases of ventilatory failure with progressive hypercarbia, acidosis, muscle fatigue, and/or altered mental status.
- **Noninvasive mechanical ventilation (BiPAP)** may be helpful but is not as well established as in CHF and COPD. Patients must be alert with intact airway reflexes.
- **Mechanical ventilation:** Use low tidal volumes (6-8 mL/kg ideal body weight), low respiratory rates (10-12 bpm), and high inspiratory flow rates to allow maximum time for expiration. Moderate hypercapnia ($Paco_2$ < 100 mm Hg) should be allowed while maintaining a pH 7.15-7.2.
- Beware of auto-PEEP and breath stacking leading to barotraumas or hypotension as asthma is primarily a **disease of prolonged expiratory phase**!

KEY FACT

Ketamine has bronchodilator effects and is the preferred induction agent for RSI in severe asthma exacerbation.

Chronic Obstructive Pulmonary Disease

This disease state is characterized by chronic airflow limitation that is no longer fully reversible. COPD is usually progressive and results from a combination of chronic bronchitis and emphysema.

- **Chronic bronchitis** is characterized by excess mucous production in the bronchial tree and defined clinically as chronic productive cough for 3 months in in the year for 2 consecutive years.
- **Emphysema** is defined pathologically as permanent abnormal enlargement of the airspaces distal to the terminal bronchioles with wall destruction.
- The most important risk factor for developing COPD is cigarette smoking. No pack-year cutoff exists for development of COPD, but it is unlikely in a person with 10-15 pack-years and is very likely with > 40 pack-years. Environmental and occupational exposures should also be taken into account. α_1-Antitrypsin (AAT) deficiency is a well-characterized genetic abnormality that predisposes individuals to the development of early onset COPD, but it accounts for < 1% of COPD.

KEY FACT

Confusion is a marker of worsening hypoxia, hypercarbia, and/or acidosis.

Pathophysiology

- Inhalation of irritants → inflammatory cells (neutrophils, lymphocytes, and macrophages) in large and small airways → ↑ in mucous secreting goblet cells in large airways, ↑ in edema, mucus and narrowing of small airways and release of proteinases causing loss of lung alveoli and elasticity.

Symptoms/Examination

- Chronic COPD: Patients present with exertional dyspnea and cough. Tachypnea, expiratory wheezes, accessory muscle use, chest wall hyperinflation and distant breath and heart sounds are often seen on examination.
- Acute exacerbation of COPD: There are often symptoms suggestive of URI or respiratory irritant as a trigger. Tachypnea, tachycardia, hypertension, cyanosis, altered mental status, increased work of breathing, diminished breath sounds, and cyanosis can be seen on examination.
- Neck vein distention, a tender liver, and lower extremity edema suggest cor pulmonale.

KEY FACT

Clubbing is not a sign of COPD. If present, look for lung malignancy.

Differential

Acute bronchitis, asthma, bronchiectasis, CF, CHF

DIAGNOSIS

Along with a history and physical examination, testing modalities that are useful in diagnosing COPD and evaluating the disease progression include CXR, pulmonary function tests (PFTs), and ABG analysis.

- **Spirometry:** Essential for diagnosis as well as for the evaluation of treatment and disease progression. A postbronchodilator FEV_1 to forced vital capacity ratio (FEV_1/FVC) of < 0.7 confirms the presence of airflow limitation that is not fully reversible and is essential for the diagnosis.
- **CXR:** Typically demonstrates ↓ lung markings, ↑ retrosternal airspace, and flattened diaphragms. Mainly used to evaluate for complications and comorbidities.
- **ABG analysis:** Acute exacerbations show hypoxemia and hypercarbia, with acute respiratory acidosis. Routine use is not recommended.
- **BODE index**: This is more effective than FEV_1 at predicting the risk of death from any cause in patients with COPD and can predict hospitalizations. The **BODE** index consists of:
  - **B**MI
  - **O**bstruction of airflow (FEV_1)
  - **D**yspnea (as measured by the modified Medical Research Council dyspnea scale)
  - **E**xercise capacity (6-minute walk)

TREATMENT

- **Acute exacerbations:** Where possible, the cause of the exacerbation should be treated.
- **β_2-Adrenergic** and **anticholinergic agents** are first-line therapy.
- Treatment includes **O_2 therapy** titrated to maintain an O_2 saturation of around 90%.
- **Systemic corticosteroids** in oral or IV form help decrease the length of exacerbations and improve FEV_1 in hospitalized patients.
- **Antibiotics** are recommended by the American Thoracic Society for patients with moderate to severe acute exacerbation who have a **change in sputum amount, consistency, or color.**
- **Noninvasive positive pressure ventilation** (**NPPV**) is of benefit for patients with **severe** acute exacerbations of COPD as it reduces in-hospital mortality, decreases the need for intubation, and diminishes hospital length of stay. It should be considered for all patients with moderate to severe dyspnea and/or respiratory rate > 25 breaths/min. Patients must be alert with intact airway reflexes.
- **Mechanical ventilation** is used when NPPV fails or is contraindicated, cardiovascular complications, failure of therapy, severe acidosis or hypoxemia, severe dyspnea, and respiratory arrest.

> **KEY FACT**
>
> Mild COPD: $FEV_1 \geq 80\%$ predicted
> Moderate COPD: $FEV_1 < 80\%$ predicted
> Severe COPD: $FEV_1 < 50\%$ predicted

> **KEY FACT**
>
> Long-term O_2 therapy is the only intervention known to ↑ life expectancy in hypoxemic COPD patients.

Acute Upper Airway Obstruction

The upper airway extends from the lips and nares to the first tracheal ring. When upper airway obstruction is present, patients typically develop stridor when the diameter is < 5 mm.

CAUSES

- **Infection:** Epiglottitis, croup, retropharyngeal abscess, peritonsillar abscess, Ludwig angina
- **Medical conditions:** Anaphylaxis, angioedema, laryngospasm, neoplasm
- **Trauma:** Blunt or penetrating trauma; tongue in presence of altered mental status
- **Physical and chemical agents:** Foreign body, burn, caustic ingestion

> **KEY FACT**
>
> **Inspiratory** stridor is associated with obstruction above the glottis. **Expiratory** stridor is more likely to result from intrathoracic obstruction.

SYMPTOMS/EXAMINATION

- The patient will typically appear anxious or agitated and will often prefer to sit upright.
- Dyspnea, stridor, drooling, or spitting secretions.
- Other symptoms depend on underlying cause (eg, fever and sore throat with epiglottitis).

DIAGNOSIS

- Often based on clinical presentation alone.
- **Soft-tissue neck x-ray:** May reveal foreign body or inflammation (**steeple sign,** which is supraglottic swelling on the AP view typically found in croup; **thumbprint sign** in epiglottitis; or an **irregular tracheal margin** in bacterial tracheitis).
- Other diagnostic modalities as indicated for suspected etiology: CXR, CT neck, laboratory work.
- **Direct laryngoscopy:** Can define degree of obstruction.

TREATMENT

- Treatment depends on the underlying cause of the obstruction.
- Allow the patient to maintain a position of comfort (typically a sniffing position) and provide supplemental O_2.
- Immediate procedures to control the airway are needed if the obstruction is severe or progressing.
- If foreign body is present or suspected:
  - Heimlich maneuver if patient is awake (see Chapter 1, Resuscitation).
  - Direct laryngoscopy and removal with Magill forceps if patient is unconscious.

Spontaneous and Iatrogenic Pneumothorax

Pneumothorax is defined as the presence of air in the pleural space.

- **Spontaneous pneumothorax:** Not caused by any obvious external factor (eg, trauma).
  - **1° spontaneous pneumothorax:** No clinically apparent lung disease; usually tall, thin males.
  - **2° spontaneous pneumothorax:** Occurring in patients with underlying pulmonary disease process (Table 10.18).
- **Iatrogenic pneumothorax**: The result of diagnostic (thoracentesis) or therapeutic intervention (central venous catheter placement).

TABLE 10.18. Common Causes of Secondary Spontaneous Pneumothorax

COPD (most common)
Asthma
Pneumonia (eg, *Pneumocystis jiroveci*, TB)
Interstitial lung disease
PE
Cystic fibrosis
Malignancy
Endometriosis

COPD, chronic obstructive pulmonary disease; PE; TB, Tuberculosis.

SYMPTOMS/EXAMINATION

- Most patients present with unilateral chest pain (either sharp or steady pressure) and acute shortness of breath.
- Patients with significant underlying lung disease may present with significant distress, even with a small pneumothorax.
- The physical examination may be normal if the pneumothorax is small.
- If the pneumothorax is large, examination may reveal ↓ chest movement, hyper-resonance, ↓ fremitus, and ↓ breath sounds.
- Tachycardia, hypotension, and tracheal deviation should raise suspicion of tension pneumothorax.

DIFFERENTIAL

Acute PE, myocardial infarction (MI), pleural effusion, pneumonia, pericardial tamponade

DIAGNOSIS

- **CXR** is usually confirmative. A **deep sulcus sign** (deep lateral costophrenic angle) suggests pneumothorax on the supine radiograph.
- Bedside ultrasound can rapidly diagnose pneumothorax. Sensitivity approaches 100%. The absence of lung sliding and loss of the comet tail artifact are consistent with pneumothorax.
- CT can be used to assess the stable patient with underlying lung disease when the diagnosis is in question (eg, differentiating bleb from pneumothorax).

TREATMENT

- **Small 1° pneumothoraces:** This usually can be resolved with simple observation and O_2 therapy. Supplemental O_2 accelerates the reabsorption of gas from the pleural space from 1% to 1.25% per day to about 8%-9% per day.
- **Larger, more symptomatic primary spontaneous pneumothoraces:** May be drained either with simple aspiration or with placement of a small-bore chest tube.
- **2° spontaneous pneumothorax:** Treat with a larger-bore chest tube attached to a water-seal device. Small-bore tube or needle aspiration may be appropriate in select patients.
- Persistent air leaks and recurrences are more common with 2° than with 1° spontaneous pneumothorax.
- For those with 2° spontaneous pneumothorax, recurrence is often prevented with instillation of sclerosing agents (eg, talc) through the chest tube, video-assisted thoracoscopic surgery, or limited thoracotomy.
- Interventions to prevent recurrence in patients with 1° spontaneous pneumothorax are usually recommended only after the second ipsilateral pneumothorax. Often, pilots and divers with 1° spontaneous pneumothorax will have an intervention at the first occurrence due to the risk to self and/or others should the pneumothorax recur.

Pneumomediastinum

Results from ↑ intra-alveolar pressures → small alveolar ruptures → gas moves along vascular sheaths into the mediastinum. The air is less often originating from the GI tract, upper airways, or intrathoracic airways. Generally, this is a benign, self-limiting condition unless associated with esophageal perforation or mediastinitis.

Q

A 45-year-old man presents to the ED for evaluation of pleuritic chest pain that started after returning home from upper endoscopy for evaluation of possible peptic ulcer disease. The patient is well-appearing with normal vital signs. Examination is remarkable for a crunching sound over the precordium and a CXR confirms your diagnosis of pneumomediastinum. What next?

KEY FACT

Tension pneumothorax is a medical emergency requiring immediate decompression of the pleural space with a 14-gauge needle in the second intercostal space at the midclavicular line.

A

Even without clinical evidence to suggest mediastinitis, the onset of symptoms following upper endoscopy makes esophageal rupture a possibility. A fluoroscopic evaluation of the esophagus using water soluble contrast should be obtained and broad-spectrum antibiotics initiated until the diagnosis is excluded.

Causes

Usually occurs spontaneously in young, healthy patients in their second to fourth decades but has been associated with acute asthma exacerbations, heavy physical exertion (eg, coughing, weight lifting, vomiting), inhaling recreational vapors ("huffing"), Valsalva maneuvers, iatrogenic procedures, mechanical ventilation, and trauma.

Symptoms/Examination

- Chest pain worsened by inspiration, often radiating to back, neck, or shoulders; dyspnea; dysphagia; and dysphonia.
- Crepitus suggestive of subcutaneous air is the most common finding.
- **Hamman sign** is a crunching sound that is synchronous with the heartbeat. It is uncommonly seen, but when present, it is highly suggestive of pneumomediastinum.
- Often there is no physical abnormality.
- Suspect esophageal perforation and/or mediastinitis if evidence of systemic toxicity.

Diagnosis

- CXR: Most easily seen on lateral view; a thin line of radiolucency that outlines the heart and mediastinal structures
- CT: More sensitive than CXR; may also provide the etiology of the air, eg, esophageal perforation
- Bronchoscopy if tracheobronchial perforation is suspected
- Contrast esophagography with water soluble contrast if esophageal rupture is suspected

Treatment

- Most cases resolve spontaneously.
- Admission or observation is indicated if symptoms are severe or if there is suspicion for pneumothorax, tension pneumothorax, esophageal perforation, or mediastinitis.
- Antibiotics are indicated if mediastinitis is suspected.
- Surgery is rarely needed.

Complications

Pneumothorax, tension pneumothorax, mediastinitis, tension pneumomediastinum.

Mediastinitis

A very serious, life-threatening condition that usually occurs after a medical procedure (eg, cardiac surgery, endoscopy, or bronchoscopy). Risk factors include malignancy, immunocompromise, autoimmune disease, diabetes, and illicit drug use. Pathogens vary with underlying cause (eg, *S aureus* and *S epidermidis* after cardiac surgery and *Peptostreptococcus* and *Bacteroides* if extending from oral or retropharyngeal spaces).

Causes

- Cardiac or mediastinal surgery/procedure
- .Esophageal perforation
- Trauma
- Odontogenic infection (descending necrotizing mediastinitis)

- Inhalational anthrax
- Chronic granulomatous disease (most commonly TB or histoplasmosis) may lead to a fibrosing mediastinitis

SYMPTOMS/EXAMINATION

- Chest pain often worsened by inspiration radiating to the neck or upper back, dyspnea, confusion, and symptoms related to diagnosis (eg, sore throat or dental pain if odontogenic).
- Fever, tachycardia, and systemic toxicity are common.
- Hamman sign (systolic crunching sound) and subcutaneous emphysema with esophageal perforation.
- Redness and swelling around surgical site.

DIFFERENTIAL

Cellulitis, necrotizing fasciitis, pharyngitis, pneumonia, Ludwig angina.

DIAGNOSIS

- Mainly a clinical diagnosis.
- CT may reveal findings of pneumomediastinum, mediastinal air fluid levels or precervical, retropharyngeal, and paratracheal soft tissue swelling.
- An esophagogram using water soluble contrast is the preferred study to diagnose esophageal perforation. Barium should not be used as an initial study as it can worsen mediastinitis.

TREATMENT

- Ensure adequate airway protection, supportive care
- Broad-spectrum antibiotics, including coverage for MRSA, *Pseudomonas*, and oral and GI flora
- Surgical consultation

COMPLICATIONS

Sepsis, pneumoperitoneum, pneumothorax.

Pulmonary Irritants

PNEUMOCONIOSIS

Pneumoconiosis is a lung disease caused by inhalation of organic or inorganic dusts. It usually develops over long periods of time and is often occupation related. The chronic inflammation caused by these dust particles eventually leads to pulmonary fibrosis.

CAUSES

Common dusts include asbestos, silica minerals, talc, and carbon materials (Table 10.19), and rarely, beryllium and hard metals (cobalt, tungsten carbide, aluminum).

SYMPTOMS/EXAMINATION

Often asymptomatic for 20-30 years from time of initial exposure. Illness depends on severity and duration of exposure. It typically presents with insidious onset of shortness of breath or dyspnea on exertion that is made worse with cigarette smoking. **Cough, sputum production, and wheezing are unusual.** Fine bibasilar and end-expiratory crackles as well as clubbing can be seen.

TABLE 10.19. Common Pneumoconiosis

SUBSTANCE/DISEASE	SOURCE	OCCUPATIONS
Asbestos/Asbestosis	Home insulation, fireproof materials, tiles for floors	Construction workers, miners, demolition workers, ship builders, and auto mechanics
Silicon dioxide/Silicosis	Sand, sandstone, slate, clay, granite	Sandblasters, miners, tunnel builders, quarry workers, masonry workers
Carbon/Coal worker's lung	Coal, graphite	Coal miners
Talc/Talcosis	Paint, cosmetics, rubber, plastics	Miners and millers, IDU
Kaolin/Kaolinosis (china clay)	Ceramics, papers, medicines, cosmetics, toothpaste, rubber	Miners and millers
Iron/Siderosis	Iron metal or dust	Welders or silver polishers, foundry workers

IDU, injection drug users.

DIFFERENTIAL

COPD, TB, fungal infection, interstitial lung disease, cancer, rheumatoid nodules, sarcoidosis.

DIAGNOSIS

- Reliable exposure history.
- CXR: Generally signs of interstitial fibrosis.
  - Asbestosis: Coarse honeycombing in advanced disease; **pleural plaques**
  - Silicosis: **Nodular opacities** in the upper lobes with sharp margins in simple silicosis; **large upper- or midzone opacities** ("angel wings") due to progressive massive fibrosis in complicated silicosis; **basilar alveolar filling pattern** in acute silicosis
  - Carbon (coal miners lung): Small, rounded opacities first seen in the upper lobes
- PFTs reveal **reduced lung volumes**, particularly vital capacity and total lung capacity, diminished single breath diffusing capacity of the lungs for carbon monoxide (DLCO), ↓ compliance, often **absence of obstruction.**
- Absence of other causes of interstitial fibrosis.

TREATMENT

- Mainly prevention and supportive
- Smoking cessation
- Supplemental O_2 as needed
- Pneumococcal and influenza vaccination
- Corticosteroids may be helpful
- Bronchodilators may be helpful

COMPLICATIONS

- Respiratory failure, especially with concomitant pulmonary infection
- Cancer (malignant mesothelioma in asbestosis, bronchogenic carcinoma in asbestosis + smoking)
- TB in cases of silicosis

TOXIC GASES, FUMES, VAPORS

Chemical irritants in the form of gases, fumes, and vapors are readily absorbed by the lung lining and can cause inflammation and edema that can lead to acute injury as well as delayed manifestations. Toxicity depends on concentration and duration of exposure.

Common substances are found in Table 10.20.

Diagnosis

- Clinical diagnosis primarily from history of exposure.
- Helpful studies may include ABG with COHb and MetHb levels, lactate, red blood cell (RBC) cyanide levels, ECG, and CXR.

Treatment

- Removal from source.
- 100% O_2.

TABLE 10.20. Common Toxic Gases, Fumes, and Vapors

Substance	Source	Odor	Toxicity
Phosgene	Plastics, textiles, pharmaceuticals	Newly mowed hay	Hydrolyzes to CO_2 and HCl in lower airway → acid burn with acute lung injury/ARDS.
Chlorine	Water purification, paper manufacturing	"Swimming pool"	Forms acids and oxidants causing mostly ocular and upper airway irritation and nausea/vomiting. ARDS is possible. Yellow-green gas.
Nitrogen dioxide	Combustion, silo gas (Silo Fillers disease)	Household bleach	Converts to nitric acid; triphasic reaction: initial dyspnea, improvement, delayed alveolar injury, pulmonary edema and ARDS.
Ammonia	Fertilizers, plastics, explosives	Cleaning products	Forms ammonium hydroxide causing severe mucus membrane irritation.
Hydrocarbons	Fuels, paint, glue, cleaning solvents	Hydrocarbons	Intentional inhalation (huffing) → CNS stimulation followed by ↓ alertness and seizures. Arrhythmias, hypoxia, aplastic anemia, sudden death possible.
Hydrogen sulfide	Anaerobic organic decomposition	Rotten eggs	Disrupts oxidative phosphorylation causing cellular asphyxia and anaerobic metabolism → rapid loss of consciousness and seizures. **Similar to cyanide.**

ARDS, acute respiratory distress syndrome; CNS, central nervous system.

- Irrigation of exposed areas, especially eyes and skin.
- Early intubation if signs of airway edema and obstruction.
- Bronchodilators may be helpful.
- Antibiotics are not helpful.
- Steroids may be helpful in nitrogen oxide poisoning to prevent bronchiolitis obliterans.
- Cyanide antidote kit in hydrogen sulfide poisoning.

COMPLICATIONS

- **Pulmonary edema** (often delayed) from a chemical pneumonitis is a common complication among most toxic gases, fumes, and vapors.

Other possible complications include:

- **Nitrogen oxides:** Methemoglobinemia, bronchiolitis obliterans
- **Ammonia:** Corneal burns
- **Hydrocarbons:** Persistent airway irritation, CNS depression, peripheral neuropathy, dysrhythmias, hepatic toxicity (eg, CCl_4), renal failure, blood dyscrasias

Cystic Fibrosis

This is the most common lethal autosomal-recessive disorder in Caucasians, affecting 1 in 3500 births. It is classically characterized by multisystem involvement of the sinuses, lungs, pancreas, liver, gallbladder, intestines, bones, and in males, the vas deferens.

> **KEY FACT**
>
> Most CF patients are diagnosed in childhood, and all 50 states instituted newborn screening by 2010, but a few mild cases are diagnosed as adults and tend to have upper-lobe bronchiectasis.

CAUSES

CF is caused by mutations in the CF transmembrane conductance regulator (CFTR) → chloride channel dysfunction → thickened secretions and decreased clearance of secretions.

SYMPTOMS/EXAMINATION

- Most CF patients are diagnosed during childhood prior to age 1. A history of failure to thrive as a child, persistent respiratory infections (*Pseudomonas*), nasal polyposis, sinusitis, intestinal obstruction, malabsorption, recurrent pancreatitis, hepatobiliary disease, and male infertility are suggestive of CF.
- 7% CF patients are diagnosed as adults, and these patients tend to present with upper lobe bronchiectasis.
- **Examination** may reveal ↑ chest AP diameter, upper lung field crackles, nasal polyps, hepatomegaly, and clubbing.
- Acute pulmonary exacerbations are typically characterized by ↑ sputum production, dyspnea, fatigue, weight loss, and a decline in FEV_1.

DIFFERENTIAL

Immunodeficiency, asthma, allergic bronchopulmonary aspergillosis (ABPA)

DIAGNOSIS

Diagnosis requires both clinical and laboratory evidence of CFTR dysfunction.

- All 50 states instituted newborn screening for CF by 2010. It typically involves serum immunoreactive trypsinogen assay followed by a confirmatory DNA assay if positive. Those screening positive for both will have confirmation with a sweat test.

- **Sweat chloride concentration:** The best screening test for CF for a patient with a suggestive clinical picture; normal sweat chloride is < 40 mmol/L.
- **Genotyping:** Screening for the presence of two CFTR mutations known to cause CF; newer tests screen for > 1000 different known mutations.
- **CXR:** Shows hyperinflation, bronchiectasis, and upper lobe infiltrates; nodules often represent mucoid impaction in the airways.

Treatment

- **Acute pulmonary exacerbations:** Treat with chest physical therapy, bronchodilators, DNase, and usually two antipseudomonal antibiotics.
- **Chronic stable CF**
  - **Inhaled tobramycin:** Slows the decline in FEV_1 and is used for long-term therapy.
  - **Nebulized DNase:** Improves clearance of secretions, improves FEV_1, and should be offered to patients with daily cough, sputum production, and airflow obstruction.
  - **Azithromycin:** Improves FEV_1, reduces inflammation and reduces pulmonary exacerbations in those infected with *Pseudomonas*.
  - **Aerobic exercise, flutter devices, external percussive vests:** Help with regular airway clearance.
  - **Pancreatic enzymes** and the **fat-soluble vitamins A, D, E, and K:** Given for malabsorption.
  - **Nutritional counseling:** Essential for proper health maintenance and to help prevent diabetic complications, osteoporosis, and weight loss.
  - **Double-lung transplantation:** Remains an option for severe progressive pulmonary disease.

Sarcoidosis

This is a systemic granulomatous disease of unknown etiology that primarily affects the lungs and lymphatics and is characterized by noncaseating granulomas. It is primarily a self-limited disease of young and middle-aged adult Black Americans or those of Scandinavian descent.

Symptoms/Examination

- Nonspecific constitutional symptoms such as fever, fatigue, anorexia, weight loss, and arthralgias.
- Physical examination may reveal dry crackles and extrapulmonary manifestations such as lymphadenopathy, **parotid enlargement**, splenomegaly, uveitis, or skin changes (erythema nodosum).

Differential

TB, fungal infections, rheumatoid arthritis, lymphoma, Wegener granulomatosis

Diagnosis

- Suspect based on findings of bilateral hilar adenopathy, pulmonary infiltrates, and skin lesions.
- Diagnosis is made by a combination of clinical, radiographic, and histologic findings along with exclusion of other diseases that have a similar clinical picture.

Treatment

Systemic corticosteroids.

Pulmonary Hypertension

Defined as an abnormally elevated pulmonary artery pressure, pulmonary hypertension is usually an indicator of an advanced underlying disease. It is classified into five groups based on cause and response to treatment:

1. Group 1: Pulmonary *arterial* hypertension (eg, idiopathic, portal hypertension, rheumatologic diseases, drug- or toxin-induced, genetic)
2. Group 2: pulmonary *venous* hypertension (eg, left heart failure, mitral stenosis)
3. Group 3: Chronic hypoxemic lung disease (eg, COPD, interstitial lung disease, obstructive sleep apnea, bronchiectasis)
4. Group 4: Chronic thromboembolic disease
5. Group 5: Miscellaneous other causes (eg, sarcoidosis, lymphatic obstructions, metabolic disorders)

Symptoms/Examination

- Along with symptoms of the underlying disease process, patients may present with progressive dyspnea, fatigue, and right upper quadrant (RUQ) pain from hepatic congestion.
- Findings of R ventricular failure (elevated jugular venous pressure, hepatomegaly and lower extremity edema).

Diagnosis

- ECG showing signs of right ventricular hypertrophy.
- Echocardiography: Can estimate the pulmonary artery pressure and provide information about L heart function.
- Right heart catheterization: Resting mean pulmonary artery pressure > 25 mm Hg confirms diagnosis.
- Further evaluation of the patient with pulmonary hypertension is focused on determining an underlying cause (eg, V/Q for chronic thromboembolism, PFTs for COPD, overnight oximetry for sleep apnea).

Treatment

- No consensus guidelines for treatment.
- Supplemental oxygen therapy titrated to > 90%.
- Anticoagulation for those with idiopathic, drug-induced, and chronic thromboembolic causes.
- Diuretics should be used with care for fluid retention.
- More advanced therapy (eg, phosphodiesterase inhibitors, prostanoids) are selected based on vasodilatory response testing, underlying cause, and functional classification.

Solitary Pulmonary Nodule

This is defined as an isolated round lesion < 3 cm in diameter that is surrounded by pulmonary parenchyma. Abnormalities > 3 cm are termed masses and are usually malignant. Cancer affects 10%-70% of those with solitary pulmonary nodules. Most benign lesions are infectious granulomas.

Causes

Granuloma (old TB, histoplasmosis, foreign body reaction), bronchogenic carcinoma, metastatic disease, bronchial adenoma.

Symptoms/Examination

- Patients are often asymptomatic but may present with cough, hemoptysis, and dyspnea.
- Older age and a history of cigarette smoking raise the suspicion of cancer.
- Patients should be questioned about prior TB and histoplasmosis.
- Physical examination of the lungs is frequently normal. However, examination of the lymphatic system may demonstrate lymphadenopathy.

Diagnosis

- Solitary pulmonary nodules are usually discovered incidentally.
- **Comparison of serial CXRs:** The **initial** step in determining the progression and extent of the nodule; stability of findings on CXR for 2 years is considered a sign that the lesion is benign.
- **Chest CT:** This offers improved estimation of nodule size, characteristics (eg, pattern of calcification), and interval growth. Contrast enhancement allows for the simultaneous evaluation of the mediastinum for lymphadenopathy.
- Positron emission tomography (**PET**) **scan:** This may help provide staging information in the case of lung cancer. The diagnostic accuracy of detecting mediastinal involvement among patients with lung cancer is 65% by CT, 90% by PET, and > 95% using a combination of CT and PET.

Treatment

- When the probability of cancer is low (age < 35 years, nonsmokers, smooth nodules with a diameter < 1.5 cm), the lesion should be monitored with serial high-resolution CT at 3-month intervals. Low threshold for excision or biopsy if it persists.
- When the probability of cancer is high (age > 35, smokers, spiculated nodules with a diameter > 2 cm), the lesion should be resected if preoperative risk is acceptable and there are no other contraindications to surgery.
- When the probability of cancer is intermediate, additional testing (PET, transthoracic needle biopsy) may be warranted.

KEY FACT

Lesions that ↑ in size or change in character are likely malignant and should be resected, assuming low surgical risk and no evidence of metastatic disease.

REVIEW QUESTIONS

QUESTIONS

1. A patient with diabetic ketoacidosis and a pH of 6.9 is paralyzed and intubated for altered mental status. After intubation, a repeat blood gas shows a pH of 6.7. What intervention should occur immediately?
   A. Administer IV sodium bicarbonate
   B. Increase peak end expiratory pressure
   C. Decrease Fio_2
   D. Increase respiratory rate

2. A previously healthy 22-year-old man presents to an emergency department (ED) in New Mexico with 3 days of fever and malaise and now shortness of breath. His O_2 saturation on room air is 82%. He has been cleaning out some cabins. His chest x-ray (CXR) shows interstitial pneumonia. What is the most likely diagnosis:
   A. Legionella
   B. Hanta virus
   C. Histoplasmosis
   D. Coccidiomycosis

3. Following intubation, a patient with altered mental status is mildly hypoxic despite 100% Fio_2. Decreased breath sounds are heard in the left chest. What problem should you suspect?
   A. Pneumothorax
   B. Pulmonary embolism
   C. Right mainstem intubation
   D. Esophageal intubation

4. A patient with a history of alcohol use presents with fever, cough, and shortness of breath. CXR shows a consolidation in the right lower lung and a larger right pleural effusion. What additional diagnostic test should be performed?
   A. CT chest
   B. Right upper quadrant (RUQ) U/S
   C. Lower extremity ultrasound
   D. Thoracentesis

ANSWERS

1. **D.** Increase respiratory rate. Patients with DKA breath fast spontaneously in order to lower their Pco_2 in compensation for their metabolic acidosis. Paralysis blocks this compensation. It is essential that you maintain a high minute ventilation after paralysis in these patients, and the usual way to do this is to maintain a high respiratory rate. Sodium bicarbonate will usually raise a patient's pH but has been associated with cerebral edema. Changes in PEEP and Fio_2 can increase oxygenation but do not direct raise pH.

2. **B.** Hanta virus. Hanta virus is found in the Western United States and is transmitted to humans via the excretion of respiratory excreta, especially deer mouse. Patients develop interstitial pneumonia which often results in profound hypoxia. Mortality is 50%-75%. Legionella is a gram-negative bacteria found in water systems. It can cause pneumonia but typically this illness is only serious in immunocompromised and the elderly. Histoplasmosis is a fungal infection that typically infects the lungs but is found in the United States predominantly in the Ohio River valley and lower Mississippi River. Coccidiomycosis is a fungal infection that occurs in the Western United States, but typical symptoms are headache, rash, muscle pain, and joint pain.

3. **C.** Right mainstem intubation. Right mainstem intubation is common. It results from placement of the tip of the ET below the level of the carina and into right mainstem bronchus. A pneumothorax can occur following positive pressure ventilation but is less likely. Pulmonary embolism would not result in reduced breath sounds in the left chest. One should always be alert to the possibility of an esophageal intubation, but this would result in profound hypoxia and no breath sounds in either chest.

4. **D.** Thoracentesis. A pleural effusion in a patient with pneumonia should raise suspicion for empyema which can only be excluded with a thoracentesis. If emphyema is present, a patient will likely require a chest tube to clear the infection. The other tests do not excluded empyema.

CHAPTER 11

Abdominal and Gastrointestinal Emergencies

C. Scott Forsythe, MD, MPH

Esophageal Disorders

ESOPHAGITIS

Esophagitis is defined as inflammation of the esophagus. The most common cause is gastroesophageal reflux disease (GERD). Other causes include infection, retained pill, caustic ingestion, radiation, autoimmune, and eosinophilic esophagitis.

Infectious esophagitis is usually seen in immunosuppressed patients. It is primarily caused by *Candida albicans*, though viral (primarily cytomegalovirus [CMV], herpes simplex virus [HSV]) and fungal infections are also seen.

Pill esophagitis occurs when a pill fails to pass through the esophagus causing focal esophageal inflammation. Structural or functional disorders of the esophagus make this more likely. Common offending pills include potassium chloride, ferrous sulfate, bisphosphonates, nonsteroidal anti-inflammatory drugs (NSAIDs), and tetracycline antibiotics.

KEY FACT

Advanced *acquired immune deficiency syndrome* (AIDS) (CD4 count < 200) should make you more aware of the potential for esophageal candidiasis. However, 25% of patients with esophageal candidiasis will not have evidence of thrush on oral examination.

SYMPTOMS/EXAMINATION

Substernal **chest pain, odynophagia, dysphagia**, and **drooling** are common symptoms. Oral lesions are not reliable diagnostic indicators. Some patients may be severely **dehydrated** from poor oral intake.

DIFFERENTIAL

Includes functional dyspepsia, esophageal stricture, mass lesion, motility disorders, esophageal spasm, and cardiac disease.

DIAGNOSIS

Endoscopy ± biopsy

TREATMENT

- **Pill esophagitis:** Instruct patients to drink 8 oz of water with each pill and then remain upright for at least 30 minutes. Full symptom relief may take up to 6 weeks.
- ***C albicans:*** Clotrimazole troches or nystatin swish and swallow for 1-2 weeks in patients with mild disease limited to the oropharynx and a normal immune state. Advanced cases and immunocompromised patients should be treated with an oral antifungal agent such as fluconazole or itraconazole for 3-4 weeks.
- **CMV:** Intravenous (IV) ganciclovir or foscarnet.
- **HSV:** Oral antiviral, such as acyclovir or valacyclovir.

COMPLICATIONS

Include **dehydration** requiring IV resuscitation, stricture, **perforation/** mediastinitis, **malnutrition**, and **hemorrhage**. Viral or fungal cases may lead to disseminated infection.

GASTROESOPHAGEAL REFLUX DISEASE

Affects approximately 10% of adults daily; often related to **incompetence of the lower esophageal sphincter**, hiatal hernia, increased intragastric pressure (pregnancy, obesity), or incomplete emptying of the stomach. Medications that relax smooth muscle (eg, nitrates, calcium channel blockers [CCBs], anticholinergics, or albuterol) can contribute.

Symptoms/Examination

- Typical presentation is subxiphoid **burning sensation** that radiates upward toward the neck within 1 hour of a meal, during exercise, or when lying recumbent. Symptoms are at least **partially relieved by antacids**. **Water brash** (excess salivation), bitter taste, **globus sensation** (throat fullness), odynophagia, dysphagia, halitosis, and otalgia are also commonly seen.
- Atypical symptoms (up to 50%) include nocturnal cough, asthma, hoarseness, and noncardiac chest pain associated with diaphoresis, pallor, nausea, and vomiting.
- Examination is often normal; patients may present with **poor dentition** or wheezing.

Diagnosis

- Diagnostic testing is rarely necessary in the ED for **typical symptoms;** treat with an empiric trial of proton pump inhibitor (PPI) for 4-6 weeks.
- If the patient is **unresponsive** to therapy or has **alarm symptoms** (dysphagia, odynophagia, weight loss, anemia, long-standing symptoms, blood in stool, age > 50), proceed as follows:
  - **Upper endoscopy with biopsy:** Standard workup in the presence of **alarm symptoms;** normal in > 50% of patients with GERD (most have nonerosive reflux disease) or may reveal endoscopic esophagitis grades 1 (mild) to 4 (severe erosions, strictures, Barrett esophagus); strictures can be dilated.
  - **Barium esophagography:** Limited role but can identify strictures.
  - **Ambulatory esophageal pH monitoring:** The gold standard, but often unnecessary; indicated for correlating persistent symptoms with pH parameters despite medical therapy and normal endoscopy.

Treatment (Table 11.1)

- **Behavior modification**: Only elevating the head of the bed and weight loss are directly evidence based. Avoiding tobacco and alcohol use, eating smaller meals, and avoiding recumbency after eating are often advised, as is avoiding certain foods (eg, mint, chocolate, coffee, tea, carbonated drinks, citrus, and tomato juice). Older guidelines recommended initial treatment with behavioral changes alone, though new evidence suggests they are rarely helpful without simultaneous medical management.
- **Antacids** are used for mild GERD and provide short-term relief.
  - **H_2-receptor antagonists** are used for mild to moderate GERD or as an adjunct for nocturnal GERD while the patient is on PPIs; they are effective in 50%-60% of cases and thought to be safe in pregnancy.
  - **PPIs**: The mainstay of therapy for mild to severe GERD; generally safe and effective in relieving and preventing symptoms. Recently associated with pneumonia, atrophic gastritis (hypergastrinemia), enteric infections (*Clostridium difficile*), and hip fractures. Avoid in patients with acute coronary syndrome (ACS) on clopidogrel as new evidence suggests an association with increased reinfarction. Daily dosage effective in 80%-90% of patients; **fewer than 5%** of patients are **refractory** to twice-daily dosage.

Complications

Include **Barrett esophagus**, in which metaplastic columnar epithelium replaces normal stratified squamous epithelial cells and predisposes to development of adenocarcinoma. **Peptic strictures** and resultant dysphagia may develop.

Q

A father brings his 6-year-old child to the emergency department (ED) for evaluation of drooling after "getting into something" under the sink. Examination reveals mild drooling and stridor, but no evidence of perioral or oropharyngeal burns or injury. What is the likely diagnosis?

KEY FACT

Both ACS and GERD or esophageal spasm may be exertional in nature and relieved by nitroglycerin.

A

Alkali ingestion

TABLE 11.1. Treatment of GERD/Peptic Ulcer Disease

Agent	Mechanism	Example
Antacid	Neutralizes gastric acid, promote ulcer healing, may also bind to bile and inhibit pepsin	Calcium carbonate, aluminum hydroxide, magnesium hydroxide
Histamine antagonist (H_2 blocker)	Competitive inhibitor of histamine for H_2 receptor on parietal cells, inhibiting gastric acid production	Cimetidine, ranitidine, famotidine, nizatidine
Proton pump inhibitor	Inhibits H^+/K^+ ATPase enzyme in parietal cells by irreversibly binding to proton pumps, preventing acid secretion	Omeprazole, lansoprazole, pantoprazole
Prostaglandins	Indicated only for prevention of NSAID-induced ulcers	Misoprostol
Sucralfate	Binds ulcer site, absorbs / inactivates bile salts. Useful for GERD in pregnancy	Sucralfate
Bismuth	Diminishes pepsin activity, used with triple therapy for *Helicobacter pylori* eradication	Bismuth subsalicylate
H pylori eradication	Causative agent in 95% of duodenal ulcers and 70% of gastric ulcers, Gram-negative, spiral-shaped organism; eradication with triple therapy treatment for 10-14 d	Amoxicillin, clarithromycin, omeprazole or bismuth, tetracycline, metronidazole, omeprazole; other PPIs acceptable to substitute for omeprazole

GERD, gastroesophageal reflux disease; NSAID, nonsteroidal anti-inflammatory drugs; PPI, proton pump inhibitor.

CAUSTIC INGESTIONS—ACIDS AND ALKALIS

Degree of injury following caustic ingestion of a strong alkali or acid is related to **concentration**, volume, and **contact time** with tissue. While **acids produce coagulation necrosis** that limits tissue injury, alkalis cause a **liquefactive** necrosis, allowing continued tissue contact and damage. Most ingestions occur accidentally in children and involve small volumes. Ingestions in adults are often intentional and therefore involve higher volumes and result in more significant injury.

Causes

Strong acids include toilet bowl cleaners, rust removers, and automotive batteries. Ingestion of **household bleach** (5%-10% sodium hypochlorite, alkali) is unlikely to cause serious problems unless > 100 mL has been ingested.

Symptoms

Presentation ranges from minor symptoms to severe chest pain, odynophagia, **dysphagia**, **respiratory distress**, and **drooling**.

Examination

May reveal **local burns** and edema to the oropharynx, with **respiratory distress** and/or stridor if upper airway edema has developed. **The absence of oropharyngeal burns does not preclude significant esophageal and/or gastric injury.**

Diagnosis

Chest x-ray (**CXR**) and/or computed tomography (**CT**) if perforation suspected; upper endoscopy to evaluate extent of injury.

Treatment

- Give IV fluids, pain medication, and PPI; add broad-spectrum **antibiotics** if significant injury is suspected. **Do not** induce vomiting, administer anything by mouth (including charcoal or neutralizing, agent such as water or milk) or place a nasogastric (NG) tube.
- Asymptomatic patient with low volume, low concentration/accidental ingestion should be observed with serial examinations and may be discharged home with outpatient follow-up.
- Otherwise, **admit** for monitoring and **endoscopy**. Severe burns may require **emergent esophagectomy.**

Complications

Airway compromise, perforation, stenosis, strictures.

KEY FACT

Alkali burns cause liquefaction necrosis (much more serious), whereas acidic burns cause coagulation necrosis and eschar formation, which is protective.

DYSPHAGIA

The sensation of difficulty swallowing is termed dysphagia. Causes of dysphagia can be broadly grouped into **neuromuscular**, **motility**, and **structural** problems (Table 11.2).

TABLE 11.2. Dysmotility Syndromes

	Oropharyngeal Dysphagia	Esophageal Dysphagia
Etiology	Neuromuscular disorders (eg, CVA, polymyositis, myasthenia gravis), malignancy, inflammation, inadequate saliva	Motility disorders (achalasia, diffuse esophageal spasm), intrinsic obstruction (mass, strictures), extrinsic obstruction (thyroid, aorta)
Historical Clues	Symptoms immediately upon swallowing, positioning to improve swallow, gagging and drooling, liquids more difficult than solids; other neuromuscular symptoms	Chest pain, food sticking Solid more difficult than liquids in obstruction Solids = liquids in motility d/o
Treatment	Treat underlying condition	Relieve obstruction, where possible Nitrates and Ca^{2+} channel blockers for achalasia

CVA, cerebral vascular accident.

Oropharyngeal dysphagia: Abnormality in transferring **food** from the pharynx to the esophagus occurring within the first 2 seconds of swallowing. Difficulty swallowing **liquids**, particularly of extreme temperatures, suggest underlying neuromuscular disorder; of these, cerebral vascular accident (CVA) is the most common.

Esophageal dysphagia: Difficulty in transfer to the stomach from the upper esophagus. Most often caused by obstructive lesions, although achalasia and diffuse esophageal spasm are well-defined esophageal motility disorders.

Diagnosis

- Careful history and physical examination alone often reveal diagnosis.
- For suspected neuromuscular condition consider central nervous system (CNS) imaging (eg, CVA) and/or laboratory studies (eg, inflammatory myopathy) as indicated by history. For structural lesions, consider laryngoscopy and/or esophagoscopy.
- **Swallow study** (oropharyngeal dysphagia or motor disorder) or **barium swallow** (esophageal dysphagia) are imaging studies of choice, but are often obtained in outpatient gastrointestinal (GI) follow-up. Manometry may be useful in that setting to diagnose motility disorders.
- Admit patients at high risk for aspiration; otherwise, most patients without clear cause of dysphagia can be referred for outpatient GI management.

STRUCTURAL ABNORMALITIES

Mallory-Weiss Tear

A 1- to 4-cm-long tear of the mucosa and submucosa of the stomach (75%) or gastroesophageal junction, typically resulting from retching or vomiting. Most cases are mild and self-limited.

Symptoms

Hematemesis after forceful retching and vomiting.

Examination

Rule out **crepitus of the neck** or peritonitis, which would suggest complete esophageal perforation.

Diagnosis

History or endoscopy.

Treatment

Supportive and symptomatic care is adequate for most cases.

Esophageal Perforation

Esophageal perforation involves all layers of the esophagus and the overlying pleura leading to leakage of nonsterile gastric contents into the mediastinum and thorax. Most noniatrogenic cases are in middle-aged men after ingestion of alcohol or large meal (**termed** *Boerhaave syndrome*); it is classically considered a surgical emergency that can cause rapid, overwhelming sepsis and significant mortality. Conservative management has been described.

Causes

- **Iatrogenic** perforations account for most cases. **Boerhaave syndrome** results from forceful retching leading to increased intraesophageal pressure and a tear of the **posterolateral aspect** (most commonly) of the distal esophagus.

- Additional causes include blunt or penetrating trauma to the neck, esophagitis, and foreign body.

SYMPTOMS/EXAMINATION

- Variable, but **most common** presentation is chest or midepigastric **pain** that **radiates to the neck** and occasionally the back. Pain may migrate from upper abdomen to chest.
- **Most reliable** presentation is pleuritic pain in the esophageal region that is **worsened by neck flexion and swallowing**.
- Often associated with pneumothorax, hydrothorax, or empyema.
- Mediastinal crunch (**Hamman sign**) may be heard during systole with auscultation of the heart (not respiration). **Mackler triad** of subcutaneous emphysema, chest pain, and vomiting is pathognomonic, but all 3 are present in less than half of cases.
- Fever or hypotension with rapid progression to cardiopulmonary collapse.

DIAGNOSIS

- **Plain CXR** and/or **lateral neck film** may reveal pneumomediastinum, subcutaneous emphysema, pleural effusion, pneumothorax, or widened mediastinum; these findings are often absent initially, so **normal plain films do not fully exclude perforation**.
- An **esophagram** using **water-soluble contrast** and **EGD** are the studies of choice to diagnose and locate a perforation. **Barium** should not be used as an initial study as it can worsen mediastinitis, but should be considered following a negative water-soluble study, which may miss up to 10% of cases.
- **CT** should be considered if contrast study is negative or unavailable, and may show mediastinal air, esophageal wall edema and thickening, periesophageal fluid, or mediastinal widening.
- Pleural fluid from thoracentesis showing high amylase levels should raise suspicion for esophageal perforation.

TREATMENT

- Keep **NPO**, administer broad-spectrum **antibiotics**, and obtain immediate **surgical consultation**. NG tubes should never be placed blindly, but can be placed during endoscopy.
- Well-contained perforations without mediastinal involvement or sepsis may be managed conservatively with IV antibiotics and NPO for 72 hours; most patients will require operative repair and ICU care.

Achalasia

Condition characterized by markedly elevated lower esophageal sphincter pressures and lack of esophageal peristalsis. Etiology is unknown.

SYMPTOMS

Dysphagia (with solids and liquids equally), odynophagia, **regurgitation** of undigested food **without** acidic taste, and **chest pain** that worsens with stress and rapid eating. Symptoms are not improved by PPIs.

DIFFERENTIAL

Spasm, stricture, rings, webs, aortic aneurysm, mediastinal masses/tumors.

DIAGNOSIS

Bird's beak on barium swallow (dilation of upper esophagus with narrowing at gastroesophageal junction, see Figure 11.1). Refer to GI for endoscopy and confirmatory manometry.

Q

A 55-year-old woman presents with epigastric and chest pain radiating to her neck, vomiting, fever, and hypotension. She had an unremarkable Esophogastroduodenoscopy (EGD) earlier this morning, and has otherwise been well without prior vomiting. On examination, she has abdominal tenderness with guarding and cervical crepitus. What is the likely diagnosis?

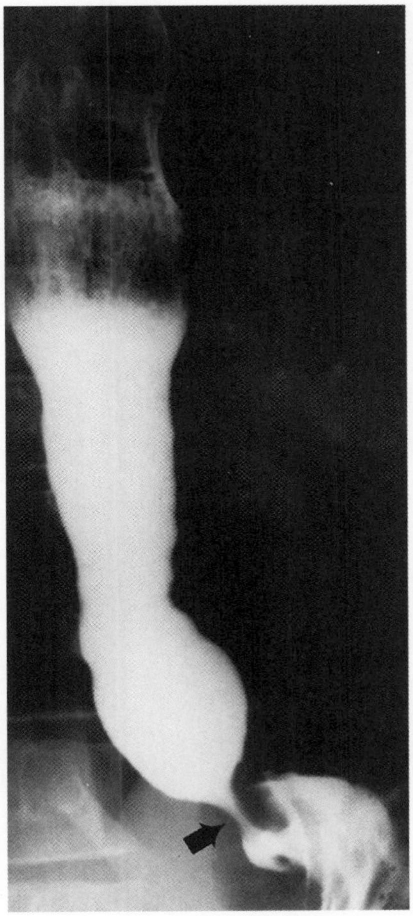

FIGURE 11.1. Achalasia seen on barium swallow (arrow). (Reproduced, with permission, from Chen MY, Pope TL, Ott DJ, eds. *Basic Radiology*. 2nd ed. New York, NY: McGraw-Hill; 2011.)

A

Iatrogenic esophageal perforation.

Treatment

Typically outpatient GI referral for surgical **myotomy** vs **dilation** vs **botulinum** toxin injections. Medical options include **nifedipine** or **nitrates** before meals to decreases LES pressure.

Complications

Dehydration, weight loss, laryngotracheal aspiration (particularly at night).

Esophageal Rings and Webs

Rings and webs are the most common structural abnormalities of the esophagus. A ring is a concentric band of normal esophageal tissue containing all 3 tissue layers. They are typically found in the lower esophagus. A web is an eccentric, thin extension of normal esophageal tissue containing mucosa and submucosa (no muscle layer). They are primarily located in middle or upper esophagus. Webs are seen alone or in **Plummer-Vinson syndrome** (triad of dysphagia, glossitis, and iron-deficiency anemia).

Symptoms

Dysphagia of **solids** greater than liquids is hallmark; symptoms are typically intermittent rather than progressive.

Diagnosis

Barium swallow or EGD.

Treatment

Disruption/dilation by endoscopy. Treat iron deficiency.

FOREIGN BODIES

80% esophageal foreign bodies (FBs) are in children. More than 50% are coins. Obstruction in adults is most often due to food impaction (usually meat). Proximal obstructions can compromise the airway and cause pain, cyanosis, and collapse (**café coronary**); more distal impactions cause severe discomfort and difficulty swallowing (**steakhouse syndrome**).

Button batteries are problematic due to the alkali contents and may cause burns and liquefactive necrosis within 2 hours and perforation of the esophagus within 4-6 hours.

Pathophysiology

Obstruction occurs in places of **physiological narrowing** in the normal esophagus. In children < 4 years, this is the level of the cricopharyngeus muscle (C6). In adults, this is just above the lower esophageal sphincter/diaphragmatic hiatus (T10-T11). However, **90%** of obstructions in adults are associated with **underlying anatomic obstruction** (eg, peptic stricture, esophageal web, or ring).

Symptoms

- **Children** may present with tracheal compression (cough, stridor, wheezing, dyspnea); other symptoms include refusal to eat, vomiting, drooling, or gagging.
- **Adults** commonly present with dysphagia and chest pain; they may localize proximal obstructions while distal obstructions typically present with visceral, epigastric pain.

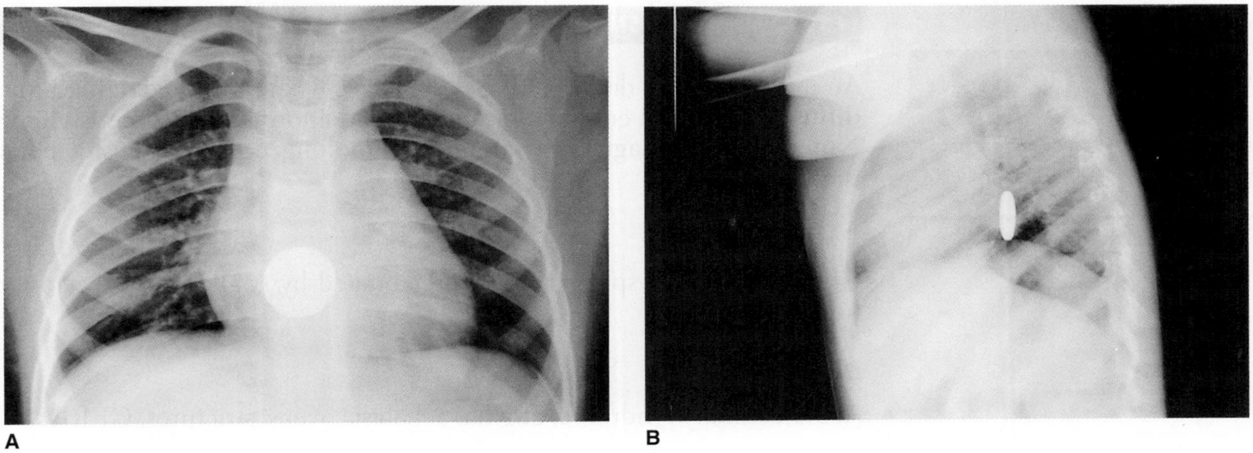

FIGURE 11.2. Posteroanterior (A) and lateral (B) chest x-rays, showing esophageal foreign body. (Reproduced, with permission, from Stone CK, Humphries RL, eds. *Current Diagnosis & Treatment: Emergency Medicine*. 6th ed. New York, NY: McGraw-Hill; 2008.)

EXAMINATION

Neck **crepitus** or **subcutaneous air** suggests esophageal perforation. Listen for **asymmetric breath sounds** or **wheeze** suggesting airway involvement. **Peritonitis** is indicative of GI perforation.

DIAGNOSIS

- Imaging is often not necessary for **food boluses**, but CXR or CT can be used to look for evidence of perforation.
- In **children**, begin with **plain radiographs** of neck and chest; **CT** or **water-soluble contrast study** can be obtained if the object is not identified, but consider that any oral contrast may limit an ensuing endoscopy.

TREATMENT

- **Direct laryngoscopy** for immediate removal if **airway compromise**; no treatment if asymptomatic and no FB visualized on imaging.
- **Expectant management** with discharge and follow-up serial imaging for: smooth objects < 5 by 2 cm and for objects that pass the pylorus (usually arrives at rectum within 3-5 days). **No foreign body of any kind should be left in the esophagus for > 24 hours.**
- **Glucagon** is thought to relax smooth muscle and can be tried in distal esophageal food impaction. Nausea and vomiting are common, and little evidence supports this practice.
- Using **Foley catheters** to remove upper esophageal foreign bodies in children carries the risk of aspiration and esophageal injury and is therefore controversial.
- **Meat tenderizers** are **not** recommended for food impaction and can cause severe damage to esophageal mucosa.
- **Endoscopic removal**
  - **Emergent endoscopy** for sharp objects or disc batteries in the esophagus, or for objects causing obstruction with inability to handle secretions
  - **Urgent endoscopy** (within 24 hours) for smooth objects or food impaction in the esophagus, sharp or large (> 6 cm) objects in the stomach/duodenum, or magnets
- **Nonurgent endoscopy** may be indicated for **asymptomatic patients.** Esophageal coins can be observed for 12-24 hours, disc/standard batteries in stomach for up to 48 hours, and blunt objects in the stomach for up to 3 weeks.
- Esophageal perforations or any signs of peritonitis require emergent surgery.

KEY FACT

On a posteroanterior (PA) film, esophageal coins appear "head on" (Figure 11.2); tracheal coins appear sideways and thin.

KEY FACT

Disc batteries appear as a "stack of coins" or with "double density" sign on plain films.

KEY FACT

90% of esophageal foreign bodies pass spontaneously.

KEY FACT

Objects longer than 5 cm or wider than 2.5 cm are unlikely to pass the stomach.

KEY FACT

IV antibiotics can reduce the absolute mortality associated with an upper GI bleed in cirrhotic patients.

MNEMONIC

Upper GI bleeds:

GUM BLEED

Gastritis
Ulcers
Mallory-Weiss tears
Biliary
Large esophageal varices
Esophagitis
Enteric-aortic fistula (seen in patients with aortic grafts)
Dieulafoy lesions (gastric vessel aneurysm)

KEY FACT

Black stool may be seen after ingestion of Bismuth or iron but will be hemoccult negative.

ESOPHAGEAL SPASM

An intrinsic motor disorder of the esophagus where **prolonged**, high-intensity, **diffuse** esophageal contractions occur in addition to normal peristaltic waves. **Nutcracker esophagus** is a variant with prolonged, high-intensity, **peristaltic** waves.

Symptoms

Chest pain and dysphagia, often precipitated by swallowing very hot or cold liquids.

Differential

Acute coronary syndrome, angina, achalasia, webs, strictures, GERD.

Diagnosis

Barium swallow shows "corkscrewing;" **manometry** shows prolonged, strong esophageal contractions interspersed over normal peristaltic waves. Most patients can be evaluated as outpatients.

Treatment

Medical therapy is limited. **Ca^{2+} channel blockers** such as diltiazem and **anticholinergics** such as hyoscyamine and dicyclomine may decrease amplitude of esophageal peristalsis. **Botulinum toxin** and **nitric oxide contributing drugs** (eg, sildenafil) are often used with mixed results, as are certain antidepressants.

GI Bleeding

GI bleeding is a relatively common and potentially life-threatening disease with significant overall mortality. It is classified as an upper or lower source by its relationship to the ligament of Treitz (located in the fourth section of the duodenum).

UPPER GI BLEEDING

Upper GI bleeding (UGIB) is defined as bleeding originating proximal to the ligament of Treitz.

Causes

Peptic ulcer disease (most common), erosive **gastritis**, and esophageal **varices** account for most adult cases of UGIB. **Mallory-Weiss tears**, **stress ulcers**, **arteriovenous malformation (AVM)**, and **malignancy** are also possible etiologies. A history of aortic graft should raise concern for **aortoenteric fistula**. In 10% of patients, **no source** is identified.

Symptoms

Patients may present with **hematemesis** or "coffee-ground" emesis. **Melena** is seen in 70% of patients with UGIB and may result from as little as 60 mL of blood in the upper GI tract; blood must remain for approximately 8 hours before turning black. Alternatively, patients may present solely with symptoms of **hypovolemia** (dizziness, weakness, chest pain, dyspnea, syncope, confusion).

EXAMINATION

Liver disease and/or **coagulopathy** are suggested by jaundice, telangiectasia, bruises, petechiae, organomegaly, ascites, or hemangiomas. Consider signs of **hypovolemia,** including hypotension, tachycardia, tachypnea, decreased peripheral perfusion, and altered mentation.

DIAGNOSIS

Is primarily based on history and rectal examination. Laboratory studies for anemia, coagulation, and liver function may be helpful. **NG lavage**, when positive, confirms the presence of an UGIB, but is no longer routinely indicated for diagnosis and has poor sensitivity to detect UGIB.

TREATMENT

- See Figure 11.3.
- Begin volume resuscitation with **crystalloid**, but consider early blood replacement; failure to achieve adequate resuscitation after 2 L of crystalloid is an indication for blood replacement. For older patients or those with history of coronary artery disease (CAD), **transfuse** to keep hemoglobin > 10 g/dL (though newer studies suggest benefit to transfusion thresholds as low as 7 g/dL).

Q

A 47-year-old man presents with massive hematemesis, hypotension, and altered mental status. On examination, he has scleral icterus, a distended abdomen, and spider telangiectasias on his chest. What is the likely diagnosis?

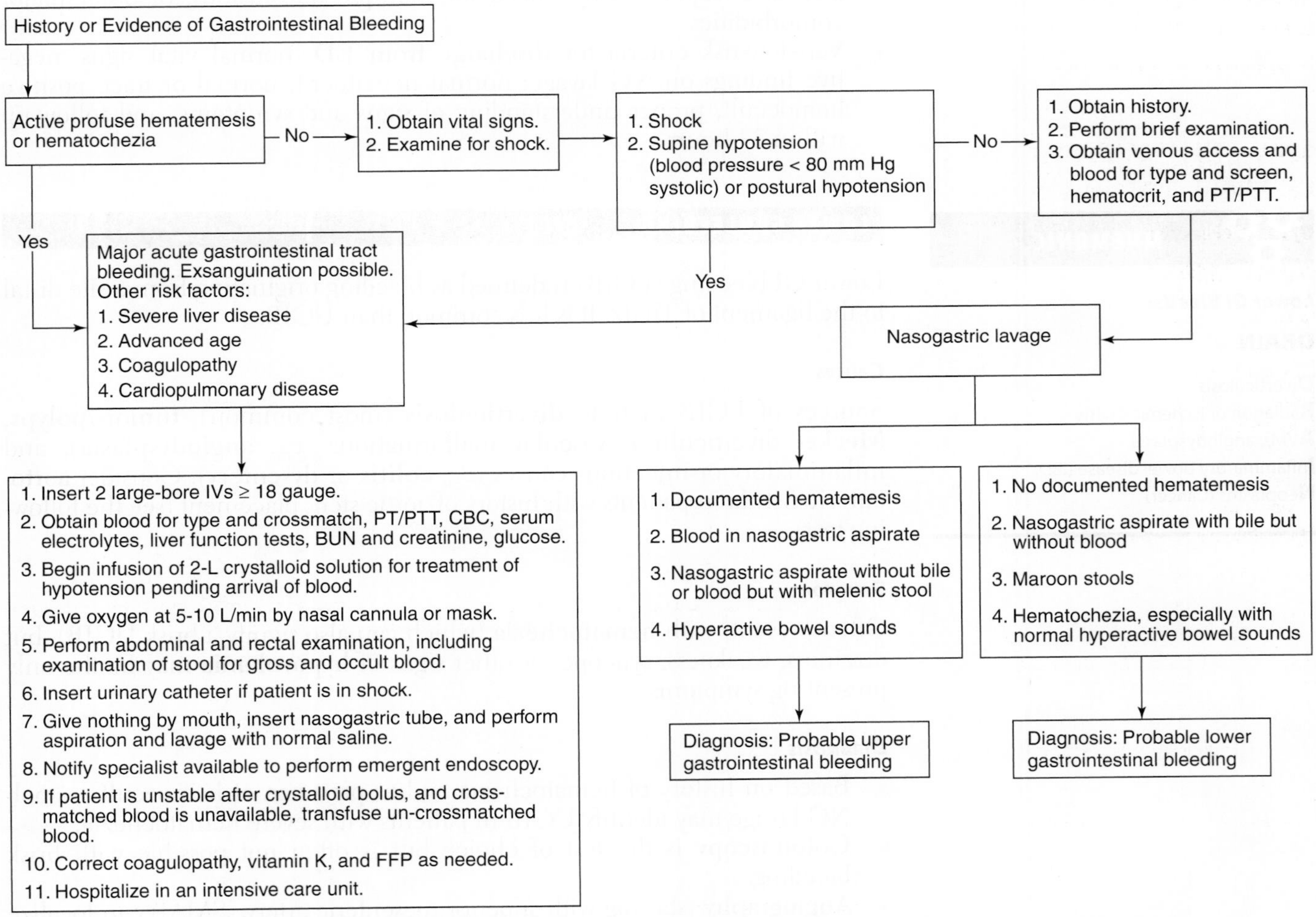

FIGURE 11.3. Management of GI bleeds. (Reproduced, with permission, from Stone CK, Humphries RL, eds. *Current Diagnosis & Treatment: Emergency Medicine*. 6th ed. New York, NY: McGraw-Hill; 2008.)

A

Esophageal varices.

- Use caution in patients with variceal bleeds as over-resuscitation and transfusion to hematocrit > 30% can increase portal pressures.
- Patients on warfarin or with liver dysfunction require **coagulation replacement** with vitamin K and/or FFP; prothrombin complex concentrates (PCCs) are indicated for life-threatening bleeds.
- **PPIs** are routinely administered as an IV bolus and drip for undifferentiated UGIB. (A recent review concluded that PPIs administered prior to endoscopy reduced evidence of bleeding and need for intervention at time of endoscopy, but showed no reduction in mortality.)
- **Octreotide** is indicated in known or suspected variceal bleeding or as adjunctive treatment in undifferentiated UGIB while awaiting endoscopy.
- **IV antibiotics** (third-generation cephalosporin or fluoroquinolone) have shown a mortality benefit in patients with cirrhosis.
- **Early endoscopy** for direct interventions (focal cautery, epinephrine injection, banding, and sclerotherapy); consult GI early.
- **Balloon tamponade** is indicated as a temporizing measure in uncontrolled hemorrhage from esophageal varices when definitive management is not immediately available. **Intubate** prior to placement.

KEY FACT

Predictors of high mortality include initial HCT < 30, age > 60 years, persistent Spontaneous bacterial peritonitis (SBP) < 100 or persistent shock, transfusion required > 4 units, and physical examination consistent with decompensated liver disease.

Disposition

- **Admit** all moderate- and high-risk patients for continued monitoring and therapy. **ICU** admission for patients with persistent tachycardia, actively bleeding varices, evidence of decompensated liver disease (coagulopathy, ascites, encephalopathy), need for multiple transfusions, or other major comorbidities.
- Very-low-risk criteria for **discharge from ED**: normal vital signs, negative findings on NG lavage, normal hematocrit, normal or trace positive hemoccult, proper understanding of signs and symptoms, and follow-up within 24 hours.

LOWER GI BLEEDING

Lower GI bleeding (LGIB) is defined as bleeding originating from a site distal to the ligament of Treitz. It is less common than UGIB.

MNEMONIC

Lower GI Bleeds:

DRAIN

Diverticulosis
Radiation or Ischemic Colitis
AVMs, angiodysplasia
Inflammatory bowel disease (IBD)
Neoplasms (Cancer)

Causes

Sources of LGIB include **diverticulosis** (most common), **tumors/polyps**, **Meckel** diverticulum, vascular malformations (eg, **angiodysplasia**), and inflammatory or infectious causes (eg, **colitis** or **dysentery**). Consider **aorto-enteric fistula** in patients with history of aortic stent placement (see the following text).

Symptoms

Often presents with **hematochezia** (which can also signify a brisk UGIB), but dizziness, weakness, syncope, or other signs of **hypovolemia** may be the only presenting symptoms.

Diagnosis

- Based on history of hematochezia and/or presence of hemoccult + stool. NG lavage may identify UGIB in patients with severe hematochezia.
- **Colonoscopy** is the test of choice but is often not possible with brisk bleeding.
- **Angiography** (starting with superior mesenteric artery [SMA]) can localize site of bleeding if rate > 0.5 mL/min and allows for direct intervention with embolization or vasopressin infusion.

- **Tagged red blood scan** can detect bleeding if rate > 0.1 mL/min but is not as good at localizing exact site of bleeding compared to angiography.

TREATMENT

- Fluid resuscitation; consider **transfusion** if patient has ongoing bleeding or is symptomatic after 2 L of intravenous fluid (IVF). Recommended **transfusion thresholds** vary, but generally transfuse for Hgb < 7 in healthy patients or < 10 in those with significant comorbidities. Patients with an elevated international normalized ratio (INR) can be given **Vitamin K ± FFP** (**PCCs** are indicated for life-threatening bleeding.) Consider transfusing **platelets** if count is < 50,000/µL.
- Definitive treatments include selective embolization, endoscopic coagulation, and surgical resection.
- **Increased morbidity** is associated with significant or ongoing bleeding, aspirin use, and the presence of comorbid conditions. Otherwise low-risk patients may be **safely discharged** if they have adequate follow-up care.

KEY FACT

Around 10%-15% apparent lower GI bleeds are actually caused by upper GI bleeds.

AORTOENTERIC FISTULA

Occur when there is a direct communication between the aorta and the GI track. Most commonly occur in patients with prosthetic aortic grafts, but may also result from aortic aneurysms, aortitis, postradiation, tumors, or trauma. The third or fourth portion of the duodenum is most commonly involved, followed by the jejunum and ileum.

SYMPTOMS/EXAMINATION

A mild GI bleed may signify impending rupture with massive bleeding. Because most involve the duodenum, patients may present with **melena** and/or **hematemesis**, as well as **abdominal pain**, **back pain**, or **fever**.

DIAGNOSIS

Is primarily based on high index of suspicion in appropriate clinical setting; known **abdominal aortic aneurysm (AAA) and GI bleeding is presumed aortoenteric fistula (AEF) until proven otherwise**. **CT** or **angiography** may confirm the diagnosis in hemodynamically stable patients.

TREATMENT

Fluid and blood resuscitation. Obtain **emergent surgical consultation**; do not wait for further diagnostic studies if the patient is unstable. Perioperative hypotension is the strongest predictor of mortality. **Emergent laparotomy** is the only life-saving treatment for massive bleeding.

Stomach

GASTRITIS

Inflammation of gastric mucosa.

CAUSES

Helicobacter pylori bacterial infection (most common), stress, burns, sepsis, drugs (ASA [aminosalicylic acid] and **NSAIDs**), **alcohol**, autoimmune conditions, ingestion of corrosive agents, or any condition causing hypotension or hypovolemia.

Q

A 55-year-old woman with a history of chronic arthritis presents with burning epigastric pain that worsens at night has been recently waking her up from sleep. She has mild tenderness in the epigastrium, but the examination is otherwise reassuring. What is the likely diagnosis?

Symptoms

Abdominal pain, nausea and vomiting, anorexia, but may be asymptomatic.

Differential

Cardiac disease, ulcers, hernia, GERD, gastroparesis, functional dyspepsia, pancreatitis, hepatitis, AAA, cholelithiasis.

Examination

Epigastric pain on palpation.

Diagnosis

Endoscopy with gastric biopsy is definitive, but diagnosis is often made empirically. Ancillary tests may be needed to rule out complications or other possible diagnoses.

Treatment

Discontinue NSAID or alcohol use and start acid suppression therapy (**PPI**, H_2 blocker). Refer for outpatient testing for *H pylori*; treat with triple therapy if present (see Table 11.1).

Complications

Include ulcers or GI **bleeding**, **perforation**, and **obstruction**. **Chronic atrophic gastritis** → loss of gastric parietal cells (and intrinsic factor production) → **vitamin B_{12} deficiency, and pernicious anemia.**

> **KEY FACT**
>
> *H pylori* serologic tests are useful for past exposure but cannot be used for test of cure. Urea breath test, endoscopic biopsy, and stool antigen may be used for diagnosis and to confirm adequate treatment.

GASTRIC AND DUODENAL ULCERS

The term peptic ulcer disease (PUD) encompasses both gastric and duodenal ulcers. Agents that damage the gastric mucosal barrier and increase risk of PUD include tobacco, alcohol, ***H pylori***, **NSAIDs**, shock, and steroid use. About 70% of PUD is attributable to *H Pylori*, 25% to NSAID use, and 1% to Zollinger-Ellison syndrome (ZES) (gastrin-secreting tumors).

Symptoms/Examination

- Burning **epigastric pain** is the most common symptom. Classically, **gastric ulcers worsen with food** while **duodenal ulcers improve with food** and worsen 2-5 hours after eating. However, these historical features correlate poorly with endoscopic findings.
- Pain that **worsens at night** and awakens the patient from sleep is a classic finding of duodenal ulcers; colicky pain or pain lasting weeks to months is atypical of PUD.
- Other symptoms may include early satiety, nausea and vomiting, postprandial belching, and epigastric fullness.
- **Infants** and **children** may present with PUD; look for poor feeding, vomiting, GI bleeding, and abdominal pain.
- The most common examination finding is **epigastric tenderness** to palpation.

Differential

Cardiac disease, hernia, gastritis, GERD, irritable bowel disease, mesenteric ischemia

Diagnosis

Endoscopy with biopsy to confirm diagnosis and to rule out *H pylori* infection and carcinoma.

> **A**
>
> Peptic ulcer disease due to NSAID use.

TREATMENT

- Uncomplicated PUD: Discontinue ASA, NSAID, and alcohol use, and start **PPI. Endoscopy**, *H pylori* testing, and/or triple therapy are typically pursued outpatient.
- If concern for bleeding ulcer, treat as upper GI bleed.
- Upright CXR or CT scan if concern for perforation (free intra-abdominal air present only with anterior perforations).

COMPLICATIONS

- Ulcer **penetration** into an adjacent structure (pancreas most common), or **perforation** (anterior duodenum most common) heralded by the abrupt onset of severe abdominal pain and peritoneal findings.
- Gastric outlet obstruction, characterized by the development of bloating, early satiety, and vomiting.

> **KEY FACT**
>
> Duodenal ulcers classically present with pain 2-5 hours after eating or nighttime pain.

> **KEY FACT**
>
> If a patient has received *H pylori* treatment but has persistent symptoms, test for eradication. If not eradicated, treat again with a different regimen. If eradicated, refer for endoscopy.

GASTRINOMA (ZOLLINGER-ELLISON SYNDROME)

Gastrinomas are gastrin-secreting endocrine tumors that arise primarily in the duodenum, pancreas or lymph nodes. Over two-thirds are malignant and one-third will have metastasized to the liver by the time of diagnosis.

SYMPTOMS

- Recurrent and intractable peptic ulcer disease.
- Diarrhea is common with Zollinger-Ellison syndrome (ZES).

EXAMINATION

Epigastric tenderness on palpation.

DIAGNOSIS

- Elevated fasting serum gastrin level (off H_2-blocker or PPI) with gastric pH < 2
- Multiple ulcers in abnormal locations on endoscopy
- Imaging to identify tumor ± mets (somatostatin receptor scintigraphy with SPECT [single-photon emission computed tomography])

TREATMENT

- PPIs
- Surgical resection ± cryoablation of liver mets

GASTRIC CANCER

Gastric adenocarcinoma is one of the most common cancers worldwide. It is a highly aggressive cancer often spreading to lymph nodes and liver. Risk factors include chronic inflammation due to atrophic gastritis (pernicious anemia), *H pylori* infection, and partial gastrectomy.

SYMPTOMS

Though usually asymptomatic until advanced, many patients have vague upper GI symptoms for 6-12 months prior to diagnosis. **Dyspepsia** symptoms with **weight loss** in a patient > 40 years old is classic. May see **anemia** from GI bleeding.

DIFFERENTIAL

PUD, GERD, gastritis

> **KEY FACT**
>
> 80% ZES is sporadic, whereas 20% is associated with multiple endocrine neoplasia type 1 (MEN 1).

> **Q**
>
> A 25-year-old woman presents with copious foul-smelling diarrhea, crampy abdominal pain, and flatus. She recently returned from a camping trip in the mountains where she drank from a stream. What is the likely diagnosis?

A

Giardia lamblia.

Examination

- Classic findings include **Virchow node**, a large rock-hard supraclavicular node, and **Sister Mary Joseph nodule**, a firm, red, nontender nodule palpable at the umbilicus.
- **Krukenberg tumors** are mucinous signet cells that metastasize to the ovaries and may lead to palpable ovarian masses. A **Blumer shelf** is a palpable nodule on rectal examination due to metastatic disease.

Diagnosis

Upper GI **endoscopy** with systematic, nontargeted biopsies

Treatment

Mostly palliative, surgery, chemotherapy (~5% survival at 5 years)

Complications

Gastric-outlet obstruction, anemia, dehydration, bowel obstruction.

Gastroenteritis

Gastroenteritis is characterized by the acute onset of vomiting and diarrhea. Peak incidence of infection occurs during winter months. It is often difficult to identify the causative agent or pathogen in the acute setting; however, up to 70% of cases are caused by viruses (Table 11.3). The remaining cases are largely caused by bacteria, with a small subset due to parasites. Infectious gastroenteritis may be termed *invasive* (inflammatory diarrhea, dysentery) that causes systemic illness, or *noninvasive* that causes secretory diarrhea and few systemic symptoms (Table 11.4).

Symptoms/Examination

See Tables 11.3 and 11.4.

TABLE 11.3. Common Causes of Noninvasive Gastroenteritis

Causative Agent	Incubation and Transmission	Description	Therapy
Viral gastroenteritis	11-72 h; person-to-person, fecal-oral, contaminated food or water, particularly poorly cooked or raw shellfish	Norovirus and Rotavirus (declining since advent of vaccine in 2006) are most common agents; nausea, vomiting, and watery diarrhea, low-grade fever; may have mild abdominal cramps and myalgias. URI symptoms or PNA may occur with rotavirus	Self-limited; supportive care with PO or IV hydration and antiemetics
Giardia lamblia	1-4 wk; contaminated food or water, particularly water from remote streams and wells. Person-to-person, fecal-oral transmission also occurs	Most common intestinal parasitic infection in the United States, backpackers, campers, the elderly; also homosexual males, persons in institutions abdominal cramping, bloating, flatus, malabsorptive chronic diarrhea. Trophozoites or cysts in stool	Metronidazole
Staphylococcus aureus	1-6 h; previously cooked food (ham, egg salad, potato salad often sitting at room temperature for several hours)	Nausea, severe vomiting, diarrhea, mild abdominal cramps; symptoms caused by preformed enterotoxins	Supportive care with IV fluids and symptomatic treatment; antibiotics ineffective

(Continued)

TABLE 11.3. Common Causes of Noninvasive Gastroenteritis (*Continued*)

Causative Agent	Incubation and Transmission	Description	Therapy
Bacillus cereus	Emetic toxin: 2-4 h following ingestion (classically fried rice) Diarrheal toxin: 6-24 h after ingestion, usually contaminated meat	Emetic syndrome: Abrupt onset of nausea, vomiting Diarrheal syndrome: diarrhea; with abdominal cramps Both syndromes caused by preformed enterotoxins	Supportive care with IV fluids and symptomatic treatment; antibiotics ineffective
Clostridium perfringens	8-24 h; previously cooked or reheated meats and poultry	Relatively large outbreaks common, abdominal cramps, nausea, minimal vomiting, and watery diarrhea; caused by enterotoxins produced in gut	Supportive care with IV fluids and symptomatic treatment
Vibrio cholerae	2-6 d; raw or undercooked seafood, fecal–oral, contaminated water, often raw oysters, large inoculum required	Explosive rice–water diarrhea; vomiting, fever, abdominal cramps, dehydration, lactic acidosis; enterotoxins are formed before and after bacterial colonization	Fluid resuscitation is critical; significant electrolyte imbalance can occur. doxy or macrolide may shorten course
Enterotoxigenic *Escherichia coli*	11-72 h; fecally contaminated water	Traveler's diarrhea; profuse watery diarrhea; caused by both heat-labile and heat-stabile enterotoxins	Self-limited; supportive care. If severe, ciprofloxacin
Antibiotic- associated enteritis	Temporally associated with antibiotic use	Mild severity without cramps, fever, or fecal leukocytes	Withdrawal of antibiotic
Cryptosporidium	1-2 wk, fecal–oral route, cysts from human or animal sources	Most common cause of chronic diarrhea in AIDS patients, profuse watering diarrhea, abdominal cramping, anorexia, nausea, flatulence. High risk: immunocompromised, animal handlers, children in day care, recent travel to Russia	Immunocompetent: Supportive care, ± nitazoxanide Immunodeficient: Restore immune status, HARRT. Nitazoxanide, paromomycin, and azithromycin are no longer recommended
Scombroid fish poisoning	20-60 min after ingestion of fish, often mahi mahi or tuna that has been preserved or refrigerated improperly; Swiss cheese also implicated	Signs and symptoms of histamine intoxication: facial flushing, throbbing headache, nausea, vomiting, diarrhea, abdominal cramps, bronchospasm (severe). Heat-stabile toxin with histamine like property, not due to allergic reaction	H_1/H_2 blockers; albuterol for wheezing. Rarely may require Tx as anaphylaxis
Ciguatera fish poisoning	2-6 h after ingestion of ciguatoxin found in carnivorous fish (eg, grouper, snapper, barracuda, king fish, jack)	Late spring and summer months; vomiting, diarrhea, myalgias, weakness, paresthesias, reversal of hot and cold sensation (pathognomonic, worsen with alcohol consumption)	Supportive care. Amitriptyline effective for dysesthesias. Single dose mannitol in stable, fluid-resuscitated pts. Abstinence from alcohol, nuts, seafood for 6 mo

AIDS, acquired immunodeficiency syndrome; HARRT, highly active antiretroviral therapy; IV, intravenous; PNA, pneumonia; PO, by mouth; URI, upper respiratory infection.

TABLE 11.4. Common Causes of Invasive Gastroenteritis

Causative Agent	Incubation and Transmission	Description	Treatment
Salmonella spp	8-72 h; contaminated food (eggs or poultry) or water, pet turtles, chicks, or lizards	Fever, abdominal pain, vomiting, diarrhea, myalgia, headache; many fecal WBCs and few RBCs. Risk of sepsis in infants, elderly, sickle cell pts, immunocompromised **Typhoid fever:** Intractable fever, bradycardia, "rose spots;" caused by distinct, "typhoidal" spp	Ciprofloxacin if severe illness, or immunocompromise; Alt: ceftriaxone or azithromycin. Antidiarrheals may cause prolonged carrier state
Shigella spp	1-3 d; fecal–oral, person-to-person, contaminated food. Few as 50-100 organisms can cause disease	Ranges from mild, self-limited diarrheal illness to frank dysentery with fever, headache, abdominal pain, nausea/vomiting and bloody diarrhea. Common in kids 1-5 y; febrile seizure may occur; many fecal WBCs and RBCs	Ciprofloxacin if severe illness, sepsis, or immunocompromise; Alt: ceftriaxone or azithromycin
Campylobacter j	1-7 d; fecally contaminated water, food (poultry, eggs), animals or pets	Common in children and young adults; acute onset fever and abdominal pain followed by diarrhea, vomiting, myalgias, and/or headache. Fecal RBCs and WBCs common; stools may become bloody or melanotic. Examination may mimic appendicitis. Complications: Reiter syndrome, Guillain Barré	Azithromycin if severely ill or septic; Alt: erythromycin or ciprofloxacin
Yersinia enterocolitica	1-5 d; contaminated food or water (milk, pork), fecal–oral, person-to-person, exposure to pets or wild animals	Children and young adults; often presents with fever, nausea/vomiting/diarrhea (bloody stools in 25%), abdominal pain; diarrhea may persist 10-14 d; many fecal WBCs and RBCs. May present as ileocecitis or mesenteric adenitis, mimicking appendicitis. Complications: Reactive arthritis, erythema nodosum	Usually self-limiting; if severe, treat with ciprofloxacin; Alt: TMP-SMX. Ceftriaxone if bacteremic
Vibrio parahaemolyticus	4-48 h; ingestion of raw or undercooked fish or shellfish	Acute diarrhea with abdominal cramping; nausea/vomiting, fever may occur; may also present as rapidly progressive wound infection	If severe: Doxy; Alt: ciprofloxacin, azithromycin. For proven bacteremia, add ceftriaxone
Clostridium difficile (*pseudomembranous enterocolitis*)	1-12 wk; recent hospitalization or antibiotic use; clindamycin, cephalosporins, quinolones most commonly implicated	Fever, abdominal pain copious foul-smelling diarrhea, rarely vomiting; fecal WBCs and RBCs; stool *C difficile* toxin confirms diagnosis	Stop offending antibiotic, treat with PO metronidazole for mild to mod cases; PO vancomycin for more severe cases. IV vancomycin ineffective; IV metronidazole may be beneficial

(*Continued*)

TABLE 11.4. Common Causes of Invasive Gastroenteritis (*Continued*)

Causative Agent	Incubation and Transmission	Description	Treatment
Entamoeba histolytica	1-11 wk; cysts transmitted through contaminated food or water, poor sanitation, anal–oral sexual practices, travel to developing countries	80% of carriers are asymptomatic Acute amoebic dysentery: abrupt onset of fever, abdominal pain, tenesmus, and bloody diarrhea Chronic dysentery: malaise weight loss, bloating, and bloody diarrhea May develop hepatic abscess; fecal RBCs, WBCs common, trophozoites/cysts in stool	Metronidazole acutely, then iodoquinol or paromomycin to clear intestinal cysts; antibiotics will usually sufficiently treat abscess as well
EHEC O157:H7	1-4 days; contaminated food or water; undercooked meats, person-to-person, fecal–oral	Fever, abdominal pain, vomiting, grossly bloody diarrhea; fecal WBCs common. **Shiga toxins**-cytotoxic to intestinal vascular endothelium. Complications: HUS (5%-10% of pts) or TTP	Supportive care; antibiotics not recommended as they may increase the incidence of HUS, especially in children

EHEC, enterohemorrhagic *Escherichia coli*; HUS, hemolytic uremic syndrome; IV, intravenous; PO, by mouth; RBC, red blood cell; TTP, thrombotic thrombocytopenic purpura; WBC, white blood cell.

Noninvasive

Mild systemic symptoms, including nausea, vomiting, and diarrhea; generally not associated with fever. Examination with mild, diffuse abdominal tenderness and signs of dehydration.

Invasive

More severe symptoms, including **fever**, **bloody diarrhea**, abdominal pain, myalgias, headache, anorexia, and weight loss. Patients have evidence of **systemic illness** and more significant **abdominal tenderness**.

Diagnosis

- Diagnosis is most often based on **history and physical** alone. Cases of noninvasive diarrhea causing only mild dehydration, minimal systemic symptoms, and lasting < 14 days are generally self-limited and do not require specific testing. Consider travel history, immunosuppression, health care/day care exposure, antibiotic use, and specific/known food exposures.
- The presence of gross **or occult blood** and **fecal leukocytes suggests** a bacterial cause but does not reliably determine those who would benefit from empiric antibiotics.
- **Stool culture** is labor intensive and low-yield; reserve for severely ill patients, immunocompromised patients, outbreaks, and patients recently on antibiotics or those with symptoms persisting > 14 days.
- Consider **ova and parasite analysis** in patients who travel to developing countries, the immunocompromised, the institutionalized, and patients with a prolonged course not responsive to traditional therapy.
- ***C difficile* toxin assay** is indicated in setting of recent antibiotic use. Diarrhea from *C difficile* usually occurs during or shortly after antibiotic use, but can occur as late as 12 weeks postexposure and sometimes in patients without recent antibiotic use. Acid suppression medication is also a risk factor for *C difficile*.

Treatment

Oral rehydration is the treatment of choice in patients with mild to moderate dehydration who tolerate oral intake. These patients may be discharged with instructions to return if symptoms persist or worsen. Give **IV fluids** and antiemetics for severely dehydrated patients unable to tolerate PO. Consider **hospitalization** for the severely dehydrated patient. Other treatment considerations depend on suspected etiology (see Tables 11.3 and 11.4).

Perforated Viscus

ESOPHAGEAL PERFORATION

Please refer to structural abnormalities in Esophageal Disorders.

GASTRIC, SMALL BOWEL, AND LARGE BOWEL PERFORATIONS

Causes

- **Gastric and duodenal perforations**: Most often due to erosion of benign gastric and duodenal ulcers through wall with leakage of air and digestive contents into the peritoneal cavity.
- **Small bowel perforation:** Causes include infection (typhoid, tuberculosis [TB]), tumors both benign and malignant, strangulated hernias, inflammatory bowel disease, ischemic colitis, necrotizing vasculitis, foreign bodies, or medications (eg, enteric-coated potassium tablets). Penetrating or blunt trauma to lower chest and abdomen may also cause perforation.
- **Large bowel perforation:** Rare but severe. Most often due to colorectal cancer and diverticulitis, but may also be secondary to colitis, foreign body, and diagnostic instrumentation.

Symptoms

- Sudden onset of **severe abdominal pain,** unrelated to eating and unrelieved with antacids. Pain is typically appreciated in epigastrium but quickly becomes generalized. Pain may also localize to right upper quadrant (RUQ), left upper quadrant (LUQ), or chest; lower thoracic or upper lumbar **back pain** is suggestive of erosion of a posterior duodenal ulcer into the pancreas.
- Large bowel perforations may present with more gradual onset of pain.
- Unilateral or bilateral shoulder pain may occur due to referred pain from the accumulation of air under the diaphragm.

Examination

Diffuse **abdominal tenderness**, **distension**, and/or **rigidity**. Patients may prefer to remain immobile. Listen for **reduced/absent bowel sounds.**

Diagnosis

Abdominal or chest **radiographs** may identify free air. **Left lateral decubitus** is the most sensitive position for detecting pneumoperitoneum. **CT** may be necessary because negative radiographs do not rule-out perforation.

Treatment

Obtain **immediate surgical consultation**. Start NG suction, pain control, **IV fluid replacement**, and Foley catheter placement to monitor urine output. Administer broad-spectrum **antibiotics**. Give **PPI** if concerned for perforated peptic ulcer.

Inflammatory Bowel Disease

Inflammatory bowel disease (IBD) is a chronic, relapsing inflammatory GI disease comprising 2 similar but distinct entities, Crohn disease and ulcerative colitis (UC). In both, the general goals of ED care are to identify possible new cases, screen for and treat complications, and identity patients who require inpatient treatment.

CROHN DISEASE

Crohn disease is a chronic, recurrent, inflammatory disease that may affect any segment of the GI tract from mouth to anus. The disease is discontinuous, with normal areas of bowel (skip lesions). It has a propensity for the ileum and proximal colon (Table 11.5). Malignancy of small and large intestine

TABLE 11.5. Distinguishing Features of Inflammatory Bowel Disease

Feature	Crohn Disease	Ulcerative Colitis
Age at onset	Bimodal: 15-30, 50-80 y	Bimodal: 15-30, 50-80 y
Abdominal pain	Sharp, focal	Crampy, associated with bowel movement
Bowel obstruction	Common	Rare
Gross hematochezia	Occasionally, + hemoccult more common	Common
GI involvement	Mouth to anus; typically terminal ileum/proximal colon; perianal involvement common	Colon only; always begins in the rectum with continuous and uniform progression proximally; perianal involvement uncommon
Abscesses	Common	Uncommon
Pattern	Segmental, transmural, eccentric	Uniform, continuous
Ulceration	Superficial to deep, linear, serpiginous	Superficial
Histology	Noncaseating granulomas, helpful but not necessary in making diagnosis	Crypt abscesses, epithelial necrosis, mucosal ulceration
Fistula/stricture	Common	Uncommon
Toxic megacolon	Uncommon, but associated with massive GI bleed	Common
Extraintestinal manifestations	Uncommon, 25%-33% of cases	Common
Surgery curative	Never	Often

GI, gastrointestinal.

are 3 times more common in patients with Crohn disease than in the general population.

Incidence is higher among Ashkenazi Jews, smokers, and those with a family history. It has a bimodal age distribution (peaks at age 20 and 60).

Pathophysiology

Transmural inflammation of all layers of bowel wall causes deep ulcerations of the bowel wall that can lead to **fistulas, strictures,** and **abscesses.** The bowel wall is often thickened, causing luminal narrowing and **obstruction.**

> **KEY FACT**
>
> 25%-30% patients with Crohn disease will manifest extraintestinal complications, but they are more common in ulcerative colitis.

Symptoms

Abdominal pain, anorexia, diarrhea, fever, weight loss, malaise, and extraintestinal complications (Table 11.6). The presence of **nocturnal diarrhea** may differentiate Crohn disease from irritable bowel syndrome.

Examination

Findings depend on location and extent of disease, but may include **abdominal tenderness** (often right lower quadrant [RLQ] due to terminal ileitis), **anal fissures** and **fistulas.**

Diagnosis

- **Colonoscopy** with biopsy is confirmative (skip lesions, linear ulcerations, and noncaseating granulomas).
- **CT scan** is useful if extraluminal complications are suspected (fistulas, abscess, obstruction). Plain films are not helpful in diagnosis of uncomplicated disease.
- Nonspecific laboratory findings include anemia, leukocytosis, elevated erythrocyte sedimentation rate (ESR) and C-reactive protein (CRP), B_{12} deficiency, electrolyte abnormalities, and fecal leukocytes.

Treatment

- First-line therapy for mild to moderate disease is 5-aminosalicylic acid (5-ASA) (sulfasalazine, or the newer, less toxic mesalamine) with steroids added for symptom flares.
- Antibiotics for primary treatment of IBD is controversial, with more evidence in Crohn disease than UC.

TABLE 11.6. Extraintestinal Manifestations of Ulcerative Colitis and Crohn Disease

Arthritic	Peripheral arthritis, ankylosing spondylitis
Vascular	Vasculitis, arteritis, thromboembolic disease
Ophthalmologic	Uveitis, episcleritis
Dermatologic	Pyoderma gangrenosum, erythema nodosum, oral aphthous ulcers
Hepatobiliary	Pericholangitis, chronic active hepatitis, cirrhosis, cholelithiasis, bile duct carcinoma
Miscellaneous	Growth retardation, delayed sexual development, hyperoxaluria with renal stones

- Patients with severe or refractory disease should be treated with immunomodulating agents (azathioprine, 6-MP, methotrexate) and anti-TNF (tumor necrosis factor) therapies.
- Small bowel obstruction (SBO) will usually respond to conservation therapy with IVF and NGT suction, ± glucocorticoids.

COMPLICATIONS

Lactose intolerance, SBO, fistulas ± abscess formation, strictures, hemorrhage (rarely severe), toxic megacolon, colorectal cancer.

ULCERATIVE COLITIS

Chronic, recurrent, ulcerative disease characterized by mucosal and submucosal inflammation of the colon. Inflammation is continuous. One-third of patients have disease confined to the rectosigmoid, one-third have disease that extends to the splenic flexure, and one-third have even more proximal disease. (See Table 11.5 for a comparison with Crohn disease.)

UC is more common among **non**smokers, Ashkenazi Jews, and those with a family history. Bimodal distribution: onset is typically from 15 to 30 years old, but another spike occurs at 50-80 years of age.

PATHOPHYSIOLOGY

Mucosal and **submucosal** inflammation primarily involving the **rectum and sigmoid** causes ulceration. **Mild** disease is present in 60% of cases with fewer than 4 bowel movements per day and few extraintestinal manifestations; **severe** disease (fulminant colitis) occurs in 15% of cases.

SYMPTOMS/EXAMINATION

Bloody diarrhea, crampy **abdominal pain**, fecal urgency, and **tenesmus**. **Abdominal tenderness** and grossly **bloody stools** are common on examination. **Extraintestinal manifestations** are also common (see Table 11.6).

DIAGNOSIS

Sigmoidoscopy or **colonoscopy** demonstrates continuous, circumferential ulceration; **biopsy** shows acute and chronic inflammation and crypt abscesses **without** granulomas. **Plain films** are adequate for diagnosis of toxic megacolon.

TREATMENT

- **Mild to moderate** disease: **5-ASA** derivatives (sulfasalazine, mesalamine) are the mainstay of therapy with **corticosteroids** (PO ± rectal) indicated for persistent symptoms or flare while on 5-ASA.
- **Severe colitis: corticosteroids** (PO/IV ± rectal) and **immunosuppressants** (eg, anti-TNF, cyclosporine).
- **Avoid NSAIDs,** which may worsen IBD. Refractor cases may require **colectomy**.
- **Loperamide**, an opioid antimotility drug, is safe for symptom control in patients with IBD.

COMPLICATIONS

Lower **GI bleeding, colorectal cancer,** and **toxic megacolon** (colon dilated > 6 cm on radiographs with signs of systemic toxicity; high risk of perforation; treat with IVF resuscitation, broad-spectrum antibiotics, IV corticosteroids, and/or anti-TNF therapy). See Table 11.6 for **extraintestinal manifestations.**

Q

A mother brings her 2-year-old boy to the ED for evaluation of bloody stools. Recently the child has been having bright red blood in his stool, though not complaining of pain or other symptoms. What is the likely diagnosis?

KEY FACT

Avoid sigmoidoscopy and colonoscopy in patients with UC if there is a severe flare because they increase the risk of perforation.

KEY FACT

Surgery can be curative and can eliminate the risk of colorectal cancer in patients with UC.

KEY FACT

There is a 10- to 30-fold increase in the risk of developing colorectal cancer with UC. Risk increases with duration and extensiveness of disease.

A

Meckel diverticulum.

TABLE 11.7. Causes of Mechanical Small Bowel Obstruction

Adhesions (most common in adults)
Neoplasms (second most common; eg, lymphoma, adenocarcinoma)
Hernias: Inguinal, femoral, internal (third most common)
Crohn disease
Volvulus
Intussusception (most common in children < 2 y)
Strictures
Gallstone ileus
Foreign body

Small Intestine

SMALL BOWEL OBSTRUCTION/ILEUS

KEY FACT

Closed-loop obstruction occurs at 2 points and often results in strangulation.

KEY FACT

Intussusception is the most common cause of SBO in early childhood.

Mechanical small bowel obstruction results from a physical interruption of the bowel lumen that prevents passage of intestinal contents and is the most common surgical emergency of the small intestine. Obstruction may be partial or complete and occur at 1 or 2 points. Simple obstruction blocks the lumen only, while strangulation impairs the blood supply to the intestine eventually leading to infarction and necrosis.

Adynamic or paralytic ileus implies failure of peristalsis to propel intestinal contents through the bowel in the absence of a mechanical barrier.

Etiology

See Table 11.7 for causes of SBO and Table 11.8 for causes of ileus.

Symptoms

- **Mechanical SBO** presents with crampy, intermittent, poorly localized abdominal pain and vomiting; **bilious** emesis is classically associated with proximal obstructions distal to the pylorus. **Feculent emesis** may occur with distal ileal obstruction. **Abdominal distention** is often more pronounced with more distal obstructions. **Stool/flatus passage** may continue for as long as 24 hours after even complete SBO formation.
- **Ileus** is associated with nausea, vomiting, obstipation, abdominal pain, and distention.

Examination

- **Early SBO** shows mild abdominal distention, increased high-pitched bowel sounds, tympany to percussion, and mild abdominal tenderness. **Late SBO** is suggested by more significant distention, decreased peristaltic

TABLE 11.8. Causes of Adynamic Ileus

Postoperative or trauma
Acute intra-abdominal inflammatory process (peritonitis)
Electrolyte abnormalities (eg, Hypokalemia)
Medications
Severe medical illness

waves, and diminished bowel sounds. The presence of an **acute abdomen** (severe tenderness, rebound, guarding) suggests a **strangulated SBO.**
- **Ileus** shows mild abdominal tenderness, minimal distention, and diminished bowel sounds.

Diagnosis

- **Upright abdominal films** classically show **dilated loops** of small bowel with **air fluid levels** and decompressed colon, though gas in the colon may be seen in early or partial SBO. If bowel is fluid-filled, may see **"string of pearls"** sign (gas trapped between valvulae conniventes). Plain films are diagnostic in only 50%-60% of cases and do not identify the underlying cause or many common complications (Figure 11.4).
- **Contrasted CT** is highly accurate for making the diagnosis. It delineates ileus vs partial vs complete obstruction, the level and type of obstruction, and may also demonstrate the underlying cause. **Decreased bowel wall enhancement** on CT is 96% specific for **strangulation**, which may otherwise be difficulty to detect. Administration of both **IV and PO contrast** remains the gold standard, though IV contrast alone is often sufficient and can be considered if circumstances require.
- Laboratory **findings** include leukocytosis, hemoconcentration, and electrolyte abnormalities. **Metabolic alkalosis** may develop from excessive GI losses; **metabolic acidosis** can develop from hypoperfusion/shock. Elevated serum **lactate** is sensitive—but not specific—for bowel ischemia in SBO.

KEY FACT

Pain from adynamic ileus is usually more diffuse, constant, and less intense than mechanical small bowel obstruction.

KEY FACT

Plain abdominal radiographs are 70%-80% sensitive for detection of SBO as ileus may mimic abdominal x-ray (AXR) findings. CT is 80%-90% sensitive.

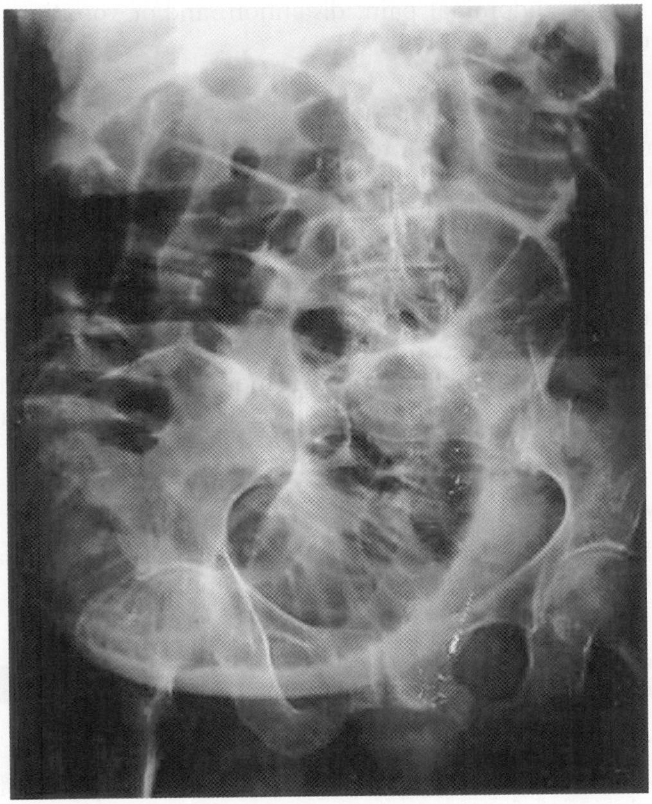

FIGURE 11.4. Small bowel obstruction. Plain AXR demonstrates dilated small bowel loops and paucity of air in the colon. (Reproduced, with permission, from Brunicardi FC, Andersen DK, Billiar TR, Dunn DL, Hunter JG, Matthews JB, Pollock RE, eds. *Schwartz's Principles of Surgery*. 8th ed. New York, NY: McGraw-Hill, 2004:1027.)

TREATMENT

- **Partial SBO** and **ileus** may be managed expectantly with **bowel rest**, **fluid resuscitation** and **electrolyte replacement**. **Complete SBO** more often requires surgical intervention; in all cases, **early surgical consultation** and **hospital admission** are warranted.
- **NG tube suction** was once recommended for all obstructions, but limited evidence supports this practice. Consider for patients who are persistently symptomatic, altered, at risk for aspiration, or have high-grade/complete obstructions.

COMPLICATIONS

Strangulation, perforation, peritonitis, hypovolemic or septic shock.

MECKEL DIVERTICULUM

> **KEY FACT**
>
> Rule of 2s for Meckel diverticulum: 2% prevalence, 2% symptomatic, 2:1 male-to-female ratio, 2 ft proximal to ileocecal valve, and half of those symptomatic are < 2 years of age.

Caused by the incomplete obliteration of the fetal omphalomesenteric duct, Meckel diverticulum is the most common congenital abnormality of the GI tract. Approximately 2% of the population is affected, but only 2% of affected patients become symptomatic. Males < 2 years are most commonly affected. Most are found in the ileum within 2 ft of the ileocecal valve. Around 60% (about 1 in 2) contain heterotopic tissue (usually gastric), which may lead to erosion with perforation or bleeding.

SYMPTOMS/EXAMINATION

Acute onset of massive, painless, "brick red" **rectal-bleeding**. Some patients may have crampy abdominal pain, distention, and/or vomiting. Older children may present like appendicitis.

DIAGNOSIS

Often an incidental diagnosis. A **technetium scan** ("Meckel scan") is the test of choice; it is 90% accurate when ectopic gastric mucosa is present. Consider CT if diagnosis is unclear. Definitive diagnosis is made surgically.

TREATMENT

- Begin **fluid/blood resuscitation** and **consider admission** to pediatric GI or surgery if needed. **Resection** of the diverticulum is indicated in patients with complications. **Expectant management** with close outpatient follow-up is appropriate for patients with minor bleeding and normal laboratory test results.

COMPLICATIONS

Intussusception, SBO, bleeding from heterotopic gastric mucosa, strictures from diverticulitis, obstruction, perforation, peritonitis.

MALABSORPTION

ETIOLOGY

Malabsorption refers to impaired digestion and absorption of nutrients, most often due to infection, pancreatic insufficiency or diffuse disorders such as celiac or Crohn disease. An increased osmotic load due to inability of the small intestine to absorb nutrient elements often causes majority of symptoms.

Symptoms

- **Watery diarrhea** from an increased osmotic load is the most common symptom. **Steatorrhea** (pale, bulky, malodorous stools) results from fat malabsorption. **Flatulence** and **abdominal distention** result from fermentation of unabsorbed food.
- **Malnutrition** causes **weight loss**, fatigue, and variable deficiencies leading to **anemia** (B_{12}, folate, iron), **edema** (hypoalbuminemia), **paresthesias** and/or bone pain (calcium, magnesium, vitamin D), **bleeding disorders** (vitamin K), or **night blindness** (vitamin A).

Examination

Varies depending on resultant deficiencies and underlying cause of malabsorption

Diagnosis

Quantitative stool fat determination is the gold standard to confirm steatorrhea, though the workup should be based on underlying clinical suspicion and is generally pursued outpatient.

Treatment

ED treatment is **supportive** (fluids and electrolyte replacement) and symptomatic (eg, **loperamide**). Severely malnourished patients may require cocktail of thiamine, multivitamins, and folate. Most can be discharged for outpatient workup and treatment of underlying cause.

Large Bowel

COLONIC DIVERTICULAR DISEASE

Diverticula are sac-like appendages of the colonic mucosa that have herniated through the intestinal mucosa. The frequency of diverticular disease is directly correlated with age. Over 80% of patients > 85 years of age have diverticula. The majority of diverticula occur in the **left colon**, usually within the sigmoid. Right-sided diverticular disease is more common in patients of Asian and African descent.

Pathophysiology

Diverticula are thought to result from low-fiber diets and resultant increased colonic pressure. **Uncomplicated diverticulitis** results from diverticular obstruction with stool that causes pain and inflammation limited to the pericolonic fat. **Complicated diverticulitis** involves inflammation extending beyond pericolonic fat with abscess formation and/or microperforation. **Diverticular bleeds** result from erosion of diverticula into the mucosal wall; they are typically painless, account for approximately 40% of lower GI bleeds, and are associated with NSAID use.

Symptoms/Examination

Uncomplicated diverticulitis presents with focal abdominal tenderness and pain (usually left sided); fever, anorexia, nausea, vomiting may be present. **Complicated diverticulitis** involves more significant tenderness and/or evidence of peritonitis. **Elderly patients** may present with relatively minor symptoms and are at increased risk for perforation with greater mortality.

Diagnosis

Uncomplicated diverticulitis may be a clinical diagnosis, given the appropriate setting. **CT** is preferred method to confirm diagnosis and evaluate for complications. **Barium enema** should be avoided in possible diverticulitis due to risk of perforation, but may diagnose asymptomatic diverticula.

Treatment

- **Uncomplicated diverticulitis** is treated with oral antibiotics with gram-negative and anaerobic coverage (quinolone + metronidazole, OR amox-clavulanate), NSAIDs, and narcotics for pain relief. Liquid diet provides some relief of symptoms but is not required.
- **Complicated diverticulitis** requires IV antibiotics. Keep NPO, and obtain surgical consultation for all patients with peritonitis or perforation.
- **Elective resection** of diverticula is generally reserved for patients with > 1 episode of diverticulitis once acute inflammation has resolved.
- **Colon cancer** may occur in as many as 9% of patients; screening is indicated after the acute episode resolves.

Complications

Perforation, obstruction, strictures, fistulas, abscess formation, sepsis.

KEY FACT

Appendiceal obstruction can result from fecalith, food, adhesions, or enlarged lymph tissue, but one-third of cases have no clear source.

APPENDICITIS

Appendicitis is the most common indication for emergent surgery and the most common surgical emergency in pregnancy. Its presentation can be highly variable, and missed appendicitis remains the third-leading cause of emergency medicine (EM) malpractice suits.

KEY FACT

The obturator sign, associated with a pelvic appendix, is induced by passively flexing and internally rotating the right hip. An inflamed appendix may irritate the obturator internus muscle.

Pathophysiology

Obstruction of the appendiceal lumen (most commonly with a fecalith) blocks venous/lymphatic drainage, causing increased pressure, **bacterial invasion of the appendiceal wall,** and acute inflammation. Ongoing inflammation eventually causes arterial stasis and **tissue infarction** with **perforation** typically occurring in 24-36 hours.

KEY FACT

The psoas sign, associated with retrocecal appendix, is elicited in the left lateral decubitus position by extension of the right hip. The maneuver will cause pain by stretching the psoas muscle, which may be inflamed by an adjacent mass.

Symptoms

Diffuse **periumbilical (visceral) pain** with migration to the right lower quadrant is followed by anorexia, nausea, and vomiting; **migratory pain** is the most predictive historical finding. One-third to one-half of patients present **atypically**, with symptoms varying by location of the tip of the appendix. **Fever** is present in only 20% of cases.

KEY FACT

Rosving sign is positive when palpation to the left lower quadrant (LLQ) causes RLQ pain; it's indicative of right-sided peritoneal irritation.

Examination

- Classically, **diffuse abdominal tenderness** progressing to tenderness over **McBurney point**. **Guarding** (typically voluntary) may be present; **rebound** tenderness is a late finding. Examination findings most strongly predictive of acute appendicitis are **RLQ tenderness** and **rigidity**.
- Many **clinical signs** are described in the literature (eg, Rovsing, Obturator, and Psoas signs), but they demonstrate highly variable and **generally poor reliability** when studied. Isolated **tenderness on rectal examination** may be seen in retrocecal appendicitis. **Cervical motion tenderness** is present in up to 25% of women with acute appendicitis.

DIAGNOSIS

- **White blood cell (WBC) count** is elevated in 80%-90% of cases, but is nonspecific. **C-reactive protein (CRP)** has poor sensitivity and specificity in isolation, but may be helpful when considered in conjunction with WBC count. **Urinalysis** may show mild, sterile pyuria, but frank pyuria (> 20 WBC/hpf) and hematuria are highly suggestive of a urinary source.
- **Graded compression ultrasound** is the test of choice in pregnant patients and children; a positive test demonstrates an appendix that is noncompressible or > 6 mm in diameter. It is 75%-90% sensitive and 85%-95% specific, but has poor sensitivity in perforation.
- **CT scan** is the test of choice in nonpregnant adults. It has excellent sensitivity (87%-100%) and specificity (89%-90%). The presence of **periappendiceal fat stranding** is the most specific finding; other findings include an inflamed appendix that does not fill with contrast, pericecal inflammation, abscess, phlegmon, or fluid collection. Multiple recent studies suggest that **CT scans without oral contrast** are sufficient to evaluate appendicitis but results vary by institution and radiologist experience. Plan radiographs are not useful.
- **CT with rectal contrast** has the highest specificity and avoids oral contrast but may be impractical.
- **Magnetic resonance imaging (MRI)** is typically reserved for pregnant patients with equivocal ultrasounds.

TREATMENT

- **Early surgical consultation** for appendectomy is the standard of care. Delayed diagnosis and intervention may lead to development of gangrene, perforation, and sepsis; however, clinical observation with serial abdominal examinations may be warranted if diagnosis is not clear.
- High-risk patients (eg, men with classic presentations) should have prompt **surgical evaluation prior to imaging** to reduce radiation exposure.
- Keep **NPO**, give fluids, **antibiotics** (eg, Pip-Tazo or Ertapenem), and **pain medication**; opiates do not obscure surgical evaluation and should never be withheld for this reason.

COMPLICATIONS

Perforation (20% of cases) with resultant peritonitis, abscess formation, and progressive systemic infection

RADIATION PROCTOCOLITIS

Radiation proctocolitis is a **common** toxicity of radiation therapy to the abdomen or pelvis, occurring in **50%-75%** of treated patients. It may be acute (during or shortly after treatment) or chronic (delayed by 2 years or longer). Symptoms result from colonic inflammation and edema associated with cell death. Fibrosis and ischemia may also occur.

PATHOPHYSIOLOGY

- **Acute disease**: Oxygen-free radicals cause cellular DNA damage and slowed replacement of normally sloughed intestinal epithelium, leading to ulcerations. Submucosal inflammation causes increased secretions and bleeding.
- **Chronic disease:** Progressive endarteritis causes decreased perfusion. Worsening bowel ischemia causes ulceration, scarring, narrowing and possibly perforation.

Q

A 65-year-old man with distant history of colon cancer presents with progressively worsening diarrhea, mucinous and bloody stool, and pain with defecation. What is the likely diagnosis?

KEY FACT

Appendicitis remains the most common extrauterine surgical emergency in pregnancy. The diagnosis should be considered in pregnant women with abdominal pain and GI symptoms.

Symptoms

- **Acute**: Onset of bleeding, abdominal pain, and tenesmus during course of radiation therapy.
- **Chronic**: Slower onset of GI symptoms months to years after radiation therapy; symptoms include diarrhea, tenesmus, fistulas (anywhere, but rectovaginal most common), and strictures.

A

Radiation proctocolitis (chronic, delayed presentation).

Examination

As with other types of colitis, patients may have abdominal tenderness to palpation and gross or microscopic blood in stool.

Differential

UC, Crohn disease, infectious colitis, ischemic colitis, radiation enteritis (small bowel).

Diagnosis

- **Acute** form is diagnosed clinically given appropriate symptoms with a history of radiation therapy. Specific testing is generally not required in the ED, but consider testing to **exclude causes of infectious enteritis**. Endoscopy is typically pursued outpatient.
- **Chronic disease** is a diagnosis of exclusion; neither endoscopy nor biopsy is diagnostic, but they may show suggestive changes and/or exclude alternative diagnoses.
- Consider **CT** for patients with **obstructive** symptoms to evaluate recurrent malignancy; **MRI** is the test of choice for **suspected fistula**.

Treatment

Steroids or sucralfate enemas, decreased radiation doses, and stool softeners may help. Limited evidence supports topical steroids + metronidazole in chronic disease.

Complications

Stricture formation can be treated with endoscopic dilation; **large bowel obstruction (LBO)** and **fistula** formation may rarely require surgical intervention.

IRRITABLE BOWEL SYNDROME

A chronic functional bowel disorder of uncertain etiology characterized by abdominal pain or discomfort and alterations in stool frequency and form. Once thought a purely psychological disorder, current theories associate symptoms with disordered gut motility/sensation. By definition, there is no structural GI abnormality or underlying medical disease. It is more common in women; average age of onset is 20 years.

Symptoms

- In the absence of **alarm symptoms** (see the following text), the **Rome III Criteria** define *irritable bowel syndrome (IBS)* as recurrent **abdominal pain/discomfort** for ≥ 3 days/month in the last 3 months AND at least two of the following: **improvement with defecation**, change in **stool frequency**, and/or change in **stool form**.
- Additional suggestive symptoms include **urgency**, passing of **mucus**, bloating, and an association with emotional upset/**stress**. **Dyspepsia** and **nausea** may also be present.

- **Alarm symptoms** argue against IBS and include onset after age 50, weight loss, anorexia, bloody stools, and nocturnal diarrhea.

Examination

Abdominal examination is generally benign but may reveal mild, diffuse, or localized tenderness, commonly in the LLQ (associated with sigmoid colon).

Diagnosis

Exclude urgent pathology; there are no specific or confirmatory laboratory/imaging tests for IBS, and the diagnosis should be made in the primary care setting.

Treatment

Provide reassurance, primary care referral, and return precautions; avoid formally diagnosing IBS from the ED. Medical management varies by predominant symptoms but may include **dietary/behavioral** modifications, **antispasmodics, antidepressants, laxatives** or **antidiarrheals**.

LARGE-BOWEL OBSTRUCTION

Mechanical colonic obstruction is due to a physical barrier that prevents the passage of bowel contents through the GI tract. Unlike SBO, the cause is rarely adhesions or hernias. The common causes are listed in Table 11.9.

> **KEY FACT**
>
> Psuedo-obstruction ("Ogilvie syndrome") is an LBO without an identified obstructing lesion; it is thought to result from disordered autonomic control of the bowel.

Pathophysiology

Increasing intraluminal pressure due to mechanical obstruction compromises blood flow to the bowel wall, leading to edema, transudative fluids losses, and dehydration. Decreased arterial flow causes ischemia and eventual perforation. Bacterial translocation may lead to sepsis.

> **KEY FACT**
>
> Colon cancer is the most common cause of LBO; up to 20% of patients with colon cancer will develop an obstruction.

Symptoms/Examination

- Symptoms include abdominal pain, distention, nausea, vomiting (sometimes feculent if the obstruction is distal), and inability to pass flatus or stool.
- Examination shows abdominal distention, tenderness, and/or tympany. Classically, high-pitched, increased bowel sounds are heard early followed by decreased or absent bowel sounds later in the course.

Diagnosis

- **Abdominal x-ray (AXR)**: Unlikely to reveal specific location or cause of an LBO, but may demonstrate air fluid levels or free air; cecal diameter > 12 cm is associated with higher risk of perforation.
- **CT**: Contrast-enhanced examination may delineate location of obstruction, etiology, and partial vs complete obstruction.
- **Contrast enema/sigmoidoscopy**: Consider for poor surgical candidates with unknown cause of obstruction; more accurately rules out pseudo-obstruction than imaging.

Treatment

- **Fluid/electrolyte** replacement, **pain control**, and **NG tube** if significant vomiting and/or distension. Definitive management varies by etiology (See Table 11.9).
- **Antibiotics** are indicated for suspected perforation or signs of toxicity.
- **Emergent surgical consultation** is warranted in call cases.

TABLE 11.9. Common Causes of Large Bowel Obstruction

Etiology	Pathophysiology/Notes	Diagnosis/Treatment (Dx/Tx)
Colorectal cancer	Most common cause of LBO; history may reveal change in bowel habits, rectal bleeding, weight loss.	Dx: contrast enema or colonoscopy. CT may reveal extension/mets. Tx: resection.
Diverticulitis	Second most common. Diverticular infection → edema → obstruction. Occurs in 10%-25% of pts with diverticula; incidence increases with age.	Dx: CT. Tx: Conservative; NPO, antibiotics, NG tube decompression, fluid/electrolyte repletion.
Sigmoid volvulus	Rotation of a bowel segment on an axis formed by its mesentery. ↑ risk in elderly, bedridden, and psychiatric pts. Triad of abdominal pain, distention and constipation. Presents with variable acuity; can be relatively mild/gradual.	AXR: Usually diagnostic. A single distended loop rising out of the pelvis with a central stripe, giving a "coffee bean" appearance. May show gas in surrounding bowel (see Figure 11.5). Contrast enema: dilated loop with "bird's beak" shape. CT is also diagnostic. Tx: Attempt decompression with scope or rectal tube; resection and fixation are indicated for unsuccessful attempts and strangulation.
Cecal volvulus	Congenital defect in cecal mesentery → twisting of mobile cecal segment. A/w younger pts, institutionalized pts, and gravid women.	Dx: AXR is diagnostic in ~50% of cases; shows distended ovoid cecum with paucity of gas in distal colon; this finding may also be described as "coffee" or "kidney bean" shaped. Contrast enema may clarify if AXR is equivocal. Tx: Surgical.
Intussusception	Most common abdominal emergency in children < 2. Proximal bowel segment invaginates into distal segment; most are ileocolic. Mostly pediatric. Most childhood cases are idiopathic; most adult cases have underlying pathology.	Dx: Ultrasound usually diagnostic; shows "target sign." Contrast enema is diagnostic and therapeutic. Can also be seen on CT. Unsuccessful reduction with enema or evidence of perf warrant surgery.
Acute colonic pseudo-obstruction (Ogilvie syndrome)	Usually seen in elderly pts hospitalized with severe illness/multiple comorbidities. Dilatation usually of the cecum and right colon in the absence of a mechanical obstruction. A/w trauma, infection, electrolyte abnormalities, medications.	Dx: CT or water-soluble enema is diagnostic. Tx; Conservative management initially (bowel rest, rectal tube, hydration, correct electrolytes avoid medications that slow colonic motility). Neostigmine may aid decompression. Surgical intervention is reserved for refractory cases or perforation.

AXR, abdominal x-ray CT, computed tomography; LBO, large bowel obstruction; NG, nasogastric; NPO, nothing by mouth; LLQ, left lower quadrant.

COMPLICATIONS

Bowel **perforation** (with 40% mortality rate). Acute **colitis** may occur due to bowel ischemia.

Anorectal

ANORECTAL ABSCESS

Includes the more limited perianal abscess (**simple anorectal abscess**) as well as the more extensive perirectal abscesses (**complex anorectal abscess**). Patients present with anorectal pain, fevers, and palpable perirectal mass.

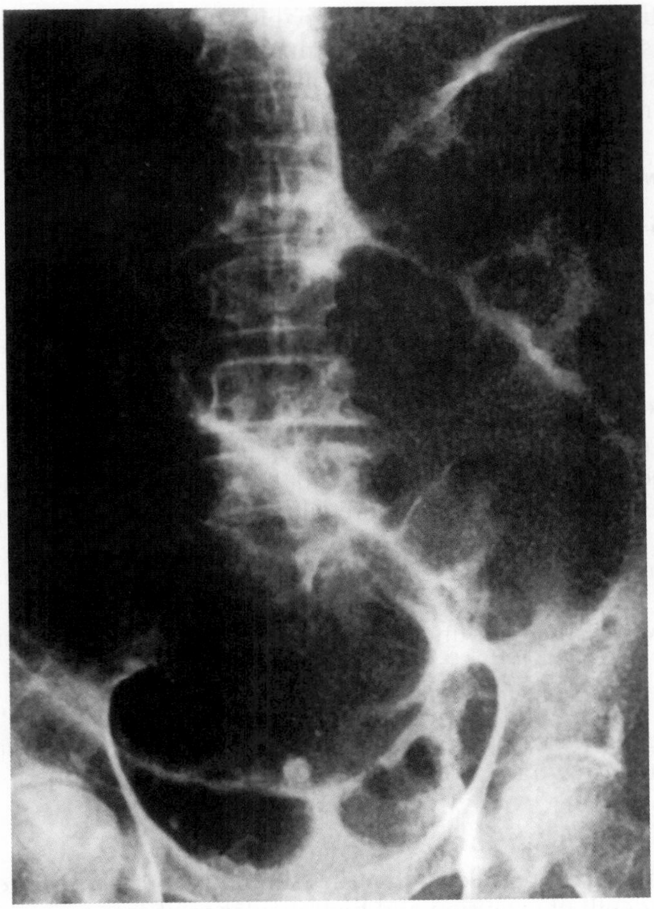

FIGURE 11.5. Sigmoid volvulus. Note distention of large bowel and central stripe, giving a "coffee bean" appearance. (Reproduced, with permission, from Tintinalli JE, Stapczynski JS, Ma OJ, et al. *Tintinalli's Emergency Medicine*. 7th ed. New York, NY: McGraw-Hill; 2011.)

Q

A mother brings her 9-month-old child to the ED for evaluation of bloody stools. Recently the infant has been having less frequent stools with scant bright red blood and has been crying inconsolably during and immediately after bowel movements. What is the likely diagnosis?

Pathophysiology

- Obstruction of anal gland → local abscess formation (polymicrobial) → spread to local potential spaces (perianal, ischiorectal, intersphincteric, supralevator, postanal)
- Other causes: Crohn disease, trauma, cancer, radiation, TB

Perianal Abscess

Symptoms/Examination

- Easily palpable tender mass, close to the anal verge, usually posterior midline
- Pain may be worse before defecation and with Valsalva maneuvers.

Diagnosis

Simple perianal abscess is a clinical diagnosis; **CT** can exclude suspected perirectal involvement.

Treatment

- Small, uncomplicated, isolated abscesses may be drained in the ED; all other abscesses and febrile/toxic appearing patients require **surgical consultation**. Use a cruciate or elliptical incision as close to the anus as possible to minimize fistula formation. Simple linear incisions may be used but require packing and 24-hour follow-up.

A

Anal fissure.

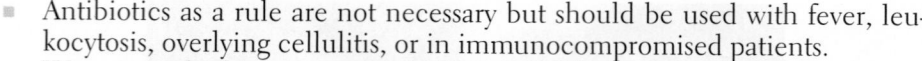

- Antibiotics as a rule are not necessary but should be used with fever, leukocytosis, overlying cellulitis, or in immunocompromised patients.
- Warm sitz baths starting at 24 hours, 48-hour wound check, referral for colorectal surgery follow-up. Advise patients of high recurrence rate.

COMPLICATIONS

Recurrence, fistulas, sphincter injury, sepsis.

Perirectal Abscess

Includes ischiorectal, intersphincteric, supralevator, and postanal abscesses.

SYMPTOMS/EXAMINATION

- See Figure 11.6 for common locations of perirectal abscesses.
- **Ischiorectal abscess**: Dull pain with few outward signs; when present, tenderness and induration is more lateral to anal verge than with perianal abscess.
- **Intersphincteric abscess:** Pain with defecation, rectal discharge, fever, mass on rectal examination.
- **Supralevator abscess:** Buttock or perirectal pain; few outward signs.

KEY FACT

All perirectal abscesses should be drained in the operating room.

DIAGNOSIS

CT will identify large pelvic abscesses but is inadequate for small perianal abscesses and fistula tracts; **MRI** and **ultrasound** may be required.

TREATMENT

Surgical consult; all perirectal abscesses should be **drained in the operating room** given depth of extension and high incidence of recurrence. **Antibiotics** are indicated if complicated by valvular heart disease, immunocompromise, surrounding cellulitis, leukocytosis, or fever.

COMPLICATIONS

Recurrence, fistulas, sphincter injury, sepsis.

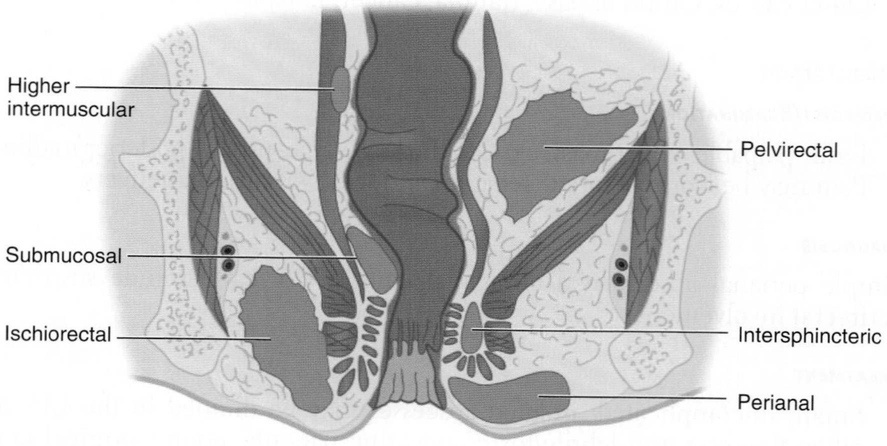

FIGURE 11.6. Anatomical classification of common anorectal abscesses. (Reproduced, with permission, from Tintinalli JE, Stapczynski JS, Ma OJ, et al. *Tintinalli's Emergency Medicine*, 7th ed. New York, NY: McGraw-Hill; 2011.)

ANAL FISTULA

Anal fistulas most commonly result from perianal/perirectal abscesses and present similarly with the addition of persistent, blood-stained, malodorous **discharge**. When intermittently obstructed/inflamed, recurrent abscesses form.

DIAGNOSIS/TREATMENT

Transrectal **ultrasound**/endosonography or **MRI** preferred. **CT** and **fistulography** have limited capacity to define small abscesses and tracts. Treatment is surgical.

PILONIDAL ABSCESS

Pilonidal abscesses are acquired, chronic infections of gluteal cleft hair follicles over the sacral/perianal region that occur more commonly in obese, hirsute, young men (rare > age 40). Pilonidal abscesses are not related to the anorectum in any way and should not be confused with perirectal abscesses, fistulae, or sacrococcygeal sinuses.

SYMPTOMS/EXAMINATION

Tender, **fluctuant mass** along superior gluteal fold, with or without draining sinus tract. Located in **posterior midline** over the sacrum/coccyx.

TREATMENT

Lateral longitudinal **I&D**, ± packing and referral for **surgical follow-up** for possible wide excision given high rate of recurrence. Antibiotics not routinely indicated.

COMPLICATIONS

Recurrence (~40%) and **fistula** formation are common; rare case reports of associated squamous cell carcinoma. Perianal **hidradenitis suppurativa** presents similarly and is often misdiagnosed as pilonidal disease.

> **KEY FACT**
>
> Pilonidal abscesses/sinus tracts form in the midline; perirectal abscesses are usually not midline.

PROCTITIS

Proctitis—inflammation of the rectal mucosa—is most often caused by sexually transmitted infections (STIs), but can also be due to enteric pathogens, radiation treatments, or UC. STIs of the anus are typically caused by anal sex, but are occasionally spread from the vagina or scrotum (eg, lymphogranuloma venereum, gonorrhea). If a patient has one of these STIs, assume that others are present as well. Table 11.10 lists STIs that commonly cause proctitis.

PRURITUS ANI

Painless, uncontrollable itching/scratching of perianal area. It is more common in men, during summer months, and is typically worse at night.

- Consider poor **hygiene**, **systemic disease**, parasitic and fungal **infections**. History and examination alone generally identifies the cause.
- Treatment requires improved **hygiene** and identification/treatment of underlying cause (eg, permethrin for pinworms/scabies, antifungals, sitz baths).

TABLE 11.10. STIs That Cause Proctitis

	Symptoms/Examination	Treatment	Complications
Condyloma acuminata (HPV)	Perianal soft fleshy growths (see Figure 11.7); may spread from vagina/scrotum; pain, itching, bleeding	Topicals (podophyllin, trichloroacetic acid, 5-FU); refer for cryotherapy, laser ablation, or excision	40% recurrence; associated with squamous cell carcinoma
Gonorrhea	Asymptomatic to rectal itching, pain and discharge; Gram stain/cultures for diagnosis	Ceftriaxone	Dissemination to heart, liver, CNS, joints
Chlamydia (including LGV)	Asymptomatic to rectal pain and discharge; ulcerations with unilateral inguinal adenopathy with LGV	Azithromycin, doxycycline; 21-d course for LGV	Rectal scarring, abscesses, fistulas
Syphilis	Primary: classic painless chancre, painful anal chancre. mucoid drainage, tenesmus, inguinal adenopathy Secondary: Perianal condyloma lata	Penicillin	Good prognosis if treated
Chancroid (*Haemophilus ducreyi*)	Indurated lesion/pustule → painful ulcer; painful adenitis	Azithromycin, ceftriaxone	
Herpes	Pruritus → pain; discrete vesicles on erythematous base progressing to ulcers	Acyclovir	Recurrent bouts; intense pain may prevent BM → constipation, fecal impaction

CNS, central nervous system; 5-FU, fluorouracil; HPV, human papillomavirus; LGV, lymphogranuloma venereum; STI, sexually transmitted infection.

KEY FACT

Anal fissures are the most frequent cause of rectal bleeding in infants and children.

ANAL FISSURE

Superficial, linear tear in the anal canal after passage of hard feces. Common in young adults, but it is also the most common cause of rectal bleeding in infants and children.

Symptoms

Sharp, **intense pain** during and immediately after bowel movements and **scant, bright red bleeding**, especially on toilet paper.

Examination

Fissures occur in the anterior (less common) or **posterior midline** in women; they are midline but rarely anterior in men (1%). Fissures that occur **off midline** are often associated with **systemic disease** (eg, Crohn, human immunodeficiency virus [HIV], TB, anal carcinoma, syphilis). May see classic "**fissure triad**" of sentinel pile, deep ulcer, and enlarged anal papillae.

Treatment

- Begins with meticulous anal **hygiene** and the **WASH** regimen: **W**arm water, **A**nalgesics, **S**tool softeners, **H**igh-fiber diet. **Hot sitz baths** relieve sphincter spasm.

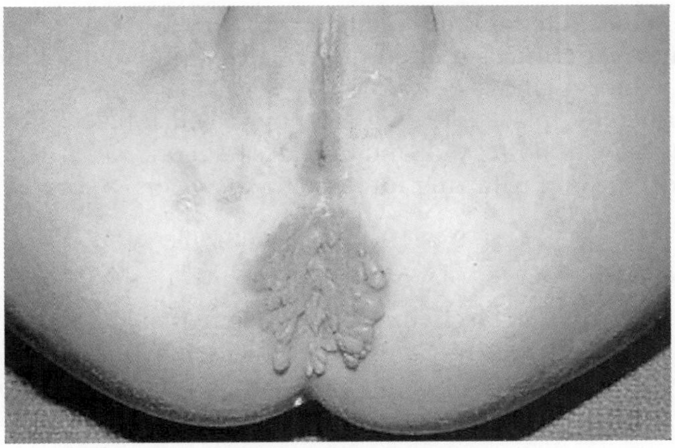

FIGURE 11.7. Perianal condylomata acuminata.

- For chronic/recurrent cases, topical nitroglycerin ointment or nifedipine gel with lidocaine, and botulinum toxin injections decrease anal canal resting pressure. Surgery is reserved for failures of medical therapy.

RECTAL FOREIGN BODIES

Symptoms/Examination

Patients may be reluctant to provide a history and describe only rectal pain, bleeding, or constipation. May present with perforation (ie, peritonitis, shock, fever).

Diagnosis

- **AXR** to delineate the size, location, and number of foreign bodies (and any signs of perforation).
- **Digital rectal examination** and/or **anoscope** will localize most foreign bodies.

Treatment

- **Surgical or colonoscopic removal** for foreign bodies that are large or have sharp edges; simple foreign bodies may be removed in ED. Recommendations vary regarding the role of sedation; awake patients can assist removal with Valsalva, but will have relatively more muscle tension. At a minimum, give a benzodiazepine for anxiolysis/muscle relaxation. All patients should undergo **sigmoidoscopy** after removal to look for mucosal injury and/or perforation.

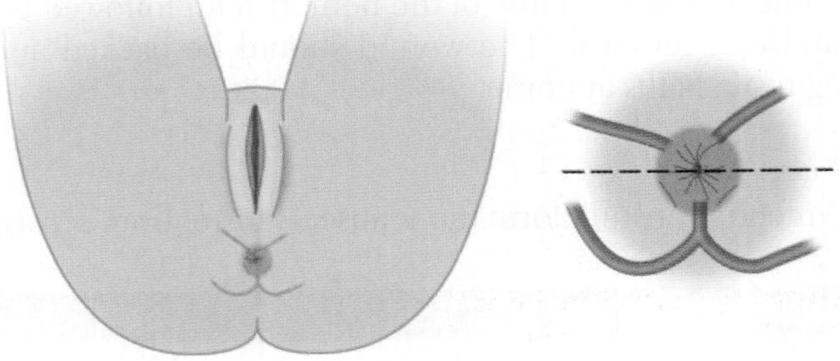

FIGURE 11.8. Goodsall's rule. (Reproduced, with permission, from Tintinalli JE, Stapczynski JS, Ma OJ, et al. *Tintinalli's Emergency Medicine*. 7th ed. New York, NY: McGraw-Hill; 2011.)

KEY FACT

Goodsall's rule: Fistulas with anterior openings follow a direct line to the anal canal, whereas fistulas with posterior openings tend to deviate and curve. See Figure 11.8.

- **Possible removal techniques** include:
- **Local anesthetic** injected circumferentially in internal sphincter to relax muscle, reduces pain.
- **Foley catheter**(s) placed beyond the object and inflated; this breaks vacuum tension with bowel wall and provides traction.
- Pull object forward with **ring forceps** and/or fingers. **Suprapubic pressure** may aid removal.

COMPLICATIONS

Perforation, obstruction, ischemic bowel segments; if suspected, administer antibiotics, consult surgery, and obtain imaging. **Mucosal lacerations** are suggested by increased pain or rectal bleeding after removal; sigmoidoscopy is diagnostic.

KEY FACT

Visceral perforation is the most serious complication of rectal foreign bodies.

HEMORRHOIDS

Hemorrhoids are vascular complexes that line and protect the anal canal; they become symptomatic with activities and disorders that increase venous pressure, causing engorgement. Engorged, prolapsed, or thrombosed hemorrhoidal veins/arterioles cause symptoms.

- **Internal:** Located proximal to dentate line; covered with **insensate** mucosal epithelium
- **External:** Located distal to dentate line; covered with **richly innervated** squamous epithelium

KEY FACT

In the adult patient, portal hypertension may cause rectal varices but not hemorrhoids.

SYMPTOMS/EXAMINATION

- **Internal**: Painless, bright-red bleeding, ± mucous discharge. They become painful when **prolapse** occurs (second degree = temporary prolapse during defecation; third degree = prolapse requiring manual reduction; fourth degree = irreducibly prolapsed). Persistent fourth degree prolapse and can lead to strangulation, thrombosis, and gangrene/significant infection (Figure 11.9).
- **External**: Can be seen with visual inspection, and may be painful with even minimal thrombosis; when acutely thrombosed, they are blue, bulging, and extremely painful.

TREATMENT

- **Uncomplicated** hemorrhoids (nonthrombosed external and nonprolapsed internal): Warm sitz baths, bulk laxatives/high-fiber diet, over-the-counter (OTC) topicals; avoid prolonged topical corticosteroid use.
- **Prolapsed internal** hemorrhoids: Surgical referral for: band ligation, sclerotherapy, or hemorrhoidectomy. Emergent hemorrhoidectomy is indicated for nonreducible, thrombosed or gangrenous internal hemorrhoids.
- **Thrombosed external hemorrhoids** < 48 hours old may be excised in the ED to relieve pain. Lidocaine with epinephrine (to minimize bleeding) should be injected at the dome of the hemorrhoid, followed by an elliptical incision and clot removal. The wound should be packed and the patient should begin sitz baths at home.

COMPLICATIONS

Recurrence, infection, fistula formation, abscess formation, sepsis.

RECTAL PROLAPSE (PROCIDENTIA)

Incomplete prolapse involves only the **rectal mucosa**, usually in children with simple constipation or diarrheal illness (though it can be associated with cystic fibrosis [CF], malnutrition, or parasitic infections). **Complete prolapse** involves

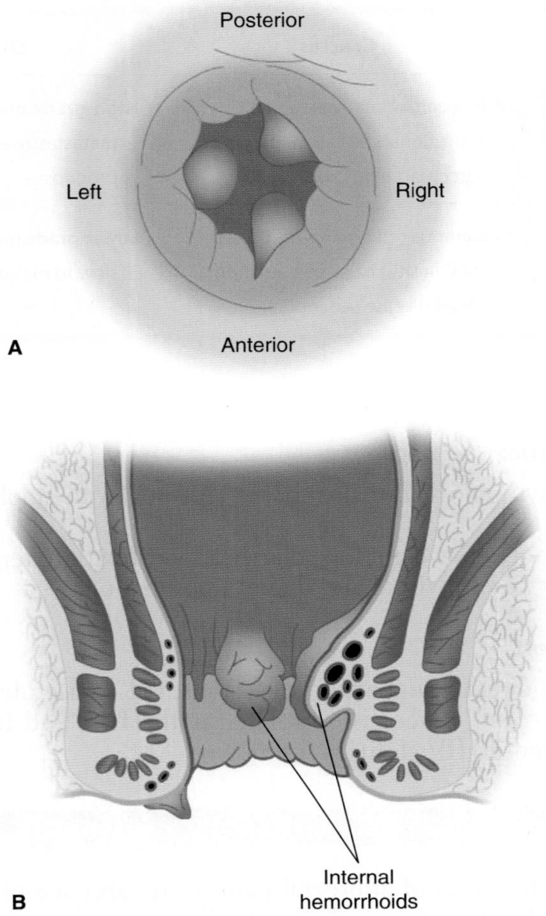

FIGURE 11.9. Common locations of internal hemorrhoids. (Reproduced, with permission, from Tintinalli JE, Stapczynski JS, Ma OJ, et al. *Tintinalli's Emergency Medicine*. 7th ed. New York, NY: McGraw-Hill; 2011.)

all layers of the rectum due to laxity of attachment structures, usually elderly women with chronic constipation.

Symptoms/Examination

A **rectal mass** is noted following defecation or straining; it may be reduced manually by the patient or seen as a swollen, ulcerated mass on examination. Other symptoms include **bloody mucous** discharge, fecal **incontinence**, dull **pain**, and foul **odor**.

Treatment

Attempt **manual reduction** with gentle, continuous pressure, ± sedation; **surgery** is necessary if reduction fails. **Treat constipation**. Refer all adults for **endoscopy** to rule out underlying lesion/lead point (eg, IBD, tumor, polyps, rectal ulcer).

KEY FACT

The anus is the third most common site for melanoma metastasis, after the eye and the skin.

ANORECTAL TUMORS

See Table 11.11.

TABLE 11.11. Classification of Anorectal Tumors by Location

Type	Location	Cell Type	Cancers	Outcome
Anal canal	Proximal to dentate line	Transition zone between squamous cell and columnar epithelium of rectum	Adenocarcinoma, melanoma, transitional cell carcinoma, Kaposi sarcoma, villous adenoma	**High-grade malignant potential;** metastasize early; poor prognosis
Anal margin	Distal to dentate line	Squamous cell	Squamous cell carcinoma, Bowen (SCC in situ) basal cell carcinoma, Paget disease (AdenoCa)	**Lower grade malignant potential,** slow to metastasize

KEY FACT

All ulcers and skin lesions that have failed to improve for 30 days should be **biopsied**.

Symptoms/Examination

- Nonspecific symptoms: Pruritus, pain, bleeding with stool, sensation of a lump
- Progressive anorexia, weight loss, diarrhea, constipation, tenesmus
- Detectable by careful visual and digital examination

Diagnosis/Treatment

Anoscopy allows direct visualization of lesions; **CT** is useful in assessing the extent of disease. Anal cancer is correlated with **HIV**, and testing is generally recommended if HIV status is unknown.

PROCTALGIA

Poorly defined syndromes of anorectal pain in the absence of an identifiable organic disorder. **Levator ani syndrome** (dull pressure brought on by defecation and prolonged sitting) and **proctalgia fugax** (intense, painful anorectal spasms lasting < 30 minutes) are the two most common.

Symptoms/Examination

- **Levator ani syndrome:** Dull, aching pain. Tender, contracted levator muscles on examination.
- **Proctalgia fugax:** Abrupt onset, brief, consistent symptoms with each episode.

Differential

Causes of chronic pelvic pain (tumors/masses, endometriosis), cauda equine syndrome.

Treatment

Limited/anecdotal evidence for sitz baths, levator massage, topical nitrates, and/or diazepam.

Liver Disorders

JAUNDICE

Jaundice is a yellow discoloration of the eyes (sclera icterus), mucosal surfaces, and skin due to an accumulation of bilirubin (> 3 mg/dL) and deposition in body tissues. Hyperbilirubinemia results from either **over-production**,

inadequate metabolism, or **decreased excretion** of bilirubin (ie, prehepatic, hepatic, and posthepatic causes). Determining the underlying cause begins with determining whether the hyperbilirubinemia is conjugated (direct) or unconjugated (indirect). See Table 11.12 for the differential diagnosis of jaundice.

Q

A 35-year-old injection drug user presents with RUQ pain, vomiting, and jaundice. A viral hepatitis panel returns with HBsAg+, anti-HBc IgM+, and HBeAg+. What is the most likely diagnosis?

Symptoms

- Ask about alcohol use, IV drug use, history of blood transfusion, viral prodrome, fever, abdominal pain, malignancy, ingestion, and pregnancy.
- Symptoms depend on the underlying etiology. May include pruritus, change in urine or stools, nausea/vomiting, abdominal pain (hepatic inflammation, biliary obstruction), increased abdominal girth (ascites), and confusion (encephalopathy).

Examination

- Jaundice appears first under the tongue → conjunctiva → spreads caudally; however, degree of spread does not accurately predict serum bilirubin levels.

TABLE 11.12. Differential Diagnosis of Jaundice

	Associated Labs	Pattern	Etiology
Unconjugated (indirect) hyperbilirubinemia	Normal AST/ALT, alkaline phosphatase, and PT/PTT	Hematologic/ pre-Hepatic (↑ production)	Hemolytic disorders Hematoma resorption Gilbert disease Crigler-Najjar type I, II Drugs (ribavirin, probenecid) Ineffective erythropoiesis (thalassemia, folate or B_{12} deficiency)
Conjugated (direct) hyperbilirubinemia	AST/ALT elevated > alkaline phosphatase	Hepatocellular (↓ metabolism)	Viral hepatitis Alcoholic hepatitis Autoimmune hepatitis
	Alkaline phosphatase elevated > AST/ALT	Obstructive/ posthepatic (↓ excretion)	Shock liver (ischemic) Toxins (APAP, INH) Wilson disease
	Isolated direct hyperbilirubinemia		Obstructive tumors Choledocholithiasis Biliary strictures AIDS cholangiopathy Primary biliary cirrhosis Primary sclerosing cholangitis Cholestatic drugs Dubin-Johnson syndrome Rotor syndrome

AIDS, acquired immune deficiency syndrome; APAP, *N*-acetyl-p-aminophenol; AST/ALT, aspartate aminotransferase/alanine transaminase; HELLP, hemolysis, elevated liver enzymes, and low platelets; INH, isoniazid; PT/PTT, prothrombin time/partial thromboplastin time.

A

Acute hepatitis B infection.

- Unconjugated hyperbilirubinemia: Normal stool and urine color, mild jaundice; splenomegaly may be present with hemolysis.
- Conjugated hyperbilirubinemia: RUQ abdominal pain, dark urine and light-colored stools if due to biliary obstruction; pruritus is common with cholestasis; stigmata of liver disease are seen with hepatocellular causes.

Diagnosis

- Prothrombin time/partial thromboplastin time (PT/PTT) may be elevated in hepatic dysfunction.
- Lipase may be elevated in choledocholithiasis.
- Complete blood count (CBC) may show thrombocytopenia in chronic liver disease, anemia in hemolysis.
- Alkaline phosphatase (ALP) elevation suggests obstruction; elevated γ-glutamyl transferase (GGT) confirms hepatic source of the ALP.
- Arterial blood gas (ABG) is useful to assess for acidosis if fulminant hepatic failure is suspected.
- Acetaminophen level for suspected ingestions.
- Ultrasound is the imaging modality of choice unless malignancy is suspected.

HEPATITIS

KEY FACT

Hepatitis C is the number 1 reason patients require liver transplantation in the United States.

The term *hepatitis* refers broadly to inflammation of the liver. Viral hepatitis is the most common cause in the United States. Hepatitis B and C can progress to chronic hepatitis, and hepatitis C is the leading cause of liver transplantation in the United States. Other causes of hepatitis include bacterial and parasitic infection, immune disorders, and prescription drugs or toxic exposures.

Hepatitis A

The hepatitis A virus (HAV) (RNA picornavirus) is endemic worldwide. In the United States, nearly one-half of all urban-dwelling adults are seropositive for the anti-HAV antibody; up to 70% of cases are asymptomatic. Routine vaccination of children in the United States has shifted the burden of new cases predominantly to adult international travelers and men who have sex with men (MSM). Most patients recover completely in 2 months, nearly all in 6 months.

Transmission

- Incubation period is 30 days.
- **Fecal-oral** via contaminated food and water and sexual practices.
- No chronic carrier state after infection.

Symptoms

- Most cases are subclinical, especially in children. May present with **flulike illness** and RUQ pain, followed by onset of **jaundice** and pruritus.
- The most common examination findings are **hepatosplenomegaly** and **jaundice**.
- **Atypical presentations** include fulminant liver failure and cholestasis (prolonged, deep jaundice). Relapsing disease is rare with HAV infection alone.

Diagnosis

- **History:** Inquire about ill contacts, substandard water supply, travel, and potentially contaminated foods (eg, **shellfish and green onions**), and sexual history—particularly MSM.

- **Labs:** Elevated Anti-HAV IgM is diagnostic in the symptomatic patient. Anti-HAV IgM and anti-HAV immunoglobulin G (IgG) titers rise during acute infection. Immunoglobulin M (IgM) titers peak during the first week of clinical illness and disappear within 3-6 months; IgG titers remain elevated for life.

TREATMENT

- Supportive; rarely progresses into fulminant infection.
- Unvaccinated patients with HAV exposure: prophylaxis with HAV vaccine **or** immune globulin (IG); vaccination is preferred. Immunosuppressed patients or those with other liver disease should receive both the vaccine and immunoglobulin (Ig).
- Avoid alcohol and any easily avoidable hepatotoxic meds (eg, acetaminophen) during acute infection; except in cases of marked liver dysfunction, hepatically metabolized medications should not be routinely discontinued.
- **Food handlers** should not return to work until jaundice clears.

Hepatitis B

Hepatitis B is a partially double-stranded DNA virus. 10% of infected persons will develop chronic hepatitis B infection. Age at infection is **inversely related** to the risk of chronic infection. Of all patients with chronic hepatitis B virus (HBV), 15%-20% develop cirrhosis and 10%-15% develop hepatocellular carcinoma. HBV is far **more infectious** than HIV or Hep C.

TRANSMISSION

- Incubation period is 6 weeks to 6 months.
- Maternal → fetal (most common cause worldwide)
- Primarily by parenteral exposure/IV drug use. Sexual transmission is possible. Transmission through blood transfusion is rare.

SYMPTOMS

Symptoms similar to Hepatitis A.

DIAGNOSIS (TABLE 11.13)

- **HBsAg:** Hepatitis B surface antigen; indicates **active** infection (acute or chronic).

TABLE 11.13. Serologic Patterns for Hepatitis B Infection

Hepatitis B surface antigen	Hepatitis B surface antibody	Hepatitis B core antibody	Hepatitis B e antigen	Hepatitis B e antibody	Interpretation
+	–	IgM	+	–	Acute hepatitis B
+	–	IgG	+	–	Chronic hepatitis B with active viral replication
+	–	IgG	–	+	Chronic hepatitis B with low viral replication
–	+	IgG	–	+ or –	Recovery from hepatitis B (immunity)
–	+	–	–	–	Vaccination (immunity)
–	–	IgG	–	–	False-positive; less commonly, infection in remote past

IgG, immunoglobulin G; IgM, immunoglobulin M.

- **Anti-HBs:** Antibody to HBsAg; indicates past viral infection or immunization.
- **Anti-HBc:** Antibody (IgM or IgG) to hepatitis B core antigen; IgM is an early marker of infection while IgG is the best marker for prior HBV exposure. IgM may also become detectable in reactivation of HBV.
- **HBeAg:** Hepatitis Be antigen; proportional to the quantity of intact virus and, therefore, infectivity. Some HBV variants (called *precore mutants*) cannot make HBeAg.
- **Anti-HBe:** Antibody to HBeAg; resolving HBV infection and decreasing infectivity.

TREATMENT

- Treatment of acute hepatitis is primarily supportive with avoidance of hepatotoxic agents; transfer to transplant-capable center should occur in fulminate hepatitis.
- **Chronic hepatitis B**: Antivirals are often used to suppress viral replication in those with evidence of ongoing infection and injury.
- **Postexposure prophylaxis**
  - **HBsAg positive source:** Completely vaccinated persons should receive booster. Partially vaccinated persons should receive hepatitis B immune globulin (HBIG) within 24 hours and complete their vaccination series. Unvaccinated persons should receive HBIG and hepatitis B vaccine.
  - **HBsAg unknown/negative source:** Initiate or complete the vaccination series.

Hepatitis C

Hepatitis C is the most common blood-borne infection and the leading cause of chronic liver disease in the United States; 75%-85% of infected persons will develop chronic hepatitis C infection. There is currently no vaccine for hepatitis C.

TRANSMISSION

- Incubation period averages 6-7 weeks.
- **Injection drug** use or blood product **transfusion prior to 1992** are the predominant causes in the United States and Europe. (Needle stick, dialysis, and other parenteral exposures are also implicated.)
- Sexual transmission is possible, but rare; multiple partners and/or MSM remain risk factors.

SYMPTOMS/EXAMINATION

- **Acute Hepatitis C virus (HCV):** Most patients are asymptomatic; may have mild flulike symptoms and jaundice.
- **Chronic HCV:** Usually asymptomatic until cirrhosis develops. Also may present with cryoglobulinemia associated with a vasculitic skin rash (**leukocytoclastic vasculitis**), **arthralgias**, sicca syndrome, and **membranoproliferative glomerulonephritis.**

DIAGNOSIS

- **Acute hepatitis:** RNA polymerase chain reaction (PCR) and HCV Ab
- **Screening:** HCV antibody (positive 4-6 weeks after infection) and qualitative PCR (positive 1-2 weeks after infection); screen patients with risk factors or persistently elevated transaminases
- **Confirmatory:** Qualitative PCR or recombinant immunoblot assay (RIBA)

TREATMENT

- **Acute infection/needlestick prophylaxis**: Currently not recommended.
- **Chronic HCV:** Treatment with sofosbuvir, peginterferon, and/or ribavirin can be curative in selected patients.

Hepatitis D

Hepatitis D is a defective RNA virus that requires simultaneous presence of host hepatitis B virus to replicate. Transmission is similar to hepatitis B and may carry higher risk of fulminant disease. Diagnosis is by positive anti-HDV. Treatment is with interferons.

Hepatitis E

Hepatitis E virus (HEV) infection is uncommon in the United States, but may be considered in patients returning from endemic areas (Asia, Africa, Russia). It is associated with fecal–oral transmission and the clinical course is similar to hepatitis A, but is generally more severe. The mortality rate is high in pregnant patients (10%-20%). Diagnosis is by positive anti-HEV IgM (acute infection) and anti-HEV (prior exposure). Treatment is supportive.

Drug-Induced Hepatitis

Drug-induced hepatitis ranges from subclinical disease with abnormal liver function tests (LFTs) to fulminant hepatic failure. Though typically mild, it accounts for half of the cases of fulminant liver failure in the United States. It can be characterized as intrinsic (direct toxic effect) or idiosyncratic (immunologically mediated injury) and as necroinflammatory (hepatocellular), cholestatic, or mixed; see Table 11.14 for a list of common toxins that cause liver injury.

Risk factors include advanced age, female gender, use of an increasing number of prescription drugs, underlying liver disease, renal insufficiency, and poor nutrition.

Autoimmune Hepatitis

A chronic immune-mediated hepatitis, most commonly seen in **young females**. It is divided into 2 types (Types 1 and 2) based on the presence of specific circulating antibodies. Presentations vary from incidental findings of **elevated LFTs** to **advanced cirrhosis**. It may be accompanied by signs of **other autoimmune** disease (eg, arthritis, Sjögren syndrome, thyroiditis), and is often "triggered" by **viral infections** such as HAV.

Diagnosis is made by characteristic serologic and histologic findings after excluding other causes. **Treatment** varies by case, but is typically with steroids and/or azathioprine.

CIRRHOSIS

Cirrhosis is the final common pathway of many liver diseases, defined as hepatocellular injury leading to fibrosis and nodular regeneration. Hepatocyte destruction causes metabolic and synthetic dysfunction; fibrosis restricts blood flow and leads to portal hypertension. Reversal may occur with treatment of some chronic liver diseases (eg, HBV, HCV).

Q

A 40-year-old woman with a history of latent tuberculosis but no history of alcohol use or prior liver disease presents with jaundice and transaminases in the thousands. What is the most likely etiology?

KEY FACT

Aspartate aminotransferase/alanine transaminase (AST/ALT) elevations > 3.5 times normal represent "moderate hepatotoxicity." Elevations > 5 times normal are considered "severe."

A

Hepatitis due to isoniazid toxicity.

TABLE 11.14. Toxins Causing Liver Injury

Toxic	Toxic and Idiosyncratic	Idiosyncratic	Primarily Cholestatic
Alcohol	Methyldopa	Volatile anesthetics (halothane)	Chlorpromazine
Acetaminophen	Isoniazid	Phenytoin	Cyclosporine
Salicylates	Sodium valproate	Sulfonamides	Oral contraceptives
Tetracyclines	Amiodarone	Rifampin	Anabolic steroids
Trichloroethylene		Indomethacin	Erythromycin estolate
Vinyl chloride			Methimazole
Carbon tetrachloride			
Yellow phosphorus			
Poisonous mushrooms (Amanita, Galerina)			

Symptoms

Chronic fatigue and **poor appetite** are common. Also muscle wasting, loss of libido, impotence, dysmenorrhea, sleep disturbance. **Often asymptomatic** until the development of an acute complication.

Examination

- Stigmata of chronic liver disease: Palmar erythema, spider telangiectasia, Dupuytren contractures, gynecomastia, testicular atrophy, **Terry nails** (white opacification of proximal two-third of the nail)
- Portal hypertension: Caput medusae, splenomegaly, ascites, varices
- Hepatic encephalopathy: Fetor hepaticus, asterixis, confusion

Differential

Congestive heart failure (CHF), nephrotic syndrome.

Diagnosis

- **Liver biopsy** is the gold standard and **CT** may reveal characteristic liver/spleen changes, but both can generally be **deferred to outpatient setting**.
- Laboratory test results may show thrombocytopenia (splenic sequestration), elevated INR, and low albumin (↓ synthetic function); **LFTs** are usually normal or only mildly elevated.
- Consider **diagnostic paracentesis** if ascites and fever or abdominal pain are present (SBP).

Treatment

- Correct electrolyte, nutritional, and/or clinically significant coagulation deficiencies. Abstain from alcohol, treat underlying disease when possible. Avoid NSAIDs (renal impairment).

- If ascites is present, restrict dietary sodium and consider diuretic therapy (spironolactone ± loop diuretic). If significant respiratory impairment, consider large-volume paracentesis.

Complications

Hepatic encephalopathy, varices, GI bleeding, ascites/SBP, hepatorenal syndrome, hepatopulmonary syndrome, hepatocellular carcinoma (see the following text)

Q

A 54-year-old man with a history of cirrhosis presents with fever, abdominal pain, and ascites. Diagnostic paracentesis reveals ascitic fluid with 320 PMNs/mm^3. What is the diagnosis?

SPONTANEOUS BACTERIAL PERITONITIS

Spontaneous bacterial peritonitis (SBP) is a spontaneous bacterial infection of ascites, probably due to translocation of bacteria from the intestines to the ascitic fluid. The most common organism implicated is *Escherichia coli*. Other organisms include *Streptococcus* and *Enterococcus* spp.

Symptoms/Examination

- Ascites may be characterized by shifting dullness, fluid wave, and bulging flanks. It is easily seen on ultrasound.
- SBP may have minimal physical findings or present with severe abdominal tenderness or altered mental status. Fever is often, but not always, present.

Diagnosis

Diagnostic paracentesis is indicated in any patient with ascites and abdominal pain, encephalopathy, or fever. (Many authors recommend correcting INR prior to paracentesis; data to support this practice are limited.) Positive for SBP if PMNs > 250 cells/mm^3.

Treatment

- Third-generation cephalosporin (eg, cefotaxime); initiate based on cell count.
- **SBP prophylaxis**: Fluoroquinolones or TMP-SMX once daily; indicated for cirrhotic patients hospitalized with GI bleed (3 days); ascites with total protein < 1.5 g/dL (while hospitalized); or ascites present in a patient with a history of prior SBP.
- Well-appearing patients with reassuring cell counts but at high risk for SBP should be started on prophylaxis and referred for PCP or GI follow-up.

HEPATIC ENCEPHALOPATHY

Hepatic encephalopathy is caused by accumulation of nitrogenous waste products in liver failure. Neuropsychiatric changes in the setting of liver disease constitute hepatic encephalopathy until proven otherwise. Look for precipitating factors, including infection, GI bleeding, dehydration, metabolic derangements, sedating medications, hypoglycemia, and nonadherence with hepatic encephalopathy treatment.

Symptoms/Examination

- Insomnia with sleep-wake reversal, personality change, confusion, frank coma
- **Asterixis** (wrist flaps rhythmically when held in extension); **fetor hepaticus** (musty breath)

Diagnosis

Diagnosis is **clinical**. Blood **ammonia** levels are typically elevated but do not correlate with degree of encephalopathy.

A

Spontaneous bacterial peritonitis.

TREATMENT

- Correct precipitating factors and anticipate treatment-related adverse effects.
- **Lactulose**, given PO, PR, or by NGT (adverse effects include dehydration and hypokalemia from diarrhea). Oral **neomycin**, **rifaximin**, or **metronidazole.**
- Patients with very mild encephalopathy and adequate home care/supervision can be discharged with lactulose or rifaximin; most will require admission.

HEPATORENAL SYNDROME

HRS is a type of subacute or **acute kidney injury** in patients with severe cirrhosis. The exact pathophysiology is multifactorial and incompletely understood. Generally, worsening portal hypertension causes splanchnic vasodilation that leads to renal artery vasoconstriction and resultant renal failure, with or without cardiac dysfunction. The **prognosis is poor**; median survival is 10-14 days. 2-month mortality is 90%. Often insidious in onset, but precipitants include GI bleeding and infection.

DIFFERENTIAL

Prerenal azotemia, acute tubular necrosis, drug-induced disorders (NSAIDs, antibiotics, radiographic contrast, diuretics), glomerulonephritis, vasculitis.

DIAGNOSIS

Diagnosis of exclusion; an otherwise unexplained elevation in Cr or BUN in the appropriate clinical setting suggests developing HRS.

TREATMENT

- The immediate goal of therapy is stabilization to allow sufficient recovery of liver function or to bridge to liver transplant. Identify and treat precipitants. Stop all unnecessary medications and diuretics.
- Treat critical hypotension with **norepinephrine** and **albumin** for volume expansion.

KEY FACT

Renal failure from hepatorenal syndrome reverses with liver transplant.

HEPATIC ABSCESS

Hepatic abscesses may be pyogenic or amebic. In the United States, most cases are due to biliary obstruction or cholangitis, although any inflammatory or infectious GI process can lead to abscess and many cases have no identifiable cause. Most pyogenic abscesses are polymicrobial. Primary amebic liver abscesses are due to the organism *Entamoeba histolytica*.

SYMPTOMS/EXAMINATION

Ill-appearing with **fever**, jaundice (if underlying biliary obstruction), **abdominal pain;** tender **hepatomegaly** may be present on examination.

DIFFERENTIAL

Hepatocellular carcinoma, ascending cholangitis.

DIAGNOSIS

- **CT** or RUQ **ultrasound**. CXR may reveal right-sided pleural effusion or elevation of right hemidiaphragm.
- Abscess aspiration and culture definitive. Serology and antigen studies for *E histolytica* are limited by false-positives, but may help exclude amoebic abscess if negative. Stool culture may aid diagnosis.

Treatment

Start empiric therapy **covering both pyogenic** and **amoebic** abscess (metronidazole, and either ceftriaxone or piperacillin-tazobactam). Frequently require percutaneous or surgical drainage; consider early surgical and/or interventional radiology consultation.

Complications

Sepsis, rupture into adjacent structure (lung, pericardium).

HEPATOCELLULAR CARCINOMA

Hepatocellular carcinoma (HCC) is the most common malignant tumor of the liver. It is usually asymptomatic until disease is advanced. The major risk factor for HCC is cirrhosis. Other associated factors include aflatoxin exposure, α_1-antitrypsin deficiency, and hemochromatosis.

Symptoms/Examination

- Deterioration in previously stable cirrhotic.
- Enlarged palpable liver and an occasional palpable mass.
- Bruit over the tumor (6%-25%).

Differential

Other malignancies of the liver (intrahepatic cholangiocarcinoma, hepatoblastoma, hemangiosarcoma, epithelioid hemangioendothelioma), benign liver tumors, metastatic cancer, liver abscess, or cyst.

Diagnosis

- **Ultrasound** is suggestive; **CT** or **MRI** in the appropriate clinical setting (cirrhosis and/or chronic HBV) can establish the diagnosis.
- Tissue biopsy may be required for confirmation or atypical cases.
- Associated with elevation in α-fetoprotein (AFP), but can be nonspecific.

Treatment

- Local regional therapy (radiofrequency ablation, chemoembolization) is not curative but often is performed as a bridge to liver transplantation.
- Liver transplant or surgical resection can be curative for limited stages without extrahepatic metastasis.
- Systemic chemotherapy is used for palliation only.
- Without liver transplantation or surgical resection the prognosis is poor, with 1- and 5-year survival rates of 25% and 5%, respectively.

BENIGN LIVER NEOPLASMS

Hemangioma

- Most common benign neoplasm.
- More common in females.
- Increases in size with use of exogenous hormones.
- Biopsy may be needed to rule out malignancy.

Focal Nodular Hyperplasia

- Hypervascular mass of hepatocytes.
- Typically asymptomatic, may have mild pain if necrosis or bleeding occurs.
- Only symptomatic patients undergo resection.

Q

A 39-year-old woman on oral contraceptive therapy presents with sudden onset of severe abdominal pain. On examination she is tachycardic and has a peritoneal abdomen. Her urine pregnancy test is negative and upright CXR shows no free air under the diaphragm. CT scan of the abdomen reveals copious free fluid and acute hemorrhage from a liver mass. What is the most likely diagnosis?

KEY FACT

80% of hepatocellular carcinoma is associated with cirrhosis.

A

Ruptured hepatocellular adenoma.

Hepatic Adenoma (Hepatocellular Adenoma)

- Common in women in their 30s and 40s, strongly linked to oral contraceptive use.
- Increased size with hormone use.
- May cause pain if necrosis develops; most serious complication is rupture with hemoperitoneum.
- Resection advised to prevent necrosis and rupture.

MNEMONIC

Risk factors for gallstones:

The 4 Fs

Fat
Female
Fertile
Forty years old

Gallbladder and Biliary Tract Diseases

CHOLELITHIASIS

Gallstones are common and often asymptomatic (up to 80% of patients). Biliary colic—a misleading term as patients often present with constant, steady pain—results from transient cystic duct blockage from impacted stones.

Causes

- **Cholesterol stones** (most common) are associated with increased age, female gender, obesity, rapid weight loss, CF, parity, certain drugs, and family history.
- **Pigment stones** contain calcium and are associated with chronic intravascular hemolysis (eg, sickle cell disease, spherocytosis) and biliary infection.

Symptoms/Examination

- Patients most commonly present with postprandial, RUQ, or generalized upper abdominal pain that may radiate to the right subscapular area (biliary colic).
- Pain is abrupt, lasts minutes to hours, and is followed by gradual relief. Symptoms are often associated with nausea, vomiting, fatty-food intolerance, dyspepsia, and flatulence.
- Examination may reveal mild RUQ tenderness.

Diagnosis

RUQ ultrasound is 85%-90% sensitive for stones; **LFTs** are normal in isolated cholelithiasis.

Treatment

Provide **pain relief** and supportive care. Refer for **elective cholecystectomy**. Poor surgical candidates are treated with diet modification, **oral bile acids**, and/or percutaneous **lithotripsy**.

KEY FACT

In children, biliary colic is uncommon and usually associated with hemolytic disorders (eg, sickle cell).

Complications

Recurrent biliary colic, acute cholecystitis, choledocholithiasis, acute cholangitis, gallstone ileus, gallstone pancreatitis.

CHOLEDOCHOLITHIASIS

Gallstones in the common bile duct.

Symptoms/Examination

Often presents with **RUQ abdominal pain, jaundice**, episodic colic, and **pancreatitis**. The presence of fever and jaundice suggests cholangitis (see the following text).

Diagnosis

- Hallmark is increased **alkaline phosphatase** and **total bilirubin**, which may be the only abnormal laboratory values.
- **Ultrasound** may reveal a dilated common bile duct or intrahepatic ducts; **MRCP** can visualize extrahepatic, intrahepatic, and pancreatic ducts.

Treatment

Endoscopic retrograde cholangiopancreatography (ERCP) with **sphincterotomy** for removal of stone, followed by semielective cholecystectomy

> **Q**
>
> A 36-year-old woman presents with sharp abdominal pain. She reports that she ate a fatty meal 2 hours before symptom onset and has had 3 previous episodes of similar pain. She does not drink alcohol. On examination, she has epigastric abdominal tenderness. Laboratory test results show a lipase of 4400. What is the most likely cause of her pancreatitis?

CHOLECYSTITIS

Prolonged blockage of the cystic duct, usually by an impacted stone, causes obstructive distention, inflammation, superinfection, and possible gangrene of the gallbladder (acute gangrenous cholecystitis). **Acalculous cholecystitis** occurs in the absence of cholelithiasis in chronically debilitated patients, classically those on total parenteral nutrition (TPN) and trauma or burn victims.

Symptoms

Presents with **RUQ abdominal pain,** nausea, vomiting, and fever. Symptoms are typically **more severe** and longer lasting than those of biliary colic.

Examination

RUQ tenderness, inspiratory arrest during deep palpation to the RUQ (**Murphy sign**), **fever**, **leukocytosis**, mild icterus, and possibly guarding or rebound tenderness.

Diagnosis

- CBC, amylase, lipase, and LFT panel should be obtained.
- **Ultrasound** may demonstrate stones, biliary sludge, pericholecystic fluid, a thickened gallbladder wall (≥ 3 mm), gas in the gallbladder, and an ultrasonographic Murphy sign (Figure 11.10).

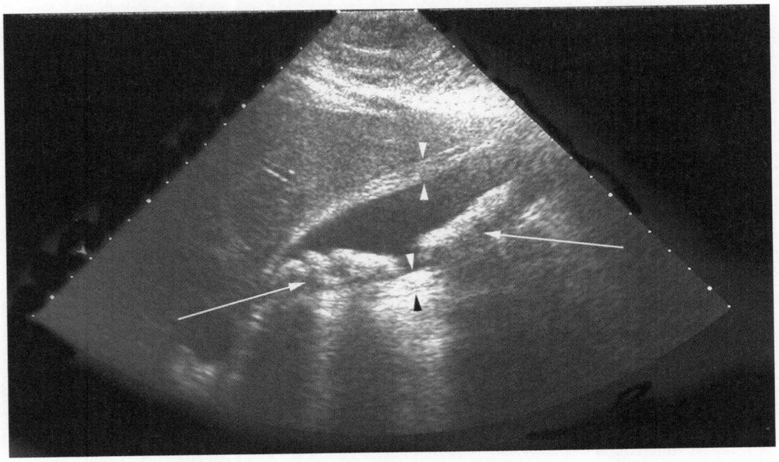

FIGURE 11.10. Acute cholecystitis. The arrowheads indicate the thickened gallbladder wall. There are several stones in the gallbladder (arrows) throwing acoustic shadows. Also seen is pericholecystic fluid. (Reproduced, with permission, from Brunicardi FC, Andersen DK, Billiar TR, Dunn DL, Hunter JG, Matthews JB, Pollock RE, eds. *Schwartz's Principles of Surgery*. 9th ed. New York, NY: McGraw-Hill; 2010.)

A

Gallstones.

- Obtain **HIDA (hepatobiliary iminodiacetic acid) scan** when ultrasound is equivocal (Figure 11.11).
- AXR or CT may demonstrate a fluid-filled gallbladder with gas in the gallbladder wall indicative of **emphysematous cholecystitis**, a rare but life-threatening complication found in older men classically with associated diabetes and caused by gas-producing organisms (eg, *Clostridium perfringens*).

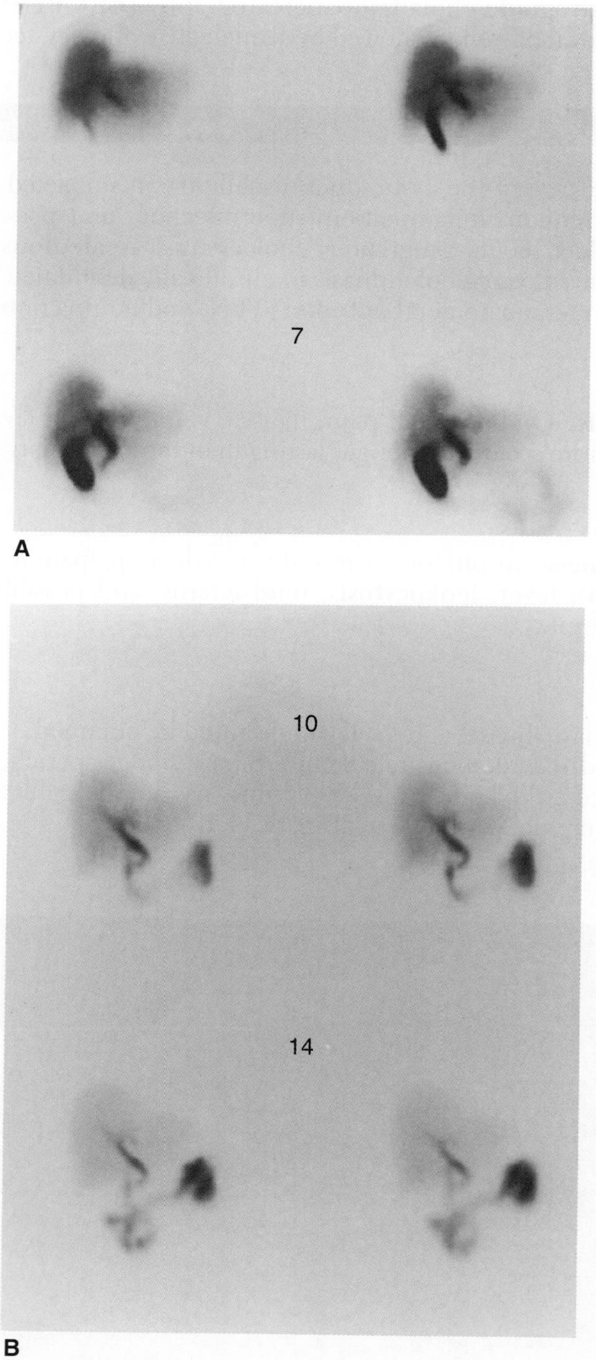

FIGURE 11.11. (A) Normal HIDA scan. IV dye is taken up by hepatocytes, conjugated, and excreted into the common bile duct. **(B) Positive HIDA scan.** Tracer appears in the duodenum, liver, and common duct but not the gallbladder, suggesting cystic duct obstruction due to acute cholecystitis. (Reproduced, with permission, from Hall J, et al. *Principles of Critical Care*. 3rd ed. New York, NY: McGraw-Hill; 2005:1258.)

TREATMENT

- Obtain **surgical consultation** and give **antibiotics** (piperacillin-tazobactam or ertapenem; beware increasing *E coli* resistance to quinolones; broad-spectrum carbapenem for life-threatening infections).
- Definitive therapy is cholecystectomy, typically after period of inpatient antibiotics; percutaneous drain placement is an alternative in the unstable patient.
- Because 50% cases resolve spontaneously, hemodynamically stable patients with significant medical problems can be managed medically with a 4- to 6-week delay in surgical treatment.

COMPLICATIONS

Gangrene, empyema, perforation, gallstone ileus, fistulization, sepsis, abscess formation.

Q

A 62-year-old woman with a history of gallstones presents with fever, hypotension, RUQ abdominal pain, and jaundice. What is the most likely diagnosis?

ACUTE CHOLANGITIS

Acute bacterial cholangitis is an infection of the biliary tree resulting from biliary obstruction and stasis. Gram-negative enterics (eg, *E coli*, *Enterobacter*, *Pseudomonas*) are commonly identified pathogens. Risk factors include gallstones (85% of cases), bile duct stricture, ampullary carcinoma, and pancreatic pseudocyst.

Note that **primary sclerosing cholangitis** (PSC) is a different entity. It is an indolent and most likely autoimmune process characterized by progressive inflammation of the biliary tree, often associated with UC.

SYMPTOMS/EXAMINATION

- **Charcot triad**—RUQ pain, jaundice, and fever—is classic, present in 70% of patients.
- **Reynolds pentad,** Charcot triad plus hypotension and altered mental status, may be present in severe cholangitis (often termed *acute suppurative cholangitis*) and suggests sepsis.

KEY FACT

Charcot triad is fever, jaundice, and RUQ pain. Reynolds pentad also includes decreased mental status and hypotension.

DIAGNOSIS

- Leukocytosis (80% of patients), increased bilirubin (80% of cases), and increased alkaline phosphatase. Obtain blood cultures.
- **Ultrasound** or **CT**; **ERCP** is both diagnostic and therapeutic.

TREATMENT

- Broad-spectrum **antibiotics** as discussed earlier. Patients often require ICU admission for monitoring, hydration, and vasopressors.
- Acute suppurative cholangitis requires **emergent bile duct decompression** via ERCP sphincterotomy, percutaneous transhepatic drainage, or open decompression.

PORCELAIN GALLBLADDER

Porcelain gallbladder is characterized by linear or punctuate calcifications within the gallbladder, often seen on AXR; diagnosis should be confirmed with ultrasound or CT. It is associated with carcinoma (~3%), so referral for cholecystectomy is necessary.

A

Cholangitis.

AIDS CHOLANGIOPATHY

Collectively describes several pathological processes associated with biliary obstruction and resultant inflammation/cholangitis seen in AIDS patients, typically with CD4 counts < 200/mm^3. Presentation is similar to other obstructive processes but varies by location and extent of obstruction. It is thought to be associated with one or more AIDS-associated infections (eg, CMV, mycobacterium avium complex [MAC], *cryptosporidium*).

Pancreas

PANCREATITIS

In the United States, > 80% of acute pancreatitis cases result from alcohol or biliary stones; however, only 5% of heavy drinkers develop pancreatitis. 20% cases are complicated by necrotizing pancreatitis. Pancreatitis can be classified as either acute or chronic (Table 11.15).

ETIOLOGY

- Ethanol (**EtOH**) and **gallstones** and, to a much lesser extent, trauma, account for about 90% cases of adult pancreatitis; in children, trauma is the most common cause.
- **Drugs:** Azathioprine, pentamidine, sulfonamides, thiazide diuretics, 6MP, valproic acid, dideoxyinosine.
- **Metabolic:** Hyperlipidemia or hypercalcemia.
- **Mechanical:** Pancreas divisum, sphincter of Oddi dysfunction, mass.
- **Infectious:** Viruses (eg, mumps, coxsackievirus B) and, to a lesser extent, bacteria and parasites (eg, *Ascaris lumbricoides*).
- **Other:** Scorpion bites, hereditary pancreatitis (an autosomal-dominant mutation of the trypsinogen gene), CF, pregnancy.

MNEMONIC

Etiologies of Pancreatitis:

I GET SMASHED

Idiopathic
Gallstones
Ethanol
Trauma
Steroids
Mumps
Autoimmune
Scorpion/spider bites
Hyperlipidemia (triglycerides)
ERCP
Drugs

SYMPTOMS

Acute: Sudden onset, persistent, **deep epigastric pain**, often radiating to the back that classically **worsens when supine** and **improves when leaning forward.** Severe nausea and vomiting are the norm; fever and leukocytosis may be seen if complications occur.

EXAMINATION

Upper **abdominal tenderness** with guarding, ± rebound. **Mild fever** is present in 50% cases with or without infection. In **severe cases,** distention, ileus, and/or hypotension may be present. **Rarely,** retroperitoneal hemorrhage manifests as umbilical (**Cullen sign**) or flank (**Grey Turner sign**) ecchymosis.

DIFFERENTIAL

Biliary colic, cholecystitis, mesenteric ischemia, intestinal obstruction/ileus, perforated hollow viscus, inferior MI, dissecting aortic aneurysm, ectopic pregnancy.

DIAGNOSIS

- **Labs:** Serum **lipase** has supplanted pancreatic amylase as the test of choice; a lipase level > 3 times normal is diagnostic. Degree of lipase/amylase elevation does NOT correlate with severity of disease. AST/ALT ratio > 2 suggests alcohol abuse. **Hyperglycemia** and **hypocalcemia** may be present; check **lactate dehydrogenase** (**LDH**) to calculate **Ranson score** (Table 11.16).

TABLE 11.15. Acute Versus Chronic Pancreatitis

	Acute Pancreatitis	Chronic Pancreatitis
Pathophysiology	Leakage of pancreatic enzymes into pancreatic and peripancreatic tissue, often secondary to gallstone disease or alcoholism	Irreversible parenchymal destruction → pancreatic dysfunction
Time course	Abrupt onset of severe pain	Persistent, recurrent episodes of severe pain
Risk factors	**Gallstones, alcoholism,** hypercalcemia, hypertriglyceridemia, trauma, drug side effects (thiazide diuretics, steroids), viral infections, post-ERCP, scorpion bites	**Alcoholism** (90%), gallstones, hyperparathyroidism, congenital malformation (pancreas divisum); may also be idiopathic
History/PE	**Severe epigastric pain (radiating to the back),** nausea, vomiting, weakness, fever, shock; flank discoloration (Grey Turner sign) and periumbilical discoloration (Cullen sign)	Recurrent episodes of **persistent epigastric pain,** anorexia, nausea, constipation, flatulence, **steatorrhea,** DM
Diagnosis	**Increased amylase and lipase, decreased calcium** if severe; **"sentinel loop" or "colon cutoff"** sign on AXR; ultrasound or CT may show enlarged pancreas with stranding, abscess, hemorrhage, necrosis, or pseudocyst	Increased or normal amylase and lipase; stool studies for pancreatic insufficiency; CT scan showing **pancreatic calcifications** and sequelae of prior episodes of pancreatitis
Treatment	Removal of offending agent if possible; standard supportive measures: IV fluids/electrolyte replacement, analgesia, bowel rest, nutritional support, O_2. IV antibiotics, respiratory support and surgical debridement if necrotizing pancreatitis is present	Analgesia, exogenous lipase/trypsin, and medium chain fatty acid diet, avoidance of causative agents (EtOH), celiac nerve block, surgery for intractable pain or structural causes
Prognosis	85%-90% mild, self-limited; 10%-15% severe, requiring ICU admission; mortality may approach 50% in severe cases	Can have chronic pain and pancreatic exocrine and endocrine dysfunction
Complications	**Pancreatic pseudocyst, fistula formation,** hypocalcemia, renal failure, ARDS, pleural effusion, chronic pancreatitis, sepsis; mortality secondary to acute pancreatitis predicted with Ranson criteria	**Chronic pain,** malnutrition/weight loss, pancreatic cancer

ARDS, acute respiratory distress syndrome; AXR, abdominal x-ray; CT, computed tomography; DM, diabetes mellitus; ERCP, Endoscopic retrograde cholangiopancreatography; EtOH, ethanol; IV, intravenous; NG, nasogastric; PE, physical exam.

- Consider **ultrasound** to evaluate for gallstones. **Routine CT is not required,** but consider for uncertain diagnosis or severe/toxic clinical presentations.

Treatment

- Anticipate **NPO** status for > 3-5 days (severe disease may require nasojejunal tube feeds or TPN). Aggressive **IV hydration**, pain, and nausea control. **NG tube** may be placed for intractable vomiting, but is no longer considered a therapeutic intervention.
- The role of **antibiotics** remains controversial; generally, prophylactic antibiotics are NOT indicated, but give severe necrotizing-pancreatitis or septic/unstable patients broad-spectrum coverage (eg, carbapenems).
- For **gallstone pancreatitis** (elevated serum bilirubin, signs of biliary sepsis), perform **ERCP** for stone removal and cholecystectomy following recovery but prior to discharge.

KEY FACT

CT is prognostic in severe pancreatitis and is used to evaluate for necrotizing pancreatitis. Necrotizing pancreatitis warrants empiric antibiotics (eg, imipenem).

Q

A 60-year-old man presents with several weeks of very mild, dull aching abdominal pain, decreased appetite, and fatigue. Today, family noticed a yellow discoloration to his eyes. What is the likely diagnosis?

TABLE 11.16. Ranson Criteria for Acute Pancreatitis[a]

On Admission	After 48 Hours
GA LAW:	**C HOBBS:**
Glucose > 200 mg/dL (> 220 mg/dL)	**C**a^{2+} < 8.0 mg/dL
Age > 55 (> 70)	**H**ematocrit decrease by > 10%
LDH > 350 IU/L (> 400 IU/L)	**O**$_2$ Pao_2 < 60 mm Hg (omitted)
AST > 250 IU/L	**B**ase deficit > 4 mEq/L (> 6 mEq/L)
WBC > 16,000/mm^3 (> 18,000/mm^3)	**B**UN increase > 5 mmol/L (> 2 mmol/L)
	Sequestered fluid > 6 L (> 4 L)

AST, aspartate aminotransferase; BUN, blood urea nitrogen; LDH, lactate dehydrogenase; WBC, white blood cell.

[a]The changes in criteria for gallstone pancreatitis are in parenthesis.

KEY FACT

The risk of mortality in pancreatitis is < 1% if 1-2 of Ranson criteria; 20% with 3-4; 40% with 4-5; near 100% with 6.

KEY FACT

The classic presentation of pancreatic cancer is painless, progressive jaundice.

COMPLICATIONS

- **Necrotizing pancreatitis:** Suspect in setting of a persistently elevated WBC count (7-10 days), high fever, and shock (organ failure); has a poor prognosis (up to 30% mortality and 70% risk of complications). If infected necrosis is suspected, perform percutaneous aspiration. If organisms are present on smear, surgical debridement is indicated.
- **Pancreatic pseudocyst:** A collection of pancreatic fluid walled off by granulation tissue; occurs in approximately 30% of cases but resolves spontaneously in about 50%. Drainage not required unless the pseudocyst is present for > 6-8 weeks and is enlarging and symptomatic.
- **Other:** Pseudoaneurysm, renal failure, **acute respiratory distress syndrome (ARDS)**, splenic vein thrombosis (which can lead to isolated gastric varices), hypocalcemia.

PANCREATIC CANCER

Roughly 90% are pancreatic ductal adenocarcinomas, mostly in the pancreatic head. Risk factors include smoking, chronic pancreatitis, a first-degree relative with pancreatic cancer, obesity, and DM. Pancreatic cancer is most commonly seen in men in their 60s. The remaining cases are neuroendocrine tumors, which carry a better prognosis.

SYMPTOMS

Presentation is variable. Most common complaint is **weight loss** due to anorexia. May present with dull, constant abdominal pain radiating toward the back as well as jaundice, anorexia, nausea, vomiting, weight loss, weakness, fatigue, and indigestion. The classic presentation is ***painless, progressive*** **jaundice**.

EXAMINATION

Examination may reveal a palpable, nontender gallbladder (**Courvoisier sign**) or migratory thrombophlebitis (**Trousseau sign**).

A

Pancreatic cancer.

DIAGNOSIS

- Use CT to detect a pancreatic mass, dilated pancreatic and bile ducts, the extent of vascular involvement, and metastases.

- If a mass is not visualized, use ERCP or endoscopic ultrasound for better visualization and consider fine-needle aspiration.

TREATMENT

- Most patients present with advanced disease, and treatment is palliative.
- 10%-20% of pancreatic head tumors have no evidence of metastasis and may be resected using the Whipple procedure (pancreaticoduodenectomy). 5-year survival varies greatly but is generally still poor after resection.
- Biliary stenting may improve jaundice and associated pruritus.

Q

A 70-year-old woman with a history of atrial fibrillation presents with severe diffuse abdominal pain but a benign examination. Serum lactate is markedly elevated. What is the likely diagnosis?

Mesenteric Ischemia

Mesenteric ischemia can be divided into arterial and venous disease as well as occlusive versus nonocclusive disease (Table 11.17). Full-thickness gut necrosis can occur in as little as 6 hours. Morbidity and mortality are high (30%-100%), so early identification and treatment are important. **Acute mesenteric ischemia** (AMI) is most commonly (> 50%) due to occlusive embolism involving the SMA. AMI is distinct from **chronic mesenteric ischemia** ("intestinal angina"), which is characterized as recurrent bouts of abdominal pain during periods of increased metabolic demand (eg, after eating). **Ischemic colitis** is a nonocclusive process involving the inferior mesenteric artery (IMA) secondary to low-flow states.

KEY FACT

Consider acute mesenteric ischemia in patients with abdominal pain out of proportion to examination or with a persistently elevated lactate without other underlying causes.

SYMPTOMS

- **Acute** disease presents with abdominal pain **out of proportion** to clinical examination. Pain is severe, colicky, and poorly localized. May be associated with vomiting and/or diarrhea.

TABLE 11.17. Causes of Mesenteric Ischemia

OCCLUSIVE DISEASE	
Embolism	**Atrial fibrillation**, myxoma, valvular disease
Arterial thrombosis	Atherosclerosis, low-flow state
Venous thrombosis	Hypercoagulable state
Arterial disease	AAA, aortic dissection, fibromuscular dysplasia, atherosclerosis
Iatrogenic	Drug-induced (pressors), postprocedure (dissection or embolism)
Trauma	Penetrating or blunt
NONOCCLUSIVE DISEASE	
Shock	Sepsis, cardiogenic, hypovolemic
Low-flow	Myocardial infarction, arrhythmia, CHF
Drug-induced	Vasoactive drugs, cocaine, digitalis

AAA; abdominal aortic aneurysm; CHF, congestive heart failure.

A

Mesenteric ischemia.

- **Chronic** disease can present as pain after eating ("intestinal angina"), weight loss, or change in bowel pattern.

Examination

Initially **soft abdomen** progresses with development of peritoneal signs once complete transmural infarct develops. Fecal **occult blood** develops in only 25% of patients and is often a late finding. Chronic mesenteric ischemia may present with an abdominal bruit.

KEY FACT

Elderly patients often present atypically with presentations that mimic other diseases.

Diagnosis

- **CT angiography** or conventional angiography remains the diagnostic test of choice for acute occlusive disease.
- **AXR** may show **"thumb-printing"** or **pneumatosis intestinalis,** which are late, rare, poorly sensitive findings. Early findings include ileus and bowel wall thickening.
- **CT** may reveal indirect signs such as **bowel wall edema**, ascites, and **intramural gas** in an arterial distribution. In rare cases an actual arterial or venous occlusion may be seen.
- Colonoscopy with biopsy is preferred method for diagnosing colonic ischemia.
- Serum lactate is sensitive for bowel infarction but is nonspecific.
- Diagnostic laparotomy if the patient is unstable.

Treatment

- Resuscitation with **IV fluids** and treat any precipitating cause. Start broad-spectrum **antibiotics**, **anticoagulation** with heparin, and obtain general or vascular **surgery consult**; immediate surgery is indicated for evidence of necrotic bowel.
- Nonocclusive ischemia may be treated with catheter-direct intra-arterial **papaverine**; angiography with stenting can also be therapeutic.

Complications

Bowel necrosis, perforation, shock, sepsis.

Abdominal Hernias (Excluding Inguinal)

Hernias are abnormal protrusions of tissue or organs through a defect in the surrounding structures that contain them. External hernias protrude through the abdominal wall. Internal hernias protrude through defects within the peritoneal cavity; they are rare in the general population but associated with bariatric surgery.

A hernia is **reducible** if it can be pushed back into the peritoneal cavity and **incarcerated** if it cannot. Incarcerated hernias may become **strangulated** if their blood supply is compromised, resulting in ischemia. See Table 11.18 for a discussion of different types of hernias.

Symptoms/Examination

- External hernias present as abdominal wall masses while internal hernias may have no obvious outward signs.
- Reducible hernias commonly cause mild or no discomfort. Worsening pain may indicate incarceration and even strangulation.
- If the hernia contains bowel, incarceration may be accompanied by obstructive symptoms such as vomiting and inability to pass stool or flatus.
- Strangulation may progress to lactic acidosis, sepsis, death.

TABLE 11.18. Classification and Management of Abdominal Wall Hernias

Type	Location	Risk Factors	Treatment/Complications
Femoral	Femoral canal	Women > men	High incarceration rate; usually repaired
Umbilical	Umbilical ring	Congenital: 8 times more common in African Americans Acquired: Due to increased intra-abdominal pressure (pregnancy, obesity, ascites, etc)	Incarceration rare **Infants:** Surgery if persist beyond 5 y old **Adults:** Surgery for symptoms only
Epigastric	Between xiphoid and umbilicus	2-3 times more common in men	Usually contain fat only, commonly strangulated; usually repaired
Incisional	Prior abdominal incision sites	Age, malnutrition, diabetes, immunosuppressive agents, conditions that increase intra-abdominal pressure	Enlarge over time, sometimes incarcerate; usually repaired although recurrence is common
Spigelian	Between rectus muscle and semilunar line; often not palpable	Middle to advanced age	High incarceration rate; usually repaired
Obturator	Obturator canal; not palpable		Obturator nerve compression (medial thigh pain) Almost half present with bowel obstruction; usually repaired
Sciatic	Greater sciatic foramen	Extremely rare	Occasional sciatica, often presents with obstruction

TREATMENT

- **Attempt reduction** in the ED; discharge with surgical follow-up for elective repair if successful. Ice packs, adequate pain medications, Trendelenburg positioning, and firms, steady pressure assist in reduction.
- Indications of strangulation, bowel obstruction, or systemic illness warrant aggressive resuscitation, **antibiotic** coverage, and immediate **surgical consult**.

Splenic Disorders

Although located in the abdominal cavity, the spleen is an organ of the reticuloendothelial system. Disorders of the spleen generally relate to its role in immune surveillance, destruction of erythrocytes, and recycling of iron.

ASPLENIA AND HYPOSPLENIA

Asplenia may be congenital (often associated with cyanotic heart disease) or acquired due to splenectomy or splenic infarction. Splenic infarction is most commonly due to sickle cell disease.

SYMPTOMS

Patients are generally asymptomatic although they are at risk of infection due to **encapsulated organisms** (eg, *Neisseria meningitidis*, *Haemophilus influenzae*, and *Streptococcus pneumoniae*), and gram-negatives (eg, *E coli*, *Pseudomonas aeruginosa*). Pneumococcal sepsis is more common and more severe in this population.

Q

A 17-year-old boy presents with over 1 week of severe sore throat, fever, and fatigue. A rapid strep test is negative. Examination reveals posterior cervical lymphadenopathy and marked splenomegaly. What is the likely diagnosis?

EXAMINATION

There may be no findings on examination because most healthy patients do not have a palpable spleen.

DIAGNOSIS

- CT may reveal infarction; CT or ultrasound may show asplenia or atrophy.
- Peripheral blood smear may show **Howell-Jolly bodies** or **pocked erythrocytes**, both normally removed by the spleen.

TREATMENT

All asplenic or hyposplenic patients should be vaccinated against encapsulated organisms. Asplenic patients presenting with fever are at increased risk for developing sepsis; collect **blood cultures** and give **antibiotics** targeting *S pneumoniae* (eg, ceftriaxone ± vancomycin).

SPLENOMEGALY AND HYPERSPLENIA

Splenomegaly refers to enlargement of the spleen while hypersplenism refers to increased destruction of blood cells by the enlarged spleen. Both are sequelae of various diseases rather than primary disorders.

SYMPTOMS

Patients may have symptoms related to the underlying cause of their splenomegaly, and occasionally may have a sense of fullness in the LUQ or early satiety.

EXAMINATION

Splenomegaly may be detected by percussion or bimanual palpation of the LUQ during inspiration, although physical examination is not very sensitive.

DIFFERENTIAL

See Table 11.19. Massive splenomegaly (spleen weighs >1000 g and/or extends > 8 cm below the costal margin) has a more limited differential, outlined in Table 11.20.

DIAGNOSIS

Ultrasound is the imaging modality of choice. Length > 13 cm constitutes splenomegaly.

TREATMENT

Indications for splenectomy depend on the underlying pathologic process. Splenectomy may be employed for symptom relief in patients with massive splenomegaly and for correction of certain hemolytic anemias.

COMPLICATIONS

- Thrombocytopenia due to splenic sequestration is often seen in hypersplenism due to portal hypertension, hematologic malignancies, and hemolytic anemias.
- Splenic rupture is a rare but potentially life-threatening complication of massive splenomegaly, and can occur with even minor trauma. Patients should avoid contact sports.

A

Infectious mononucleosis.

TABLE 11.19. Diseases Associated with Splenomegaly Grouped by Pathogenic Mechanism

Enlargement Due to Increased Demand for Splenic Function	Enlargement Due to Abnormal Splenic or Portal Blood Flow
Reticuloendothelial system hyperplasia (for removal of defective erythrocytes)	Cirrhosis
Spherocytosis	Hepatic vein obstruction
Early sickle cell anemia	Portal vein obstruction, intrahepatic or extrahepatic
Ovalocytosis	Cavernous transformation of the portal vein
Thalassemia major	Splenic vein obstruction
Hemoglobinopathies	Splenic artery aneurysm
Paroxysmal nocturnal hemoglobinuria	Hepatic schistosomiasis
Pernicious anemia	Congestive heart failure
Immune hyperplasia	Hepatic echinococcosis
Response to infection (viral, bacterial, fungal, parasitic)	Portal hypertension
Infectious mononucleosis	**Infiltration of the Spleen**
AIDS	Intracellular or extracellular depositions
Viral hepatitis	Amyloidosis
Cytomegalovirus	Gaucher disease
Subacute bacterial endocarditis	Niemann-Pick disease
Bacterial septicemia	Tangier disease
Congenital syphilis	Hurler syndrome and other mucopolysaccharidoses
Splenic abscess	Hyperlipidemias
Tuberculosis	Benign and malignant cellular infiltrations
Histoplasmosis	Leukemias (acute, chronic, lymphoid, myeloid, monocytic)
Malaria	Lymphomas
Leishmaniasis	Hodgkin disease
Trypanosomiasis	Myeloproliferative syndromes (eg, polycythemia vera, essential thrombocytosis)
Ehrlichiosis	Angiosarcomas
Disordered immunoregulation	Metastatic tumors (melanoma is most common)
Rheumatoid arthritis (Felty syndrome)	Eosinophilic granuloma
Systemic lupus erythematosus	Histiocytosis X
Collagen vascular diseases	Hamartomas
Serum sickness	Hemangiomas, fibromas, lymphangiomas
Immune hemolytic anemias	Splenic cysts
Immune thrombocytopenias	**Unknown Etiology**
Immune neutropenias	Idiopathic splenomegaly
Drug reactions	Berylliosis
Angioimmunoblastic lymphadenopathy	Iron-deficiency anemia
Sarcoidosis	
Thyrotoxicosis (benign lymphoid hypertrophy)	
Interleukin-2 therapy	
Extramedullary hematopoiesis	
Myelofibrosis	
Marrow damage by toxins, radiation, strontium	
Marrow infiltration by tumors, leukemias, Gaucher disease	

AIDS, acquired immunodeficiency syndrome.

(Adapted with permission from Longo DL, Fauci AS, Kasper DL, Hauser SL,, Jameson JL, Loscalzo J. *Harrison's Principles of Internal Medicine*. 18th ed. New York, NY: McGraw-Hill; 2011.)

TABLE 11.20. Diseases Associated with Massive Splenomegaly[a]

Chronic myeloid leukemia
Lymphomas
Hairy cell leukemia
Myelofibrosis with myeloid metaplasia
Polycythemia vera
Gaucher disease
Chronic lymphocytic leukemia
Sarcoidosis
Autoimmune hemolytic anemia
Diffuse splenic hemangiomatosis

[a]The spleen extends > 8 cm below left costal margin and/or weighs > 1000 g.

(Adapted with permission from Longo DL, Fauci AS, Kasper DL, Hauser SL,, Jameson JL, Loscalzo J. *Harrison's Principles of Internal Medicine*. 18th ed. New York, NY: McGraw-Hill; 2011.)

REVIEW QUESTIONS

QUESTION

1. A 3-year-old child is brought to the ED after being found playing with his grandfather's hearing aids. Mom reports pulling 1 small battery out of his mouth, but does not know if more were present. He is asymptomatic with a benign examination. What is the best next step?
   A Discharge home with instructions to monitor his stool for foreign bodies and return for any abdominal pain or gastrointestinal (GI) symptoms
   B. Plain films of the chest and abdomen
   C. Emergent endoscopy to rule out battery ingestion or remove battery if present
   D. Administer glucagon to aid propulsion of any foreign body into the stomach

2. A 65-year-old man with a history of hypertension, coronary artery disease, and distant abdominal aortic aneurysm (AAA) repair presents complaining of "hemorrhoids." He reports 2 days of painless, maroon-colored stools, and 24 hours of vague, dull abdominal pain. Examination reveals normal vital signs, a soft abdomen, and a small, nonbleeding external hemorrhoid. What is the best next step?
   A. Start a bowel regimen, increased fiber diet, and daily sitz baths
   B. Place a nasogastric (NG) tube to rule out brisk upper GI bleed and consult general surgery
   C. Check complete blood count (CBC) and coagulation studies, and refer for prompt colonoscopy if reassuring
   D. Obtain contrasted computed tomography (CT) of the abdomen

3. A 40-year-old woman presents with 3 days of nausea, vomiting, and nonbloody diarrhea. Her vomiting has improved, but the diarrhea persists. Her examination reveals normal vital signs, minimal diffuse abdominal tenderness, mild dehydration, and guaiac negative stools. She is otherwise healthy. Her husband recovered from a similar illness several days ago. What is the best next step in management?
   A. Check CBC, chemistries, send stool culture, and give intravenous (IV) fluids.
   B. Offer reassurance and oral rehydration therapy; if tolerated, discharge with strict return precautions.
   C. Keep NPO, give IV fluids, and admit for colonoscopy with biopsy.
   D. Offer supportive care and send stool for ova and parasite analysis.

4. Which of the following descriptions is most consistent with irritable bowel syndrome (IBS)?
   A. Chronic, intermittent abdominal pain with bloody diarrhea and mucinous discharge
   B. Episodic abdominal pain associated with both nonbloody diarrhea and constipation
   C. Sharp pain during defecation with scant bright red bleeding that resolves between bowel movements
   D. Nausea, vomiting, abdominal pain and distension, and decreased bowel movements

5. Which of the following findings is most specific for acute appendicitis?
   A. Fever and leukocytosis
   B. Migratory pain and right lower quadrant (RLQ) tenderness
   C. Pain with passive flexion and internal rotation of the right hip
   D. Elevated C-reactive protein (CRP)

6. A 40-year-old man with recent travel to Mexico presents with progressive right upper quadrant (RUQ) abdominal pain, fever, and jaundice. CT shows a poorly defined, fluid-filled hepatic mass. Which of the following therapies is the most appropriate?
   A. Supportive care now; initiate antibiotics after percutaneous aspiration and culture
   B. Metronidazole
   C. Ertapenem and metronidazole
   D. Piperacillin-tazobactam

7. A well-appearing woman is incidentally found to have small calcifications about the gallbladder on an abdominal plain film; a diagnosis of "porcelain gallbladder" is subsequently confirmed on abdominal CT. Which is the best next step in management?
   A. Obtain emergent surgical consultation for cholecystectomy due to risk of perforation
   B. Admit for Endoscopic retrograde cholangiopancreatography (ERCP) to remove suspected calcified stones
   C. Refer for palliative treatment of advance cholangiocarcinoma
   D. Advise her of the increased risk of gallbladder cancer and refer for elective cholecystectomy

ANSWERS

1. **B.** Evaluation of foreign body ingestion without evidence of airway compromise should begin with plain films. Disc batteries can cause irreversible damage quickly if left in the esophagus and require prompt endoscopic removal but are easily seen on plain films.

2. **D.** Even minor GI bleeding in a patient with a known or repaired AAA should be considered aortoenteric fistula until proven otherwise. Fistula can progress quickly from minor GI bleeding on presentation to massive, life-threatening hemorrhage. External hemorrhoids should not cause maroon bleeding.
3. **B.** The vast majority of noninvasive gastroenteritis is caused by viruses (most common: Norovirus). Nontoxic patients with benign examinations, symptoms < 7-14 days, and no particular risk factors do not routinely require specific testing. Oral rehydration is the treatment of choice.
4. **B.** IBS causes recurrent abdominal pain, classically improves with defecation, and can be associated with diarrhea, constipation, or both in the same patient. Bloody diarrhea and discharge are concerning for inflammatory bowel disease. Sharp pain with defecation is associated with anal fissures. Vomiting, distension, and decreased bowel movements suggest small bowel obstruction.
5. **B.** Leukocytosis, elevated CRP, and fever are commonly found with appendicitis, but are nonspecific. The obturator sign is associated with an inflamed appendiceal tip in the pelvis, but is also nonspecific.
6. **C.** Liver abscess in patients from/with travel to endemic areas is concerning for *Entamoeba histolytica*, which is treated with metronidazole. Most pyogenic abscesses are caused by gram-negative and anaerobic infections. Initial therapy should begin immediately and cover both until the diagnosis is confirmed.
7. **D.** Though there is little risk of acute obstruction or perforation, about 3% of patients with porcelain gallbladder will develop cancer of the gallbladder. Patients should nonemergently consult a general surgeon for elective removal.

CHAPTER 12

Obstetrics and Gynecology

Sabrina A. Adams, MD

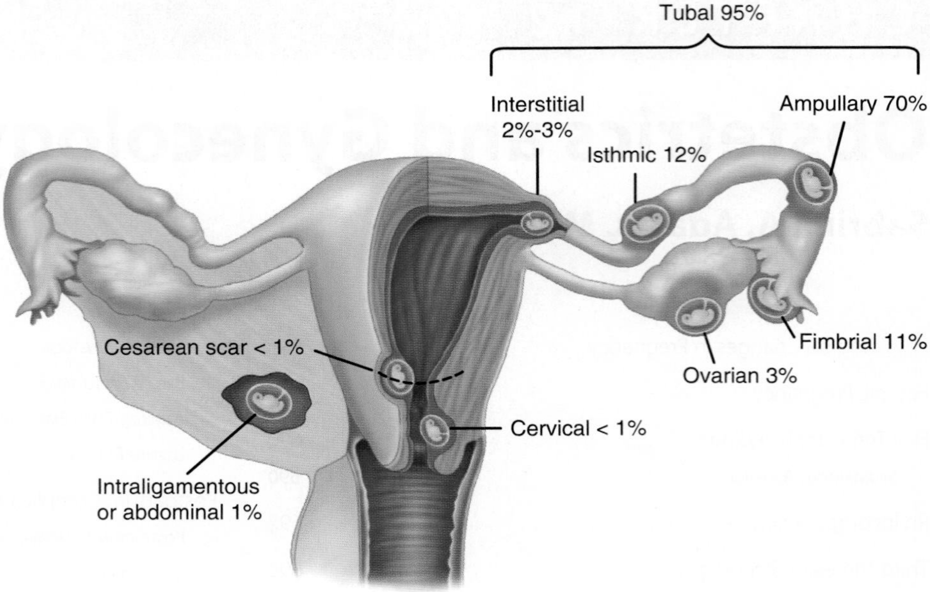

FIGURE 12.1. Various sites and frequency of ectopic pregnancies. (Reproduced, with permission, from Cunningham FG, Leveno KJ, Bloom SL, et al. *Williams Obstetrics*. 24th ed. New York, NY: McGraw-Hill Education; 2010. Figure 19.1.)

Physiological Changes in Pregnancy

Physiologic changes begin in early pregnancy and continue throughout. Major changes are listed in Table 12.1.

TABLE 12.1. Maternal Physiological Changes in Pregnancy

Cardiovascular	↑ Cardiac output ↓ Systemic vascular resistance ↑ HR 10-15 bpm
Respiratory	↓ Functional residual capacity ↑ Tidal volume and RR ↑ Minute ventilation Respiratory alkalosis
Hematology	↑ Blood volume > ↑ RBC volume Physiologic anemia Hypercoagulable state
Musculoskeletal	↑ Ligament laxity
Gastrointestinal	↓ Esophageal sphincter tone

HR, heart rate; RBC, red blood cell; RR, respiratory rate.

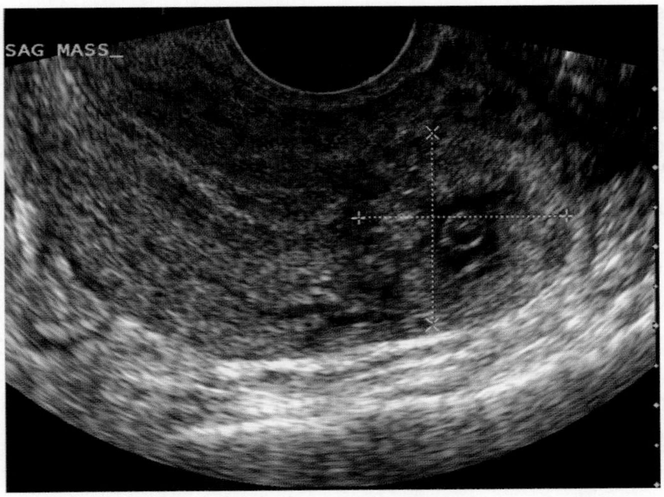

FIGURE 12.2. Interstitial ectopic pregnancy. Parasagittal long-axis ultrasound imaging showing empty uterus with ectopic mass that is located cephalad and lateral to the uterine fundus in the region of the interstitium of the fallopian tube. (Reproduced with permission from Cunningham FG, Leveno KJ, Bloom SL, et al. *Williams Obstetrics*. 24th ed. New York, NY: McGraw-Hill Education, 2010. Figure 19.9A.)

Ectopic Pregnancy

Extrauterine pregnancy is common in the emergency department, occurring in up to 10% of patients with first trimester bleeding. The vast majority are located in the **fallopian tube**; other sites include the ovary, abdominal cavity, and cervix (Figures 12.1 and 12.2). A simultaneous intrauterine pregnancy (IUP) and ectopic pregnancy, or *heterotopic pregnancy*, is rare, occurring in only 1 in 30,000 naturally-conceived pregnancies. The incidence is much higher with assisted reproduction.

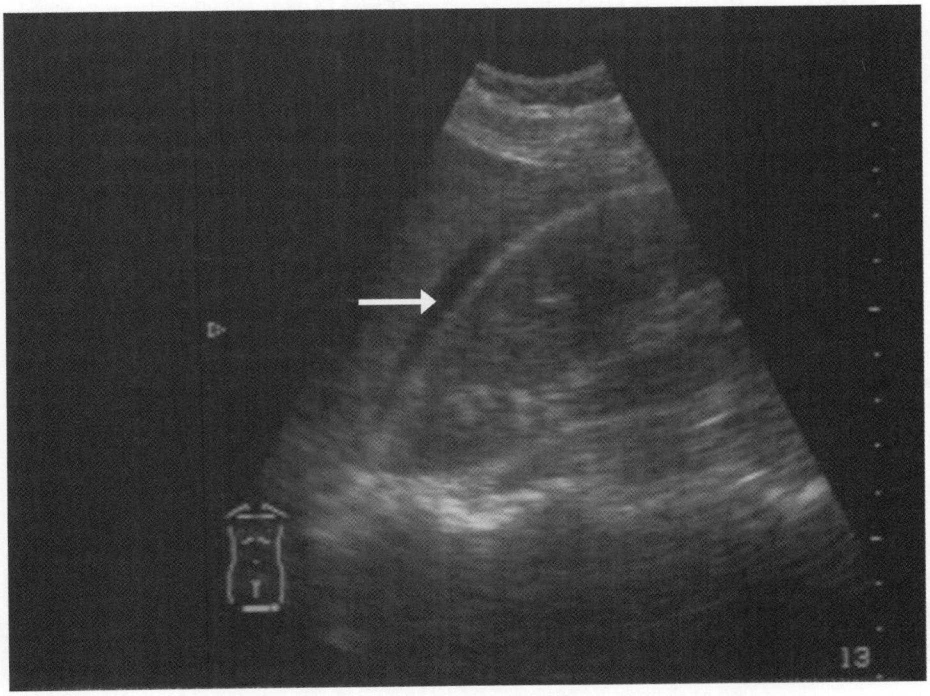

FIGURE 12.3. Ultrasound showing free fluid in Morison's pouch (arrow).

Q

A 33-year-old woman presents to the emergency department with abdominal pain. Her last menstrual period was 2 months ago. Vital signs are BP 90/60 mm Hg, HR 130 bpm, and RR 18 breaths/min. Urine pregnancy test is positive. An ultrasound is done (Figure 12.3). What is the next appropriate step?

KEY FACT

Heterotopic pregnancy occurs in 1-3% of patients with assisted reproduction.

A

Emergent consultation of OB/GYN for surgical treatment of ectopic pregnancy.

KEY FACT

All other forms of contraception besides IUD decrease the incidence of ectopic.

KEY FACT

Classic triad for ectopic pregnancy:
Abdominal pain
Vaginal bleeding
Positive pregnancy test

KEY FACT

The first definitive sign of an IUP is the presence of a yolk sac within the gestational sac.

Risk Factors

History of previous ectopic pregnancy (most common), prior tubal infection, abnormal fallopian tubes, previous tubal surgery, intrauterine device (IUD) use, smoking, advanced age, elective abortion, and fertility treatments. Over half of patients have no identifiable risk factors at time of diagnosis.

Symptoms/Examination

- Most patients present with vaginal bleeding and/or abdominal pain, although symptoms range from isolated amenorrhea to dizziness and syncope.
- Vital signs may be normal or hypotension/tachycardia may be present due to hemorrhagic shock.
- The abdominal and pelvic examinations may be normal, show localized tenderness or diffuse peritonitis. An adnexal mass is felt in less than half of patients.

Diagnosis

- Ectopic pregnancy should be considered in all women of childbearing age who present with vaginal bleeding or abdominal/pelvic pain, especially those with unexplained signs or symptoms of hypovolemia.
- Positive pregnancy test is an almost universal finding in the diagnosis of ectopic. Very dilute urine or switched urine samples may lead to a false negative!
- Ultrasound (US) is the test of choice (Table 12.2). Correlation with the β-hCG level is often required. The **discriminatory zone** is the β-hCG level above which a **normal** IUP should be visualized by US. This is institution (machine and ultrasonographer) dependent. For transvaginal ultrasound, it is between 1000-1500 mIU/mL and for transabdominal ultrasound between 4000-6500 mIU/mL.
  - **Diagnostic for IUP**: The presence of an intrauterine gestational sac with yolk sac or embryo. An isolated gestational sac or double decidual sac is not diagnostic for IUP because it may be confused with a pseudosac, which is often present in patients with ectopic pregnancy.
  - **Diagnostic for ectopic pregnancy**: The presence of an extrauterine gestational sac with yolk sac or embryo.
  - **Strongly suspicious for ectopic**: Extrauterine mass, echogenic intraperitoneal fluid, or a lack of definitive IUP with β-hCG level above the discriminatory zone.
  - **Nondiagnostic**: A β-hCG level below the discriminatory zone with ultrasound that fails to show an IUP or extrauterine pathology.
- Always check Rh factor to determine need for Rh(D) immunoglobulin (RhoGAM).

TABLE 12.2. Ultrasound Findings in Suspected Ectopic Pregnancy

IUP	Ectopic	Suggest Ectopic	Nondiagnostic
Intrauterine gestational sac with yolk sac (Figure 12.4)	Ectopic gestational sac with yolk sac	Extrauterine mass	β-hCG < discriminatory zone with no IUP or ectopic pathology
Intrauterine gestational sac with fetal pole	Ectopic gestational sac with fetal pole (Figure 12.5)	Echogenic intraperitoneal fluid	Gestational sac without yolk sac or fetal pole (Figure 12.6)
Intrauterine fetal heart tones	Ectopic fetal heart tones	β-hCG above discriminatory zone with no IUP	

IUP, intrauterine pregnancy.

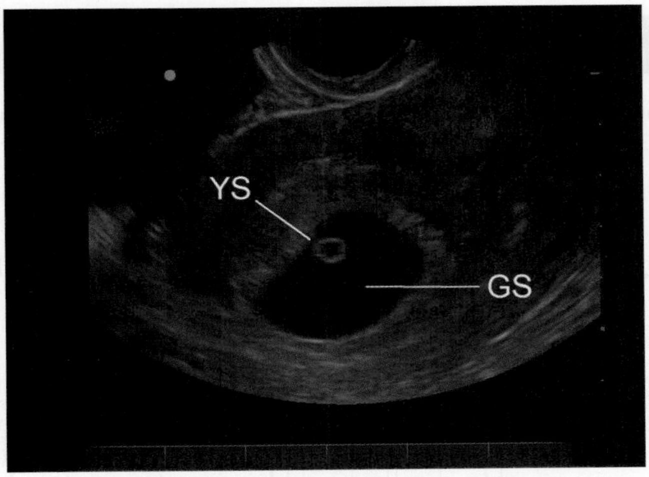

FIGURE 12.4. Intrauterine gestational sac with yolk sac indicating an intrauterine pregnancy. (Reproduced, with permission, from Stone CK, Humphries RL. *Current Diagnosis & Treatment: Emergency Medicine*. 7th ed. New York, NY: McGraw-Hill Education; 2011. Figure 6.36.)

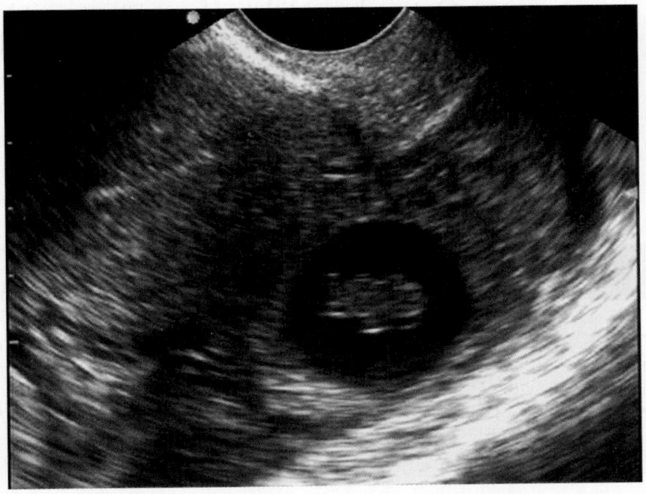

FIGURE 12.5. Ectopic gestational sac with fetal pole indicating an ectopic pregnancy. Note presence of thin bright endometrial stripe along with embryo in adnexa. (Reproduced with permission from Ma OJ, Mateer JR, Reardon RF, et al: Ma & Mateer's *Emergency Ultrasound*, 3rd ed. New York, NY: McGraw-Hill Education, 2014. Figure 14.30.)

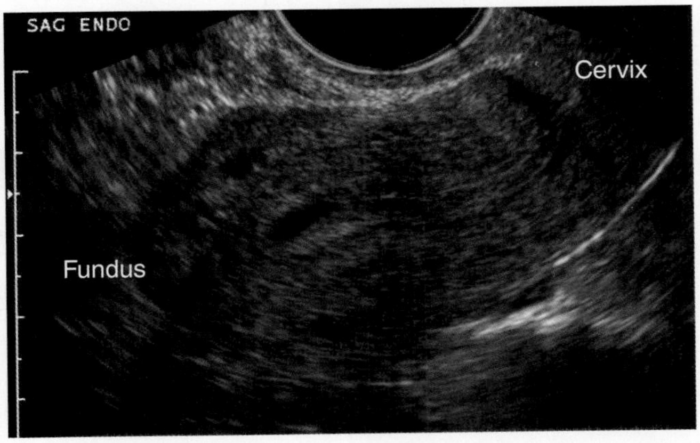

FIGURE 12.6. Single gestational sac or "pseudosac" within the endometrial cavity in a patient with ectopic pregnancy. (Used with permission from Dr. Elysia Moschos.)

KEY FACT

Expect to visualize a normal IUP using:

1. Transvaginal ultrasound if β-hCG > 1500 mIU/mL
2. Abdominal ultrasound if β-hCG > 4000 mIU/mL

- Heterotopic pregnancy must be considered in unstable patients with findings diagnostic for IUP. Look at the adnexa and for signs of simultaneous ectopic pregnancy.
- Culdocentesis (placement of a needle through the posterior wall of the vagina to aspirate blood in the cul-de-sac) is rarely performed. It is indicated only in settings where sonography is not available and ruptured ectopic is suspected. Aspiration of nonclotting blood is considered positive and indicative of an ectopic pregnancy.
- Laparoscopy is extremely accurate and can be both diagnostic and therapeutic.

TREATMENT

- **Unstable patient with suspected ectopic pregnancy**: Two large-bore intravenous lines with rapid infusion of crystalloid and/or packed red blood cells should be given to maintain blood pressure. OB/GYN should be consulted immediately (even before the US is performed).
- **Stable patient with definite ectopic pregnancy**: Definitive treatment is determined by the OB/GYN consultant but may consist of laparoscopy, expectant management, or treatment with methotrexate.
  - Optimal candidates for methotrexate therapy include patients with a β-hCG < 5000 mIU/mL, no fetal cardiac activity, and an ectopic mass < 3-4 cm.
  - Contraindications to methotrexate include free peritoneal fluid outside the pelvic cavity, immunodeficiency, active pulmonary disease or peptic ulcer disease; hypersensitivity to methotrexate, coexistent viable IUP, breast-feeding, and noncompliance risk with post-therapeutic monitoring.
- **Stable patients with nondiagnostic US**: OB/GYN consultation for follow-up in 2-3 days for repeat β-hCG level. Women with viable pregnancies should double their serum β-hCG in 48-72 hours. Patients with persistent symptoms or whose β-hCG rises by < 66% over 48 hours require further evaluation.
- Rh-negative women should receive RhoGAM.

KEY FACT

β-hCG levels in ectopic pregnancy are often below the discriminatory zone!

First Trimester Bleeding

Causes of first trimester bleeding include ectopic pregnancy, spontaneous abortion, gestational trophoblastic disease, implantation bleeding, and vaginal, cervical or uterine pathology (eg, vaginal trauma, cervicitis, cancer, warts, fibroids).

SPONTANEOUS ABORTION

Spontaneous abortion (SAB) or miscarriage is defined as a loss of pregnancy before 20 weeks of gestation. Studies show a rate of pregnancy loss after implantation of up to 30%. Chromosomal abnormalities are found in about half of the cases.

RISK FACTORS

Advanced maternal age, previous SAB, smoking, trauma, alcohol or drug abuse, and extremes of weight

SYMPTOMS

Women usually present with a history of amenorrhea followed by vaginal bleeding and pelvic pain.

EXAMINATION

Pelvic examination is necessary to document volume of bleeding, degree of cervical dilation, and presence of purulent drainage (suggesting septic abortion). Visualization of products of conception confirms a miscarriage but can be hard to identify at the bedside in early pregnancies.

DIAGNOSIS

- Bedside ultrasound showing:
  - Gestational sac ≥ 25 mm diameter without yolk sac or embryo (empty sac) (Figure 12.7)
  - Loss of previously identified IUP
  - Absence of cardiac activity in an embryo with crown rump length (CRL) > 7 mm. A fetal HR of < 70 bpm is an ominous sign that warrants follow up ultrasound.
  - Lack of development of embryo with heartbeat 2 weeks after ultrasound (US) showing gestational sac **without** yolk sac
  - Lack of development of embryo with heartbeat 11 days after US showing gestational sac **with** yolk sac
- Rh factor blood test to determine need for RhoGAM.
- Suspect septic abortion if fevers/chills, purulent discharge, or boggy and tender uterus.
- SAB is a dynamic process. The postdiagnostic classification is listed in Table 12.3.

TREATMENT

- Rh-negative women should receive RhoGAM 300 μg, or 50 μg if < 12 weeks gestation.
- Most patients with threatened abortion may be discharged with expectant management and return precautions with OB/GYN follow-up, as long as ectopic pregnancy has been excluded.
- Patients with incomplete or complete abortion with persistent bleeding should have OB/GYN consult and be offered dilation and curettage.

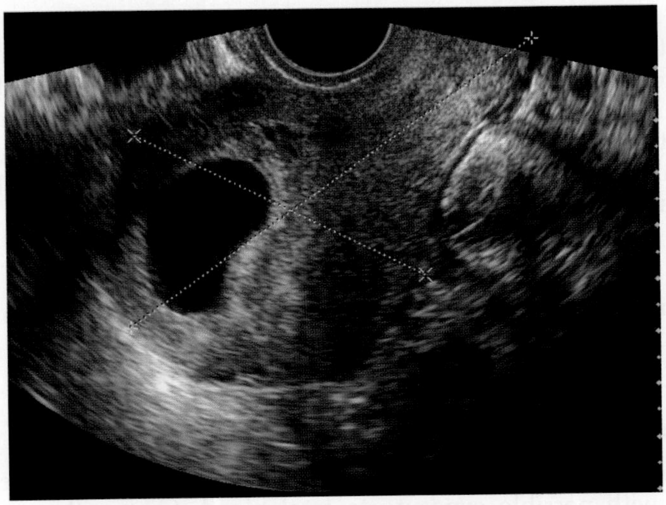

FIGURE 12.7. Gestational sac > 25 mm diameter without yolk sac or embryo indicating an empty sac and failed pregnancy. (Reproduced, with permission, from Cunningham FG, Leveno KJ, Bloom SL, et al. *Williams Obstetrics*. 24th ed. New York, NY: McGraw-Hill Education, 2010. Figure 18.4).

KEY FACT

Complications of a missed abortion include infection and coagulopathy.

KEY FACT

A SAB cannot be diagnosed until ectopic pregnancy has been excluded by US or serial quantitative β-hCG levels.

TABLE 12.3. Postdiagnostic Classification of Abortion

Diagnosis	Description
Threatened abortion	Vaginal bleeding in the first 20 wk of gestation without fetal loss, closed cervix on examination, no passage of fetal tissue by history or examination
Inevitable abortion	Vaginal bleeding with open cervix but no passage of products
Incomplete abortion	Incomplete passage of products of conception, open cervix, pain, and vaginal bleeding
Complete abortion	Complete passage of products of conception, closed cervix, uterus contracted
Missed abortion	In utero death of the fetus prior to 20 wk of gestation with retention of the products for a prolonged period of time
Empty sac	Previously called anembryonic pregnancy or blighted ovum. Defined as the presence of a gestational sac > **25 mm** without presence of yolk sac or embryo (see Figure 12.7)
Septic abortion	Infection of the uterus during a miscarriage, usually due to *Staphylococcus aureus*; fever, chills, purulent cervical discharge, and uterine tenderness

KEY FACT

Septic abortion is a leading cause of maternal mortality in the developing world, mostly because of illegal and unsterile abortions.

- Septic abortion mandates dilation and curettage and broad-spectrum antibiotics (cefoxitin and doxycycline or clindamycin and gentamycin).
- Inform patients that miscarriage is common, grieving is normal, and counseling may be needed.

Rh Incompatability

Approximately 15% of individuals are Rh negative. This percentage varies among different ethnic groups. In Rh-negative women with an Rh-positive fetus, maternal exposure to even small amounts of fetal blood can result in the production of maternal antibodies to the foreign Rh "D" antigen. The formation of maternal Rh antibodies exposes the current and subsequent pregnancies to antibody-induced hemolytic disease of the newborn.

Causes

Causes of maternal exposure to fetal blood include trauma, vaginal bleeding, ectopic, SAB, and obstetric procedures. Transfusion of Rh-positive blood may sensitize an Rh-negative woman, even if she is not pregnant.

Diagnosis/Treatment

- Rh(D) immunoglobulin (RhoGAM) 300 μg for Rh-negative pregnant patients with possible exposure to fetal blood. Give within 72 hours of exposure. Half-life is 24 days.
- "Mini-RhoGAM" (50 μg) can be used for patients < 12 weeks of gestation, however there is no harm in giving the larger dose of 300 μg.

- RhoGAM is given routinely at 28 weeks of gestation for patients who are Rh negative.
- In the setting of maternal abdominal trauma at > 20 weeks, large amounts of fetomaternal hemorrhage (> 15 mL) may occur, and the **Kleihauer-Betke test** should be used to quantify the volume and guide the administration of extra vials of RhoGAM.

Q

A 28-year-old G2P1 at 36 weeks by dates presents to the emergency room with abdominal tenderness and vaginal bleeding for 1 hour. What do you NOT want to do?

Third Trimester Bleeding

PLACENTAL ABRUPTION

Placental abruption is a premature separation of the implanted placenta from the uterine wall. It occurs in about 1% of all pregnancies. Bleeding between the placenta and uterine wall can result in significant blood loss with maternal and fetal compromise. Separations > 50% result in fetal death and DIC.

KEY FACT

300 μg dose of RhoGAM covers up to 15 mL of fetomaternal hemorrhage.

RISK FACTORS

Risk factors for abruption include previous abruption, abdominal trauma, cocaine or other drug use, smoking, hypertension, polyhydramnios, advanced maternal age, and multiparity.

SYMPTOMS

- Vaginal bleeding with abdominal/back pain is the most common presentation.
- If the blood is contained within the uterus ("concealed abruption"), the patients can present with symptoms of preterm labor only with minimal to no bleeding.

KEY FACT

Painful third trimester vaginal bleeding = abruption

EXAMINATION

- Uterine tenderness with hypertonic/hyperactive contractions
- Fetal distress/demise can occur with large abruptions.
- Pelvic examination should NOT be performed until placenta previa has been ruled out!

DIFFERENTIAL

Placenta previa, preterm or term labor, bloody show, and lower genital tract lesions.

DIAGNOSIS

- Clinical diagnosis, ultrasound has low sensitivity for identifying retroplacental blood.
- Ultrasound should still be obtained to rule out placenta previa and to look for signs of fetal distress.
- Disseminated intravascular coagulation (DIC) studies: Fibrinogen, D-dimer, PT/PTT, complete blood cell

KEY FACT

Ultrasound is not sensitive for identifying abruption, but should be used to rule out previa or fetal distress.

TREATMENT

- Assess hemodynamics and fluid/blood resuscitate if needed.
- Emergent OB/GYN consultation should be obtained.

- Initiate continuous monitoring of uterine contractions and fetal HR. Fetal distress warrants emergent delivery and is suggested by HR < 120 bpm, or > 160 bpm, decelerations after uterine contractions, or loss of beat-to-beat variability.
- RhoGAM prophylaxis if Rh negative

A vaginal examination can cause massive hemorrhage if bleeding is secondary to placenta previa.

PLACENTA PREVIA

Placenta previa occurs when the placenta overlaps or lies within 2-3 cm of the internal cervical os. Bleeding occurs due to shearing forces on the placenta because the lower uterine segment changes shape in the third trimester, or from local trauma to the cervix (intercourse, bimanual examination).

RISK FACTORS

Risk factors include previous previa as well as any pathology that changes the inner surface of the uterus: prior C-section, fibroids, multiparity, multiple induced abortions, advanced maternal age, and smoking.

SYMPTOMS

Painless, bright red vaginal bleeding is the most common presentation.

EXAMINATION

Abdominal examination reveals a soft, nontender uterus. DO NOT perform a pelvic examination.

KEY FACT

Painless, bright red, third trimester vaginal bleeding = placenta previa

DIAGNOSIS

Ultrasound is the key to the diagnosis! Transvaginal ultrasound is safe and more accurate than transabdominal.

KEY FACT

Do not perform pelvic examination on patients with third trimester vaginal bleeding.

TREATMENT

- Emergent OB consult for maternal/fetal monitoring
- Do not encourage vaginal delivery; most cases require C-section.
- RhoGAM prophylaxis if Rh negative

PREMATURE RUPTURE OF MEMBRANES

Premature rupture of membranes (PROM) is defined as rupture of membranes prior to the onset of labor. Furthermore, **preterm premature rupture of membranes** (PPROM) refers to rupture of membranes occurring prior to labor in a patient < 37 weeks of gestation. PPROM occurs in 3% of all pregnancies and is responsible for one-third of preterm births.

RISK FACTORS

Genital tract infections, antepartum bleeding, and cigarette smoking

SYMPTOMS

Rush of fluid or a continuous leak of fluid from the vagina

KEY FACT

Blue Nitrazine paper + ferning = amniotic fluid

DIAGNOSIS

Confirm PROM with a sterile speculum examination showing pool of fluid in the posterior fornix, fluid pH > 6.5 (Nitrazine paper turns blue!), and ferning of fluid as it dries on a slide.

TREATMENT

- Immediate OB consultation and admission
- Test patients for chlamydia, gonorrhea, and group B *Streptococcus*.

Complication

Chorioamnionitis: An ascending intraamniotic infection with normal vaginal flora (genital mycoplasma most commonly isolated). Risk increases with duration of rupture of membranes. Can also be due to placental infection or invasive procedures. Fever and uterine tenderness are common findings along with evidence of fetal distress. Treatment is with ampicillin plus gentamicin and delivery of the fetus.

Q

A 20-year-old, 10-weeks pregnant woman presents with severe nausea and vomiting. Her BP is 160/100 mm Hg and her fundus is palpable at her umbilicus. What test do you perform to confirm your diagnosis?

Gestational Trophoblastic Disease

Gestational trophoblastic disease (GTD) occurs when a nonviable embryo implants and trophoblastic cells proliferate in the uterus. The noninvasive (no invasion of uterine wall) and nonmalignant form of GTD is the hydatidiform mole. The presence of persistent, relapsed, or invasive GTD is termed *gestational trophoblastic neoplasia* and includes choriocarcinoma and trophoblastic tumors. These malignancies are extremely sensitive to chemotherapy.

KEY FACT

Higher β-hCG and larger uterine size than expected by dates should raise suspicion of molar pregnancy.

Hydatidiform moles are defined as either partial or complete.

- Partial mole: Triploid (two sets of paternal chromosomes/one set of maternal), fetal tissue present, has higher tendency to progress to choriocarcinoma
- Complete mole: Diploid (two sets of paternal chromosomes) with the absence of fetal tissue

Symptoms/Examination

- Severe nausea/vomiting
- Intermittent vaginal bleeding during early pregnancy or passage of "grape-like" material
- Uterus larger than expected for dates
- **Preeclampsia** prior to 20 weeks of gestation and eclampsia prior to 24 weeks of gestation

Diagnosis

- β-hCG higher than expected for dates and a characteristic snowstorm or cystic appearing on ultrasound (Figure 12.8)

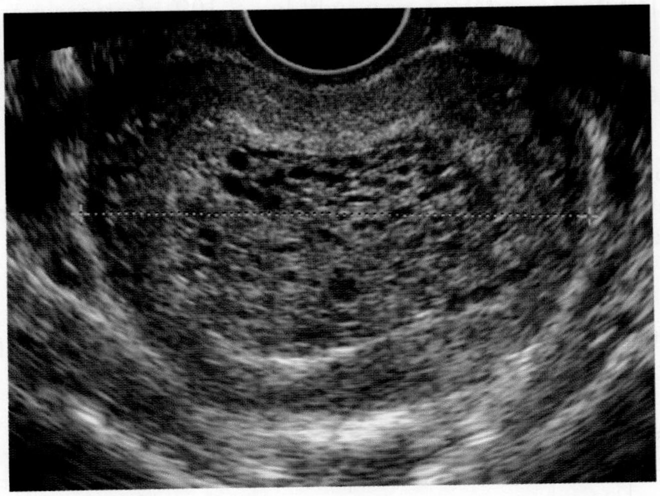

FIGURE 12.8. Transverse ultrasound of uterus showing classic "snowstorm" patter of a complete hydatidiform mole. (Reproduced, with permission, from Hoffman BL, Schorge JO, Schaffer JI, et al. *Williams Gynecology*. 2nd ed. New York, NY: McGraw-Hill Education; 2012. Figure 37.5.)

A

US to look for a molar pregnancy, and β-hCG.

- Obtain chest x-ray if any pulmonary symptoms or chest pain. Trophoblastic tumors metastasize to lung, liver, and brain.

Treatment

Consult OB/GYN for dilation and curettage and subsequent monitoring of β-hCG levels; failure of β-hCG to decrease to zero suggests gestational trophoblastic neoplasia.

Hyperemesis Gravidarum

A severe form of morning sickness, with excessive pregnancy-related nausea and/or vomiting that prevents adequate intake of food and fluids. Typical onset at 6 weeks of gestation peaking at 9 weeks and resolving by 16-20 weeks.

Symptoms/Examination

- Intractable nausea/vomiting, weight loss (from prepregnancy weight; > 5% = severe)
- Hypokalemia, ketonuria
- No abdominal tenderness on examination

Differential

Obstetric (eg, gestational trophoblastic disease) and nonobstetric causes of nausea/vomiting (eg, pyelonephritis, appendicitis, cholelithiasis, pancreatitis, gastroenteritis, and bowel obstruction)

Diagnosis

Because nausea and vomiting during pregnancy exist on a continuum, there is no clear boundary between common morning sickness and hyperemesis.

KEY FACT

Zofran has recently been associated with an increased risk of birth defects though causation has not been established.

Treatment

- Fluid resuscitation with 5% glucose-containing fluids
- Antiemetics (eg, antihistamines, metoclopramide)
- Consider thiamine (vitamin B_1) 100 mg IV for patients with prolonged symptoms to prevent Wernicke encephalopathy.
- Admit patients with persistent vomiting, electrolyte abnormalities, and ketosis despite resuscitation, or weight loss > 10% of prepregnancy weight.

Incarcerated Uterus

Typically occurs as a growing **retroflexed gravid uterus** (20% of women) fails to convert to an anteverted position and becomes trapped in the pelvis between the sacrum and pubic symphysis.

Risk factors

Adhesions from prior pelvic surgery, endometriosis or pelvic inflammatory disease, fibroids.

Symptoms/Examination

- Classic presentation is abdominal pain with difficulty urinating or retention at 14-16 weeks of gestation.
- Cervix is very anteriorly displaced on examination and difficult to find on speculum examination or palpate bimanually.

DIAGNOSIS/TREATMENT

- Suspicious findings on ultrasound include an elongated and anterior cervix with a superiorly displaced and elongated bladder.
- Treatment is manual reduction by OB/GYN.

Gestational (Pregnancy-Induced) Hypertension

Gestational hypertension is defined as BP > 140/90 mm Hg or an increase in systolic BP > 20 mm Hg (or diastolic > 10 mm Hg) above baseline. It can be divided into 3 types: chronic hypertension (hypertension before pregnancy or developing in early pregnancy), gestational hypertension (hypertension that develops after week 20 and resolves postpartum), and preeclampsia.

> **KEY FACT**
>
> Eclampsia = preeclampsia plus seizures

PREECLAMPSIA/ECLAMPSIA

Preeclampsia is defined as the presence of new-onset hypertension along with proteinuria or end-organ dysfunction after 20 weeks of gestation. It can be superimposed upon chronic hypertension and can progress to eclampsia. The hallmark of eclampsia is seizures. Up to one-third of eclamptic seizures occur postdelivery and can occur up to 6 weeks postpartum.

RISK FACTORS

Risk factors for preeclampsia include prior or family history of preeclampsia, first pregnancy, advanced maternal age, pregestational diabetes mellitus, multiple gestations, obesity, chronic kidney disease, and chronic hypertension.

SYMPTOMS

- Headache with or without visual disturbances
- Peripheral edema
- Upper abdominal pain, nausea/vomiting
- Chest pain and/or shortness of breath

> **KEY FACT**
>
> Never ignore an elevated BP in a pregnant patient. Eclampsia can kill both the mother and the fetus.

EXAMINATION

- Severe and persistent hypertension
- Peripheral edema is often present.
- Right upper quadrant tenderness may be present in the setting of HELLP syndrome.

DIAGNOSIS

- Presence of new-onset HTN and either proteinuria or end-organ dysfunction after 20 weeks of gestation
- Proteinuria: ≥ 0.3 g in 24 hours or urine protein-to-creatinine ratio ≥ 0.3
- End-organ dysfunction: Thrombocytopenia, rising creatinine, AST, or ALT, congestive heart failure, etc.
- Check CBC, liver function tests, electrolytes, renal function, magnesium, coagulation panel, and urine protein and creatinine.
- Eclampsia: Preeclampsia + seizures

> **KEY FACT**
>
> Eclampsia can occur up to 6 weeks postpartum.

TREATMENT

- Medical management should be initiated immediately and includes:
  - Magnesium sulfate (6-g IV bolus, then 2 g/h). Watch for signs of magnesium toxicity: Hyporeflexia, loss of deep tendon reflexes, respiratory depression, and bradydysrhythmias.

KEY FACT

Antihypertensives do not prevent eclamptic seizures, magnesium does.

  - Antihypertensive drugs: Labetalol is considered first-line therapy but hydralazine may also be used.
- Emergent OB consultation should be obtained. The cornerstone of treatment for severe preeclampsia or eclampsia is delivery of the fetus.
- Expectant management can be attempted in a monitored setting for preeclamptic patients < 34 weeks of gestation with only mild proteinuria.

HELLP SYNDROME

HELLP (hemolysis, elevated liver enzymes, low platelet count) syndrome is an uncommon but severe variant of preeclampsia. It typically occurs at 28-36 weeks of gestation but may occur earlier and in the postpartum period.

Symptoms/Examination

Epigastric/RUQ abdominal pain with nausea and vomiting is the most common presentation and tenderness. Patients may (or may not) have other signs/symptoms of preeclampsia.

Differential

Fatty liver of pregnancy, cholecystitis, gastritis, pancreatitis, appendicitis, thrombotic thrombocytopenic purpura, hemolytic uremic syndrome.

Diagnosis

- Primarily a laboratory diagnosis requiring the following to be present:
  - Microangiopathic hemolytic anemia (schistocytes) on peripheral smear
  - Total bilirubin > 1.2 mg/dL
  - Thrombocytopenia (< 150,000/mm^3 at nadir)
  - Hepatic dysfunction with lactate dehydrogenase > 600 IU/L or AST or ALT > 40 IU/L

MNEMONIC

HELLP syndrome

Hemolysis
Elevated **L**iver enzymes
Low **P**latelets

Treatment

- Treat preeclampsia, as earlier.
- Obtaine emergent OB consultation. The cornerstone of treatment is delivery of the fetus.
- Correct coagulopathy, as needed (fresh frozen plasma, platelets, blood transfusion).
- Dexamethasone has **not** been shown to be helpful in the treatment of HELLP syndrome.

Infections in Pregnancy

URINARY TRACT INFECTIONS

Asymptomatic bacteriuria, defined as a positive urine culture in an asymptomatic patient, can be seen in up to 10% of pregnant patients. *Escherichia coli* is responsible for most infections. Bacteriuria is associated with an increased risk of preterm birth, low birth weight, and perinatal mortality. Approximately 30% of patients will go on to develop pyelonephritis. Screening urinalysis is typically performed at 12-16 weeks of gestation.

TREATMENT

Cephalosporins and nitrofurantoin are recommended antibiotics. Fluoroquinolones and sulfonamides are contraindicated secondary to teratogenic effects. Always send urine cultures.

APPENDICITIS

The most common general surgical emergency in pregnancy. Overall, pregnant women are less likely to have a classic presentation of appendicitis, leading to a frequent delay in diagnosis and higher incidence of rupture.

> **KEY FACT**
>
> Appendicitis is the most common nonobstetrical surgical emergency in pregnancy.

SYMPTOMS/EXAMINATION

- Similar to the nonpregnant patient in early pregnancy
- Later in pregnancy, the enlarging uterus may shift the appendix slightly upwards causing the location of pain to shift upwards as well. Pain is located in the RUQ in 20% of pregnant patients.

DIAGNOSIS

- US is the initial modality of choice. Findings that support appendicitis are the presence of a noncompressible, blind-ending tubular structure arising from the cecal tip that measures > 6 mm in diameter and lacks peristalsis.
- Magnetic resonance imaging (MRI) is also an excellent choice and has excellent sensitivity and specificity for diagnosing appendicitis.

Medications During Pregnancy

See Tables 12.4 and 12.5. In no way is this a comprehensive list, but it includes the medications you are likely to encounter on a daily basis.

> **KEY FACT**
>
> Adenosine is the drug of choice in pregnant patients with supraventricular tachycardia. Avoid electricity if possible because of potential harm to the fetus.

TABLE 12.4. Vaccines and Medications Contraindicated During Pregnancy

Vaccines (any live vaccines)	MMR Live, attenuated influenza vaccine (FluMist) Varicella TDaP (but Td is safe after first trimester)
Antibiotics	Tetracyclines Fluoroquinolones Sulfonamides Chloramphenicol
Antiepileptic drugs	Phenytoin Valproic acid Phenobarbital
Other	Oral hypoglycemic (glyburide is safe, metformin and acarbose are acceptable) Warfarin

MMR, measles, mumps, and rubella; TDaP, tetanus diphtheria acelluar pertussis.

TABLE 12.5. Vaccines and Medications Considered Safe During Pregnancy

Vaccines	Td (okay after first trimester) Influenza (inactivated) Pneumococcal
Antimicrobials	Penicillin Cephalosporins Azithromycin Nitrofurantoin INH Rifampin Nystatin Clotrimazole
Analgesics	Acetaminophen
Antidysrhythmics	Digoxin Adenosine
β-Adrenergics	Albuterol
GI agents	Promethazine Prochlorperazine Metoclopramide Ondansetron (after 1st trimester) Cimetidine Ranitidine
Antihistamines	Benadryl

GI, gastrointestinal; INH, isonicotinic acid hydrazide; Td, tetanus diphtheria.

Normal Labor and Delivery

Normal labor proceeds through three basic stages (Table 12.6).

Emergency delivery often proceeds rapidly and requires minimal help from the ED provider. If time allows, the ideal option is to get the patient rapidly to the obstetric suite. Have the supplies ready for neonatal resuscitation including warmer and airway management.

- Delivery of the fetal head should be controlled by applying moderate upward pressure on the fetal chin through the perineum while holding the fetal head against the pubic symphysis.

TABLE 12.6. Stages of Labor

Stage 1: Cervical stage	Onset of regular contractions to complete cervical dilation/effacement
Stage 2: Expulsion stage	Complete dilation/effacement to delivery of fetus
Stage 3: Placental stage	Delivery of fetus to delivery of placenta

- If meconium is present, suction the mouth followed by the nose at the perineum. If there is no meconium, there is no indication for suctioning. Proceed to palpate for a nuchal cord, and reduce it when possible.
- The anterior shoulder should be delivered first by placing hands on either side of fetal head and applying gentle downward traction. The posterior shoulder typically follows spontaneously.

Delivery Complications

NUCHAL CORD

Occurs in approximately 30% of all cephalad presenting deliveries; can result in fetal asphyxia if not identified and treated promptly.

KEY FACT

A tight nuchal cord must be cut and clamped as soon as possible.

TREATMENT

- Loose nuchal cord: Slip over head of fetus in between contractions.
- Tight nuchal cord: If the cord is preventing the fetus from delivery, then cut and clamp the cord and immediately deliver the fetus. If the cord is tight but not preventing the delivery, then allow the fetus to deliver and cut and clamp the cord after delivery.

CORD PROLAPSE

Occurs when the umbilical cord precedes a fetal presenting part that doesn't fill the birth canal completely; most likely to occur with abnormal fetal presentations and with fetal prematurity.

KEY FACT

First step in treatment of cord prolapse? Elevate presenting part off cord.

DIAGNOSIS

Visualization or palpation of pulsating umbilical cord at or through the cervical os

TREATMENT

- Elevate the presenting fetal part to reduce compression of the cord. The mother should not push.
- This is an obstetrical emergency and a **C-section** is indicated. The examiner's hand should stay in the vagina elevating the presenting part until the patient undergoes surgery. Mortality can be reduced from 15% to 5% if C-section performed within 10 minutes of presentation.
- Other adjunctive maneuvers include knee chest position with Trendelenburg position and manually filling bladder with fluid (via Foley catheter).

SHOULDER DYSTOCIA

A failure of the fetal shoulders to deliver after delivery of the fetal head; occurs when the anterior shoulder impacts behind or above the pubic symphysis; most likely to occur with large fetal size or in the presence of abnormal pelvic anatomy. It is the second most common malpresentation (after breech). It can lead to asphyxia, traumatic brachial plexus injury, and humeral or clavicular fracture.

RISK FACTORS

- Maternal factors: Diabetes, obesity, prolonged second stage of labor
- Fetal factors: Macrosomia, postmaturity, erythroblastosis fetalis

SYMPTOMS/EXAMINATION

Turtle sign: Fetal head pulled tight against perineum and retracted back into the birth canal with each contraction

TREATMENT

- Obtain immediate OB backup. The mother should not push and traction should not be applied to the fetal head. Empty the bladder.
- The following maneuvers should be tried in order:
- **McRoberts maneuver:** Sharply flexing maternal hips and legs, which (results in straightening of sacrum and is successful alone about half the time). See Figure 12.9.
- Apply firm maternal suprapubic (**not fundal**) pressure to dislodge the impacted fetal shoulder.
- Deliver the posterior arm: With fetal elbow flexed, pull posterior arm out the vagina.
- Place hand behind posterior shoulder and push shoulder forward 180° (Woods corkscrew maneuver).
- Push a fetal shoulder anteriorly to adduct shoulders (Rubin maneuver).
- Episiotomies are no longer recommended by the OB literature.
- Fracture of fetal clavicle or symphysiotomy is last resort.

KEY FACT

First maneuver in treatment of shoulder dystocia? McRoberts.

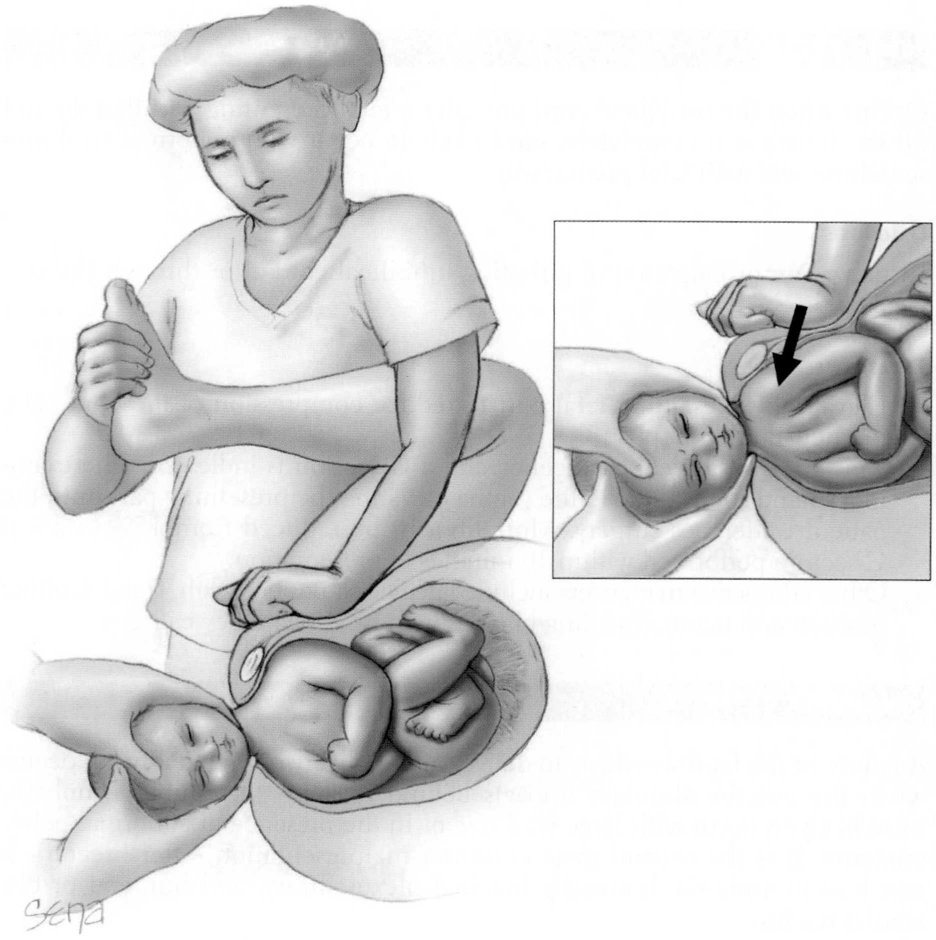

FIGURE 12.9. McRoberts maneuver consists of sharply flexing the thighs up onto the abdomen. The assistant is simultaneously providing suprapubic pressure to relieve the obstructing shoulder. (Reproduced, with permission, from Cunningham FG, Leveno KJ, Bloom SL, et al. *Williams Obstetrics*. 24th ed. New York, NY: McGraw-Hill Education; 2010. Figure 27.7.)

BREECH PRESENTATION

The major risk of breech delivery is cord prolapse, entrapment of the fetal head, and resultant fetal hypoxia. Breech presentation occurs in about 4% of all deliveries and is the most common malpresentation.

Possible breech presentations: Frank (fetal hips flexed with knees extended), complete (hips and knees flexed), incomplete (hips flexed, one knee flexed), footling (hips extended, feet as presenting part). Footling breech has the highest incidence of complications because of the smaller presenting part.

KEY FACT

Footling breech presentation has the highest incidence of breech complications.

Risk Factors

Prematurity, multiparity, fetal abnormalities, polyhydramnios, uterine abnormalities, prior breech deliveries

Treatment

- Obtain immediate OB consultation in case operative intervention is required.
- The delivery should be allowed to progress as spontaneously as possible until the fetal umbilicus appears. At this point provider assistance and fetal rotation will be needed for delivery of fetal legs and arms.
- If the fetal head becomes entrapped, administer a uterine relaxant (eg, terbutaline), apply suprapubic pressure, and insert fingers to draw the fetal chin to the fetal chest. Persistent entrapment requires symphysiotomy or an attempt to push the body of fetus back into uterus (Zavanelli maneuver) and emergent C-section.

KEY FACT

Sudden change in maternal respiratory status during labor?
- Pulmonary embolism
- Sepsis
- Anaphylaxis
- Myocardial infarction
- Amniotic fluid embolism

AMNIOTIC FLUID EMBOLISM

Results from release of amniotic fluid into the maternal circulation causing a rapid maternal pulmonary arterial obstruction and biochemical mediator release. Typically occurs during labor or shortly after delivery, but may also be seen following uterine trauma. Fortunately rare (1 in 8000-80,000 deliveries), as mortality is as high as 90% with the majority of survivors suffering from severe neurologic impairment due to hypoxia.

Symptoms/Examination

- Sudden catastrophic dyspnea, hypoxia, altered mental status, seizures, and hemodynamic collapse
- Disseminated intravascular coagulation frequently follows

Diagnosis/Treatment

- A clinical diagnosis after consideration and evaluation for pulmonary embolism, sepsis, anaphylaxis, and myocardial infarction
- Treatment is rapid delivery of infant and intensive supportive care.

UTERINE RUPTURE

Rupture of uterine wall during labor, typically in patients undergoing trial of labor after prior C-section. Can also be seen in the setting of trauma. It is rare in the "unscarred" uterus.

Symptoms/Examination

Sudden or worsening abdominal pain with fetal distress, decreased contractions, and change in fetal station

DIAGNOSIS/TREATMENT

Primarily a clinical diagnosis. Fetal distress is indication for emergent C-section where definitive diagnosis is made.

Postpartum Complications

POSTPARTUM HEMORRHAGE

> **KEY FACT**
>
> Causes of postpartum hemorrhage 4 Ts:
> Tone
> Trauma
> Tissue
> Thrombin

Postpartum hemorrhage (> 500 mL for vaginal birth) is divided into **early** (< 24 hours) and **late** (24 hours-6 weeks) hemorrhage. Early postpartum hemorrhage can have brisk bleeding, and shock can develop rapidly. Maternal vital signs may remain normal while large volumes (> 1.5 L) of blood accumulate in the uterus. This is the most common postpartum complication and accounts for up to 25% of obstetric death.

CAUSES

- Early postpartum hemorrhage: **Uterine atony** (most common), laceration of the lower genital tract, retained placenta, placenta accreta, uterine rupture, uterine inversion, coagulopathy
- Late postpartum hemorrhage: Retained placenta (most common), infection, uterine inversion, coagulopathy, sloughing of the placental site eschar

EXAMINATION/DIAGNOSIS

- Physical examination is the cornerstone to the diagnosis.
- An enlarged and "boggy" uterus is seen with uterine atony.
- A vaginal mass is seen with uterine inversion.
- Vaginal bleeding despite good uterine tone and size is likely due to retained products.

TREATMENT

- Depends on suspected underlying cause. Intervene early.
- Manage blood loss aggressively; initiate rapid transfusion protocol if any evidence of shock.
- Emergent OB consultation for consideration of surgical management.
- Initial treatment of uterine atony is with **vigorous bimanual massage** and IV oxytocin (10-40 U in 1-L normal saline). Additional treatments include methylergonovine and prostaglandins.

ENDOMETRITIS

Polymicrobial postpartum infection of the endometrium, usually gram-positive cocci and gram-negative coliforms. Usually presents on day 2 or 3 postpartum.

RISK FACTORS

Cesarean delivery (most important), chorioamnionitis, prolonged rupture of membranes, frequent vaginal examinations during labor, presence of high-virulence organisms, use of an internal monitoring device, lack of prenatal care, prolonged second stage of labor

Symptoms/Examination/Diagnosis

- Fever, uterine tenderness, and foul-smelling lochia
- Clinical diagnosis, excluding other causes of fever; ultrasound is not diagnostic.

Treatment

- Hospitalization and IV antibiotics (clindamycin plus gentamicin first line of treatment). Tetracyclines are not recommended in nursing mothers.
- A search for retained products of conception is indicated if bleeding is ongoing.
- Consider removal of IUD, if present.

> **Q**
>
> A 29 year old presents to the emergency room 3 days after discharge from the hospital after a course of IV antibiotics for postpartum endometritis with continued fever and pelvic pain. What diagnosis do you need to consider and how is it treated?

SEPTIC PELVIC THROMBOPHLEBITIS

Develops from an infection of the placental site along with thrombophlebitis of the ovarian or deep pelvic veins (iliac veins, inferior vena cava). Incidence is increased after C-section or other pelvic surgery. Presentation is that of unexplained delayed fever. Computed tomography is imaging of choice. Treatment includes anticoagulation and antibiotics.

MASTITIS

Mastitis is localized infection of breast tissue. Typical risk factors include a blocked milk duct, failure to empty breast completely, and irritation or cracking of the mother's breast tissue. It is most commonly due to S *aureus* (including methicillin-resistant S *aureus*).

Symptoms/Examination

Focal area of breast erythema, edema and tenderness; malaise, and often fever

Differential

- Breast abscess: Confirmed by US; requires incision and drainage
- Inflammatory breast cancer: Skin often has classic orange-peel appearance in addition to warmth, tenderness, and redness; confirmed by biopsy

Diagnosis

The physical examination is the key for diagnosis. If concern for an abscess exists, a breast ultrasound or needle aspiration can be helpful.

Treatment

- Anti-inflammatory pain medication, cold compresses/ice packs
- Breast-feeding should be continued with frequent complete breast emptying.
- Antistaphylococcal antibiotics (dicloxacillin or cephalexin)

PERIPARTUM CARDIOMYOPATHY

The onset of heart failure due to left ventricular systolic dysfunction in late pregnancy or the postpartum period (most common). Most common in African American women.

Symptoms/Examination

Range from mild fatigue to dyspnea on exertion, orthopnea, and pulmonary edema

> **KEY FACT**
>
> Patients with peripartum cardiomyopathy have an ejection fracture of <45% without another identifiable cause.

A

Septic pelvic thrombophlebitis; treat with anticoagulation and antibiotics.

Treatment

- Similar to other types of heart failure with diuretics, ACE inhibitors (postpartum only), oxygen, and vasodilators.
- Cardiac function returns to normal in 50% of patients is within 6 months.

Emergency Contraception

Emergency contraception refers to contraceptive measures taken after sex to prevent a pregnancy. Pregnancy should be excluded prior to prescribing.

- **Copper IUD placement**: Probably the **most effective** method if placed within 5 days of unprotected intercourse.
- Levonorgestrel (Plan B): A progestin-only treatment. Most effective when taken in the first 72 hours after unprotected intercourse. Reduces likelihood of pregnancy from about 8% to 1%, can cause nausea and vaginal bleeding. Less effective if patient's weight is > 75 kg.
- Ulipristal (Ella): Progesterone receptor modulator. Highly effective if taken within 5 days of unprotected intercourse.
- Mifepristone (RU-486): A steroid that blocks progesterone receptors. A dose of 600 mg is approved for up to 49 days gestation in the United States. It is highly effective.

KEY FACT

Plan B is less effective if patient weighs >75 kg.

Cervicitis and Pelvic Inflammatory Disease

CERVICITIS

Inflammation/infection of the cervix. Most common infectious agents are chlamydia and gonorrhea. Herpes simplex virus, *Trichomonas vaginalis*, *Mycoplasma genitalium*, group A strep, and bacterial vaginosis are less common causes. Inflammatory etiologies include mechanical and chemical irritants (eg, douching).

Symptoms/Examination

- Vaginal discharge and intermenstrual bleeding are the most common symptoms, though many patients are asymptomatic.
- Examination shows a red and friable cervix with mucopurulent discharge.
- In trichomonal infection, a "strawberry" cervix characterized by punctate hemorrhages can be seen (Figure 12.10).

Diagnosis

- Clinical diagnosis based on examination findings
- Laboratory testing should be performed to rule out infectious cause:
  - Nucleic acid amplification test of vaginal fluid for gonorrhea and chlamydia
  - Wet prep evaluation of vaginal fluid for bacterial vaginosis (BV)
  - Wet prep microscopy and (if negative) culture or nucleic acid amplification test of vaginal fluid for *T vaginalis*

Treatment

- Empiric therapy for chlamydia and gonorrhea is warranted in most women, especially a high-risk individual. Ceftriaxone plus azithromycin or doxycycline is currently recommended by the Centers for Disease Control and Prevention (CDC).

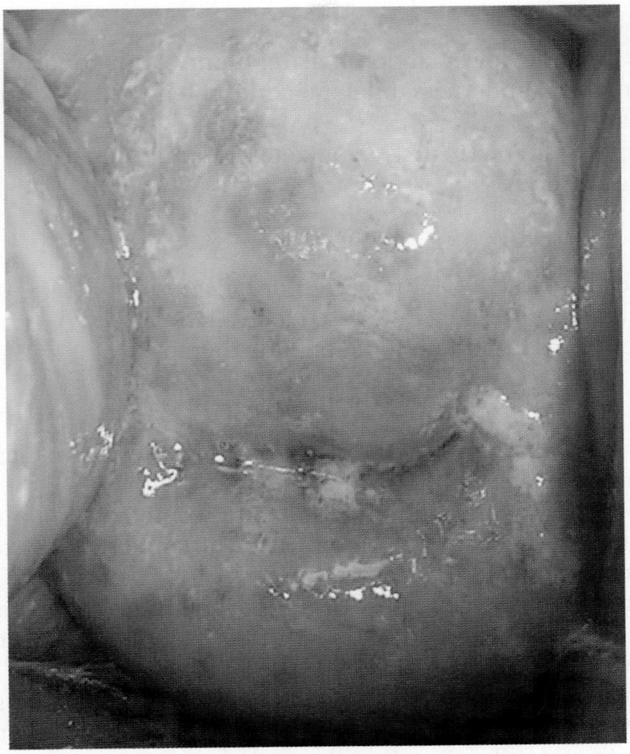

FIGURE 12.10. Strawberry cervix of trichomonal cervicitis, characterized by punctate hemorrhages. (Reproduced with permission from Usatine RP: *The Color Atlas of Family Medicine*. 2nd edition. New York, NY: McGraw-Hill Education; 2013. Photographer: Richard P. Usatine.)

- Other treatment (BV, trichomonas) should be based on test results.
- Sexual partners should also be tested and/or treated.
- Discharge instructions should recommend use of condoms, and further testing for HIV, hepatitis, and syphilis.

PELVIC INFLAMMATORY DISEASE

Pelvic inflammatory disease (PID) is an ascending infection from the lower genital tract that makes up a spectrum of disease that ranges from endometritis to salpingitis and tubo-ovarian abscess (TOA). *Neisseria gonorrhoeae* and *Chlamydia trachomatis* are the most common causes. Simultaneous infection occurs.

KEY FACT

Although STD's are the most common trigger for ascending genital infection, the infection is often polymicrobial when cultured.

Risk Factors

Multiple sexual partners, history of sexually transmitted disease, young age, nonbarrier contraception, and IUD. Half of the patients have no identifiable risk factors.

Symptoms

- Most common presenting complaint is lower abdominal pain.
- Often associated with abnormal vaginal discharge, vaginal bleeding, postcoital bleeding, dyspareunia, fever, malaise, and nausea and vomiting.
- Symptom onset is usually 2-5 days after menstruation.

KEY FACT

Chandelier sign = severe cervical motion tenderness seen with PID

KEY FACT

Use transvaginal ultrasound to rule out TOA in patients with PID and unilateral pelvic tenderness.

KEY FACT

PID admission indications:

Pregnancy
Immunosuppression
TOA or pelvic abscess
Presence of IUD
Severe vomiting
SIRS/sepsis
Failed outpatient management

EXAMINATION

- Findings include lower abdominal tenderness, mucopurulent cervicitis, cervical motion tenderness, bilateral adnexal tenderness; fever is present in 50% of cases.
- Evidence of systemic toxicity, unilateral adnexal tenderness, or unilateral mass suggests TOA.

DIAGNOSIS

- See Table 12.7 for CDC Guidelines for Diagnosis of PID.
- Transvaginal ultrasound can be used to evaluate for TOA.
- Pregnancy test is important to help guide therapy.

TREATMENT

- All patients meeting minimum criteria with no alternative diagnosis identified should receive empiric treatment.
- Hospitalization is indicated in pregnant women, immunosuppression, documented or suspected pelvic or tubo-ovarian abscess, systemic inflammatory response syndrome/sepsis, presence of IUD, severe vomiting, or failed outpatient management. Therapy consists of IV cefotetan or cefoxitin, plus PO or IV doxycycline. IV clindamycin and gentamycin is an alternative.
- Outpatient therapy for mild-to-moderate disease not meeting criteria for hospitalization: Ceftriaxone 250 mg IM plus doxycycline 100 mg PO bid × 14 days with our without metronidazole bid.
- Other treatment (BV, trichomonas) should be based on test results.
- Sexual partners should also be tested and/or treated.
- Discharge instructions should recommend use of condoms and further testing for HIV, hepatitis, and syphilis.

COMPLICATIONS

Fitz-Hugh-Curtis syndrome, infertility, ectopic pregnancy secondary to scarring of the fallopian tubes, chronic pain

TABLE 12.7. 2015 CDC Guidelines for Diagnosis of PID

Minimum criteria needed for PID diagnosis:
Pelvic or lower abdominal pain **with**
Cervical motion tenderness
or
Uterine tenderness
or
Adnexal tenderness
Additional criteria that increase the specificity of the diagnosis:
Fever > 38.3°C (100.9°F)
Abnormal mucopurulent discharge or cervical friability
+ WBCs on saline microscopy of vaginal fluid
Elevated ESR
Elevated CRP
+ Chlamydia or gonorrhea testing

CDC, Centers of Disease Control and Prevention; CRP, C-reactive protein; ESR, erythrocyte sedimentation rate; PID, pelvic inflammatory disease; WBC, white blood cell.

FITZ-HUGH-CURTIS SYNDROME

An ascending pelvic infection due to chlamydia (most common) or gonorrhea which results in perihepatitis with inflammation of the liver capsule and peritoneal surfaces. It is a rare complication of PID.

SYMPTOMS/EXAMINATION

Presents with RUQ pain that may mimic cholecystitis. May present with referred pain to the right shoulder. May or may not be associated with symptoms of PID.

DIAGNOSIS

- Definitive diagnosis requires direct visualization of the liver capsule via laparoscopy.
- RUQ US, CT abdomen, and CXR may be used to exclude other causes of RUQ pain. CT abdomen may show a perihepatic fluid collection.
- The combination of RUQ pain, fever and/or elevated markers of infection (WBC, ESR), positive cervical cultures for chlamydia or gonorrhea, and the absence of other cause of RUQ pain (eg, pneumonia, cholecystitis, pyelonephritis, hepatitis) allows a presumptive diagnosis of Fitz-Hugh-Curtis syndrome.

TREATMENT

- Treatment is the same as for PID.

VAGINITIS/VULVOVAGINITIS

Trichomoniasis

A sexually transmitted disease caused by *T vaginalis*, a flagellated protozoan. Women are affected more often than men. It is a frequent cause of vaginitis and an uncommon cause of cervicitis.

SYMPTOMS/EXAMINATION

- Vaginal discharge, perineal itching, dysuria, spotting, and pelvic pain
- Physical examination shows vaginal erythema and a frothy thin malodorous discharge.
- Strawberry cervix characterized by punctate hemorrhages can be seen (see Figure 12.10).
- Half of infected female and most males are asymptomatic. Males usually present as partners of infected female.

DIFFERENTIAL

BV, candidal vaginitis, cervicitis, PID

DIAGNOSIS

- Wet prep microscopy showing motile, pear-shaped, flagellated trichomonads (Figure 12.11) and (if negative) culture or nucleic acid amplification test of vaginal fluid for *T vaginalis*.

TREATMENT

- Oral metronidazole or tinidazole
- Partners need to be treated.

KEY FACT

Wet prep is positive in only 60% of culture proven trichomonas infections.

KEY FACT

Cure rates of vaginal therapy for trichomonas infections are low.

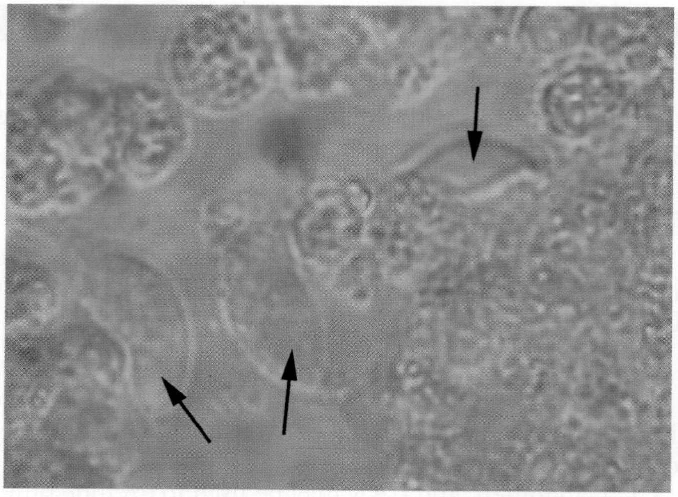

FIGURE 12.11. ***Trichomonas vaginalis*** **(arrows) under high power on wet prep.** (Reproduced with permission from Usatine RP: *The Color Atlas of Family Medicine.* 2nd edition. New York, NY: McGraw-Hill Education; 2013. Photographer: Richard P. Usatine.)

Bacterial Vaginosis

Bacterial vaginosis (BV) is secondary to high concentrations of anaerobic bacteria and *Gardnerella vaginalis* replacing the normal lactobacilli flora. It is the most common cause of vaginal discharge and vaginitis in premenopausal women. Risk factors include sexual activity, douching, and smoking.

KEY FACT

Clue cells = epithelial cells coated by bacteria

Symptoms/Examination

"Fishy smelling" vaginal discharge (accentuated after coitus), itching, and increased discharge.

KEY FACT

Amsel criteria for BV:

At least 3 present:
Gray-white discharge
Vaginal pH > 4.5
Positive whiff test
Clue cells on wet mount

Diagnosis

- Physical examination shows a malodorous gray/white discharge.
- Vaginal pH > 4.5
- Wet mount shows clue cells (Figure 12.12).
- Addition of 10% KOH to a smear of the discharge reveals same fish smell, referred to as a "positive whiff test."

Treatment

- First line is metronidazole PO or intravaginal gel. When prescribing metronidazole, warn patients about the disulfarim-like reaction when co-ingested with alcohol.
- Clindamycin PO or intravaginal suppository/gel is a reasonable alternative.
- Oral therapy is preferred over intravaginal therapy in pregnancy due to the possibility of subclinical upper genital tract infection.

CANDIDA VULVOVAGINITIS

This is caused by *Candida albicans*, which have filamentous forms that penetrate the mucosal surface, causing inflammation and lysis of tissue.

Risk Factors

Diabetes mellitus, HIV, recent antibiotic use, and pregnancy (Table 12.8).

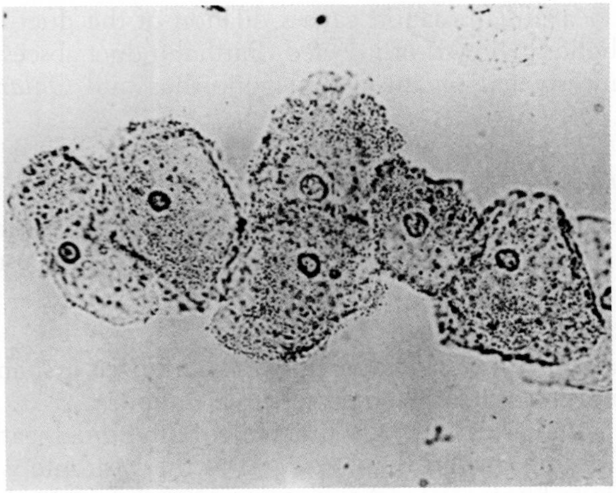

FIGURE 12.12. Clue cells on wet mount in patient with bacterial vaginosis. (Reproduced, with permission, from DeCherney AH, Nathan L, Laufer N, et al. *Current Diagnosis & Treatment: Obstetrics & Gynecology*. 11th ed. New York, NY: McGraw-Hill Education; 2013. Figure 39.9.)

Q

A 50-year-old woman presents to the ED with the third visit in 2 months for *Candida* vulvovaginitis that seems resistant to treatment. What do you want to check?

Symptoms/Examination

- Itching is a significant complaint along with dysuria and dyspareunia.
- Exam shows white "cottage cheese" vaginal discharge along with red/swollen vaginal mucosa and labia.

Diagnosis

- Usually, visualization of the vagina allows a clinical diagnosis.
- Confirm diagnosis based on the presence of pseudohyphae and spores ("spaghetti and meatballs") on wet mount examination with 10% KOH prep.

Treatment

Consists of fluconazole PO or intravaginal antifungals

BARTHOLIN DUCT ABSCESS

Bartholin glands are tiny mucus producing glands located bilaterally at the posterior introitus. They drain through ducts into the vaginal orifice at approximately the 4-o'clock and 8-o'clock positions. Obstruction of the duct

TABLE 12.8. Vaginal Discharge

Discharge	Normal	Candidiasis	Trichomoniasis	Bacterial Vaginosis
Color	Clear/white	White	Green/yellow	Gray/white
pH	< 4.5	< 4.5	> 5.0	> 5.0
Amine odor with KOH	Negative	Negative	Positive	Positive
Wet mount	Epithelial cells, lactobacilli	WBC, spores, pseudohyphae	WBC, motile trichomonads	Few WBCs, clue cells

WBC, white blood cell.

A

Glucose check to rule out underlying diabetes.

opening from local inflammation causes dilation of the duct that can either be sterile (Bartholin duct cyst) or infected (Bartholin duct abscess). *E coli* is the most commonly isolated organism, but gonorrhea and *Chlamydia* are also known causes.

Symptoms/Examination

Pain, tenderness, and dyspareunia are acute symptoms. Surrounding tissue becomes edematous and inflamed. A tender, fluctuant mass is usually palpable.

Treatment

- Primary treatment consists of drainage of the infected cyst/abscess followed by insertion of a Word catheter or marsupialization.
- The Word catheter is a small inflatable bulb-tipped catheter used to develop a fistula from the Bartholin cyst to the vestibule which can take up to 8 weeks to form.
- Incision and drainage alone without use of the Word catheter to keep the wound open is associated with recurrent disease.
- Broad-spectrum antibiotic therapy is warranted **only** when significant cellulitis is present.

Ovarian Torsion

Most cases of ovarian torsion result from a mass or large cyst on the affected ovary or fallopian tube that stretches the pedicle and causes a rotation on its axis. It can, however, occur in the structurally normal ovary (especially in children). Torsion leads to decreased blood flow and ovarian ischemia. The right ovary is more frequently affected.

Symptoms/Examination

- Acute, severe pain with nausea, vomiting, and low-grade fever. Pain may be intermittent and radiate to flank, back, or groin.
- Examination is variable depending on degree of necrosis and size of ovary. Tenderness may be absent and an ovarian mass is not always palpable.

KEY FACT

Torsion can occur in the structurally normal ovary.

Differential

Appendicitis, ruptured ovarian cyst, ovarian tumor, TOA, renal stone, ectopic pregnancy

Diagnosis

- Transvaginal ultrasound with color flow Doppler. Because the ovary has dual blood supply, Doppler flow may be present in the setting of torsion. Additional findings that suggest torsion include:
  - Abnormal anterior location of ovary
  - Increased ovarian size with heterogenous stroma (due to edema)
  - Ovarian mass or cyst (more likely to torse)
- Maintain a high index of suspicion. A consistent story and lack of alternative diagnosis warrant gynecology consultation for consideration of laparoscopy.
- Definitive diagnosis is by direct surgical visualization.

KEY FACT

Dual ovarian blood supply:
Ovarian artery
Uterine artery

Treatment

Surgical detorsion with possible salpingo-oophorectomy if ovary deemed nonviable.

TABLE 12.9. Causes of Primary Amenorrhea With Normal Genital Examination

	Uterus Present	Uterus Absent
Breast development present	Hypothalamic Pituitary Ovarian Uterine	Congenital (uterovaginal agenesis) Androgen insensitivity (testicular feminization)
Breast development absent	Gonadal failure CNS (hypothalamic, pituitary disorders)	17,20-Desmolase deficiency Agonadism 17-Hydroxylase deficiency (46, XY)

Amenorrhea

Defined as absence of menstruation for ≥ 3 months during the reproductive years. This is a symptom and not a diagnosis! It is divided into 2 broad categories:

- **Primary amenorrhea**: Failure of menses by age 16 or within 2 years of full secondary sexual characteristic development; see Table 12.9. This is usually caused by a genetic (eg, hypothalamic hypogonadism) or anatomic abnormality (eg, absence of uterus).
- **Secondary amenorrhea**: Lack of menses for > 3 months in a woman who previously had normal menstruation. Most common cause is pregnancy. Other causes include endocrine pathology (eg, hypothyroidism, pituitary disease) or ovarian disorders (eg, polycystic ovaries, premature ovarian failure).

KEY FACT

Rule out pregnancy as a cause of amennorhea.

Symptoms/Examination

Symptoms and findings vary broadly with the underlying cause of the disease.

Diagnosis

Careful history and physical will help determine which organ is primarily responsible for amenorrhea. Check levels of thyroid-stimulating hormone, luteinizing hormone, follicle-stimulating hormone, prolactin, and estradiol.

Treatment

Management of the amenorrheic patient depends on the individual's desire to ovulate and the etiology of the amenorrhea.

Vaginal Bleeding

One of the most common female chief complains presenting to the ED. See Table 12.10 for common definitions of vaginal bleeding.

Causes

Causes of abnormal vaginal bleeding in nonpregnant, reproductive age females include:

TABLE 12.10. Definitions of Vaginal Bleeding

Abnormal vaginal bleeding	Occurs outside menstrual cycle
Menorrhagia	Menses > 7 d, or > 60-mL blood loss or occurring < every 21 d
Metrorrhagia	Bleeding at irregular times
Menometrorrhagia	Heavy irregular vaginal bleeding
Dysfunctional uterine bleeding	Abnormal vaginal bleeding due to anovulation
Postcoital bleeding	Vaginal bleeding after intercourse suggesting cervical pathology
Postmenopausal bleeding	Any bleeding that occurs > 1 y after cessation of menses, unless on hormone therapy

- **Ovulatory bleeding**: Associated with regular menses; typically a heavy or prolonged bleeding in the otherwise healthy patient that suggests a uterine structural problem such as leiomyoma (fibroid), uterine polyp, or adenomyosis.
- **Anovulatory bleeding**: Also called dysfunctional uterine bleeding. Common in perimenopausal and perimenarchal patients due to unopposed estrogen production. Also seen with polycystic ovary syndrome, obesity, eating disorders, and hyper/hypothyroidism.
- **Bleeding disorders:** Consider von Willebrand disease or other coagulation disorders in the perimenarchal patient with heavy menses or those with frequent bruising and gum bleeding.
- **Extrauterine source:** Cervicitis, vaginal tears, cervical cancer, etc.
- **Medication use:** Especially hormone contraceptive pills/devices or anticoagulants
- **Malignancy**
- **Postmenopausal vaginal bleeding** is most commonly due to atrophy. Other causes include polyps, endometrial hyperplasia, endometrial cancer, and hormonal effect.

KEY FACT

Consider possible sexual abuse in children presenting with vaginal bleeding.

DIAGNOSIS

- Pregnancy test and CBC are needed in most cases of vaginal bleeding. Other laboratory test results should be obtained based on clinical suspicion.
- Vaginal ultrasound can be useful to characterize the uterus and endometrium and determine the presence of leiomyomas (fibroids), tumors, and endometriosis. In stable patients, ultrasound may be deferred to the outpatient setting.
- Gynecology referral for endometrial biopsy should be obtained for women > 35 years with abnormal vaginal bleeding and for women < 35 years with risk factors for endometrial cancer (obesity, chronic anovulation).

KEY FACT

All patients of childbearing age with vaginal bleeding need a pregnancy test.

TREATMENT

- Treatment depends on hemodynamic stability and underlying cause.
- Unstable patients with uterine bleeding require fluid and blood replacement along with emergent OB/GYN consultation for interventions to stop bleeding which may include intrauterine tamponade, D&C, uterine artery embolization, and administration of high-dose IV estrogen and rarely, hysterectomy.

- Stable patients with uterine bleeding can be treated with hormone therapy. Options include high-dose oral estrogen therapy, high-dose oral progestin therapy, and high-dose oral contraceptive therapy. Numerous formulations are available.
- Referral to OB/GYN is warranted for further evaluation of the stable patient.

KEY FACT

Endometrial biopsy is warranted for women >35 years with abnormal vaginal bleeding.

Endometriosis

Disease is defined by the presence of endometrial glands/stroma outside the uterus and seen exclusively in women of reproductive age. The size of the lesions varies from microscopic to large invasive masses that erode into underlying organs and cause extensive adhesions.

Symptoms

- Infertility, dysmenorrhea, dyspareunia
- Pelvic pain or low sacral pain that occurs premenstrually and resolves after the onset of menses is common.

Examination

Pelvic examination may reveal tender nodules in the posterior vaginal fornix and pain with movements of the uterus.

Diagnosis

The diagnosis should be suspected in any woman of reproductive age complaining of pain or infertility. Confirmation requires direct visualization of the implants with laparoscopy or laparotomy.

Treatment

- Treatment is directed based on the woman's desire for future fertility.
- Nonsteroidal anti-inflammatory drugs are the analgesic therapy of choice.
- Hormonal therapy is used to interrupt the cycles of stimulation and bleeding of endometrial tissue.
- Oral contraceptive pills and progestational agents (eg, oral medroxyprogesterone acetate or Depo-Provera IM). Also consider gonadotropin-releasing hormone agonists and antagonists.
- Surgical treatment is indicated in women with infertility or with severe disease or adhesions.

Uterine Leiomyoma

The most common pelvic tumor in women. Arise from the smooth muscle of the myometrium and are benign. More common in African American women. They naturally shrink after menopause.

Symptoms/Examination

- Heavy or prolonged menstrual bleeding, pelvic pain, infertility
- An enlarged and irregularly contoured uterus may be palpated on bimanual examination.

Diagnosis/Treatment

Ultrasound is diagnostic. Treatment depends on degree of symptoms and desire for fertility and ranges from observation to surgical myomectomy or hysterectomy.

REVIEW QUESTIONS

QUESTIONS

1. A 24-year-old woman G1P1 starts to experience profuse vaginal bleeding shortly after vaginal delivery of a full-term baby. What is the next step in managing this patient?
   A. Administer platelets and fresh frozen plasma for presumed disseminated intravascular coagulation.
   B. Obtain ultrasound to look for retained products of conception.
   C. Perform vigorous bimanual massage and administer intravenous (IV) oxytocin.
   D. Give methylergonovine intramuscularly.
2. A 32-year-old woman is brought to the emergency department via emergency medical services actively seizing. Her vitals are as follow: temperature 37.8°C (100°F), HR 120 bpm, BP 205/115 mm Hg, RR 30 breaths/min, and on examination you notice a gravid abdomen with a fundal height of 36 cm. Fetal heart tones are present. What is the next step?
   A. Administer Ativan 2 mg IV.
   B. Emergently deliver the baby in the ED.
   C. Administer magnesium sulfate 4-6 g IV.
   D. Give the patient a loading dose of intravenous phenytoin.
3. A 24-year-old woman G4P3, 34-week pregnant presents to the ED in active labor after she felt a rush of water at home. On examination you see protrusion of the umbilical cord and the baby's foot. What is the next step in managing this patient?
   A. Admit to L+D for further monitoring.
   B. Reduce the prolapsed cord and fetal parts back into the uterus.
   C. Clamp the prolapsed cord, cut it, and attempt delivery.
   D. Elevate the presenting part off the prolapsed cord.
4. You are seeing a 21-year-old woman G1P0 who is 10-week pregnant presenting to the ED complaining of malodorous vaginal discharge. On pelvic examination you confirm a thin white discharge, with a vaginal pH of 6 and a positive whiff test. What therapy should be avoided in this patient?
   A. Metronidazole vaginally
   B. Metronidazole PO
   C. Clindamycin PO
   D. All of the above
5. A patient presents to the ED 2 days postpartum complaining of foul-smelling discharge and abdominal pain. On examination she has a temperature of 38.9°C (102°F), HR 110 bpm, and BP 100/70 mm Hg, and you noticed significant uterine tenderness on examination. Patient most likely had which of the following during delivery?
   A. Premature rupture of membranes
   B. Cesarean section
   C. Internal fetal monitoring
   D. Prolonged labor
6. Which of the following meets criteria for methotrexate administration in ectopic pregnancy?
   A. Ectopic mass = 5 cm
   B. Presence of fetal cardiac activity
   C. Presence of free fluid within the pelvis and high suspicion for rupture
   D. Quantitative β-hCG = 4000 mIU/L
7. A 15-year-old woman presents with acute onset of severe left lower quadrant (LLQ) pain. She is afebrile, mildly tachycardic, and normotensive. On pelvic examination she has no cervical motion tenderness (CMT), no discharge, and has severe left adnexal tenderness. β-hCG is negative. Ultrasound shows an abnormal anterior location of the ovary with increased ovarian size and heterogenous stroma. Doppler flow is present. Which of the following is the most appropriate management?
   A. Computed tomography scan to look for alternative diagnosis
   B. Emergent gynecology consultation for laparoscopy
   C. Pain management and observation
   D. Empiric treatment for pelvic inflammatory disease

ANSWERS

1. **C.** This patient is experiencing early postpartum hemorrhage which can be life threatening. The most common cause is uterine atony which is treated with vigorous bimanual massage and IV oxytocin (10-40 U in 1-L NS). Methylergonovine and prostaglandins are additional treatments that can be used. Maternal resuscitation should occur simultaneously, starting with normal saline fluid boluses and packed red blood cell resuscitation, though massive transfusion protocols should be implemented as needed. Other less common causes of early postpartum hemorrhage include lacerations of the lower genital tract, retained placenta, uterine rupture, and uterine inversion.

2. **C.** This patient has eclampsia given her hypertension and seizures with gestational age > 20 weeks. The initial treatment for eclampsia is the administration of magnesium rather than antiepileptic drugs. The dose of magnesium is 4-6 g IV followed by a 2 g/h gtt. The definite treatment of eclampsia is delivery of the baby, but magnesium should be given first to manage active seizures.

3. **D.** This patient has umbilical cord prolapse, which is life threatening to the fetus. Risk factors include multiparity, premature rupture of membranes, and breech presentation. The mainstay of management is manual elevation of the presenting part off the cord followed by patient transfer to L&D for C-section. Retrograde filling of bladder can also help reduce pressure on the cord. Reduction of the cord or clamping/cutting the cord prior to delivery should not be performed.

4. **A.** This patient has bacterial vaginosis based on the presence of at least 3 of the 4 Amsel criteria: Thin, white discharge, vaginal pH > 4.5, a positive whiff test, and the presence of clue cells on microscopic examination. The recommendation is to treat all symptomatic infections in pregnancy. Topical metronidazole should be avoided in pregnancy because oral treatment is more effective against potential subclinical upper genital tract infection. Both oral clindamycin and metronidazole are indicated. Some clinicians prefer clindamycin over metronidazole, given the possible teratogenic effects of metronidazole in the first trimester, although studies have not found any relationship between metronidazole exposure during the first trimester of pregnancy and birth defects, and the CDC no longer discourages the use of metronidazole in the first trimester.

5. **B.** This patient has postpartum endometritis. The strongest risk factor for postpartum endometritis is cesarean delivery. Premature rupture of membranes, internal fetal monitoring, and prolonged labor are also risk factors, but less likely causes when compared to cesarean delivery. Treatment includes admission and broad-spectrum IV antibiotics.

6. **D.** Methotrexate has replaced surgery for many patients with ectopic pregnancy. The optimal candidates for methotrexate include patients with a β-hCG < 5000 mIU/L, no fetal cardiac activity, and an ectopic mass < 3-4 cm. Contraindications to methotrexate include free peritoneal fluid outside the pelvic cavity, immunodeficiency, active pulmonary disease or peptic ulcer disease, hypersensitivity to methotrexate, coexisting viable intrauterine pregnancy, breast-feeding, and noncompliance risk with posttherapeutic monitoring.

7. **B.** This patient has ovarian torsion and needs urgent laparoscopy in attempt to preserve the ovary. Given the dual blood supply to the ovary, Doppler flow may be present in torsion. Most cases result from a mass or cyst on the affected ovary, but torsion can occur in the structurally normal ovary, especially in children.

CHAPTER 13

Environmental Emergencies

Leah Jacoby, MD

Bites and Stings

MAMMALIAN BITES

The vast majority of mammalian bite wounds seen in the ED are due to domesticated animals. Infecting organisms vary based on the oral flora from the biting animal (Table 13.1).

Wounds With Increased Risk of Infection (High-Risk Wounds)

- Puncture wounds
- Intraoral, hand, below knee, or over joints
- Cat bites > human bites > dog bites
- Immunocompromised (eg, asplenic, alcoholic, diabetic) or elderly patient
- Presence of peripheral vascular disease or prosthetic valve
- Delayed presentations

Diagnosis

- X-ray to rule out foreign body (particularly tooth fragments) or fracture.
- Check blood sugar to see if diabetic.

General Treatment

- Anesthetize, clean and irrigate, and debride devitalized tissue.
- Explore in full flexion and extension for ligamentous or tendon injury.
  - If present, surgical consultation and admission are warranted.

TABLE 13.1. Common Infecting Organisms in Mammalian Bites

Cat	*Pasteurella multocida* *Staphylococcus aureus*
Dog	*Staphylococcus aureus* *Pasteurella multocida* *Bacteroides* sp *Fusobacterium* sp *Capnocytophaga canimorsus*
Human	Polymicrobial *Streptococcus viridans* *S aureus* *Bacteroides* sp *Corynebacterium* sp *Eikenella corrodens* *Fusobacterium* sp
Rodent	*Streptobacillus moniliformis* *Spirillum minus* Other transmitted diseases: Leptospirosis Tularemia Sporotrichosis Plague

TABLE 13.2. Indications for Prophylactic Antibiotics in Mammalian Bites

Cat and human bites
Immunocompromised or elderly patients
Presence of peripheral vascular disease
Presence of prosthetic valve
Deep puncture wounds or extensive crush injuries
Intraoral, hand, below knee, or joint wounds
Delayed presentation

- Tetanus prophylaxis.
- Consider rabies prophylaxis (animal bites).
- No evidence for infection:
  - Okay to close wound **unless** high-risk wound.
  - Give antibiotic prophylaxis if high-risk wound (Table 13.2).
- Evidence of infection:
  - Admit for intravenous (IV) antibiotics if high-risk wound or patient, otherwise treat with oral antibiotics.
- Arrange follow-up in 48 hours for discharged patients.

Human Bites

Infections are commonly **polymicrobial**.

- *Streptococcus viridans*.
- *Staphylococcus aureus*.
- *Bacteroides* sp.
- *Corynebacterium* sp.
- ***Eikenella corrodens*** (a gram-negative rod found in dental plaque).
- *Fusobacterium* sp.
- Other transmitted infections include syphilis and herpes.
- HIV and hepatitis transmission should be considered if exposure to blood occurred.

A special concern is the closed-fist injury ("fight bite"), which is associated with joint infection, osteomyelitis, and tenosynovitis.

Treatment

- General treatment, as given earlier.
- Antibiotic of choice for prophylaxis = amoxicillin/clavulanate (ciprofloxacin + metronidazole or clindamycin + TMP-SMX for penicillin [PCN]-allergic).
- Closed-fist injury requires aggressive irrigation and wound exploration. If there is evidence for deeper structure involvement, surgical consultation and admission are indicated.
- Consider human immunodeficiency virus (HIV) and hepatitis B prophylaxis.

Cat Bites

The majority of untreated cat bites become infected.

Common organisms:

- ***Pasteurella multocida***: A highly virulent gram-negative nonmotile coccobacillus; a rapidly progressive cellulitis develops within 24 hours.
- The other common organism is *S aureus*.

Q

A 31-year-old man presents to the emergency department (ED) for evaluation of hand pain after an altercation outside a bar. On examination there is pain, swelling, and a laceration present over the third metacarpal phalangeal joint. The extensor tendon sheath is visible through the wound. What is the risk if this injury is left untreated?

KEY FACT

All wounds at high risk for infection should be left open and treated with antibiotic prophylaxis.

KEY FACT

Most human bite wound infections are polymicrobial, including gram-positive, gram-negative, and anaerobic organisms.

KEY FACT

Rapid onset of infection < 24 hours after a cat bite = *P multocida*

A

This patient has sustained a "fight bite" or closed-fist injury from striking a person's tooth with a closed fist. If left untreated, tenosynovitis, osteomyelitis, and septic arthritis can occur, requiring surgical intervention.

KEY FACT

All cat bite wounds should receive antibiotic prophylaxis.

KEY FACT

Gangrenous wound or overwhelming sepsis following dog bite = *C canimorsus*

KEY FACT

Antibiotic prophylaxis of choice for bite wounds = amoxicillin/clavulanate

KEY FACT

Rat-bite fever is associated with brain, myocardial, and soft-tissue abscesses.

TREATMENT

- General treatment, as given earlier.
- Most wounds are puncture wounds and should be left open.
- Antibiotic prophylaxis is recommended for **all** cat bite wounds: Amoxicillin/clavulanate or doxycycline (Clindamycin + TMP-SMX or clindamycin + ciprofloxacin in PCN-allergic) (usually a 3-5 day treatment course for prophylaxis).
- *P multocida* is highly sensitive to PCN.

Dog Bites

Approximately 5%-10% of dog bites become infected.

Common organisms:
- *S aureus*
- *P multocida*
- *Bacteroides* sp
- *Fusobacterium* sp
- ***Capnocytophaga canimorsus***
  - Gram-negative rod → overwhelming sepsis, disseminated intravascular coagulation (DIC), and cutaneous gangrene at bite site. Treatment is PCN or a cephalosporin.

TREATMENT

- General treatment, as given earlier
- Antibiotic prophylaxis of choice: Amoxicillin/clavulanate, doxycycline (clindamycin + TMP-SMX or clindamycin + ciprofloxacin in PCN-allergic)

Rodent Bites

Usually these are small puncture wounds at low-risk for local wound infection.
- Rat-bite fever
  - Results from infection with *Streptobacillus moniliformis* and *Spirillum minus*

SYMPTOMS/EXAMINATION

- Abrupt onset of fevers/chills, headache, and subsequent rash 1-3 days after the bite
- Associated with brain, myocardial, and soft-tissue abscesses

TREATMENT

PCN or tetracycline

Multiple other diseases can be transmitted via rodent bites including leptospirosis, tularemia, sporotrichosis, and plague. Hantavirus pulmonary syndrome can be transmitted by bites or inhalation of aerosolized viral material. It is characterized by fever, bilateral pulmonary infiltrates, respiratory collapse, and is usually fatal.

SPIDER BITES

Black Widow Spider (*Latrodectus* sp)

The black widow spider can be found throughout the United States (except Alaska) and Southern Canada in woodpiles, sheds, barns, and outhouses. It is classically identified by a yellow-red hourglass shape on its belly (Figure 13.1). The venom is a neurotoxin.

MECHANISM OF TOXICITY

Envenomation → release of acetylcholine and norepinephrine at nerve terminals → muscle cramping and systemic effects.

SYMPTOMS/EXAMINATION

- Bite site: Target lesion with local redness and pain. Sometimes bite site cannot be seen.
- Prominent muscle cramping and pain most notably of abdominal, back, and leg muscles, starting locally and then progressing diffusely.
- Tachycardia, hypertension.
- Diaphoresis.
- Nausea/vomiting.
- Symptoms may wax and wane, but generally disappear over 2-3 days.
- Can cause cardiac failure and respiratory collapse in children.

TREATMENT

- Local wound care.
- Tetanus prophylaxis.
- **Symptomatic treatment** is the mainstay of therapy.
  - **Opioid analgesia**
  - **Benzodiazepines** to reduce muscle spasm
  - Antihypertensives as needed (nitroprusside = agent of choice)
- **Black widow antivenom** is indicated if severe symptoms or high-risk patient (Table 13.3).
  - Antivenom is derived from horse serum; therefore, administer a test dose first; risk of anaphylaxis immediately and serum sickness at 7-10 days.

Brown Recluse Spider (*Loxosceles Reclusa*)

The brown recluse spider is identified by the brown violin shape on its cephalothorax ("**fiddle back**") (Figure 13.2). It is found primarily under rocks, woodpiles, and in attics in the southern Midwestern United States (from central Texas to Georgia and north to Nebraska and Ohio).

MECHANISM OF TOXICITY

Venom contains a variety of cytotoxic enzymes → local **necrotic wound** and (rarely) systemic toxicity.

TABLE 13.3. Indications for Antivenom in Black Widow Spider Bite

Children and elderly patients
Severe pain despite symptomatic treatment
Severe envenomation (seizures, uncontrolled HTN, respiratory failure)
Significant comorbidities (HTN, atherosclerotic disease)
Pregnancy

HTN, hypertension.

Q

A 30-year-old man presents to the ED with severe abdominal, back, and leg muscle cramping after being "bit by a spider" 2 hours earlier while cleaning his basement. On examination, he appears anxious, sweaty, and is mildly hypertensive. What is the most definitive treatment for this patient?

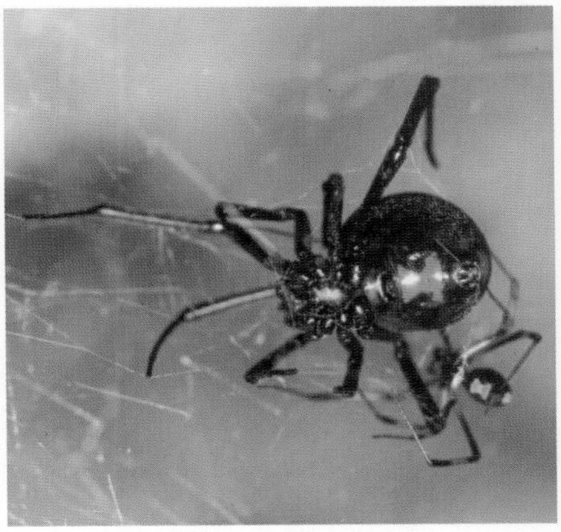

FIGURE 13.1. Black widow spider (Latrodectus mactans) with offspring. Note characteristic hourglass marking on abdomen. (Reproduced, with permission, from Knoop KJ, Storrow AB, Stack LB, and Thurman RJ. *Atlas of Emergency Medicine*. 3rd ed. New York, NY: McGraw-Hill; 2010. Figure 16.42. Photographer: Lawrence B. Stack, MD.)

KEY FACT

Black widow spider envenomation → severe cramping of abdominal, back, and leg muscles.

For black widow bites, symptomatic treatment with opioids and benzodiazepines is the mainstay of therapy.

A

This patient has likely been bitten by a black widow spider. Black widow spider venom is a neurotoxin that causes release of acetylcholine and norepinephrine at nerve terminals. Symptoms should be controlled with opioids and benzodiazepines. If his symptoms become severe or he has hemodynamic instability, he should also be treated with black widow spider antivenom.

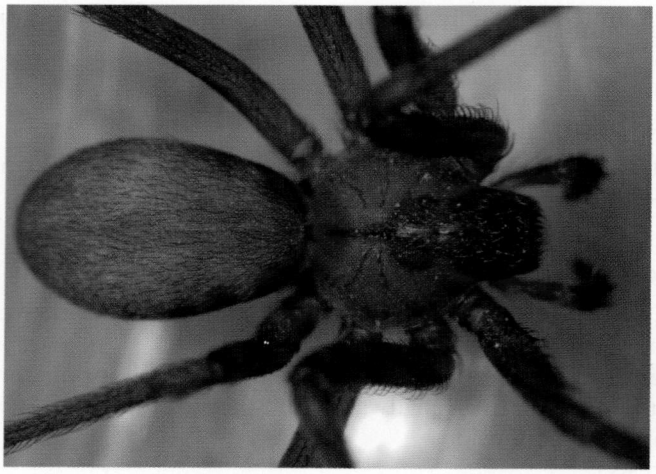

FIGURE 13.2. Fiddle back marking. A close-up look at the characteristic fiddle back marking of the brown recluse spider. (Reproduced, with permission, from Knoop KJ, Stack LB, Storrow AB. *Atlas of Emergency Medicine*. 3rd ed. New York, NY: McGraw-Hill; 2010. Figure 16.46. Photographer: R. Jason Thurman, MD.)

Symptoms/Examination

- The initial bite is **painless** and causes a localized red lesion that usually heals.
- If severe:
  - A target lesion or pustule forms.
  - Bullae and necrotic tissue develop over 3-4 days → eschar formation.
  - Systemic effects (in 24-72 hours) with fevers, chills, nausea/vomiting.
  - Hemolysis, seizures, renal failure, DIC, and pulmonary edema are possible.

Treatment

- Supportive therapy as needed.
- Local wound care and tetanus prophylaxis.
- An antivenom is **not** available in the United States.
- Nitroglycerin, phentolamine, heparin, hyperbaric O_2, cyproheptadine, and steroids have all been used but show no clear evidence for efficacy.
- **Dapsone** (a leukocyte esterase inhibitor) is still recommended in some texts, but has limited benefit and is associated with hemolysis (in patients with G6PD) and methemoglobinemia.
- **Delayed** (**not early**) excision, debridement, and possible skin grafting.

KEY FACT

Brown recluse spider bite wounds should undergo delayed excision and debridement.

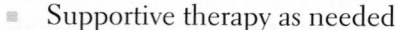

HYMENOPTERA STINGS

The class hymenoptera include the following stinging insects:

- **Bees**
- **Wasps**
- Hornets
- Yellow jackets
- **Fire ants**

Bees

- Barbed stingers → stinger remains in victim (one sting/bee).
- The process kills the bee.
- Killer bees have similar toxin potency but attack in large numbers → greater overall venom load.
- Venom contains proteins and enzymes (histamine, bradykinin, etc).
- Honeybee venom can induce a larger histamine release and cause more severe symptoms.

Wasps

- Nonbarbed stinger → can sting multiple times
- Similar venom to bees

Fire ants

- Small and light reddish-brown to brown
- Contain unique alkaloid venom

In general, three types of reactions are possible:

1. **Local toxic reaction**
2. **Allergic reaction**
3. **Serum sickness**

Mechanism of Toxicity

- Local reaction to venom
- Exposure to venom in sensitized individual → mast cell degranulation → allergic reaction; each species has unique antigens
- Development of delayed (type III) immune response → systemic symptoms and rash (serum sickness)

Symptoms/Examination

- Local reaction:
  - Bees and wasps: Irritation, itching, and redness at sting site that may last for 2-3 days
  - Fire ants: Intense burning, papules that may turn to sterile pustules in 24 hours
- Allergic reaction: Ranging from diffuse pruritus and urticaria to anaphylaxis; vast majority occur within 30 minutes
- Serum sickness: Onset of symptoms 7-10 days after the sting with fever, arthralgias, malaise (flulike symptoms), and rash (most commonly angioedema/urticaria)

Treatment

- Local wound care and tetanus prophylaxis.
- Remove stingers by fastest means possible to reduce venom exposure, preferably by scraping gently parallel to the skin, taking care not to squeeze the venom sac.
- Oral antihistamine.
- Treat anaphylaxis and provide Rx for EpiPen (up to 60% recurrence with future exposure).

BARK SCORPION STINGS

Most US scorpion species are not highly toxic and stings result in local pain only. Pancreatitis is associated with one species (*Tityus trinitatis*).

KEY FACT

Three possible reactions to hymenoptera envenomation:

1. **Local toxic reaction**
2. **Allergic reaction**
3. **Serum sickness**

KEY FACT

Serum sickness is a delayed immune response occurring 7-10 days after antigen exposure.

The bark scorpion (*Centruroides sculpturatus*), however, can cause systemic toxicity. Children < 5 years old have a higher mortality rate than adults. It is found in the southwestern United States.

> **KEY FACT**
>
> Serious bark scorpion envenomations are more common in children.

Mechanism of Toxicity

Envenomation → ↑ Na^+ channel permeability → ↑ depolarization → sympathetic, parasympathetic, and neuromuscular activation

Symptoms/Examination

> **KEY FACT**
>
> Bark scorpion envenomation → roving eye movements, muscle spasms, and excessive secretions

- Sensitivity to touch at site
- Numbness, tingling
- Blurred vision or **roving eye movements**
- Muscle spasms or weakness
- Hyperthermia
- Anxiety, nausea/vomiting
- Respiratory distress with **excessive secretions**
- May cause cardiopulmonary arrest

Treatment

> **KEY FACT**
>
> Atropine may be needed to treat excessive secretions.

- Local wound care and tetanus prophylaxis.
- Symptomatic treatment with:
  - **Opioids** for muscle pain
  - **Benzodiazepines** for neuromuscular symptoms
  - **Atropine** for excessive secretions
- Scorpion antivenom is available only in Arizona; indicated in severe bark scorpion envenomation.

Marine Animal Envenomations

Can be divided into three groups based on mechanism of venom delivery:

1. **Stingers**
2. **Nematocysts**
3. **Bites**

STINGERS

> **KEY FACT**
>
> Marine animals with a stinger apparatus include stingrays, sea urchins, cone shells, and venomous fish.

Marine animals with specialized sting apparatus include (Table 13.4):

- Stingrays
- Venomous fish (catfish, zebra fish, scorpion fish, stonefish)
- Sea urchins
- Cone shells

Mechanism of Toxicity

Special stinger apparatus punctures skin and introduces venom → severe local symptoms and (rarely) systemic effects

Symptoms/Examination

- Vary with species.
- Most commonly, intense local pain.
- Systemic symptoms may include nausea/vomiting, hypotension, muscle cramps, paralysis, and cardiac arrest.

TABLE 13.4. Marine Animals That Sting

MARINE ANIMAL	VENOM DELIVERY APPARATUS
Stingrays	Barbed stinger at end of whip-like tail
Bony fish: Catfish, zebra fish (eg, lionfish), scorpion fish, stonefish	Spines located on their fins
Sea urchins	Toxin-coated spines
Cone shells	Venom gland and teeth at end of proboscis

TREATMENT

- Supportive therapy.
- Remove spines and stinger (use x-ray to verify).
- **Immediately immerse wound in hot water** (45°C for 90 minutes or until pain is relieved as this breaks down venom).
- Aggressive cleaning.
- Tetanus prophylaxis.
- Consider antibiotics if deep puncture wound or high-risk patient.
- Antivenom exists for stonefish toxicity.

NEMATOCYSTS

Marine animals with nematocysts include:

- Jellyfish (Cnidaria)
- Portuguese man-of-war
- Corals
- Fire corals
- Sea anemones
- Sea wasp (*Chironex fleckeri*, aka box jellyfish)

MECHANISM OF TOXICITY

Physical contact or osmotic gradient → discharge of nematocysts ("spring loaded with venom") → local and (rarely) systemic symptoms

SYMPTOMS/EXAMINATION

- Vary with species.
- Most commonly, intense local pain.
- Systemic symptoms may include nausea and vomiting, tachycardia, hypertension, respiratory paralysis, and cardiac arrest.

TREATMENT

- **Immerse in 5% acetic acid (vinegar)** to inactivate nematocysts. Alternatives include immersion in rubbing alcohol (isopropyl 40%) or covering with slurry of baking soda.
- No fresh or tap water rinsing because this causes nematocysts to discharge via osmotic gradient.
- If the nematocyst is still embedded in the skin, apply flour or shaving cream and shave.

Q

A 50-year-old woman presents to the ED complaining of severe pain to her right forearm 10 minutes after being stung by a zebra fish while cleaning her saltwater aquarium. Her vitals are normal. Physical examination shows a small puncture wound to the forearm with mild surrounding swelling. What can you do to inactivate the venom?

KEY FACT

Marine animals with nematocysts include jellyfish, the Portuguese man-of-war, fire corals, and sea anemones.

KEY FACT

Stinger injury → Immerse in hot water

Nematocyst injury → Immerse in acetic acid

- Provide adequate analgesia.
- Treat any allergic reaction.
- Tetanus prophylaxis.
- **Antivenom is available for severe box-jellyfish sting.**

Zebra fish are venomous fish that cause envenomation through a specialized sting apparatus. Symptoms will primarily consist of intense local pain. The venom can be inactivated by immersing the wound in hot (45°C [113°F]) water for 90 minutes or until the pain subsides.

OCTOPUS BITES

All octopuses are venomous; only one subgroup, blue-ringed octopuses (Hapalochlaena maculosus), has been documented as lethal to humans.

KEY FACT

Octopus bites can cause flaccid paralysis and respiratory failure via tetrodotoxin.

MECHANISM OF TOXICITY

Venom contains tetrodotoxin → inhibition of voltage-gated Na^+ channels → paralysis/respiratory failure.

SYMPTOMS/EXAMINATION

- Bites are typically small and may initially be painless; local erythema may be present.
- Paresthesias, flaccid paralysis.
- Respiratory failure.

TREATMENT

- Supportive therapy and local wound care; survival likely if supported through paralysis.
- No known antivenom exists.

Reptile Envenomations

There are five families of venomous snakes worldwide. Two of these families, Viperidae (subfamily Crotalidae) and Elapidae, cause the majority of envenomations in the United States. Envenomations may be characterized by either local toxicity ± coagulopathy or neurotoxicity.

VIPERIDAE FAMILY

Envenomation is characterized by local tissue toxicity and, less commonly, systemic effects. Approximately 25% of bites with fang marks are "dry" bites.

The Viperidae are the largest family of venomous snakes in the world and are characterized by:

- **Pit or depression** (heat-sensitive thermoreceptor) **between the eye and nostril** on either side of head
- Vertical or elliptical pupils
- Triangular-shaped head
- Retractable fangs

Viperidae family includes:

- Rattlesnakes (eg, Mojave, diamondback) (See Figure 13.3.)
- Copperheads
- Water moccasin (aka cottonmouth)

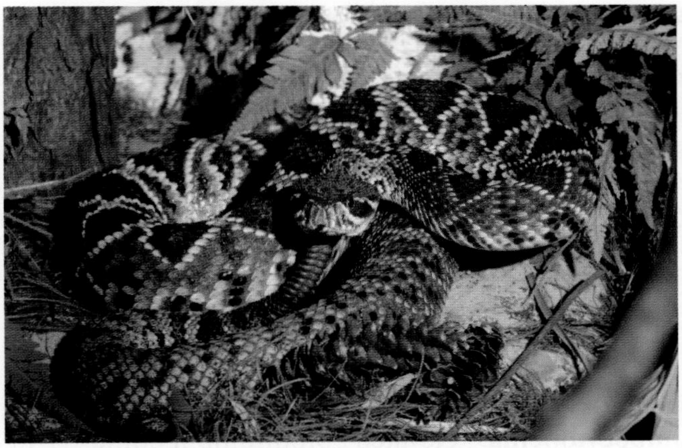

FIGURE 13.3. Eastern diamondback rattlesnake. The eastern diamondback is the largest US rattlesnake and has a characteristic diamond-shaped pattern on its dorsal aspect. Note the triangular head, which is characteristic of pit vipers. (Reproduced, with permission, from Knoop KJ, Stack LB, Storrow AB. *Atlas of Emergency Medicine*. 3rd ed. New York, NY: McGraw-Hill; 2010. Figure 16.32. Photographer: R. Jason Thurman, MD.)

Q

A 30-year-old man presents to the ED after sustaining a snake bite while on a hunting trip in North Carolina. The patient complains of some localized paresthesias and swelling around a small puncture wound to his left leg, which has been progressively spreading up his leg over the past few hours. Does this patient need antivenom?

Mechanism of Toxicity

The venom has digestive enzymes and proteins → local tissue edema and toxicity and (less commonly) systemic toxicity and coagulopathy. Venom concentrations vary with species.

KEY FACT

Most US snakebites are inflicted by pit vipers (rattlesnakes, cottonmouths, copperheads).

Symptoms/Examination

- Local tissue toxicity (Figure 13.4)
  - **Pain** (within 15-30 minutes)
  - Swelling (may be marked, but compartment syndrome is rare)
  - Local petechiae or ecchymosis
  - Bullae (may be hemorrhagic)
- Systemic toxicity
  - Oral paresthesias and metallic taste
  - Fasciculations
  - Tachycardia and hypotension
  - Anaphylaxis

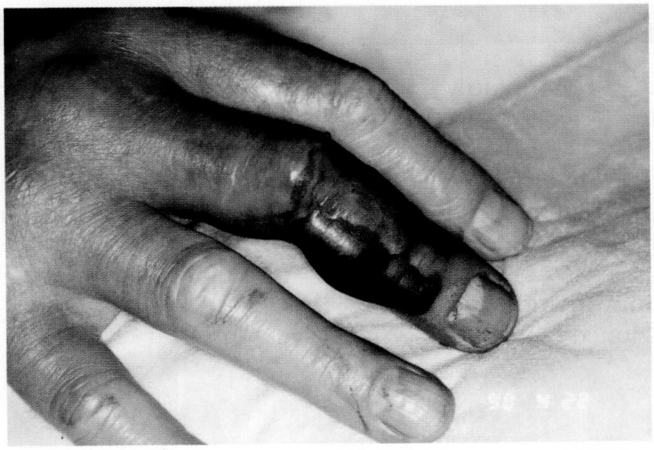

FIGURE 13.4. Local toxicity from rattlesnake envenomation. (Reproduced, with permission, from Knoop KJ, Stack LB, Storrow AB. *Atlas of Emergency Medicine*. 2nd ed. New York, NY: McGraw-Hill; 2002:528. Figure 16.37. Photographer: Sean P. Bush, MD.)

A

Yes. Progressive spreading of erythema proximally is an indication for the antivenom (CroFab). Most US snakebites are inflicted by pit vipers, and their venom can cause local tissue necrosis, systemic toxicity, and coagulopathies. If there is concern for an eastern coral snake bite, antivenom should be given even if the patient is asymptomatic because it can cause respiratory paralysis.

KEY FACT

Viperidae envenomation → marked local tissue toxicity, minimal systemic effects

TABLE 13.5. Indications for Antivenom in Snake Envenomations

Severe localized pain or throbbing
Moderate local edema and/or erythema
Progressive spreading of erythema proximally
Any coagulopathy
Any systemic symptoms
Concern for compartment syndrome
All eastern coral snake bites

- Coagulopathy
  - **Thrombocytopenia**, elevated prothrombin time (PT), decreased fibrinogen

TREATMENT

- Prehospital:
  - Immobilize extremity in neutral position.
  - No incision and suction (no benefit).
  - No tourniquet.
  - Minimize physical activity, if possible, but seek medical care immediately even if it means hiking out of deep wilderness.
  - Mark leading edge of tenderness/swelling to follow progression.
- Aggressive supportive care, wound care, tetanus prophylaxis.
  - Prophylactic antibiotics are **not** indicated.
  - Correct coagulopathy as needed.
- Elevate extremity and immobilize.
- Treat anaphylaxis aggressively.
- **Antivenom.**
  - A newer sheep-derived antivenom (CroFab) is available (less antigenic than the polyvalent horse serum antivenom).
  - Watch closely for **allergic reaction**.
  - Indications include severe local effects or systemic illness (Table 13.5).
  - Serum sickness can sometimes occur following administration.
- Avoid fasciotomy, which likely causes more harm than good.

ELAPIDAE FAMILY

KEY FACT

Elapidae envenomation → marked systemic neurotoxicity, minimal local reaction

Coral snakes are primarily found in the southeastern and southwestern United States.

In the United States, Elapidae are characterized by red/yellow/black bands with red bands touching yellow bands. This does not hold true for other parts of the world.

KEY FACT

Pattern of bands on poisonous coral snakes vs nonpoisonous milk and king snakes (applies to the United States only): "Red on yellow, kill a fellow" "Red on black, venom lack."

Elapidae family includes:

- Corals (United States)
- Cobras
- Kraits
- Mambas

MECHANISM OF TOXICITY

Coral snake venom → irreversibly binds acetylcholine receptors → systemic toxicity.

Symptoms/Examination

- Minimal local reaction
- Weakness, numbness, fasciculations, tremor
- Diplopia and bulbar palsies with slurred speech, dysphagia
- **Respiratory paralysis** (immediate cause of death)

Treatment

- Prehospital treatment similar to Viperidae envenomation, as given previously.
- Aggressive supportive care, wound care, tetanus prophylaxis.
- **No** prophylactic antibiotics.
- **Antivenom** (see Table 13.5).
  - For all eastern coral snake bites (even if asymptomatic!)
  - Otherwise, if any systemic symptoms
  - No antivenom available for Arizona coral snake (less toxic)
  - A horse-serum antivenom—administer test dose and watch for allergic reactions
- All coral snake bites require admission for observation.

> **KEY FACT**
>
> Respiratory-muscle paralysis is the immediate cause of death in most coral snake envenomations.

LIZARD BITES

The Mexican beaded lizard and the Gila monster are venomous lizards. Approximately 70% of their bites are complicated by envenomation.

Mechanisms of Toxicity

- Venom is delivered by glands in the lower jaw into the laceration created by the teeth → local and (rarely) systemic effects.
- The lizard's teeth may break and be left in the wound as a foreign body and cause infection.

Symptoms/Examination

- Crush/puncture wounds with local erythema, ecchymosis, and severe pain
- Systemic effects: Weakness, hypotension, and diaphoresis
- Progressive edema, lymphadenopathy, angioedema

Treatment

- Supportive therapy.
- Remove animal if still attached and obtain x-ray to identify any foreign body/retained teeth.
- Irrigate copiously; consider antibiotics depending on degree of tissue destruction.
- Tetanus prophylaxis.

Heat-Related Illness

Heat-related illness is a continuum of disease extending from minor heat illness to heat exhaustion and heat stroke.

Mechanisms of Heat Loss/Gain

- **Conduction**: Direct physical contact with another surface → heat loss or gain (eg, ice packs, heating pad)
- **Convection**: Heat transfer via circulating air or water molecules (eg, wind chill)

TABLE 13.6. Risk Factors for Heat Illness

Increased Heat Production	Decreased Heat Loss	Impaired Mobility
Thyroid storm	High ambient temperature and humidity	Infants and young children
Seizures	Infants	Physical or mental impairment
Severe agitation	Advanced age	Acute CNS process
Exercise	Volume depletion	Alcoholism
Acute toxicological process	Impaired cardiac function	Tranquilizer/sedative use
Neuroleptic malignant syndrome	Skin conditions	Elderly or severely disabled
Malignant hyperthermia	Medications:	
	Anticholinergics	
	Neuroleptics	
	β-Blockers	
	Diuretics	
	Phenothiazines	
	Ca^{2+} channel blockers	
	Amphetamines	
	MAO inhibitors	

CNS, central nervous system; MOI, monoamine oxidase.

- **Radiation**: Heat transfer by electromagnetic waves (eg, heat from the sun, poor insulation in cold environment)
- **Evaporation**: Heat transfer as water is vaporized (eg, sweating)

KEY FACT

What is the difference between hyperthermia and fever? Hyperthermia = hypothalamus overwhelmed by heat production. Fever = ↑ hypothalamic set point from circulating cytokines.

Pathophysiology

- The **anterior hypothalamus** is the body's thermostat and regulates body temperature.
- ↑ Core body temperature → peripheral vasodilation (to dissipate heat via convection) → perspiration and respiration (for evaporative heat loss).
- Acclimatization to hot environment = earlier and greater sweating, more dilute sweat. Occurs over a period of 1-2 weeks; mediated by aldosterone.

Risk factors for heat illness can be divided into three groups (Table 13.6):

- Increased heat production
- Decreased heat loss
- Impaired ability to move to a cool environment

Malignant hyperthermia deserves special mention. It is due to a genetic instability of skeletal muscle that allows for excessive calcium release in the muscle cell when exposed to certain anesthetic agents (including succinylcholine) → muscle rigidity and profound hyperthermia. Can be treated with dantrolene.

Prevention of Heat Illness

- Keep hydrated (drink solutions that replete electrolytes).
- Wear loose, light-colored clothing.
- Stay indoors with air conditioning on hot and humid days.

MINOR HEAT ILLNESS

- **Heat rash (miliaria rubra)**: "Prickly heat" due to blocked sweat pores.
- **Heat cramps**: These are painful contractions of large muscles that occur AFTER exertion 2° to relative hyponatremia. Individuals replace evaporative losses by drinking hypotonic fluids such as free water without replacing salt. Measured electrolytes are often normal. It is usually self-limited; treatment is supportive.
- **Heat edema**: Secondary to peripheral vasodilation and orthostatic pooling of blood.
- **Heat tetany**: Carpal–pedal spasm due to hyperventilation and ↓ P_{CO_2}.
- **Heat syncope**: Syncope during heat stress 2° to peripheral vasodilation in the setting of dehydration.

HEAT EXHAUSTION

This is the most common form of heat-related illness. It is characterized by volume and/or salt depletion under conditions of heat stress. **Mental status is normal**.

Symptoms/Examination

- Dizziness, weakness, irritability.
- Headache.
- Perspiration.
- Nausea and vomiting.
- Core temperature is typically normal, but may be elevated (38°C-40°C).

Diagnosis

- Based on clinical presentation.
- Electrolytes **may** be abnormal: Hyponatremia, hypochloremia, and elevated blood urea nitrogen (BUN).
- Liver function tests (LFTs) are normal.

Treatment

Remove patient from heat source and replete fluids with electrolyte solutions (oral or intravenous, depending on severity).

HEAT STROKE

Heat stroke is a severe form of heat injury with a high mortality rate in which homeostatic thermoregulatory mechanisms fail, leading to hyperthermia and multisystem organ dysfunction.

It is historically classified as **classic** or **exertional**:

- Classic heatstroke: Elderly or debilitated patients without access to air conditioning; sweating is often absent; may be on medications that affect heat dissipation.
- Exertional heatstroke: Younger individuals exercising in a hot environment.

This classification has no clinical bearing because the treatment is the same.

Symptoms/Examination

- **Altered mental status and central nervous system (CNS) dysfunction**
- Possible seizure

Q

A 2-year-old boy is brought to your ED after being found unconscious in his car seat. His mother left him in the locked car while shopping. His field blood sugar is normal. His rectal temperature on arrival is 105°F (40.6°C). What is the preferred mechanism to rapidly lower this child's core temperature while still allowing for monitoring of vital signs?

KEY FACT

Heat stroke = Hyperthermia with CNS dysfunction

A

This child has sustained heat stroke. Rapid lowering of his core body temperature is essential for a good neurologic outcome. Many cooling techniques are available. Direct immersion in an ice water bath is most rapid but often logistically complicated in a critically ill patient. Evaporative technique using cold water sprayed on the patient's skin with a fan blowing on the patient allows for access to the patient.

KEY FACT

Hepatic damage is nearly always present in heat stroke.

KEY FACT

Antipyretics are **not** effective (and may be harmful) in treatment of heat stroke!

- Anhidrosis: Hot/dry skin (not reliable)
- Core body temperature usually > 40.5°C rectal (may be lower)
- Jaundice 24-72 hours later
- Cardiovascular dysfunction: Hypotension, pulmonary edema

Diagnosis

- Based on clinical presentation.
- Marked elevation of aspartate aminotransferase (AST)/alanine transaminase (ALT) is expected with peak in 24-72 hours. Complete recovery is expected.
- Renal injury is common and may be due to volume depletion, direct thermal injury, or rhabdomyolysis.
- Fluid, electrolyte, and hematologic disorders vary.

Treatment

- Supportive therapy with continuous temperature monitoring.
- Correct electrolyte imbalances.
- **Rapid cooling** (within 1 hour) to core temperature of 39°C-40°C. Remove clothing and initiate either:
  - **Evaporative cooling** (moisten skin with tepid water and fan skin with warm air) **or**
  - **Cold water immersion** (downside = less access to patient)
- Adjuncts: Include ice packs to groin, axillae, and neck and cooling blanket.
- Administer IV benzodiazepines (or paralysis) to prevent shivering (which generates heat); treat seizures.
- If refractory, consider invasive methods including gastric, pleural, or bladder lavage.
- IV fluids to central venous pressure (CVP) of 12 cm H_2O or urine output = 0.5 mL/kg/h. Fluid requirements vary with underlying cause and can worsen underlying pulmonary edema from heatstroke.
- Dopamine for persistent hypotension despite adequate fluid resuscitation.
- Dantrolene: If suspected malignant hyperthermia.
- **Avoid:**
  - Antipyretics—**not** effective and may be harmful!
  - Prophylactic steroids—**not** effective
  - Norepinephrine—causes vasoconstriction and decreases cutaneous heat exchange
- Poor prognostic indicators:
  - Coma
  - AST > 1000 IU/L
  - Delay in rapid cooling (morbidity and mortality are directly related to the duration of hyperthermia)
  - DIC
  - Hypotension
  - Renal failure in < 48 hours
  - Lactic acidosis

Complications

- Acute respiratory distress syndrome (ARDS), electrolyte abnormalities, renal failure, rhabdomyolysis, hepatic injury, DIC.
- If left untreated, cerebral edema and multisystem organ failure will develop.

TABLE 13.7. Mechanisms of Heat Loss/Gain

Conduction	Direct physical contact with another surface → heat loss or gain (eg, ice packs, heating pad)
Convection	Heat transfer via circulating air or water molecules (eg, wind chill)
Radiation	Heat transfer by electromagnetic waves (eg, poor insulation in cold environment)
Evaporation	Heat transfer as water is vaporized (eg, sweating, breathing)

Q

A 60-year-old homeless man presents to your ED after walking > 3 miles in snow. He is complaining of numbness and swelling to both feet. On examination, the patient has diffuse erythema, edema, and both clear and hemorrhagic blisters affecting the toes on bilateral feet. How will you treat this man's feet?

Cold-Related Injuries

There are four physiologic mechanisms of heat loss/gain (Table 13.7). Radiation is responsible for the majority of **normal** heat loss.

PATHOPHYSIOLOGY

- ↓ Core body temperature → peripheral vasoconstriction (to decrease convection) and ↓ HR (to decrease blood flow to periphery) → peripheral ischemia and cold injury
- Risk factors include: Extremes of age, homelessness, altered mental status, substance abuse, nicotine use, peripheral vascular disease, atherosclerosis, and diabetes

CHILBLAINS

Chilblains (pernio) is a mild tissue injury from repetitive exposure to dry cold at **nonfreezing** temperatures. It characteristically involves the dorsum of hands and feet, but may also involve face, ears, and thighs. Raynaud phenomenon carries a high risk of chilblains.

SYMPTOMS/EXAMINATION

- Painful/inflamed skin lesions that are pruritic and erythematous.
- May evolve to plaques, blue nodules, and ulcerations.
- Lesions develop 12-24 hours after exposure.

TREATMENT

- Rewarming and symptomatic treatment

TRENCH FOOT (IMMERSION FOOT)

Trench foot, a nonfreezing injury, occurs with exposure to wet cold at freezing temperatures (0°C-10°C) over several hours to days. (Figure 13.5)

SYMPTOMS/EXAMINATION

- Before rewarming (**prehyperemic stage**): Feet appear cold, mottled, and pale
- After rewarming (**hyperemic stage**): Feet are red, painful, and swollen

TREATMENT

- Carefully wash and dry feet, then wrap with warm clothing.
- Elevate feet.
- Non–weight bearing until improved.

A

Once there is no risk of refreezing, rapidly warm affected areas (40°C water). With frostbite, damaged tissue releases arachidonic acid breakdown products (prostaglandins and thromboxane). These released products promote platelet aggregation, leading to thrombosis and ischemia. Blisters should be left intact or sterilely aspirated. Avoid early debridement of tissue.

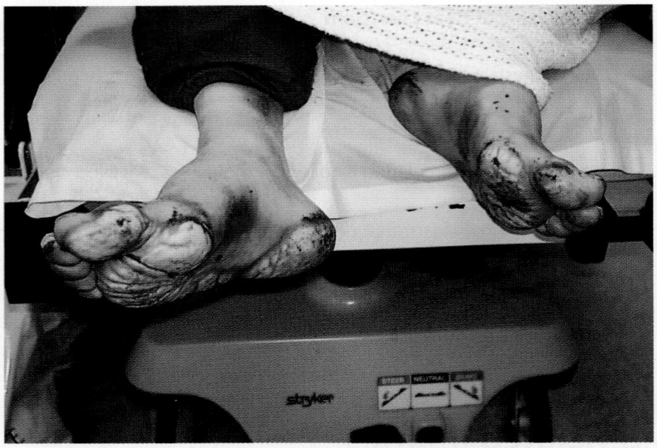

FIGURE 13.5. Immersion foot. Early appearance of immersion foot in a mentally ill homeless patient. (Reproduced, with permission, from Knoop KJ, Stack LB, Storrow AB. *Atlas of Emergency Medicine*. 3rd ed. New York, NY: McGraw-Hill; 2010. Figure 16.15. Photographer: Ken Zafren, MD.)

Complications

- Wet gangrene, if untreated.
- Late sequelae (**posthyperemic stage**): Cold sensitivity, pain and numbness, atrophy, weakness.
- Tissue loss is uncommon.

FROSTNIP

Frostnip is a superficial freezing injury without tissue loss or tissue destruction. It typically involves exposed surfaces (face, hands).

Symptoms/Examination

- Transient numbness and tingling, resolves with rewarming.
- Affected skin appears firm, cold, and white.
- Superficial blistering and peeling may occur.

Treatment

Rewarm and prevent further cold exposure.

FROSTBITE

The most common freezing injury of tissue that occurs when tissue temperatures drop < 0°C (32°F). Ice crystal formation damages cellular architecture leading to microvascular thrombosis, ischemia, and eventual tissue necrosis.

Only after rewarming of tissue can depth of injury can be assessed.

Traditional classification of frostbite:

- **First degree**: Central white plaque with surrounding hyperemia.
- **Second degree**: Clear blisters.
- **Third degree**: Hemorrhagic blisters → eschar and tissue loss (Figure 13.6).
- **Fourth degree**: Full thickness injury affecting skin, muscle, and bone → tissue loss.

However, the above classification has no impact on treatment, so a simpler classification is often used.

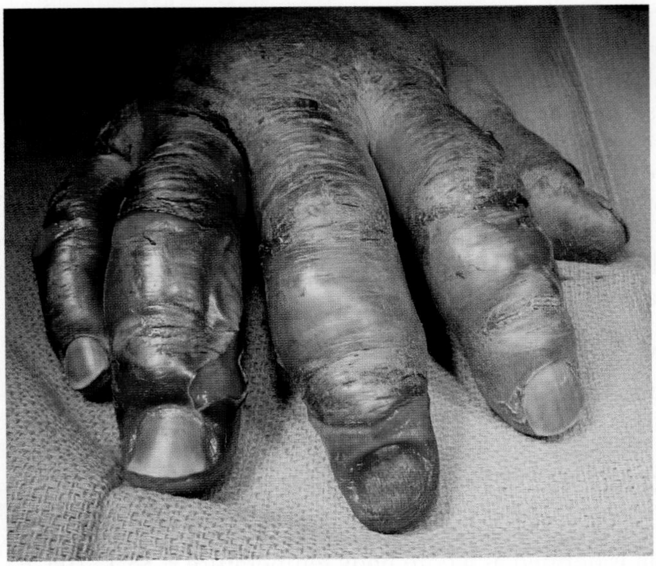

FIGURE 13.6. Frostbite-ruptured blebs. Frostbite injury to the hand with ruptured blebs. (Reproduced, with permission, from Knoop KJ, Stack LB, Storrow AB. *Atlas of Emergency Medicine*. 3rd ed. New York, NY: McGraw-Hill; 2010. Figure 16.10. Photographer: R. Jason Thurman, MD.)

- **Superficial frostbite**: No evidence for tissue loss; underlying skin and tissues are soft.
- **Deep frostbite**: Evidence for tissue loss; underlying tissues are often rock hard.

PATHOPHYSIOLOGY

- Tissue freezing → release of arachidonic acid breakdown products (prostaglandins and thromboxane) → thrombosis and ischemia

SYMPTOMS/EXAMINATION

- Before rewarming affected area appears mottled, pale, firm, and waxy, and extremity may feel numb or "wooden."
- After rewarming, blisters and focal necrosis develop.
- Dead tissue demarcates in anywhere from 3-5 weeks.

TREATMENT

- Treat any associated hypothermia **first**.
- **Rapid rewarming** with immersion in **40°C-42°C** (104°F-107°F) circulating water until tissue feels pliable. Opioid analgesia is often needed.
- **Avoid:**
  - Friction or rubbing of skin
  - Dry heat
  - Refreezing (disastrous!)
- Tetanus prophylaxis.
- Intra-arterial thrombolytics can be considered in subjects presenting within 24 hours of injury (not widely available).
- Blisters:
  - **Aspirate clear blisters only or leave intact**; avoid debridement or aspiration of hemorrhagic blisters.
  - Debridement of skin overlying hemorrhagic blister may result in marked desiccation of the underlying tissues.

KEY FACT

Never rewarm tissue in the field if there is a possibility it will refreeze.

KEY FACT

Rewarm by immersion in 40°C-42°C circulating water.

- Prevent further tissue loss:
  - Splint and elevate limb to minimize edema formation.
  - Smoking cessation.
  - Nonsteroidal anti-inflammatory drugs (NSAIDs) (inhibit arachidonic acid cascade).
  - Topical aloe vera (inhibits thromboxane).
- **Many** other therapies have been proposed: Nifedipine, topical corticosteroids, prednisone, hyperbarics, etc, but none has been proven beneficial.
- Delayed surgical debridement and escharotomy; early debridement **only** if severe gangrene or sepsis develops.

Complications

- Secondary bacterial/fungal infections

Accidental Hypothermia

Hypothermia is defined as a core body temperature < 35°C (95°F).

Risks for hypothermia can be divided into three groups (Table 13.8):

- Decreased heat production
- Increased heat loss
- Impaired ability to move to warm environment

Hypothermia is clinically defined as mild, moderate, or severe.

- **Mild hypothermia (32°C-35°C)**: **Excitation stage**: Characterized by physiologic responses to generate heat such as shivering, peripheral vasoconstriction, and increased metabolic rate.
- **Moderate hypothermia** (30°C-32°C): As temperature drops < 32°C, shivering ceases and victims enter a stage of general slowing of metabolism = **adynamic stage**.
- **Severe hypothermia** (< 30°C): Patient appears dead. Ventricular fibrillation (VFib) risk increases.

KEY FACT

With temperatures < 30°C (severe hypothermia), the patient appears dead and the risk of VFib increases.

Pathophysiology

- As core temperature ↓ → peripheral vasoconstriction (to limit further radiant heat loss) and shivering (to increase heat production)
- Further decrease in temperature → generalized slowing of body functions

TABLE 13.8. Factors Predisposing to Accidental Hypothermia

Decreased Heat Production	Increased Heat Loss	Impaired Mobility
Hypothyroidism	Inadequate clothing	Infants and young children
Hypoadrenalism	Vasodilation	Physical or mental impairment
Malnutrition	Alcohol	Acute CNS process
Hypoglycemia	Medications	Alcoholism
Dehydration	Spinal cord injury	Tranquilizer or sedative use
Physical exhaustion	Neuropathies	
Extremes of age	Skin disorders	
Inactivity	Burns	
Impaired shivering	Exfoliative dermatitis	
	Infants	

CNS, central nervous system.

- **Leftward shift of oxyhemoglobin dissociation curve** → decreased release of O_2 to tissues
- Renal dysfunction and peripheral vasoconstriction (central **hyper**volemia) → **cold diuresis** → dehydration

SYMPTOMS/EXAMINATION

- **Mild hypothermia:**
  - Tachycardia and tachypnea
  - Hyperactive reflexes
  - Shivering
- **Moderate-to-severe hypothermia:**
  - Mental status change ranging from poor judgment to lethargy to coma.
  - Pupils may become fixed and dilated.
  - Poor coordination, dysarthria.
  - Bradycardia or ANY atrial/ventricular dysrhythmia.
  - Hypoactive reflexes, muscular rigidity.
  - Paradoxical undressing may occur, thought to be due to a loss of vasomotor tone leading patient to feel warm.

DIAGNOSIS

- Based on history of exposure and core body temperature
- Electrocardiogram (ECG):
  - Classic ECG = Osborne ("J") waves appear at junction of QRS complex (Figure 13.7).
  - ST segment and QT interval are often prolonged.
  - **Any** dysrhythmia may occur.
- Arterial blood gas (ABG)
- Laboratory studies:
  - Hemoconcentration is common.
  - Clotting factor dysfunction.
  - Thrombocytopenia.
  - Hyperglycemia or hypoglycemia may be present.

TREATMENT

- Start with ABCs.
- Continuous core temperature measurement (esophageal probe if available; bladder or rectal thermometers most commonly used).

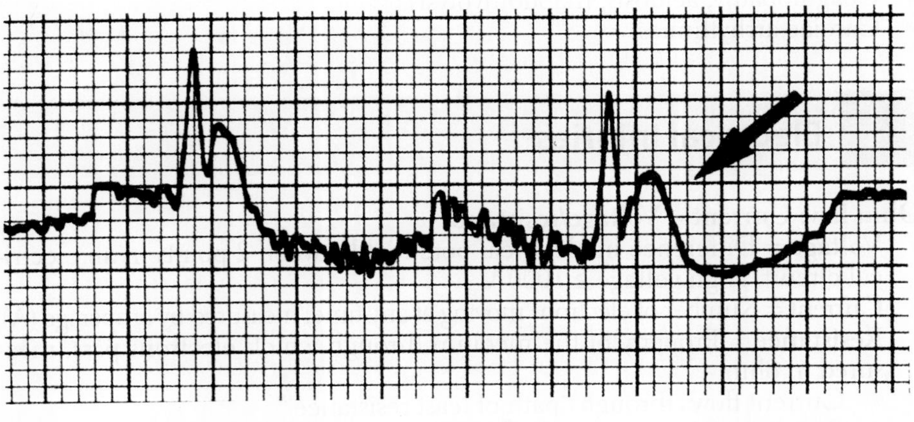

FIGURE 13.7. Osborne ("J") waves (arrow). (Reproduced, with permission, from Tintinalli JE, Kelen GD, Stapczynski JS. *Emergency Medicine: A Comprehensive Study Guide*. 6th ed. New York, NY: McGraw-Hill; 2004:1180.)

Q

A 70-year old homeless man is found down outside during a snowstorm in upstate New York. On arrival he is altered but protecting his airway, bradycardic, and cold to the touch. A rectal temperature reads 31°C. What are the initial steps you will take to correct his hypothermia?

KEY FACT

Patients with exposure to cold develop a "cold diuresis" secondary to peripheral vasoconstriction and increased blood flow to kidneys. This can result in dehydration.

KEY FACT

Osborne "J" waves are classic for moderate-to-severe hypothermia, but may be seen in other conditions.

KEY FACT

Three general methods of rewarming: Passive (noninvasive) rewarming, active external rewarming, active core rewarming.

A

This patient would classify as moderate hypothermia. Start active external rewarming by removing wet clothes, using heating lamps, forced-air warming blankets to the torso, warm blankets, warm IV fluids, and increasing the temperature of the room. It is important not to apply heat only to the extremities as you can cause core afterdrop.

KEY FACT

If VFib develops with severe hypothermia: Defibrillate once, then hold until core temperature > 32°C.

KEY FACT

Failure to rewarm? → consider underlying endocrine failure.

KEY FACT

"The patient is not dead until he is warm and dead."

KEY FACT

Core afterdrop: Cold peripheral blood returns to core → further decrease in core temperature.

- **Passive rewarming:**
  - For mild hypothermia; blankets, dry clothes, move from cold environment.
- **Active external rewarming** for severe **hypothermia without cardiovascular instability:**
  - Heating lamps (radiation).
  - Bair huggers (convection) placed on torso, not limbs.
  - Avoid applying heat to extremities only in order to avoid core afterdrop.
  - Warm blankets (conduction).
  - Warm IV fluids at 40°C-42°C (104°F-107°F).
  - Warm humidified O_2 by mask (↓ evaporative loss).
- **Active core rewarming** for severe **hypothermia with cardiovascular instability:**
  - Warmed gastric, bladder, peritoneal, and pleural lavage
- The best treatment for dysrhythmias, coagulopathy, and hyperglycemia = rewarming.
- Rehydrate with warmed IV fluids (most patients are dehydrated from "cold diuresis").
- Many medications, including insulin, are ineffective until core temperature is > 30°C.
- **Cardiac arrest:**
  - Administer cardiopulmonary resuscitation (CPR).
  - Consider surgical approaches to rewarming including cardiopulmonary bypass, continuous arteriovenous and venovenous rewarming, extracorporeal membrane oxygenation (ECMO), and hemodialysis.
  - Defibrillation and medications may not be effective at or < 30°C; therefore, continue CPR while the patient is warmed.
  - If in VFib, only 1 defibrillation attempt (2 J/kg) is indicated until the core temperature exceeds 32°C.
  - Patient may be pronounced dead if core temperature is **32°C-35°C** and no vital signs are present.
- **Avoid**:
  - Suppressing shivering response.
  - Rough handling (may induce VF).
  - Transvenous pacing (may induce VF): Use transcutaneous pacing instead.

COMPLICATIONS

- **Core afterdrop** occurs when skin or extremities are warmed before the core → cold peripheral blood returns to core → core temperature drops further. Key is to rewarm core **before** periphery in all cases of hypothermia.
- Coagulopathy, acidosis, rhabdomyolysis.
- Cardiac arrhythmias.

Electrical Injuries

Ohm law: Current = Voltage/resistance

- **Voltage** = Difference in electrical potential between 2 points in an electrical circuit. High voltage ≥ 1000 V
- **Current** = Number of electrons moving at any time, measured by amperage (A)
- **Resistance** = Property of the medium through which electrons pass, measured in ohm
  - Current flows through "path of least resistance."
  - Resistance decreases with ↑ fluid content (eg, nerves, blood vessels, wet skin).
  - Increases with calloused skin.

There are two basic types of electrical circuits:

- **Alternating current (AC)**
  - Typical household current
  - Changes its direction of current flow at a given frequency
  - More dangerous than DC at any given voltage
    - 1-4 mA → tingling sensation
    - 6-9 mA (the **"let go" threshold**) → tetanic muscle contraction → above this level one cannot release the electrical source, resulting in prolonged contact
    - > 70 mA → cardiac depolarization and possible VF
- **Direct current (DC)**
  - Batteries, electronics, high-voltage electrical power transmission, lightning.
  - Tends to throw the victim from the source → secondary traumatic injuries.
  - Overall, high-voltage electrical injury is characterized by minimal external findings hiding extensive internal tissue damage.

Q

An 18-month-old girl presents after sustaining an electrical injury while chewing on a power cord. On examination, there is a burn present to the corner of her mouth without marked tissue loss or evidence of other intraoral burns. What is the most feared complication in this patient?

KEY FACT

AC is more dangerous than DC at any given voltage.

KEY FACT

Decreasing order of electrical resistance: Bone, fat, tendon, skin, muscle, mucous membranes, blood vessels, nerves

Symptoms/Examination

- Immediate cardiac arrest may occur from asystole or VFib (primary cause of death).
- Patients who survive the initial electrical shock present with a variety of injuries depending on path of current flow and associated trauma.
- Loss of consciousness, confusion, amnesia.
- Paresthesias.
- Seizure.
- Thermal source contact burns, most commonly on hand. Size of burn does not correlate with underlying tissue injury.
- **Arc burns** (kissing burns) = arc of extremely high voltage current across areas of different electric potential → extensive tissue damage.
- Visual changes from corneal burns, retinal detachment, and uveitis.
- Tinnitus, hearing loss, ruptured tympanic membranes (TMs).
- Muscular pain.
- Traumatic injuries (blunt or blast), most notably **posterior shoulder dislocations** from being "thrown from source."

Diagnosis

- Diagnosis of electrical injury is typically based on the history.
- Virtually any organ can be injured; therefore, detailed evaluation is warranted.
- ECG and monitoring: Dysrhythmias, heart block, QT prolongation, nonspecific ST-T changes are all possible.
- Laboratory tests include: Complete blood cell (CBC), electrolytes, Urinalysis (UA), creatine kinase (CK).
- Standard trauma evaluation, as necessary.

KEY FACT

Primary cardiac arrest in electrical injuries = asystole or VFib

Treatment

- ABCs.
- IV fluids with monitoring of urine output (goal 1-2 mL/kg/h).
- Treat rhabdomyolysis, if present.
- Trauma management, as necessary.
- Wound (burn) care and tetanus prophylaxis.
- Low-voltage injuries that are initially asymptomatic can often be safely sent home.

A

This child has sustained a local arc burn to the commissure of the mouth. There is a risk for delayed bleeding in 3-14 days because of injury to the labial artery.

KEY FACT

Pediatric oral burns can have life-threatening labial artery bleeding 2-3 weeks after injury when the eschar falls off.

Complications

- Renal failure from rhabdomyolysis.
- DIC (uncommon).
- Arterial and venous thrombosis.
- Labial artery burns can present with delayed severe bleeding.
- Cataracts.

Lightning Injuries

Lightning is a **direct current** of **extremely high voltage**. Fortunately, the duration of exposure is **very brief** and the majority of the current is transmitted via external "**flashover**."

Lightning strike victims who reach the hospital often have many external findings, but minimal (excluding associated trauma) internal injuries.

A comparison between lightning and high-voltage electrical injuries can be found in Table 13.9.

Pathophysiology of Lightning Injury

- **Direct contact**: Current travels directly to victim.
- **Side flash**: Current traverses through air from first object to victim.
- **Step or ground current**: Lightning hits ground → current travels via ground to nearby victims.
- **Blunt trauma**: 2° to fall or falling objects.
- **Blast trauma:** Victims suffer from pulmonary contusions, TM rupture, and conductive hearing loss.
- **Thermal burns**: 2° to fires or steam burns from vaporized cutaneous sweat, burning clothes.

Pathophysiology of Lightning Death

- Intense electrical stimulus → **asystole** ("**primary death**") and apnea from inhibition of brainstem respiratory centers.

TABLE 13.9. Key Differences in Lightning and High-Voltage Electrical Injuries

	Lightning	High Voltage
Duration	Short	Prolonged contact
Volts	10 million-2 billion	1000-10,000
Current	DC	AC
Side flash	Present	Absent
Cardiac	Asystole	Ventricular fibrillation
Burns	Minor and superficial	More extensive
Myoglobinuria	Infrequent	Common
Fasciotomy	Rarely indicated	Common

AC, alternating current; DC, direct current.

- Asystole often resolves spontaneously **but** if apnea persists → "**secondary death" from respiratory paralysis leading to hypoxia and VFib**.

SYMPTOMS/EXAMINATION

- Cardiac arrest.
- Respiratory arrest.
- The patient who survives the immediate strike may present with a variety of findings.
- Seizures, confusion, amnesia.
- Anisocoria or dilated pupils.
- TM rupture, tinnitus, and hearing loss.
- **Keraunoparalysis**: A transient paralysis with blue, mottled, pulseless lower and/or upper extremities. Results from sympathetic activation and resultant extreme vasoconstriction; resolves spontaneously over several hours.
- Skin:
  - **Lichtenberg figures** (Figure 13.8): Superficial fern or feather pattern from "electron shower"
  - **Linear burns**: From sweat converting to steam
  - **Punctuate burns**: Multiple small, round burns
  - **Thermal burns**
- Associated traumatic injuries.

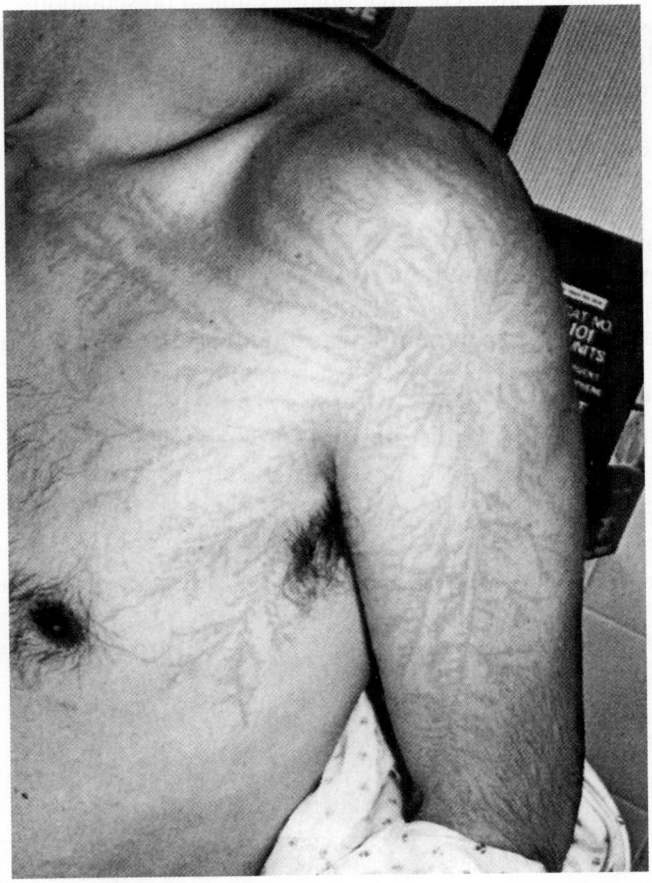

FIGURE 13.8. Lichtenberg figures. (Reproduced, with permission, from Tintinalli JE, Kelen GD, Stapczynski JS. *Emergency Medicine: A Comprehensive Study Guide*. 6th ed. New York, NY: McGraw-Hill; 2004:1238.)

Q

A 55-year-old man is brought to the ED for evaluation after being found down on a golf course after a thunderstorm. He has no recollection of events. He is complaining of ringing in his ears and states that he is unable to move his extremities. What physical examination findings would help you determine if he was struck by lightning?

KEY FACT

Lichtenberg figures are pathognomonic for lightning injury.

A

Fernlike markings (also known as Lichtenberg figures) are pathognomonic for lightning injuries and usually fade in a few hours. Other findings consistent with lightning injury include TM rupture, tinnitus, hearing loss, and paralyzed, cold, and pulseless extremities (keraunoparalysis, a temporary condition due to sympathetic nervous system activation).

KEY FACT

Reverse triage applies in lightning injuries → treat those that appear dead first.

KEY FACT

Duration of lightning is extremely brief: Asystole is common but internal burns and rhabdomyolysis aren't typically seen.

KEY FACT

Cataracts can occur acutely or several years after lightning injury.

Diagnosis

- Typically obvious based on clinical presentation
- ECG and cardiac monitor
- Useful laboratory tests include: CBC, electrolytes, BUN, creatinine (Cr), UA

Treatment

- ABCs.
- If on scene treat those in cardiac arrest (appear dead) **first**. This is unlike other mass-casualty incidents.
- Trauma precautions and evaluation as indicated.
- Tetanus prophylaxis.
- IV fluids.
- Admit all patients with cardiac findings (examination or ECG), neurologic abnormalities, or significant trauma/burns.

Complications

- If pregnant: Fetal mortality rate can be as high as 50%.
- Neurologic sequelae are common but extremity paralysis is usually only temporary.
- Cataracts (delayed).

High-Altitude Illness

High-altitude illness consists of three unique clinical presentations: Acute mountain sickness (AMS), high-altitude pulmonary edema (HAPE), and high-altitude cerebral edema (HACE). AMS can occur after several **hours** of exposure to altitude, whereas HAPE and HACE typically take **days** to develop.

Risk factors for developing high-altitude illness:

- Adolescents and adults > elderly (age > 50 years decreases risk)
- Rapid ascent
- Elevation attained
- Heavy exertion
- Cold exposure (exacerbates pulmonary hypertension)
- Comorbid pulmonary or neurologic conditions (hypoventilation)

Pathophysiology (Table 13.10)

- As altitude increases, partial pressure of O_2 decreases.

TABLE 13.10. Altitude Classification and Pathophysiology

Classification	Elevation Attained (ft)	Pathophysiology
Moderate altitude	8000-10,000	↓ Exercise performance ↑ Ventilation to ↑Po_2
High altitude	10,000-18,000	Maximal Sao_2 < 90% Maximal Pao_2 < 60 mm Hg Hypoxemia
Extreme altitude	> 18,000	Severe hypoxemia Severe hypocapnia Physiologic deterioration with time

- Periodic breathing → alternating tachypnea and apnea
- Pulmonary artery hypertension
- Fluid retention
- Cerebral hypoxia → cerebrovascular changes and damage

High-altitude acclimatization is the body's ability to **gradually** adjust to lower O_2 concentrations by the following methods:

- Carotid body hypoxemia → hypoxic ventilatory response that stimulates ventilation to ↓ $Paco_2$ and ↑ Pao_2.
- In response to the acute respiratory alkalosis, the kidneys excrete bicarbonate (to normalize pH).
- Erythropoietin production is ↑ within 2 hours of ascent → ↑ red cell mass and ↑ O_2-carrying capacity.
- ↑ 2,3-DPG → rightward shift of oxyhemoglobin dissociation curve → improved O_2 release to tissues.

Q

A 25-year-old man presents to the ED with shortness of breath and cough. He has an oxygen saturation of 86% and rales on examination. Chest x-ray (CXR) shows bilateral patchy infiltrates and a normal heart size. On further history he just flew from San Diego to Vail, Colorado for 3 days of strenuous hiking. He has been feeling unwell since arriving in Colorado and now his breathing has gotten worse. What is his most likely diagnosis and how would you best treat him?

ACUTE MOUNTAIN SICKNESS

Develops several hours after arrival to altitude > 8000 ft in unacclimatized individuals.

KEY FACT

Best prevention for all types of high-altitude illness:

- Ascend slowly and spend time at each altitude for acclimatization.
- Avoid alcohol and other sedatives.
- Avoid overexertion.

SYMPTOMS/EXAMINATION

Symptoms are similar to viral syndrome or hangover: Anorexia, headache, nausea/vomiting, fatigue, weakness, insomnia.

TREATMENT

- Usually self-limited and resolves with acclimatization in 24-48 hours
- **No further ascent** until symptoms abate
- Descend if severe/unrelenting symptoms
- Acetazolamide: To speed acclimatization (may start prior to ascent); may be used for prevention as well as treatment of AMS
- For symptomatic relief:
  - Supplemental O_2
  - Dexamethasone (use with caution: can mask symptoms of worsening AMS if taken on ascent)
  - Tylenol, aspirin
- **Avoid:** All CNS and respiratory depressants (narcotics, alcohol, benzodiazepines)

KEY FACT

The best definitive treatment for all high-altitude syndromes is immediate descent.

HIGH-ALTITUDE PULMONARY EDEMA

High-altitude pulmonary edema (HAPE) is a form of noncardiogenic pulmonary edema. It typically occurs 2-4 days after arrival to high altitude.

KEY FACT

Acetazolamide can be used for AMS prevention and treatment; dexamethasone can mask symptoms of worsening AMS and should be used with caution and in conjunction with descent.

PATHOPHYSIOLOGY

- Pulmonary vasoconstriction → ↑ pulmonary hypertension → endothelial damage and capillary leak.
- Patients with a patent foramen ovale may experience right-to-left shunting at altitude resulting in more severe arterial hypoxemia. This condition may exacerbate symptoms of HAPE.

SYMPTOMS/EXAMINATION

- AMS symptoms (common)
- Cough (dry or productive)

A

This patient likely has high-altitude pulmonary edema (HAPE). This is the most common cause of death related to high altitude. Treatment includes descent to a lower altitude, supplemental oxygen, hyperbaric O_2, and nifedipine.

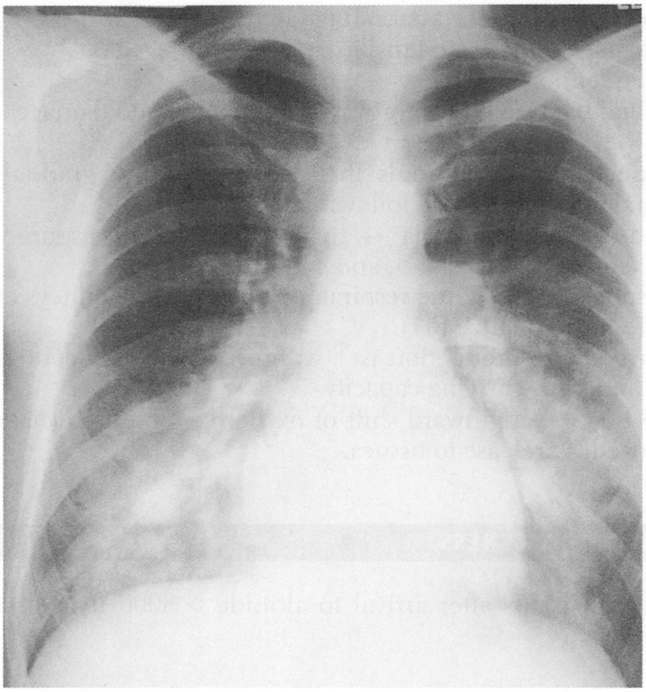

FIGURE 13.9. Chest x-ray (CXR) of patient with high-altitude pulmonary edema. (Reproduced, with permission, from Knoop KJ, Stack LB, Storrow AB. *Atlas of Emergency Medicine*. 2nd ed. New York: McGraw-Hill; 2002:515. Photographer: Peter Hackett, MD.)

- **Dyspnea at rest**
- Tachypnea and tachycardia
- Rales
- Fever

DIAGNOSIS

- Primarily clinical, but can be confirmed with chest x-ray (CXR) showing bilateral patchy infiltrates (may be asymmetric, right more commonly involved than left) and **normal** heart size (Figure 13.9)

TREATMENT

- **Descent**.
- Mild-to-moderate cases may recover with bed rest ± O_2 at altitude.
- Supplemental O_2.
- Minimize exertion.
- Portable hyperbaric O_2 therapy.
- Nifedipine.
- Bronchodilators (salmeterol) or phosphodiesterase inhibitors (sildenafil) have been used experimentally for HAPE prevention.
- Morphine, diuretics, and antibiotics are controversial regarding benefit vs harm and are not routinely recommended.

KEY FACT

HAPE is the most common cause of death related to high altitude.

HIGH-ALTITUDE CEREBRAL EDEMA

High-altitude cerebral edema (HACE) is the most severe form of high-altitude illness. As with HAPE, onset is typically 2-4 days after arrival to altitude > 12,000 ft.

SYMPTOMS/EXAMINATION

- AMS symptoms (severe headache, nausea/vomiting).
- HAPE symptoms may also be present.
- Cerebellar ataxia: **Most sensitive sign**.
- MS changes: Stupor to coma; seizures may occur.
- Third/sixth cranial nerve palsies (rare).

> **KEY FACT**
>
> Ataxia is the most sensitive sign of HACE.

DIAGNOSIS

- Clinical diagnosis: AMS **plus** ataxia = HACE
- Magnetic resonance imaging (MRI), if diagnosis in question (rarely available)

> **KEY FACT**
>
> Monge disease (chronic mountain polycythemia) is a late effect of high altitude characterized by headache, trouble sleeping, and mental sluggishness.

TREATMENT

- Immediate descent/evacuation.
- Supplemental O_2.
- Acetazolamide for prevention and treatment of mild AMS.
- Dexamethasone for moderate-to-severe AMS.
- Portable hyperbaric therapy (Gamow bag) if descent not available.
- Furosemide or mannitol may be used with caution (downside = volume depletion) (Table 13.11).

TABLE 13.11. Medications Used For Treatment of High-Altitude Illness

MEDICATION	MECHANISM OF ACTION	INDICATION
Acetazolamide	Carbonic anhydrase inhibitor → bicarbonate diuresis and metabolic acidosis → compensatory hyperventilation	AMS prophylaxis AMS treatment Disturbing periodic breathing
Dexamethasone	↓ Vasogenic edema ↓ Intracranial pressure Antiemetic	Moderate-to-severe AMS HACE
Tylenol Aspirin Antiemetics	Symptomatic treatment	AMS HACE
O_2 (to $Sao_2 > 90\%$)	Improves hypoxemia	Moderate to severe AMS HAPE HACE
Hyperbaric O_2	Improves hypoxemia	Severe AMS HAPE HACE
Nifedipine	Decreases pulmonary artery pressure	HAPE

AMS, acute mountain sickness; HACE, high-altitude cerebral edema; HAPE, high-altitude pulmonary edema.

TABLE 13.12. Types of Dysbarism

Descent dysbarism ("the squeeze")
Dysbarism at depth
Nitrogen narcosis
O_2 toxicity
Alternobaric vertigo
Ascent dysbarism
Ascent barotrauma
Decompression sickness
Arterial air embolism

Dysbarism

Dysbarism refers to diving injuries from underwater pressure changes. It is easiest to think of dysbarism regarding timing of symptom onset (Table 13.12).

- **Descent dysbarism** ("the squeeze")
- **Dysbarism at depth**
  - Nitrogen narcosis
  - O_2 toxicity
  - Alternobaric vertigo
- **Ascent dysbarism**
  - Ascent barotrauma
  - Decompression sickness (DCS)
  - Arterial air embolism

KEY FACT

Boyle law (for any given air space): PV = k, where P = pressure, V = volume, k = constant; if P increases, V must decrease).

Physiology of Gases

- **Boyle law** states that as the pressure (P) on a given air space increases, the volume of gas (V) decreases (PV = constant).
- **Henry law** states that the amount of a gas dissolved in a liquid is directly proportional to the partial pressure of that gas.
- Atmospheric pressure at sea level = 760 mm Hg or 1 atm. As one descends to 33 ft (in seawater), the atmospheric pressure ↑ to 2 atm and the volume of air-filled spaces decreases by 50%. For each gas within the space, both the partial pressure and the amount dissolved in solution (eg, blood) will ↑ accordingly.

DESCENT DYSBARISM

Descent dysbarism can occur in any air-filled space in the body (Table 13.13).

Middle ear squeeze is the most common manifestation.

Pathophysiology

↑ Dive depth → increased ambient pressure and "squeeze" (barotrauma) of air-filled spaces in body → symptoms if body unable to equalize pressures

Treatment

- Depends on location and severity of injuries.
- Most injuries respond to conservative therapy (rest) alone.
- Prophylactic antibiotics if ruptured TM.
- Oral steroids if seventh nerve palsy.

TABLE 13.13. Descent Dysbarism

LOCATION OF "SQUEEZE"	UNDERLYING CAUSE	SYMPTOMS
External ear	Obstruction of external ear canal (**no** ear plugs!)	Ear pain
Middle ear (most common)	External pressure on TM not equalized by Eustachian tube	Ear pain Hearing loss TM rupture → nystagmus and vertigo Seventh nerve palsy
Inner ear	Transmission of middle ear pressure → rupture of round window	Ear pain Hearing loss Severe nystagmus and vertigo → ataxia and vomiting
Sinus	Obstruction of sinus ostia	Facial pain Epistaxis
Lung	Holding breath during descent	Shortness of breath Hemoptysis Pulmonary edema
Equipment	Tight-fitting mask or wet suit	Petechiae

TM, tympanic membrane.

- Topical nasal decongestants for ear and sinus squeeze.
- Recompression therapy is **not** indicated.
- No further diving (until injuries have healed).

DYSBARISM AT DEPTH

Nitrogen Narcosis

Nitrogen narcosis occurs when scuba tank air (containing nitrogen and O_2) is breathed at depth. Symptoms of nitrogen narcosis typically occur after the diver has descended to ≥ 100 ft.

PATHOPHYSIOLOGY

Increasing dive depth → increased ambient pressure → ↓ volume of tank air (Boyle law) and ↑ partial pressure of nitrogen in inspired tank air → increased nitrogen dissolved in blood (Henry law) → symptoms

SYMPTOMS/EXAMINATION

- Altered behavior, poor judgment, hallucinations, diminished motor control. Similar to alcohol or benzodiazepine intoxication.
- Loss of consciousness may occur.

TREATMENT

- Ascend slowly with assistance; slow ascent is essential to prevent ascent dysbarism (discussed in the next section).
- Use mixtures with less nitrogen in the inspired tank for dives > 100 ft.

Q

A 50-year-old man complains of a headache, and then abruptly loses consciousness 3 minutes after surfacing from a dive. What is the most likely diagnosis?

A

This patient has likely experienced an arterial gas embolism (AGE). Any diver who develops CNS symptoms within 10 minutes of surfacing should be assumed to have an AGE. Treatment includes administering 100% O_2 by mask, placing victim supine, administering IV fluids, and rapid transport for hyperbaric therapy.

Oxygen Toxicity

Results from breathing elevated partial pressures of O_2 for extended periods of time; primarily affects the CNS and lungs.

Symptoms/Examination

- Tunnel or blurred vision
- Tinnitus
- Nausea/vomiting
- Dizziness and paresthesias
- Confusion, agitation, anxiety
- Twitching, seizures

Treatment

- Ascend slowly with assistance; slow ascent is essential to prevent ascent dysbarism (discussed in the next section).
- Can be prevented by limiting duration of deep dives or using air with < 21% oxygen by adding helium.

ASCENT DYSBARISM

Ascent Barotrauma

Ascent barotrauma is caused by expansion of gas during ascent from diving.

Pathophysiology

- ↓ In ambient pressure → ↑ in size of air-filled spaces.
- Failure of air to passively exit middle ear due to blocked Eustachian tube → **alternobaric vertigo**. Risk factors include otitis media and Eustachian tube dysfunction.
- Breath-holding during ascent → air dissects into pulmonary tissue (sub-cutaneous emphysema to pneumomediastinum to pneumothorax).

KEY FACT

Asthma patients have a significantly increased risk of pulmonary barotrauma.

Symptoms/Examination

- **Alternobaric vertigo**
  - Ear pain and possible TM rupture.
  - Severe but transient nystagmus and vertigo.
  - Nausea/vomiting may occur.
  - Transient hearing loss.
- **Pulmonary barotrauma**
  - Shortness of breath
  - Hemoptysis
  - Chest pain

Treatment

- Supplemental O_2 as needed
- Typically resolves with rest
- Chest tube for large pneumothorax

Arterial Gas Embolism

Arterial gas embolism (AGE) is a form of pulmonary barotrauma that occurs during or **within 10 minutes** of ascent.

Pathophysiology

Expanding gas ruptures alveoli → air enters pulmonary venous circulation and travels to left heart and systemic circulation → obstruction to flow and symptoms depending on location of embolization.

Can also result from a right-to-left shunt in a diver with a patent foremen ovale.

SYMPTOMS/EXAMINATION

Air bubbles can embolize to any organ.

- **Cerebral embolization (most common)**
  - Sudden stroke-like symptoms, seizure, loss of consciousness, confusion
- **Coronary artery embolization**
  - Symptoms and findings consistent with acute coronary syndrome

TREATMENT

- 100% O_2 by mask
- Recumbent/supine position
- IV fluids to increase perfusion
- Rapid recompression in hyperbaric O_2 chamber

Decompression Sickness

Symptoms result from formation of nitrogen bubbles in tissues or vessels. Nitrogen is highly fat soluble leading to CNS symptoms (Table 13.14 for risk factors).

PATHOPHYSIOLOGY

As diver ascends → ambient pressure decreases and nitrogen bubbles come out of solution → precipitate and coalesce in blood and tissues

SYMPTOMS/EXAMINATION

- Symptoms depend on tissues involved. Typically symptoms begin > 10 minutes after surfacing.
- **Type I DCS** = **"the bends"** (skin, joint, and extremities).
  - Pruritus, erythema, and skin marbling
  - Limb and joint pain—shoulder most commonly affected
  - Lymphedema
- **Type II DCS** = other organ involvement (CNS, inner ear, lungs).
  - More serious manifestations
  - Mental status changes, headache, visual changes
  - Upper lumbar spine particularly susceptible → weakness, paralysis
  - **"The Staggers"**—inner ear involvement with vertigo, nystagmus, and nausea/vomiting
  - **"The Chokes"**—dyspnea, cough, chest pain

TREATMENT

- Rapid recompression in a hyperbaric chamber
- 100% O_2 by mask
- Recumbent/supine position
- IV fluids

TABLE 13.14. Risk Factors for Decompression Sickness

Older age
Fatigue or heavy exertion
Dehydration
Obesity
Increased total length and depths of dive(s)
Diving at altitude
Rapid ascent
Flying after diving

KEY FACT

AGE and DCS require hyperbaric therapy.

Submersion Injuries

KEY FACT

The effect on electrolyte status is the same regardless of seawater (oceans and some lakes) or freshwater (lakes, rivers, pools) drowning.

The submersion victim is defined as any person who requires medical evaluation after a submersion event. Drowning is now defined as fatal drowning or nonfatal drowning. Terms such as "near drowning," "dry or wet drowning," or "secondary drowning" are no longer used.

To contradict earlier beliefs, there appears to be no difference between freshwater and saltwater submersion without massive volumes of salt or fresh water aspiration, which rarely occurs in drowning. Precipitating injuries include spinal cord injury, hypothermia, seizure, and syncope.

Pathophysiology

- In the majority of submersion events: Aspiration of water into the lungs → loss of surfactant and alveolar collapse → hypoxia → brain cell death after 3 minutes.
- In 10%-15% victim maintain laryngospasm and bronchospasm while submerged, significantly limiting the amount of aspirated water.
- **Diving reflex**: (in young infants and other mammals) → transiently protective bradycardia, apnea, and peripheral vasoconstriction with maintenance of brain and cardiac perfusion.
- **Immersion syndrome**: Immersion in very cold water → vagally mediated asystolic cardiac arrest.

Risk Factors

- Toddlers and male teenagers
- Swimming pools, bathtubs, buckets → unsupervised children
- Boating without personal floatation devices (PFDs); under the influence of alcohol/drugs

KEY FACT

Following submersion, respiratory deterioration can be delayed for up to 6 hours.

Symptoms/Examination

- Respiratory distress with wheezes, rales, or rhonchi on examination
- May be delayed up to 6 hours ("secondary drowning")
- AMS ranging from confusion to coma
- Hypothermia if cold water submersion
- Cardiac dysrhythmias

Diagnosis

- CXR—if patient symptomatic.
- ECG ± cardiac monitoring if abnormal.
- Electrolyte studies are rarely helpful.
- Trauma evaluation (as indicated, consider c-spine injury).

KEY FACT

Poor prognostic factors: Age < 3 years, delay in initiation of CPR > 5 minutes, prolonged submersion time, acidosis, Glasgow Coma Scale (GCS) 3, need for ongoing CPR.

Treatment

- ABCs and supportive care.
- Warm to 32°C-35°C.
  - Temperature 30°C-35°C → passive or active external rewarming
  - Temperature < 30°C → active core rewarming
- Treat associated injuries or trauma.
- **Not** shown to improve outcome: hyperventilation, steroids, induced coma, prophylactic antibiotics.
- Asymptomatic patients can be discharged home after 4-6 hours of observation.

COMPLICATIONS

- Numerous pulmonary complications—pneumonia, pulmonary edema, pneumonitis, ARDS
- Hemolysis and DIC
- Hypoxia-associated complications—CNS injury, multiorgan injury

> **Q**
>
> A 3-year-old boy is brought in to the ED after falling into his family's pool. On arrival he is awake, alert, with mild tachypnea and wheezing. How long do you want to watch him in the ED?

Poisonous Plants

Hundreds of poisonous plants exist. This section will focus on those more commonly encountered (Table 13.15).

CASTOR BEAN AND JEQUIRITY BEAN

The castor bean plant (*Ricinus communis*) and jequirity bean (*Abrus precatorius*) plant seeds are from the same family and contain potent toxalbumins (**ricin and abrin**, respectively). They are used for ornamental purposes, such as in prayer beads or musical instruments (maracas). In part because it is so easy to obtain, ricin is a potential biological warfare agent.

> **KEY FACT**
>
> Castor beans contain ricin. Jequirity beans contain abrin.

MECHANISM OF TOXICITY

- Chewing of bean → toxin absorption → inhibition of protein synthesis → cytotoxic cellular effects.
- Chewing and swallowing as little as one bean may be lethal.

SYMPTOMS/EXAMINATION

- **Fever** is the major presenting feature.
- **Delayed gastrointestinal (GI) symptoms** (6 hours to days).
  - Nausea/vomiting, abdominal pain, bloody diarrhea
- Followed by delirium, seizures, liver and renal failure, coma, and death.
- Castor beans are antigenic and may cause severe cutaneous hypersensitivity or systemic allergic reactions.

DIAGNOSIS

Based on history of ingestion/exposure and clinical presentation

TREATMENT

- Supportive therapy.
- Gastric decontamination (consider whole-bowel irrigation).
- Replace GI fluid losses with IV fluids.
- Electrolyte replacement.

> **KEY FACT**
>
> In water hemlock toxicity, seizures are often refractory to standard treatment.

WATER HEMLOCK

Water hemlock (*Cicuta maculata*) grows throughout North America in wetlands or near streams. It is tall (up to 2.5 m) with small white flowers. The root contains the highest concentration of toxin, and a single bite can be lethal. It is occasionally mistaken for parsnips.

Toxin = **cicutoxin.**

MECHANISM OF TOXICITY

Ingestion of plant → noncompetitive GABA receptor antagonist and CNS stimulant.

A

Respiratory deterioration can be delayed for up to 6 hours. Given that he is already starting to show signs of respiratory distress, this patient needs to observed for at least 6 hours for any clinical deterioration. He is at high risk for pulmonary complications such as pneumonia, pulmonary edema, pneumonitis, and ARDS.

TABLE 13.15. Common Poisonous Plants

Plant	Toxin Mechanism of Toxicity	Major Toxic Effects
Castor bean/jequirity bean	Ricin/abrin: Cytotoxic cellular effects	Fever Delayed severe GI symptoms
Water hemlock	Antagonism of GABA	Severe status epilepticus
Azalea	Andromedotoxins: Increased permeability of Na^+ channels	Bradycardia Progressive paralysis
Cardiac glycosides Foxglove Common oleander Yellow oleander Lily of the valley	Inhibition of Na^+-K^+ ATPase pump	Symptoms of digoxin toxicity
Cyanogenic fruit seeds	Amygdalin: Metabolized to hydrocyanic acid	Cyanide poisoning
Nicotine-Containing		
Tobacco plant	Nicotine: Stimulation of nicotinic receptors	Early stimulation Later weakness, paralysis, bradycardia
Poison hemlock	Coniine alkaloids: Stimulation of nicotinic receptors	As given previously
Anticholinergic		
Jimsonweed	Atropine-like alkaloids: Competitive inhibition of cholinergic receptors	Anticholinergic toxidrome
Deadly nightshade	Atropine-like substance: Inhibition of cholinergic receptors	Anticholinergic toxidrome
Hallucinogenic		
Marijuana	Δ-9-THC	Low level: Euphoria High level: Lethargy
Mexican peyote cactus	Mescaline: Similar to LSD	Euphoria, altered perception High doses: sympathomimetic toxicity
Morning glory	D-Lysergic acid amide: Similar to LSD	Hallucinations, dilated pupils

GI, gastrointestinal; LSD, lysergic acid diethylamide; THC, tetrahydrocannabinol.

Symptoms/Examination

- Rapid onset of symptoms after ingestion
- Nausea/vomiting, abdominal pain
- Hypersalivation, mydriasis, delirium, agitation

- Tachycardia, dysrhythmias, hyper/hypotension
- **Severe status epilepticus**
- Death

TREATMENT

- Supportive care plus aggressive gastric decontamination
- Standard treatment for status epilepticus

AZALEA

Rhododendron species: Exposure from ingestion of plant or honey made from these plants: "mad honey disease."
Toxin = **Andromedotoxins (grayanotoxins)**.

MECHANISM OF TOXICITY

Ingestion → increased permeability of Na^+ channels → prolonged depolarization and excitation → increased permeability of Ca^{2+} channels → digitalis-like effect.

SYMPTOMS/EXAMINATION

- Nausea/vomiting, diarrhea
- Salivation
- Bradycardia, hypotension, atrioventricular (AV) blocks
- Progressive paralysis
- Death (rare)

TREATMENT

- GI decontamination.
- Supportive care.
- Atropine as needed for bradycardia; AV blocks may require pacing.

CARDIAC GLYCOSIDES

Cardiac glycosides are found in a large number of plants including:

- Foxglove (*Digitalis purpurea*) (Figure 13.10)
- Common oleander (*Nerium oleander*)
- Yellow oleander (*Thevetia peruviana*)
- Lily of the valley (*Convallaria majalis*)

Foxglove contains digoxin; the others are structurally similar to digoxin.

MECHANISM OF TOXICITY

Inhibit the Na^+-K^+ ATPase pump.

Cardiac glycoside toxicity is covered in detail in Chapter 6, Toxicology.

CYANOGENIC PLANTS

Cyanide poisoning may result after ingesting large numbers of pits/seeds of a variety of fruits, including:

- Peach pits
- Apricot pits
- Pear seeds
- Crab apple seeds
- Cassava roots/leaves

Q

A 37-year-old woman is brought into the ED hyperthermic, tachycardic, unable to urinate, and actively hallucinating. She adamantly denies using illicit drugs but does admit to eating some flowers growing along the side of the road. What type of plant did she likely ingest?

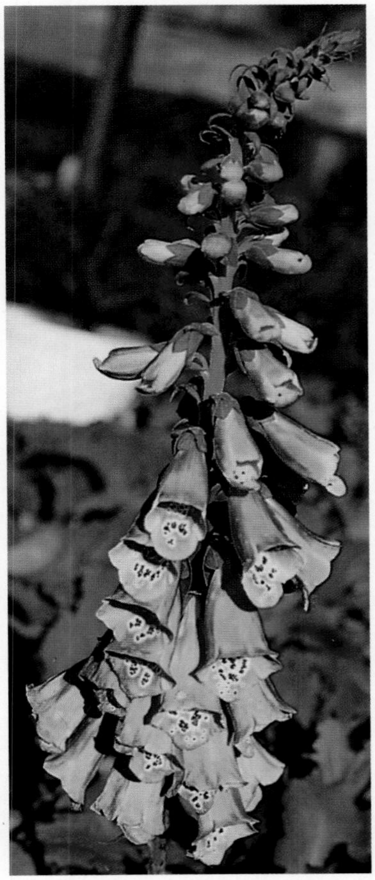

FIGURE 13.10. *Digitalis purpurea* (purple foxglove). The ornamental plant. (Reproduced, with permission, from Knoop KJ, Stack LB, Storrow AB. *Atlas of Emergency Medicine*. 3rd ed. New York, NY: McGraw-Hill; 2010. Figure 17.65. Photographer: Lawrence B. Stack, MD.)

A

This patient likely ingested jimsonweed (*Datura stramonium*). It is a light purple trumpet-like flower that is found along roadsides. Ingestion can cause an anticholinergic toxidrome. Treatment consists of supportive care, benzodiazepines, and physostigmine if the benzodiazepines are ineffective.

Mechanism of Toxicity

- Amygdalin and linamarin, cyanogenic glycosides, are metabolized into **hydrocyanic** acid.
- Hydrocyanic acid may lead to acute cyanide toxicity.

Symptoms/Examination

- Acute toxicity = Cyanide poisoning (see Chapter 6, Toxicology)
- Delayed symptom onset because cyanide is released by metabolism
- Nausea/vomiting
- Shortness of breath
- Headache, ataxia, altered mental status
- Cardiovascular collapse
- Chronic ingestion → polyneuropathies

Treatment

- GI decontamination
- Hydroxycobalamin or cyanide antidote kit (amyl nitrite or sodium nitrite plus sodium thiosulfate) for acute toxicity

NICOTINE-CONTAINING PLANTS

Tobacco Plant

Tobacco plants contain the toxin **nicotine**. Common methods of use include cigarette smoking, cigar smoking, pipe smoking, and smokeless tobacco (snuff).

Mechanism of Toxicity

Ingestion or large skin exposure → stimulation of nicotinic receptors and symptoms.

Symptoms/Examination

- Characterized by early stimulation, followed by inhibition
- **Early stimulation**
  - Abdominal pain, nausea/vomiting
  - Salivation, bronchorrhea
  - Hypertension, tachycardia
  - Fasciculations, seizures
- **Inhibition**
  - Weakness
  - Respiratory muscle paralysis
  - Bradycardia and death

Treatment

- GI decontamination with activated charcoal
- **Atropine** as needed to control secretions
- **Benzodiazepines** to control agitation and seizures
- Supportive care

Poison Hemlock (*Conium Maculatum*)

Poison hemlock grows along roads, ditches, and in damp areas throughout the United States. It is tall (1.5-2.5 m) with small white flowers and appears similar to water hemlock.

Toxin = **Coniine alkaloids,** which are structurally similar to nicotine.

Mechanism of Toxicity

Ingestion of plant → stimulation of nicotinic receptors and symptoms.

Presentation and treatment as with tobacco plant exposure, given previously.

ANTICHOLINERGIC PLANTS

Jimsonweed (*Datura Stramonium*)

Also known as Jamestown weed and locoweed, jimsonweed is commonly found along roadsides and in cornfields and pastures. It has broad green leaves, light purple trumpet-like flowers, and large spiny seeds. It is used intentionally for its hallucinogenic properties. Related species containing similar alkaloids include henbane (*Hyoscyamus niger*), deadly nightshade (*Atropa belladonna*), and mandrake root (*Mandragora officinarum*).

Toxins = **Atropine, scopolamine, and hyoscyamine (belladonna) alkaloids**.

Mechanism of Toxicity

Ingestion → competitive inhibition of cholinergic receptors → anticholinergic toxidrome.

Symptoms/Examination

- **Anticholinergic toxidrome**
  - Hallucinations
  - Hyperthermia
  - Flushed skin, dry skin, and mucous membranes
  - Mydriasis
  - Tachycardia
  - Urinary retention

Treatment

- Supportive (IV fluids, external cooling)
- Gastric decontamination (charcoal or whole-bowel irrigation)
- Sedation with **benzodiazepines**
- **Physostigmine** if benzodiazepines are not effective; a cholinesterase inhibitor, complications include AV block, asystole

Deadly Nightshade (*Atropa belladonna*)

Deadly nightshade is a black-cherry-like fruit that contains an atropine-like substance. Its Latin name means "pretty woman"—drops of belladonna were once used cosmetically to dilate the pupils.

Mechanism of Toxicity

Ingestion → inhibition of cholinergic receptors → anticholinergic toxidrome.

Presentation and treatment are similar to jimsonweed.

HALLUCINOGENIC PLANTS

Marijuana: Hemp Plant (*Cannabis Sativa*)

The active ingredient of marijuana is Δ-9-tetrahydrocannabinol. It can be smoked or eaten.

Symptoms/Examination

- **Low-level exposure**
  - Somnolence, euphoria, heightened sensory awareness, feelings of well-being, alteration of time perception, and paranoia
- **High-level exposure**
  - Lethargy, decreased coordination, and ataxia
- Abstinence syndrome
  - Agitation, apprehension, and insomnia

Diagnosis

- May be detected on urine toxicology screen

Treatment

Supportive care and benzodiazepines for agitation.

Complications

Postural hypotension, tachycardia, paranoia, agitation.

Mescaline

Mescaline is a hallucinogenic alkaloid found in the **Mexican peyote cactus** *Lophophora williamsii*.

Symptoms/Examination

- Similar to LSD
- Euphoria, alerted perception, nystagmus, and ataxia
- Nausea/vomiting, abdominal pain
- In high doses: Sympathomimetic toxicity (see Chapter 6, Toxicology)
  - Diaphoresis
  - Hypertension, tachycardia
  - Mydriasis
  - Hyperthermia

Treatment/Complications

As with marijuana, given earlier.

Morning Glory (*Ipomoea Violacea*)

Seeds of this plant contain D-lysergic acid amide, a compound related to LSD.

Symptoms/Examination

- Hallucinations
- Dilated pupils
- Nausea/vomiting, diarrhea
- Numbness of extremities and muscle tightness

Treatment/Complications

As with marijuana, given previously.

Gastrointestinal Irritants

- **Holly (*Ilex* sp)**—toxic berries
- **Pokeweed (*Phytolacca americana*)**—entire plant is toxic

Symptoms/Examination

- Abdominal pain, nausea/vomiting, diarrhea
- Death (rare)

Treatment

GI decontamination and supportive care.

Mushrooms

Mushroom toxicity may occur during experimental ingestions by patients looking for a "high" or more commonly in foragers who misidentify the species. The toxic dose is unknown, and the amount of toxin varies widely among mushrooms.

Mushroom toxicity can be divided into two groups based on the onset of symptoms: Early-onset toxicity and delayed-onset toxicity.

EARLY-ONSET TOXICITY

Symptom onset 0-4 hours after mushroom ingestion typically indicates a benign course. The presentation varies with the type of mushroom ingested (Table 13.16).

Q

A 54-year-old man presents to the ED with nausea/vomiting and abdominal pain. He reports eating some "unusual" mushrooms while out in the woods earlier in the day, but felt fine until about 7 hours later when the GI symptoms started. What can you tell this patient about his likelihood of having a serious mushroom poisoning?

KEY FACT

Amanita sp causes most deaths.

TABLE 13.16. Mushroom Toxicity

Clinical Symptoms	Representative Mushroom	Toxin	Treatment
Early Onset (0-4 h)			
Gastrointestinal	Many species		Supportive and symptomatic
Muscarinic (SLUDGE)	*Cytocybe* sp *Inocybe* sp	Muscarine	Atropine for bradycardia and bronchorrhea
CNS excitation	*Amanita muscaria*	Muscimol, ibotenic acid	Supportive and symptomatic
Hallucinations	*Psilocybe* sp	Psilocybin	Supportive Benzodiazepines
Disulfiram-like reaction	*Coprinus* sp	Coprine (with EtOH)	Supportive Benzodiazepines
Delayed Onset (6-24 h)			
Gastroenteritis followed by hepatotoxicity	*Amanita phalloides* *Gyromitra* sp	Amatoxins, phallotoxins Gyromitrin	Supportive and symptomatic May require transplant Supportive
Gastroenteritis followed by seizures	*Gyromitra* sp		Benzodiazepines **Pyridoxine for seizures**
Gastroenteritis followed by renal failure	*Cortinarius orellanus*	Orellanine	Supportive May require hemodialysis

CNS, central nervous system.

A

Assuming his symptoms are due to ingestion of mushrooms, the onset of symptoms are > 6 hours since the time of ingestion, indicating a potential for serious toxicity. Depending on the species, hepatotoxicity, renal toxicity, or seizures could develop. Consultation with a local mycologist may help determine the likely species.

Gastrointestinal Irritant Mushrooms

- Seen with many mushroom species
- Sx/examination: Nausea/vomiting, diarrhea, abdominal pain usually within 0.5-2 hours of ingestion

Muscarine-Containing Mushrooms

- Seen with *Clitocybe* sp, *Inocybe* sp which contain the toxin **muscarine**
- Sx/examination: Symptoms of cholinergic (SLUDGE) syndrome: Salivation, lacrimation, urination, defecation, ↑ GI motility, and emesis, as well as bradycardia

Ibotenic Acid and Muscimol-Containing Mushrooms

- Seen with *Amanita muscaria Amanita pantherina*, *Amanita gemmata*.
- Caused by toxin **muscimol**, a toxic metabolite of ibotenic acid that stimulates GABA receptors.
- Sx/examination: Intoxication, dizziness, and anticholinergic effects (dry mouth/skin, mydriasis, tachycardia). Children may have myoclonus and seizures.

Psilocybin-Containing Mushrooms

- Seen with *Psilocybe*, *Gymnopilus*, *Conocybe*, *Panaeolus* sp
- Caused by toxin **psilocybin**, an LSD-like serotonin stimulator
- Sx/examination: Visual hallucinations, ataxia, hyperkinesis, seizures, tachycardia

Coprine-Containing Mushrooms: Disulfiram-Like Reaction (*with Co-Ingestion of ETOH*)

- Seen with *Coprinus atramentarius* ("inky cap")
- Caused by toxin **coprine**, which inhibits acetaldehyde dehydrogenase
- Sx/examination: Headache, flushing, tachycardia, hyperventilation with EtOH ingestion within 72 hours of mushroom ingestion

DELAYED-ONSET TOXICITY

KEY FACT

Mushroom toxicity: Early onset of GI symptoms → benign course. Delayed onset of GI symptoms → potential for serious toxicity

Delayed-onset toxicity is a marker for ingestion of mushrooms with potential for serious toxicity. In these cases, GI symptoms (nausea/vomiting, diarrhea) do not begin until 6-24 hours after ingestion and are followed by liver, CNS, or renal toxicity.

Gastrointestinal Effects Followed by Hepatotoxicity

- Seen with *A phalloides*
- Caused by **cyclopeptides** (amatoxins and phallotoxins)
- Sx/examination: Delayed nausea/vomiting and diarrhea followed by hepatic failure in 72 hours (LFTs begin to rise at 24-48 hours); acute renal failure; seizures, coma

Gastrointestinal Effects Followed by Seizures

- Seen with *Gyromitra esculenta* ("false morel")
- Caused by gyromitrin toxin, which **inhibits pyridoxine-dependent (vit. B_6) pathways and depletes GABA (similar to INH overdose)**
- Sx/examination: Delayed nausea/vomiting and diarrhea followed by seizures and hepatorenal failure

GI Effects Followed by Renal Failure

- *C orellanus*
- Caused by orellanine toxin, a nephrotoxin
- Sx/examination: Delayed (24-36 hours) nausea/vomiting and diarrhea followed days to weeks later by thirst, chills, flank pain, and oliguric renal failure

Treatment

- Observe for development of early-onset symptoms (4-6 hours).
- If no early-onset symptoms, have patient return if delayed symptoms develop.
- Mainstay of therapy is supportive care.
- **Monitor *glucose*** (hypoglycemia is common).
- Atropine if symptomatic bradycardia or bronchorrhea from muscarinic syndrome.
- Benzodiazepines to control agitation.
- Pyridoxine: For delayed-onset seizures (inhibition of pyridoxine-dependent pathways) with *Gyromitra* sp.

REVIEW QUESTIONS

QUESTIONS

1. A 60-year-old man with history of ethanol abuse presents after a physical altercation with a laceration over his third metacarpophalangeal (MCP) joint with no evidence of tendon involvement or fracture. Management of his injury includes:
   A. Irrigation only
   B. Laceration repair
   C. Irrigation, wound exploration, antibiotics
   D. Immediate surgical consultation
2. An 82-year-old woman arrives to the emergency department altered with a rectal temperature of 40°C. The most likely cause of her presentation is:
   A. Heat exhaustion
   B. Heat tetany
   C. Heat stroke
   D. Stroke
3. A 50-year-old homeless man presents to the emergency department with decreased mentation, a rectal temperature of 30°C, heart rate of 45 bpm, and a blood pressure of 100/60 mm Hg. Initial efforts to rewarm him should include:
   A. Room temperature intravenous (IV) fluids
   B. Warm blankets to his extremities
   C. Cardiopulmonary bypass
   D. Heating lamps
4. Which of the following is true regarding high-altitude pulmonary edema (HAPE)?
   A. Usually occurs within 4 days after arrival at altitude.
   B. Patients with a patent foramen ovale are at decreased risk of developing HAPE.
   C. Chest x-ray will show an enlarged cardiac silhouette.
   D. Diuretics are the mainstay of treatment for HAPE.
5. Match the plant with the major toxic effect.

A. Water hemlock	1. Fever, delayed gastrointestinal (GI) symptoms
B. Jimsonweed	2. Status epilepticus
C. Foxglove	3. Hallucinations, hyperthermia
D. Castor bean	4. Dysrhythmias, visual changes

ANSWERS

1. **C.** This is a case of a human bite to the hand, often referred to as a "fight bite." These wounds are at high risk for infection and can lead to septic arthritis, osteomyelitis, and tenosynovitis. These wounds need extensive irrigation and exploration. If there is any evidence of tendon or bone involvement, surgical consultation is indicated. All these wounds require antibiotic prophylaxis. Generally, laceration repair is not recommended because it may increase risk of infection.
2. **C.** This patient has an elevated core temperature and evidence of central nervous system (CNS) dysfunction, which defines heat stroke. Heat stroke occurs due to failure of the homeostatic thermoregulatory mechanisms of the body. This classically occurs in an elderly or debilitated population although can also been seen in younger individuals who are exercising in a hot environment. Heat exhaustion is the most common form of heat-related illness and can have a normal or elevated core temperature. What differentiates heat exhaustion from heat stroke is that the mental status is normal in heat exhaustion and abnormal in heat stroke. Heat tetany is characterized by carpal–pedal spasms due to hyperventilation.
3. **D.** This patient is suffering from moderate hypothermia. Hypothermia can be classified as mild (temperature > 32°C with no changes in mentation) or moderate to severe (temperature < 32°C with mental status changes, cardiovascular instability, electrocardiogram [ECG] changes). Active external rewarming is the mainstay of treatment for moderate-to-severe hypothermia without cardiovascular instability. This includes heating lamps, bair huggers to torso, warm IV fluids, and warm blankets. In these patients, it is important that rewarming should be focused on the core because extremity-only rewarming can cause core afterdrop. If patients develop cardiovascular instability (arrhythmias, severe hypotension), active core rewarming with gastric, bladder, peritoneal, and pleural lavage should be considered. Warming via cardiopulmonary bypass should be initiated only in patients in cardiac arrest or persistent malignant arrhythmias.
4. **A.** HAPE is a form of noncardiogenic pulmonary edema that usually occurs 2-4 days after arrival to altitude. This is thought to be due to pulmonary vasoconstriction, which leads to pulmonary hypertension causing endothelial damage and capillary leak. Patients with a patent foramen ovale may experience right-to-left shunting and therefore be at higher risk of HAPE symptoms. HAPE is a clinical diagnosis but can be confirmed with a chest x-ray showing bilateral patchy infiltrates and a normal heart size. Treatment of HAPE includes descent, supplemental oxygen, and calcium channel blockers such as nifedipine. Diuretic therapy is controversial in the treatment of HAPE and not routinely recommended.

5. **A.** 2, **B.** 3, **C.** 4, **D.** 1. Water hemlock is a tall plant with small white flowers that grows throughout North American wetlands and near streams. It is a GABA antagonist and therefore can cause severe and often intractable status epilepticus.

Jimsonweed is commonly found along roadsides and used intentionally for its hallucinogenic properties. It is a competitive inhibitor of cholinergic receptors and causes an anticholinergic toxidrome (hallucinations, hyperthermia, flushed skin, mydriasis, tachycardia, urinary retention).

Foxglove is a cardiac glycoside from which digoxin is derived and it works by inhibiting the Na^+-K^+ ATPase pump. Ingestion can cause symptoms similar to digoxin toxicity such as dysrhythmias, nausea, vomiting, abdominal pain, confusion, and visual disturbances (blurred or yellow vision).

The castor bean plant contains the potent toxalbumin ricin, which inhibits protein synthesis causing cytotoxic cellular effects. Fever and delayed GI symptoms are the major presenting features. As little as one bean may be lethal.

CHAPTER 14

Head, Eyes, Ear, Nose, and Throat, and Dental Emergencies

W. Gannon Sungar, DO

Facial Trauma

While motor vehicle accidents used to account for the majority of facial trauma, increased use of safety belts and the prevalence of air bags have made interpersonal violence the most common cause of facial injuries. After assessing for airway compromise, the care of facial trauma is focused on identifying threats to vision and optimizing function and cosmesis. Traditional teaching has shown correlation between facial fractures and associated injuries (10% incidence of associated cervical spine injury); however, newer data show that intracranial and spinal injuries should be evaluated outside the influence of facial trauma.

NASAL FRACTURE

Nasal fracture is the most common maxillofacial fracture (mandibular fracture is second) and generally occurs in the setting of blunt trauma.

Symptoms/Examination

- Examine for swelling, tenderness, mobility, crepitus, deformity, and step-offs.
- Look for **septal hematoma**, appearing as a dark purple/blue mass coming off of the septum (Figure 14.1).

Diagnosis

- Clinical diagnosis; radiographs are insensitive and computed tomography (CT) is unnecessary unless concerned for additional facial fractures.
- If alignment is acceptable, epistaxis is controlled, there is no septal hematoma, and the patient can breathe out of each individual naris, no further management is required.

Treatment

- Ice to reduce swelling
- If markedly displaced can attempt reduction using scalpel handles in each nare with anterior and midline pressure.
- Follow-up with plastic surgery, ENT, or oral and maxillofacial surgery (OMS) in 3-5 days for further reduction, only if alignment is unacceptable once swelling decreases.

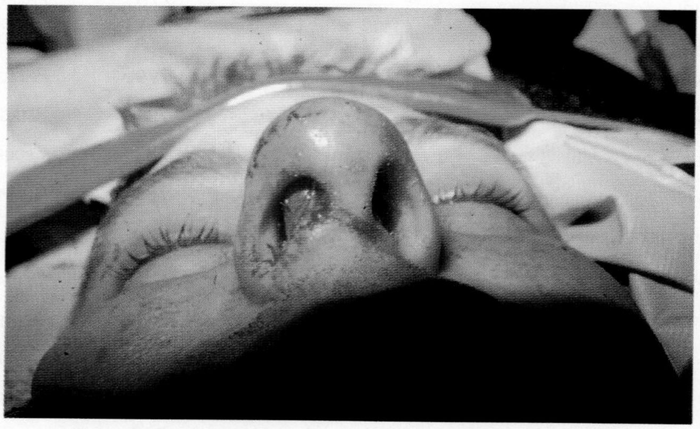

FIGURE 14.1. Septal hematoma. (Reproduced, with permission, from Knoop KJ, Stack LB, Storrow AB. *Atlas of Emergency Medicine*. 2nd ed. New York, NY: McGraw-Hill Education; 2002. Photographer: Lawrence B. Stack, MD.)

COMPLICATIONS

- **Septal hematoma** = Blood accumulation separating the septal cartilage from the perichondrial blood supply; requires recognition and prompt drainage as follows:
  - Anesthetize the septum with topical, atomized, or injectable anesthetic.
  - Make an elliptical incision in the mucosa overlying the hematoma, being careful not to incise the cartilage.
  - Evacuate the clot with pressure and/or suction.
  - Place a small Penrose drain into the incision.
  - Pack both nostrils as in anterior epistaxis to reapproximate perichondrium and septal cartilage.
  - Follow-up with ENT in 48 hours.
- Untreated septal hematomas can lead to abscess, necrosis, and septal perforation.

> **KEY FACT**
>
> Evaluate all patients with nasal trauma for septal hematoma. Drain septal hematoma to prevent abscess formation and cartilage necrosis.

ORBITAL FRACTURE

Orbital floor or "blowout" fractures are the most common and are often isolated. They result from a direct blunt force to the globe, usually from a fist or a ball, increasing intraocular pressure enough to fracture the weakest, inferior portion, of the orbit causing herniation of orbital contents into the maxillary sinus. **Medial orbital fractures** occur through the lamina papyracea into the ethmoid sinus and are commonly associated with nasal and midface fractures.

SYMPTOMS/EXAMINATION

- Swelling, orbital tenderness, or deformity
- Ecchymosis, numbness over cheek and upper lip (infraorbital nerve compression)
- Enophthalmos can be seen with orbital blowout fractures as the globe sinks back within the orbit, whereas exophthalmos should raise concern for retrobulbar hematoma.
- Assess extraocular movements and evaluate for diplopia.

DIAGNOSIS

CT orbit showing fracture line and air fluid level indicating blood in the affected sinus

COMPLICATIONS

- Entrapment of the extraocular muscles; **inferior rectus** is most common resulting in limitation or diplopia with upward gaze.
- Ocular injury including iritis, hyphema, ruptured globe, retrobulbar hematoma

TREATMENT

- Analgesia, ice to reduce swelling, sinus precautions
- Prophylactic antibiotics to cover sinus pathogens (amoxicillin-clavulanate or azithromycin)
- Muscle entrapment, diplopia, or limitation of extraocular movements necessitates urgent follow-up within 24 hours with a specialist, either ophthalmology, plastic surgery, or OMS.
- Surgical repair is generally delayed for 1 or 2 weeks to allow swelling to resolve.

> **KEY FACT**
>
> Blowout fracture can result in entrapment of the **inferior rectus muscle** within the orbital floor causing limitation of, or diplopia with, upward gaze.

MANDIBLE FRACTURE

The second most common maxillofacial fracture. Forced occlusion often results in fracture to the condyle, whereas a lateral blow results in fracture to the body or angle. Traditional teaching states that due to the U shape of the mandible, ≥ 2 sites are often fractured, but more recent studies have shown that 42% may be unifocal.

SYMPTOMS/EXAMINATION

- Malocclusion, trismus, step-off, intraoral bleeding/deformity, ear pain
- Lower lip and chin anesthesia from injury to mental nerve
- **Sublingual or buccal ecchymosis** is considered pathognomonic.

DIAGNOSIS

- Tongue blade test: The ability to maintain the bite on a tongue blade being twisted with enough force that it cracks has a negative predictive value of 95% for mandibular fracture.
- Panorex x-ray will likely reveal fracture, but CT of face is often preferred by specialists to evaluate associated injuries and assist in surgical planning.

COMPLICATIONS

- Airway compromise from intraoral swelling or lack of tongue support in the case of multifocal fractures (flail mandible)
- If forced occlusion by history, consider hyperextension injury to cervical spine, including fracture or vascular injury.

TREATMENT

- All open fractures (blood in mouth) require antibiotic coverage with penicillin, cephalosporin or clindamycin, tetanus booster, and urgent ENT or OMS consultation.
- Patients with closed, nondisplaced fractures may be discharged home with appropriate analgesia, soft diet, and ENT or OMS follow-up within 1-2 days.

KEY FACT

If mandible deviates toward the side with pain = fracture. If mandible deviates away from side with pain = unilateral dislocation

MANDIBULAR DISLOCATION

Mandibular dislocation is generally because of **excessive mouth opening** that occurs during laughing, yawning, eating, or dental procedures. The mandibular condyles are displaced **anterior and superior** relative to their articulating surface resulting in inability to open or fully close the mouth and a protruding chin. Dislocations are most often bilateral and symmetric, but can occur unilaterally with the jaw deviating **away** from the injury.

TREATMENT

- Eliciting a gag reflex inhibits the muscles of mouth closure and may result in autoreduction, but if this is unsuccessful, reduction often requires procedural sedation.
- Firmly grasp the mandible with both hands with the thumbs resting inside the mouth in the buccal sulcus of the mandible; press the angle of the mandible downward while rotating the chin upward and backward.
- Postreduction x-ray is used to verify reduction and rule out fracture.
- Avoid extreme jaw opening for 3 weeks, soft diet, nonsteroidal anti-inflammatory drugs (NSAIDs) for pain, and OMS follow-up in 1-3 days.

ZYGOMATICO-MAXILLARY-ORBITAL COMPLEX (TRIPOD) FRACTURES

A "tripod" fracture is usually caused by a direct blow to the face resulting in a classic fracture pattern involving the zygoma, the lateral orbital wall, and the maxilla (Figure 14.2).

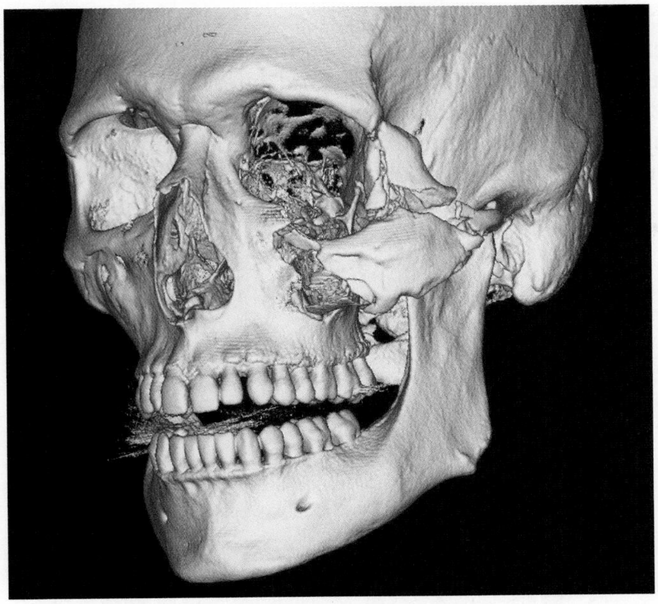

FIGURE 14.2. Tripod fracture. (Reproduced, with permission, from Knoop KJ, Stack LB, Storrow AB, Thurman RJ. *Atlas of Emergency Medicine*. 3rd ed. New York, NY: McGraw-Hill Education; 2010. Figure 1.16. Photographer: David Effron, MD.)

Q

A 22-year-old man is brought in by ambulance following an altercation where he was punched in the face with no loss of consciousness. The patient complains of his teeth "not matching up normally," but denies numbness, weakness, nausea, or vomiting. Examination is unremarkable except for a bit of blood in his oropharynx, but no clear lacerations. What is the diagnosis and the next step in management?

Symptoms/Examination

- Facial asymmetry and flattening of the cheek bone
- Malocclusion of the maxillary teeth
- Maxillary teeth paresthesias due to **dentoalveolar nerve** injury
- Palpation of the zygoma from within the mouth may allow better evaluation of the bony structures without being confused by overlying soft tissue swelling or tenderness.

Diagnosis

Clinical suspicion confirmed by facial CT (1-3 mm coronal and axial cuts)

Treatment

- Sinus precautions, prophylactic antibiotics, and appropriate analgesia
- Tripod fractures are often displaced and require operative fixation to avoid sinking of the cheek bone and facial asymmetry.

MIDFACE FRACTURES

Midface fractures are due to blunt trauma and are described using the **Le Fort** classification (Figure 14.3). These fractures can be differentiated by pulling the central incisors anteriorly during the secondary survey and noting what part(s) of the face is mobile.

- **Le Fort I**
  - Unilateral or bilateral fracture through the inferior maxilla just above the roots of the teeth
  - Dental arch is mobile with anterior displacement of the central incisors.
- **Le Fort II**
  - Bilateral pyramidal fracture extending superiorly from the maxilla through the orbital floor and rim, medially through the lacrimal bones, and across the nasal bridge
  - The nasal complex moves as a unit when the central incisors are grasped and rocked.

A

Malocclusion, or the sensation of the teeth not lining up, is one of the most sensitive symptoms for mandibular fracture. Given the blood in the oropharynx, this fracture is likely open and should be treated with antibiotics, an update of tetanus status, CT scan of the face to assist in surgical planning, and OMS consult.

- **Le Fort III**
  - Rare injury with fractures spreading laterally from the nasal bridge through the medial wall, floor, and lateral wall of the orbit and then the zygoma resulting in complete craniofacial dissociation
  - Intranasally, the fracture extends posteriorly to the sphenoid and is frequently associated with a cerebrospinal fluid (CSF) leak.
  - The entire face pulls anteriorly with rocking of the central incisors.

Diagnosis

Facial CT (1-3 mm coronal and axial cuts)

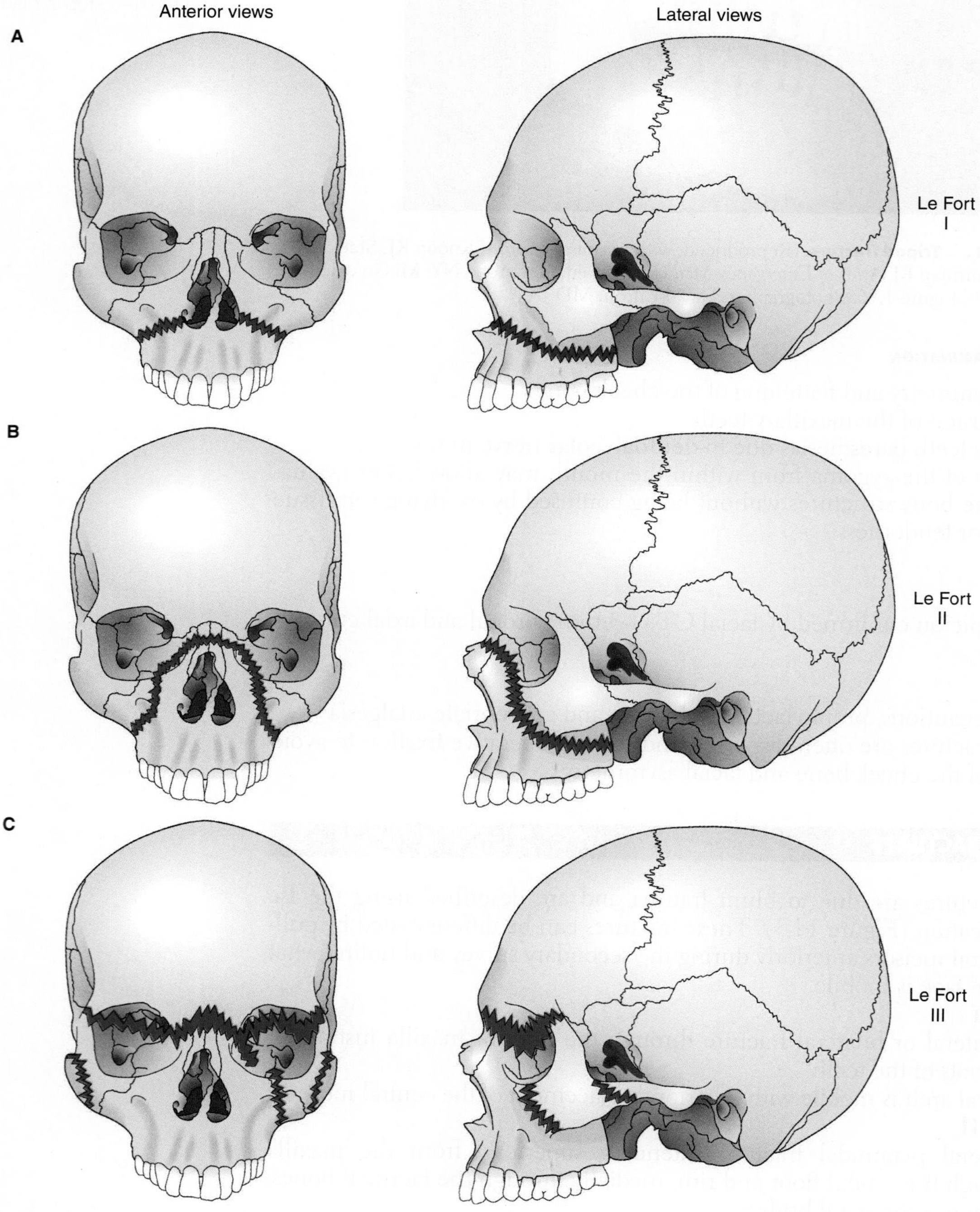

FIGURE 14.3. Le Fort classification of midface fractures. (Reproduced, with permission, from Stone CK, Humphries RL. *Current Diagnosis & Treatment: Emergency Medicine*. 7th ed. New York, NY: McGraw-Hill Education; 2010. Figure 23.6.)

TREATMENT

- Airway protection as these fractures can result in collapse of airway supporting structures and significant bleeding
- Massive, uncontrolled bleeding from arterial injuries: Immediate airway control, reduction, and packing of the nares and oropharynx followed by definitive management with arterial embolization
- Neurosurgery consult if CSF leak is present.
- Prophylactic antibiotics covering sinus pathogens (eg, amoxicillin-clavulanate or clindamycin)
- Le Fort fractures require urgent OMS consultation because early surgical repair is preferred.

Ear

AURICULAR HEMATOMA

Results from blunt trauma directly to the auricle typically related to sports (eg, boxing, wrestling, rugby).

SYMPTOMS/EXAMINATION

Tender, tense, fluctuant mass, most commonly seen on the anterior pinna within the scaphoid fossa (Figure 14.4)

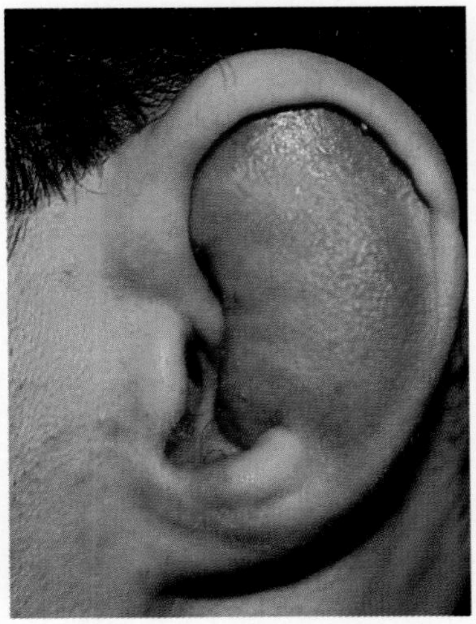

FIGURE 14.4. Auricular hematoma. (Reproduced, with permission, from Knoop KJ, Stack LB, Storrow AB Thurman RJ. *Atlas of Emergency Medicine*. 3rd ed. New York, NY: McGraw-Hill Education; 2010. Photographer: C. Bruce MacDonald, MD.)

TREATMENT

- Needle aspiration of small (< 2 cm) hematomas may be successful, while larger lesions (> 2 cm) warrant incision and drainage.
- A pressure dressing should be placed following hematoma evacuation to prevent reaccumulation
- Daily follow up should be scheduled until the wound is healed.
- Undrained hematomas > 7 days old have likely formed granulation tissue and should be referred to ENT.

COMPLICATIONS

- **Cauliflower ear:** Cartilage necrosis, fibrosis, and neocartilage formation with permanent deformity from untreated auricular hematoma separating the underlying cartilage from the perichondrial blood supply

EAR FOREIGN BODY

Most common in children with any variety of small objects placed in the external canal. Additionally, campers and people with poor living conditions are at risk for insects crawling into the external ear canal.

SYMPTOMS/EXAMINATION

- Adults: Ear pain or decreased hearing and history of foreign body insertion
- Children: Ear pain and secondary signs of foreign body, including malodorous discharge
- Patients with an insect in their external canal will complain of movement or a buzzing sensation.

TREATMENT

- Proper anesthesia with topical lidocaine or with local anesthesia by injecting the external canal in all 4 quadrants.

- Foreign bodies may be removed with forceps, a small suction catheter, or an adhesive tipped cotton applicator.
- Alternatively, room temperature water can be instilled with a 14-guage catheter to flush out the object. Irrigation should **not** be attempted in the following scenarios:
  - Concern for tympanic membrane (TM) perforation
  - Potential for swelling of foreign bodies (eg, vegetables)
  - Button batteries because irrigation can increase current flow and tissue damage
- Insects in the canal should be killed or immobilized prior to attempts at removal. This can be achieved by immersion with liquid or viscous lidocaine, mineral oil, or alcohol.
- Topical antibiotics are recommended postextraction if the canal has been damaged.
- Immediate ENT consultation should be obtained for embedded button batteries or foreign bodies that cannot be removed with concern for TM rupture or infection.

COMPLICATIONS

- Complications are generally minor including bleeding and pain, but may include secondary otitis externa and TM perforation.
- Button batteries can cause rapid erosion by alkaline tissue necrosis.

VESTIBULAR NEURITIS AND LABYRINTHITIS

KEY FACT

Vestibular neuritis = inflammation of vestibular branch of CN VIII

Labyrinthitis = inflammation of vestibular *and* cochlear branches of CN VIII

KEY FACT

Cochlear branch involvement leads to hearing loss.

Closely related disorders characterized by inflammation of the vestibular branch (vestibular neuritis) or both the vestibular and cochlear branches (labyrinthitis) of CN VIII, the vestibulocochlear nerve. Most commonly viral or reactive, but other causes include acute suppurative bacterial infection and ototoxicity from aminoglycosides, chemotherapeutics, salicylates, loop diuretics, etc.

SYMPTOMS/EXAMINATION

- **Vertigo** (often continuous)
  - Reactive: Upper respiratory infection symptoms, mild vertigo
  - Acute suppurative: Acute otitis media with signs of systemic toxicity
  - Toxic: Gradually progressive in a patient on medication causing toxicity
- **Hearing loss** if cochlear branch involved

DIAGNOSIS

- Physical examination and history point to a peripheral cause of vertigo ± associated hearing loss.
- Head impulse testing will show a corrective saccade when the patient tries to focus on the examiner's nose during head thrust, indicating vestibular nerve dysfunction.

DIFFERENTIAL

- **Acoustic neuroma:** A slow-growing schwannoma of CN VIII that can cause hearing loss, tinnitus, and gradual onset of vertigo. Diagnosis confirmed by magnetic resonance imaging.
- **Benign paroxysmal positional vertigo:** A peripheral vertigo due to calcium debris (otoconia) within the semicircular canals of the inner ear. Characterized by vertigo worse with head movement. See also Chapter 15, Neurology.

TREATMENT

- Acute suppurative labyrinthitis requires emergent ENT consultation, intravenous antibiotics, and hospital admission.
- Nontoxic patients may be managed as outpatient with a trial of meclizine.

MÉNIÉRE DISEASE

An idiopathic excess of fluid in the endolymphatic spaces of the inner ear.

SYMPTOMS/EXAMINATION

- Classic triad: Sensorineural hearing loss, peripheral vertigo, **tinnitus**
- Attacks occur in clusters with long symptom-free intervals.

DIFFERENTIAL

As with all etiologies of acute vestibular syndromes, including labyrinthitis, must rule out central cause by examination and/or imaging.

TREATMENT

- Antiemetics, antihistamines (eg, meclizine), and benzodiazepines for acute attacks.
- Chronic therapy includes low-sodium diet, diuretics, smoking and caffeine cessation, and chemical ablation of vestibular function with aminoglycosides in extreme cases.

OTITIS EXTERNA

Inflammation of the external auditory canal, generally due to bacterial infection, most commonly *Pseudomonas aeruginosa* and *Staphylococcus aureus*. Fungal infection (otomycosis), most commonly due to *Aspergillus*, can be seen in diabetics and immunosuppressed. Risk factors include local trauma, prolonged moisture exposure ("swimmer's ear"), and high humidity and temperature climates.

SYMPTOMS/EXAMINATION

- Initially pruritic, advancing to ear pain, drainage, and fullness with conductive hearing loss
- Erythema and edema of the external auditory canal along with reproduction of pain with manipulation of the auricle or tragus

DIFFERENTIAL

- **Furunculosis** is a well-circumscribed infection of the cartilaginous portion of the external canal caused by *S. aureus* that requires incision and drainage and oral antibiotics.
- **Ramsay-Hunt syndrome**, or herpes zoster oticus:
  - Reactivation of herpes zoster in the geniculate ganglion
  - Presence of vesicles on the auricle, ear canal, or mucus membranes of oropharynx
  - Neurologic symptoms are common including seventh nerve palsy, vertigo, and hearing loss.
  - Treatment consists of acyclovir or valacyclovir.

TREATMENT

- Clean the external canal to remove cerumen, debris, and purulent material.

> **KEY FACT**
>
> Acute suppurative (bacterial) labyrinthitis is the only peripheral cause of vertigo that requires emergent management with IV antibiotics and ENT consultation.

> **Q**
>
> A 4-year-old girl with no medical history, up-to-date on all immunizations presents with the complaint of left ear pain and fever. The patient was seen by her pediatrician 6 days ago and diagnosed with an ear infection and was treated with amoxicillin without improvement. On examination, the child is febrile, and the left ear is more prominent than the right. What is the diagnosis and management?

- Treat inflammation and infection:
  - Topical antibiotic/glucocorticoid combination is recommended for most cases: Polymyxin B/neomycin/hydrocortisone or ciprofloxacin/hydrocortisone.
  - Consider placement of a wick to facilitate antibiotic delivery and drainage in cases of severe swelling.
  - Mild cases can be treated with acidifying agent/glucocorticoid combination alone (eg, acetic acid/hydrocortisone).
- If TM is ruptured, use oral antibiotics and avoid Cortisporin otic solution or suspension.
- Topical anesthetics (benzocaine/antipyrine) should be provided.

KEY FACT

New recommendations suggest avoiding both Cortisporin otic solution *and* suspension in cases of tympanic membrane rupture.

NECROTIZING (MALIGNANT) OTITIS EXTERNA

An aggressive infection of the external auditory canal and skull base at the temporal bone, typically due to ***P. aeruginosa***. The typical patient is an elderly diabetic, but it may also be seen in younger patients with acquired immunodeficiency syndrome or other immunocompromised states.

Symptoms/Examination

- Otalgia, drainage, periauricular pain, and swelling are common.
- Granulation tissue at the floor of the ear canal is the hallmark physical finding.
- Facial nerve palsy is common, due to extension to the stylomastoid foramen.
- May progress to meningitis, brain abscesses, and sigmoid sinus thrombosis

Diagnosis/Treatment

- CT and MRI may be valuable in characterizing the spread of the disease.
- Admission for IV antibiotics is required in most cases.
- Nontoxic patients may be treated with oral ciprofloxacin, often for 6-8 weeks, and ENT referral.

ACUTE OTITIS MEDIA

Defined as signs and symptoms of acute infection with middle ear effusion. Eustachian tube dysfunction, usually in setting of viral URI, results in poor drainage of the middle ear and a middle ear effusion, termed otitis media with effusion (OME). When this effusion becomes infected, AOM results. Risk factors include male gender, day care attendance, parental smoking, pacifier use, and family history.

Causes

- Bacterial etiologies include *Streptococcus pneumoniae*, *Haemophilus influenzae*, *Moraxella catarrhalis*, *Streptococcus pyogenes*, and *S. aureus*.
- Viral etiologies include respiratory syncytial virus, parainfluenza, influenza, rhinovirus, and adenovirus.

A

Mastoiditis may complicate AOM with infection spreading to involve the mastoid air cells. Examination may show a protruding auricle and the mastoid may be exquisitely tender to percussion. A CT temporal bone will confirm the diagnosis. Patients require parenteral antibiotics and may require surgical drainage.

Symptoms/Examination

- URI symptoms including cough, congestion, fever (rarely high-grade), ear pain or pulling, and decreased hearing.
- **Lack of mobility of the** TM on pneumatic otoscopy is the most sensitive finding.
- May also see erythema, cloudiness, bulging TM, and loss of the normal light reflex (Figure 14.5).

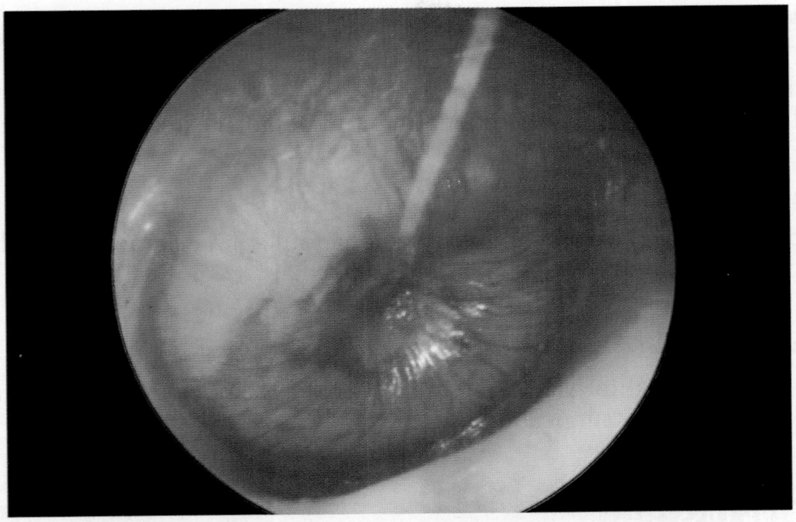

FIGURE 14.5. Acute otitis media. (Reproduced, with permission, from Knoop KJ, Stack LB, Storrow AB. *The Atlas of Emergency Medicine*. 3rd ed. New York: McGraw-Hill Education, 2010. Figure 5.3. Photographer: Richard A. Chole, MD, PhD.)

- **Bullous myringitis** is seen in a small subset of patients with AOM and is characterized by more severe ear pain and formation of bullae on the TM and medial canal wall. Classically associated with *Mycoplasma* infection, current teaching is that pathogens are the same as other types of AOM.

Complications

Rare in the setting of widespread antibiotic use, but include TM perforation (most common complication), **mastoiditis, otic meningitis** (most common intracranial complication), intracranial abscess, and venous sinus thrombosis

Treatment

- Analgesia with acetaminophen and/or ibuprofen; may add topical anesthesia with benzocaine-antipyrine
- > 80% of cases of AOM resolve spontaneously.
  - Delayed antibiotic administration or "watchful waiting" for 48 hours can be used in children > 6 months with presumed AOM.
- Amoxicillin is the recommended first-line agent.
- In the setting of tympanostomy tubes with an acutely draining ear, topical fluoroquinolone otic drops (oflaxacin or ciprofloxacin) should be used to cover *P. aeruginosa*.

KEY FACT

Significant fever is rare in AOM, so other causes of fever should be investigated in a febrile, toxic-appearing child.

MASTOIDITIS

Mastoiditis is a suppurative infection of the mastoid air cells, most commonly in children < 2 years. It is a complication of AOM due to extension of a middle ear infection into the adjacent mastoid air cells. *S. pneumonia* is the most common organism. It is also seen with Kawasaki disease, leukemia, and mononucleosis.

Symptoms/Examination

- Fever, headache, otalgia
- Postauricular erythema, mastoid tenderness, abnormal TM, and protrusion of the auricle **outward and down**

Diagnosis

- CT will show opacification of the mastoid air cells and may show skull osteomyelitis.
- MRI is preferred if there is concern for intracranial extension of infection.

Complications

Occipital (calvaria) osteomyelitis, intracranial infection, sigmoid sinus thrombosis, extension to sternocleidomastoid (Bezold abscess)

Treatment

Most cases respond to parenteral antibiotics (eg, ceftriaxone or clindamycin) without the need for surgical drainage.

HEARING LOSS

There are 2 types of hearing loss: **conductive**, involving the outer ear, TM, or middle ear; and **sensorineural**, involving the inner ear, CN VIII, and brain. A sudden sensorineural hearing loss (SSNHL) is considered an otolaryngologic emergency.

Causes

- Conductive: AOM, OME, cerumen impaction, foreign body, Eustachian tube dysfunction, cholesteatoma
- Sensorineural: >70% of SSNHL is idiopathic; other causes include infection, malignancy, autoimmune, multiple, sclerosis, trauma and vascular disease.

Symptoms/Examination

- Sudden unilateral hearing loss.
- **Rinne test** is used to evaluate for conductive hearing loss. A tuning fork is placed against the mastoid until the patient can no longer hear the vibrations and then moved toward the ear. Normally air conduction is better than bone, so a patient with no conductive hearing loss should continue to hear the tuning fork after bone conduction has ceased.
- **Weber test:** A tuning fork is placed on the patient's forehead and sound should be heard equally in both ears. In sensorineural hearing loss, the sound will localize to the unaffected ear. In conductive hearing loss, the sound will localize to the affected ear.

Treatment

If a cause is identified, treat appropriately, otherwise oral steroids for 10-14 days and ENT follow-up.

CHOLESTEATOMA

An accumulation of epithelial cells resulting from chronic Eustachian tube dysfunction or middle ear infection with retraction of the TM that can lead to bone erosion of the middle ear.

SYMPTOMS/EXAMINATION

- Recurrent or persistent purulent otorrhea with hearing loss is common.
- Whitish mass of epithelial debris may be visible behind the TM.

DIAGNOSIS/TREATMENT

- Usually a clinical diagnosis, but CT can be obtained to determine extent of erosion.
- Treatment is by reversing the underlying process—treating middle ear infection, improving Eustachian tube function.
- Surgical intervention may be required.

OTOTOXICITY

Inner ear dysfunction with symptoms of sensorineural hearing loss and/or dizziness due to a chemical or pharmacologic agent. Damage may be temporary or permanent.

Common agents include:
- Aminoglycosides
- Loop diuretics
- Salicylates (usually chronic toxicity)
- Erythromycin
- Quinine and related drugs
- Chemotherapeutics

TYMPANIC MEMBRANE PERFORATION

CAUSES

- Otitis media is the most common cause.
- Others include penetrating object, barotrauma, and blast injury.

SYMPTOMS/EXAMINATION

- Pain and decreased hearing; may complain of discharge
- Exam with visible perforation

TREATMENT

- Keep ear dry; provide analgesia and topical antibiotic suspension if contaminated or at risk for contamination.
- Most (90%) heal within a few months, but should follow-up with ENT.

KEY FACT

Pars tensa (anterior and inferior) is the thinnest part of the TM and most prone to perforation.

KEY FACT

Use topical antibiotics suspension not solutions in setting of TM perforation.

Slit Lamp Examination

- Allows a magnified binocular (3-dimensional) view of anterior eye structures for delicate procedures and diagnosis (Figure 14.6)
  - Eyelid: Foreign body, blepharitis, hordeolum, dacryocystitis
  - Conjunctiva/sclera: Injuries or inflammation (conjunctivitis)
  - Cornea: Abrasions, ulcers, foreign bodies, and the depth of these lesions
  - Anterior chamber: Depth, cell and flare as seen in iritis, and also for blood (hyphema) or pus (hypopyon)
  - Iris (injuries) or lens (dislocation)

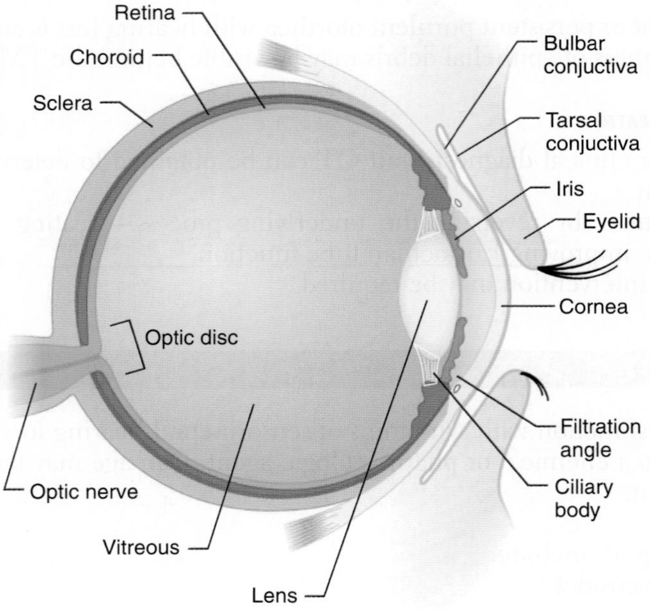

FIGURE 14.6. Eye general anatomy. (Reproduced, with permission, from Reichman EF. *Emergency Medicine Procedures*. 2nd ed. New York, NY: McGraw-Hill Education, 2013. Figure 155-1.)

> **KEY FACT**
>
> Viral conjunctivitis typically has a clear or mucoid discharge.

Red Eye

The complaint of a red eye, with or without pain, is a common one with a very broad differential. The following stepwise diagnostic approach can be useful to identify time-sensitive injuries and organize potential diagnoses.

- Chemical exposure?
  - Caustic keratoconjunctivitis requires rapid and extensive irrigation
- External swelling around the eye?
  - Blepharitis, chalazion, dacryocystitis, hordeolum, periorbital and orbital cellulitis, retrobulbar hematoma
- Pain, foreign body sensation, or limbal injection?
  - Keratitis (corneal abrasion/ulceration), keratoconjunctivitis, episcleritis, uveitis, acute angle-closure glaucoma, hypopyon, hyphema, endophthalmitis
- Focal redness?
  - Inflamed pinguecula/pterygium, scleral injury, subconjunctival hemorrhage
- Purulent discharge?
  - Bacterial conjunctivitis

Occular Trauma

> **KEY FACT**
>
> Any eyelid laceration that involves the tarsal plate should be repaired by plastic surgery or ophthalmology.

EYELID LACERATION

- Two-thirds of patients with eye lid lacerations have associated ocular injury; carefully evaluate the eye for signs of ruptured globe, foreign body, and corneal injury.
- Simple superficial eyelid lacerations can be repaired with 6-0 nonabsorbable suture.

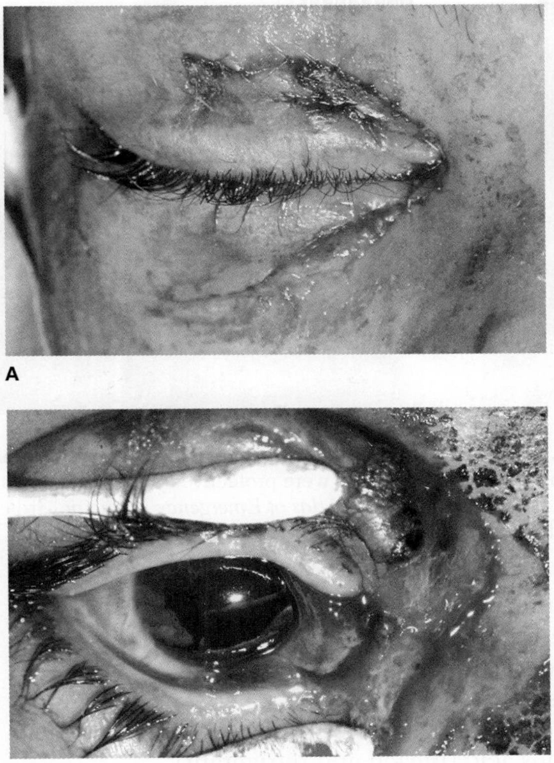

FIGURE 14.7. Lacrimal duct injury. Note laceration with extension medial to lacrimal punctum. (Reproduced, with permission, from Riordan-Eva P, Cunningham E. *Vaughan & Asbury's General Ophthalmology*. 18th ed. New York, NY: McGraw-Hill Education; 2011. Figure 19.1.)

- Because of the risk of scaring and loss of eyelid function, plastic surgery or ophthalmology should repair any complex wound including full-thickness wounds, tarsal plate injury, orbital fat prolapse, poor alignment or avulsion, and wounds involving the lid margin or lacrimal system.

Lacrimal Duct Injury

- Lacerations **medial to the punctum** (medial canthus) should raise high suspicion for lacrimal system injury (Figure 14.7).
- Lacrimal system injuries may be evaluated by instilling fluorescein into the eye and seeing if dye is present in the wound.
- Plastic surgery or ophthalmology should repair any wounds with damage to the lacrimal system to prevent duct dysfunction and permanent tearing.

CORNEAL BURN

Burns may be thermal, chemical, or due to ultraviolet radiation. Thermal burns generally affect the eyelids more than the cornea due to reflex blinking. Chemical burns are most dangerous, particularly **alkali burns** because they can rapidly penetrate the cornea (5-15 minutes) by **liquefactive necrosis** (Figure 14.8). Acid burns cause coagulation necrosis and eschar formation and are therefore limited in their depth of penetration.

Causes

- Alkali burns:
  - Ammonia (fertilizers, cleaning agents, refrigerants)
  - Sodium hydroxide/lye (drain cleaners, airbags)

Q

A 42-year-old male accidentally sprays himself in the eye with oven cleaner (pH 13) while cleaning his kitchen at home. He calls the hospital nurse line. What advice should be given?

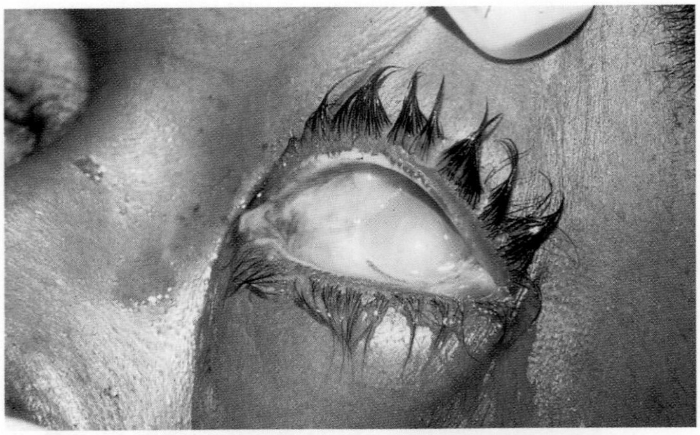

FIGURE 14.8. Corneal alkali burn causing diffuse corneal opacification. Note the absence of fluorescein uptake where the eyelids were protective. (Reproduced, with permission, from Knoop KJ, Stack LB, Storrow AB. *The Atlas of Emergency Medicine*. 3rd ed. New York, NY: McGraw-Hill Education, 2010. Figure 4-32. Photographer: Stephen W. Corbett, MD.)

    - Calcium hydroxide/lime (cement, plaster)
    - Magnesium hydroxide (fireworks)
    - Potassium hydroxide (detergents)
- Acid burns:
    - Sulfuric acid (car batteries)
    - Sulfurous acid (bleach and refrigerant)
    - Hydrofluoric acid (glass polishing)
    - Hydrochloric acid (swimming pools)
- Ultraviolet (UV) radiation:
    - Sun lamps, welding
    - Snow or water reflection, high-altitude environment

Symptoms/Examination

- Patients typically present with eye pain and decreased vision of the affected eye.
- UV keratitis is characterized by severe eye pain **6-12 hours** after UV exposure. Examination shows punctuate areas of fluorescein uptake with linear edge where eyelids were protective (Figure 14.9).

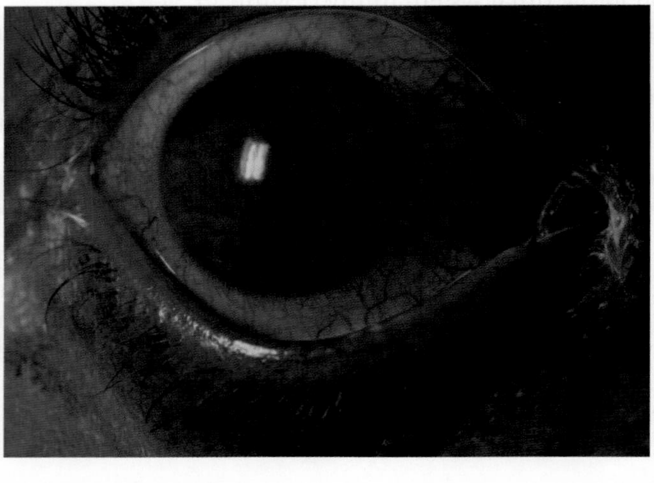

FIGURE 14.9. Ultraviolet keratitis. Note absence of fluorescein uptake where the eyelids were protective. (Reproduced, with permission, from Knoop KJ, Stack LB, Storrow AB. *Atlas of Emergency Medicine*. 3rd ed. New York, NY: McGraw-Hill Education; 2010. Figure 16.21. Photographer: Lawrence B. Stack, MD.)

A

The nurse should advice the man to immediately rinse his eye with a steady stream of tap water for 15-30 minutes continuously. The man should then be instructed to present to the emergency department where irrigation should continue until pH testing of the patient's tear film is neutral.

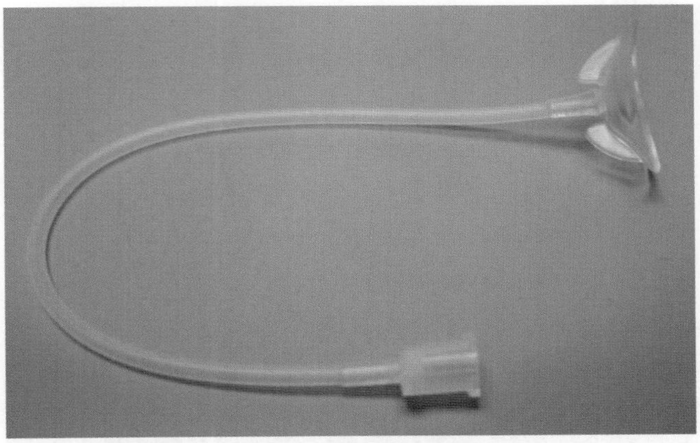

FIGURE 14.10. Morgan lens. (Reproduced, with permission, from Reichman EF. *Emergency Medicine Procedures*. 2nd ed. New York, NY: McGraw-Hill Education; 2013. Figure 155.4A.)

- For chemical exposures:
  - **Treat first** with immediate and copious irrigation starting on scene and lasting at least 30 minutes; consider use of a Morgan lens (Figure 14.10).
  - After irrigation, check the pH of the tear film by inserting a strip of Nitrazine paper into the inferior fornix; continue irrigation until the tear pH is neutral (7.0).
  - After pH is neutralized, topical analgesics (proparacaine) may be applied and careful examination under slit lamp with fluorescein should be conducted to establish the depth of the corneal injury and to evaluate for perforation.
  - Once perforation has been ruled out, intraocular pressure (IOP) should be checked, because pressure can spike, particularly after alkali burns; if elevated treat with acetazolamide.

KEY FACT

In setting of suspected chemical burn, irrigate FIRST then check pH.

Treatment

- Obtain emergent ophthalmology consult for all serious chemical exposures ($pH < 2$ or > 12), significant injuries, or elevated IOP.
- Standard treatment of chemical burns includes topical steroids (with ophthalmology consultation), cycloplegics, artificial tears, and antibiotic ointment (eg, erythromycin) along with oral pain medication.
- UV keratitis treatment is similar, but topical steroids are usually not required.

Complications

Permanent vision loss, perforation, corneal scarring (opacification), cataracts, adhesions to the lid (symblepharon), glaucoma, and retinal damage

CORNEAL ABRASION

Most commonly due to mechanical injury from a retained eyelid foreign body, repetitive eye rubbing, or direct trauma.

Symptoms/Examination

- Eye pain, foreign body sensation
- Redness, photophobia
- Decreased visual acuity if the injury involves the central visual axis

Differential

- **Infectious keratitis** (including herpes simplex keratitis)
- Corneal foreign body or ulcer
- Glaucoma and iritis may also cause eye redness and pain.

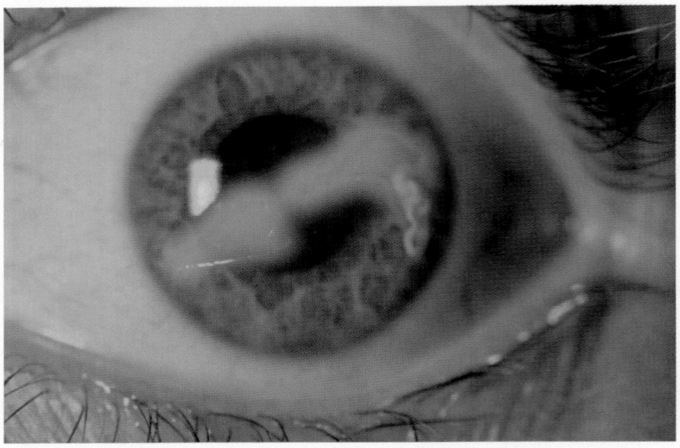

FIGURE 14.11. Large corneal abrasion involving the visual axis. (Reproduced, with permission, from Knoop KJ, Stack LB, Storrow AB. *Atlas of Emergency Medicine*. 3rd ed. New York, NY: McGraw-Hill Education; 2010. Figure 4.3. Photographer: Lawrence B. Stack, MD.)

KEY FACT

Postive Seidel test = globe rupture

Diagnosis

- Relief of pain with topical anesthesia (eg, proparacaine) can be used as a diagnostic test to identify corneal injury as opposed to other causes of acute eye pain.
- Slit lamp examination will show corneal epithelial defect and increased fluorescein uptake (Figure 14.11).
  - Horizontal defects point to repetitive eye rubbing, whereas vertical suggest a retained foreign body under the lid.
  - Both upper and lower lids should be fully everted to evaluate for foreign bodies (Figure 14.12).
- **Seidel test** (Figure 14.13): In the case of full-thickness corneal injuries or lacerations with an open globe, a clear stream of actively flowing fluid parting the fluorescein dye will be noted, resulting from aqueous humor leaking from the anterior chamber.

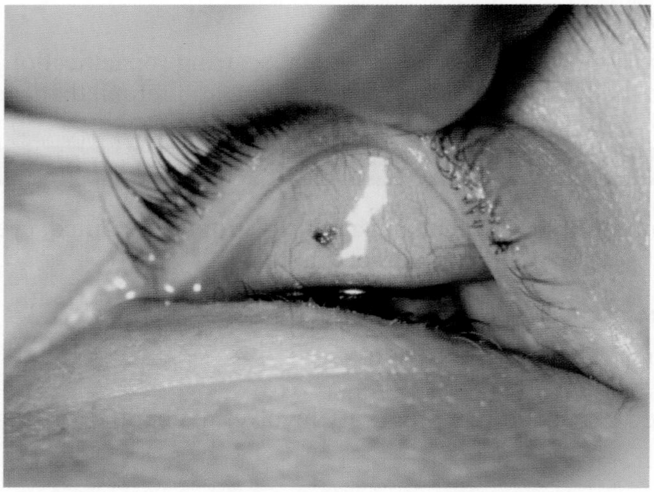

FIGURE 14.12. Lid eversion with foreign body. (Reproduced, with permission, from Knoop KJ, Stack LB, Storrow AB. *Atlas of Emergency Medicine*. 3rd ed. New York, NY: McGraw-Hill Education; 2010. Figure 4.4. Photographer: Lawrence B. Stack, MD.)

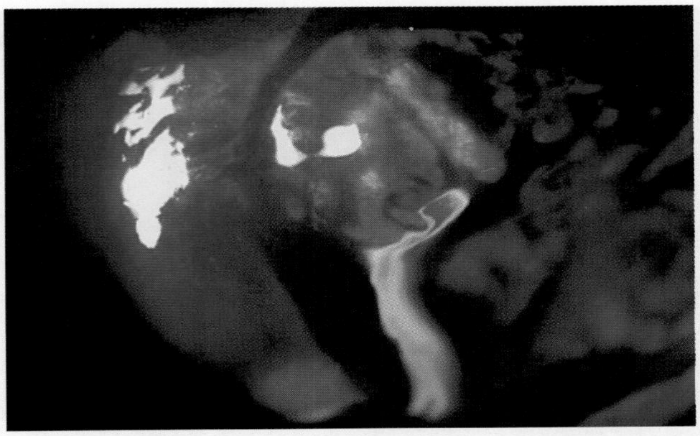

FIGURE 14.13. Seidel sign. Note the stream of aqueous humor flowing from the anterior chamber. (Reproduced, with permission, from Tintinalli JE, Stapczynski JS, Ma OJ, et al. *Tintinalli's Emergency Medicine*, 8th ed. New York, NY: McGraw-Hill; 2016. Figure 241-17.)

TREATMENT

- Pain control with topical NSAIDs (eg, ketorolac 0.5% qid) or oral analgesics and topical antibiotics (eg, erythromycin ointment qid) are the mainstay of treatment for any corneal injury.
- Contact lens wearers should be instructed not to wear their contacts until their symptoms completely resolve and should be given topical antibiotics to cover for *Pseudomonas* (eg, levofloxacin).
- Corneal abrasions typically heal in 3-5 days and patients should follow-up in 24 hours if their symptoms have not significantly improved.

KEY FACT

Topical anesthetics should not be prescribed to patients with eye pain because there are some data to suggest increased risk of further corneal injury and scarring.

KEY FACT

With the exception of globe injuries when used for protection, eye patching is generally not recommended for any acute eye injury.

CORNEAL FOREIGN BODY

SYMPTOMS/EXAMINATION

Pain, foreign body sensation, tearing

DIAGNOSIS/TREATMENT

- Visualized on slit lamp examination
- Attempt at removal may first be made with sterile saline irrigation or a moistened cotton-tipped applicator rolled over the foreign body.
- Lastly, a 25-gauge needle may be used to scoop the foreign body off of the cornea.
- Deeply embedded foreign bodies should be removed by ophthalmology.
- **Rust ring** (Figure 14.14)
  - Removal of iron-containing foreign bodies may leave behind a residual rust ring that migrates to the surface as the cornea softens over time; this should be **removed at 24-hour follow-up** in the emergency department (ED) or with ophthalmology.
- Discharge with topical NSAIDs, oral analgesics, and topical antibiotics.

Globe Rupture/Penetrating Globe Injury

Blunt trauma more commonly causes rupture at the limbus or at the insertion of the extraocular muscles where the sclera is thinnest, whereas penetrating injuries most commonly occur through the cornea and are often occupational injuries in the setting of inadequate eye protection. The risk of an intraocular foreign body increases with high-energy mechanisms, explosions, or high-velocity projectiles (drills or grinders).

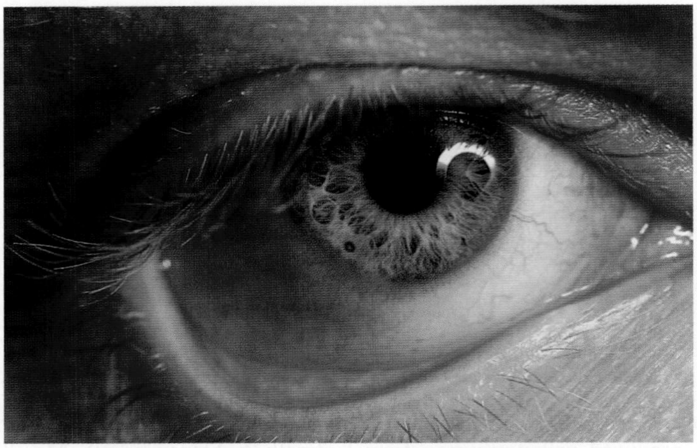

FIGURE 14.14. Small corneal rust ring. (Reproduced, with permission, from Knoop KJ, Stack LB, Storrow AB. *Atlas of Emergency Medicine*. 2nd ed. New York, NY: McGraw-Hill Education; 2002.)

KEY FACT

New data suggests that succinylcholine and ketamine are safe to use in the setting of globe injury.

Symptoms/Examination

- History of high-velocity projectile or significant blunt force with complaint of eye pain and decreased vision
- Evidence of afferent pupillary defect, eccentric or teardrop pupil (Figure 14.15), extrusion of vitreous, Seidel sign, and uveal prolapse (brown/black discoloration)
- 360° bullous subconjunctival hemorrhage should raise suspicion for posterior globe rupture.

Diagnosis

CT orbit (1-2 mm axial and coronal cuts) has poor sensitivity, but may be used to complement clinical findings in diagnosing globe rupture and can evaluate for intraocular foreign bodies.

Complications

Vitreous extrusion, loss of vision, intraocular foreign body, enucleation, and endophthalmitis

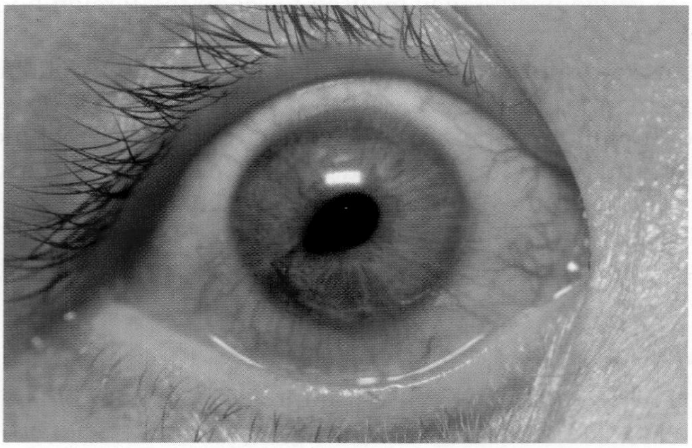

FIGURE 14.15. Teardrop pupil. Note the anterior chamber foreign body and small hyphema. (Reproduced, with permission, from Knoop KJ, Stack LB, Storrow AB et al. *The Atlas of Emergency Medicine*. 3rd ed. New York, NY: McGraw-Hill Education, 2010. Figure 4.13. Photographer: Lawrence B. Stack, MD.)

Treatment

- Shield eye immediately; avoid any pressure on the globe itself.
- Provide aggressive pain control and antiemetics to limit increases in IOP.
- Update tetanus and give prophylactic IV antibiotics (eg, vancomycin plus ceftazidime).
- Obtain mergent ophthalmology consult for surgical repair

> **KEY FACT**
>
> Do NOT check IOP in the case of a suspected open globe injury as any pressure on the globe may further expel contents.

TRAUMATIC HYPHEMA

Hyphema is a blood collection in the anterior chamber due to injury to the blood vessels of the iris or ciliary body. Trauma is the most common cause, but it can also occur spontaneously (eg, hemophilia, anticoagulant use).

Symptoms/Examination

- Pain, photophobia, and decreased visual acuity
- Hyphemas may be graded by the extent of the anterior chamber that is occupied when the patient is **upright** (Figure 14.16), ranging from minimal to the "eight ball" with blood completely filling the anterior chamber.
- Elevation in IOP is common, but is usually mild and self-limited.

Complications

- Rebleeding, which occurs 2-5 days after initial injury as blood clot retracts; higher risk with **sickle cell disease**, clotting disorders, or anticoagulant use
- Anterior or posterior synechiae (adherence of the iris to the cornea or lens, respectively)
- Acute or chronic glaucoma
- Corneal blood staining and vision loss are also seen.

Treatment

- Eye shield, elevation of the head of bed to > 30°, antiemetics
- Patients with bleeding disorders should be treated with appropriate therapy to restore clotting capabilities.
- Urgent ophthalmology consultation

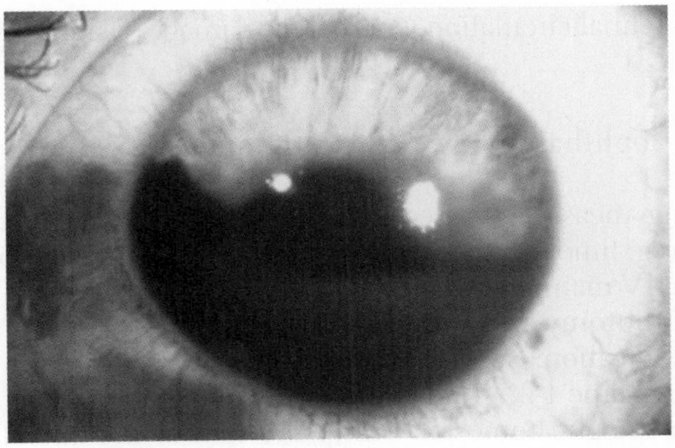

FIGURE 14.16. Hyphema. (Reproduced, with permission, from Riordan-Eva P, Cunningham E. *Vaughan & Asbury's General Ophthalmology*. 18th ed. New York, NY: McGraw-Hill Education; 2011 Figure 19.9.)

KEY FACT

Carbonic anhydrase inhibitors should not be used in sickle cell patients as they can precipitate sickling.

- Further treatment should be guided by an ophthalmologist but may include topical β-blockers (eg, timolol), topical or systemic glucocorticoids, cycloplegics (eg, cyclopentolate) and carbonic anhydrase inhibitors (eg, dorzolamide), mannitol or surgical intervention.
- Inpatient management is recommended for hyphemas > 50%, decreased visual acuity, increased IOP, bleeding dyscrasias, and sickle cell patients.

TRAUMATIC IRITIS/IRIDOCYCLITIS

Blunt trauma to the globe can contuse and inflame the iris and ciliary body resulting in inflammation to the anterior chamber and ciliary spasm.

Symptoms/Examination

- Recent history of blunt eye trauma with deep aching eye pain and both direct and consensual photophobia
- Small poorly dilating pupil with perilimbal conjunctival injection (ciliary flush) and cell and flare in the anterior chamber on slit lamp examination

KEY FACT

Mydriatics block pupillary muscle function resulting in persistent pupillary dilation. Cycloplegics block ciliary muscle function blocking accommodation.

Treatment

- Long-acting mydriatics/cycloplegics (eg, homatropine) for symptom control and to prevent synechiae
- Ophthalmology follow-up; generally resolves within 1 week

RETROBULBAR HEMATOMA

Blunt trauma causing injury to the orbital vessels and hemorrhage into the potential space surrounding the globe, resulting in an acute rise in intraorbital pressure that can be transmitted to the globe, compress the retinal artery, and put tension on the orbital nerve.

Symptoms/Examination

Proptosis, chemosis, limitation of extraocular movements, decreased visual acuity, and **increased IOP**

Diagnosis

- Clinical diagnosis aided by tonometry with IOP > 40 mm Hg
- CT orbit will show a hematoma in the retrobulbar space (Figure 14.17), but treatment should not be delayed awaiting imaging.

Complications

Compromised retinal circulation, optic nerve damage, **vision loss** in 2 hours

Treatment

- Emergent ophthalmology consultation for definitive hematoma evacuation
- Temporizing measures to decrease IOP may be taken including topical β-blockers (eg, timolol), systemic carbonic anhydrase inhibitor (eg, acetazolamide), and IV mannitol.
- **Lateral canthotomy and cantholysis**
  - Contraindication: Suspected globe rupture
  - Inject lidocaine 1-2% with epinephrine into the lateral canthus.
  - Using a straight hemostat, crimp the skin at the lateral corner of the eye and hold pressure for 1-2 minutes to minimize bleeding.
  - Using iris or Stevens scissors, make an incision from the lateral canthus to the lateral orbital rim to gain exposure.

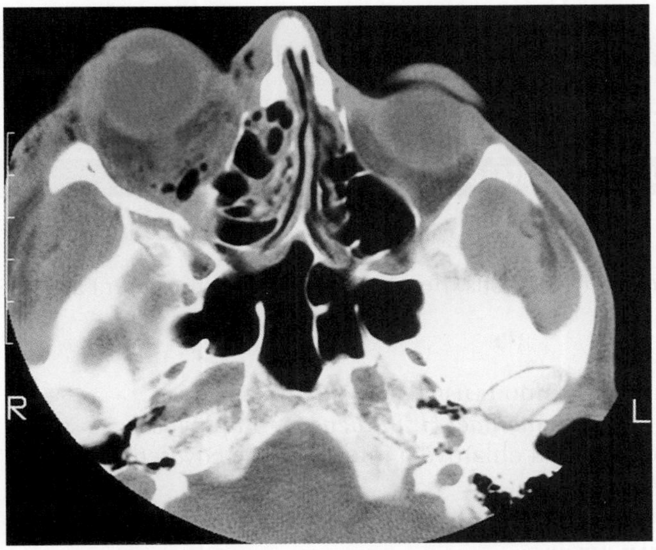

FIGURE 14.17. Retrobulbar hematoma. (Reproduced, with permission, from Knoop KJ, Stack LB, Storrow AB. *Atlas of Emergency Medicine*. 3rd ed. New York, NY: McGraw-Hill Education; 2010. Figure 1.43. Photographer: Frank Birinyi, MD.)

- Taking precautions to avoid injuring the globe, palpate along the orbital rim with the scissor tip until you can "strum" the inferior crux and cut it from the orbital rim.
- If this procedure is insufficient, using the same technique, release the superior crux.
- Lateral canthotomy incisions generally heal well without suturing or significant scarring.

KEY FACT

Retrobulbar hematoma, causing orbital compartment syndrome, is a rapidly progressive vision-threatening emergency. Lateral canthotomy is indicated as soon as the condition is diagnosed.

External Eye

PTERYGIUM

A fibrovascular proliferation that extends, generally from the nasal side of sclera, onto the cornea. Risk factors include sun exposure ("surfer's eye"), low humidity, and dust.

KEY FACT

Pterygium extends onto the cornea, pinguecula does not

Symptoms/Examination

- Eyes are dry and chronically irritated.
- Bird's wing-shaped growth that **extends onto the cornea**

Treatment

Surgical removal if interfering with vision

PINGUECULA

A common benign conjunctival nodule in persons > 35 years. Often bilateral, sun exposure and dryness appear to play an important role in their development.

Symptoms/Examination

Yellowish patch on conjunctiva **near limbus** that does not grow or extend onto cornea

Q

A 4-day-old infant, born full term via vaginal delivery, is brought in by his parents for right eye redness and discharge. The patient is afebrile, the right eye is noted to be red with conjunctival injection and white discharge, but the patient is otherwise well appearing. What is appropriate ED management and disposition?

TREATMENT

Artificial tears to prevent dryness. Topical steroids if acutely inflamed (pinguecultitis)

INFECTIOUS/INFLAMMATORY DISORDERS

Conjunctivitis

Inflammation of the mucus membranes that line the sclera and lids.

CAUSES

- Viral is most common (usually adenovirus).
- Bacterial: *S. pneumoniae, H. influenzae, Staphylococcus* sp, *M. catarrhalis*
  - Gonorrhea and chlamydia infections are covered separately.
- Allergic/irritant.

SYMPTOMS/EXAMINATION

- **Viral:** Preceding or concurrent URI symptoms, itching, slowly spreads bilaterally, mucoid/watery discharge, preauricular lymphadenopathy, and follicular reaction with cobblestone appearance to inferior palpebral conjunctiva
- **Bacterial:** Abrupt onset, quickly spreads bilaterally, more painful, thick purulent discharge, morning crusting
- **Allergic:** Itching predominates, bilateral clear watery discharge, rhinorrhea

DIAGNOSIS/TREATMENT

- It is OK to prescribe topical antibiotics if there is uncertainty about possible bacterial infection.
  - Ophthalmic ointments have a soothing effect and are preferred for children or at nighttime, while ophthalmic drops are preferred for adults because they do not interfere with vision.
    - Polymyxin-trimethoprim ophthalmic drops
    - Erythromycin ophthalmic ointment
- Contact lens wearers are at risk for ***Pseudomonas*** infection and should immediately remove lenses, discontinue lens wear until symptoms completely resolve, be treated with topical fluoroquinolone drops (eg, levofloxacin) and should have close follow-up with ophthalmology in 1-2 days.
- Cultures should be obtained if symptoms are severe or unresponsive to antibiotics.

KEY FACT

Contact lens wearers are at risk for ocular *Pseudomonas* infections and should be covered with a topical fluoroquinolone such as levofloxacin.

Gonococcal Conjunctivitis

Caused by *Neisseria gonorrhoeae*, gonococcal infection is often severe and vision threatening.

SYMPTOMS/EXAMINATION

Termed **hyperacute conjunctivitis** due to severity of symptoms: Pain, conjunctival injection, chemosis, and **copious purulent discharge** (Figure 14.18)

DIAGNOSIS/TREATMENT

- Gram stain showing gram-negative intracellular diplococci and/or culture (Thayer-Martin medium)
- Treatment with saline irrigation, topical antibiotics, and ceftriaxone IM; treat for concomitant chlamydial infection.

A

Ophthalmia neonatorum, or neonatal conjunctivitis, can be divided by the time of onset and the severity of the infection. Gonorrheal infections typically occur 2-5 days after birth. Gram stain and culture of the discharge should be sent to confirm the diagnosis, and the patient should be empirically treated with ceftriaxone 25-50 mg intramuscularly once and both erythromycin topical and systemic formulations.

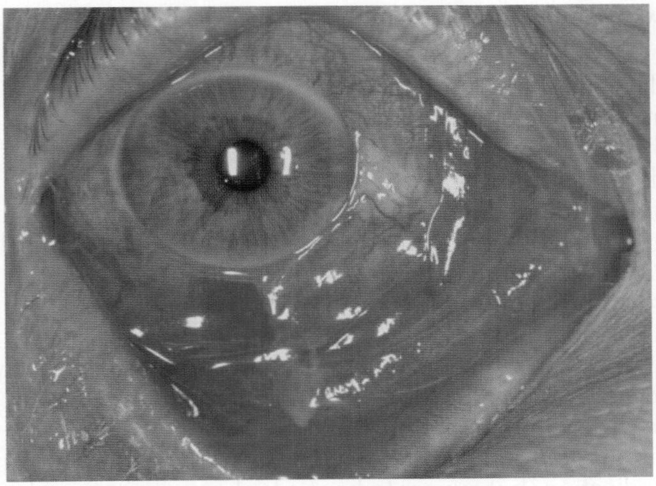

FIGURE 14.18. Hyperacute (gonococcal) conjunctivitis. Note degree of chemosis. This patient also had copious purulent exudate. (Reproduced, with permission, from Knoop KJ, Stack LB, Storrow AB. *Atlas of Emergency Medicine*. 3rd ed. New York, NY: McGraw-Hill Education; 2010. Figure 9.11. Photographer: Lawrence B. Stack, MD.)

- High risk for sight-threatening complications including ulceration and perforation; any corneal involvement warrants admission, and urgent ophthalmology follow-up is indicated for all cases.

> **KEY FACT**
>
> Gonococcal conjunctivitis can rapidly lead to corneal perforation.

Chlamydial Conjunctivitis

In developed countries, chlamydial conjunctivitis is an inclusion conjunctivitis caused by certain serotypes of *Chlamydia trachomatis* and transmitted via genital secretions. In underdeveloped countries chlamydial conjunctivitis is typically a follicular conjunctivitis, called Trachoma. It is caused by different non-sexual serotypes of the same organism and with repeat exposures leads to inward rotation of the eyelids and corneal scarring and blindness.

> **KEY FACT**
>
> Trachoma is the most common cause of blindness worldwide.

Symptoms/Examination

- Inclusion conjunctivitis
  - Unilateral conjunctivitis with chronic low-grade injection and scant discharge that is resistant to topical antibiotics.
  - May become bilateral over days to weeks
  - Follicles are present on conjunctiva lining the lids (palpebral surface).
- Trachoma begins as a follicular conjunctivitis that leads to eyelid scarring and entropion with resultant repeated corneal trauma and eventual blindness.

Diagnosis/Treatment

- Culture is gold standard.
- Nucleic acid amplification test (NAAT) of conjunctival stainings is not approved for this indication, but has a high sensitivity/specificity.
- Treat with azithromycin 1 gm PO or doxycycline 100 mg PO BID; consider treatment for gonorrhea as well.

Ophthalmia Neonatorum

Ophthalmia neonatorum is conjunctivitis occurring within the first month of life. Causes include chemical, bacterial (gonorrhea and/or chlamydia), and viral etiologies.

Symptoms/Examination/Diagnosis

- Chemical
  - 1-2 days after birth, minimal discharge
  - From antibiotic ointment applied postdelivery
- Gonorrhea
  - 2-5 days after birth
  - Profuse purulent discharge with associated swelling of eyelids
  - Diagnosed by Gram stain showing gram-negative intracellular diplococci and/or culture (Thayer-Martin medium)
- Chlamydia (most common)
  - 5-14 days after birth
  - Watery discharge that becomes purulent and possibly bloody
  - Associated with chlamydial pneumonia; obtain chest x-ray if cough or other URI symptoms are present.
  - Culture is gold standard for diagnosis; NAAT tests are not approved for this indication, but appear to have a high sensitivity/specificity.
- Herpes simplex virus
  - 1-2 weeks after birth
  - Injection with nonpurulent discharge
  - Diagnosed by culture

KEY FACT

Time frame of symptom onset is important in determining etiology of ophthalmia neonatorum.

Onset 1-2 days = chemical
Onset 2-5 days = gonorrhea
Onset 5-14 days = chlamydia

Treatment

- Chemical conjunctivitis requires no specific treatment.
- Gonorrhea:
  - Saline washes, ceftriaxone IM, topical antibiotic drops (eg, polymyxin-bacitracin).
  - Treat for concurrent chlamydial infection (below).
  - Corneal involvement or systemically ill patients require hospitalization, blood and CSF studies, and parenteral antibiotics.
- Chlamydia: Topical erythromycin ointment and oral erythromycin syrup
- Herpes simplex virus: Acyclovir IV plus vidarabine ointment

Corneal Ulcer

A type of keratitis that is most commonly a bacterial infection associated with prolonged or inappropriate contact lens use. Fungal infections can also occur, typically when the corneal epithelial integrity is breached (eg, trauma, steroids). A true ocular emergency as it may progress to corneal scarring, vision loss, corneal perforation, or hypopyon.

Symptoms/Examination

- Scooped out epithelial defect with underlying or surrounding corneal opacification due to edema (Figure 14.19)
- Large area of intense fluorescein uptake

Treatment

- Topical fluoroquinolone drops (eg, levofloxacin q2h while awake)
- Pain control with NSAIDs or narcotics
- Because of risk for permanent corneal damage and vision loss, close ophthalmology follow-up is required.

Herpes Simplex Keratitis

Corneal epithelial infection caused by herpes simplex virus, either primary infection or reactivation of latent disease. Most often seen in young adults.

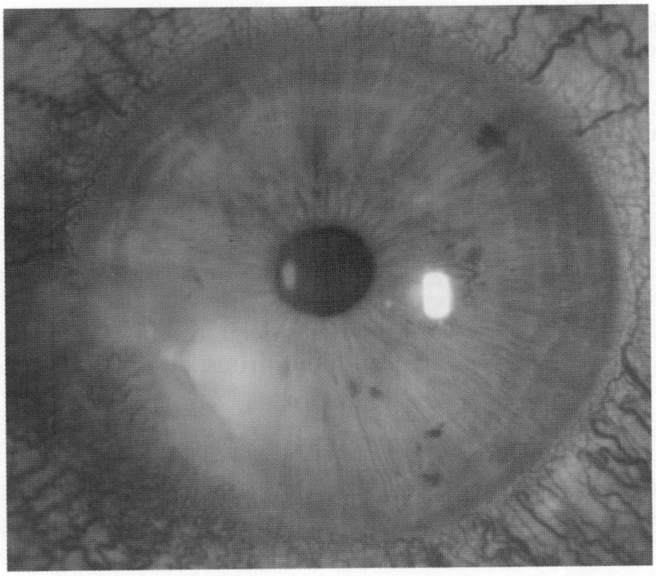

FIGURE 14.19. Corneal ulcer in 7 o'clock position on this unstained cornea. (Reproduced, with permission, from McKean S, Ross JJ, Dressler DD, et al. *Principles and Practice of Hospital Medicine*. New York, NY: McGraw-Hill Education; 2012. Figure 81.1.)

Symptoms/Examination

- Foreign body sensation, pain, decreased visual acuity, tearing, and photophobia
- Injection and **dendritic** lesions that evolve to form a central ulcer with dendritic extensions (Figure 14.20)

Treatment

- Urgent ophthalmology consult and treatment with topical antiviral (eg, trifluridine 1% every 2 hours)
- 97% heal completely within 2 weeks on topical antivirals alone.
- Topical steroids are contraindicated.

Herpes Zoster Ophthalmicus

Reactivation of varicella-zoster virus (VZV) in the ophthalmic division of the trigeminal nerve (CN V1). It is most common in patients > 60 years.

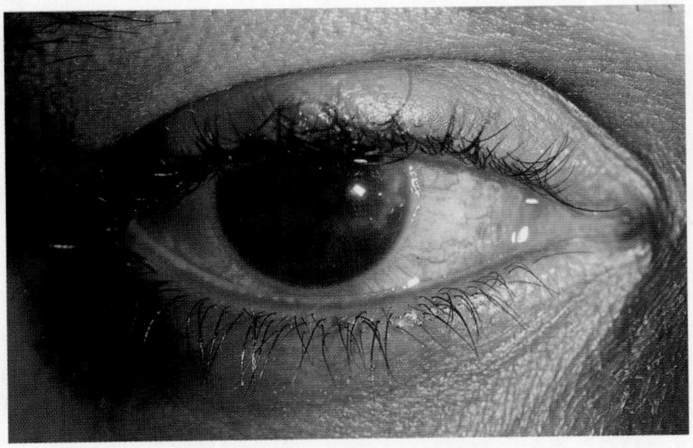

FIGURE 14.20. Herpes simplex keratitis. Note the dendritic-shaped ulcerations on this stained cornea. (Reproduced, with permission, from Knoop KJ, Stack LB, Storrow AB. *Atlas of Emergency Medicine*. 3rd ed. New York, NY: McGraw-Hill Education; 2010. Figure 2.37. Photographer: Kevin J. Knoop, MD, MS.)

KEY FACT

Due to high risk of complications, corneal ulcers must be differentiated from simple corneal abrasions. Ulcers require topical antibiotics and close ophthalmology follow-up.

Prompt diagnosis and emergent ophthalmology consultation is critical because corneal involvement may progress to **acute necrotizing retinitis** and complete vision loss.

Symptoms/Examination

- Severe pain, hyperesthesia, redness, decreased vision, and typically unilateral dermatomal vesicular rash involving the forehead and upper eyelid
- **Hutchinson sign:** Vesicular lesions on the tip of the nose indicate involvement of the **nasociliary branch of the trigeminal nerve** and are associated with a high risk (76%) of ocular involvement.
- Examination may show conjunctival injection, episcleritis, ptosis, and/or fluorescein uptake revealing **pseudodendrites**, described as branches without end bulbs.

KEY FACT

Herpes zoster ophthalmicus is associated with corneal perforation.

Treatment

- Oral antivirals (acyclovir, valacyclovir), topical steroids, and topical prophylactic antibiotics after consultation with an ophthalmologist

Blepharitis

Chronic eyelid inflammation with acute exacerbations that involves the meibomian glands. Associated with seborrheic dermatitis and rosacea, but can be due to *Staphylococcus epidermis* colonization.

Symptoms/Examination

- Bilateral dry red eyes, gritty foreign body sensation, increased blinking, crusting of eyelashes, blurred vision
- Lid margins are pink and irritated with crusting at the base of the eyelashes.

Treatment

- Initial treatment is warm compress for 15 minutes 4 times a day as well as scrubbing of lid margin with a washcloth and mild shampoo.
- Artificial tears may help with dry eye symptoms.

Hordeolum and Chalazion

Hordeola (Figure 14.21) and chalazia (Figure 14.22) are inflammatory lesions of the sebaceous glands that open on the margin of the eyelid.

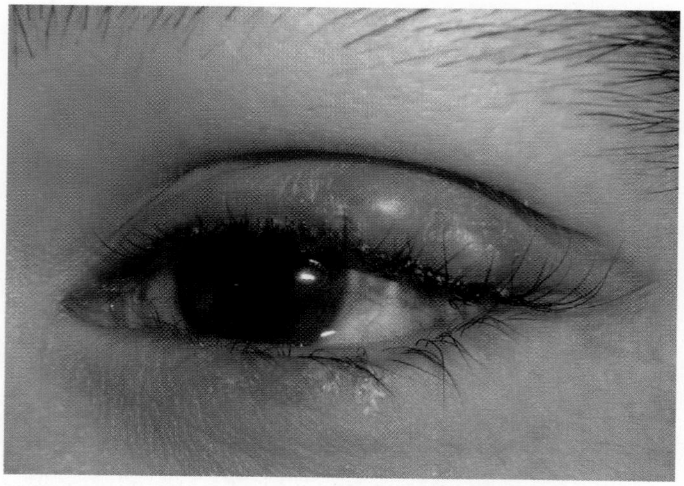

FIGURE 14.21. Hordeolum. (Reproduced with permission from Usatine RP: *The Color Atlas of Family Medicine*. 2nd edition. New York, NY: McGraw-Hill Education; 2013. Photographer: Richard P. Usatine.)

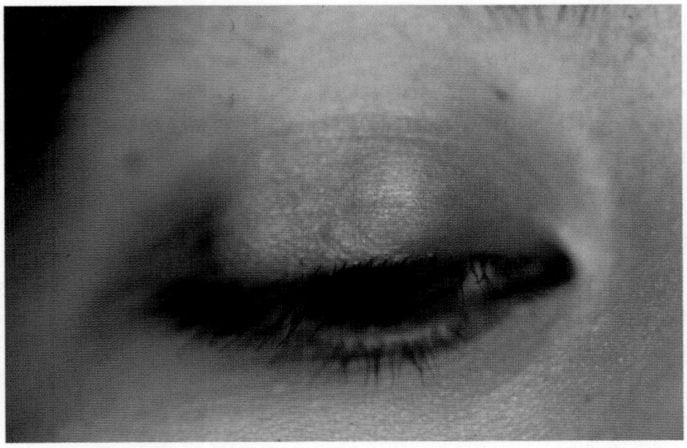

FIGURE 14.22. **Chalazion.** (Reproduced, with permission, from Knoop KJ, Stack LB, Storrow AB. *Atlas of Emergency Medicine*. 3rd ed. New York, NY: McGraw-Hill Education; 2010. Figure 2.17. Photographer: Kevin J. Knoop, MD, MS.)

- A hordeolum (**stye**) is an **acute** purulent infection most often caused by *S. aureus*. It can be internal, involving the meibomian gland, or external, involving the gland of Zeis.
- A chalazion is a **chronic** granulomatous inflammation of an obstructed meibomian gland that often results from the progression of a hordeolum.

SYMPTOMS/EXAMINATION

- Hordeolum: Erythematous and tender eyelid nodule.
- Chalazion: Hard, rubbery and painless; lid margin is normal.

TREATMENT

- Initial treatment for a hordeolum/chalazion includes warm compresses to the eye for 15 minutes 4 times a day.
- Persistent symptoms despite warm compresses warrant ophthalmology referral for surgical drainage.
- Topical antibiotics are not indicated; however, oral antibiotics may be necessary if associated with a preseptal cellulitis.

KEY FACT

Meibomian glands are located on the interior of the eyelid in the tarsal plate; glands of Zeis are located at the lid margin at the base of the eyelashes.

Periorbital (Preseptal) Cellulitis

Infection in the superficial structures of the eyelids, anterior to the orbital septum. Preseptal cellulitis can be caused by extension from sinusitis, but more commonly results from superinfection of minor local trauma. Both preseptal and orbital cellulitis are much more common in children than adults.

CAUSES

Most often caused by *S. aureus* and *Streptococcus* species

SYMPTOMS/EXAMINATION

- Low-grade fever, eyelid erythema, warmth, swelling, and tenderness
- Normal visual acuity and painless full ocular motility

DIFFERENTIAL

- Must be differentiated from orbital cellulitis (discussed next) based on systemic toxicity, pain or limitation with extraocular movements and, if there is any doubt, CT orbits

Q

a 10-year-old male presents to the ED with complain of L eye swelling and pain. He has a low grade fever with eyelid redness, warmth and swelling and pain with extra-ocular movement. What is the next step in the management of this patient.

TREATMENT

- Nontoxic patients with preseptal cellulitis may be treated as outpatient with amoxicillin-clavulanate for 10-14 days and next day follow-up.
- Coverage for MRSA should be considered based on risk factors and local prevalence and may include clindamycin.

Orbital Cellulitis

In contrast a preseptal cellulitis, orbital cellulitis is almost always caused by extension of sinus infection, most commonly from the ethmoid sinus through the lamina papyracea, into the postseptal orbit.

CAUSES

- *S aureus* and *Streptococcus* species, or *milleri* increasing incidence of *Streptococcus anginosis* (milleri), are the common bacterial pathogens.
- Fungal infection (Mucormycosis and Aspergillus) should be considered in diabetics and the immunocompromised.

SYMPTOMS/EXAMINATION

KEY FACT

Pain with or restriction of extraocular movement distinguishes orbital cellulitis from periorbital (preseptal) cellulitis.

- Preceding or concomitant symptoms of sinus infection (86%-98% of cases)
- Toxic appearing, systemically ill
- Eyelid swelling extending beyond the eyelid margin, erythema, and tenderness
- Inflammation of the fatty tissues and the extraocular muscles may cause **proptosis**, pain or limitation with extraocular movements, and diplopia.

DIAGNOSIS

- Any clinical suspicion for orbital cellulitis warrants emergent evaluation with a CT of the orbits.
- Elevated IOPs (> 20 mm Hg) should be considered a surgical emergency.

COMPLICATIONS

- Subperiosteal or orbital abscess, increased IOP, vision loss, cavernous venous sinus thrombosis, meningitis

TREATMENT

- Blood cultures and initiation of broad-spectrum IV antibiotics, including vancomycin and ceftriaxone, piperacillin-tazobactam, or ampicillin-sulbactam
- Emergent ophthalmology consultation, inpatient admission

LACRIMAL SYSTEM DISORDERS

A

This patient has orbital cellulitis based on the pain with extra-ocular movement. Blood cultures should be obtained and he should be started on broad-spectrum IV antibiotics. A CT scan of the orbits should also be performed to further evaluate the extent of the infection and look for associated sinusitis or abscess.

Nasolacrimal Duct Obstruction (Dacryostenosis).

Dacryostenosis occurs most commonly at the distal aspect of the duct. It is seen in 20% of normal newborns.

SYMPTOMS/EXAMINATION/TREATMENT

- Excessive tearing and ocular discharge
- Initial treatment involves frequent lacrimal massage.
- Recalcitrant cases may need referral to ophthalmology for lacrimal duct probing or stenting.

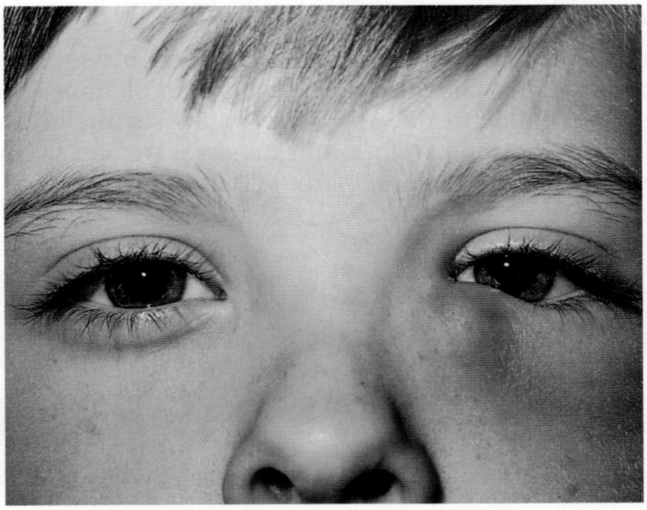

FIGURE 14.23. Dacryocystitis. (Reproduced, with permission, from Knoop KJ, Stack LB, Storrow AB. *Atlas of Emergency Medicine*. 3rd ed. New York, NY: McGraw-Hill Education; 2010. Figure 2.10. Photographer: Kevin J. Knoop, MD, MS.)

Dacryocystitis

A bacterial infection of the lacrimal sac, most commonly with *S. aureus*, *S. epidermis*, and alpha-hemolytic streptococci, due to nasolacrimal duct obstruction. Dacryocystitis has a bimodal distribution in infants and adults > 40 years.

KEY FACT

Dacryocystitis can extend to orbital cellulitis, meningitis and cavernous sinus thrombosis.

Symptoms/Examination

- Erythema, swelling, warmth, and tenderness at the lacrimal sac (Figure 14.23).
- Severe infections may present with systemic toxicity and sepsis.
- Pressure applied over the lacrimal sac may produce purulent discharge from the puncta (tear duct).

Treatment

- Warm compress and gentle massage to express purulent material
- Mild-to-moderate infections should be treated with **topical** (eg, erythromycin ophthalmic ointment) **and oral antibiotics** (eg, amoxicillin-clavulanate, clindamycin, cephalexin) and referred for outpatient ophthalmology follow-up.
- Severe cases require urgent ophthalmology consultation and systemic antibiotics covering methicillin-resistant *Staphylococcus aureus* (MRSA), usually vancomycin and a third-generation cephalosporin.

Dacryoadenitis

Inflammation of the lacrimal gland most commonly due to a viral or bacterial infection. Common bacterial organisms include *S. aureus* and *S. pneumoniae*. Other causes include sarcoidosis and Wegener granulomatosis.

Symptoms/Examination

- Erythema, swelling, warmth, and tenderness extending to the lacrimal gland (superior lateral orbit) with acute infection
- More indolent presentation with underlying inflammatory causes

DIAGNOSIS/TREATMENT

- CT should be obtained if the diagnosis is in question.
- Warm compress and gentle massage to express purulent material
- Treatment is similar to dacryocystitis (above) with mild cases managed with oral and topical antibiotics and severe cases requiring ophthalmology consultation and parental antibiotics including MRSA coverage.

Anterior/Posterior Eye

VISION LOSS

Acute monocular vision loss is generally divided by painful and painless causes (Table 14.1).

GLAUCOMA

KEY FACT

Normal IOP is 10-20 mm Hg.

Optic neuropathy caused by increased IOP (> 20 mm Hg) due to an imbalance in aqueous humor production and drainage. Aqueous humor is produced in the posterior chamber, flows through the pupillary aperture, and is drained via the trabecular meshwork at the angle of the anterior chamber.

Acute Angle-Closure Glaucoma

Pupillary dilation bulges the iris anteriorly against the peripheral cornea obstructing the anterior chamber angle and blocking aqueous outflow resulting in rapidly increasing IOP. Risk factors include a shallow anterior chamber, plateau (flat) iris, hyperopia (farsightedness), and age > 60 years.

SYMPTOMS/EXAMINATION

- Pupillary dilation is always the trigger so patients will give a history of onset with dim lighting, emotional upset, or use of anticholinergic/sympathomimetic agents.

TABLE 14.1. Acute Vision Loss

PAINFUL	PAINLESS
Acute angle-closure glaucoma	Open-angle glaucoma
Temporal arteritis[a]	Retinal detachment
Optic neuritis	Central retinal artery/vein occlusion
Corneal ulcer/abrasion	Vitreous hemorrhage
Iritis/uveitis	Amaurosis fugax
Keratitis	Hyphema

[a]Temporal arteritis causes headache, jaw pain, but not ocular pain.

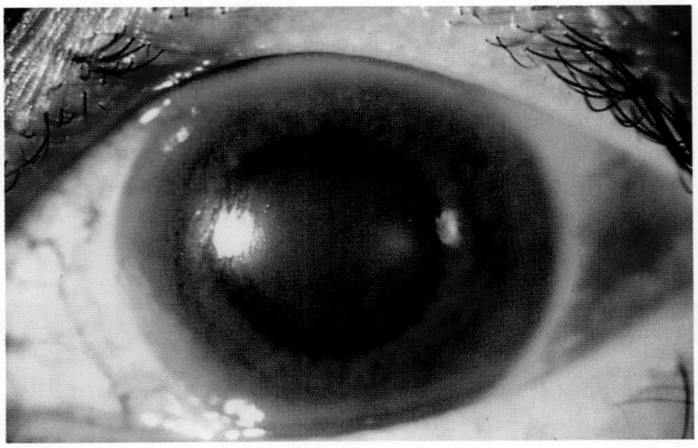

FIGURE 14.24. Acute angle-closure glaucoma. (Reproduced, with permission, from Knoop KJ, Stack LB, Storrow AB. *Atlas of Emergency Medicine*. 3rd ed. New York, NY: McGraw-Hill; 2010. Figure 2-25. Photographer: Gary Tanner, MD.)

- Acute onset severe unilateral eye **pain**, blurred vision with halos around lights, headache, nausea, and vomiting
- Examination will show conjunctival injection and a steamy cornea with a midposition to dilated pupil (Figure 14.24) that is fixed or sluggishly reactive; the globe may be tender and firm compared to the unaffected side.

KEY FACT

The classic presentation for acute angle closure glaucoma is onset of headache, eye pain and nausea/vomiting shortly after entering a dark room.

DIFFERENTIAL

- **Open-angle glaucoma**: The most common form of glaucoma and the leading cause of blindness in the United States
  - Caused by increased resistance to aqueous outflow in the absence of physical obstruction
  - Chronic condition characterized by insidious slowly progressive bilateral **painless** vision loss
  - Treatment includes topical β-blockers and topical carbonic anhydrase inhibitors (eg, dorzolamide) to temporize prior to ophthalmologic intervention.

KEY FACT

Acute angle closure glaucoma is an ocular emergency and systemic therapies in addition to topical medications are indicated for IOP > 50 mm Hg.

DIAGNOSIS

- Visual acuity may be markedly decreased and diagnosis is confirmed with IOP > 20 mm Hg on tonometry.

TREATMENT

- Aggressive pain and nausea control.
- Immediate administration of topical pressure lowering agents including:
  - β-Blockers: Timolol 0.5% 1 drop once; reduces aqueous humor production, but is contraindicated in patients with chronic obstructive pulmonary disorder, asthma, or congestive heart failure
  - Miotic agent: Pilocarpine 1%-2% 1 drop every 15 minutes for 2 doses; forces pupillary constriction, opening the trabecular meshwork and increasing outflow
  - α_2-Agonist: Apraclonidine 1 drop once; decreases aqueous humor production and increases outflow
  - Topical steroids may be indicated but should be administered under the guidance of an ophthalmologist.

KEY FACT

Agents that decrease aqueous humor production:
- Topical β-blocker (timolol)
- Topical α-agonist (apraclonidine)
- Carbonic anhydrase inhibitor (acetazolamide)

- Severe visual deficits (hand motion or less) or IOP > 50 mm Hg warrants systemic medications to reduce IOP including:
  - Carbonic anhydrase inhibitor: Acetazolamide 250-500 mg IV; reduces aqueous humor production; avoid with sulfa allergy.
  - Osmotic agents: Mannitol 1.5 g/kg over 45 minutes; reduces IOP.
- Emergent ophthalmology consultation as definitive treatment is laser iridotomy.

ANTERIOR UVEITIS/IRITIS

Inflammation of the anterior segment of the eye that may include the anterior chamber, iris, and ciliary body (iridocyclitis).

Causes

- **Infection**
  - Cytomegalovirus (CMV) is common in immunocompromised patients, particularly AIDS.
  - Reactivation of congenitally acquired toxoplasmosis may be seen in immunocompetent patients.
  - Syphilis and tuberculosis are other possible causes.
- **Systemic autoimmune disease**
  - Highly associated with **HLA-B27**–related spondyloarthropathies (eg, ankylosing spondylitis, reactive arthritis)
  - Also seen with sarcoidosis, inflammatory bowel disease, psoriatic arthritis, Behçet, etc.

Symptoms/Examination

- Sudden onset **painful** red eye exacerbated by eye movement, photophobia, blurred vision
- Limbic inflammation, constricted and sluggish pupil, both consensual and direct photophobia
- The diagnosis of anterior uveitis is confirmed with the findings of **cell and proteinaceous flare** on slit lamp examination.

KEY FACT

Cell and flare refers to inflammation in the anterior chamber and is described as dust particles moving through a movie projector beam.

Differential

- **Posterior uveitis:** Also known as choroiditis/chorioretinitis, presents without pain and redness, but with floaters; most often caused by CMV or toxoplasmosis in immunocompromised patients
- **Sympathetic ophthalmia:** A form of uveitis seen in patients with a history of contralateral penetrating eye trauma caused by autoimmune response to retinal antigens

Complications

- **Hypopyon:** Layering of inflammatory cells in the anterior chamber (Figure 14.25).
- Other complications include vision loss, intraocular hypertension, synechiae formation, as well as systemic complications associated with autoimmune disease.

Treatment

- Analgesics, mydriatics, and cycloplegics for symptom control and to prevent synechiae formation
- Ophthalmology follow-up within 24 hours to rule out infection followed by initiation of topical steroids

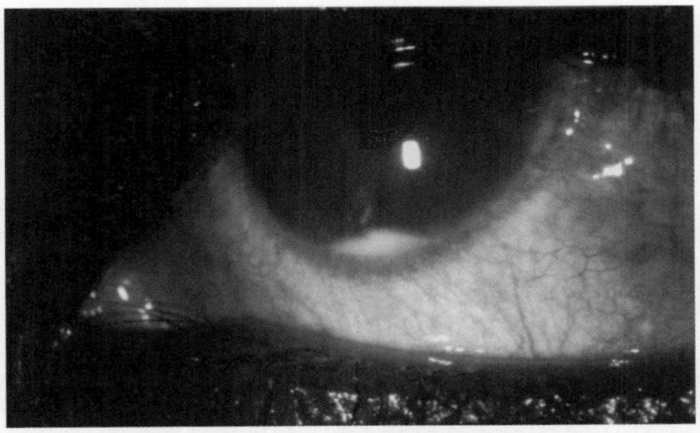

FIGURE 14.25. Hypopyon. (Reproduced, with permission, from Riordan-Eva P, Cunningham Jr ET. *Vaughan & Asbury's General Ophthalmology*. 18th ed. New York, NY: McGraw-Hill Education; 2011. Figure 3.4.)

Q

A 49-year-old man with history of diabetes presents with painless right eye vision loss that occurred acutely 12 hours prior to presentation. The patient describes his vision loss as "a curtain coming down" and denies any trauma. Visual acuity in the right eye is light perception only. What imaging modality can be used to confirm the diagnosis?

ENDOPHTHALMITIS

Bacterial or fungal infection involving the anterior, posterior, and vitreous chambers most often associated with penetrating eye injury, foreign body or ocular surgery, but may also be seen in the setting of bacteremia.

Symptoms/Examination

- Acute onset red and **painful** eye with decreased visual acuity and afferent pupillary defect
- Distinguished from uveitis due to presence of eyelid erythema/edema, proptosis, and often purulent discharge
- Anterior chamber will be hazy or opaque with cell and flare on slit lamp examination; hypopyon may be present.

Treatment

- Emergent ophthalmology consult for intravitreal aspiration for culture and intraocular antibiotics.
- Hospital admission may be required for adjunctive systemic antibiotics and close monitoring.
- Rule out bacteremia in cases with no history of ocular trauma or surgery.

KEY FACT

Postcataract surgery endophthalmitis is the most common form in the United States and generally presents in the first postoperative week.

RETINAL DETACHMENT

Separation of the neurosensory retina from its underlying retinal pigment epithelium.

Pathogenesis

- Rhegmatogenous detachment (most common): Full-thickness retinal tear that allows fluid to separate the tissue layers
  - **Posterior vitreous detachment (PVD)** due to the natural aging process is the most common cause of retinal tears. The aging vitreous liquefies and pulls away from the retina, leading to tears. Symptoms include flashes of light and floaters that may appear like a cobweb due to vitreal blood.
  - Risk factors include age > 50 years, myopia (nearsightedness), history of retinal detachment, and history of cataract surgery
- Traction: From the formation of fibrous bands within the vitreous from retinal neovascularization, as with diabetes or sickle cell disease.
- Exudative: Uncommon, due to inflammatory conditions.

A

Bedside emergency ultrasound is an excellent tool for the evaluation of many ocular complaints. On ophthalmic ultrasound, retinal detachment appears as a continuous linear density arising from the fundus and protruding into the posterior chamber (Figure 14.2).

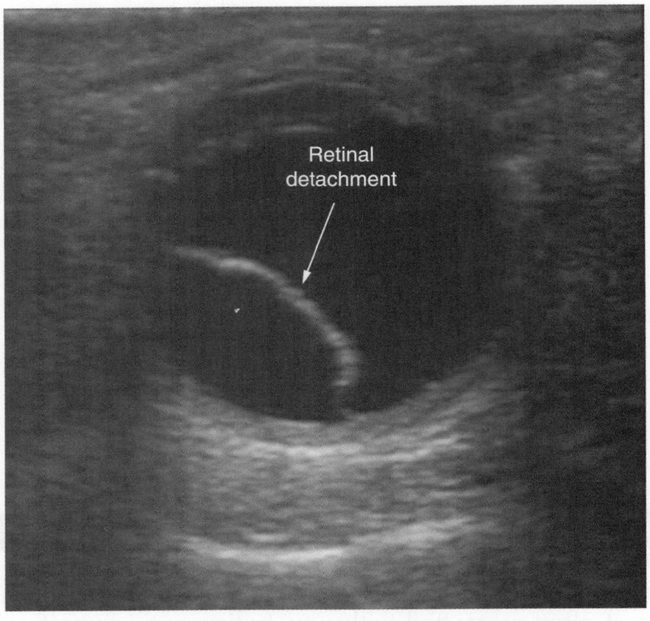

FIGURE 14.26. Ocular ultrasound showing retinal detachment. Note the continuous linear density arising from the fundus and protruding into the posterior chamber. (Reproduced, with permission, from Knoop KJ, Stack LB, Storrow AB. *Atlas of Emergency Medicine*. 3rd ed. New York, NY: McGraw-Hill Education; 2010. Figure 24.83. Photographer: Stephen J. Leech, MD, RDMS.)

Symptoms/Examination

- Preceding increase in floaters and flashes of light (from PVD) with rhegmatogenous detachment
- **Painless** vision loss generally described in a **curtain-like** distribution

Diagnosis

- Direct funduscopy is insensitive, therefore indirect funduscopy is needed to completely evaluate for retinal detachment.
- Bedside ED ultrasound can easily confirm the diagnosis (Figure 14.26).

Treatment

- Emergent ophthalmology consult because most will progress to complete vision loss if not treated.
- Timing of surgical repair depends on the involvement of the macula at presentation. If the macula is still attached, urgent surgery is recommended to prevent macular detachment. If the macula is detached, repair is less urgent (5-7 days).

CENTRAL RETINAL ARTERY OCCLUSION

Ischemic stroke of the retina caused by central retinal artery embolism, most commonly from the carotid arteries. Central retinal artery occlusion (CRAO) is seen in patients 50-70 years old with the following risk factors: Hypertension, cardiac disease, diabetes, collagen vascular disease, vasculitis, cardiac valvular abnormalities, sickle cell disease, and patients with increased IOP (eg, glaucoma, endocrine exophthalmos).

KEY FACT

Central retinal artery occlusion is an ischemic stroke of the eye!

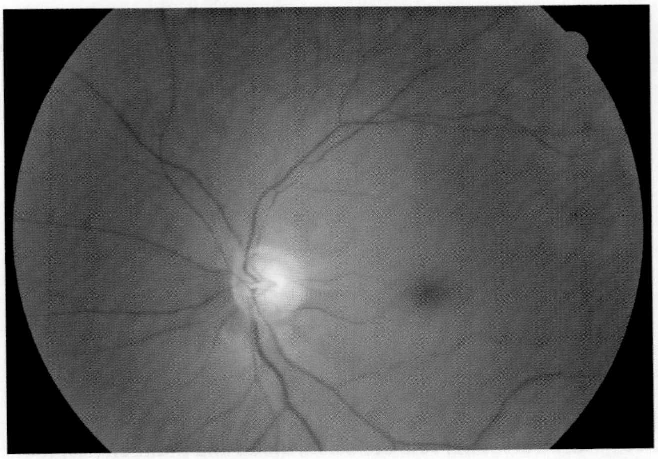

FIGURE 14.27. Central retinal artery occlusion. Note the pale retina with cherry red fovea. (Reproduced, with permission, from Knoop KJ, Stack LB, Storrow AB. *Atlas of Emergency Medicine*. 3rd ed. New York, NY: McGraw-Hill Education; 2010. Figure 3.9. Photographer: Aaron Sobol, MD.)

Symptoms/Examination

- Severe **painless** monocular vision loss that occurs over a few seconds
- Afferent pupillary defect and funduscopic examination showing an edematous pale gray-white retina with a **cherry red fovea** (Figure 14.27)

Treatment

- Attempt to displace the embolus distally and limit infarct size with digital ocular massage with direct pressure over the eyelids for 10-15 seconds followed by a sudden release.
- True ocular emergency necessitating immediate ophthalmology consultation because ischemia time > 2 hours produces massive irreversible damage. Treatment options include:
  - Anterior chamber paracentesis by ophthalmologist to dislodge embolus
  - Carbogen inhalation (95% O_2 5% CO_2 mix) to vasodilate vessels and increase retinal artery blood flow
  - Topical timolol or systemic acetazolamide to decrease IOP and increase the flow gradient
- Response to treatment is rare and some studies are suggesting systemic or intra-arterial thrombolytics, but data at this point are insufficient.
- Because CRAO is an embolic ischemic stroke, medical workup should focus on identifying the source of the embolus and optimal medical therapy should be initiated to reduce future risk.

CENTRAL RETINAL VEIN OCCLUSION

Central retinal vein occlusion (CRVO) is the second most common cause of vision loss from retinal vascular disorders, behind diabetic retinopathy.

Pathogenesis

- Thrombotic disease caused by atherosclerotic build up causing occlusion of the central retinal vein leading to edema, hemorrhage, and vascular leakage
- Risk factors include age, hypertension, diabetes, smoking, obesity, hypercoagulable states (factor V Leiden, activated protein C resistance), and glaucoma.

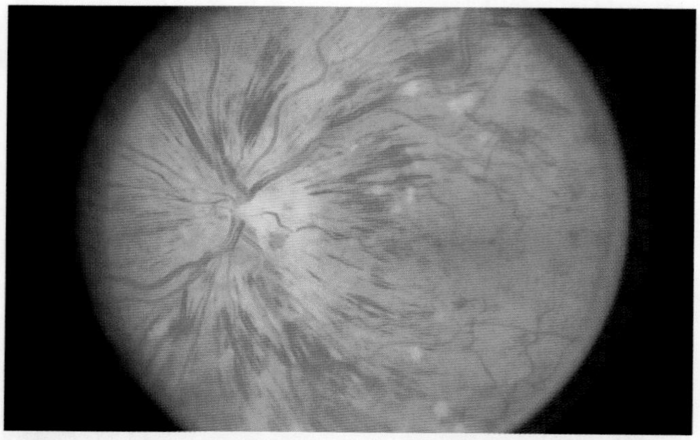

FIGURE 14.28. Central retinal vein occlusion, blood and thunder. (Reproduced, with permission, from Knoop KJ, Stack LB, Storrow AB. *Atlas of Emergency Medicine*. 3rd ed. New York, NY: McGraw-Hill Education; 2010. Figure 3.11. Photographer: Department of Ophthalmology, Naval Medical Center, Portsmouth, Virginia.)

Symptoms/Examination

- **Painless** monocular vision loss that gradually develops, afferent pupillary defect
- Funduscopic examination with disk edema, dilated and tortuous veins, and hemorrhage that may cover the entire fundus giving a **"blood and thunder"** appearance (see Figure 14.28).

Complications

Untreated CRVO leads to neovascular glaucoma and macular edema.

> **KEY FACT**
>
> Blood and thunder = CRVO
>
> Cherry red fovea = CRAO

Treatment

Treatment should be guided by an ophthalmologist and may include lowering of IOP, topical steroids, cyclocryotherapy, photocoagulation, intraocular antivascular growth factor, and low-molecular-weight heparin.

OPTIC NEURITIS

Pathogenesis

- Autoimmune demyelinating inflammation of the optic nerve that may be idiopathic, but also strongly associated with multiple sclerosis (MS).
  - 50% of patients with MS will develop optic neuritis in their lifetime, and 25% of cases of optic neuritis are due to MS.

Symptoms/Examination

- Monocular vision loss progressive over several hours to days; central visual field deficit (scotoma)
- Periocular **pain** exacerbated by eye movement
- **Afferent pupillary defect**
- Funduscopic examination can show a normal or swollen disk
- Vision loss peaks at about two weeks, then gradually improves; progressing symptoms beyond two weeks suggest another etiology.

Differential

Other optic neuropathies including ischemic (temporal arteritis), infectious (West Nile, toxoplasmosis, tuberculosis, *Cryptococcus*, syphilis), autoimmune (sarcoidosis, Behçet), toxic (ethylene glycol, methanol), and compressive (glaucoma, tumor, aneurysm, Graves' disease)

DIAGNOSIS

Clinical examination confirmed by MRI of brain and orbits with gadolinium, showing optic nerve inflammation and possibly sequelae of MS

TREATMENT

- Optic neuritis is generally self-resolving, though return of visual acuity may be somewhat incomplete.
- Neurology consult with treatment focused on improving vision and preventing/delaying the development of MS
  - Parenteral corticosteroid therapy is controversial and may hasten visual recovery but has no effect on long-term visual acuity.

> **KEY FACT**
>
> Patients presenting with optic neuritis must be evaluated for MS.

PAPILLEDEMA

The subarachnoid space of the brain is contiguous with the optic nerve sheath so that elevated intracranial pressures are transmitted to the optic nerve, resulting in swelling of the optic disc and visual changes from transient fluctuations in optic nerve perfusion.

CAUSES

- Intracranial tumor
- Idiopathic intracranial hypertension (pseudotumor cerebri)
- Intracranial hematoma, subarachnoid hemorrhage
- Cerebral edema
- Brain abscess, meningitis, or encephalitis

SYMPTOMS/EXAMINATION

- Vision changes include brief obscurations, enlargement of the physiologic blind spot, and **nasal visual field loss.**
- Swelling of the optic disk, blurring of the disk margin, and loss of physiologic cupping on funduscopic examination (Figure 14.29)
- Bedside ED ultrasound can be used to objectively quantify papilledema by measuring the **optic nerve sheath diameter** 3 mm posterior to the globe (Figure 14.30); width > 5 mm suggests papilledema.

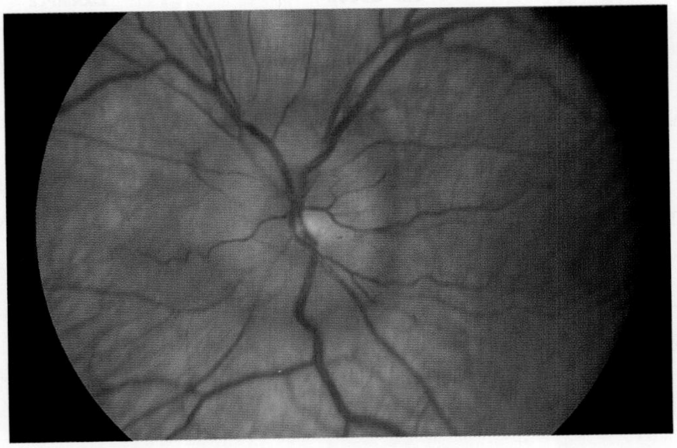

FIGURE 14.29. Papilledema. Note the blurring of the optic disc margin (Reproduced, with permission, from Knoop KJ, Stack LB, Storrow AB. *Atlas of Emergency Medicine*. 3rd ed. New York, NY: McGraw-Hill Education; 2010. Figure 3.24. Photographer: Arun D. Singh, MD.)

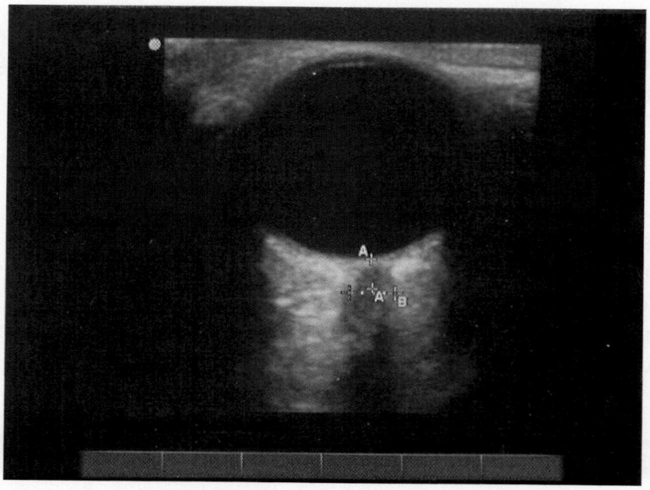

FIGURE 14.30. Optic nerve sheath diameter on ocular ultrasound. (Reproduced, with permission, from McKean S, Ross JJ, Dressler DD, et al. *Principles and Practice of Hospital Medicine*. New York, NY: McGraw-Hill Education; 2012. Figure 114.1B.)

Diagnosis/Treatment

Depends on suspected underlying cause.

Topical Ophthalmologic Medications

In the United States, all prescription topical eye drops have a color-coded cap to differentiate between classes of medication (Table 14.2). Topical ocular medications are absorbed and are capable of producing systemic side effect.

TABLE 14.2. Ophthalmologic Medications

Class	Cap Color	Example
Antibiotic	TAN	Trimethoprim/polymyxin, levofloxacin, erythromycin
Antiviral	TAN	Trifluridine, ganciclovir
Cycloplegic/mydriatic	RED	Tropicamide, homatropine, cyclopentolate
β-Blocker	YELLOW	Timolol
Carbonic anhydrase inhibitor	ORANGE	Dorzolamide, brinzolamide
Anesthetic	WHITE	Proparacaine, tetracaine
NSAID	GRAY	Ketorolac

NSAID, nonsteroidal anti-inflammatory drug.

Nose

NASAL FOREIGN BODY

The nose is the most common site of foreign body insertion, seen most in children < 5 years. With the exception of button batteries and paired disc magnets, the complications and risk of aspiration of nasal foreign bodies are low.

SYMPTOMS/EXAMINATION

Subtle presentations include epistaxis, unilateral malodorous purulent discharge, mouth breathing, or even sinusitis refractory to antibiotics.

TREATMENT

- Foreign body removal:
  - "Mother's kiss" technique in which a parent insufflates a short burst of air into the child's mouth while occluding the unaffected naris
  - Mechanical retrieval after pretreatment with vasoconstrictive agents (oxymetazoline or nebulized racemic epinephrine) and topical anesthetic

KEY FACT

Anterior epistaxis:
- 90% of epistaxis
- Kiesselbach plexus
- Anterioinferior nasal septum

Posterior epistaxis:
- 10% of epistaxis
- Sphenopalatine artery
- Posterior nasal septum and lateral wall

EPISTAXIS

Epistaxis has a bimodal distribution occurring primarily in ages 2-10 and 50-80 years. Coagulopathies, whether inherited, acquired (eg, liver or renal disease), or pharmacologic, increase the risk of epistaxis.

CAUSES

- Anterior epistaxis (90%)
  - Typically from Kiesselbach plexus in the anterior nasal septum; a vascular plexus of 5 arteries (sphenopalatine, greater palatine, anterior and posterior ethmoidal, and superior labial)
  - Results from damage to the nasal mucosa from digital trauma, sinus infection, cold dry climate, or oxygen supplementation.
- Posterior epistaxis (10%)
  - Arises from branches of the sphenopalatine artery.
  - Arteriosclerotic disease is a common contributor.

SYMPTOMS/EXAMINATION

- The source of bleeding may be directly visualized with anterior epistaxis; the inability to visualize a source or control bleeding with anterior packing suggests a posterior source.
- Patients with profound bleeding may require a complete blood count (CBC) to evaluate need for transfusion.
- Routine coagulation studies are NOT indicated unless there is a clinical concern for coagulopathy.

TREATMENT

- Assess airway, breathing, and circulation (ABCs) as significant bleeding can result in aspiration, airway obstruction, and hemodynamic compromise.
- Initial management includes the following three steps:
  - Have patient blow their nose to remove clots.
  - Apply topical vasoconstrictive medication (eg, oxymetazoline, cocaine, lidocaine-epinephrine).

- Have patient hold direct pressure by pinching the nasal alae against the septum constantly for 10-15 minutes.
- Topical thrombin can be sprayed into the naris with a special applicator.
- Anterior epistaxis:
  - Chemical cautery by placing a silver nitrate stick around the identified source (4-5 seconds at a time) until an eschar develops; avoid cautery to the bilateral septum due to risk of perforation.
  - Persistent bleeding requires anterior packing with Vaseline gauze, prefabricated nasal tampon, or epistaxis balloon.
  - Bilateral packing may be required if there is significant septal deviation with unilateral packing.
- Posterior epistaxis:
  - Requires more invasive posterior packing with the use of a 10- to 14-French Foley catheter or a double-balloon catheter that is inserted into the naris until visualized in the oropharynx followed by inflation of the distal balloon, gentle traction to seal off the postnasopharyngeal space, and then proximal balloon inflation or anterior packing to achieve tamponade.
- Persistent bleeding following anterior and posterior packing requires emergent ENT evaluation and/or interventional radiology-guided arterial embolization.

KEY FACT

Digital trauma is the most common cause of epistaxis.

COMPLICATIONS

- Hypertension is often a **result** of epistaxis due to the associated discomfort and anxiety, and not a cause of continued bleeding. Antihypertensive medications have no role in the management of epistaxis.
- Patients with packing in place are at risk for secondary sinus infection as well as toxic shock syndrome. It is customary to prescribe prophylactic antibiotics (second-generation cephalosporin, amoxicillin/clavulanate), though there are no data to support this practice.

KEY FACT

Profound hemorrhage may result from epistaxis, particularly posterior sources, and can be life threatening.

DISPOSITION

- Patients with anterior nasal packing can be safely discharged home with prophylactic antibiotics and follow-up in 48-72 hours for packing removal.
- Posterior nasal packing should remain in place for 72-96 hours and requires hospital admission to a telemetry bed due to risk of respiratory suppression due to the nasopulmonary reflex as well as bradycardia and dysrhythmias.

SINUSITIS

Due to ostial obstruction and ciliary immobility leading to poor mucus drainage. It is classified based on duration of symptoms as acute (< 4 weeks), subacute (4-12 weeks), chronic (> 12 weeks), or recurrent (> 4 acute episodes per year).

CAUSES

- The vast majority (90%-98%) of cases of acute sinusitis are viral in etiology caused by spread of viral pathogens from the nasal mucosa to the sinus.
- Bacterial superinfection by *S. pneumoniae, H. influenzae*, and *M. catarrhalis; P. aeruginosa* occurs in a small percentage of patients.
  - Predisposing factors include allergic rhinitis, trauma, structural abnormalities, cocaine abuse, foreign bodies, or nasogastric tubes.
- Fungal infections (*Aspergillus, Candida, Mucor, Rhizopus*) may occur in patients with diabetes or immunocompromised.

SYMPTOMS/EXAMINATION

- Classic symptoms include headache, sinus pressure, congestion, and mucopurulent nasal discharge.
- May also see hyposmia, maxillary dental pain, and ear fullness.
- Patients may have tenderness to percussion over affected sinuses and inflamed nasal passages.

DIAGNOSIS

- Acute viral sinusitis progresses over 7-10 days and then spontaneously resolves.
- Symptoms beyond 10 days or "double sickening" where symptoms initially improve only to worsen suggests bacterial sinusitis and are an indication for antibiotic treatment.
- CT of face is sensitive but has poor specificity and is only recommended for chronic sinusitis (> 12 weeks) in conjunction with ENT referral, recurrent sinusitis (> 4 episodes per year) or for investigation of complications of acute sinusitis.

COMPLICATIONS

Periorbital/orbital cellulitis, abscess, optic neuritis, blindness, Pott puffy tumor (frontal bone subperiosteal abscess and osteomyelitis), epidural or subdural empyema, meningitis, cavernous sinus thrombosis, and brain abscess

TREATMENT

- Acute viral sinusitis should be treated symptomatically with topical decongestants (eg, oxymetazoline) limited to a maximum of 5 days (due to rebound vasodilation) and sinus self-irrigation.
- Systemic decongestants have no advantage over topical agents and have significant systemic effects.
- Amoxicillin/clavulanate for 5-7 days is the recommended treatment for acute bacterial sinusitis; azithromycin if penicillin allergic.

> **KEY FACT**
>
> The osteomeatal complex, located between the inferior and middle turbinates, drains the frontal, maxillary, and anterior ethmoid sinuses.

RHINOCEREBRAL MUCORMYCOSIS

Invasive fungal infection caused by *Rhizopus* or related species of the Mucorales order of fungi, occurring exclusively in poorly controlled diabetics and the immunocompromised.

> **KEY FACT**
>
> Mucorales order of fungi:
> *Mucor*
> *Rhizopus*
> *Absidia*

SYMPTOMS/EXAMINATION

- Initial symptoms are that of an acute sinusitis.
- Patients subsequently develop symptoms of invasive disease including cranial nerve palsies, proptosis, orbital inflammation and edema, restricted eye movement, or loss of vision.
- Fungal angioinvasion results in tissue infarction manifested by **black eschars** of the face, nasal mucosa, or palate.

DIAGNOSIS/TREATMENT

- Diagnosis should be suspected based on clinical presentation and is confirmed by biopsy/culture specimens.
- CT can help determine the extent of disease.
- Prompt treatment with IV amphotericin B and emergent ENT consultation for surgical debridement are critical, though mortality remains high.

> **Q**
>
> A 44-year-old woman with no significant medical problems presents with a headache and fever for the past 2 days. The patient denies any neck pain and has no history of headaches. On examination, the patient is febrile, ill appearing, and is noted to have a 3-mm pustule just lateral to her right nare. She is neurologically intact. What test can confirm the diagnosis, and what is the appropriate ED management?

Cavernous Sinus Thrombosis

The cavernous sinuses are dural sinuses that lie just lateral to the sella turcica and contain the internal carotid with its surrounding sympathetic plexus as well as cranial nerves III, IV, VI, and the ophthalmic (V1) and maxillary (V2) branches of the fifth cranial nerve. Sinus and midface infections may extend into the cavernous sinuses along the drainage of the facial and ophthalmic veins resulting in **septic thrombosis** of the sinus.

Etiology/Causes

S aureus is the most common pathogen.

Symptoms/Examination

- Preceding **sinusitis or midface infection**, most commonly a furuncle
- Headache, fever, periorbital edema
- Cranial nerve palsies (most common **CN VI lateral gaze palsy**)

Diagnosis

Noncontrast head CT is insensitive and diagnosis requires CT venography, or preferably MR venography.

Treatment

- Early broad-spectrum IV antibiotics covering MRSA, gram-negative, and anaerobic organisms.
- Although controversial, anticoagulation with heparin should be considered to prevent further thrombosis and septic emboli.
- ENT consultation for drainage or management of facial infection

KEY FACT

Meningitis is not the only cause of headache and fever. Cavernous sinus thrombosis must be considered in patients with severe headache preceded by a facial or sinus infection.

Oropharynx/Throat

GINGIVOSTOMATITIS

Causes

- Most commonly viral due to Coxsackie virus, causing **herpangina** and **hand-foot-and-mouth disease** (Figure 14.31), or HSV-1
- Can also be idiopathic (aphthous stomatitis) related to stress, nutrition and hormone imbalance

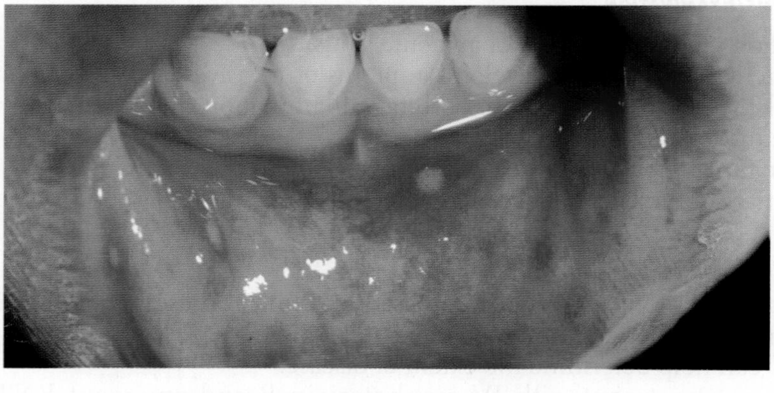

FIGURE 14.31. Gingivostomatitis in hand-foot-and-mouth disease. (Reproduced, with permission, from Wolff K, Johnson RA, Saavedra AP. *Fitzpatrick's Color Atlas and Synopsis of Clinical Dermatology*. 7th ed. New York, NY: McGraw-Hill Education; 2013. Figure 27.26.)

A

Facial soft tissue and sinus infections may extend along the facial veins into the cavernous sinus, causing cavernous sinus thrombosis. This diagnosis must always be considered in a patient with headache and a fever, and evaluation of risk factors (recent sinus infection, etc) must be examined. The diagnosis is confirmed with CT or MR venogram of the head, and treatment consists of parenteral antibiotics and frequently anticoagulation.

SYMPTOMS/EXAMINATION

- Small painful oral mucosal ulcers that can coalesce to form larger plaques
  - Coxsackie virus classically involves the palate and the posterior oropharynx.
  - HSV-1 results in the classic herpetic vesicular lesions generally involving the lips and the anterior oropharynx.

TREATMENT

- Supportive care using oral rinses and topical analgesia with "magic mouthwash" formulation including some combination of topical anesthetic, antihistamine, and/or antacid (eg, viscous lidocaine/diphenhydramine/magnesium-hydroxide)
- Treatment with antivirals (acyclovir) for oral herpes should be considered for immunocompromised patients, healthy patients with frequent outbreaks, or severe cases of primary infection.

THRUSH

Infection of the oral mucosa with *Candida* species, most commonly *Candida albicans*. Thrush is common in newborns and the immunocompromised. It is an AIDS-defining illness in HIV.

> **KEY FACT**
>
> Thrush can be differentiated from other intra-oral conditions as plaques can be easily scraped off.

SYMPTOMS/EXAMINATION

Characterized by friable gray/white plaques on an erythematous base located on the buccal mucosa, gingiva, tongue, palate, or tonsils (Figure 14.32); plaques are **easily scraped off.**

DIFFERENTIAL

Leukoplakia: A hyperkeratotic response to oral mucosal irritation manifested as white patches or plaques that do not scrape off. It is more common in smokeless tobacco users and can be a precancerous lesion, especially when located on the floor of the mouth or ventral tongue.

DIAGNOSIS/TREATMENT

- Microscopy showing yeast with pseudohyphae
- Topical nystatin swish and swallow (4-6 mL qid) continued for 5-7 days after lesions disappear

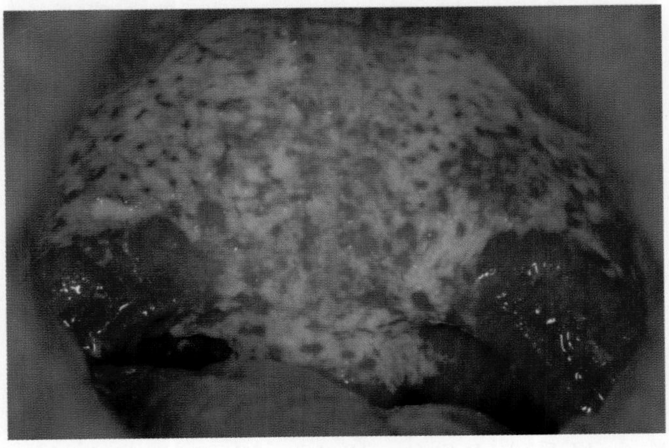

FIGURE 14.32. Thrush. (Reproduced, with permission, from Knoop KJ, Stack LB, Storrow AB. *Atlas of Emergency Medicine*. 3rd ed. New York, NY: McGraw-Hill Education; 2010. Figure 6.41. Photographer: Lawrence B. Stack, MD.)

SIALOADENITIS

Acute inflammation or infection of the salivary glands. The parotid and submandibular glands are most commonly affected.

Causes

- Bacterial infections (suppurative) tend to be unilateral, secondary to obstruction from stones or dehydration, and caused by *S. aureus*, *Streptococcus sp*, and *H. influenzae*.
  - Risk factors for bacterial infection include age > 65 years, diabetes, dehydration, poor oral hygiene, and duct obstruction from stone or neoplasm.
- Bilateral parotid infection (parotitis) is generally viral, most commonly **mumps virus**.

Symptoms/Examination

- Painful swelling of the affected salivary glands
- Purulent discharge expressed from the duct with massage of gland suggests a bacterial infection.
- Because of the close proximity of the facial nerve to the parotid gland, parotitis may result in facial nerve palsy.

Differential

- **Sialolithiasis** (Figure 14.33): Salivary duct stones occur in 1% of the population, most commonly in patients 30-50 years old. The submandibular duct is most commonly affected (> 80% of cases) resulting in painful swelling of the gland that is worse when eating. Physical examination may reveal a hard mass on palpation of the duct.
- **Sarcoidosis** can cause painless, usually bilateral, swelling of the parotid gland.

Treatment

- Mainstay is rehydration, moist heat, gentle massage of the affected gland, and sialogogues (lemon or tart candy to promote secretions)
- Antibiotics (eg, amoxicillin/clavulanate, clindamycin, cephalexin) if suspected bacterial infection
- IV antibiotics and ENT consultation for surgical drainage if infection is severe

KEY FACT

The parotid gland drains via Stensen duct at the buccal mucosa lateral to the maxillary second molar; Wharton duct at the base of the tongue drains the submandibular gland.

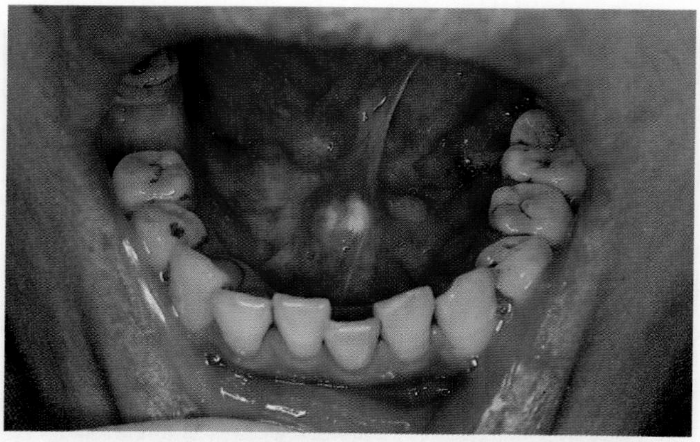

FIGURE 14.33. Sialolithiasis with stone visible at Wharton duct. (Reproduced, with permission, from Knoop KJ, Stack LB, Storrow AB. *Atlas of Emergency Medicine*. 3rd ed. New York, NY: McGraw-Hill Education; 2010. Figure 5.55. Photographer: David P. Kretzschmar, DDS, MS.)

LUDWIG ANGINA

A rapidly spreading cellulitis of the bilateral submandibular, sublingual, and submaxillary spaces that can quickly lead to airway obstruction, asphyxiation, and death.

KEY FACT

Ludwig's angina is most commonly caused by dental disease with extension of polymicrobial aerobic and anaerobic flora into the sublingual space.

Etiology/Causes

- Dental disease is the most common cause with infection or recent extraction of a mandibular molar noted in most cases.
- Polymicrobial with mixed aerobic and anaerobic oral flora

Symptoms/Examination

- Patients may present with neck pain/stiffness, fevers, dysphonia, dysphagia, odynophagia, or tongue swelling.
- Bilateral submandibular swelling with elevation and/or protrusion of the tongue with a "woody" or indurated consistency of the floor of the mouth
- "Bull neck" (tense edema and brawny induration of the upper portion of the neck)
- Stridor, tachypnea, dyspnea, inability to handle secretions, and altered mentation suggest impending airway failure.

Diagnosis

Clinical diagnosis that may be confirmed via CT with IV contrast, but only in a patient with a stable or secure airway

Treatment

- Airway management is paramount. Early awake fiberoptic nasal or oral intubation with topical anesthesia is recommended with surgical cricothyrotomy as a rescue measure.
- IV antibiotics with ampicillin/sulbactam, penicillin plus metronidazole, or clindamycin if penicillin allergic.
- ICU admission and ENT consultation as surgery may be necessary for patients who do not respond promptly to antibiotics

Complications

- The infection may spread to surrounding tissue causing empyema, mediastinitis, pericarditis, or **Lemierre's syndrome (internal jugular septic thrombophlebitis).**
- Aspiration may result in pneumonia or lung abscess.

KEY FACT

Lemierre's syndrome (internal jugular septic thrombophlebitis) is most commonly caused by *Fusobacterium necrophorum*.

PHARYNGITIS/TONSILLITIS

Inflammation of the oropharynx and tonsils.

Etiology/Causes

- Most commonly caused by respiratory viruses
- Group A β-hemolytic *Streptococcus* (GABHS) is the most common bacterial cause of pharyngitis, but only accounts for 30% of cases in children and 15% in adults.
- Other bacterial pathogens responsible for pharyngitis include gonorrhea, *Diphtheria*, *Chlamydia*, and anaerobes.

Q

A 22-year-old female presents with limited mouth opening and right sided throat and ear pain 5 days after onset of a sore throat. Physical exam shows fullness to the right posterior oropharynx and deviation of the uvula to the left side. What is the most feared complication from aspiration of this lesion?

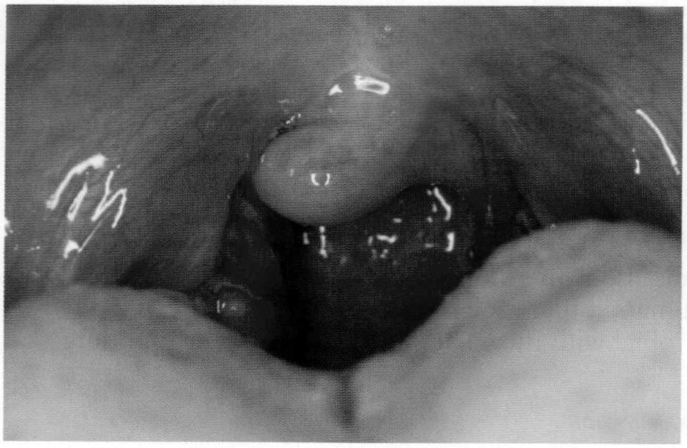

FIGURE 14.34. Group A β-hemolytic *Streptococcus* (GABHS) pharyngitis. (Reproduced, with permission, from Knoop KJ, Stack LB, Storrow AB. *Atlas of Emergency Medicine*. 3rd ed. New York, NY: McGraw-Hill Education; 2010. Figure 5.35. Photographer: Kevin J. Knoop, MD, MS.)

Symptoms/Examination

- Pharyngeal pain, worse with swallowing
- Pharyngeal erythema, tonsillar swelling, and exudate (Figure 14.34)
- Viral pharyngitis is more frequently associated with cough, rhinorrhea, myalgias, headache, stomatitis, and conjunctivitis.

> **KEY FACT**
>
> Centor Criteria for strep pharyngitis:
> - Fever
> - Absence of cough
> - Anterior cervical lymphadenopathy
> - Tonsillar exudate

Differential

- **Mononucleosis:** Caused by Epstein-Barr virus (EBV) and presents with fever, creamy or cheesy white tonsillar exudate, posterior cervical lymphadenopathy, and possible hepatosplenomegaly. Diagnosis is confirmed with monospot testing, and treatment is supportive with care to avoid contact sports due to risk of splenic rupture.
- **Diphtheria:** Potentially lethal cause of pharyngitis caused by *Corynebacterium diphtheriae* that presents with fever, malaise, and a gray or white pharyngeal pseudomembrane. Some strains produce a systemic toxin that causes myocarditis, polyneuritis, vascular collapse, and diffuse focal organ necrosis. Empiric treatment with antitoxin (horse serum product) should be initiated if suspicion for diphtheria is high.
- **Gonorrhea:** STI that is most common in patients that practice receptive oral sex; highly variable clinical presentation that can progress to gonococcemia; NAAT testing or culture on Thayer-Martin agar confirms diagnosis. Treatment is similar to other STIs with antibiotics covering both gonorrhea and chlamydia.

Diagnosis

- Clinical differentiation of the causative organism is nearly impossible.
- The Centor Score (1 point per category met) may be helpful in risk stratifying patients for GABHS pharyngitis:
  - Fever
  - Tonsillar exudates
  - Tender anterior cervical lymphadenopathy
  - Absence of cough
- Some guideline recommend empiric therapy for a score of 4, no testing for scores ≤ 1, and treatment based on the results of rapid strep testing or throat culture for scores of 2-3.

> **A**
>
> Aspiration or incision and drainage are the mainstay of treatment for peritonsillar abscesses, but careful attention must be paid to avoid injuring the carotid artery, which lies posterior and lateral to most peritonsillar abscesses. Puncture should be made in line with or medial to the maxillary teeth and depth of puncture should be approximately 1 cm. Depth can be limited by using a scalpel or needle guard.

Treatment

- Both viral and GAHBS pharyngitis are self-limited illnesses that last 3-5 days.

- Supportive care with acetaminophen and NSAIDs, throat lozenges, and oral hydration.
- Glucocorticoids therapy with dexamethasone 10 mg IM/PO once has been shown to speed the time to onset of pain relief and shorten the overall duration of symptoms.
- The treatment of GABHS is primarily for reduction of transmission and the prevention of rheumatic fever and suppurative complications as antibiotics do little to provide symptom relief or shorten the course of illness.
  - Benzathine penicillin 1.2 million units IM once *or*
  - Penicillin V 500 mg bid × 10 days
  - Erythromycin or azithromycin for penicillin allergies

COMPLICATIONS

- **Scarlet fever:** GABHS pharyngitis associated with "strawberry tongue" and a desquamating sandpaper erythematous rash.
- **Suppurative complications:** Peritonsillar abscess, otitis media, sinusitis, rarely bacteremia, meningitis, deep space neck infections, necrotizing fasciitis.
- **Rheumatic fever:** Complicates 0.3% of cases of GABHS pharyngitis, a combination of carditis, arthritis, and dermatologic findings occurring 2-6 weeks following a GABHS pharyngitis.
  - Acute rheumatic fever is diagnosed by the Jones Criteria, requiring 2 major or 1 major and 2 minor criteria along with evidence of a recent *Streptococcus* infection
    - Major criteria: Carditis, migratory arthritis, chorea, erythema marginatum, subcutaneous nodules
    - Minor criteria: Fever, arthralgia, previous rheumatic fever, elevated acute phase reactants (erythrocyte sedimentation rate, C-reactive protein), prolonged PR interval
- **Poststreptococcal glomerulonephritis:** Incidence is unaffected by antibiotic therapy.

PERITONSILLAR ABSCESS

The most common deep space infection of the neck, classically a complication of streptococcal pharyngitis. Risk factors include dental infection, mononucleosis, smoking, and tonsilloliths.

CAUSES

Most often polymicrobial due to invasion of the tonsillar pits with bacteria resulting in tonsillar cellulitis and then abscess.

SYMPTOMS/EXAMINATION

- Development of **trismus**, odynophagia, dysphagia, foul breath, and referred otalgia 2-5 days after the initial onset of sore throat
- Examination may be limited by trismus, but will show an inflamed and erythematous tonsil, most often unilateral, displaced medially and inferiorly with contralateral **deviation of the uvula**.

DIFFERENTIAL

Patients with peritonsillar abscess have a 20% incidence of mononucleosis, and monospot testing should be done on any patients with systemic symptoms suspicious for EBV infection.

DIAGNOSIS

- Diagnosis is made clinically and confirmed with aspiration or drainage of pus from the abscess.

- Ultrasound may be useful in identifying the abscess pocket.
- CT with IV contrast can rule out deeper extension of infection as needed.

TREATMENT

- As with all abscesses, drainage is the mainstay of treatment either via needle aspiration or stab incision and drainage.
- A single dose of dexamethasone can help decrease swelling and pain.
- Patients should be discharged with antibiotics to cover oral flora—ampicillin/clavulanate or clindamycin.

EPIGLOTTITIS

A supraglottic cellulitis involving the base of tongue, vallecula, aryepiglottic folds, arytenoids, lingual tonsils, and epiglottis. The incidence of pediatric epiglottitis has decreased due to *H. influenzae* vaccine, but there is an increased incidence of adult cases.

CAUSES

- Most commonly due to *H. influenzae* type b.
- Other infectious agents include viruses, *Streptococcus*, *Staphylococcus*.
- Noninfectious causes include thermal injury, toxic inhalation/ingestion, and angioedema.

SYMPTOMS/EXAMINATION

- Muffled "**hot potato voice**," dysphagia, odynophagia, and sore throat
- Fever is absent in 50% of cases.
- Epiglottitis should be suspected in patients with severe sore throat but with minimal signs of pharyngeal inflammation on examination.

DIAGNOSIS

- Diagnosis is made by laryngoscopy, preferably with a fiberoptic scope in the operating room, showing a cherry red epiglottis. Pretreatment with a drying agent (eg, glycopyrrolate 0.2 mg IV), topical anesthesia (eg, atomized 4% lidocaine), and light sedation is recommended.
- Lateral soft tissue neck radiographs have a sensitivity of 90%, showing the classic "thumbprint sign" (Figure 14.35).

> **KEY FACT**
>
> Due to the high risk of airway collapse in epiglottitis, all airway interventions should be made in the safest possible environment—ideally in an operating room.

COMPLICATIONS

Rapid and unpredictable airway obstruction is the most feared complication. An inability to tolerate secretions, holding the head in the classic sniffing position, and rapid onset of symptoms are signs of impending airway collapse.

TREATMENT

- Airway management is critical. Any stimulation of the inflamed airway can lead to laryngospasm and complete airway obstruction. Laryngoscopy should therefore be performed in the safest environment possible, ideally in an operating room with a "double setup" providing the ability to proceed immediately to cricothyrotomy.
- Nebulized racemic epinephrine may be used as a temporizing measure to decrease airway edema only until definitive airway management can be achieved.
- Immediate IV antibiotics with ceftriaxone, cefotaxime, or ampicillin/sulbactam and emergent ENT consultation.

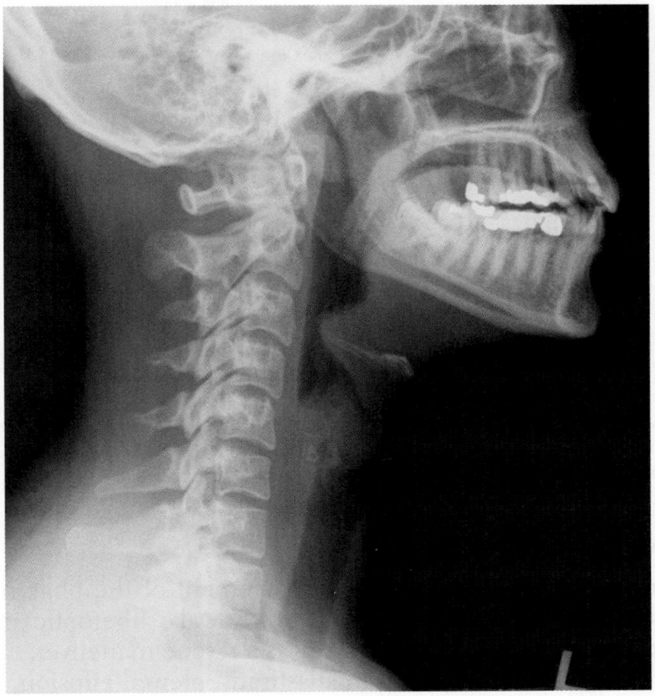

FIGURE 14.35. Epiglottitis thumbprint sign. (Reproduced, with permission, from Knoop KJ, Stack LB, Storrow AB. *Atlas of Emergency Medicine*. 3rd ed. New York, NY: McGraw-Hill Education; 2010. Figure 5.46. Photographer: Kevin J. Knoop, MD, MS.)

Q

A 30-month-old, full-term, previously healthy boy is brought in by his parents for rapid breathing and a barky cough that woke the child from sleep. On examination, the child is afebrile, tachypneic with a coarse dry cough, subcostal retractions, and stridor that can be heard from the doorway. What is the diagnosis and appropriate ED management?

RETROPHARYNGEAL ABSCESS

Classically a disease of childhood due to the presence of large retropharyngeal lymph nodes—96% occurring in children < 6 years—but there is increasing incidence in adults. Risk factors include diabetes, immunocompromise, extension of common ENT infections, trauma, foreign bodies (eg, fish bones), vertebral infections (osteomyelitis or diskitis), and bacteremia.

Causes

- Polymicrobial mixed aerobes and anaerobes with *Streptococcus* and *Staphylococcus* species being the most common pathogens isolated
- Tuberculosis can cause subacute "cold" retropharyngeal abscess.

Symptoms/Examination

- Sore throat, dysphagia, odynophagia, neck pain/stiffness, and fever
- Toxic appearance, neck held in extension
- Drooling, muffled voice, dysphonia (duck "quack" —cri du canard)
- Pain with lateral manipulation of the larynx and trachea
- Trismus, posterior pharyngeal erythema/edema

Diagnosis

- Lateral soft tissue neck radiograph obtained during inspiration shows widening of the prevertebral space (Figure 14.36).
  - C2: > 7 mm in adults or children
  - C6: > 14 mm in children; > 22 mm in adults
- CT neck with IV contrast or MRI may help delineate the extent of the infection and may assist with surgical planning, but should only be performed in patients with stable or controlled airways.

KEY FACT

A positive "tracheal rock sign" with pain on lateral manipulation of the larynx and trachea can be seen in patients with retropharyngeal abscess.

A

Croup, or laryngotracheobronchitis, is a viral illness most commonly caused by parainfluenza that results in subglottic inflammation and is characterized by a seal-like barky cough. All patients presenting to the ED with croup should be given dexamethasone 0.6 mg/kg once, and patients with significant stridor should be treated with nebulized racemic epinephrine.

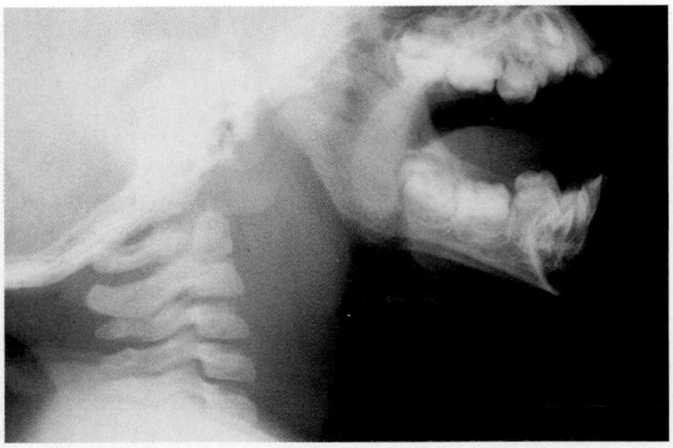

FIGURE 14.36. Retropharyngeal abscess. (Reproduced, with permission, from Knoop KJ, Stack LB, Storrow AB. *Atlas of Emergency Medicine*. 3rd ed. New York, NY: McGraw-Hill Education; 2010. Figure 14.60. Photographer: Richard Ruddy, MD.)

KEY FACT

Patients with concern for impending airway obstruction should not be given paralytics for intubation, rather awake fiberoptic intubation is preferred.

Complications

- **Airway obstruction** from anterior displacement of the pharyngeal wall is the most acute and feared complication; awake fiberoptic intubation is preferred with surgical cricothyrotomy as a rescue maneuver.
- **Extension of infection** causing mediastinitis, pleural effusion, pericarditis, empyema, epidural abscess, transverse myelitis, and atraumatic atlantoaxial separation may occur.

Treatment

- Early airway assessment and management
- High-dose IV antibiotics with clindamycin or ampicillin/sulbactam, ENT consultation, and ICU admission

CROUP (LARYNGOTRACHEOBRONCHITIS)

Croup is a viral infection causing inflammation, exudate and edema of the subglottic airway. It is most common in in patients 6 months-3 years (peak 2 years) and is rare beyond age 6 years. It is seen in late fall and early winter and ED presentation is more common at night.

Causes

Most commonly **parainfluenza** viruses, but also respiratory syncytial virus, influenza, and rhinovirus

Symptoms/Examination

Barky **seal-like cough**, hoarse voice, high-pitched inspiratory stridor, following a viral prodrome

Diagnosis

- The Westley croup score can assist in determining the severity of disease (mild ≤ 2, moderate 3-7, severe > 7). It uses 5 clinical features:
  - Level of consciousness: Normal = 0, disoriented = 5
  - Cyanosis: None = 0, with agitation = 4, at rest = 5
  - Stridor: None = 0, with agitation = 1, at rest = 2
  - Air entry: Normal = 0, decreased = 1, markedly decreased = 2
  - Retractions: None = 0, mild =1, moderate = 2, severe = 3
- Anteroposterior (AP) neck x-ray showing subglottic narrowing (**"steeple sign"**) is only useful when the diagnosis is in doubt (Figure 14.37).

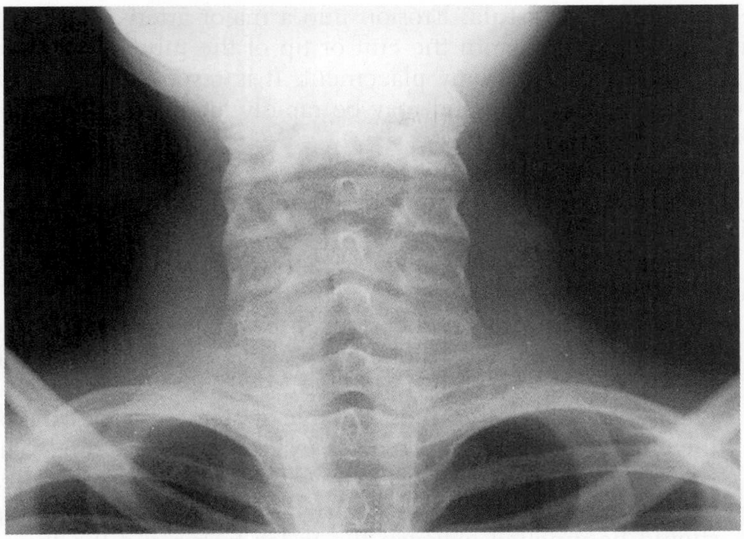

FIGURE 14.37. Croup, steeple sign. (Reproduced, with permission, from Stone CK, Humphries RL, eds. *Current Diagnosis & Treatment: Emergency Medicine*. 7th ed. New York, NY: McGraw-Hill Education; 2011. Figure 32.10B.)

Treatment

- Cool mist or humidified air is a classic home remedy, but has no evidence to support its efficacy.
- Glucocorticoid therapy with dexamethasone 0.6 mg/kg oral/IM/IV is the mainstay of treatment and is indicated in almost all patients presenting to the ED with croup.
- Nebulized racemic epinephrine should be added for any patient with stridor at rest (moderate-to-severe symptoms).
- Children with severe croup should be made as comfortable as possible because anxiety may worsen airway obstruction.
- Endotracheal intubation is required in < 1% of ED presentations of croup, but if necessary an endotracheal tube at least a half size smaller than expected should be used due to likely subglottic narrowing.
- Cases of moderate croup who have received aerosolized epinephrine may be safely discharged home after a 2- to 4-hour observation period **IF** they are free of stridor and retractions and have access to close follow-up care.

Differential

- **Bacterial tracheitis:** Bacterial infection of the trachea most commonly caused by *S. aureus* or mixed flora resulting in sloughing of the tracheal lining.
  - Can be difficult to differentiate from croup, but patients are generally older (3-5 years), toxic appearing, do not respond to general treatment for coup, and are more likely to acutely decompensate.
  - Neck and chest radiographs may show subglottic narrowing, a ragged edge of the tracheal air column, a hazy density within the tracheal lumen, and coexisting pneumonia.
  - Treat with broad-spectrum antibiotics (eg, vancomycin and ceftriaxone); patients frequently require intubation and bronchoscopy.

COMPLICATIONS OF TRACHEOSTOMY

Patients with tracheostomies can have multiple complications including increased risk of infection (tracheitis), plugging, dislodgment and creation of a false track, and bleeding.

KEY FACT

Be able to identify retropharyngeal abscess (wide retropharyngeal space), croup (steeple sign), and epiglottitis (thumbprint sign) on lateral soft tissue neck x-rays.

- **Tracheoinnominate fistula:** Erosion into a major artery (most commonly the innominate artery) from the cuff or tip of the tube is the most feared complication of tracheostomy placement. It is responsible for 10% of all tracheostomy hemorrhage and may be rapidly fatal (mortality approaches 100%).
  - A single episode of hemoptysis or tracheal bleeding should be taken very seriously because this may be the only warning of impending massive hemorrhage.
  - Treatment involves emergent ENT consultation and hemostatic measures that may include:
    - Hyperinflation of the tracheostomy tube cuff to tamponade bleeding.
    - Replacement of tracheostomy tube with cuffed endotracheal tube if the source of bleeding is more distal.
    - Digital pressure is the most reliable strategy for hemostasis and in the emergent setting may require extension of the stoma. The index finger should be placed inside the stoma and into the trachea (making sure not to fully occlude the airway), and the offending artery should be pinched between the index finger and the thumb until definitive management is available.

Dental

DENTAL INFECTIONS

Whether involving the periodontium (gingiva and tooth attachment apparatus) or the teeth, dental infections are multifactorial involving a susceptible host, cariogenic oral flora, poor hygiene, and a substrate (Figure 14.38).

Pathogenesis

- **Dental caries (pulpitis)** result from bacterial plaques that decalcify the enamel, erode the dentin, and invade the pulp eventually leading to tooth necrosis.

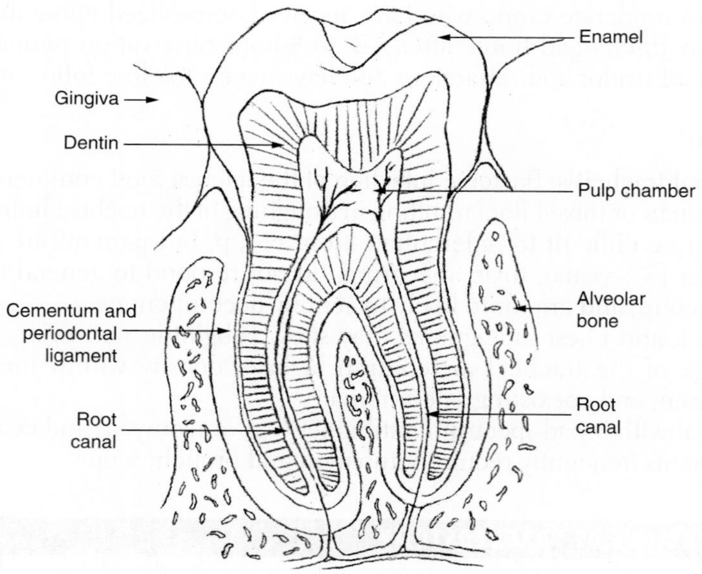

FIGURE 14.38. Tooth. (Reproduced with permission from Iserson KV. *Improvised Medicine: Providing Care in Extreme Environments*. 2nd edition. New York, NY: McGraw-Hill Education, 2016. Figure 26-3.)

- **Periapical abscesses** occur when pus leaks from the apex of a necrosed tooth to form an abscess within the alveolar bone. If this pus erodes through the alveolar bone, it will form a **dental abscess** with fluctuance under the gingiva at the base of a tooth.
- **Gingivitis** is inflammation caused by bacterial plaque that may progress to involve the alveolar bone causing **periodontitis** resulting in gingival resorption, destruction of the attachment apparatus, and creation of pockets that can trap food or plaque.
- **Pericoronitis** is an acute soft tissue swelling due to bacteria trapped under a gingival flap covering a partially erupted tooth.

Symptoms/Examination

Pain with percussion of a tooth suggests periapical abscess, whereas dental abscesses appear as a tender fluctuant mass at the base of a tooth.

Treatment

- Dental infections beyond dental caries should be treated with antibiotics (PCN or clindamycin).
- Dental abscesses should be incised and drained prior to initiation of antibiotics.
- Refer to dentist or oral surgeon for possible tooth extraction or root canal.

ACUTE NECROTIZING ULCERATIVE GINGIVITIS

Caused by overgrowth and bacterial invasion (usually ***Fusobacterium*** **and spirochetes**) of the gingiva. In developed countries it is seem primarily in young adults. Risk factors include poor dental hygiene, malnutrition, smoking, and stress.

Symptoms/Examination

- Patient complaint of foul breath, fever, malaise, and pain
- Examination shows friable gingival inflammation with gingival ulcerations and a gray pseudomembrane (Figure 14.39).

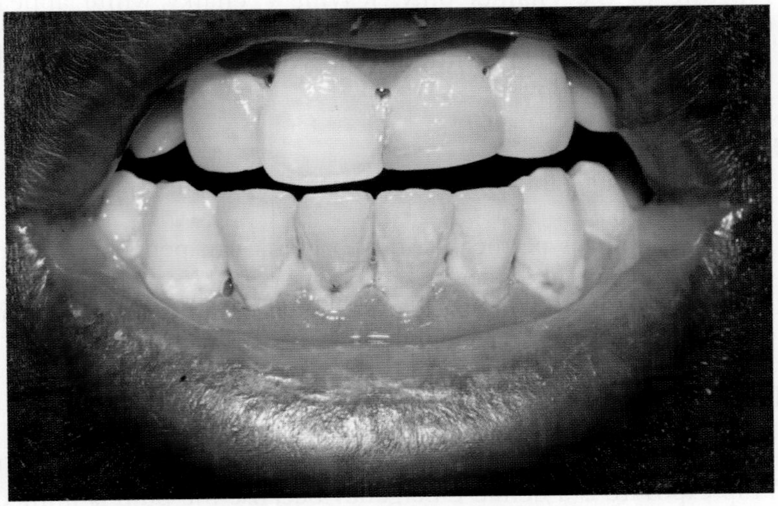

FIGURE 14.39. Acute necrotizing ulcerative gingivitis (ANUG). (Reproduced, with permission, from Wolff K, Johnson RA, Saavedra AP. *Fitzpatrick's Color Atlas and Synopsis of Clinical Dermatology*. 7th ed. New York, NY: McGraw-Hill Education; 2013. Figure 33.8.)

Treatment

Warm saline rinses, oral antibiotics (eg, penicillin or doxycycline), and improved dental hygiene

SUBLUXED AND AVULSED TEETH

Trauma can result in tooth subluxation, defined as mobility of a tooth, or complete avulsion where the tooth is expelled from its socket. Tooth avulsion is a true dental emergency with a 1% loss of successful reimplantation for every minute the tooth is out of socket.

Treatment

- Minimally subluxed teeth: Soft diet for several days
- Marked mobility:
  - Temporary stabilization with a periodontal pack—mixing a resin and a catalyst to create a mold to immobilize the affected tooth to two neighboring teeth on each side.
  - Follow-up with a dentist or oral-maxillofacial surgeon ASAP for definitive stabilization
- Tooth avulsion:
  - Reimplantation should occur as soon as possible; only permanent/secondary teeth should be reimplanted.
  - An avulsed tooth should be touched only by the crown, gently rinsed in saline or tap water (no scrubbing) and then transported in Hanks solution, milk, or placed under the patient's or parent's tongue to bathe in saliva; a tooth should never be transported in a dry medium.
  - After reimplantation, the tooth should be stabilized with a periodontal pack, tetanus status should be updated as indicated, and the patient should be discharged with antibiotics (penicillin VK) and a liquid diet with dental follow-up as soon as possible for definitive stabilization.

> **KEY FACT**
>
> Never reimplant primary (baby) teeth because this can cause fusion to the alveolar bone and block the permanent teeth from erupting.

FRACTURED TEETH

Class I

- Fracture of the enamel only, leaving a chalky white appearance (Figure 14.40).
- Smooth fracture edge with an emory board and recommend non-urgent dental follow-up.

Class II

- Fracture through the enamel and into the dentin, appearing with an ivory-yellow base
- Because dentin is permeable, oral bacteria can penetrate to the pulp causing infection and necrosis.
- Place calcium hydroxide paste over the exposed dentin, cover with dry foil, and provide next day dental follow-up.

Class III

- Full-thickness fracture through enamel and dentin exposing pulp, identified with a pink blush or a drop of blood over the fracture site
- Pulp exposure is a dental emergency because the pulp is immediately contaminated with oral bacteria and will progress to necrosis.
- Cover exposed pulp with moist cotton and dry foil and provide dental consult or dental follow-up as soon as possible for pulpectomy.

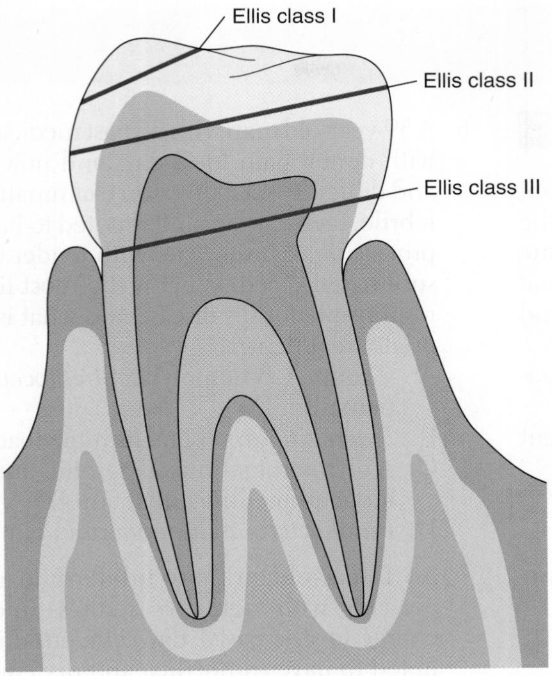

FIGURE 14.40. Ellis classification. (Reproduced, with permission, from Stone CK, Humphries RL, eds. *Current Diagnosis & Treatment: Emergency Medicine*. 7th ed. New York, NY: McGraw-Hill Education; 2011. Figure 32.7.)

COMPLICATIONS

Always consider aspiration, soft tissue entrapment, and ingestion with any dental fracture or avulsion injury.

KEY FACT

A CXR may be necessary to evaluate for aspiration of a tooth or tooth fragment in the setting of dental fracture/avulsion.

REVIEW QUESTIONS

QUESTIONS

1. A 66-year-old diabetic woman presents with ear pain, hearing loss, and discharge. On examination, the patient is nontoxic appearing with granulation tissue layering the inferior external auditory canal. What pathogen is responsible for this disease process and what is the appropriate treatment?
   A. Methicillin-resistant *Staphylococcus aureus*; intravenous (IV) vancomycin
   B. *Rhizopus* species; IV amphotericin B and emergent ENT consultation
   C. *Pseudomonas aeruginosa*; PO ciprofloxacin
   D. *Streptococcus pneumoniae*; PO amoxicillin

2. The Rinne test is used to evaluate:
   A. Sensorineural hearing loss
   B. Conductive hearing loss
   C. Central versus peripheral vertigo
   D. Both sensorineural and conductive hearing loss

3. Which of the following is an indication for the initiation of systemic therapy for acute angle-closure glaucoma?
   A. Intraocular pressure > 50 mm Hg
   B. Headache
   C. Severe eye pain
   D. Loss of pupillary reflex

4. A 22 year-old man with a history of sickle cell disease presents with painless atraumatic eye pain and decreased vision. On examination, the anterior chamber is filled with blood obscuring the inferior portion of the pupil. What is the appropriate management?
   A. Head of bed to 30° and outpatient ophthalmology follow-up
   B. Emergent ophthalmology consultation for drainage
   C. CT arteriogram of the head and orbits
   D. IOP measurement, ophthalmology consultation, and inpatient admission

5. A 66-year-old man presents with a nosebleed for the past 45 minutes. The patient denies any trauma, but states that he has lost "a lot" of blood despite applying continuous pressure to his nose for the past 15 minutes. His vital signs are stable and after blowing his nose, no site of bleeding can be seen. Despite placement of bilateral anterior nasal packing, the patient continues to have blood pooling in his posterior oropharynx. What is the most likely source of the bleeding?
   A. Kiesselbach plexus
   B. Sphenopalatine artery
   C. Anterior ethmoid artery
   D. Labial artery

6. A 59-year-old man with no past medical history presents with dental pain for 2 days and now tongue swelling and difficulty speaking. On examination, the patient is febrile, tachycardic, and is noted to have elevation and protrusion of his tongue with tender induration of the sublingual space. What is the most likely organism(s) responsible for his disease and what is the most appropriate treatment?
   A. Group A β-hemolytic *Streptococcus*; benzathine penicillin IM
   B. *P aeruginosa*; piperacillin/tazobactam IV
   C. Polymicrobial mixed aerobic and anaerobic bacteria; ampicillin/sulbactam IV
   D. *Fusobacterium necrophorum*; clindamycin PO

7. An 11-day-old girl born full term to a healthy mother presents with right eye redness and moderate discharge for the past 1 day. The child is afebrile, but is noted to have rhinorrhea and dry cough. What is the most appropriate management?
   A. Culture of eye discharge, erythromycin ophthalmic ointment, and consideration of a chest x-ray
   B. Supportive care and outpatient follow-up
   C. Antihistamine treatment
   D. IV ceftriaxone, emergent ophthalmology consult, and inpatient admission

8. Which of the following is an indication for ophthalmology consultation in the setting of eyelid laceration?
   A. Bulbar fat herniation
   B. Fluorescein uptake in the wound
   C. Full-thickness laceration
   D. All of the above

9. Mandibular dislocation is most commonly because of:
   A. Motor vehicle collisions
   B. Fist-to-face assault
   C. Excessive mouth opening (yawning, eating)
   D. Underlying collagen vascular disease

10. A 22-year-old man presents with left eye pain after getting an industrial cleaning agent splashed into his eye about 20 minutes ago. The patient is in a considerable amount of pain and his vision is "blurry" despite rinsing the eye out for 5 minutes prior to arrival. The Material Safety Data Sheet (MSDS) for the product lists a pH of 12. What is the next step in management for this patient?
    A. Immediate copious irrigation of the affected eye with 1-2 L of normal saline with or without the use of a morgan lens
    B. Topical proparacaine and fluorescein examination
    C. Measurement of IOP
    D. Testing of visual acuity

ANSWERS

1. **C.** This patient is a diabetic with a description consistent with malignant otitis externa. While these patients may require inpatient admission and parenteral antibiotics, nontoxic patients with normal vital signs may be treated with oral fluoroquinolone and close follow-up.
2. **B.** There are 2 types of hearing loss: conductive, involving the outer ear, tympanic membrane, or middle ear, and sensorineural, involving the inner ear CN VIII and brain. The Rinne test is used to diagnose conductive hearing loss when bone conduction is greater than air conduction. The Weber test can be used to diagnose both conductive and sensorineural hearing loss with vibration louder in the affected ear in the setting of conductive hearing loss and quieter in the setting of sensorineural hearing loss.
3. **A.** The diagnosis of acute angle-closure glaucoma is confirmed with IOPs > 20 mm Hg on tonometry and requires immediate administration of topical therapies. Severe visual deficits or an IOP of > 50 mm Hg warrants initiation of systemic therapy in addition to topical therapies.
4. **D.** This patient is presenting with atraumatic hyphema in the setting of sickle cell disease. These patients are considered high risk and warrant ophthalmology consultation and inpatient admission. All patients with hyphema should be instructed to elevate their head of bed to minimize synechiae formation.
5. **B.** Unlike anterior epistaxis, arising from Kiesselbach plexus, posterior epistaxis results from bleeding from branches of the sphenopalatine artery and can be much more difficult to control.
6. **C.** Ludwig angina is most commonly caused by mixed oral flora and is usually odontogenic in origin. Immunocompetent patients may be treated with IV ampicillin/sulbactam or clindamycin. *Fusobacterium necrophorum* is commonly identified as the causative pathogen in Lemierre syndrome—internal jugular vein septic thrombophlebitis.
7. **A.** This child is presenting with moderate eye discharge in the time frame typically associated with chlamydial conjunctivitis. Treatment involves topical macrolides, and providers must consider concomitant atypical pneumonia in patients with cough and other upper respiratory infection symptoms.
8. **D.** Simple eyelid lacerations can frequently be repaired in the emergency department, but full-thickness lacerations with or without herniation of bulbar fat, in addition to lacrimal system injuries, as evidenced by fluorescein uptake in the wound, are indications for specialist consultation and repair.
9. **C.** Mandibular dislocation is frequently atraumatic resulting from excessive mouth opening. Typically, the mandible deviates away from the side of pain in the setting of a dislocation—the opposite is true for mandibular fractures.
10. **A.** Chemical eye exposures are extremely time sensitive, particularly in the setting of alkali exposure, and every effort should be made to irrigate the eye as soon as possible after the exposure. Eye irrigation should be continued for 30 minutes or until the pH of the tear film is neutral. Once irrigation is complete, additional diagnostics can be performed.

CHAPTER 15

Neurology

Jessica J. Slim, MD, MPH

Stroke

A stroke is any process that disrupts the flow of oxygen and substrate-rich blood to the brain. Neurons are very sensitive to changes in cerebral blood flow, and die within minutes. Commonly, an infarcted area of brain is surrounded by a region of tenuous blood flow, the **ischemic penumbra**. The focus of stroke management is to maintain the blood supply to this region, thereby limiting infarct size. Overall, 85% of strokes are ischemic and 15% are hemorrhagic.

ANATOMY OF CEREBRAL BLOOD FLOW (FIGURE 15.1)

- Anterior circulation (from carotid arteries, 80% of cerebral blood flow [CBF])
  - Anterior cerebral: Frontal pole, anteromedial cerebral cortex, anterior corpus callosum
  - Middle cerebral: Frontoparietal lobe, frontotemporal lobe, language centers
  - Ophthalmic: Optic nerve and retina
- Posterior circulation (from vertebrobasilar arteries, 20% of CBF)
  - Posterior cerebral: Visual occipital cortex, medial temporal lobe, auditory/vestibular structures
  - Vertebral: Brainstem
  - Basilar: Thalamus, pons
  - PICA: Cerebellum
- Circle of Willis
  - Connection between anterior and posterior circulations

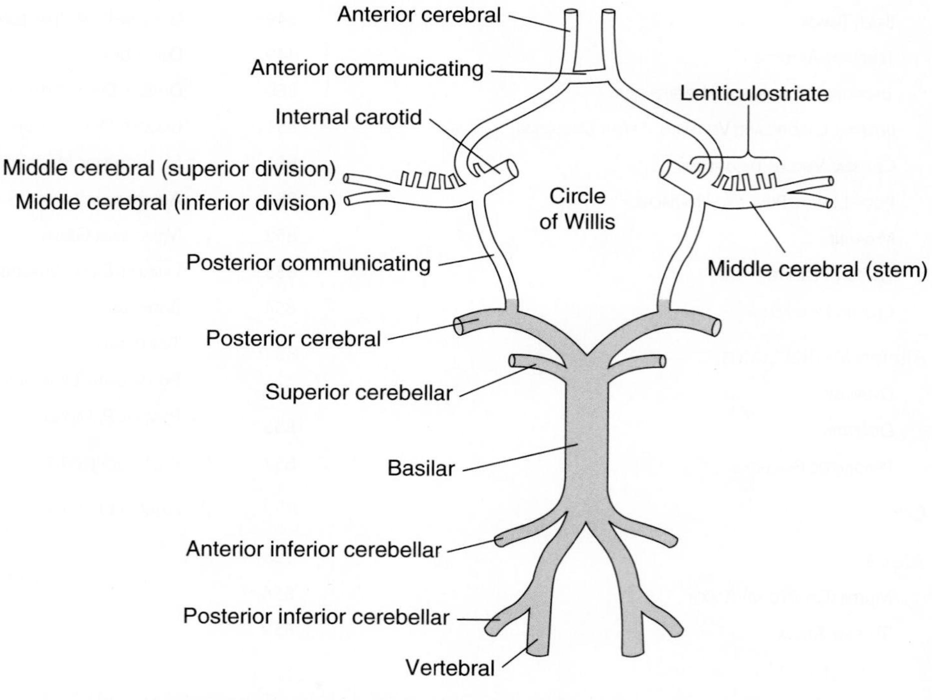

FIGURE 15.1. Anatomy of cerebral blood flow. (Reproduced, with permission, from Aminoff MJ, Greenberg DA, Simon RP. *Clinical Neurology.* 6th ed. New York: McGraw-Hill, 2005:288.)

TABLE 15.1. Comparison of Ischemic Stroke Types

	Thrombotic	Embolic	Hypoperfusion
Time course	Gradual onset/TIAs	Sudden onset	Waxing/waning
Mechanism	Vascular damage, clot formation	Mural thrombus, usually cardiac	↓ Cerebral perfusion pressure

TIAs, transient ischemic attacks.

ISCHEMIC STROKE

Ischemic stroke may be divided into three types: Thrombotic, cardioembolic, and hypoperfusion states (Table 15.1).

Thrombotic Stroke

Causes

Thrombosis is the most common cause of stroke in the United States and typically results from clot formation at the site of an ulcerated atherosclerotic plaque.

Other causes include:

- Vessel narrowing from vasculitis, dissection, infectious disease, vasospasm
- Thrombophilia from hypercoagulable states
- Sickle cell disease
- Polycythemia

Symptoms generally come on gradually and may be preceded by transient ischemic attacks (TIAs) affecting the same region as the stroke.

A subset of thrombotic stroke is the **lacunar stroke**. This is a stroke of a small terminal vessel, typically deep in the subcortical cerebrum, basal ganglia, internal capsule, thalamus, corona radiata, or brainstem. There is higher incidence in African Americans, Mexican Americans, Hong Kong Chinese, and patients with hypertension and diabetes. Patients with lacunar strokes are candidates for thrombolysis if they meet standard criteria.

Lacunar	Cortical
Small infarct	Large infarct
Better prognosis	Worse prognosis
Stuttering course	Progressively worse
Consciousness remains intact	Decreasing consciousness
Motor or sensory	MOTOR AND SENSORY
No corticol signs	CORTICOL DYSFUNCTION (aphasia, neglect)

Cardioembolic Stroke

Causes

Occurs when intravascular material (eg, clot) from a proximal source travels to the cerebral circulation, causing obstruction.

Types of emboli include:

- Cardiac (mural thrombus, valvular vegetations, cardiac tumors).
- Venous thrombosis in the presence of a ventricular or atrial septal defect. This is also known as a *paradoxical embolus*.

Q

A 58-year-old woman is brought to the emergency department (ED) as a "stroke alert." Her husband states that she woke up 1 hour prior to arrival with slurred speech and weakness in her right arm and leg. On physical examination she has aphasia, right-sided hemiparesis, and sensory deficits. Laboratory test results are drawn, and the patient is rushed to the computed tomography (CT) scanner. What blood vessel is associated with this stroke syndrome? Is this patient a thrombolysis candidate?

KEY FACT

The most common source of embolic stroke is a cardiac mural thrombus in patients with atrial fibrillation.

A

The patient is found to have an ischemic left middle cerebral artery (MCA) stroke. While the patient is presenting within 4.5 hours of perceived onset of symptoms, we do not know the actual time the stroke occurred. Thus, the patient is not a thrombolysis candidate. However, immediate discussion with neurology is recommended.

- Proximal aortic or carotid atherosclerotic plaque.
- Fat (from a broken bone).
- Air (air embolism).
- Particulate matter (eg, talc from injection drug use).
- Onset is typically sudden and maximal in severity.
- Accounts for 20% of ischemic strokes.

Hypoperfusion States

Causes

Low-flow state leading to decreased perfusion of neurons. Cerebral perfusion pressure (CPP) is dependent on mean arterial blood pressure (MAP) and intracranial pressure (ICP), and is represented by the formula: CPP = MAP − ICP. Hypoperfusion may result from either an increased ICP or decreased MAP.

Hypoperfusion stroke is a diffuse process with regional variability depending on state of vasculature and brain in any given region. Prolonged hypoperfusion will result in permanent injury, often referred to as a watershed infarction.

Stroke symptoms may wax and wane as these variables change.

Symptoms/Examination

- Symptom onset varies with stroke type
  - Sudden and maximal at onset with embolic
  - More gradual or preceded by TIA with thrombotic
  - Waxing and waning with hypoperfusion state
- **NIH stroke scale:** A method used to standardize the assessment of clinical severity of stroke. Scale ranges from 0 to 42. Scores > 22 = ↑ risk of symptomatic hemorrhage (Table 15.2).
- Location of symptoms varies with location of obstruction (Table 15.3).
- **Amaurosis fugax**: Transient monocular blindness from embolization of carotid plaque to the ophthalmic artery.
- **TIA:** Traditional definition has been an acute neurologic deficit that has complete clinical resolution within 24 hours. However, there has been a movement to change this definition to a tissue-based diagnosis: transient neurologic deficits lasting < 1 hour with no evidence of infarction on brain imaging studies (MRI).
- **Wernicke aphasia** (receptive aphasia): Ischemia/infarct in Wernicke area (temporal lobe) resulting in an inability to comprehend language input. Speech is fluent but disorganized.
- **Broca aphasia** (expressive aphasia): Ischemia/infarct of Broca area (frontal lobe) resulting in inability to communicate verbally. Speech is halting and produced with great effort.

KEY FACT

The hallmark of posterior circulation stroke is crossed deficits (eg, sensory loss on right side of face vs left side of body).

Diagnosis

- Suspect based on age, comorbidities, history and examination: unilateral weakness/numbness, confusion, aphasia, visual deficits, dizziness, ataxia, gait abnormalities, memory deficit.
- Exclude stroke mimics: Syncope, postseizure paralysis (Todd paralysis), metabolic (hypoglycemia/hyperglycemia, encephalopathy), toxicologic, Bell palsy, complicated migraine, traumatic brain injury, psychogenic.
- Determine time of onset → last known time when patient at baseline. If symptoms are waxing and waning, time of onset is at first symptom. The clock does not restart with each fluctuation in symptoms.
- Confirmed based on CT or magnetic resonance imaging (MRI). Early on, there are no visible CT changes. MRI is more sensitive for acute injury, especially diffusion weighted MRI.

KEY FACT

3%-21% patients treated with tPA are stroke mimics.

TABLE 15.2. NIH Stroke Scale

Examination	Instructions	Scale Definition
LOC	Evaluate the patient for response to verbal or painful stimuli. Full evaluation may be prevented by ETT, language barrier, trauma.	0: Alert, keenly responsive 1: Arousable by minor stimulation 2: Obtunded, requires repeated or painful stimuli 3: Totally unresponsive or reflex motor movements only
LOC Questions	"What month is it?" "How old are you?"	0: Both questions correct 1: One question correct 2: Neither question correct
LOC Commands	"Open and close your eyes." "Squeeze and release my hand."	0: Performs both correctly 1: Performs one correctly 2: Performs neither correctly
Best Gaze	Only horizontal eye movements tested. Both voluntary and reflexive eye movements scored.	0: Normal 1: Partial gaze palsy in one or both eyes 2: Forced deviation or total gaze paresis not overcome by oculocephalic maneuver
Visual	Test visual fields by confrontation (all four quadrants) using finger counting or visual threat.	0: No vision loss 1: Partial hemianopsia 2: Complete hemianopsia 3: Bilateral hemianopia (blind, including cortical blindness)
Facial Palsy	Ask patient to smile, show teeth, raise eyebrows, close eyes.	0: Normal symmetric movements 1: Minor paralysis (flattened nasolabial fold, mild asymmetry) 2: Partial paralysis 3: Complete paralysis of one or both sides
Motor Arm	Place patient's arms in extended position, palms down, at 90° if sitting or 45° if supine.	0: No drift at 10 s 1: Drifts down before full 10 s but does not hit bed 2: Some effort against gravity, but hits bed within 10 s 3: No effort against gravity 4: No movement
Motor Leg	Place patient's leg at 30° to bed in supine position.	0: No drift at 5 s 1: Drifts down before full 5 s but does not hit bed 2: Some effort against gravity, but hits bed within 5 s 3: No effort against gravity 4: No movement
Limb Ataxia	Finger-nose-finger and heel-to-shin tests performed with eyes open. Examination is for ataxia out of proportion to weakness.	0: Absent 1: Present in 1 limb 2: Present in 2 limbs

(*Continued*)

TABLE 15.2. NIH Stroke Scale (*Continued*)

Examination	Instructions	Scale Definition
Sensory	Sensation or grimace to pinprick that can be attributed to stroke.	0: Normal, no sensory loss 1: Mild to moderate sensory loss (↓ sensation) 2: Severe to total sensory loss (no sensation)
Best language	Rate patient's comprehension and language abilities. You may ask patient to describe what is happening in test picture, name items on test naming sheet, or read from list of test sentences.	0: No aphasia 1: Mild to moderate aphasia 2: Severe aphasia 3: Mute, global aphasia
Dysarthria	Rate the patient's ability to articulate speech. Patient may again be asked to read from test naming sheet or test sentences.	0: Normal 1: Mild to moderate dysarthria 2: Severe dysarthria
Extinction and inattention	Stimulate patient on one side, the other side, and then both sides. Evaluate for extinction with double simultaneous stimulation.[a]	0: No abnormality 1: Visual, tactile, auditory, spatial, or personal inattention or extinction to bilateral simultaneous stimulation 2: Profound hemi-inattention or extinction to more than one modality

(Modified with permission from National Institute of Neurological Disorders and Stroke. NIH Stroke Scale. http://www.ninds.nih.gov/doctors/NIH_Stroke_Scale.pdf. Accessed January 25, 2012.)

ETT, endotracheal tube; LOC, level of consciousness.

[a]Extinction with double simultaneous stimulation: Double simultaneous stimulation is tested by stimulating the patient on one side, the other side, or both sides at once (visual, tactile, auditory, spatial). The patient is asked which side is being stimulated, or if both sides are being stimulated. If the patient neglects one side on double simultaneous stimulation, this is an indicator of neglect (likely contralateral posterior parietal lobe lesion typically right parietal injury, yielding left-sided neglect or inattention).

    - Appears as area of hypodensity on noncontrast CT (Figure 15.2).
    - Perfusion-weighted CT angiography can identify the ischemic penumbra.
    - Ischemic stroke may not be visible on noncontrast CT until > 6 hours.
- Glucose to rule out hypoglycemia
- Electrocardiogram (ECG) to evaluate rhythm (atrial fibrillation), risk of concomitant myocardial infarction (MI)
- Coagulation studies

Treatment

- ABCs (including intubation for decreased level of consciousness)
- **Hypotension:** Restore euvolemia, then use pressors (if necessary)
- Hypertension
    - Avoid aggressive lowering of BP in chronically hypertensive patients (who have cerebral autoregulation curve shifted to right), because this may limit flow to the ischemic penumbra.
    - If considering tissue plasminogen activator (tPA) and blood pressure (BP) > 185/110 mm Hg: Consider labetalol and nicardipine as first-line agents. Nitroprusside infusion as second-line agent.
    - If patient is not a tPA candidate: Do not treat unless BP persistently elevated above 220 systolic or 120 diastolic. Same agents (labetalol, nicardipine, nitroprusside) may be used.
    - If treatment is initiated, goal = BP ≤ 185/110 mm Hg.
    - Maintain cerebral blood flow with fluids and/or vasopressor support if systolic blood pressure (SBP) < 100 or diastolic blood pressure (DBP) < 70 to prevent stroke from ↓ perfusion to brain.

KEY FACT

In stroke, treat BP if persistently elevated > 220/120 mm Hg. Persistently elevated BP > 185/110 mm Hg is contraindication for tPA use.

TABLE 15.3. Ischemic Stroke—Clinical Findings

Area of Blockage	Major Finding	Other Findings
Anterior cerebral artery	Contralateral weakness of leg > arm and face with minimal sensory findings	Altered mentation and judgment Reappearance of primitive reflexes (grasp and suck) If both arteries originate from occluded common trunk (bilateral infarct) → paraplegia and severe dysarthria
Middle cerebral artery (most common)	Contralateral weakness **and** numbness of arm and face > leg	Homonymous hemianopsia Gaze preference toward side of infarct If dominant hemisphere (usually left): Receptive/expressive aphasia Nondominant hemisphere: Inattention and neglect. Failure to identify touch (extinction) on double simultaneous stimulation
Lacunar artery	Pure motor *or* pure sensory findings	Clumsy hand—dysarthria syndrome
Posterior cerebral artery	Contralateral visual field and light touch/pinprick deficit with *minimal* weakness	Memory loss Alexia—inability to read
Vertebrobasilar artery	Crossed deficits: Ipsilateral cranial nerve deficits with contralateral weakness	Vertigo, ataxia Oculomotor palsies, limb weakness
Distal vertebral or posterior inferior cerebellar artery **Lateral medullary (Wallenberg) syndrome**	Crossed pain and temperature deficits: Ipsilateral loss on face, contralateral on body	Ipsilateral Horner syndrome and cranial nerve deficits may be present Gait and limb ataxia
Basilar artery	"Locked in" syndrome (complete paralysis of voluntary muscles except eye movement; normal level of consciousness)	Quadriplegia Coma
Cerebellar artery	Sudden inability to walk or stand with headache, vertigo, nausea/vomiting, abnormal gait, CN abnormalities	Lateralizing dysmetria (eg, finger-nose-finger) Dysdiadochokinesia (inability to perform rapid alternating movements)

- Glucose control
  - Treat hyperglycemia to keep blood glucose 100-200. Glucose level > 400 is contraindication for tPA.
  - Avoid intravenous (IV) solutions with glucose.
  - Avoid steroids if possible.
- Systemic tPA (thrombolysis)
  - Criteria (Table 15.4):
    - Symptoms < 4.5 hours duration
    - Age > 18 years

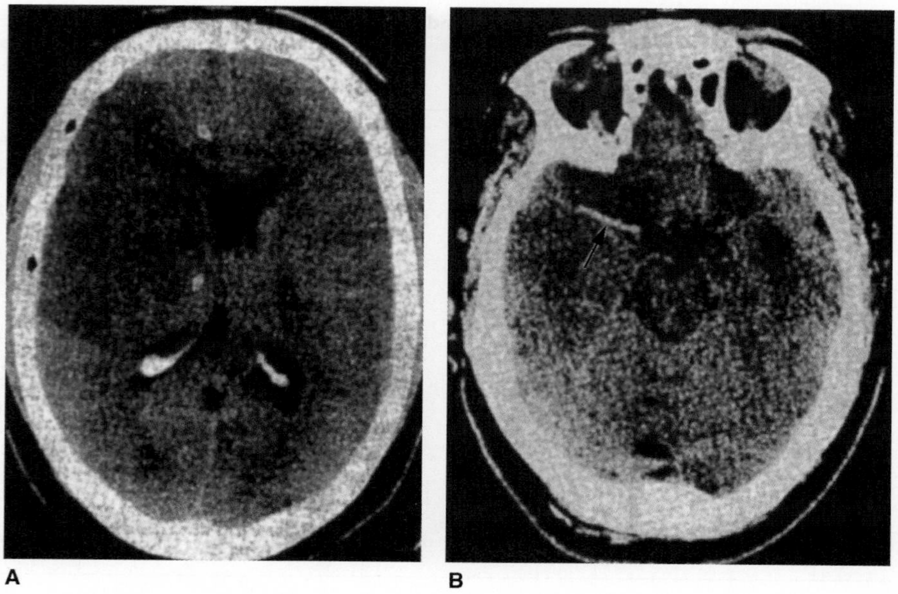

FIGURE 15.2. Noncontrast head CT demonstrating right middle cerebral artery distribution stroke. (A) Note the well-defined area of hypodensity (*arrows*) in the right middle cerebral artery (MCA) territory. (B) Acute thrombus in the right MCA (*arrow*). (Reproduced, with permission, from Chen MYM, Pope TL, Ott DJ. *Basic Radiology*. New York: McGraw-Hill, 2004:336-337.)

- BP < 185/110 mm Hg
- Meaningful neurologic deficit that is not resolving
- No finding on noncontrast CT head scan or clear ischemic penumbra on contrast perfusion images

- See Table 15.2 for summary of indications and contraindications to thrombolytics.
- Dose: 0.9 mg/kg with 10% given as bolus, remaining infused over 60 minutes.
- Time goals (from arrival time):
  - Evaluation by provider—10 minutes
  - Head CT—25 minutes
  - Interpretation of neuroimaging scan—45 minutes
- Drug delivery time—60 minutes.
- After tPA: BP and neuro checks q15 minutes × 2 hours. No antiplatelet agents for 24 hours.
- The National Institute of Neurological Disorders and Stroke (NINDS) trial showed improved outcomes at 3 months despite ↑ risk of symptomatic hemorrhage. The European Cooperative Acute Stroke Study III (ECASS III) trial provided some evidence to expand the treatment window to 4.5 hours (modest improvement in 3-month outcome although no difference in mortality, additional exclusion criteria and increased risk of intracranial bleeding).

- Complications of Systemic tPA
  - Symptomatic intracranial hemorrhage (SICH): Usually occurs within 36 hours in 6%-8% who get tPA.
    - Risk factors include older age, high National Institutes of Health (NIH) stroke scale score (> 20), radiographic evidence of stroke on CT (hypodensity or cerebral edema).
    - Signs of SICH: Acute neurologic decline, decrease in level of consciousness, sudden headache, nausea/vomiting, or sudden increase in blood pressure.

TABLE 15.4. Criteria for Intravenous Thrombolysis in Ischemic Stroke

Inclusion	Exclusion[a]
Age 18 y or older (no upper limit)	Minor stroke symptoms
Clinical diagnosis of ischemic stroke	Rapidly improving neurologic signs
Time since onset *well established* to be less than 4.5 h	Prior intracranial hemorrhage
	Blood glucose < 50 mg/dL or > 400 mg/dL
	Seizure at onset of stroke
	GI or GU bleeding within preceding 21 d
	Recent myocardial infarction
	Major surgery within preceding 14 d
	Sustained SBP > 185 mm Hg or DBP > 100 mm Hg despite initial attempt treatment
	Previous stroke within past 90 d
	Previous head injury within preceding 90 d
	Current use of oral anticoagulants or PT > 15 s or INR > 1.7
	Use of heparin within preceding 48 h and a prolonged PTT
	Platelet count < 100,000/μL

(Reproduced, with permission, from Tintinalli JE, Kelen GD, Stapczynski JS. *Emergency Medicine: A Comprehensive Study Guide,* 6th ed. New York: McGraw-Hill, 2004:1386 based on data from Adams HP, Brott TG, Furlan AJ, et al. Guidelines for thrombolytic therapy for acute stroke: A supplement to the guidelines for the management of patients with acute ischemic stroke. *Circulation* 94:1167, 1996.)

DBP, diastolic blood pressure; GI, gastrointestinal; GU, genitourinary; INR, international normalized ratio; PT, prothrombin time; PTT, partial prothrombin time; SBP, systolic blood pressure.

[a]Caution is advised before giving tPA to persons with severe stroke (NIH Stroke Scale Score > 22) or in patients with multilobar infarct on CT.

- Treatment: Immediately stop tPA infusion and obtain nocontast CT head. If SICH is confirmed, administration of agents to reverse the effects of thrombolytic and antiplatelet therapy should be considered, including fresh frozen plasma (FFP), platelets, and cryoprecipitate. No evidence-based guidelines exist for tPA reversal.

- Intra-arterial tPA
  - Some data supported for use in delayed time periods (> 3 hours). Typically, these are patients with significant occlusion of a large vessel (MCA) presenting between 3 and 6 hours. Also consider use for vertebral or basilar artery occlusions or where contraindications to intravenous thrombolytics exist.
- Antithrombotic therapy:
- **Aspirin:** 160-325 mg within 48 hours (unless thrombolysis candidate) for secondary stroke prevention. Clopidogrel or ticlopidine if aspirin allergic.
- **Aspirin and dipyridamole (Aggrenox):** A combination of two antiplatelet agents; greater risk reduction for secondary stroke prevention than aspirin alone for Asian patients with high-risk TIA (ie, ABCD^2 score ≥ 4) or minor stroke (ie, NIHSS score ≤ 3).
  - Early neurosurgical consultation for all cerebellar strokes (increased risk of herniation). Mortality is increased when obstructing hydrocephalus present.
- **Avoid:**
  - Routine seizure prophylaxis
  - Heparin: No proven benefit in acute stroke (even embolic)
  - Sublingual calcium channel blockers (unpredictable drops in BP)

KEY FACT

Consider intra-arterial thrombolysis in patients with brainstem strokes (even in delayed presentations).

KEY FACT

Heparin has no proven benefit in acute stroke.

Transient Ischemic Attack

Transient ischemic attack (TIA) is now defined as a transient episode of neurologic dysfunction caused by focal brain, spinal cord, or retinal ischemia, without acute infarction. The end point is biologic (tissue injury) rather than time based (eg, 24 hours). TIA was originally defined as a sudden onset of a focal neurologic symptom and/or sign lasting < 24 hours, caused by a transient decrease in blood supply. This prior definition of TIA is inadequate because even relatively brief ischemia can cause permanent brain injury. About 20% of clinical TIAs reveal an infarct on MRI.

Symptoms/Examination

Related to vascular distribution involved (please refer to Table 15.3)

Diagnosis

- Clinical diagnosis with neuroimaging.
- Evaluation for underlying etiology includes: ECG, carotid ultrasound, echocardiogram (in selected patients).

Treatment

- Antiplatelet agent (aspirin is first line, clopidogrel is second line, or ticlopidine is third line) is primary therapy. Combination therapy (ASA + dipyridamole) is indicated if TIA is recurrent after aspirin treatment.
- Goal is prevention of stroke, based on suspected underlying process (eg, anticoagulation if mural thrombus or history of paroxysmal atrial fibrillation).
- The **ABCD² score** can be used to predict likelihood of subsequent stroke within 2 days (Table 15.5).
- Higher ABCD² scores have been shown to correlate with increased risk of subsequent stroke, but evidence-based guidelines to determine who requires hospital admission have not been firmly established. In general, admit patient for inpatient evaluation if symptoms last > 1 hour or are concerning for crescendo TIAs. Also consider admission if patient has known internal carotid stenosis > 50%, history of atrial fibrillation, known hypercoagulable state, or if patient with ABCD² score of 0 to 2 is not able to have an outpatient work-up performed within 2 days.

MNEMONIC

ABCD² Score:

Age
Blood pressure
Clinical features
Duration
Diabetes

TABLE 15.5. ABCD² Score to Predict Subsequent Stroke in Patients with TIA

Variable	Points
Age > 60 y	1
BP ≥ 140/90 mm Hg	1
Unilateral weakness	2
Speech disturbance without weakness	1
Duration ≥ 60 min	2
Duration 10-59 min	1
Diabetes	1

Risk for subsequent stroke:
Low: 0-3 points
Moderate: 4-5 points
High: 6-7 points

BP, blood pressure; TIA, transient ischemic attack.

HEMORRHAGIC STROKE

Can be divided into intracerebral hemorrhage and subarachnoid hemorrhage.

Intracerebral Hemorrhage

Causes

Intracerebral hemorrhage (ICH) is an acute bleeding into the brain parenchyma as a result of:

- Chronic hypertension (most common)
- Cerebral amyloid angiopathy: Not associated with systemic amyloidosis
- Cocaine or methamphetamine use
- Vascular malformation
- Anticoagulation or thrombolysis

Symptoms/Examination

- Characterized by sudden onset and rapid progression of neurologic symptoms (Table 15.6)
- Headache
- Nausea, vomiting
- Patients usually present hypertensive

Differential

Hypoglycemia, Todd paralysis, complicated migraine, mass lesion, delirium

KEY FACT

The most common location for hemorrhagic stroke is the putamen, which is the outermost portion of the basal ganglia in 35%, subcortex in 30%, cerebellum in 15%, thalamus in 15%, and the pons 5%.

TABLE 15.6. Hemorrhagic Stroke—Neurologic Findings

Location	Neurologic Finding
Putamen (most common)	Contralateral hemiparesis/hemiplegia Contralateral sensory deficits Contralateral conjugate gaze paresis Homonymous hemianopsia Aphasia, neglect, apraxia Usually more lethargic than middle cerebral infarcts
Cerebellar	Severe ataxia, vertigo, nystagmus Dysarthria Decreased LOC (may occur) Ipsilateral gaze palsy, facial weakness and sensory loss NO hemiparesis
Thalamic	Contralateral hemiparesis/hemiplegia Contralateral sensory deficits Sensory loss > motor loss May cause isolated sensory symptoms
Pontine	Severe headache Pinpoint pupils Absence of oculovestibular reflexes Decerebrate posturing

LOC, level of consciousness.

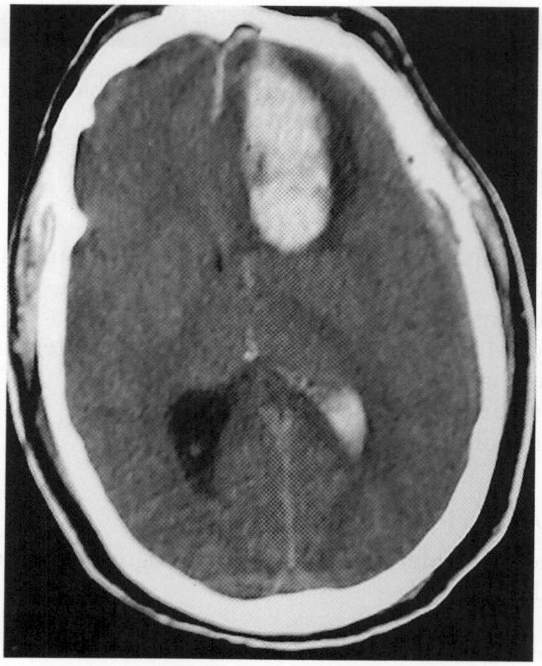

FIGURE 15.3. Noncontrast head CT demonstrating a large frontal intracerebral hemorrhage. (Reproduced, with permission, from Stone CK, Humphries, RL. *Current Emergency Diagnosis and Treatment.* 5th ed. New York: McGraw-Hill, 2004:374.)

Diagnosis

- Suspect based on history and examination.
- Confirm by noncontrast CT scan (Figure 15.3). Consider MRI if concern for underlying mass lesion.

Treatment

- Supportive therapy.
- Reverse coagulopathy (FFP, vitamin K, protamine sulfate, prothrombin complex concentrate, as appropriate).
- Elevated head of bed to 30°.
- Hyperventilation (to $Paco_2$ of 30), mannitol, and furosemide if impending herniation.
- Consider hypertonic (3%) saline for reduction of ICP.
- Seizures.
  - If seizure occurs, treat with antiepileptic drugs
- **Prophylactic** antiepileptic drugs should not be routinely administered.
- Hypertension.
  - If SBP > 200 mm Hg or MAP 150 mm Hg, consider aggressive reduction of BP.
  - If no clinical signs of ↑ ICP, aim for target BP of 160/90 mm Hg.
  - If clinical signs of ↑ ICP exist, consider ICP monitoring and maintain CPP = 60-80 mm Hg.
  - Use titratable agent—labetalol, esmolol, nicardipine, or nitroprusside.
- Neurosurgery consult
  - Especially for cerebellar hemorrhage, which is associated with rapid deterioration and herniation and is amenable to suboccipital craniotomy.

KEY FACT

The "Bs" of increased ICP: Bradycardia, blood pressure increasing, bradypnea.

Mannitol dose for increased ICP: 0.25-2 g/kg IV of 15%-25% solution over 30-60 minutes.

Seizures

CAUSES

Seizures result from excessive and disordered neuronal firing. There may be a primary disorder or secondary to an underlying medical condition (Table 15.7).

Seizures are classified based on behavioral, electrophysiologic, and clinical features of the seizure rather than on anatomic or pathophysiologic features. They can generally be broken down into partial and generalized seizures.

PARTIAL (FOCAL) SEIZURES

Partial seizures begin in localized area of the brain.

SYMPTOMS/EXAMINATION

- Simple partial
  - Brief event without alteration of consciousness
  - May manifest as isolated motor, sensory, autonomic, or psychic/ecstatic symptoms

TABLE 15.7. Secondary Causes of Seizures

Metabolic derangement
Hypoglycemia
Hyponatremia
Hypocalcemia
Drugs and toxins
Anticholinergics/cholinergics
Antidepressants
Mushrooms (*Gyromitra* sp.)
Sympathomimetics
Toxic alcohols
Isoniazid
Withdrawal syndromes
CNS infection: encephalitis or meningitis
CNS lesion or event
Neurocysticercosis
Hemorrhage
Tumors
Stroke
Vasculitis
Hydrocephalus
Febrile seizure (pediatrics)
Trauma
Eclampsia

KEY FACT

Consciousness remains normal with simple partial seizures. Consciousness is **impaired** with complex partial seizures. Consciousness is lost with generalized seizures.

    - If involving motor neurons → unilateral focal clonic movements. Medial temporal lobe focus → olfactory/gustatory hallucinations. Occipital focus → visual symptoms
- Complex partial (temporal lobe or psychomotor)
    - Partial seizure with **impairment** of consciousness and postictal state
    - Commonly manifests as mental and psychological symptoms, including changes in affect, confusion, hallucinations, automatisms (eg, lip smacking)
- **Secondary generalized:** Partial seizure that spreads to both hemispheres (eg, generalized seizure preceded by aura or unilateral motor symptoms)

GENERALIZED SEIZURES

Primary generalized seizures begin in both hemispheres and do not have an inciting focus. All except myoclonic have altered level of consciousness (LOC). Precipitating factors include missed medications, substance abuse or withdrawal, sleep deprivation, infection, and electrolyte disturbances.

Symptoms/Examination

KEY FACT

Nonconvulsive (absence) seizures typically develop in childhood.

- Nonconvulsive (absence or petit mal)
    - Alteration in mental status without motor activity
    - Most frequent in 5- to 10-year-olds
    - Rarely postictal
    - Characterized by brief 3-Hz, spike-and-wave discharges on electroencephalography (EEG)
- Convulsive (grand mal)
    - Abrupt loss of consciousness at onset (except with myoclonic)
    - Can be clonic, tonic, tonic-clonic, myoclonic, or atonic
    - Followed by postictal state
- **Todd paralysis:** Focal paralysis, typically following a generalized seizure; usually lasts 1-2 hours but may last 1-2 days

Differential

Primary considerations include syncope, dysrhythmia, psychiatric illness, decerebrate posturing, migraines, eclampsia, initial symptoms of stroke especially embolic, or subarachnoid hemorrhage.

Diagnosis

- EEG during event confirms diagnosis (if diagnosis is in question).
- Emergency department (ED) evaluation may be limited (known seizure disorder) or extensive (seizure in febrile immunocompromised patient).
- First-time seizure:
    - Check serum sodium and glucose. Consider testing of calcium and magnesium.
    - Check urine toxicology and urine pregnancy.
    - CT scan if **any** suspicion for serious structural lesion.
    - LP if **any** suspicion for meningitis, subarachnoid hemorrhage. Or if the patient has a history of a cancer that spreads to the meninges.
    - In patients with human immunodeficiency virus (HIV), consider CT head with IV contrast or MRI if no other explanation is found.
- Recurrent seizure:
    - Check glucose and anticonvulsant levels (if available).
        - Supratherapeutic levels of phenytoin and carbamazepine can result in seizures.
    - More extensive evaluation is necessary if there is a change in seizure pattern, prolonged postictal state, fever, etc.
    - Status epilepticus (see "Status Epilepticus").

KEY FACT

Serum lactate may be elevated immediately following a generalized tonic-clonic seizure, but should clear spontaneously within 1 hour.

TREATMENT

- Roll patient on side to decrease aspiration risk.
- Establish a patent airway, suction if necessary.
- Anticonvulsants not necessary for uncomplicated seizure < 5 minutes.
- First-time seizure:
  - Treat underlying cause, if identified.
  - If central nervous system (CNS) lesion is present, initiate anticonvulsant therapy.
  - Otherwise recommend outpatient follow-up for MRI and EEG if no cause found. In general, defer initiation of antiepileptics to outpatient neurology setting. Provide instructions to patient: No driving, swimming, or other high-risk activities.
  - Chronic recurrent seizures: Consider medication adjustment if there is noted change in pattern or frequency of seizures.
  - Alcohol withdrawal seizure: Treat with benzodiazepines; patients do not require chronic anticonvulsant therapy.
- Ongoing seizures (see "Status Epilepticus").

STATUS EPILEPTICUS

Seizure defined as lasting > 30 minutes or recurrent seizures without resolution of postictal state; may be generalized seizures (life-threatening, high mortality), absence seizures, or complex partial seizures. Because of clinical urgency in treating status epilepticus, a 30-minute definition is neither practical nor appropriate in practice. An accepted operational definition of status epilepticus is ≥ 5 minutes. or ≥ 2 discrete seizures without a complete recovery in between the events.

> **KEY FACT**
>
> The blood prolactin level may be elevated for 15-60 minutes following generalized seizure.

DIAGNOSIS

- EEG is confirmative (if diagnosis is in question)
- Check glucose immediately
- Check electrolytes, magnesium, toxicology screen, liver and renal function, pregnancy test (as indicated)
- Obtain head CT
- Consider lumbar puncture

TREATMENT

- Thiamine and glucose if hypoglycemic or if alcoholism suspected.
- First-line therapy = benzodiazepines—diazepam, lorazepam, or midazolam.
  - Lorazepam has a relatively longer duration of seizure suppression.
  - If no IV access, several medications can be considered: Valium (rectal), Versed (IM, intranasal, buccal), or Fosphenytoin (IM).
- Second-line therapy.
  - Phenytoin or fosphenytoin: Rapid administration of phenytoin may cause hypotension and cardiac dysrhythmias due to its propylene glycol diluent; this may be avoided with fosphenytoin (water soluble prodrug). Onset of action is 10-30 minutes.
  - Phenobarbital: Anticipate sedation, respiratory depression, and hypotension. Onset of action is 15-30 minutes. Rarely used in present day practice.
  - Valproic acid: Rates up to 5 mg/kg/min can be administered without adverse effects on blood pressure or heart rate without significant sedation.
  - Levetiracetam, lacosamide, and topiramate have also been used effectively.
- Pregnancy: Magnesium sulfate, if eclamptic. Many antiepileptics are teratogenic, but risk of seizures to fetus is often worse than side effects of medications. Carefully consider medications in consultation with neurology and obstetrics.

- Pyridoxine (vitamin B_6) if isoniazid overdose or gyromitrin toxin (mushroom) suspected.
- Drug-induced coma (pentobarbital, midazolam, propofol) or general anesthesia, if resistant to above. Continuous EEG should be instituted to monitor for the persistence or recurrence of seizures, depth of coma, burst suppression.

CNS Infections

MENINGITIS

Meningitis is bacterial, viral, fungal, or aseptic inflammation of the membranes covering the brain or spinal cord.

CAUSES

The causes of meningitis in adult patients include:

- Bacterial
  - *Streptococcus pneumoniae* (most common overall, gram-positive diplococci)
  - *Neisseria meningitides* (younger ages, gram-negative rod)
  - *Listeria monocytogenes* (adults > 60 years, gram-positive rod)
  - *Haemophilus influenzae* type B; disappearing with the HIB-vaccine
  - *Mycobacterium tuberculosis* (uncommon)
  - Group B *Streptococcus, Escherichia coli,* and *L monocytogenes* are the most common bacterial causes in neonates < 1 month
  - *S pneumoniae, Staphylococcus aureus, Pseudomonas aeruginosa,* and coliform bacteria are common following neurosurgical procedure or head trauma
- Viral
  - Enteroviruses (most common, increased in summer months)
  - Herpes simplex virus should always be suspected
  - Numerous other viruses
- Fungal (eg, *Cryptococcus*) and parasitic (eg, *Toxoplasma gondii*)—in the immunocompromised
- Noninfectious
  - Systemic lupus erythematosus (SLE)
  - Vasculitis
  - Drug induced
  - Carcinomatosis
  - Sarcoidosis
  - Behçet disease

A significant overlap exists between bacterial and viral meningitis presentations. Viral meningitis is a diagnosis that can be made only after other more serious pathogens have been excluded.

PATHOPHYSIOLOGY

- Bacterial infection usually begins with nasopharyngeal colonization → hematogenous spread (more likely with encapsulated organisms) → CNS infection.
- Viruses enter through the skin or via respiratory, gastrointestinal (GI), or genitourinary (GU) tracts.
- Fungi primarily spread from pulmonary source.

- Meningeal inflammatory response to foreign agent resulting in:
  - Increased permeability of blood–brain barrier → increased cerebrospinal fluid (CSF) proteins
  - Decreased glucose transport → decreased CSF glucose levels

SYMPTOMS

- Fever.
- Headache (most common).
- Stiff neck (seen half the time).
- Photophobia.
- Mental status changes or irritability (infants).
- Vomiting.
- Seizures.
- Initially, symptoms may be diminished/absent in immunocompromised, very young, or elderly patients.
- Absence of fever/altered mental status/stiff neck does not exclude meningitis.

EXAMINATION

- Fever.
- Nuchal rigidity.
- Increased deep tendon reflexes (DTRs).
- Altered mental status.
- Lateral gaze ophthalmoplegia.
- Petechial or purpuric rash (ominous sign).
- **Kernig sign**: Position the patient with hips and knees flexed. Extend the knees. Flexion of neck or pain in neck is positive sign.
- **Brudzinski sign**: Neck flexion results in flexion at hips (neck sign) **or** passive flexion of hip on one side results in contralateral hip flexion (contralateral sign).
- The classic signs of Kernig and Brudzinski signs are not sensitive for meningitis.
- Look for concomitant infection, such as sinusitis, otitis, pneumonia.

KEY FACT

Kernig's = Knee

DIFFERENTIAL

The differential diagnosis includes encephalitis, brain abscess, subdural, subarachnoid hemorrhage, intracranial hemorrhage, brain tumor.

DIAGNOSIS

- Meningitis should be considered in all patients presenting with a headache or stiff neck and fever.
- Head CT:
  - Recommended before LP in patients > 60 years old, the immunocompromised (eg, HIV), history of CNS disease (including stroke, mass lesions, or recent head trauma), new onset seizures within 1 week, the presence of marked CNS depression, papilledema, or focal neurologic deficits.
- Lumbar puncture (LP):
  - Contraindications:
    - Coagulopathy (relative): The international normalized ratio (INR) > 1.5. Platelets < 50 K (< 20 K absolute)
    - Infection at skin puncture site (absolute)
    - ↑ ICP or trauma to lumbar vertebrae
  - CSF findings classically vary with viral, bacterial, and fungal etiologies (Table 15.8).
    - **but**—early or partially treated bacterial infections due to recent antibiotic use may have a paucity of findings!
    - **and**—early viral infections may have increased neutrophils or ↓ glucose!

Q

A 23-year-old military recruit is brought in by ambulance with mental status changes. Naloxone was given without effect. On arrival he is noted to be minimally responsive to painful stimuli and hypotensive. D-stick is normal. While the patient is being intubated, the skin is noted to be warm and covered with a petechial rash. What is the most appropriate next step?

TABLE 15.8. Analysis of Cerebrospinal Fluid

	Normal Levels	Bacterial	Viral	Fungal
Opening pressure (cm H_2O)	5-20	Elevated	Normal or slightly elevated	Elevated
Leukocytes/mm³	≤ 5	≥ 500, although may be mildly elevated early	100-500, although may be mildly elevated early	10-500
% Neutrophils	0 (≤ 1 PMN)	> 80%	< 50%	< 50%
Protein (mg/dL)	20-45	> 200	< 200	> 200
Glucose (mg/dL)	50-80% or 60-70% of serum level	≤ 40% or < 50% of serum	Usually normal	< 50
Cultures or studies		Gram stain, culture, PCR, bacterial antigen assays	HSV or enterovirus PCR	Cryptococcal antigen, yeast

PCR, polymerase chain reaction; PMN, polymorphonuclear.

KEY FACT

Fungal meningitis is difficult to diagnose: Low-grade fevers, variable headache, possible weight loss, lassitude; CSF with very elevated protein.

KEY FACT

Do not delay antibiotics for CT or LP.

A

This patient likely has meningococcal meningitis and needs immediate antibiotic therapy with cefotaxime or ceftriaxone IV. Until the diagnosis is confirmed, vancomycin should also be given to cover resistant strains of *S pneumoniae*. Depending on season and region, doxycycline should also be given for Rocky Mountain spotted fever (RMSF). Listeria should also be considered in older adults, pregnant women, and those with cellular immunodeficiency and ampicillin should be given.

- CSF cultures may help isolate causative organism.
- Gram stain results:
  - Gram-positive diplococci suggest pneumococcal infection.
  - Gram-negative diplococci suggest meningococcal infection
  - Small pleomorphic gram-negative coccobacilli suggest *H influenzae* infection
  - Gram-positive rods and coccobacilli suggest listerial infection

Treatment

- Stabilization and supportive therapy, as needed.
- **Immediate** empiric antibiotic:
  - Vancomycin, 1 g IV,
  - Ceftriaxone or cefotaxime, 2 g IV, and
  - **Ampicillin** if neonate, > 60 years, debilitated, alcoholic or
  - **Metronidazole** if concern for extension from sinusitis or otitis.
  - Will not decrease ability to detect organism in CSF fluid if LP performed within 2 hours and antigen assays are utilized.
  - If high clinical suspicion for bacterial meningitis, admit regardless of LP results.
- Dexamethasone:
  - Appears to decrease morbidity and mortality in adults with **bacterial** meningitis (especially *S pneumoniae*) and children with *H influenzae* meningitis.
  - Give 0.15 mg/kg IV 15 minutes before or concurrent with the first dose of antibiotics, repeat every 4-6 hours (max 10 mg in adults).
- Other antibiotics are indicated if fungal infection is suspected or identified.
- Viral meningitis (diagnosis of exclusion) requires no specific treatment. If herpes simplex meningitis is suspected, empiric therapy with acyclovir can be administered.

Complications

- Sepsis
- Disseminated intravascular coagulation (DIC)

- Seizures
- Focal neurologic deficits
- Hearing loss
- Cognitive deficits
- Waterhouse-Friderichsen syndrome (adrenal hemorrhage)
- SIADH/cerebral salt wasting
- Transmission of *Neisseria meningitidis* or *H influenzae* type B
  - Seen in household contacts, day care centers, schools, barracks, and mucous membrane contacts.
  - Chemoprophylaxis with rifampin (4 doses 10 mg/kg q12h) is recommended once bacterial organism is identified. Alternatively, ciprofloxacin can be used (500 mg PO single dose).

KEY FACT

Family members and close contacts of patients with *N meningitidis* or *H influenzae* meningitis should receive antibiotic prophylaxis.

ENCEPHALITIS

Encephalitis is an infection of the brain parenchyma itself, often due to a progression of viral meningitis. Consider encephalitis in any patient with concern for meningitis coupled with the presence of altered mental status.

Causes

- Viruses cause the majority of cases (* = most common).
  - *Arboviruses
  - Mosquito and tick-borne viruses
  - Include West Nile virus, St. Louis encephalitis
  - *Herpes simplex virus (usually HSV 1)
  - Other herpes viruses (Epstein–Barr virus [EBV], cytomegalovirus [CMV])
  - Rabies virus
- Paraneoplastic and autoimmune syndromes.
- *T gondii* (immunocompromised).
- Lyme disease, Rocky Mountain spotted fever (RMSF).

Symptoms/Examination

- Often begins with nonspecific acute febrile illness.
- Headache and fever (common).
- Neurologic abnormalities:
  - Altered mental state
  - New psychiatric symptoms
  - Emotional outbursts
  - Cognitive deficits
  - Focal neurologic deficits
  - Seizures
  - Movement disorders
- Sensorimotor deficits are uncommon.

KEY FACT

HSV 1 has a predilection for the temporal lobes. Patients often present with "psychiatric symptoms" or behavioral changes.

Herpes simplex virus 1 encephalitis can also typically present with stroke-like symptoms or seizures.

Diagnosis

- Suspect diagnosis based on presenting symptoms and examination.
- Lumbar puncture
  - To exclude bacterial meningitis and help identify viral organism via polymerase chain reaction (PCR). While it is possible to have encephalitis without meningitis, it is very rare.
- MRI with contrast.
  - Can readily identify areas of involvement (focal edema).
  - Lesions in the temporal lobes = HSV encephalitis.
- CT with contrast is alternative but is less sensitive.
- EEG
  - Suggestive EEG abnormalities may be seen.
- **Brain biopsy:** Definitive.

TREATMENT

- Empiric treatment for suspected etiologic organisms
  - Acyclovir (10 mg/kg IV q8h) for HSV and herpes zoster virus.
  - Ganciclovir for cytomegalovirus.
  - Once herpes and cytomegalovirus infections have been excluded, there is no benefit from antiviral agents.

BRAIN ABSCESS

Brain abscess is an infection that becomes localized to a particular region of the brain: Intraparenchymal, epidural, or subdural locations.

MECHANISMS

Infection reaches the brain via three mechanisms:

- Contiguous infection of middle ear, sinus, or teeth
- Neurosurgery or penetrating trauma
- Hematogenous spread

Common organisms include:

- Often polymicrobial
- Streptococci
- Anaerobic bacteria (esp. *Bacteroides*)
- *Staphylococus aureus*
- Fungal and parasitic infections in the immunocompromised

SYMPTOMS/EXAMINATION

- Often mild course that progresses slowly over weeks. Patients rarely appear acutely ill.
- The vast majority of patients complain of headache.
- Classic triad of headache, fever, neurologic deficit present in less than one-third of patients.
- Focal neurologic deficits **may occur**.
- Papilledema is not uncommon.

DIAGNOSIS

- CT or MRI with contrast
  - Cannot exclude abscess with noncontrast studies or LP
  - Classic finding = ring-enhancing lesion(s)

TREATMENT

- Supportive therapy
- Treat associated seizures
- Empiric antibiotic therapy
  - Depends on suspected source (oral vs sinus or otogenic vs hematogenous spread)
  - No obvious source: Vancomycin + ceftriaxone or cefotaxime + metronidazole
- Surgical vs medical therapy
  - Surgery for large abscesses

KEY FACT

Neurocysticercosis (CNS *T solium* larvae infection) is the most common cause of secondary seizures in the developing world.

NEUROCYSTICERCOSIS

CNS infection with the larval form of the tapeworm *Taenia solium*; very common in developing countries and the most common cause of 2° epilepsy in developing world. Humans become infected by eating undercooked pork.

MECHANISMS

Forms of disease:

- Invasion of brain parenchyma (most common) → formation of cysts → inflammation and fibrosis
- Cysticerci in ventricles → obstructing hydrocephalus
- Cysticerci in basilar cisterns → arachnoiditis → meningitis or communicating hydrocephalus

SYMPTOMS/EXAMINATION

- Seizure is the most common clinical finding.
- Headache or signs of increased intracranial pressure are seen, if hydrocephalus develops.

DIAGNOSIS/TREATMENT

- Based on exposure history, CT or MRI findings, and serologic testing.
- Treatment depends on clinical manifestations (eg, antiseizure medications, shunting procedure if obstructing hydrocephalus present).
- Antiparasitic agents (praziquantel and albendazole).

SHUNT INFECTION

The majority of shunt infections present within 6 months of placement (50% within 2 weeks).

- Common infecting organisms:
  - *Staphylococcus epidermidis* (50%)
  - *S aureus*
- Other organisms include gram-negatives and anaerobes.

SYMPTOMS/EXAMINATION

- Shunt obstruction (most common): Headache, nausea/vomiting, altered mentation.
- Other findings may include fever, meningismus, and tenderness, erythema, or warmth along shunt tubing. Abdominal pain may be a symptom if ventriculoperitoneal (VP) shunt has distal obstruction or pseudocyst.

DIAGNOSIS/TREATMENT

- Shunt tap is required to exclude diagnosis as an LP may miss the CNS infection. CSF findings include ↑ leukocytes and protein, normal glucose.
- Consider abdominal CT if pseudocyst or abscess suspected.
- Immediate neurosurgical consultation and initiation of antibiotic therapy (vancomycin + third-generation cephalosporin and aminoglycoside).

Headache

Intracranially, only the arteries at the base of the brain, their main branches, the periarterial dura mater, and the venous sinuses are pain sensitive. These pain-sensitive intracranial structures are supplied by sensory axons of the trigeminal ganglion (supratentorial structures) and by the upper cervical roots (posterior fossa structures).

Headaches are classified as **primary** (vast majority of headaches) and **secondary** (Table 15.9). Secondary headaches are considered "secondary" to some underlying cause (eg, subarachnoid hemorrhage).

Q

A 54-year-old woman presents complaining of a severe headache. The headache was sudden in onset while she was moving boxes of books at work. The patient has neck stiffness and nausea but denies weakness or numbness in arms or legs. Her vital signs and neurologic examination are normal. Head CT confirms your suspicion for subarachnoid hemorrhage (SAH). What is her likely prognosis? What pharmacologic agent has been shown to prevent secondary ischemic stroke in patients with SAH?

KEY FACT

Lumbar puncture is not useful in diagnosing a shunt infection. A shunt tap is required.

A

Based on the Hunt and Hess classification, this patient has a Grade I hemorrhage and should have a good neurologic outcome. Nimodipine is used to prevent vasospasm-induced ischemic stroke. Additional treatment is aimed at preventing symptoms that might lead to further bleeding (eg, antiemetics, seizure prophylaxis).

TABLE 15.9. Etiologies of Headache

Critical Secondary Causes	Reversible Secondary Causes	Primary Headache Syndromes
Vascular	Non-CNS infections	Migraine
Subarachnoid hemorrhage	Focal	Tension
Intraparenchymal hemorrhage	Systemic	Cluster
Epidural hematoma	Sinusitis	
Subdural hematoma	Odontogenic	
Stroke	Otic	
Cavernous sinus thrombosis	Drug-related	
Arteriovenous malformation	Chronic analgesic use	
Temporal arteritis	Monosodium glutamate	
Carotid or vertebral artery dissection	Miscellaneous	
CNS infection	Post lumbar puncture	
Meningitis	Coital migraine (SAH mimic)	
Encephalitis	Reversible Cerebral	
Cerebral abscess	Vasoconstriction Syndrome	
Tumor	(cause of multiple	
Pseudotumor cerebri	thunderclap headaches)	
Ophthalmic		
Glaucoma		
Iritis		
Optic neuritis		
Drug-related		
Nitrates and nitrites		
Monoamine oxidase inhibitors		
Alcohol withdrawal		
Toxic		
Carbon monoxide poisoning		
Endocrine		
Pheochromocytoma		
Metabolic		
Hypoxia		
Hypoglycemia		
Hypercapnia		
High-altitude cerebral edema		
Preeclampsia		

(Reproduced, with permission, from Tintinalli JE, Kelen GD, Stapczynski JS. *Emergency Medicine: A Comprehensive Study Guide,* 6th ed. New York: McGraw-Hill, 2004:1376.)

SUBARACHNOID HEMORRHAGE

Subarachnoid hemorrhage is an acute bleed into the subarachnoid space. SAH can be further divided into traumatic and nontraumatic causes.

Causes

The majority of patients with nontraumatic SAH have a ruptured berry aneurysm. Other causes include mycotic aneurysms, arteriovenous malformations

(AVMs), and neoplasms. Around 2% population will have aneurysms found at autopsy.

Conditions associated with increased incidence of berry aneurysms:
- Family history of berry aneurysm
- Coarctation of aorta
- Polycystic kidney disease
- Marfan syndrome
- Ehlers-Danlos syndrome
- AVMs
- 20% patients with aneurysms have multiple aneurysms
- Risk factors for ruptured aneurysm: hypertension (2×), smoking (5×)

Symptoms

- Characterized by **sudden onset** of severe headache.
  - May be preceded by activities that increase ICP (intercourse, coughing, weight lifting)
  - Nausea/vomiting (in majority)
- Other possible symptoms include seizures, neck stiffness, preceding less severe headache ("sentinel bleed").
- Resolution of headache is not sufficient to exclude diagnosis of SAH.

KEY FACT

Mortality from SAH ↑ from 30% on first rupture to 70% on second rupture. Detection of sentinel bleed can be life saving.

Examination

- Depends on degree of hemorrhage and inflammatory response.
  - Nuchal rigidity, neurologic signs, subhyaloid retinal hemorrhage in some cases.
  - Around 50% have a completely normal examination.
- Hunt and Hess classification:
  - **Grades I and II** have good prognosis: Headache with nuchal rigidity ± third or sixth cranial nerve palsy; normal mental status.
  - Grade III is at risk for rapid deterioration (50% survival): Drowsiness, confusion, ± mild focal deficit.
  - **Grades IV and V** have poor prognosis: Stupor, hemiparesis, deep coma, decerebrate posturing.

Diagnosis

- Head CT without contrast (Figure 15.4)
  - Symptoms < 24 hours = sensitivity > 90%-95% (controversial, some sources cite 98% within 12 hours). Increasing evidence that the sensitivity of CT within the first 6 hours after a minor SAH approaches 100%.
  - Symptoms for 1 week = sensitivity < 50%.
  - Recent studies suggest that combination of CT/CTA approaches sensitivity of 99%. CTA only detects the presence of aneurysm, not rupture; LP is still indicated to determine if aneurysmal rupture occurred and is important for neurosurgical planning. However, this topic remains controversial.
- MRI/MRA (magnetic resonance angiogram): Equal to or less sensitive than CT for SAH
- LP if CT negative; positive CSF findings for SAH:
  - Grossly or persistently bloody.
  - Clearing of blood on successive collection tubes is an unreliable sign of a traumatic tap and an SAH is still possible.
  - Xanthochromia (via spectrophotometry, NOT naked eye) ≥ 12 hours after onset of headache = gold standard.

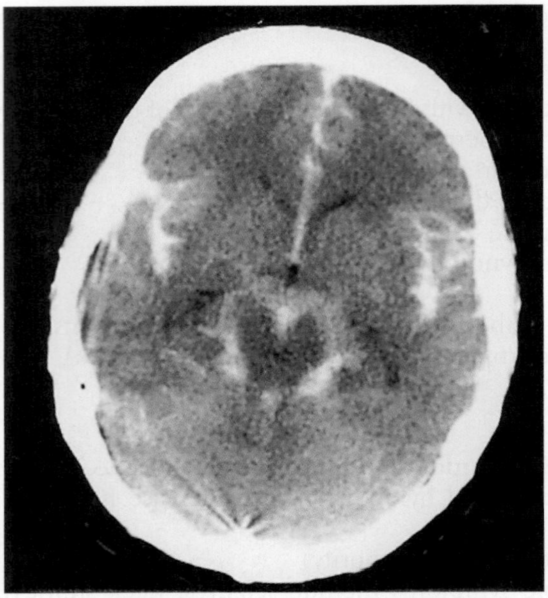

FIGURE 15.4. Noncontrast head CT demonstrating acute subarachnoid blood. (Reproduced, with permission, from Stone CK, Humphries, RL. *Current Emergency Diagnosis and Treatment.* 5th ed. New York: McGraw-Hill, 2004:372.)

TREATMENT

- Supportive therapy, prevent rebleeding (risk greatest in first 24 hours).
- Control BP (MAP < 130).
- **Nimodipine** has been shown to prevent vasospasm and ischemic stroke (initiate within 4 days of symptom onset). Administer PO rather than IV.
- Antiemetics to prevent nausea/vomiting.
- Prophylactic phenytoin or levetiracetam to prevent seizures.
- Sedation, as needed.
- Definitive therapy with endovascular coil embolization or surgical clipping.

MENINGITIS

See "CNS Infections."

CHRONIC SUBDURAL HEMATOMA

Blood clot between the dura and the brain with symptom onset > 2 weeks after trauma (some patients report minor or no injury); seen more commonly in patients with brain atrophy (elderly and alcoholics).

SYMPTOMS/EXAMINATION

- Headache
- Unilateral weakness (up to half)
- Altered consciousness, dementia

DIFFERENTIAL

Subdural hygroma: Collection of blood-tinged fluid in dural space of uncertain etiology; tends to follow trauma; on CT fluid density is same as CSF; surgical evaluation is needed, if symptomatic.

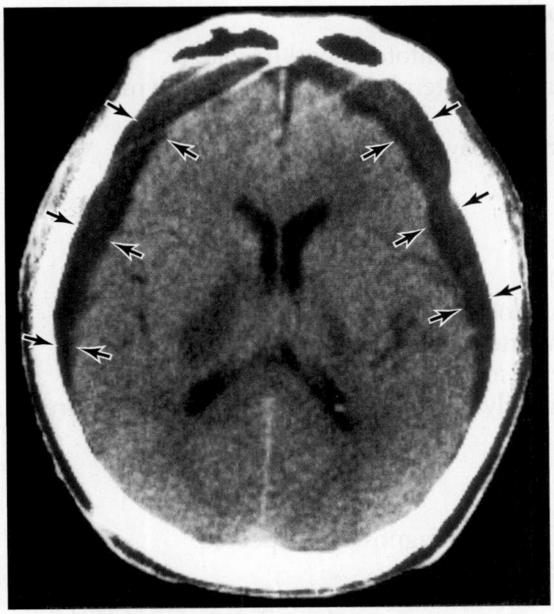

FIGURE 15.5. Noncontrast head CT demonstrating chronic subdural hematoma. (Reproduced, with permission, from Aminoff MJ, Greenberg DA, Simon RP. *Clinical Neurology*. 6th ed. New York: McGraw-Hill, 2005:61.)

DIAGNOSIS

- Noncontrast CT scan (Figure 15.5): Blood becomes isodense after about a week, then subsequently hypodense. Mass effect may also be seen.
- MRI scan: Will appear hyperdense.

TREATMENT

- Supportive therapy.
- Correct any coagulopathy, if present.
- Immediate neurosurgical consultation for surgical evacuation.

KEY FACT

Chronic subdurals appear isodense or hypodense on noncontrast CT.

BRAIN TUMOR

Headache is a common complaint in patients with brain tumor.

CAUSES

The most common cause is metastases from lung or breast carcinoma.

SYMPTOMS/EXAMINATION

- Worsening headache for weeks to months.
- May be worse upon awakening.
- The vast majority will have focal findings on detailed neurological examination.

DIAGNOSIS/TREATMENT

- CT or MRI to confirm presence of mass
- Urgent neurosurgical evaluation
- Dexamethasone if edema present on imaging or if severe symptoms

TEMPORAL ARTERITIS

Temporal arteritis is an arteritis of small- and medium-sized arteries that selectively involves arterial walls with significant amounts of elastin. The disease occurs predominantly in women and is rare in patients < 50 years old.

SYMPTOMS/EXAMINATION

- Severe, throbbing, frontotemporal headache.
- Jaw claudication, systemic symptoms, or polymyalgia rheumatica may be present.
- Temporal artery may be nonpulsatile or tender.

DIAGNOSIS

- 3 of 5 criteria:
  - Age > 50
  - New onset localized headache
  - Temporal artery tenderness or decreased pulse
  - Erythrocyte sedimentation rate > 50 mm/h
  - Refer urgently for temporal artery biopsy to confirm diagnosis if highly suspicious

TREATMENT

- Start immediately if diagnosis is suspected.
- Prednisone 40-80 mg/d.
- Nonsteroidal anti-inflammatory drugs (NSAIDs) for pain relief.

COMPLICATIONS

Severe complication → loss of vision due to ischemic optic neuritis

IDIOPATHIC INTRACRANIAL HYPERTENSION

Also known as *pseudotumor cerebri*. A disease primarily of young obese females.

Pathophysiology is uncertain, possibly due to an alteration of CSF absorption. It is also linked to oral contraceptives, vitamin A, chronic steroid use, tetracycline, and thyroid disorders.

KEY FACT

Temporal arteritis and idiopathic intracranial hypertension may both lead to loss of vision if left untreated.

SYMPTOMS/EXAMINATION

- Long-standing headache ± visual disturbances and nausea/vomiting.
- **Visual loss may occur**.
- Eye findings may include **papilledema, loss of *peripheral* vision, and CN VI palsy**.

DIAGNOSIS

- Based on finding of increased intracranial pressure (> 25 cm H_2O) with normal CSF evaluation.
- Head CT may show small ventricles and an enlarged cisterna magna.
- Consider magnetic resonance venography (MRV) for evaluation of cerebral venous thrombosis if new diagnosis of idiopathic intracranial hypertension is being made based on ↑ ICP.

TREATMENT

- Aimed at lowering intracranial pressure
  - **Acetazolamide** decreases the formation of CSF; furosemide can be used as an adjunctive.
- In the setting of acute visual loss, a short course of intravenous steroids or therapeutic lumbar punctures may be used as a temporizing measure until surgical intervention.
  - Repeated LPs or surgery (optic nerve sheath fenestration or shunt placement) for refractory cases.

INTERNAL CAROTID AND VERTEBRAL ARTERY DISSECTION

The most frequent cause of stroke in patients < 45 years, internal carotid and vertebral artery dissection may result from major head and neck trauma, but most occur spontaneously or after minor or trivial injury. Various connective tissue and vascular disorders have been associated with dissections. Diagnosis is challenging because early symptoms are often vague and nonspecific.

SYMPTOMS/EXAMINATION

Internal carotid dissection:

- Unilateral anterior neck pain or headache around the eye or frontal area, classically abrupt in onset.
- Findings include ipsilateral Horner syndrome, contralateral stroke, or TIA symptoms.

Vertebral artery dissection:

- Marked occipital or posterior neck pain with signs of brainstem TIA or stroke

DIAGNOSIS

- CTA and/or MRI/MRA to confirm diagnosis.
- Noncontrast CT is not diagnostic study of choice.

TREATMENT

- Surgical
- Anticoagulation: IV heparin → warfarin. Target INR 2-3
- Thrombolysis: IV alteplase for eligible patients with acute ischemic stroke

KEY FACT

Neck pain and neurologic symptoms? Consider internal carotid and vertebral artery dissection.

CEREBRAL VENOUS THROMBOSIS

This disorder is more common in neonates and children. Among young adults, it is more common in women. Thrombosis of cerebral veins or dural sinus may lead to cerebral edema, hemorrhage, and/or ischemia.

CAUSES

Include adjacent local infection (meningitis or ear, nose, and throat [ENT] infections), direct injury (eg, trauma) or hypercoagulable state (eg, pregnancy, Factor V Leiden, lupus anticoagulant, nephrotic syndrome, cancer).

SYMPTOMS/EXAMINATION

- Symptoms are varied and often vague.
- Headache is the most common presenting complaint. Consider this diagnosis in patients with new persistent headaches in the absence of a prior headache history. Frequently, the initial presentation is quite benign. Symptoms will steadily worsen over days to weeks.
- Altered mental status, focal neurologic deficits, papilledema, or seizures may occur.
- Consider diagnosis in patients with ↑ ICP for unclear reasons and consider in any patient with new diagnosis of idiopathic intracranial hypertension.

DIAGNOSIS

- CT and standard MRI scanning are useful only if positive (cannot exclude the diagnosis).
- **MRV combined with MRI** is imaging modality of choice and has replaced angiography.

- CT venography is a rapid, readily available, and accurate technique for detecting cerebral venous thrombosis; use may be limited because of low resolution of the deep venous system and cortical veins.

Treatment

- Heparin
- Catheter-based thrombolysis if severe symptoms

POST–LUMBAR PUNCTURE HEADACHE

Causes

A post-LP headache develops within 24-48 hours of LP due to persistent CSF leak from the LP puncture site. Occurs in 10%-30% of patients following LP. This same type of headache can develop as the result of a persistent dural leak anywhere along the neural axis. Frequently, no history of trauma can be elicited but often occurs postsurgically with any procedure where the dura is opened.

Symptoms/Diagnosis

Headache that is worse with upright posture and improved with lying flat.

Treatment

- Simple analgesics
- Intravenous fluids
- Prevention: Use small-bore needle with noncutting tip, angle needle parallel to longitudinal fibers of the dura and reinsert stylet prior to needle removal. Bed rest after LP and patient positioning have not been shown to reduce incidence
- **Caffeine IV**
- Blood patch (epidural injection of autologous blood) if no relief with above measures

> **KEY FACT**
>
> Caffeine IV can be very effective in treating post-LP headaches.

MIGRAINE

Pathophysiology

- Hypothesis is related to a slowly spreading wave of neuronal depolarization across the brain → ion dysfunction and vasoconstriction → prodrome and aura (seen in 20%).
- Trigeminovascular activation and release of peptides → inflammation of the pain-sensitive areas and vasodilation.

Many factors can directly or indirectly trigger this neurovascular activation:

- Menstruation, contraceptive estrogens, pregnancy
- Certain foods or drinks, such as chocolate, caffeine, hard cheese, alcoholic beverages (especially red wine), monosodium glutamate (MSG), nitrites
- Alterations in circadian rhythm

Symptoms

Migraine without aura ("common migraine"):

- Slow onset and lasts 4-72 hours
- Unilateral and pulsating
- Nausea, vomiting, and photo- or phonophobia

Migraine with aura ("classic migraine"):

- Headache follows aura within 60 minutes.
- Aura develops gradually over minutes, lasts < 1 hour and is fully reversible.
- Types of auras:
  - Visual is most common → scintillating scotomata or visual field deficit.
  - Motor → hemiparesis, ophthalmoplegia, aphasia.
  - Sensory → hemiparesthesia, dysesthesia.
  - Brainstem (basilar migraine) → vertigo, ataxia.
- Ophthalmoplegic migraine: Headache + CN 3, 4, 6 deficits.
- Retinal migraine: headache + sudden monocular blindness.

DIFFERENTIAL

Includes subarachnoid hemorrhage, giant cell arteritis, cerebrovascular disease, and other secondary headaches.

DIAGNOSIS

- Typically a clinical diagnosis.
- Further evaluation (CT/LP) to rule out a secondary cause is needed in patients with new onset migraine or symptoms different from their typical migraine.

TREATMENT

- Goal is to abort or decrease the neurovascular effects.
- **Triptans** (eg, sumatriptan): Selective 5-HT (serotonin) agonists.
  - Cause vasoconstriction and blocks peptide release = ↓ inflammation and pain.
  - Should not be used in patients with hypertension or other cardiovascular disease.
  - Do not use within 24 hours of other ergotamine-containing medication
- **Dihydroergotamine (DHE):** Nonselective 5-HT agonist.
  - Again contraindicated in patients with cardiovascular disease or within 24 hours of triptan use.
  - Nausea and vomiting are common side effects.
- **Antiemetics** (eg, prochlorperazine, metoclopramide).
- **NSAIDs** (eg, indomethacin, ibuprofen, ketorolac).
- Steroids: Decreases migraine recurrence.
- Opiates should be used as last resort.
- Prophylactic therapy may be indicated in patients with frequent migraines: β-Blockers, Ca^{++} channel blockers, tricyclic antidepressants.

> **KEY FACT**
>
> Triptans and DHE are vasoconstrictors and should not be used in patients with hypertension or cardiovascular disease.

TENSION-TYPE HEADACHES

PATHOPHYSIOLOGY

Thought to share a common pathophysiology with migraines.

SYMPTOMS

- Bilateral, nonpulsating, not worsened by exertion.
- Usually not associated with nausea and vomiting.

DIFFERENTIAL

Other primary or secondary headaches.

TREATMENT

- NSAIDs.
- For severe headache → treat same as migraine.

CLUSTER HEADACHES

Cluster headaches are most common in young- to middle-aged men and may be precipitated by alcohol and stress. They result from dysfunction of the trigeminal nerve.

SYMPTOMS/EXAMINATION

- Severe, unilateral orbital, supraorbital, or temporal pain.
- Episodes last for 15-180 minutes, but recur in clusters (eg, daily on same side for weeks).
- Associated ipsilateral findings:
  - Conjunctival injection, lacrimation, nasal congestion, rhinorrhea, facial swelling, miosis, or ptosis

TREATMENT

- **High-flow O_2** is effective in 70% of patients.
- IV dihydroergotamine or sumatriptan; oral preparations take too long to be effective.
- Prophylaxis with oral steroid burst, verapamil, or antiepileptic agents (carbamazepine, phenytoin).

Altered Mental Status

Confusional states can be broadly divided into **delirium, dementia,** and **psychosis** (Table 15.10).

TABLE 15.10. Features of Delirium, Dementia, and Psychiatric Psychosis

CHARACTERISTIC	DELIRIUM	DEMENTIA	PSYCHIATRIC
Onset	Over days	Insidious	Sudden
Course over 24 h	Fluctuating	Stable	Stable
Consciousness	Reduced	Alert	Alert
Attention	Disordered	Normal	May be disordered
Cognition	Disordered	Impaired	May be impaired
Orientation	Impaired	Often impaired	May be impaired
Hallucinations	Visual and/or auditory	Often absent	Usually auditory
Delusions	Transient, poorly organized	Usually absent	Sustained
Movements	Asterixis, tremor may be present	Often absent	Absent

(Data from Tintinalli, J et al. *Emergency Medicine: A Comprehensive Study Guide*, 6th ed. New York, NY: McGraw-Hill, 2004:229; based on data from Lipowski Z: Delirium in the Elderly Patient. *New Engl J Med* 320:578, 1989.)

DELIRIUM

In delirium, functions of cognition and attention (arousal) are disordered due to widespread neuronal or neurotransmitter malfunction from an underlying medical (organic) cause. The development of delirium in hospitalized patients is associated with increased mortality.

> **KEY FACT**
>
> Delirium is a medical emergency.

CAUSES

Common causes include:

- Drug intoxication or withdrawal (most common)
- Metabolic disorders (eg, endocrine disorder, hepatic encephalopathy, uremia, hypoglycemia)
- Toxins (eg, carbon monoxide)
- Infections (eg, CNS, *urinary tract infection* [UTI], sepsis)
- Hypercapnia
- Trauma
- Seizures

SYMPTOMS/EXAMINATION

- **Acute** confusional state
- Transient attention and cognition impairment
- **Waxing and waning** symptoms
- Hallucinations, if present, are visual and/or auditory

DIFFERENTIAL

Dementia, psychosis.

DIAGNOSIS

- History of acuity of change in behavior.
- General pulmonary embolism (PE) and ancillary tests to search for underlying cause.
  - Include head CT and LP, if necessary.

TREATMENT

- Treat underlying cause.
- Family presence, supporting of sensory function (eg, hearing aids, glasses), attention to needs (bathroom use, pain control), normal sleep patterns, and redirection can help prevent delirium.
- Sedate with haloperidol or benzodiazepines if severe agitation as a last resort with the knowledge that these medications may actually worsen delirium.

> **KEY FACT**
>
> The mini-mental state examination is used to screen for cognitive impairment.

DEMENTIA

Dementia results from a **gradual** loss of mental capacity with relatively preserved attention function.

CAUSES

Causes include:

- Alzheimer disease (most common)
  - Reduction of neurons in the cerebral cortex and increased amyloid deposition → neurofibrillary tangles and plaques
- Vascular (multi-infarct)

- Parkinson disease
- Viral infection: HIV, Creutzfeldt-Jakob disease
- Possible **treatable causes**:
  - Depression (most common treatable cause)
  - Vitamin B_{12} deficiency
  - Neurosyphilis
  - Hypothyroidism
  - Normal pressure hydrocephalus
  - Intracranial mass (eg, brain tumor)
  - Chronic drug use

KEY FACT

Keep in mind reversible causes when evaluating the patient with dementia.

SYMPTOMS/EXAMINATION

- **Gradual onset** confusional state
- Usually presents in the **elderly**
- Disordered cognition with normal attention
- Loss of mental capacity especially memory
  - Remote memories often preserved

DIFFERENTIAL

Delirium, psychosis

DIAGNOSIS

- Diagnosis is primarily based on history of slow, progressive change in behavior. All patients warrant neuroimaging, thyroid-stimulating hormone (TSH), and vitamin B_{12} level at minimum.
- Look for reversible cause or exacerbating comorbid condition (eg, UTI).
- **Mini-mental state examination:** Tests orientation, memory, attention, calculation, recall, and language.
- Cutoffs of < 24 or < 25 out of 30 are used to identify cognitive impairment.

TREATMENT

- Treat reversible causes, if present.
- Environmental and psychosocial interventions.
- Depends on cause: For Alzheimer, donepezil (Aricept) and tacrine (Cognex) reduce the metabolism of acetylcholine. For vascular dementia, treat risk factors (hypertension).

Normal Pressure Hydrocephalus

A potentially reversible cause of dementia; results from defective CSF uptake (either a primary process or secondary to prior infection/injury/bleed) leading to increased CSF volume; most commonly occurs in older patients, but 50% are < 60 years old.

KEY FACT

Normal pressure hydrocephalus: Wacky, wobbly, and wet.

SYMPTOMS/EXAMINATION

Triad of progressive dementia, ataxia, and urinary frequency or incontinence

DIAGNOSIS

Based on CT showing ventricular enlargement (without other pathology) and LP with normal intracranial pressure and fluid studies.

TREATMENT

Neurosurgical consultation for shunt placement.

PSYCHIATRIC PSYCHOSIS

Functional (psychiatric) cause of confusional state.

Symptoms

- Loss of contact with reality.
- Hallucinations, if present, are auditory.
- Usually not waxing and waning.
- Consciousness not clouded.

Differential

Dementia, delirium ("organic" psychosis)

Treatment

Environmental, psychosocial, and medical

Coma

Consciousness can be divided into arousal and content functions. Arousal functions reside in the reticular activating system (RAS) in the midbrain, pons, and medulla. Content functions reside in the cerebrum. Coma represents a failure in both arousal and content functions of the brain. *Bilateral* cortical involvement or brainstem pathology is necessary to cause coma.

Causes

Causes are myriad and include (Table 15.11):

- Encephalopathy—metabolic, hypertensive, hypoxic, Wernicke
- Toxins (Table 15.12)
- Drug reaction
- Infection
- Hyper-/hypothermia
- Seizure (postictal or nonconvulsive status epilepticus)
- Psychiatric
- CNS lesion or event (less common)
- Sepsis
- Endocrine: Hypo/hyperglycemia, hypothyroid, Addison
- Heme: Thrombotic thrombocytopenic purpura

TABLE 15.11. Causes of Coma

Causes of coma—**TIPS AEIOU**
Trauma, **t**emperature
Infection
Psychiatric, **p**oisonings
Space occupying lesion, **s**ubarachnoid
Alcohol
Epilepsy, **e**lectrolytes, **e**ncephalopathy
Insulin
Opioids/overdose, **o**xygen (hypoxia, CO_2 narcosis)
Uremia (metabolic)

TABLE 15.12. Common Toxicologic Causes of Coma

Alcohols
Antipsychotics
Antiseizure medications
Carbon monoxide
Muscle relaxants
Opiates
Sedative/hypnotics

SYMPTOMS/EXAMINATION

- Eyes-closed state with inappropriate response to environmental stimuli.
- Other findings vary depending on depth of coma and underlying etiology (see Table 15.10).
- Look for asymmetric findings that suggest focal or regional CNS dysfunction.
- Hypertension and bradycardia indicate ↑ ICP (Cushing reflex).

DIAGNOSIS

- Diagnosis is made based on clinical findings (Table 15.13).
- Evaluation should focus on identifying underlying cause.
- Obtain head CT, glucose, electrolytes, renal and liver function tests.
- Consider EEG to evaluate for nonconvulsive status epilepticus in all.
- With toxic-metabolic coma: Pupils continue to be reactive and reflexes and response to painful stimuli remain symmetric. Exception: Barbiturates.

MNEMONIC

Oculovestibular reflex:

Direction of fast component of nystagmus, with irrigation of cold versus warm water in patient with intact brainstem:

COWS

Cold
Opposite
Warm
Same

TREATMENT

- Supportive care.
- Coma "cocktail" (IV) for the undifferentiated patient.
  - Thiamine
  - Glucose
  - Naloxone
- Treat underlying cause once identified.
- Empiric antibiotic coverage for meningitis if cause not readily apparent.

Ataxia

Ataxia is the failure to make smooth, intentional movements. Ataxia and gait disturbances are symptoms of particular disease processes and not diagnoses in and of themselves. In general, ataxia can be divided into two groups:

MOTOR (CEREBELLAR) ATAXIA

- Disorders of cerebellum (most common).
  - Sensory receptors and afferent pathways intact, but integration of proprioceptive information is poor.
  - Usually ipsilateral to lesion. If lateral cerebellar lesion → limb incoordination. If midline cerebellar lesion (vermis) → axial incoordination.
- Far less commonly due to infarcts in the internal capsule, thalamic nucleus, or frontal lobe.

TABLE 15.13. Pertinent Neurologic Findings in Coma

EXAMINATION	FINDING	INTERPRETATION
Funduscopic examination	Absent venous pulsations	Increased intracranial pressure
Pupillary constriction	Absent response to light Unequal pupils	Midbrain structural lesion or topical cycloplegic drug use Structural lesion or normal variant
Eye position	Tonic deviation	Seizure or irritant brain lesion
Corneal reflex (tests CN V and VII)	Absent	Posterior fossa or brainstem lesions
Oculocephalic reflex (doll's eye)	Conjugate deviation of eyes in direction *opposite* to passive head rotation Conjugate deviation in same direction as head rotation	Intact brainstem No brainstem function
Oculovestibular reflex (cold caloric)	Irrigate ear canal with 10 mL *cold* water: ▪ *Horizontal nystagmus* with fast component *away* from irrigated ear ▪ Tonic deviation to side of irrigation No response	 Intact cortex and brainstem Toxic/metabolic or lesion above brainstem No brainstem function
Response to painful stimuli	Decorticate posturing (elbow/wrist/finger flexion, forearm supination, legs extended) Decerebrate posturing (elbow/wrist extension, shoulder adduction and internal rotation, forearm pronation) Asymmetric movement	Severe damage above the midbrain Damage at the midbrain or diencephalon Structural lesions

SENSORY ATAXIA

Failure of transmission of proprioception to the CNS via peripheral nerves, dorsal columns, or cerebellar input tract.

CAUSES

Common causes of ataxia are listed in Table 15.14.

SYMPTOMS/EXAMINATION

- Patients may complain of difficulty ambulating, weakness, or falls.
- Ataxia that is worse with loss of visual input (eg, walking in the dark) = sensory ataxia.
- The examination should focus on differentiating motor from sensory ataxia.
- The classic **cerebellar gait** is wide based with unsteady and irregular steps.
- A **sensory ataxic gait** is characterized by abrupt movement of legs and slapping impact of feet with each step.
- Cerebellar function testing: Observe patient perform smooth, voluntary movements, and rapidly alternating movements. Inaccurate fine movements = dysmetria. Clumsy rapid movements = dysdiadochokinesia. Breakdown of movements into parts = dyssynergia.

Q

A 44-year-old otherwise healthy man presents to the ED with sudden onset of "dizziness" that began when he rolled over in his bed this morning. Patient describes the dizziness as a sensation that "the room is spinning." He denies any weakness or numbness. On physical examination, he has worsening of his symptoms and horizontal nystagmus with Dix-Hallpike maneuver. He has no focal neurologic deficits on examination. What is the most appropriate diagnosis?

TABLE 15.14. Causes of Ataxia

Group	Example
Drug intoxications	Ethanol, dilantin toxicity
Metabolic disorders	Hyponatremia
Peripheral neuropathy	Alcoholic peripheral neuropathy
Vestibulopathy	Meniere disease
Cerebellar disorder	Infarction, mass, degenerative disorders of cerebellum
Posterior column disorder	Vitamin B_{12} deficiency

- **Romberg test:** Worsened unsteadiness with eyes closed (loss of visual input) is suggestive of sensory ataxia. If unsteadiness present with patient's eyes open, consider cerebellar pathology.

Diagnosis

Diagnosis is primarily made via history and physical examination.

Treatment

Define underlying cause. Treatment is directed toward primary disease process.

> **KEY FACT**
>
> The direction of nystagmus is named by the **fast** (cortical) component.

> **KEY FACT**
>
> Vertigo with any CNS symptoms or findings? Assume central cause!

Vertigo

Vertigo is defined as the perception of movement where no movement exists. Vertigo is typically categorized as central or peripheral.

CENTRAL VERTIGO

Causes

Results from disorders affecting the brainstem and cerebellum:
- Cerebellar hemorrhage, tumor, or infarct
- Vertebrobasilar insufficiency
- Vertebral artery dissection
- Wallenberg syndrome (lateral medullary infarction of brainstem)
- Multiple sclerosis
- Migraine

> **A**
>
> This patient clinically has benign paroxysmal peripheral vertigo (BPPV) and can be treated symptomatically. Patients with advanced age, multiple stroke risk factors, or those with gradual onset of symptoms, headache or neck pain, presence of focal neurologic deficits, or vertical nystagmus should be considered for imaging to evaluate for causes of central vertigo.

Symptoms/Examination

Onset may be sudden or gradual.
- Symptoms are often ill defined and persistent
- **Vertical and bidirectional (direction-changing) nystagmus = central cause**
- Associated with other CNS symptoms/findings indicating posterior fossa pathology—diplopia, dysarthria, visual changes

Diagnosis/Treatment

MRI is imaging of choice to visualize the posterior fossa, though CT scan may identify cerebellar mass, hemorrhage, or infarct. CT scan may miss up to 80% of posterior Cerebrovascular accidents (CVAs).

PERIPHERAL VERTIGO

Causes

Caused by disorders affecting CN VIII and the vestibular apparatus (Table 15.15).

Symptoms/Examination

- Most commonly a **dramatic and sudden** onset of intense paroxysmal vertigo
- Nausea and vomiting
- Often aggravated by position
- Rotatory-vertical or horizontal nystagmus with 1- to 5-second latency period
- Hearing loss (not with benign paroxysmal peripheral vertigo [BPPV], vestibular neuronitis)
- No central findings

Diagnosis

- Primarily a clinical diagnosis.
- A positive **Dix-Hallpike** test confirms posterior canal BPPV. This test is not useful in making any other diagnosis—only BPPV.
- MRI to visualize CN VIII lesions and detect central causes.

Treatment

- Depends on underlying etiology (eg, discontinue ototoxic agents in ototoxicity, Epley maneuver for posterior canal BPPV).
- Symptomatic treatment with antihistamines, antiemetics, or benzodiazepines.
- Consider antibiotics and ENT consult for bacterial labyrinthitis (↑ risk of meningitis).

Q

A 50-year-old man presents to the ED with a concern about possible stroke. The patient has history of hypertension and BP 180/100 mm Hg upon arrival. Physical examination reveals a left-sided facial droop that includes the forehead. There is no arm or leg weakness or other neurologic complaints. Should this patient be worked up for a CVA?

KEY FACT

Central vertigo is classically ill defined and constant with associated vertical nystagmus. Peripheral vertigo is classically dramatic and sudden with rotatory–vertical or horizontal nystagmus.

The ABCs can cause isolated vertigo: **A**cute vestibular neuronitis, **B**PPV, and **C**erebellar strokes.

TABLE 15.15. Disorders Causing Peripheral Vertigo

Disorder	Pathophysiology	Associated Findings
BPPV	Otoconia in the semicircular canals	Precipitated by sudden head movement Positive Dix-Hallpike Improvement/resolution with Epley maneuver < 1 min episodes
Meniere disease	Increased endolymph within the cochlea and labyrinth	Ear "fullness," tinnitus, *hearing loss*
Labyrinthitis	Viral or *bacterial* infection	Recent URI or otitis media. Middle-ear findings (infection, fluid), tinnitus, *hearing loss*
Acute vestibular neuronitis	Viral infection	Lasts several days, no recurrence or hearing loss
Ramsay-Hunt syndrome (vestibular ganglionitis)	Viral infection of vestibular ganglion	Hearing loss, vertigo, facial nerve palsy, grouped vesicles
Perilymph fistula	Trauma, sudden pressure change	Abrupt onset after inciting event ± hearing loss Requires surgical repair
Ototoxicity	Damage to vestibular apparatus—may be irreversible	Hearing loss, vertigo, tinnitus
CN VIII lesions	Schwannomas, meningioma	Gradual onset, preceded by *hearing loss*

BPPV, Benign paroxysmal positional vertigo; URI, upper respiratory infection.

A

No. This patient has isolated facial droop with forehead *included* which is consistent with a peripheral (not central) seventh nerve palsy ie, Bell palsy.

Cranial Nerve Disorders

OCULOMOTOR, TROCHLEAR, AND ABDUCENS PALSIES: OCULOMOTOR MOVEMENTS

Third Cranial Nerve (Oculomotor Nerve, CN3) Palsy

The third cranial nerve supplies the levator muscle of the eyelid and four extraocular muscles: medial rectus, superior rectus, inferior rectus, and inferior oblique. CN3 also constricts the pupil through its parasympathetic fibers. A CN3 palsy can result from lesions anywhere along its path (between the oculomotor nucleus in the midbrain and the extraocular muscles within the orbit). Compressive CN3 damage can result in compression of the parasympathetic fibers before any disruption of the motor fibers because the parasympathetic fibers run on the outside of the nerve resulting lid ptosis and mydriasis (a "blown" pupil) before the "down and out" position is seen.

Causes

- Congenital
- Intracranial aneurysm (posterior communicating artery)
- Ischemic (aka "diabetic third nerve palsy")—caused by diabetes or hypertension
- Trauma
- Infection or inflammatory disease
- Ophthalmoplegic migraine

Symptoms/Examination

- Sudden onset of binocular horizontal, vertical, or oblique diplopia and a droopy eyelid.
- Sudden, severe pain ("the worst headache of my life") might suggest subarachnoid hemorrhage due to a ruptured aneurysm.
- Patients have ptosis and paralysis of adduction, elevation, and depression. The eye rests in a position of abduction, slight depression, and intorsion "down and out" (Figure 15.6).
- Pupil may be dilated and minimally reactive to light (pupillary involvement), totally reactive and normal (pupillary noninvolvement), or may be sluggishly responsive (partial pupillary involvement).

KEY FACT

Isolated third nerve palsy due to ischemia will spontaneously resolve over a period of 3-6 months.

KEY FACT

Myasthenia gravis has the ability to mimic virtually any cranial neuropathy, including isolated third nerve palsies.

Diagnosis

- Based on clinical presentation. Absence of pupillary involvement suggests a benign process that can be observed over a couple of weeks.
- Third nerve palsies that are accompanied by other neurologic deficits, orbital signs, or meningismus require an evaluation that usually includes neuroimaging. An LP may also be required to evaluate for possible infectious or inflammatory process.

TROCHLEAR NERVE (CN4) PALSY

The superior oblique muscle is innervated by CN4. The patient will have **vertical** diplopia, which is apparent when the patient tries to patient tries to read or walk down stairs. The patient often tilts his head contralateral to the affected side. In adults, approximately 40% of all isolated CN4 palsies are traumatic, 30% are idiopathic, 20% are due to vascular infarct, and only 10% are due to tumor or aneurysm. The vast majority of fourth nerve palsies are benign.

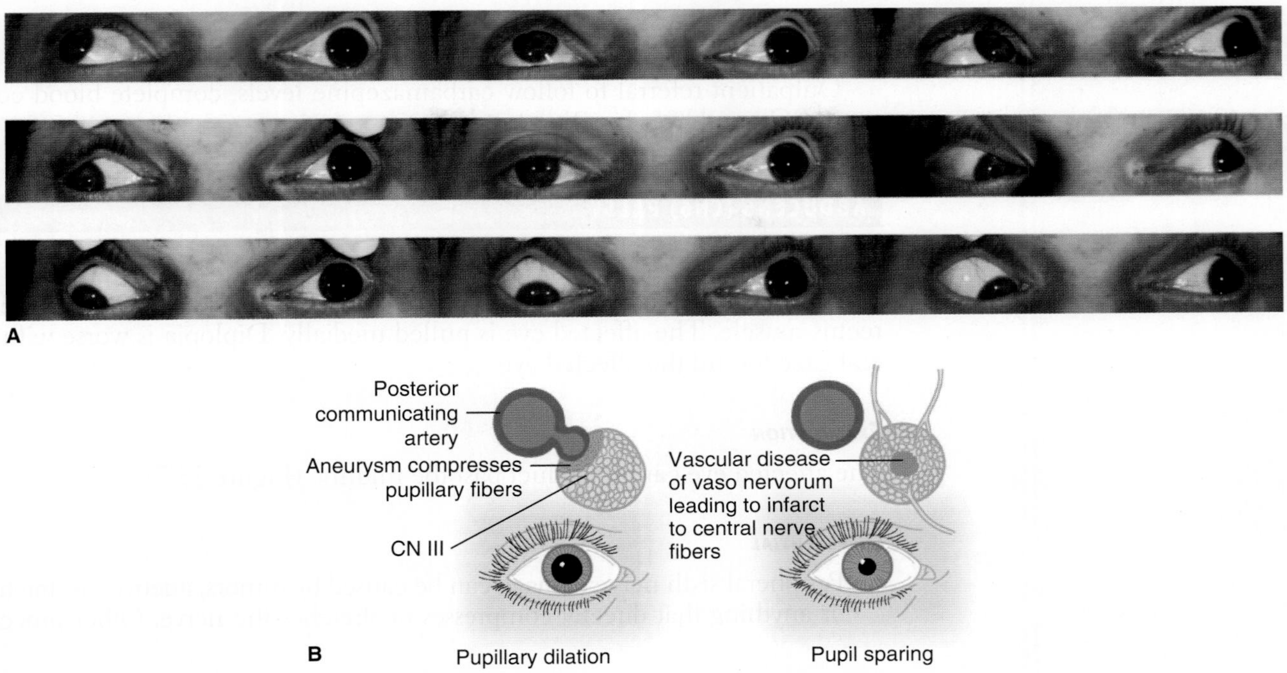

FIGURE 15.6. (A) This composite shows the classic defects of a third cranial nerve palsy in all fields of gaze. The pupil is dilated. Conjugate eye movement is present in only 1 position, when the affected eye gazes laterally to the affected side (intact lateral rectus). When gaze is directly ahead, exotropia is seen secondary to the unopposed lateral rectus muscle of the affected side. (Reproduced, with permission, from Knoop KJ, Stack LB, Storrow AB, et al. *Atlas of Emergency Medicine*. 3rd ed. New York: McGraw-Hill Education, 2010. Figure 2.48. Photographer: Frank Birinyi, MD.) **(B) Posterior communicating artery aneurysm compresses the peripherally located pupillomotor fibers of cranial nerve (CN) III, causing a nerve palsy and pupillary dilatation. Diabetes and hypertension can cause microvascular compromise of the central nerve fibers causing nerve palsy with pupil sparing.** (Reproduced, with permission, from Tintinalli JE, Stapczynski JS, Ma OJ, et al. *Tintinalli's Emergency Medicine: A Comprehensive Study Guide*. 8th ed. New York, NY: McGraw-Hill; 2016. Figure 241.55.)

TRIGEMINAL NEURALGIA

The trigeminal nerve (CN V) has three anatomic divisions, V_1-ophthalmic, V_2-maxillary, and V_3-mandibular, which innervate the cornea, the face, and the mucous membranes of the oral and nasal cavity. The motor fibers innervate the muscles of mastication.

> **KEY FACT**
>
> Treatment for trigeminal neuralgia = Tegretol (carbamazepine)

Symptoms/Examination

- Brief, recurrent episodes of excruciating, unilateral facial pain lasting only seconds
- Right more than left side predominance
- May be able to elicit pain by tapping the side of the face, otherwise there should be no demonstrable physical findings

Differential

Includes vascular or space-occupying lesions (acoustic neuroma), demyelinating diseases (multiple sclerosis), herpes zoster, sinus infection, odontogenic pathology, migraine, temporomandibular joint dysfunction

Diagnosis

- Based on clinical presentation.
- MRI should be performed to rule out other etiologies if neurological findings are present.

TREATMENT

- Initiate **carbamazepine** and analgesics in ED.
- Outpatient referral to follow carbamazepine levels, complete blood count (CBC), and liver function tests.

ABDUCENS (CN6) PALSY

CN6 innervates the lateral rectus muscle. Complete interruption of the peripheral sixth nerve causes diplopia due to unopposed action of the medial rectus muscle. The affected eye is pulled medially. Diplopia is worse with lateral gaze toward the affected eye.

EXAMINATION

The affected eye cannot abduct past the midline (Figure 15.7).

DIFFERENTIAL

- Peripheral sixth nerve damage can be caused by tumors, aneurysms, fractures or anything that directly compresses or stretches the nerve. Other processes

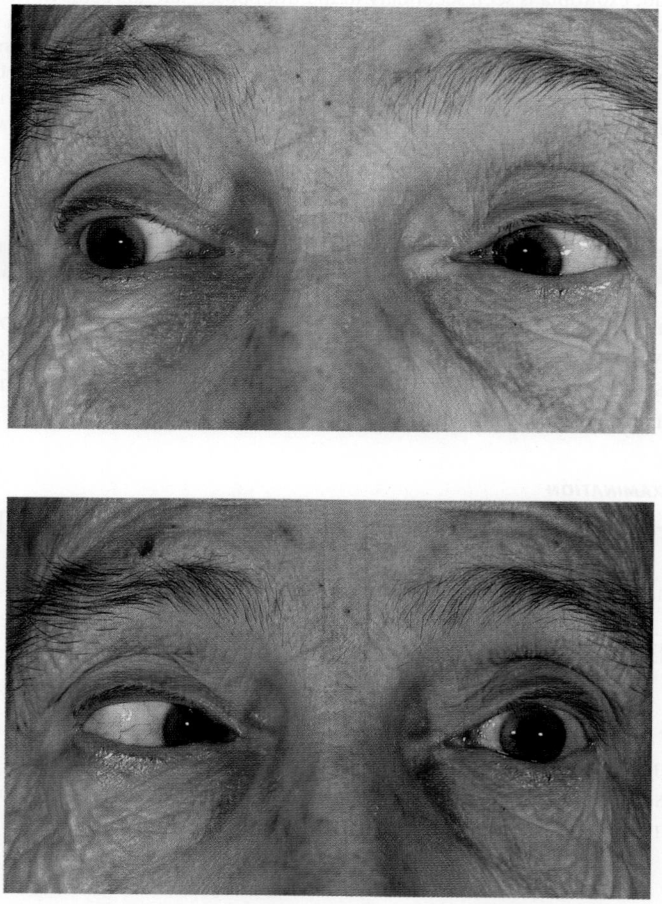

FIGURE 15.7. Loss of abduction of the left eye is seen in lateral gaze, demonstrating an isolated sixth-nerve palsy. (Reproduced, with permission, from Knoop KJ, Stack LB, Storrow AB, et al. *Atlas of Emergency Medicine.* 3rd ed. New York: McGraw-Hill Education, 2010. Figure 2.47A & C. Photographer: Frank Birinyi, MD.)

that can damage the sixth nerve include strokes, demyelination, infections, cavernous sinus diseases, and various neuropathies.
- The most common cause of sixth nerve impairment is diabetic neuropathy.

> **KEY FACT**
>
> CN6 palsy is the most common false-localizing sign of increased ICP because of its long intracranial course.

BELL PALSY

A lower motor neuron ("peripheral") CN VII palsy.

Causes

Bell palsy is most commonly due to herpes virus infection. Pregnant women are at greater risk. Other infections (HIV, Lyme disease) can also cause a CN VII palsy.

Symptoms/Examination

- Viral prodrome (50% of time)
- Abrupt onset of unilateral facial paralysis with forehead included (central causes will spare the forehead due to bilateral innervation of the upper face by upper motor neurons)
- May also have loss of taste to anterior two-thirds of tongue, hyperacusis (sound distortion or tinnitus)
- Bell phenomenon: Eye appears to roll back in head when patient attempts to close the lid

Differential

- **Ramsay Hunt syndrome**
  - Herpes zoster infection of geniculate ganglion.
  - Characterized by facial paralysis, pain, tinnitus, hearing loss, and typical zoster lesions on the affected side, including inside external auditory canal, and/or the tympanic membrane.
  - Treatment = prednisone. Many sources recommend adding antivirals (eg, acyclovir) for severe cases, but this remains controversial.
- **Lyme disease**
  - A leading cause of facial paralysis in regions where Lyme disease is endemic.
  - May be unilateral or **bilateral.**
  - Diagnosed via serologic titers.
  - Treatment = doxycycline PO.
- **Malignant otitis externa**
  - Severe otitis externa that is typically seen in diabetes or immunocompromised patients.
  - *Pseudomonas* sp often implicated.
  - Requires IV antibiotic therapy and ENT consultation.
- **Acoustic neuroma**
  - Hearing loss accompanying facial weakness.
  - MRI is diagnostic test of choice.
- Other causes include temporal bone trauma, mononucleosis, HIV seroconversion, other infectious organisms, mononeuropathy multiplex, Sjögren syndrome.

Diagnosis

- Primarily a clinical diagnosis.
- Any evidence for sparing of upper face ("central" CN VII paralysis) warrants CT or MRI to evaluate for stroke or CNS lesion.

TREATMENT

- Pharmacologic therapy should be initiated if patient presents within 1 week of symptom onset.
  - Corticosteroids
  - Antiviral therapy
- Eye protection:
  - Eye patch for sleeping and artificial tears during the day

ACOUSTIC NEUROMA

Schwannoma of CN VIII that typically causes isolated CN VIII symptoms, but if large may → mass effect on adjacent structures (CN VII, CN V, fourth ventricle).

SYMPTOMS/EXAMINATION

- Characteristic triad of sensorineural hearing loss, tinnitus, and disequilibrium

DIAGNOSIS/TREATMENT

- Audiogram to formally evaluate hearing loss.
- MRI can confirm diagnosis.
- Treatment is surgical.

Spinal Cord Disorders

> **KEY FACT**
>
> Damage to single corticospinal tract or posterior column → ipsilateral motor weakness or vibration/position loss. Damage to single spinothalamic tract → contralateral loss of pain and temperature.

Spinal cord anatomy:

- **Corticospinal tract:** Motor pathway; fibers cross in medulla then descend in cord
- **Spinothalamic tract:** Pain and temperature pathway; fibers first cross, then ascend in cord
- **Posterior (dorsal) columns:** Vibration and proprioceptive pathway; fibers ascend in ipsilateral posterior column to medulla, then cross
- **Cauda equina:** Lumbar and sacral nerve roots

CAUSES

Causes of spinal cord dysfunction include:

- Trauma
- Multiple sclerosis
- Transverse myelitis
- Spinal AVM or hemorrhage
- Compression from tumor, disc, epidural abscess, or hematoma
- Syringomyelia
- HIV (myelopathy)
- Infarction

SYMPTOMS/EXAMINATION

- Patients present with motor and sensory deficits depending on location of injury.
- Scoring motor function:
  - 5 = Full strength
  - 4 = Able to resist, but weak
  - 3 = Able to move against gravity
  - 2 = Able to move when gravity eliminated
  - 1 = Muscle fires, but no movement is generated
  - 0 = No muscle firing

TABLE 15.16. Examination Findings: Upper Motor Neuron vs Lower Motor Neuron

	Bulk	Tone	Fasciculations	Reflex	Power
Upper	Normal	Increased	No	Increased, with clonus and upgoing toes	Decreased
Lower	Normal acutely, decreased if chronic	Normal acutely, wasting if chronic	Yes	Decreased or absent, downgoing toes	Decreased

- Scoring reflexes:
  - 0 to 4 scale with 2 being normal (0 = no reflexes, 4 = hyperactive reflexes with clonus)
- In general, lower motor neuron pathology results in ↓ reflexes while upper motor neuron pathology may result in either ↑ or ↓ reflexes depending on time course. Upper motor neuron (UMN) lesions produce ↓ reflexes initially, followed by hyperreflexia after several days. See Table 15.16 for comparison.
- Complete injury results in complete loss of motor, sensory, and autonomic function below level of injury.
- Partial injury often presents as a spinal cord syndrome (Table 15.17).
- Table 15.18 summarizes the findings in specific disease processes.

DIAGNOSIS

- MRI is imaging of choice to evaluate for compression or mass lesion. Location of imaging must be carefully selected based on history and examination.
- Lumbar puncture is indicated to further define a suspected inflammatory or demyelinating process.

TABLE 15.17. Spinal Cord Syndromes

Syndrome	Characteristic Findings (Below Level of Injury)	Likely Cause	Comments
Central cord	Bilateral motor weakness of upper extremities > lower extremities and distal > proximal extremities	Hyperextension injury of narrowed cervical spinal canal	More common in elderly patients
Brown-Sequard (cord hemisection)	Ipsilateral motor weakness and vibration/ position loss Contralateral pain and temperature loss	Penetrating trauma	Often partial syndrome Best prognosis
Anterior cord	Motor weakness, pinprick and light touch loss. Preserved vibration and position sense	Infarction of anterior spinal artery	Poorest prognosis Preservation of posterior columns
Cauda equina	Urinary retention (overflow incontinence), decreased rectal tone, saddle anesthesia, motor weakness	Ruptured L4–5 disc	Peripheral nerve (nerve root) injury

TABLE 15.18. Clinical Features and Etiology of Spinal Cord Disorders

Spinal Cord Disorder	Clinical Features	Etiology
Discitis	Back pain, fever, and refusal to walk in child < 10 y	Inflammatory process in disc (viral or *Staphylococcus aureus*)
Dorsal column disorders	Loss of position sense, vibration, and light touch	Syphilis or vitamin B_{12} deficiency
HIV myelopathy (one of many myelopathies)	Weakness, gait problems, spasticity, sphincter dysfunction	Advanced HIV
Neoplasm	Severe pain with radiation down spine, signs of cord compression	Most common—lung cancer, breast cancer, lymphoma
Spinal epidural abscess	Severe pain with radiation down spine, signs of cord compression, fever	Expanding abscess (IDU or immunocompromise)
Spinal epidural hematoma	Severe pain with radiation down spine, signs of cord compression	Expanding hemorrhage (trauma or coagulopathy)
Syringomyelia	Dissociative anesthesia, weakness	Syrinx formation in central spinal cord
Transverse myelitis	Transverse level of sensory loss, paresis, sphincter dysfunction	Post-viral or toxic inflammation

HIV, human immunodeficiency virus.

SPINAL EPIDURAL HEMATOMA

More likely to occur following spinal trauma or spinal procedures but may occur spontaneously in patients with coagulopathy (eg, liver disease, anticoagulation, thrombocytopenia).

Symptoms/Examination

- Abrupt severe and radicular back pain
- Weakness, loss of bowel/bladder, and sensory deficits depending on degree of compression

Treatment

Immediate correction of coagulopathy (when present) and surgical decompression.

SPINAL EPIDURAL ABSCESS

Typically results from hematogenous spread of infection to epidural space; **most common organism is** ***S aureus*****.**

Major risk factors include:

- Injection drug use
- Chronic renal failure
- Dental abscess
- Bacterial endocarditis
- Alcoholism
- Diabetes

- Immunosuppression
- Recent back surgery, lumbar puncture, or epidural anesthesia

SYMPTOMS/EXAMINATION

- Progressive pain
- Constitutional symptoms: Fevers, sweats
- Weakness, loss of bowel/bladder and sensory deficits depending on degree of compression

DIAGNOSIS/TREATMENT

- **ESR** is almost always elevated.
- Obtain immediate MRI to confirm diagnosis.
- If MRI unavailable, a CT myelogram should be obtained.
- Antibiotics: Vancomycin and third-generation cephalosporin.
- Immediate surgical intervention.

> **KEY FACT**
>
> An elevated ESR/CRP in the patient with unexplained back pain should raise concern for spinal epidural abscess.

DISCITIS

Discitis is an inflammatory process of the intervertebral disc space, often due to viral or bacterial (*S aureus*) infection. It is usually seen in children < age 10. Risk factors include spinal surgical procedures, systemic infections (eg, UTI), and immunocompromise.

SYMPTOMS/EXAMINATION

- Moderate to severe local pain and radicular symptoms.
- Children often present with sudden onset of back pain and refusal to walk. Mean age of presentation in children is 7 years old.
- Adult presentation is more chronic and insidious.
- Fever (in most).
- Neurologic deficits are uncommon.
- Usually spreads from a hematogenous source.

DIAGNOSIS/TREATMENT

- MRI
- Intravenous antibiotics

SPINAL NEOPLASM

Most commonly due to metastasis or direct spread from lung cancer, breast cancer, and lymphoma.

SYMPTOMS/EXAMINATION

- Symptoms commonly localized to thoracic spine
- Characterized by pain that is worse at night

DIAGNOSIS

- Plain x-rays are abnormal in most patients.
- MRI is confirmative.

TREATMENT

Includes high-dose steroids, radiation and surgery, depending on suspected pathology and degree of compression.

TRANSVERSE MYELITIS

Spinal cord dysfunction due to viral infection, autoimmune or idiopathic cause.

Symptoms/Examination

- Characterized by a transverse level of sensory impairment, paraplegia, and sphincter disturbance

Differential

- Spinal cord tumors, Guillain-Barré syndrome

Diagnosis/Treatment

- MRI to exclude compressive lesion.
- Steroids (uncertain benefit).
- Only 50% have fair to good recovery.

SYRINGOMYELIA

Syringomyelia results from a CSF fluid collection (syrinx) within the spinal cord. Any location is possible, but it is most commonly seen in the cervical spine in association with Arnold-Chiari malformation.

Symptoms/Examination

- Depend on location of syrinx (most lesions are between C2 and T9)
- Asymptomatic to prominent central pain syndrome in a segmental distribution
- **Dissociative anesthesia:** Loss of pain and temperature sensation with preservation of proprioception and light touch
- Weakness, spasticity, interosseous wasting of the hands

Diagnosis/Treatment

- MRI
- Treated with surgery, if progressive symptoms

Neuromuscular Disorders

The neuromuscular unit is made up of the anterior horn cells, the peripheral nerve, the neuromuscular junction, and the muscle. Neuromuscular disorders are a large group of disorders that result in degeneration and atrophy of muscles or nerve tissue. They can be grouped based on the location of pathology (Table 15.19).

> **KEY FACT**
>
> *C jejuni* gastroenteritis is a common precursor to GBS.

GUILLAIN-BARRÉ SYNDROME (GBS)

GBS is primarily an **acute demyelinating disorder of the peripheral nerve.** Variants include early cranial nerve findings and ataxia, primary sensory involvement, and autonomic involvement.

Pathophysiology

- Antecedent illness (viral or ***Campylobacter jejuni*** gastroenteritis, upper respiratory infection [URI]) → autoimmune response → damage to myelin sheath → symptoms

TABLE 15.19. Grouping of Neuromuscular Disorders Based on Location of Pathology

Location of Pathology	Common Diseases
Anterior horn cells	Spinal muscular atrophies
Peripheral nerve	Demyelinating polyneuropathies (eg, Guillain-Barré syndrome, diphtheria) Distal symmetric polyneuropathies (eg, diabetic, alcoholic) Radiculopathies and plexopathies (eg, brachial plexopathy) Mononeuropathies (eg, Saturday night palsy) Mononeuropathy multiplex Amyotrophic lateral sclerosis
Neuromuscular junction	Myasthenia gravis Lambert-Eaton myasthenic syndrome Botulism Tick paralysis
Skeletal muscle	Myopathies Muscular dystrophies Periodic paralysis

SYMPTOMS/EXAMINATION

- Antecedent illness followed by latent period of days to weeks.
- Classic presentation is **ascending symmetric paresthesias and motor weakness** with peak symptoms within 3 weeks of onset. Often associated with coexisting back pain.
  - Miller Fisher Variant: Ophthalmoplegia, ataxia, ↓ or absent reflexes. Around 25% will have limb weakness in addition to cranial nerve/cerebellar findings.
  - Decreased deep tendon reflexes.
  - Variable sensory loss.
  - Normal rectal tone.
  - May progress to ventilatory failure.
- Less common findings (seen in half of patients):
  - Autonomic dysfunction (eg, urinary retention).
  - Cranial nerve involvement (including seventh nerve palsy).

KEY FACT

The classic CSF finding in GBS is a markedly elevated protein with up to 100 lymphocytes/μL.

DIFFERENTIAL

- Acute and chronic polyneuropathies
- Disease of the spinal cord, neuromuscular junction, or muscle

DIAGNOSIS

- Suspect based on clinical presentation.
- Electrodiagnostic testing.
- Cerebrospinal fluid analysis:
  - Classic picture = markedly elevated protein (> 45 μg/dL) with up to 100 lymphocytes/μL
  - Often normal, when early

TREATMENT

- Supportive therapy
- IVIG or plasmapheresis

Q

A 55-year-old man presents with complaint of progressive weakness of arms and legs and dry mouth. Review of systems (ROS) is positive for significant weight loss over the preceding months. Examination is significant for proximal muscle weakness that improves with repeated use. This is most consistent with which disease of the neuromuscular junction?

- Close observation of respiratory function with forced expiratory volume (FEV_1) monitoring
- Prophylactic intubation or ventilatory support if:
  - Decreased FEV_1 < 100% predicted
  - CO_2 retention
  - Negative Inspiratory Force (NIF) < –30 cm H_2O (normal is –35 or less)

DIPHTHERIA

A toxin-mediated multisystem illness caused by *Corynebacterium diphtheriae*.

PATHOPHYSIOLOGY

- Respiratory or skin (tropical climates or poor hygiene) infection with ***C diphtheriae*** → exotoxin release →
  - Local membrane formation
  - Peripheral neuropathy → neurologic symptoms

SYMPTOMS/EXAMINATION

- Respiratory infection
  - Symptoms indistinguishable from pharyngitis, tonsillitis
- Adherent, grayish white to grayish black membrane visible at site of infection
  - Sharply demarcated borders
- Skin infection
  - Clinically similar to chronic skin ulcers/wounds
    - Grayish membrane present

COMPLICATIONS

- Airway obstruction from membrane formation
- Neurologic
  - Weakness → paralysis (often starts with paralysis of the soft palate)
  - Dysphagia and dysarthria
- Myocarditis
- Nephritis

DIAGNOSIS

- Suspect and treatment based on clinical examination.
- Culture is confirmative.

TREATMENT

- Diphtheria antitoxin
- Antibiotics (penicillin or erythromycin)
- Supportive care

KEY FACT

Diphtheria: Exudative pharyngitis with progressive weakness. Treat with diphtheria antitoxin.

A

Lambert-Eaton myasthenic syndrome (LEMS), where antibodies form to the neuromuscular junction. This may be a solitary disease but has also been seen in association with underlying malignancy.

DIABETIC DISTAL SYMMETRIC POLYNEUROPATHY

The most common type of peripheral neuropathy. It is a gradually progressive disease process (years) due to microvascular injury to the nerve.

SYMPTOMS/EXAMINATION

- **Distal, symmetric**, stocking glove distribution of sensory and motor dysfunction
  - Pain and paresthesias
  - Loss of deep tendon reflexes

- Typically involves lower extremities and moves proximally
  - Before reaching knees → fingertips involved
- May involve any peripheral nerve
  - Gastrointestinal → dysphagia, diarrhea
  - Genitourinary → incontinence, impotence

DIFFERENTIAL

- Other causes of distal symmetric polyneuropathy include:
  - Alcoholic neuropathy
  - HIV neuropathy
  - Toxic and metabolic neuropathy (eg, B_{12} deficiency, medications)

DIAGNOSIS

Primarily based on clinical examination findings and exclusion of toxic-metabolic causes

TREATMENT

- Tricyclic antidepressants, carbamazepine, and/or gabapentin to control pain
- Improve glycemic control

ISOLATED MONONEUROPATHIES

Neuropathy involving a single peripheral nerve; most commonly due to compression of the nerve or trauma (Table 15.20).

Carpel tunnel syndrome is uniquely associated with multiple conditions:
- Diabetes mellitus (most common)
- Hypothyroidism
- Pregnancy
- Amyloid
- Arthritis
- Obesity
- HIV (late in course, possible relation to antiretrovirals)

DIAGNOSIS

- Mostly a clinical diagnosis
- Carpel tunnel provocative testing
  - Tinel sign: Tapping at volar wrist → symptoms
  - Phalen sign: Holding wrist in flexion for 30-60 seconds → symptoms
- Electrodiagnostic studies if confirmation needed

TREATMENT

- Once compression is relieved, most mononeuropathies will resolve spontaneously over a period of weeks.
- Radial mononeuropathy.
  - Splint wrist in **60° of dorsiflexion**.
- Ulnar mononeuropathy.
  - Corticosteroid injection may help.
  - May require surgical intervention if persistent.
- Median mononeuropathy.
  - Wrist splinting in **neutral position**
  - Corticosteroid injection into carpel tunnel
  - Oral corticosteroid burst
  - Release of flexor retinaculum for severe symptoms
- Sciatic and common peroneal mononeuropathy.
  - Splint ankle at 90° with posterior splint.

TABLE 15.20. Common Peripheral Mononeuropathies Related to Trauma or Compression

Mononeuropathy	Location of Injury	Clinical Findings
Radial ("Saturday night palsy")	Mid-humerus	Wrist and finger drop Numbness over first dorsal interosseus muscles
Ulnar	Elbow (cubital tunnel or ulnar condylar groove)—most common Wrist (Guyon's canal)	Paresthesias to fourth and fifth digits Inability to tightly adduct fingers or grasp with thumb Claw hand is the result of paralysis of the ulnar nerve
Median ("Carpal tunnel syndrome")	Wrist (carpal tunnel)	Pain and paresthesias in palmar aspect of thumb, index, third and half of fourth digits Thumb weakness Thenar atrophy and ulnar deviation
Sciatic	Buttock	Inability to flex knee Inability to flex or extend ankle (→ footdrop)
Lateral femoral cutaneous ("Meralgia paresthetica")	Inguinal ligament	Dysesthesia and numbness to upper thigh, improves over several weeks with looser clothing
Common peroneal nerve	Proximal fibula	Numbness to web space between great and second toe Footdrop

MONONEURITIS MULTIPLEX

Mononeuropathy multiplex is characterized by the presence of multiple mononeuropathies. Unlike isolated mononeuropathies, it is not due to compression/trauma.

Etiologies

- Most common = diabetes mellitus
- Most serious = vasculitis (must be considered in all cases)
- Others include inflammatory/autoimmune disorders, Lyme disease (late), HIV, toxic, neoplastic

Differential

- **Plexopathies:** On detailed examination, these can be mapped to the brachial or lumbosacral plexus.
  - Symptoms will involve distal and proximal extremity.
  - May be due to trauma, radiation, malignancy, viral infection (lumbosacral).

Symptoms/Examination

Pain and weakness in multiple peripheral nerves (eg, sciatic, common peroneal, radial, femoral)

- Asymmetric

Diagnosis

- Electrodiagnostic studies
- Sural nerve biopsy if diagnosis in question

TREATMENT

- Treat underlying disorder (eg, steroids for vasculitis).
- Treat associated neuropathic pain (eg, amitriptyline, carbamazepine, gabapentin).

AMYOTROPHIC LATERAL SCLEROSIS

Amyotrophic lateral sclerosis (ALS) is a disorder characterized by upper motor neuron disease in addition to lower motor neuron pathology.

PATHOPHYSIOLOGY

- Anterior horn cell neuronopathy → peripheral nerve findings
- Loss of Betz cells in the CNS motor cortex → upper motor neuron findings

SYMPTOMS/EXAMINATION

- Lower motor neuron involvement
  - Muscle fasciculations and atrophy
  - Muscle cramps
  - Asymmetric distal weakness
- Upper motor neuron involvement
  - Hyperreflexia and clonus
  - Spasticity
  - Positive Babinski
- Serious complications and/or death result from progressive respiratory muscle weakness (→ respiratory failure) or dysphagia (→ aspiration). ↑ risk with forced vital capacity < 25 mL/kg

DIAGNOSIS

Electrodiagnostic testing

TREATMENT

- Supportive therapy
- Riluzole: Modulates glutamate metabolism

MYASTHENIA GRAVIS

Myasthenia gravis is an autoimmune disorder of the neuromuscular junction.

PATHOPHYSIOLOGY

- Antibodies against acetylcholine receptors at the neuromuscular junction → destruction of receptors → decrease in available receptors
- Associated with thymomas (25%)

SYMPTOMS/EXAMINATION

- Fatigable muscle weakness.
  - Repeated muscle use increases weakness (vs Lambert-Eaton myasthenic syndrome where repeated muscle use improves strength).
  - Weakness is improved after rest.

Q

A 37-year-old woman presents to the ED complaining of double vision and fatigue. Patient has a history of myasthenia gravis and recently completed a course of erythromycin for bronchitis. Patient is also noted to have ptosis and proximal muscle weakness on examination. What is the likely cause of her symptoms?

KEY FACT

The hallmark of ALS is the presence of both upper motor neuron and lower motor neuron signs and symptoms.

- Ocular muscle weakness is common → ptosis, diplopia, blurred vision.
- Dysarthria and dysphagia may be present.
- Exacerbated by heat, improved by cold.
- **Acute myasthenic crisis** = respiratory failure requiring mechanical ventilation.
  - Triggers include infection, medications.

DIFFERENTIAL

- Lambert-Eaton myasthenic syndrome
- Botulism
  - Often known as "the great imitator" due to similarities with multiple neurologic disorders of different etiologies

DIAGNOSIS

- Suspect based on clinical examination.
- Edrophonium (Tensilon) test:
  - Edrophonium is a short-acting acetylcholinesterase blocking agent → increased acetylcholine available at neuromuscular junction → improvement in measured ptosis (and other symptoms).
  - Test dose must be administered first to ensure that cholinergic crisis will not be induced. Cholinergic crisis from excess anticholinesterase inhibitors can present with flaccid paralysis and is difficult to distinguish from myasthenic crisis.
  - Have atropine ready in case of excessive cholinergic symptoms.
- Serologic testing for acetylcholine receptor antibodies.
- Electromyographic testing.
- Consider medications as cause for inducing myasthenic crisis: Certain antibiotics (macrolides, fluoroquinolones, aminoglycosides), antidysrhythmics (Ca channel blockers, β-blockers), as well as many others (lithium, levothyroxine, or paradoxical reaction to steroids).

TREATMENT

- Cholinesterase inhibitors → increased circulating acetylcholine → symptom control.
  - Pyridostigmine, neostigmine.
  - Should NOT be used during myasthenic crisis!
  - Excessive administration → cholinergic crisis with **weakness**, tachycardia, excessive secretions, etc.
- Immunosuppressive agents for chronic control.
- Thymectomy:
  - May induce early or late (2-5 years) remission of disease
- Plasmapheresis (plasma exchange) and intravenous immunoglobulin (IVIG) for acute exacerbations.
- Succinylcholine is safe in myasthenic crisis, but increased doses are needed.

LAMBERT-EATON MYASTHENIC SYNDROME

Lambert-Eaton myasthenic syndrome is an autoimmune disorder of the neuromuscular junction. About half the time it is associated with cancer (small cell carcinoma of the lung, lymphoma).

PATHOPHYSIOLOGY

Antibodies → inadequate release of acetylcholine at neuromuscular junctions → symptoms

---

A

This patient likely has an acute exacerbation of her myasthenia induced by recent administration of erythromycin. Several antibiotics as well as multiple other medications have similar effects. Use caution when prescribing to patients with known myasthenia gravis.

KEY FACT

Differential of ptosis: Myasthenia gravis, CN3 palsy, Horner syndrome.

KEY FACT

Myasthenia gravis: Muscle weakness, worse with repeated use and commonly involving ocular muscles; treat with cholinesterase inhibitors and immunosuppressive agents.

Ice pack test: Ice pack on eyelid will improve ptosis in Myasthenia gravis patients.

KEY FACT

Acute myasthenic crisis: Acute ventilatory failure, requiring mechanical ventilation; treat with plasma exchange and/or IV. Often times, early use of BiPAP may decrease need for intubation and minimize complications.

Symptoms/Examination

- Proximal (primarily leg) muscle weakness that improves with repeated stimulation
- Autonomic symptoms (dry mouth, impotence)

Diagnosis

- Clinical presentation
- Electrodiagnostic testing

Treatment

- Treat underlying malignancy, when present.
- Immunosuppressive agents.
- Plasmapheresis and IVIG, if severe.

> **KEY FACT**
>
> **Lambert-Eaton myasthenic syndrome:** Proximal muscle weakness that improves with repeated stimulation; treat with immunosuppressive agents or plasmapheresis/IVIG, if severe.

BOTULISM

Botulism is a toxin-mediated disorder of the neuromuscular junction.

Pathophysiology

- Toxin produced by *Clostridium botulinum* → presynaptic inhibition of acetylcholine release at the neuromuscular junction.
  - Infants may ingest spores (**honey is a common agent**) → bacteria germinate in GI tract and produces toxin.

Symptoms/Examination

- Onset 6-48 hours after ingestion of toxin or *C botulinum* spores.
- Nausea, vomiting, abdominal cramps.
- Classic presentation = descending flaccid paralysis.
  - Diplopia, dysarthria, and dysphagia occur early.
  - Progresses to generalized weakness; ventilatory failure may occur.
  - May last for months.
  - In children, may present as constipation, feeding difficulty, and hypotonia.
- Other anticholinergic symptoms may be present (dry skin, dilated pupils, increased temperature, constipation, urinary retention).
- Infantile botulism → lethargy, weakness/floppiness, poor feeding.

Diagnosis

- Clinical suspicion
- Electrodiagnostic testing
- Botulinum toxin testing of serum and stool

Treatment

- Supportive care
- Horse serum antitoxin

TICK PARALYSIS

Tick paralysis is a toxin-mediated disorder of the neuromuscular junction. Symptoms begin approximately 2-6 days after tick attachment.

Pathophysiology

Tick toxin → decreased release of acetylcholine at neuromuscular junction → symptoms

> **KEY FACT**
>
> **Botulism:** Descending flaccid paralysis with diplopia, dysarthria, and dysphagia occurring early; treat with horse serum antitoxin.

Symptoms/Examination

Symmetric ascending paralysis

Differential

Other disorders at neuromuscular junction (GBS, botulism, myasthenia)

Diagnosis

Based on finding an attached feeding tick

Treatment

- Supportive
- Remove tick: Resolution of symptoms ranges from hours to days

POLYMYOSITIS/DERMATOMYOSITIS

Polymyositis and dermatomyositis are both **inflammatory myopathies** of autoimmune etiology that produce muscle weakness. Dermatomyositis can occur in children.

Symptoms/Examination

- Chronic symmetric proximal muscle weakness.
- Muscle pain and tenderness.
- Dermatomyositis has additional skin findings, including photosensitivity and extensor rashes.

Diagnosis

- Electromyography and muscle biopsy confirm diagnosis.
- CK may (or may not) be elevated.
- Significant rhabdomyolysis is unlikely.

Treatment

Oral prednisone or cytotoxic drugs

PERIODIC PARALYSIS

Periodic paralysis is a disorder characterized by generalized muscle weakness due to muscle ion channel abnormalities.

- Hyperkalemic and hypokalemic periodic paralysis:
  - Most common
  - Familial
- Hyperthyroid periodic paralysis:
  - Secondary to related hypokalemia

Symptoms/Examination

- Episodic muscle weakness of rapid onset.
- Flaccid paralysis of extremities.
- Limited bulbar and ocular involvement.
- Ventilatory failure is uncommon.

DIAGNOSIS

- Clinical diagnosis is based on personal and/or family history of similar episodes.
- ECG may show findings consistent with hyper- or hypokalemia.
- Serum K^+ levels.

TREATMENT

- Supportive care.
- Treat underlying electrolyte abnormalities (not overzealous potassium repletion because problem is potassium shift, not potassium depletion).
- Treat hyperthyroidism, if present.

Multiple Sclerosis

PATHOPHYSIOLOGY

Genetic and environmental factors → inflammatory reaction → regions of CNS demyelination with sparing of axons. Onset common in third decade of life. Incidence in females three times greater than in males. Twice as common in Caucasians as in African Americans.

SYMPTOMS/EXAMINATION

- Relapsing/remitting: Characterized by episodic neurologic dysfunction that begins rapidly, then slowly resolves.
- May involve any aspect of the CNS (cranial nerve findings, motor weakness, cerebellar dysfunction, cognitive changes, bowel/bladder dysfunction).
  - Lower extremities > Upper extremities
  - ↓ strength, ↓ vibration/proprioception, ↑ tone, ↑ reflexes, (+) Babinski
- **Optic neuritis** is often the presenting finding and is the most common cranial nerve finding; it is characterized by eye pain that is worse with eye movement followed by scotoma of central vision.
- **Afferent Pupillary Defect (Marcus-Gunn Pupil): Swing bright light back and forth and affected eye/pupil will paradoxically dilate.**
- **Internuclear ophthalmoplegia:** Abnormalities in eye adduction bilaterally associated with horizontal nystagmus; may also be seen (less commonly) in brainstem vascular lesions, hypertensive crisis, trauma, cocaine use, and SLE.
- **Uhthoff phenomenon:** Small increases in body temperature (eg, exercise, fever) → worsened symptoms (visual symptoms often most affected).
- **Lhermitte phenomenon:** Electric shock sensation down spine with flexion of neck (common with all cervical myelopathies (disc bulge, spinal stenosis, etc).

DIAGNOSIS

- Suspect in patients with two episodes of differing neurologic symptoms occurring at different times.
- MRI may show multiple white matter lesions (better than CT).
- Lumbar puncture: CSF cell counts, protein, and glucose are typically normal; CSF may show oligoclonal bands of IgG and/or myelin-based proteins.

TREATMENT

- High-dose methylprednisolone burst with taper for acute exacerbations
- β-Interferon, azathioprine

Q

A 30-year-old woman presents to the ED complaining of pain with eye movement and visual changes in her right eye. She denies trauma or other complaints. Upon further investigation, the patient reports transient episodes of hand or leg weakness over the past few years. She has never seen a physician for this. On examination, the pupillary response to light is decreased in the affected eye and funduscopic examination shows a blurred optic disc. What is the treatment for this patient's presenting illness?

KEY FACT

Multiple sclerosis: Neurologic symptoms separated by "space and time."

A

This patient likely has MS and is presenting with optic neuritis. IV (not oral) steroids is the recommended treatment.

Parkinson Disease

Parkinson disease is a chronic neurodegenerative disease of the elderly resulting from damage to dopaminergic neurons in the substantia nigra. Environmental and genetic factors play a role.

MNEMONIC

Parkinson disease findings:

TRAP

Tremor
Rigidity
Akinesia
Postural instability

Symptoms/Examination

- Four characteristic findings:
  - Resting tremor ("pill-rolling")
  - Cogwheel rigidity
  - Bradykinesia or akinesia
  - Postural instability
- Other common findings include depression, muscle aches/fatigue, akathisia, paresthesias.

Diagnosis

- Based on clinical findings.
- CT/MRI is not definitive.

Treatment

- Agents to increase CNS dopamine and anticholinergics to decrease central muscarinic activity; see Chapter 6, Toxicology.
- Drug "holidays" of 1 week may be used as effectiveness diminishes over time.

Complications

- Include dementia, falls, DVT/PE, aspiration
- Caution with psychotropics (haloperidol) → may cause tardive dyskinesia

REVIEW QUESTIONS

QUESTIONS

1. A patient presents with diplopia, unilateral ptosis, inability to adduct the eye, with intact pupillary responses to light. The most likely diagnosis is:
   A. Botulism
   B. Multiple sclerosis
   C. Diabetic mononeuropathy
   D. Aneurysm of posterior communicating artery

2. A 50-year-old man presents with bilateral peripheral facial nerve paralysis after 2 weeks after returning from a week long hunting trip. He has no other neurological deficits. What is the likely pathogen?
   A. Herpes virus
   B. Dermacentor andersoni
   C. *Rickettsia rickettsii*
   D. *Borrelia burgdorferi*

3. A 60-year-old man is brought in by his wife after having a seizure at home. She states he has had a sinus infection with headache and nausea and has been acting odd for the past week. Patient is obtunded and sluggish. A contrast-enhanced CT is obtained (Figure 15.8).

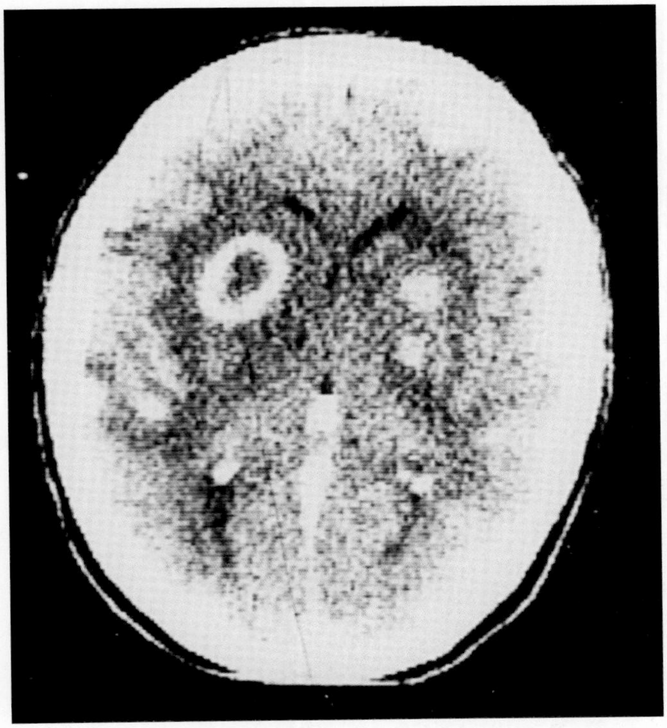

FIGURE 15.8. Contrast CT demonstrating classic ring enhancing lesions of a brain abscess. (Reproduced, with permission, from Ropper AH, Samuels MA: *Adams & Victor's Principles of Neurology*. 9th ed. New York, McGraw-Hill, 2009.)

   Which of the following statements is correct?
   A. Corticosteroids are contraindicated.
   B. Delayed surgical decompression after a 24-hour course of antibiotics is preferred.
   C. Recommended antibiotic choice is metronidazole and a cephalosporin.
   D. Less than 10% patients have long-term sequelae.

4. A 38-year-old man with diabetes presents with headache and right eye pain. His headache is sharp, isolated to the R face and is progressively worse over 2 days. He recently underwent a root canal for a complicated dental abscess. Which of the following examination findings suggest serious intracranial complication of a dental abscess?
   A. Right-sided facial paralysis
   B. Lateral gaze palsy of the right eye
   C. Right-sided ptosis, miosis, and loss of sweating
   D. The presence of an afferent pupil defect in the right eye

5. Which of the following is true about vertigo?
   A. Vertical nystagmus almost always represents peripheral vertigo
   B. Nystagmus in central vertigo can change directions
   C. Nausea and vomiting are classically associated with central vertigo
   D. Patients with either peripheral or central vertigo have similar difficulty with ataxia

ANSWERS

1. **C.** Diabetic mononeuropathy. Diabetic mononeuropathy of the third cranial nerve presents with ptosis, inability to adduct, depress, or elevate the eye. Patient presents with complaint diplopia. Pupillary sparing occurs because there is infarction of the central portion of the oculomotor nerve with sparing of the more peripheral fibers that medicate constriction. An aneurysm of the posterior communicating artery would push on the peripheral fibers of the oculomotor nerve causing pupillary dilation.

2. **D.** *B burgdorferi*. The most common cause of bilateral peripheral seventh cranial nerve palsy is infection with *B burgdorferi* which causes Lyme disease. HIV, sarcoidosis, and infectious mononucleosis can also cause bilateral facial nerve palsy. The most common cause of unilateral facial nerve palsy is herpes virus. Dermacentor andersoni causes tick paralysis. *R rickettsii* causes Rocky Mountain spotted fever.

3. **C.** The recommended antibiotic choice is metronidazole plus a cephalosporin. This head CT scan shows ring-enhancing lesions of a brain abscess. **Between** 30% and 50% of patients suffer long-term sequelae (seizures, motor deficits, cognitive delay).When signs of herniation are present (obtundation, sluggish pupils, bradycardia, bradypnea, and hypertension), aggressive treatment to decrease intracranial pressure should be undertaken. This includes hyperventilation, mannitol administration, and the use of corticosteroids to decrease swelling. This is the only situation in which corticosteroids should be used in patients with brain abscess. Use of antibiotics should not delay surgery. Empiric antibiotic coverage should be started. For this patient with an ENT or oral source, a combination of a cephalosporin and metronidazole should be used. In patients with no known source, vancomycin should be added to cover MRSA.

4. **B.** Lateral gaze palsy in the right eye. The question describes a patient with a cavernous sinus thrombosis (CST) secondary to his dental infection. Cranial nerves 2, 3, 4, and 6 run through the cavernous sinus. CN6 is the first to be affected as it floats freely in the sinus. Choice A describes Bell palsy; choice C describes Horner syndrome. An afferent pupil defect (choice D) is uncommon and unusual in CST.

5. **B.** Nystagmus in central vertigo may change direction. Both central and bidirectional nystagmus represent central vertigo. Patients with peripheral causes of vertigo classically present with significant nausea and vomiting. Patients with central nystagmus typically cannot walk or take a single step without falling. In contrast, patient with peripheral vertigo can usually walk even in the acute phase of their illness.

CHAPTER 16

Psychobehavioral Disorders

Cameron G. Isaacs, MD, HO-1

The DSM-IV Classification

The DSM-IV (*Diagnostic and Statistical Manual of Mental Disorders*, 4th edition) classification aids in making a comprehensive assessment of disease and in organizing complex clinical disorders.

Axis I: Clinical syndromes of mental disorders (eg, schizophrenia, depression)
Axis II: Personality disorders and developmental disorders
Axis III: General medical conditions (eg, diabetes, hypertension)
Axis IV: Psychosocial and environmental stressors or problems
Axis V: Global assessment of functioning

The Emergency Care of Psychiatric Patients

KEY FACT

The presence of dangerousness without severe mental illness is not sufficient to involuntarily hospitalize a patient. Such persons are the responsibility of the police, NOT the psychiatrist!

INDICATIONS FOR SECLUSION AND RESTRAINT

- To prevent clear and imminent harm to patient or others
- To decrease sensory overstimulation
- To prevent significant disruption to treatment program and physical surroundings
- To assist in treatment as part of ongoing behavioral therapy
- To comply with patient's voluntary reasonable request

INDICATIONS FOR INVOLUNTARY HOSPITALIZATION/CIVIL COMMITMENT

- Mental illness with impaired self-control, judgment, and/or discretion
- Dangerousness to self or others in the setting of mental illness
- Grave disability, ie, inability to provide basic needs of food, clothing, and shelter

KEY FACT

A patient likely to sign out against medical advice (AMA) should be involuntarily hospitalized if the clinician believes the criteria for involuntary commitment have been met.

ACUTE MANAGEMENT OF THE VIOLENT PATIENT

- Assess risk to self and staff
- Secure a safe environment (eg individual room, remove belongings and dangerous objects).
- Verbal redirection to avoid escalation of behavior
- Physical restraint (Change position frequently and monitor for neurovascular injury)
- Chemical restraint, typically with short-acting benzodiazepines (eg lorazepam, midazolam) and/or antipsychotics (eg haloperidol)
- Address underlying cause (organic vs functional) of patient behavior

The Suicidal Patient

The majority of persons who commit suicide have seen a health care provider within 2 weeks of their death, making identification of those at high risk essential for all health care providers.

Diagnosis/Treatment

- Assess risk of suicide in any patient who presents with a problem related to chronic alcoholism, substance abuse, or other psychiatric disorder.

TABLE 16.1. Risk Factors for Suicide

Demographics	Male gender, white race, adolescent or age > 65 y old
Medical history	Chronic pain or illness (eg, diabetes, coronary artery disease), terminal illness, history of physical or sexual abuse
Psychiatric history	Major depression, bipolar disorder, schizophrenia, panic disorder, borderline personality disorder, history of previous suicide attempts
Family history	Family violence, suicide attempts, substance abuse
Social history	Divorced, lives alone, unemployed, homeless, recent personal loss, lack of religious or community involvement, access to firearms

Q

A 65-year-old white man with a history of hypertension and diabetes presents to the emergency department (ED) with "depression." He is divorced, lives alone, and states he was "getting by" until recently losing his job. Since then, he has started to drink more heavily due to anxiety and difficulty sleeping, and he is feeling hopeless about finding a new job to support himself. He denies any history of mental illness but his sister suffers from depression and has had multiple previous suicide attempts. What is his risk for suicidality?

- When assessing risk of suicide, consider lethality of plan and the presence of underlying mental health, medical and psychosocial risk factors (Table 16.1).
- The SAD PERSONS mnemonic (Table 16.2) is a useful screening tool in the emergency department.
- Persons deemed high risk need further emergency psychiatric evaluation ± hospitalization.

TABLE 16.2. SAD PERSONS Scale

Factor	Points
Sex (male)	1
Age (< 19 or > 45 y)	1
Depression or hopelessness	2
Previous suicide attempts or psychiatric care	1
Excessive alcohol or drug use	1
Rational thinking loss	2
Separated, divorced or widowed	1
Organized or serious attempt	2
No social supports	1
Stated future intent	2

(Reproduced with permission from William M. Patterson, Henry H. Dohn, Julian Bird, Gary A. Patterson, Evaluation of suicidal patients: The SAD PERSONS scale. *Psychosomatics* 1983 Apr;24(4):343.)

Score of 6-8: Full emergency psychiatric evaluation/treatment.

Score of 9 or greater: Immediate psychiatric hospitalization.

A

High! He has numerous risk factors (see the following text). This patient should be screened extensively for suicidal ideation and may need urgent psychiatric evaluation.

Mood and Thought Disorders

MOOD DISORDERS

Major Depression

Major depression affects 10%-25% of women and 5%-12% of men. If untreated, the lifetime risk of suicide is 15%. Risk factors include recent stressors, postpartum state, family history, early childhood trauma, and lack of daylight exposure (seasonal affective disorder).

Pathophysiology

Decrease in central nervous system (CNS) monoamine (ie, serotonin, dopamine, and norepinephrine) activity.

Symptoms/Examination

- Depressed mood (or irritability in children and adolescents) and/or loss of interest or pleasure along with 4 or more of the following depressive symptoms (Figure 16.1):
  - Change in weight (unintentional) or appetite
  - Change in sleep (insomnia or hypersomnia)
  - Psychomotor agitation or retardation
  - Fatigue or loss of energy
  - Feelings of worthlessness or guilt
  - Decreased concentration or indecisiveness
  - Recurrent thoughts of death or suicide
- In older patients, depression may present with memory loss, inattention, social withdrawal, confusion, and poor hygiene, known as *pseudodementia*.

Differential

- Dementia, hypothyroidism, metabolic conditions, substance abuse, bereavement, adjustment disorder
- Dysthymic disorder: Persistent depressed mood for > 2 years that does not meet criteria for major depression and has no symptom-free period lasting > 2 months.

Diagnosis

Symptoms (1) must be present almost every day for at least 2 weeks; (2) must be associated with significant impairment in daily functioning; and (3) must NOT be due to general medical condition (eg, hypothyroidism) or substance abuse.

IN SAD CAGES

Interest
Sleep
Appetite
Depressed mood
Concentration
Activity
Guilt
Energy
Suicidality

FIGURE 16.1. Symptoms of Major Depression.

TREATMENT

- Screen all patients for suicide: Use SAD PERSONS scale for risk stratification (see Table 16.2).
- Important risk factors include access to firearms, previous attempts, and substance abuse.
- Admit all suicidal patients and patients at high risk for suicide. Otherwise, treat with antidepressants (starting treatment in ED is controversial) and close follow-up/therapy.

Grief Reaction

Grief and bereavement are normal after the loss of a loved one.

SYMPTOMS/EXAMINATION

- Normal grief reactions may include: shock, numbness, intense sadness, insomnia, and loss of appetite; physical sensations such as chest tightness, sighing, weakness, and fatigue; and transient hallucinations (eg, seeing or hearing loved one briefly).
- Individuals with persistent depressed mood, anhedonia, and feelings of self-worthlessness or self-loathing should be evaluated for concurrent major depression.
- Severe symptoms typically resolve after 2 months and moderate symptoms after 1 year.
- Prolonged symptoms (> 1 year) that include marked functional impairment, morbid preoccupation with the deceased, suicidal ideation, psychotic symptoms, and psychomotor retardation are abnormal and should prompt immediate psychiatric evaluation.

TREATMENT

Similar to major depression (see previously).

Bipolar Disorder

Lifelong disease characterized by periods of extreme mood episodes.

PATHOPHYSIOLOGY

Poorly understood, likely due to genetic and environmental influences.

SYMPTOMS/EXAMINATION

- Manic episode is characterized by an elevated, expansive or irritable mood with at least 3 of the following (4 if the mood is only irritable):
  - Inflated self-esteem or grandiosity
  - Decreased need for sleep
  - Frequent or pressured speech
  - Flight of ideas/racing thoughts
  - Distractibility
  - Increased goal-directed activity
  - Excessive involvement in pleasurable activities (eg, shopping, sexual indiscretion)
- Depressive episode is characterized by symptoms of major depression.
- Mixed episode is characterized by symptoms of both mania and major depression.
- Hypomanic episode is characterized by symptoms of mania without marked impairment in daily function, need for hospitalization, or psychotic features.

Differential

- Temporal lobe epilepsy, hyperthyroidism, substance abuse (eg, cocaine, phencyclidine [PCP], amphetamines), dementia, psychotic disorders
- Cyclothymia: Life-long mood swings insufficient to meet formal criteria for bipolar disorder, typically with lives of unstable relationships and uneven school or work performance

Diagnosis

- Symptoms (1) must be for at least 2 weeks; (2) must be associated with significant impairment in daily functioning; and (3) must NOT be due to general medical condition (eg, hyperthyroidism) or substance abuse.
- Bipolar I: One or more manic episode(s) cycling with depressive episodes
- Bipolar II: One or more hypomanic episode(s) cycling with depressive episodes

Treatment

- All patients with acute mania, suicidality, or psychosis require inpatient admission.
- First-line treatment is with mood stabilizers (eg lithium, valproic acid, lamotrigine).
- The use of antidepressants is controversial due to concern for precipitating mania.

THOUGHT DISORDERS

Group of disorders characterized by disorganized thinking and behavior.

Acute Psychosis

Disturbed perception of reality characterized by delusions, hallucinations, and disorganized speech or behavior.

Symptoms/Examination

- Delusions: erroneous beliefs that involve misinterpretation of perceptions or experiences
- Hallucinations: sensory experience that exists only in the mind of the person experiencing it; may be auditory, visual, olfactory, gustatory, or tactile
- Catatonic behavior: Motor immobility and unresponsiveness to external stimuli
- Disorganized speech: Loosening of associations (rapid switching from topic to unrelated topic), neologisms (nonsense words invented by patient), perseverations, word salad
- Disorganized behavior: Unpredictable agitation and absence of goal-directed behavior

Differential

Hypercarbia, hypoxia, hyponatremia, hypoglycemia, meningitis, encephalitis, hepatic encephalopathy, uremia, dementia, normal pressure hydrocephalus, hyperthyroidism

Diagnosis

- Clinical findings may help differentiate organic from functional psychosis (Table 16.3).
- If organic etiology is suspected, complete medical workup for altered mental status: complete blood count, serum electrolytes, urinalysis, consider thyroid and liver studies

TABLE 16.3. Symptoms of Organic vs Functional Causes of Psychosis

	Organic (Medical)	Functional (Psychiatric)
Memory deficits	Abrupt, recent onset	Remote onset
Activity	Psychomotor retardation, tremor	Posturing, rocking, repetitive
Distortions	Visual hallucinations	Auditory hallucinations
Feelings	Labile	Flat
Orientation	Disoriented	Oriented
Cognition	Able to focus, periods of lucidity, wax and wane during course of day	Unable to focus, continuous symptoms
Some others	Age > 35, abnormal vitals, abnormal physical examination, history of substance abuse	Age < 35, normal vital signs, awake and alert

(Modified, with permission, from Frame DS, Kercher EE "Acute psychosis: functional vs organic." *Emergency Medicine Clinic North America* 1991;9:123.)

- Head computed tomography (CT) and/or lumbar puncture for abnormal neurological examination or concern for CNS infection
- Psychiatric diagnosis is based on clinical criteria:
  - Brief psychotic disorder: Psychotic symptoms lasting > 1 day but < 1 month
  - Schizophreniform disorder: Psychotic symptoms lasting > 1 month but < 6 months
  - Schizophrenia: Psychotic symptoms present ≥ 6 months (see the following text)
  - Delusional disorder: Non-bizarre delusions (eg involving situations that occur in real life, such as being followed, poisoned, etc) lasing > 1 month without functional impairment
  - Mood disorder with psychotic features: Psychosis during mood episode only
  - Schizoaffective disorder: Mood episode plus psychosis, with psychosis present at least 2 weeks prior to onset of mood episode

Treatment

- Treat organic cause if found (nutritional replacement, antibiotics, correction of electrolytes).
- Any patient with new-onset psychosis needs to be evaluated by a psychiatrist and/or admitted after organic causes are ruled out.
- A patient who presents with psychotic disorder has a high risk of suicide and should be screened before discharge.

SCHIZOPHRENIA

Schizophrenia is characterized by periods of active psychosis and diminished personal, intellectual, and social functioning.

Pathophysiology

- Poorly understood, may be due to decreased dopamine activity in the mesocortical system (negative symptoms), and increased activity in the mesolimbic system (positive symptoms)

Q

A 21-year-old man is brought to the ED by his mother for "bizarre behavior." Over the last 7 months, the patient has gone from being an energetic, "straight A" student to failing out of his undergraduate classes and refusing to leave his room. Over the last several weeks, his mother has heard him speaking to himself about "the day of doom." She recently discovered marijuana in his room and is concerned that he is now a "drug addict." In the ED, the patient appears withdrawn, paranoid, and refuses to make eye contact. His conjunctivae are injected bilaterally and he smells of marijuana. What evaluation does this patient require?

A

Although the patient's symptoms may be related to marijuana abuse, his greater than 6-month history of functional decline and withdrawal is concerning for the prodromal stage of schizophrenia, and he is now displaying positive signs of possible auditory hallucinations and delusions. Inpatient psychiatric evaluation is appropriate.

- Associated with mild ventricular enlargement and decreased volume in medial temporal lobes
- Available evidence suggests that marijuana use is an independent risk factor for schizophrenia in genetically susceptible individuals

Symptoms/Examination

- Positive symptoms: Delusions, hallucinations, disorganized speech, or behavior
- Negative symptoms: Flat affect, poverty of speech, social withdrawal, inability to achieve goal-directed tasks
- Symptoms may vary depending on the course of illness (Table 16.4).

Differential

- Same as for acute psychosis
- Schizoid personality disorder: Voluntary social withdrawal with no signs of psychosis
- Schizotypal personality disorder: Odd, magical thinking with no signs of psychosis

Diagnosis

- Patient must have 6 months of continuous signs of disturbance with at least 1 month of 2 or more active symptoms (delusions, hallucinations, disorganized speech, disorganized behavior, or negative symptoms). Only 1 symptom is required if delusions are bizarre or hallucinations consist of a running commentary.
- Patient must have a marked deterioration from prior level of functioning and symptoms must not be caused by substance abuse, medication, or general medical condition.

Treatment

- First, ensure staff and patient safety. Rapid tranquilization with antipsychotics may be necessary. Consider adjunctive treatment with benzodiazepines for continued agitation or as first line for catatonia.
- Outpatient management varies depending on the stage of illness (see Table 16.4).

TABLE 16.4. Signs and Symptoms of Schizophrenia

Phase	Signs/Symptoms	Treatment
Prodromal phase	**"Negative" symptoms** with decline in personal, intellectual, and social functioning	Experimental studies designed to train patients in appropriate social behavior
Active phase	**"Positive" symptoms**: Active delusions and hallucinations, very disorganized; likely time of presentation to ED	Antipsychotic medications, possible inpatient admit, group therapy
Residual phase	Between episodes of psychosis: continued negative symptoms, low-level positive symptoms	Outpatient and group therapy, antipsychotics

COMPLICATIONS

- Estimated 5%-10% lifetime risk of completing suicide, often at onset of symptoms
- High prevalence of concurrent substance abuse (40%-50%), most commonly nicotine and marijuana
- Long-term use of antipsychotics can cause extrapyramidal symptoms and/or neuroleptic malignant syndrome.

Anxiety Disorders

Anxiety disorders are a group of conditions characterized by a sense of fear or apprehension accompanied by physical symptoms. They range from common phobias to disabling panic or generalized anxiety disorders.

SYMPTOMS/EXAMINATION

- The symptoms of various anxiety disorders are described in Table 16.5.
- Physical manifestations of anxiety include autonomic arousal (tachypnea, tachycardia, diaphoresis, lightheadedness), chest pain, palpitations, shortness of breath, dry mouth, difficulty swallowing, epigastric pain, tremor, muscle cramps, and headache.

DIFFERENTIAL

- Numerous medical conditions can present with symptoms of anxiety, and up to 40% of patients presenting with anxiety ultimately have an underlying medical condition.

KEY FACT

Onset of anxiety symptoms after age 35 without any personal or family history, absence of obvious trigger, and poor response to medications make an organic etiology more likely.

TABLE 16.5. Anxiety Disorders

DISORDER	SYMPTOMS/EXAMINATION	TREATMENT
Panic attack	Discrete period of sudden onset of intense apprehension, fear, terror.	Verbal deescalation/reassurance, benzodiazepines
GAD	6 mo of persistent and excessive anxiety/worry about a broad range of topics.	CBT, group therapy, **long-acting benzodiazepines**, buspirone, SSRI
Panic disorder	Recurrent, unexpected panic attacks AND at least 1 mo of worry (or behavior modification) surrounding the attacks or over subsequent attacks.	SSRI, short-acting benzodiazepines, β-blockers, desensitization, "flooding" therapy (CBT)
Phobic disorder	Significant anxiety provoked by exposure to a **specific feared object** or situation. Leads to avoidance behavior.	CBT (exposure-response prevention therapy), desensitization, SSRI, short-acting benzodiazepines, β-blockers (eg, propranolol)
OCD	Repetitive thoughts (obsessions) that cause marked anxiety or distress and lead to mannerisms (compulsions) that serve to neutralize and relieve anxiety.	CBT (exposure-response prevention therapy), SSRI, clomipramine; higher doses than those for depression usually required
Post-traumatic stress disorder	Reexperiencing an extremely traumatic event associated with symptoms of: increased arousal, hypervigilance, and avoidance of stimuli associated with the trauma. **Patients typically have no history of panic attacks.**	CBT, individual/group therapy (especially helpful), SSRI, sleep agents, long-acting benzodiazepines.

CBT, cognitive behavioral therapy; GAD, generalized anxiety disorder; OCD, obsessive compulsive disorder; SSRI, selective serotonin reuptake inhibitor.

- Etiologies may include: acute coronary syndrome, asthma, congestive heart failure, hyperthyroidism, hypoglycemia, cerebrovascular accident, sympathomimetic intoxication, alcohol, or sedative/hypnotic withdrawal.

DIAGNOSIS/TREATMENT

The diagnosis and treatment of various anxiety disorders are listed in Table 16.4.

Somatoform Disorders

Somatoform disorders are conditions in which psychological stress is expressed as physical symptoms. In contrast to factitious disorders (see in the next section), symptoms are not intentionally produced or faked.

SYMPTOMS/EXAMINATION

- Various physical complaints that are not explained by an underlying medical condition
- Patients may not be able to recall the life event precipitating their psychological stress.
- Patients are often convinced there is a physical problem despite evidence to the contrary.

DIAGNOSIS

SOMATIZATION DISORDER

- History of medically unexplained physical symptoms beginning before age 30
- Presence of all of the following at any time during disorder: (1) 4 pain symptoms (different sites or body functions), (2) 2 gastrointestinal (GI) tract symptoms, (3) 1 sexual symptom, and (4) 1 pseudoneurologic symptom

> **KEY FACT**
>
> "La belle indifference" refers to an apparent lack of concern shown by patients with conversion disorder toward their symptoms.

CONVERSION DISORDER

- Abnormalities or deficits in voluntary motor or sensory function that are not medically explained (eg, pseudoseizures, pseudoparalysis, movement disorders, blindness)
- Symptoms do not fit an anatomic distribution or diagnosis
- Most commonly occurs in young, uneducated women and is associated with comorbid mood and anxiety disorders as well as a history of physical or sexual abuse

PAIN DISORDER

Persistent pain in one or more anatomic site(s) that limits daily functioning and cannot be pathophysiologically explained

HYPOCHONDRIASIS

- Preoccupation with the belief that one has a serious medical disease despite medical evaluation and physician reassurance
- Patients typically demonstrate physical symptoms disproportionate to any apparent organic disease, conviction that they have a serious medical illness, preoccupation with their body, and relentless pursuit of medical care, often with doctor shopping.

Treatment

- Acknowledge symptoms and attempt to provide reassurance via explanation of symptoms. Refrain from formerly labeling symptoms as psychosomatic.
- Avoid prescription of unnecessary and "as needed" medications.
- Refer to outpatient psychiatrist or therapist for "stress management," as patients are often reluctant to undergo psychiatric evaluation for the symptoms they perceive as organic.
- Primary goal is to establish care with compassionate primary care physician.

> **Q**
>
> A 15-year-old girl presents to the ED after seeing a friend hit by a car and reports sudden paralysis of her left leg. She was not involved in the accident. Her neurologic examination is significant for no voluntary movement of the left leg although sensation is intact. Upon motor examination, she has a positive thigh adductor test (when the examiner places his or her hands on the patient's bilateral inner thighs and asks her to adduct against resistance, both legs adduct). What is her diagnosis?

Factitious Disorders and Malingering

Group of disorders and behaviors in which patients intentionally cause, exaggerate, or feign illness for the purpose of securing some gain. In factitious disorders, patients intentionally create or exaggerate symptoms out of desire to assume the "sick role," known as primary gain. In malingering, patients create symptoms to secure some external motivator such as disability, avoiding jail or work time, pain medication, etc., known as *secondary gain*.

MALINGERING

Symptoms/Examination

- Feigning or creating symptoms for some secondary gain, which may be obvious (eg, patient is homeless or incarcerated), or more occult (eg, difficulties at home)
- Marked discrepancy between patient's complaints and objective findings, often with poor cooperation during examination and a history of nonadherence
- Common complaints include: headache, fibromyalgia, chronic fatigue syndrome, chronic pain, and dental pain.
- In drug-seeking behavior, patients may report multiple allergies to nonnarcotic medications for goal secondary gain of obtaining narcotics for themselves or for diversion.

MUNCHAUSEN SYNDROME

Symptoms/Examination

- Feigning or creating symptoms for primary gain of adopting the "sick role," with attention from nursing staff, physicians, etc.
- Patients often view themselves as important people, have extensive knowledge of medical terminology, and pathologically lie and romanticize about their own medical history (known as "pseudologica fantastica").
- Common complaints include: bleeding disorders (eg taking warfarin to induce bleeding), headaches, hypoglycemia (eg by injecting themselves with insulin), chest pain, dyspnea, renal colic, or other complaints with high admission rates.

MUNCHAUSEN SYNDROME BY PROXY

Symptoms/Examination

- Rare disorder in which an adult, most commonly the biological mother (98%), intentionally creates symptoms in a child (or rarely elderly person) in order to have contact with health care and to assume the role of the concerned caregiver (primary gain)

A

Conversion disorder.

- Symptoms may be simulated (eg, contaminating urine samples with blood) or produced (eg, administration of drugs or toxins such as warfarin, intentional chemical burns, asphyxiation)
- By definition, symptoms are present only when the perpetrator is immediately present
- Perpetrator is often friendly, manipulative, knowledgeable of health care, and eager to have invasive procedures performed on their child

Personality Disorders

Mental disorders characterized by long-lasting, rigid patterns of thought and behavior that cause significant distress and impairment in daily functioning (Table 16.6).

TABLE 16.6. Personality Disorders

Disorder	Characteristics
Paranoid	Pervasive distrust and suspicion that others are exploiting, harming, or deceiving him or her. Reluctant to confide in others and bears grudges easily.
Schizoid	Pervasive detachment from social relationships and restricted range of emotional expression. Neither desires nor enjoys close relationships and prefers solitude.
Schizotypal	Pervasive social and interpersonal deficits with reduced capacity for close relationships along with **cognitive** or **perceptual distortions** and **eccentricities**, such as **odd** or **magical thinking**. Does NOT meet criteria for schizophrenia.
Histrionic	Pervasive and excessive emotionality and attention-seeking. Consistently uses physical appearance to draw attention to self with inappropriate provocative behavior.
Narcissistic	Pervasive inflation of self-worth, pattern of grandiosity, and need for admiration. Believes that he or she is "special" and has a strong sense of entitlement.
Borderline	Pervasive instability of interpersonal relationships, self-image, and affects, with **marked impulsivity**, emotional lability, and compromised empathy and intimacy. Often associated with **recurrent suicidal behavior**, gestures, and **self-harm**.
Antisocial	Pervasive disregard for and violation of the rights of others. Marked deceitfulness, impulsivity, aggressiveness, and reckless disregard for safety of others with lack of remorse. High prevalence of **imprisonment**.
Avoidant	Pervasive social inhibition, feelings of inadequacy, and hypersensitivity to negative evaluation. Avoids interaction due to fear of criticism, disapproval, or rejection.
Dependent	Pervasive need to be taken care of leading to submissive and clinging behavior. Has difficulty making decisions without reassurance and excessive fears of being alone.
Obsessive-compulsive	Pervasive preoccupation with orderliness. Perfectionist at the expense of flexibility, openness, and efficiency.

Eating Disorders

Eating disorders have the highest mortality rate of any mental disorder and affect 5%-10% of women and at least 1% of men the United States.

ANOREXIA NERVOSA

Symptoms

- Refusal to maintain body weight at or above 85% of the age-adjusted expected body weight
- Intense fear of gaining weight or becoming fat despite being underweight
- Misperception of body weight, size, or shape
- Primary amenorrhea or absence of at least three consecutive menstrual cycles (secondary amenorrhea)
- Subtypes: restricting (eg excessive dieting, starvation), and binge eating/ purging (eg vomiting, laxatives, diuretics, excessive exercise)

Examination

- Orthostatic hypotension, bradycardia (often pronounced), hypothermia
- Loss of subcutaneous fat and muscle atrophy due to starvation ketosis
- Dry skin with lanugo, brittle hair and nails, acral cyanosis, pedal/pretibial edema
- Parotid hypertrophy due to excessive purging
- Peripheral neuropathy

Differential

New-onset diabetes, adrenal insufficiency, hypothyroidism, chronic pancreatitis, human immunodeficiency virus (HIV), pregnancy, malignancy, other chronic inflammatory conditions

Diagnosis

- Diagnosis is clinical based on history and examination
- Initial workup should screen for etiologies and complications of anorexia, including urinalysis, urine pregnancy test, serum electrolytes (with magnesium and phosphate), electrocardiogram (ECG), and thyroid-stimulating hormone.

Treatment

- Primary goal is rehydration, correction of electrolyte imbalances, and gradual refeeding
- Admit patients with severe malnutrition (< 75% ideal body weight), physiologic instability (HR < 50 bpm, BP < 80/50 mm Hg, orthostatic hypotension, T < 35.6°5), cardiac arrhythmias or myopathy, significant electrolyte abnormalities, underlying psychiatric concerns (suicidal ideation, obsessive-compulsive disorder [OCD], etc), lack of social support, or other medical complications of disease (eg, pancreatitis).
- Outpatient therapy includes psychotherapy (both individual and group) and antidepressants.
- Screen all anorexic patients for suicidal ideation prior to discharge.

COMPLICATIONS

- Amenorrhea, osteoporosis, osteopenia due to hypothalamic-pituitary axis abnormalities
- Cardiac arrhythmias, cardiomyopathy, significant electrolyte disturbances (hypokalemia, hyponatremia, hypoglycemia, contraction alkalosis), pancreatitis, glucose intolerance
- Refeeding syndrome: Reintroduction of food triggers metabolic increase with rapid consumption of already depleted electrolytes causing profound hypophosphatemia, hypokalemia, and hypomagnesemia with severe cardiopulmonary and neurologic sequelae.

BULIMIA NERVOSA

SYMPTOMS

- Episodes of binge eating with sense of loss of control followed by compensatory behaviors, either purging type (eg, self-induced vomiting, laxatives, diuretics) or nonpurging type (eg, excessive exercise, fasting, dieting)
- Binges and compensatory behavior at least twice per week for 3 or more months
- Dissatisfaction with body shape and weight
- Must NOT occur during episode of anorexia nervosa

EXAMINATION

- Parotid and submandibular gland enlargement
- Dental enamel erosion, tooth decay, gingivitis, palatal and posterior pharyngeal abrasions
- Russell sign (callus formation over the dorsal aspect of fingers due to acidic vomit)
- Facial petechiae, scleral hemorrhage due to forced purging
- Stress fractures or overuse syndromes from excessive exercise

DIAGNOSIS

- Diagnosis is clinical based on history and examination
- Initial workup similar to that of anorexia nervosa (see previously), with particular attention to electrolyte abnormalities due to purging

TREATMENT

- First-line treatment is psychotherapy (especially cognitive-behavioral therapy) plus selective serotonin reuptake inhibitors (SSRIs).
- Admission criteria similar to those for anorexia nervosa (see previously).

> **KEY FACT**
>
> SSRIs are the antidepressants of choice for eating disorders, particularly bulimia.

COMPLICATIONS

- Similar to anorexia nervosa (see previously).
- Increased risk of profound electrolyte disturbances (eg contraction alkalosis), GI bleeding, esophageal or gastric perforation, cathartic colon, and rhabdomyolysis with myoglobinuria from compulsive exercise.

EATING DISORDER, NOT OTHERWISE SPECIFIED (NOS)

DIAGNOSIS

- All criteria for anorexia except the patient is still menstruating or is normal weight
- All criteria for bulimia but decreased frequency of binging or duration of symptoms

- Purging after consumption of **small** amounts of food in person of normal weight
- Repeatedly chewing and spitting out large amounts of food
- Binge eating disorder: Binging without other compensatory behaviors

TREATMENT

Same as for anorexia/bulimia

Violence/Abuse/Neglect

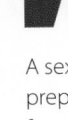

> **KEY FACT**
>
> Any cutaneous injury to nonambulatory children (< 1 year old) should raise concern for possible abuse.

CHILD ABUSE

The role of the emergency physician in caring for an abused child includes (1) recognizing complaints attributable to child abuse, (2) treating these complaints, and (3) protecting the child by reporting the suspicion of abuse to appropriate authorities.

RISK FACTORS

- Victimization: age < 4 years old, special needs with increased caregiver burden
- Perpetration: History of personal abuse/maltreatment, young age, low education, low income, social isolation, substance abuse and/or mental health disorders, family violence

SYMPTOMS/EXAMINATION

> **KEY FACT**
>
> A sexually transmitted disease (STD) in a prepubescent child is highly suspicious for sexual abuse.

- Cutaneous injuries: Bruises over locations that are not over bony prominences; patterned injuries in distribution of recognizable object (eg, hand, belt); human teeth bites with an intermaxillary distance > 3 cm, suggestive of adult bite; cigarette burns; and immersion burns with distinct margins (Figures 16.2 and 16.3).
- Skeletal injuries: See Diagnosis in the following text for more details.
- Shaken baby syndrome: Shaking of child (typically < 1 year old) leads to traumatic axonal injury and cerebral edema with lethargy, vomiting, retinal hemorrhages, skeletal injuries, and possibly death.

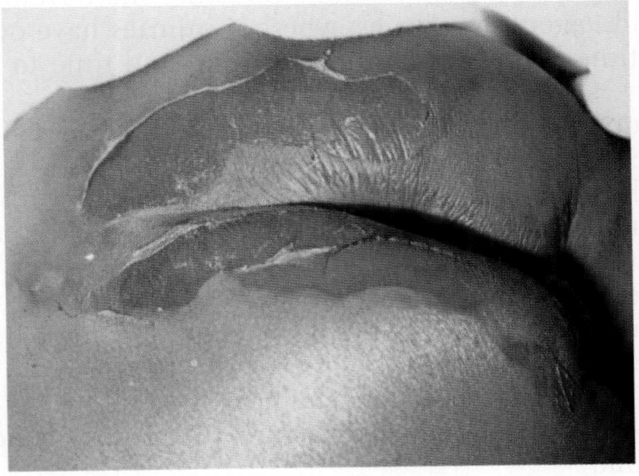

FIGURE 16.2. Burns on buttocks. (Reproduced, with permission, from Weinberg S, et al. *Color Atlas of Pediatric Dermatology*, 3rd ed. New York, NY: McGraw-Hill, 1998:240.)

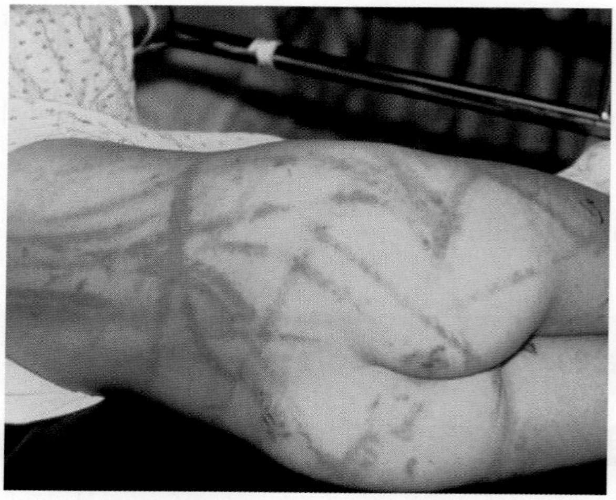

FIGURE 16.3. Loop marks from hanger. (Reproduced, with permission, from Weinberg S, et al. *Color Atlas of Pediatric Dermatology*, 3rd ed. New York, NY: McGraw-Hill, 1998)

- Sexual abuse injuries: Tears, petechiae, or hematomas of the hymen or other genital structures; anal lacerations, fissures, scars, or changes in anal tone or contour; genital warts, herpetic lesions, or other signs suggestive of sexually transmitted infections.

DIFFERENTIAL

- Accidental trauma, eg, toddler's fracture with accidental spiral fracture of tibia
- Dermal melanocytosis (formerly Mongolian spot): Blue-black discolorations normally seen over the buttocks and lower spine in children with darker complexion; due to entrapment of melanocytes
- Coagulopathy, such as hemophilia A or B
- Coining/cupping, bullous impetigo, contact dermatitis
- Osteogenesis imperfecta
- Urethral prolapse, priapism
- Straddle injuries to the perineum, lichen sclerosus et atrophicus

DIAGNOSIS

- History and physical examination. Consider the developmental stage of the child, extent of injuries, whether injuries have occurred over a period of time, witnesses to alleged event, and time to seeking medical care.
- Skeletal survey, ophthalmologic examination, head CT if indicated. Consider coagulation studies.
- Fractures that raise suspicion of abuse:
  - Any fracture in a child < 2 years old, especially nonambulatory children
  - Fractures of the ribs, scapula, vertebrae, or sternum (Figure 16.4)
  - Metaphyseal injuries, including a chip fracture or bucket-handle fracture
  - Any skull fracture, especially if multiple
  - Spiral or transverse diaphyseal fractures (or any long bone in nonambulatory child)
  - Multiple fractures in different stages of healing

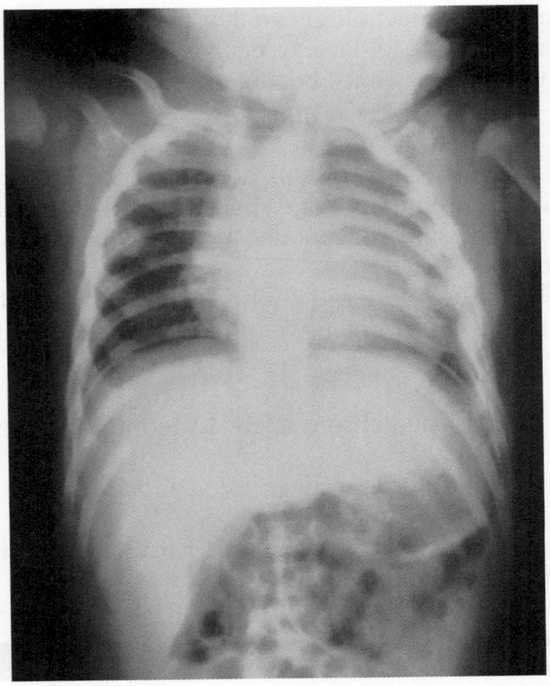

FIGURE 16.4. Rib fractures. (Reproduced, with permission, from Skinner HB, et al. *Current Diagnosis and Treatment in Orthopedics*, 4th ed. New York, NY: McGraw-Hill, 2006: 644.)

TREATMENT

- Identify, document, and treat all physical injuries and comorbidities.
- Immediately contact Child Protective Services and physician abuse specialists.
- Sexual abuse specialists should collect forensic evidence in suspected cases.

INTIMATE PARTNER VIOLENCE

Intimate partner violence (IPV) refers to the threat or infliction of physical or sexual violence by a current or former adolescent or adult intimate partner or spouse. Estimates suggest that 1%-7% of all females and increasingly large numbers of males who present to the ED for **any** reason actually do so as a result of IPV.

RISK FACTORS

- Perpetrator: Male, antisocial or borderline personality disorder, alcohol or substance abuse, recent unemployment, history of police arrest, low educational attainment, witnessed abuse as a child
- Victim: Female, younger age, exposure to violence in family of origin, presence of physical or mental disability, alcohol and substance abuse

SYMPTOMS/EXAMINATION

- Reported history may be vague, changing, and inconsistent with injuries.
- Pain is a common presenting symptom (eg, headache, pelvic pain, anal pain).
- Victims may present with suicidal ideation, depression, post-traumatic stress disorder.

- Sexually transmitted infections, genital or perineal trauma
- Physical injury to the head, face, or neck is highly suggestive of IPV.
- Any trauma in pregnancy must be screened for IPV.

DIAGNOSIS

- Suspect IPV if history is inconsistent, does not fit with physical examination, or if complaint is chronic but not responsive to any medical intervention.
- Ask patient directly and independently in a patient-only interview. Use screening tools.
- Maintain a high suspicion with injuries in central locations (eg, trunk, breasts), bilateral injuries, defensive injuries, and patterned injuries.

TREATMENT

- Assess immediate risk and ensure safety. Determine the location of abusive partner.
- Identify, document, and treat all injuries. Conduct an extensive mental health screen to identify suicidality.
- Make emergency consult to Social Work. Ensure appropriate and safe discharge plan for patient and patient's family.

ELDER ABUSE AND NEGLECT

Elder abuse is a form of family violence that is increasingly common yet often underrecognized. Elder abuse may be domestic (inflicted at home by a family member or caregiver), institutional (inflicted in a residential facility for elderly persons), or self-inflicted (elder's own behavior threatens well-being).

RISK FACTORS

- Perpetrator: Substance abuse, mental illness, financial stress, unrealistic expectations, resent
- Victim: Physical/functional impairment, dementia, aggressiveness, female, incontinence
- Environmental: Shared living situation, social isolation
- Institutional: Poor working conditions, low wages, understaffing

SYMPTOMS/EXAMINATION

- Sudden onset of behavioral symptoms (depression, confusion, anxiety)
- Lack of physical care (poor hygiene, malnutrition, soiled beddings or clothing, decubiti)
- Unexplained delay in seeking treatment or previous unexplained injuries.
- Caregiver refuses to leave patient alone with physician, never accompanis patient to the ED, exhibits indifference or anger toward the patient, and/or seems overly concerned with cost of treatment
- Patient appears fearful of caregiver with change in behavior in presence of caregiver

DIAGNOSIS

- Conduct detailed examination for any signs of physical abuse (eg, contusions, abrasions, patterned injuries, fractures), sexual abuse (genital, rectal, or oral trauma), and neglect (dehydration, soiled clothing, malnutrition, poor oral hygiene, skin breakdown)
- Directly question the patient regarding abuse, alone
- Consider chemistries and albumin to assess for metabolic or nutritional abnormalities. Check for sexually transmitted infections when indicated.
- Plain radiographs to assess for fractures

TREATMENT

- Identify, document, and treat all medical conditions.
- Patients in immediate danger should be hospitalized. Otherwise, disposition should be decided via shared decision making with the patient.
- Contact Adult Protective Services and Social Work to arrange appropriate support.

SEXUAL ASSAULT

Sexual assault refers to any sex act undertaken by force, threat of bodily injury, or with the inability of the victim to give appropriate consent.

RISK FACTORS

- Victim: Female sex, adolescent age, mentally or physically disabled, homeless, elderly, sex trade workers, in college or military service
- Perpetrator: Known by the victim in > 80% of cases, most often current or former significant others; the younger the victim, the more likely the perpetrator is a relative

SYMPTOMS/EXAMINATION

- Patients typically present with symptoms related to the psychological stress (eg, anxiety, suicidal ideation) and/or injuries sustained during the assault (eg, contusions, genital trauma).
- Important historical information includes time of assault, activities since assault (eg, washing, brushing teeth), oral/anal/rectal penetration, use of condom or weapons, physical trauma, last regular sexual activity, and use of drugs or alcohol.
- Female genital injury is most likely at the 4, 6, and 9 o'clock positions, most commonly involving the posterior fourchette.

DIAGNOSIS

- A multidisciplinary approach with trained abuse specialists using an approved rape kit is critical. Physical examination and evidence collection should occur concurrently.
- Collect patient clothing and perform complete physical examination, documenting any findings.
- Examine in detail any areas of penetration, with appropriate sample collection by abuse specialists. Pubic hair brushings should be collected. Colposcopy and/or toluidine blue dye may aid in identifying cervical and vaginal trauma.
- Use a Woods's lamp to identify and collect samples of stains or secretions.

TREATMENT

- Treat all injuries. Admit any patient with life-threatening medical or psychological illness.
- Offer pregnancy prophylaxis using emergency contraceptives. Consider progestin-only contraceptives or copper intrauterine device (IUD) in individuals with contraindications to estrogen.
- Provide prophylaxis for gonorrhea, chlamydia, trichomoniasis, and bacterial vaginosis with an appropriate regimen, such as ceftriaxone 250 mg intramuscularly once, metronidazole 2 g orally once, plus azithromycin 1 g orally or doxycycline 100 mg orally twice daily for 7 days.
- Provide hepatitis B prophylaxis via vaccination (not immune globulin) if not immunized.
- Consider postexposure prophylaxis for HIV and referral to an HIV specialist if the estimated risk is high. If patient declines, consider follow-up testing at 6 weeks, 3 and 6 months.
- Provide counseling and arrange for close follow-up.

Q

A 55-year-old woman with a history of depression presents to the ED with anxiety, palpitations, and severe headache shortly after drinking Chianti wine at dinner. What class of antidepressants was this patient likely taking, and what additional symptoms might be expected?

KEY FACT

In most states, physicians are mandated to report cases of known or suspected elder abuse.

A

The patient's symptoms are suggestive of an acute tyramine reaction while taking an MAO inhibitor. Hypertension, hyperthermia, and neuromuscular excitability would be expected. This patient is at risk for serious complications, including seizure and cardiovascular compromise.

Effects of Selected Psychotropic Medications

MONOAMINE OXIDASE INHIBITOR TOXICITY

Although once commonly used for depression, monoamine oxidase (MAO) inhibitors are now reserved for atypical or refractory depression. However, selective MAO-B inhibitors are increasingly being used in Parkinson disease. Examples include phenelzine, tranylcypromine, St. Johnlz Wort, and selegiline (selective MAO-B). Of note, the antibiotic linezolid is also a reversible inhibitor of MAO.

Pathophysiology

- MAO is a mitochondrial enzyme responsible for the breakdown of catecholamines. Type A enzymes primarily affect serotonin and norepinephrine, whereas Type B enzymes break down phenylethylamine. Both degrade tyramine and dopamine.
- Inhibition of MAO → decreased breakdown of biogenic amines → increased catecholamines
- Toxicity can result from acute overdose or as a consequence of a food or drug interaction.
  - Tyramine reaction occurs due to impaired breakdown of tyramine from MAO inhibition after consuming foods rich in tyramine (aged cheeses, red wine, smoked and aged meats).
- Serotonin syndrome may occur in patients taking other serotonergic drugs (eg meperidine, dextromethorphan, tramadol, SSRIs).

KEY FACT

Tyramine syndrome can occur up to 3 weeks after discontinuation of an MAO inhibitor.

Symptoms/Examination

- Symptoms may occur within hours (tyramine reaction) or up to 24 hours following overdose.
- Initial symptoms include tachycardia, hypertension, and hyperthermia. Subsequent depletion of catecholamine stores may lead to seizures, rhabdomyolysis, coma, and cardiovascular collapse.
- Physical examination may reveal agitation, mydriasis, myoclonus, and hyperreflexia.
- Tyramine syndrome: Headache, hypertension, diaphoresis, and neuromuscular excitation.

Differential

Sympathomimetic abuse (eg cocaine, methamphetamine), anticholinergic toxicity, meningitis, pheochromocytoma, thyroid storm, neuroleptic malignant syndrome, sedative withdrawal

Diagnosis

Diagnosis is based on clinical history and examination.

KEY FACT

Complications of MAO inhibitors toxicity, although rare, include intracranial hemorrhage and myocardial infarction. Obtain a noncontrast head CT on any patient with severe headache or focal neurological findings, and an ECG on all patients with chest pain!

Treatment

- Consider activated charcoal early in overdose.
- Mainstay is supportive care:
  - Benzodiazepines for CNS excitation, rigidity, and seizures
  - External cooling for hyperthermia
  - Short-acting antihypertensives (eg, phentolamine, nitroprusside) for hypertensive emergency, particularly intracranial hemorrhage. Avoid β-blockers.

- Treat hypotension with direct-acting catecholamines (eg, norepinephrine or epinephrine).
- All patients with MAO inhibitor overdose should be admitted or observed for 24 hours.

SEROTONIN SYNDROME

Serotonin syndrome is a potentially lethal condition caused by excess serotonin.

PATHOPHYSIOLOGY

- Impaired breakdown, reuptake, or increased production of serotonin → excess serotonin in the synaptic cleft → overstimulation of 5-HT_{1A} and 5-HT_{2A} postsynaptic receptors
- Most commonly occurs by combining drugs that raise serotonin levels by different mechanisms, but may also occur with overdose of a single serotonergic agent
- Commonly implicated agents include:
  - Antidepressants: SSRIs, serotonin and norepinephrine reuptake inhibitors (SNRIs), tricyclic antidepressants (TCAs), MAO inhibitors
  - Drugs of abuse: Cocaine, amphetamine derivatives, lysergic acid diethylamide (LSD)
  - Analgesics: Tramadol, meperidine, pentazocine
  - Miscellaneous: Dextromethorphan, lithium, metoclopramide, St. John's wort

SYMPTOMS/EXAMINATION

- Autonomic dysfunction: Hyperthermia, diaphoresis, tachycardia, tachypnea
- Neuromuscular symptoms: rapid onset of muscle rigidity (greater in lower extremities), tremor, ataxia, clonus/hyperreflexia
- CNS dysfunction: confusion/disorientation, agitation, seizures, coma

DIFFERENTIAL

Similar to MAO inhibitor toxicity (see previously).

DIAGNOSIS

Diagnosis is clinical and requires a high index of suspicion. There are numerous but no gold-standard criteria for diagnosis, and the condition should be suspected in any patient developing symptoms in the setting of known exposure to a serotonergic agent.

TREATMENT

- Primary treatment is removal of the offending drug.
- Supportive care: Benzodiazepines for muscle rigidity, agitation, and seizures; sodium bicarbonate for QRS widening > 100 milliseconds; and intravascular (IV) fluids for rhabdomyolysis.
- Consider cyproheptadine (5-HT_{2A} antagonist) in severe cases.
- Up to 25% of cases will require intubation and mechanical ventilation. In hyperthermic patients, use a nondepolarizing agent.

NEUROLEPTIC MALIGNANT SYNDROME

Neuroleptic malignant syndrome (NMS) is a serious, potentially lethal drug reaction that often occurs within two weeks of initiation of typical or atypical antipsychotics, although the reaction may occur at any time during treatment.

PATHOPHYSIOLOGY

- Dopamine receptor blockade in hypothalamus → hyperthermia, dysautonomia
- Dopamine receptor blockade in nigrostriatal pathway → rigidity, tremor, Parkinsonism

RISK FACTORS

- Rapid loading or increasing dosages of antipsychotics, use of high dose or high potency antipsychotics (eg droperidol, haloperidol, loxapine), administration via parenteral form, patient dehydration, personal history of NMS, concurrent use of lithium, and withdrawal from dopaminergic agents used for Parkinson disease

SYMPTOMS/EXAMINATION

- Fever and muscle rigidity (cogwheel or lead-pipe) developing over hours to days
- Altered mental status: Lethargy, agitation, coma
- Autonomic dysfunction: Diaphoresis, labile blood pressures, tachycardia
- CNS dysfunction: Tremor, dysphagia, mutism, incontinence

DIAGNOSIS

Muscle rigidity **and** hyperthermia along with two or more minor criteria, including those mentioned earlier (eg diaphoresis, tachycardia, tremor, agitation) or laboratory evidence of leukocytosis or elevated creatine kinase.

DIFFERENTIAL

Similar to that of MAO inhibitor toxicity. Consider serotonin syndrome, malignant hyperthermia, malignant catatonia, and intrathecal baclofen withdrawal based on history.

> **KEY FACT**
>
> NMS can be distinguished from serotonin syndrome by its **lack of hyperreflexia/clonus** and usually normal, rather than dilated, pupil size.

TREATMENT

- Primary treatment is removal of the offending drug and aggressive supportive care with IV fluids, external cooling, antihypertensive agents (consider vasodilators to facilitate cooling), benzodiazepines for aggression, prophylactic anticoagulation, and mechanical ventilation and/or antiarrhythmic agents as needed.
- The use of dantrolene and dopaminergic agents such as bromocriptine and amantadine is controversial. Electroconvulsive therapy is also being studied for possible utility in NMS.

COMPLICATIONS

Dysrhythmias, renal failure, coagulopathy, acidosis, seizures, pneumonia, disseminated intravascular coagulation (DIC), death.

EXTRAPYRAMIDAL SYMPTOMS

Blockade of dopamine receptors in the basal ganglia due to antipsychotic medications can lead to a variety of extrapyramidal and dystonic reactions.

SYMPTOMS/EXAMINATION/DIAGNOSIS

- Acute dystonia: Intermittent, involuntary motor tics and spasms of the face, neck, back, and extremities that begins within hours of starting antipsychotic treatment.

- Examples include oculogyric crisis (blepharospasm, periorbital twitches, protracted staring episodes) and laryngeal dystonia (potentially life-threatening laryngospasm).
- Akathisia: Sensation of restlessness associated with objective motor hyperactivity that begins within days of starting treatment.
- Parkinsonian syndrome: Bradykinesia, masked faces, muscular rigidity, resting tremor that begins within months of starting treatment.
- Tardive dyskinesia: Chronic movement disorder involving involuntary tics of the face, extremities, or trunk that begins after years of antipsychotic treatment.

Q

A 64-year-old man comes to the ED complaining of "feeling shaky." He is anxious appearing, tachycardic, and exhibits tremulousness. He states that he normally drinks a "pint or two" of liquor daily. He says that his last drink was > 10 hours ago. BAC is 80 mg/dL. How would you treat his symptoms?

TREATMENT

- Stop or decrease the dose of offending antipsychotic. Consider switching to alternative class.
- Use anticholinergic agents (eg diphenhydramine, benztropine) to control acute symptoms.
- Tardive dyskinesia is often permanent and not responsive to therapy.

DISULFIRAM REACTION

The disulfiram reaction is an unpleasant, potentially life-threatening reaction due to elevated serum acetaldehyde that occurs in patients who consume alcohol while taking disulfiram or similar drugs, most notably metronidazole.

PATHOPHYSIOLOGY

Disulfiram inhibits aldehyde dehydrogenase, preventing the breakdown of the acetaldehyde generated by the metabolism of ethanol.

SYMPTOMS/EXAMINATION

- Skin flushing, nausea/vomiting, headache, chest pain, abdominal discomfort, diaphoresis, vertigo, palpitations, and confusion may occur within 15-30 minutes after alcohol use.
- Severe reactions may cause hypotension, seizures, and dysrhythmias.

TREATMENT

Supportive care with IV fluids, antiemetics, and rarely dopamine for hypotension

Substance Abuse Disorders/Addiction

DEFINITIONS

- Intoxication: Reversible substance-specific syndrome due to recent ingestion of a substance.
- Abuse: Persistent substance use despite recurrent and significant negative consequences related to this use, without the additional physical or psychological signs of dependence (see the following text).
- Dependence: Adaptive state to chronic substance abuse characterized by tolerance and production of withdrawal symptoms or extreme psychological craving and seeking behavior in response to cessation or reduction of substance ingestion.
- Tolerance: Physiological adaptation to chronic exposure to a substance, such that repeated exposure requires increasing dosages to produce intoxication.

A

The patient is manifesting initial symptoms of alcohol withdrawal, despite his elevated BAC. This patient has likely developed a high tolerance to alcohol, with 80 mg/dL significantly below his baseline level. He should be given benzodiazepines for acute withdrawal.

- Withdrawal: Development of substance-specific maladaptive behavioral, physiological, or cognitive changes as the result of cessation of or reduction in prolonged substance use.

ALCOHOL

Alcohol is the most common recreational drug taken by Americans, with an estimated 18 million alcoholics in the United States alone. The standard drink equivalent is 12 oz of beer, 5 oz of table wine, or 1.5 oz shot of 80-proof spirits.

Alcohol Intoxication

Pathophysiology

- Ethanol is rapidly absorbed from the stomach and small intestine.
- Blood alcohol concentration (BAC) typically peaks within 30 minutes of consumption of a standard drink. Resulting BAC is determined by gender and weight (eg, 2 standard drinks will typically raise the BAC to 50 mg/dL in a 70-kg man, higher in women).
- Ethanol is metabolized to acetaldehyde in the liver by alcohol hydrogenase via zero-order kinetics (eg, at a constant rate independent of concentration).
- The average rate of metabolism is 10-20 mg/dL/h (up to 40 mg/dL/h in alcoholics).

Symptoms/Examination

- A nontolerant patient's BAC typically correlates with symptoms of intoxication (Table 16.7). Chronic drinkers can function at much higher BACs due to tolerance.
- Intoxicated patients display maladaptive behavior such as sexual or aggressive behavior, impaired judgment, labile mood, and impaired social/occupational functioning.
- Physical signs include slow or slurred speech, incoordination, unsteady gait, nystagmus, impairment of attention or memory, stupor, or coma.

Differential

Hypoglycemia, hypoxia, hypercapnia, mixed alcohol-drug overdose, toxic alcohol poisoning (methanol, ethylene glycol, isopropanol), hepatic encephalopathy, psychosis, vertigo, CNS infections or intracranial pathology, postictal state

TABLE 16.7. BAC Correlated with Typical Presentation in Nontolerant Alcohol-Intoxicated Patient

BAC (mg/dL)	Clinical Presentation
30	Attention difficulties, mild euphoria
50	Coordination problems
100	Typical drunk-driving parameter, ataxia
200	Confusion, decreased consciousness
> 400	Seizure, coma, could result in death

(Reproduced, with permission, from Hillard R, et al. *Emergency Psychiatry*. New York: McGraw-Hill, 2004:140.)

BAC, blood alcohol concentration.

DIAGNOSIS/TREATMENT

- Complete primary survey for any intoxicated patient. Secure airway if needed.
- Evaluate for alternative etiologies of altered mental status. Consider naloxone if opioid use is suspected and head CT if there is any concern for trauma.
- Check BAC if alternative etiology is suspected or to assess time required for metabolism prior to psychiatric consultation.
- Supportive care with IV fluids as needed (clinically dehydrated and unable to tolerate PO intake), thiamine (100 mg IV), dextrose (25-50 g IV), folate, and a multivitamin. Chronic alcohol users may benefit from magnesium supplementation.
- For agitated patients, avoid additional respiratory depressants. Consider antipsychotics.
- Discharge should only be considered once a patient is clinically sober and able to dress, walk, and function independently.

Alcohol Dependence

- The lifetime risk of alcohol abuse for the general population is 15%. The CAGE screening tool can be used to identify patients with alcohol dependence (Figure 16.5).
- "At risk" drinking is defined as: > 14 drinks per week or > 4 drinks per occasion for men; > 7 drinks per week or > 3 drinks per occasion for women.
- Risk factors include male sex, age 25-34 years old, family history of substance abuse, mental illness, and homelessness.
- Alcoholics have at least a 10- to 15-year shorter life span than nonalcoholics due to the multiple medical comorbidities associated with alcohol (see Table 16.8).

KEY FACT

Alcoholic cirrhosis is the most common cause of liver failure in the United States and worldwide.

Wernicke Encephalopathy

Wernicke encephalopathy is an acute, life-threatening disorder (10%-20% mortality) caused by thiamine (vitamin B_1) deficiency, most often seen in chronically malnourished patients such as heavy alcohol drinkers.

SYMPTOMS/EXAMINATION

- Confusion, memory impairment, lethargy, inattentiveness, abulia (lack of will or initiative)
- Cerebellar dysfunction (ataxia, incoordination)
- Nystagmus and ophthalmoplegia (lateral rectus muscle weakness, conjugate gaze palsies)
- Korsakoff syndrome: Neurological disorder with persistent anterograde and retrograde memory impairment, apathy, and often confabulation (pathologic lying about invented memories)

KEY FACT

Remember to give magnesium! Magnesium is a cofactor required for utilization of thiamine.

CAGE: Have you ever felt:

The need to **Cut down** on your drinking?

Annoyed by criticism of your drinking?

Guilty about your drinking?

The need to drink an **Eye opener** in the morning?

A positive answer to 2 or more questions is highly sensitive for alcohol dependence.

FIGURE 16.5. The CAGE Questionnaire.

TABLE 16.8. Effects of Chronic Heavy Alcohol Consumption

Cardiac	Hypertension Dilated cardiomyopathy Dysrhythmia
Pulmonary	Higher incidence of pneumonia and TB
Gastrointestinal	Alcoholic hepatitis and cirrhosis Gastritis Gastric or duodenal ulcers Pancreatitis Higher incidence of gastric and esophageal cancer
Neurologic	Symmetric sensorimotor polyneuropathy Wernicke–Korsakoff syndrome Intracranial hemorrhage and CVA Myopathy Cerebellar degeneration
Metabolic	Thiamine, vitamin B_{12}, folic acid deficiencies Coagulopathy Hyperlipidemia Hypoglycemia Immunocompromise
Endocrine	Increased ACTH Decreased testosterone synthesis Glucocorticoid or catecholamine release

ACTH, adrenocorticotropic hormone; CVA, cerebrovascular accident; TB, tuberculosis.

DIAGNOSIS/TREATMENT

- Clinical diagnosis based on history and physical examination
- Treat with abstinence, adequate diet, and aggressive IV magnesium and thiamine repletion. Theoretically, one should give thiamine before glucose supplementation to avoid precipitating acute thiamine deficiency.
- Preventative treatment with daily oral thiamine for any alcoholic/malnourished patient

Alcohol Ketoacidosis

Alcohol ketoacidosis (AKA) is an anion gap metabolic acidosis most commonly seen in chronic alcoholics following an alcohol binge with subsequent vomiting, decreased food intake, and dehydration.

PATHOPHYSIOLOGY

- Low glycogen stores from malnutrition + NAD [nicotinamide adenine dinucleotide] depletion due to alcohol metabolism → anaerobic metabolism, ketogenesis, impaired gluconeogenesis → hypoglycemia + wide anion gap acidosis
- NAD depletion also drives acetoacetic acid toward β-hydroxybutyric acid, making this the primary ketoacid in AKA.

SYMPTOMS/EXAMINATION

- History of chronic alcoholism, often with recent alcoholic binge followed by protracted nausea, vomiting, abdominal pain, and poor PO intake
- Typically clear sensorium
- Examination: Acetone odor, tachypnea (Kussmaul respirations), tachycardia, dehydration

DIFFERENTIAL

- Diabetic ketoacidosis, starvation, toxic alcohol ingestion, salicylate toxicity, lactic acidosis, sepsis, acute renal failure

DIAGNOSIS/TREATMENT

- AKA is a diagnosis of exclusion. Evaluate for alternative etiologies with serum electrolytes, ketone levels, urinalysis, lactic acid, blood gas analysis, salicylate level if overdose is suspected, or serum osmolality toxic alcohol levels if ingestion is suspected.
- Evaluate for comorbidities, including alcohol withdrawal, hepatitis, pancreatitis, GI bleed
- Primary treatment is rehydration with normal saline and glucose administration (IV or PO) to stop ketogenesis. Replete thiamine, potassium, phosphate, and magnesium.

> **KEY FACT**
>
> The nitroprusside test used to measure serum and urine ketones detects acetoacetate but NOT β-hydroxybutyrate, which may lead to false negatives and underestimation of ketonemia in AKA.

Alcohol Withdrawal

Alcohol withdrawal presents as a continuum of symptoms ranging from mild to severe.

PATHOPHYSIOLOGY

- Ethanol directly binds to inhibitory γ-aminobutyric acid (GABA) receptors and inhibits glutamate-induced excitation. Chronic use leads to decreased sensitivity of GABA receptors and upregulation of glutamate N-methyl-D-aspartate (NMDA) receptors.
- Cessation of alcohol → activation of previously-inhibited NMDA receptors in absence of alcohol-related GABA inhibition → CNS hyperexcitability

> **KEY FACT**
>
> Unlike delirium tremens, alcoholic hallucinosis is NOT associated with global clouding of the sensorium and vital signs are often normal.

SYMPTOMS/EXAMINATION

- See Table 16.9 for a summary of common clinical signs of alcohol withdrawal.

TABLE 16.9. Findings Associated with Alcohol Withdrawal

	ONSET AFTER LAST DRINK	SYMPTOMS/SIGNS
Minor withdrawal	6-36 h	Nausea, anorexia, coarse tremor, tachycardia, hypertension, hyperreflexia, insomnia
Seizures	6-48 h	Brief **generalized tonic-clonic seizures**. If untreated, 60% of patients will have additional seizures within 6 h
Alcoholic hallucinosis	12-48 h	Visual, auditory, and/or tactile, with **intact orientation** and normal vital signs
Delirium tremens	48-96 h	**Altered sensorium** with confusion, hallucinations, paranoia, and profound autonomic hyperactivity

- Delirium tremens (DT) is the most severe complication of alcohol withdrawal.
  - Occurs in 5% of individuals with alcohol withdrawal and carries a 5% mortality rate
  - Risk factors: History of DT, age > 30 years old, persistent heavy alcohol abuse with presence of withdrawal symptoms despite an elevated BAC, longer period since last drink

DIFFERENTIAL

Sympathomimetic intoxication (eg, cocaine), metabolic abnormalities (hypoglycemia, hypo/hypernatremia, hypocalcemia), encephalitis, meningitis, intracranial trauma, cerebrovascular accident (CVA), benzodiazepine/barbiturate withdrawal, noncompliance with anticonvulsants

DIAGNOSIS/TREATMENT

> **KEY FACT**
>
> An alcohol-abusing patient with a first seizure should be treated and evaluated as any patient with a first-time seizure.

- Rule out all other medical causes. If alcohol intake is not known and patient is unable to provide history, pursue work-up for altered mental status. Consider CT imaging if trauma is suspected.
- Benzodiazepines are the mainstay of treatment.
  - Consider benzodiazepines with short half-lives and inactive metabolites, such as lorazepam or oxazepam, in patients with liver failure.
  - Example: Lorazepam 2-4 mg IV every 15-20 minutes for acute withdrawal, followed by symptom-triggered therapy (eg Clinical Institute Withdrawal Assessment for Alcohol Scale, or CIWAS).
- Secondary agents for refractory withdrawal include barbiturates and propofol.
- Adjunctive therapy includes: Thiamine and magnesium supplementation, β-blockers or clonidine for autonomic hyperactivity and withdrawal symptoms, butyrophenones for hallucinations or aggressive behavior.
- Admit any patient with severe withdrawal, persistent autonomic instability, or > 2 seizures in ED.
- Outpatient candidates should be referred to substance abuse specialist with a short course of outpatient benzodiazepines (eg, lorazepam 1-2 mg 3 times daily in a tapering dose).

Cocaine

Cocaine has both local anesthetic and CNS stimulant effects.

> **KEY FACT**
>
> Cocaine is primarily metabolized by **plasma cholinesterase.** Cocaine use can be fatal in patients with a relative deficiency of this enzyme!

PATHOPHYSIOLOGY

- In the CNS, cocaine triggers release and inhibits reuptake of dopamine, epinephrine, norepinephrine, and serotonin, triggering sympathetic activation and reward (dopamine effect).
- Topically, cocaine blocks fast sodium channels in neuronal membranes, inhibiting conduction.
- Time of onset and duration of effect vary by route of administration (Table 16.10).

SYMPTOMS/EXAMINATION

- Intoxication triggers an addictive euphoria and general sense of well-being.
- Sympathomimetic effects: Mydriasis, tachycardia, hypertension, diaphoresis, hyperthermia
- Acute cocaine toxicity has profound systemic effects (Table 16.11).

DIFFERENTIAL

Other sympathomimetic abuse (eg amphetamine, phencyclidine) hypoglycemia, alcohol or other sedative/hypnotic withdrawal, serotonin syndrome, NMS, thyrotoxicosis, meningitis, encephalitis, seizures, primary psychiatric disease

TABLE 16.10. Pharmacokinetics of Cocaine

Route of Exposure	Onset of Action	Peak Action	Duration of Action
IV	< 1 min	3-5 min	30-60 min
Nasal insufflation (snorting)	1-5 min	20-30 min	60-120 min
Inhalation (smoking)	< 1 min	3-5 min	30-60 min
GI	30-60 min	60-90 min	Unknown

(Reproduced, with permission, from Flomenbaum NE, Goldfrank LR, Hoffman RS, et al: *Goldfrank's Toxicologic Emergencies*, 9th ed. New York: McGraw-Hill, 2006.)

GI, gastrointestinal; IV, intravascular.

Q

A 28-year-old pregnant woman presents with hypertension, anxiety, and diaphoresis. On further interview, she admits to snorting cocaine prior to the onset of symptoms. What obstetrical complications might be expected, and what is your first-line treatment for this patient?

Diagnosis

- Acute intoxication is primarily a clinical diagnosis.
- Urine drug screen remains positive for up to 3 days after single use and 7-12 days after repeated high doses.
- In significant toxicity:
  - ECG to evaluate for ischemia, hyperkalemia, QRS prolongation, other abnormalities
  - Creatine kinase, serum chemistries, liver function tests if there is significant hyperthermia or concern for rhabdomyolysis or end-organ dysfunction
  - Troponin if patient is complaining of chest pain
  - Head CT with lumbar puncture in patients with headache

KEY FACT

Cocaine-induced hyperthermia can be life threatening with subsequent multisystem organ failure and DIC. Treat aggressively to reduce core temperature to < 102°F within 20 minutes.

Treatment

- Primary treatment is benzodiazepines, which restore inhibitory tone to the CNS
- Aggressively treat hyperthermia with rapid evaporative cooling and IV fluids

TABLE 16.11. Acute Cocaine Toxicity

Organ System	Effects
Cardiovascular	Hypertensive emergency, dysrhythmias, myocarditis, myocardial ischemia and infarction, aortic dissection
Neurological	Psychomotor agitation, seizure, coma, intracranial hemorrhage, acute cerebrovascular accident, dystonia, dyskinesias
Pulmonary	Angioedema, pulmonary hemorrhage, pulmonary infarction, acute lung injury, pneumonitis, bronchospasm, barotrauma
Gastrointestinal	Ischemic colitis, intestinal infarction, splenic infarction
Renal	Renal infarction, hypertensive renal disease, myoglobinuria
Placental	Abruptio placentae, spontaneous abortion, growth retardation
Ophthalmologic	Acute closed-angle glaucoma

Cocaine use in pregnancy is associated with decreased uteroplacental blood flow. Complications include abruptio placentae, spontaneous abortion, fetal prematurity, and intrauterine growth retardation. First-line treatment for cocaine toxicity is the same as for the nonpregnant patient—benzodiazepines.

- Use nitroglycerin, nitroprusside, or phentolamine for uncontrolled hypertension.
- Avoid β-blockers, which may precipitate unopposed α-blockade with worsening of hypertension. Also avoid butyrophenones (eg haloperidol, droperidol), which can lower seizure threshold and cause dysrhythmias and hyperthermia
- Percutaneous intervention in patients with persistent chest pain or ECG changes despite benzodiazepines, aspirin, nitroglycerin, and morphine

Complications

- IV or subcutaneous use ("skin popping") may result in cutaneous abscess, cellulitis, endocarditis, brain abscess, epidural abscess.
- Levamisole, an agent used to "cut" cocaine, may cause life-threatening agranulocytosis and vasculitis.
- Cocaine withdrawal: dysphoria, irritability, hypersomnolence, anergia

Amphetamines

As a class, amphetamines enhance release of catecholamines with subsequent CNS stimulation and sympathomimetic effects similar to cocaine. Management is similar to cocaine toxicity (see previously).

3,4-Methylenedioxy-N-Methamphetamine

- A.k.a. ecstasy, E, XTC, X, or Adam. *Molly* refers to purified 3,4-methylenedioxy-N-methamphetamine (MDMA), although street samples reveal increasing contamination with other synthetic sympathomimetic drugs.
- Molecular structure also confers serotonergic effects, leading to hallucinogenic properties
- MDMA-induced hyponatremia shares features with the syndrome of inappropriate antidiuretic hormone secretion (SIADH) and can be life threatening.
- Cathinone salts, or "bath salts," are synthetic chemicals with both amphetamine and hallucinogenic properties similar to MDMA.

Methamphetamine

- A.k.a. crystal meth, ice, crank, chalk, speed
- Illicit production requires metal salts, causing heavy metal toxicity (eg lead poisoning).
- "Meth mouth" is common due to bruxism, decreased saliva production, and poor hygiene.

Ephedrine

- Sympathomimetic found in cold remedies, decongestants, and weight loss supplements
- Acts primarily at α- and β-adrenergic receptors, with greater cardiovascular and fewer CNS effects.

KEY FACT

Pupils may not be constricted despite opioid use due to coingestion of stimulants or anoxia. Moreover, opioids such as meperidine and propoxyphene dilate, rather than constrict, the pupils.

Prescribed Stimulants

- Methylphenidate (Ritalin, Concerta), dextroamphetamine (Dexedrine), amphetamine mixed salts (Adderall), and other prescribed stimulants have high abuse potential.
- Toxicity may occur at prescribed dosages, especially in amphetamine-naïve patients.
- Abuse is common in adolescent and college-age individuals.

Opioids

Opioid refers to any natural, synthetic, or semisynthetic agent with morphine or opium-like effects.

PATHOPHYSIOLOGY

- Opioid receptors are G protein-coupled receptors located in the CNS, sensory nerve endings, endothelial cells, and throughout the GI tract.
- There are 3 established opioid receptors:
  - Mu receptors: Primary receptor for analgesia, euphoria, and addiction
  - Delta receptors: Additional spinal analgesia and respiratory depression
  - Kappa receptors: Same as delta, with possible dysphoria upon activation

SYMPTOMS/EXAMINATION

- Classic toxidrome is CNS depression, respiratory depression, and miosis
- Additional effects may include mild hypotension, relative bradycardia, nausea/vomiting, constipation, urinary retention, and pruritus
- Examination may reveal track marks in IV opioid abusers

DIFFERENTIAL

Alcohol intoxication, sedative/hypnotic abuse, toxic overdose (clonidine, organophosphates, phenothiazines), carbon monoxide poisoning, hypoglycemia, hypoxia, CNS infections, postictal state, myxedema coma, CNS trauma.

DIAGNOSIS/TREATMENT

- Diagnosis is clinical. Assess airway, breathing, and circulation (ABCs) with airway protection and ventilation as needed.
- Naloxone (Narcan) is a pure opioid antagonist and antidote for opioid overdose.
  - Onset in 1-2 minutes, duration is 20-60 minutes. Redose and consider infusion as needed.
  - Initial dose is 0.4-2 mg. Titrate to respiratory effort and airway protection. Consider lower starting doses (0.04-0.2 mg) in chronic users to avoid acute withdrawal.
  - For continuous infusion, administer two-third of the effective initial dose per hour.
- Supportive care with airway support and IV fluids for hypotension
- Disposition depends on type and dosage of opioid. Admit any patient who requires repeated boluses or infusion of naloxone. Always assess for suicidality.

> **KEY FACT**
>
> Remember to check an acetaminophen level on patients with possible ingestion of an opioid-acetaminophen combination.

COMPLICATIONS

- Acute lung injury may occur with acute opioid overdose (often heroin).
  - Acute onset of dyspnea, tachypnea, rales, and hypoxia. Chest x-ray may show bilateral infiltrates with normal cardiac silhouette.
  - Often occurs as patient is recovering from opioid-induced respiratory depression, but may occur immediately after use or after naloxone administration.
  - Manage with positive pressure ventilation and intubation as needed.
- Opioid withdrawal is characterized by sympathetic discharge and adrenergic hyperactivity.
  - Symptoms include: anxiety, insomnia, yawning, diaphoresis, nausea, vomiting, diarrhea, lacrimation, rhinorrhea, mydriasis, and piloerection
  - Onset depends on type of opioid (within 12 hours of last heroin use, up to 30 hours or more after long-acting opioid use)

- Refer for outpatient treatment with methadone, buprenorphine, or other substitution
- Adjuncts include clonidine for withdrawal symptoms, antiemetics (eg, promethazine), antihistamines (eg, diphenhydramine, hydroxyzine), antidiarrheals (eg, loperamide), NSAIDs for myalgia, and baclofen for cramping.

Phencyclidine

Phencyclidine (PCP) is a dissociative anesthetic that is structurally related to ketamine.

Pathophysiology

- Acts as a noncompetitive antagonist of N-methyl-D-aspartate (NMDA) receptors; inhibits reuptake of dopamine, norepinephrine, and serotonin; and acts as an anticholinergic.
- Peak effects occur 5-10 minutes after inhalation and up to 2 hours after oral intake.

Symptoms/Examination

- Tachycardia, hypertension, hyperthermia
- CNS effects range from bizarre behavior, agitation, violent behavior, and seizures to sedation, unresponsiveness, and coma.
- Vertical, horizontal, and rotatory nystagmus is often present. Pupil size is variable.

Differential

Alcohol withdrawal/intoxication, dextromethorphan abuse, trauma, meningitis, catatonia, heat stroke, hypoglycemia, hypoxia, sedative/hypnotic withdrawal, acute psychosis, sympathomimetic abuse (eg, cocaine, methamphetamine).

Diagnosis

- Diagnosis is clinical. Alternative etiologies and complications should be ruled out with basic chemistries, creatine kinase level, and imaging as indicated.
- Urine drug screening can detect PCP but is not useful in acute setting (chronic PCP users can test positive for up to 1 week after last use).

Treatment

- Treatment is primarily supportive with IV fluids and evaporative cooling for hyperthermia.
- Chemical sedation with benzodiazepines is preferred to physical restraint.
- Manage hypertension with nitroprusside or nitroglycerin. Avoid β-blockers.
- Most patients will recover within 4-6 hours. Admit patients with coingestion or persistent intoxication.

Hallucinogens

Hallucinogens are drugs that impair cognition and perception. See Table 16.12 for a description of common hallucinogens.

Sedative Hypnotics

Sedative hypnotics are a broad class of drugs used for sedation, seizures, and treating anxiety. Examples include benzodiazepines, barbiturates, and related drugs such as chloral hydrate and zolpidem.

TABLE 16.12. Common Hallucinogens

Drug(s)	Duration of Action (hours)	Clinical Features	Complications
MDMA	4–6	Mydriasis, sympathomimetic symptoms, bruxism, ataxia, dry mouth, nausea	Hyperthermia, rhabdomyolysis, dehydration, excessive water drinking and hyponatremia, seizures, arrhythmias
LSD (derived from fungus *Claviceps purpurea*)	8–12	Mydriasis, sympathomimetic symptoms, anxiety, muscle spasm	Coma, hyperthermia, coagulopathy, persistent psychosis, "flashbacks" or hallucinogen persisting perception disorder
Psilocybin (derived from mushrooms of *Psilocybe* genus)	4–6	Mydriasis, sympathomimetic symptoms, nausea/vomiting, muscle tension	Seizures (rare), hyperthermia (rare)
Mescaline (a phenylethylamine found in Mexican peyote cactus)	6–12	Mydriasis, sympathomimetic symptoms, abdominal pain, nausea/vomiting, dizziness, nystagmus, ataxia	Rare
Marijuana	2–4	Tachycardia, conjunctival injection, impaired motor coordination	Rare

(Adapted with permission from Tintinalli JE, Stapczynski JS, Ma OJ, et al. *Tintinalli's Emergency Medicine: A Comprehensive Study Guide*. 8th ed. New York: McGraw-Hill; 2016.)

LSD, lysergic acid diethylamide; MDMA, 3,4-methylenedioxy-*N*-methamphetamin.

Pathophysiology

- Both benzodiazepines and barbiturates bind directly to GABA receptors to increase GABA-mediated inhibitory tone.
- Barbiturates increase duration of channel opening, whereas benzodiazepines increase frequency of channel opening.

Symptoms/Examination

- Mild sedative intoxication mimics ethanol intoxication (see previously), with drowsiness, slurred speech, incoordination, nystagmus, and impaired cognition.
- Severe toxicity may result in hypotension, bradycardia, respiratory depression, and coma.

Differential

Similar to acute alcohol intoxication (see previously). Coma or severe respiratory failure suggests coingestion, particularly with opioids.

Diagnosis

- Diagnosis is clinical. Rule out alternative etiologies for altered mental status with point-of-care blood glucose and basic chemistries.
- Urine and blood toxicology are rarely helpful in the acute setting, as these tests can be positive for up to 1 week with long-acting sedatives and/or chronic abuse.

Treatment

- Immediate stabilization with intubation and mechanical ventilation as needed

KEY FACT

Barbiturates act centrally to directly depress respiratory drive, whereas benzodiazepine-mediated depression is typically due to oversedation with increased upper airway obstruction and resistance.

Q

A 30-year-old woman with panic disorder presents with worsening anxiety and tremulousness after running out of her "nerve pill." Shortly after arrival to the ED, she has a grand mal seizure lasting several minutes. What is your first step?

- Supportive care with IV fluids, close monitoring. Consider empiric treatment for coingestion and substance abuse with naloxone, glucose, and thiamine.
- Flumazenil is a nonspecific competitive antagonist of the benzodiazepine receptor.
  - It is NOT recommended for routine reversal as it may cause generalized seizures (due to reversal of the benzodiazepine's anticonvulsant properties and/or precipitation of acute withdrawal), cardiac dysrhythmias, and increased intracranial pressure.
  - Specific indications may include small children with accidental poisoning or accidental overdose during procedural sedation.
- Admit any patient with severe toxicity. Patients that remain asymptomatic after 4-6 hours may be medically cleared. Always assess suicidality and intentional overdose.

Complications

KEY FACT

Unlike other benzodiazepines, **oxazepam**, **temazepam**, and **lorazepam** are excreted renally and are safe in liver failure patients.

- Chloral hydrate, a once commonly prescribed sedative, has particularly erratic GI absorption with a low therapeutic ratio and is associated with dysrhythmias such as torsades de pointes. Chloral hydrate-induced torsade can be treated with β-blockers.
- Accumulation of active metabolites may cause toxicity in patients with liver failure.
- Benzodiazepine withdrawal is potentially life threatening and clinically similar to alcohol withdrawal (anxiety, insomnia, tremor, tachycardia, delirium, seizures). Treat by restarting benzodiazepines and outpatient follow-up for long taper.

Special Populations

KEY FACT

Packaged drugs may contain > 10 times the lethal dose of substance, making rupture a dangerous and life-threatening event.

- Body packer: Individual who intentionally ingest large amounts of well-packaged product, typically for smuggling purposes.
  - Place all patients on continuous monitoring with large-bore IV access.
  - Treat asymptomatic patients with polyethylene glycol to expedite passage. If rupture is suspected, obtain immediate surgical consult for laparotomy.
- Body stuffer: Individual who swallows a poorly wrapped quantity of drug, usually in an attempt to avoid arrest or detection.
  - Treat with activate charcoal (1 g/kg), close monitoring, and symptomatic treatment as in acute intoxication. Consider whole-bowel irrigation if severe toxicity is suspected.

A

This is most likely benzodiazepine withdrawal, and benzodiazepine administration is indicated. This patient can be very tolerant and may require large doses for treatment of her symptoms.

REVIEW QUESTIONS

QUESTIONS

1. A 25-year-old woman with a history of anorexia nervosa, currently at 70% of her ideal body weight, presents with generalized weakness and myalgias. She admits to recently taking her mother's furosemide in order to lose weight. Her vitals are as follows: HR 55, BP 90/52 mm Hg, temperature of 36.4°C. You perform a general physical examination and laboratory analysis. Which of the following laboratory results would *not* be expected in this patient?
   A. Hypokalemia
   B. Hypophosphatemia
   C. Metabolic acidosis
   D. Hypomagnesemia

2. A 42-year-old man with a history of refractory depression presents to the emergency department with altered mental status and extreme agitation. The patient's roommate, who called emergency medical services (EMS), states the patient appeared fine before leaving to attend a large dinner party at a local vineyard. On arrival, his vital signs are as follows: temperature 103.7°F (39.8°C), HR 140 bpm, BP 210/104 mm Hg, RR 24 breaths/min. He has no known history of hypertension or other medical problems. Which of the following treatments is *contraindicated* in the initial management of this patient?
   A. Lorazepam
   B. External cooling
   C. Phentolamine
   D. Metoprolol

3. A 22-year-old man with known schizophrenia presents with acute agitation, hallucinations, and homicidal ideation. He admits that he stopped taking his antipsychotic because it made him "feel funny." Attempts to verbally redirect and physically restrain the patient are unsuccessful, so you administer haloperidol 5 mg intramuscularly (IM). The patient de-escalates over several minutes. However, despite initially responding well to the haloperidol, he becomes acutely restless, pacing the room and stating he "just need(s) to keep on moving." What is the next best step in the management of this patient?
   A. Additional haloperidol
   B. Diphenhydramine
   C. Lorazepam
   D. Hydroxyzine

4. A 63-year-old man with Parkinson disease presents to the emergency department with acute onset of hallucinations, agitation, and aggression. He is confused and oriented only to person. He becomes agitated with attempts to start intravascular (IV) access and does not respond to nonpharmacologic attempts at de-escalation. Which of the following drugs is *contraindicated* in this patient?
   A. Hydroxyzine
   B. Lorazepam
   C. Haloperidol
   D. Ketamine

ANSWERS

1. **C.** Metabolic acidosis. Patients with anorexia nervosa often have profound serum and total body electrolyte deficiencies, including hypokalemia, hypophosphatemia, and hypomagnesemia. Anorexic patients that abuse diuretics often demonstrate a significant contraction alkalosis, whereas those that abuse laxatives may exhibit a metabolic acidosis due to gastrointestinal (GI) losses of bicarbonate.

2. **D.** Metoprolol. This patient's history and examination suggest acute tyramine syndrome due to ingestion of tyramines (wine, aged cheeses) at his dinner party while taking a monoamine oxidase (MAO) inhibitor, such as phenelzine, which is indicated for atypical or refractory depression. Tyramine syndrome is caused by an excess of catecholamines causing sympathetic overload. Consequently, β-blockers are contraindicated due to the risk of worsening hypertension and tachycardia due to unopposed α-adrenergic activity.

3. **B.** Diphenhydramine. This patient is exhibiting symptoms of akathisia, a sensation of restlessness associated with objective motor hyperactivity. This typically occurs within days of starting antidopaminergic antipsychotic therapy, and may be the reason this patient stopped his medications. Extrapyramidal symptoms such as akathisia induced by antipsychotics are best treated with anticholinergics, such as diphenhydramine or benztropine. Attributing the patient's restlessness to worsening psychosis, with subsequent administration of haloperidol, would likely worsen this patient"s akathisia.

4. **C.** Haloperidol. The symptoms of Parkinson disease are caused by a relative dopamine deficiency within the substantia nigra. Antidopaminergic drugs such as haloperidol may worsen the symptoms of Parkinson disease and are contraindicated in these patients.

CHAPTER 17

Dermatology

Jeremy Voros, MD

TABLE 17.1. Primary Lesions

Lesion	Description
Macule	Flat, nonpalpable, circumscribed lesion < 5 mm in diameter
Patch	Flat, nonpalpable, circumscribed lesion > 5 mm in diameter
Papule	Palpable, circumscribed lesion < 5 mm in diameter, raised above skin surface
Plaque	Palpable lesion > 5 mm in diameter, raised above skin surface
Nodule	Firm lesion arising in subcutaneous tissue < 2 cm in diameter
Tumor	Firm lesion arising in subcutaneous tissue > 2 cm in diameter
Vesicle	Raised, fluid-filled, superficial lesion < 5 mm in diameter
Bulla	Raised, fluid-filled, superficial lesion > 5 mm in diameter
Pustule	Pus-filled superficial lesion < 5 mm in diameter
Abscess	Pus-filled lesion arising in subcutaneous tissue > 5 mm in diameter
Wheal	Evanescent, raised, round, or flat-topped lesion caused by edema

Table 17.1 describes the names and descriptions of primary dermatological lesions.

Erythema Multiforme

An immune-mediated self-limited rash most commonly triggered by herpes simplex virus infection. Rash without mucosal involvement is termed *erythema multiforme (EM) minor* while that with mucosal involvement, **EM major**. It is now considered to be distinct from and **not** on a continuum with Stevens-Johnson syndrome (SJS) and toxic epidermal necrolysis (TEN). Additional triggers include other viral, bacterial or fungal infection and medications.

KEY FACT

Four erythemas:

1. Erythema marginatum: Migratory annular and polycyclic erythematous eruption, cutaneous manifestation of acute rheumatic fever.
2. Erythema migrans: Expanding red lesion with central clearing at site of tick bite, Lyme disease.
3. Erythema multiforme: Target lesions, ± mucosal involvement, many causes.
4. Erythema nodosum: Tender, raised red nodules on legs, many causes.

Symptoms/Examination

- Erythematous, papular rash (Figure 17.1) appears over 72 hours, most commonly on palms and dorsal surface of forearms but also on feet, face, and lower extremities, usually < 10% BSA. There is great variation, but typically > 100 lesions are present.
- Papules may evolve to **target lesions** with a characteristic central dusky or purple zone surrounded by a pale ring and then third erythematous halo.
- Lesions may have a vesicular or bullous appearance.
- Discrete **oral lesions** are present in approximately 50% of patients.

Differential

- Stevens-Johnson syndrome/toxic epidermal necrolysis: Skin and oral lesions are more severe and progress to skin necrosis and sloughing.
- Urticaria: Lesions migrate (EM lesions are fixed, persists > 24 hours).
- See Table 17.2 for differential diagnosis of rashes on the palms.

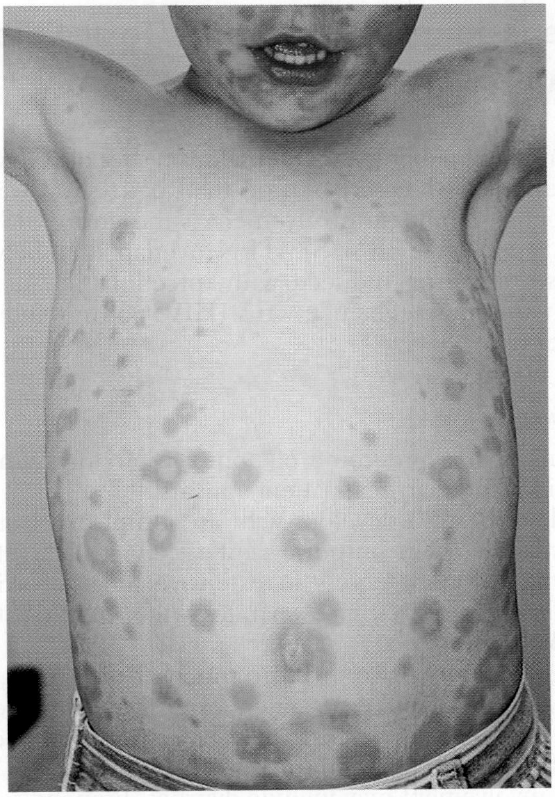

FIGURE 17.1. Erythema multiforme with characteristic target lesions with central dusky or purple zone surrounded by pale ring and third erythematous halo. (Reproduced, with permission, from Knoop KJ, Storrow AB, Stack LB, et al. *The Atlas of Emergency Medicine*. 3rd ed. New York, NY: McGraw-Hill; 2010. Figure 13.5. Photographer: Michael Redman, PA-C.)

Q

A 50-year-old woman, recently started on antibiotics for a mild urinary tract infection, presents to the emergency department with complaint of fever, chills, malaise for a few days, and now with redness to her body (50% TBSA) and sores inside her mouth. Her examination shows a positive Nikolsky sign with sloughing of skin, and ulcerations inside her mouth and vaginal canal. Where should she be admitted? Should she continue her antibiotics?

TREATMENT

- Symptomatic treatment and topical steroids are mainstay of therapy.
- Short course of oral prednisone for those with mucosal involvement.
- Hospitalize patients with impaired intake due to extensive oral involvement.
- Antiviral prophylaxis can prevent recurrent EM due to HSV reactivation.

TABLE 17.2. Differential Diagnosis for Rashes on the Palms

Name	Clinical Features
Erythema multiforme	Target lesions evolve over 72 h
Rocky Mountain spotted fever	Erythematous/hemorrhagic macules and papules
Drug eruption	Lesions occur minutes to several hours after drug administration and recur in the same area with re-exposure. circular, violaceous, or edematous plaques that resolve with macular hyperpigmentation
Secondary syphilis	Scaling papular eruptions
Scabies	Papules and burrows, mainly in web spaces; intensely pruritic
Hand, foot, and mouth disease	Small, discrete vesicles; patients usually < 10 y old

A

This patient's history and examination are consistent with toxic epidermal necrolysis (TEN). She should be admitted to a burn center intensive care unit for fluid resuscitation, close monitoring of her airway, and pain management. She should NOT continue the antibiotic, as this is likely the inciting cause of her symptoms.

Stevens-Johnson Syndrome/Toxic Epidermal Necrolysis

SJS and TEN are desquamating, erythematous rashes distinguished from each other only by extent of disease based on total body surface area (TBSA). In both cases mucous membrane involvement is the norm. SJS involves < 10% TBSA and TEN > 30% TBSA (SJS/TEN overlap is in-between). The vast majority of cases are drug induced with infections a much less common trigger. Human immunodeficiency virus (HIV)-positive individuals are at a 1000-fold higher risk.

Symptoms/Examination

- Illness begins with a prodrome of upper respiratory symptoms, malaise, fever, vomiting, and diarrhea; patient appears ill.
- After 1-14 days the rash develops with an abrupt onset of symmetric erythematous macules with purpuric centers (atypical target lesions) or diffuse erythema, which progress to extensive areas of skin necrosis and sloughing (Figure 17.2). Skin separates when gentle lateral pressure is applied (**Nikolsky sign**).
- There is involvement of **two or more mucosal sites** (eyes, mouth, vagina, urethra, anus). Oral mucosa is often extensively denuded with hemorrhagic crust on lips and mucosa; may have compromised airway due to sloughing of respiratory epithelium.
- Multisystem involvement may include diarrhea, bronchitis, arthritis, arthralgias, hepatitis, myocarditis, and nephritis.

KEY FACT

"Target lesion" classically refers to the bright red borders and central petechiae of erythema multiforme and Stevens-Johnson syndrome, but is also used to describe erythema migrans, the primary lesion in Lyme disease.

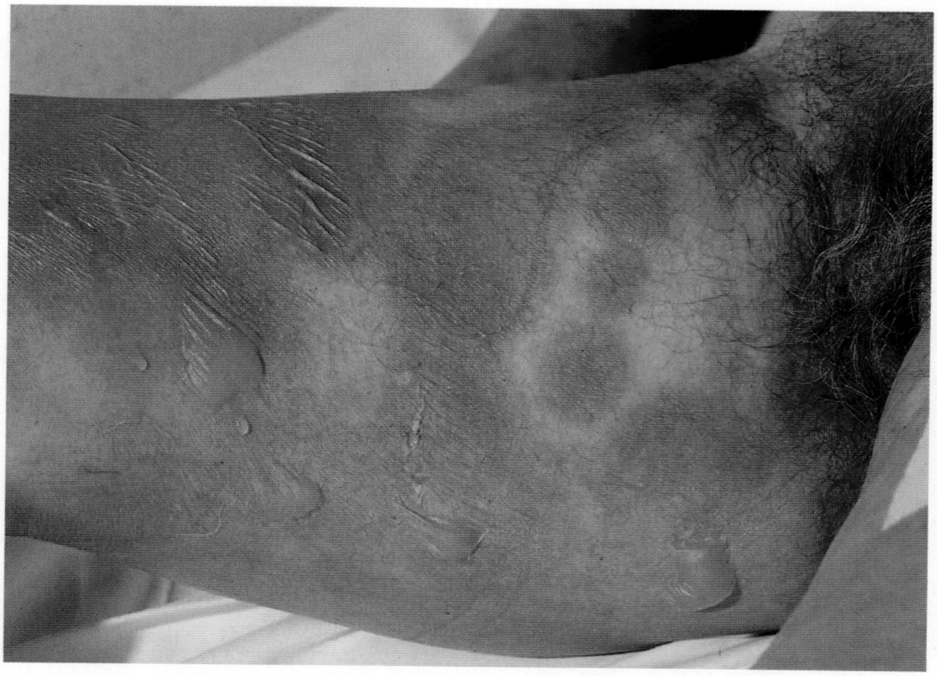

FIGURE 17.2. Stevens-Johnson syndrome. Note the diffuse erythema with skin necrosis and sloughing. A few atypical target lesions are present. (Reproduced, with permission, from Tintinalli JE, Stapczynski S, Ma OJ, et al. *Tintinalli's Emergency Medicine*. 7th ed. New York, NY: McGraw-Hill Education, 2011. Figure 245.2.)

TREATMENT

- Admit to ICU or burn unit for skin care fluid/electrolyte correction.
- Withdraw offending drug.
- Ophthalmology evaluation is mandatory for patients with eye involvement.
- Intravenous immunoglobulin (IVIG) and steroids are controversial.

COMPLICATIONS

- Mortality is up to 40% related to sepsis, gastrointestinal (GI) hemorrhage, fluid/electrolyte imbalances.
- Long-term morbidity is due to scarring, blindness, renal tubular necrosis and renal failure.

KEY FACT

Five dangerous rashes:
Hives associated with anaphylaxis
Petechiae due to meningococcemia
Erythema due to SJS/TEN or SSSS
Macules starting on wrists/ankles due to Rocky Mountain Spotted Fever
Woody induration and pain due to necrotizing fasciitis

KEY FACT

Painful and tender symmetric erythematous rash? Think SJS/TEN or SSSS.

Staphylococcal Scalded Skin Syndrome

Staphylococcal scalded skin syndrome (SSSS) usually occurs in neonates and young children < 6 years old with *Staphylococcus aureus* infections of the conjunctiva, nasopharynx, or umbilicus. Caused by an **exotoxin** produced by *S. aureus* that is released into the bloodstream causing superficial separation of the skin and widespread painful erythema and blistering.

SYMPTOMS/EXAMINATION

- Sudden appearance of **tender erythema** with sandpaper-like texture prominent in perioral, periorbital, and groin regions and in skin creases of the neck, axilla, popliteal, and antecubital regions; mucous membranes are not affected.
- Exfoliative phase begins on second day of illness. Minor trauma causes skin to wrinkle and peel off. There is **positive Nikolsky sign**. Large flaccid, fluid-filled bullae and vesicles appear, which easily rupture and are shed in large sheets. Underlying skin resembles scalded skin (Figure 17.3).
- After 3-5 days the skin desquamates, leaving normal skin in 10-14 days.

DIFFERENTIAL

- TEN
- Toxic shock syndrome
- Exfoliative drug eruptions
- Localized bullous impetigo
- Pemphigus

TREATMENT

- Admission to ICU for fluid resuscitation, wound care and electrolyte correction if extensive involvement.
- Identify and treat source of staph infection with penicillinase-resistant penicillins, such as oxacillin or vancomycin (depending on prevalence of community-acquired methicillin-resistant S. *aureus*).
- Steroids are not recommended.

COMPLICATIONS

- 3% mortality in children
- Disease is very rare in adults, is associated with renal failure and immunosuppression, and a higher mortality rate > 50%.

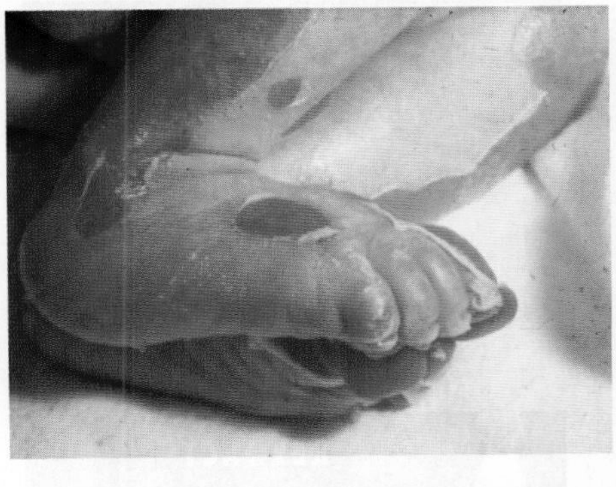

FIGURE 17.3. Staphylococcal scalded skin syndrome in a young child with characteristic involvement of skin folds. (Reproduced, with permission, from Ryan K, Ray CG. *Sherris Medical Microbiology*. 6th ed. New York, NY: McGraw-Hill Education, 2014. Figure 24.7B.)

Exanthematous Drug Eruptions

The vast majority of cutaneous drug reactions are exanthematous with a smaller percentage urticarial. Exanthematous reactions are a type-IV immune reaction, appearing within 1-2 weeks after an offending drug is taken for the first time, sooner in a sensitized individual. Antibiotics are a common culprit.

Symptoms/Examination

- Widespread symmetric maculopapular eruption that resembles a viral exanthem.
- Pruritus is common while pain suggests a more serious problem such as SJS or TEN.

Treatment

- Discontinuation of inciting agent
- Symptom control with antihistamines, high potency topical corticosteroids, Domeboro or Burow's solution

KEY FACT

High-potency corticosteroids should never be used on the face, groin, or axilla.

Urticaria (Hives)

Urticaria is due to activation of cutaneous mast cells with resultant mediator release. The most frequent causes are drugs (eg, penicillin cephalosporins, vancomycin, morphine, NSAIDs), infection (especially viral infections in children), and food (eg, shellfish, fish, eggs, nuts). Emotional stress, exercise, and excess heat or cold exposure are other known causes.

KEY FACT

The standard epinephrine dose for anaphylaxis is 0.3 mg intramuscularly (IM) (usually given as 0.3 mL of 1:1000).

Symptoms/Examination

Pruritic, erythematous plaques of varying size that are **transient and migratory**, usually lasting < 24 hours. Urticaria becomes chronic when recurrent eruptions occur for > 6 weeks.

Treatment

- Avoid cause and administer a H_1-receptor antagonist (eg, Benadryl).
- Prednisone can be added when symptoms are severe or unresponsive to first-line treatment.
- Epinephrine 0.3 mg IM for adults, 0.15 mg IM for children when associated with anaphylaxis (ie, hypotension, wheezing, or difficulty breathing).
- H_2-receptor blockers are of uncertain benefit.

Exfoliative Dermatitis (Erythroderma)

KEY FACT

Exfoliative dermatitis is distinguished from other desquamating diseases by a feeling of skin tightness, scaly skin, and large areas of involvement.

A diffuse and potentially life-threatening skin disorder characterized by severe inflammation and increased epidermal cell turnover. Causes include exacerbation of an existing dermatitis (psoriasis or atopic), hypersensitivity drug reaction and underlying malignancy. In many cases, a cause is not identified.

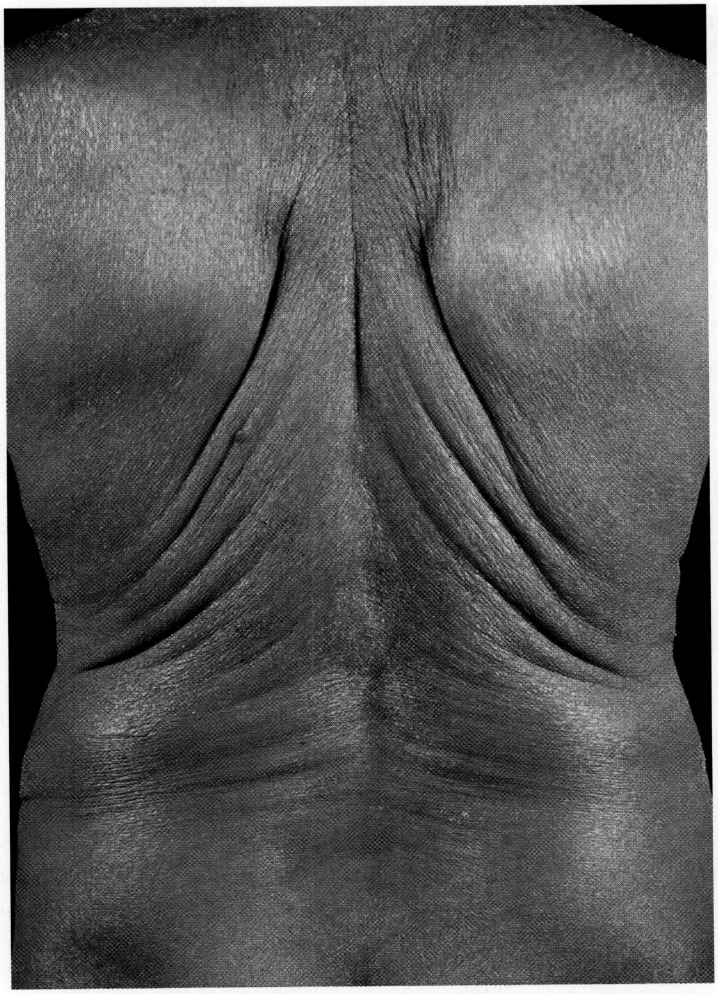

FIGURE 17.4. Exfoliative dermatitis, characterized by diffuse erythema and scaling. (Reproduced with permission from Wolff K, Johnson RA, Saavedra AP: *Fitzpatrick's Color Atlas and Synopsis of Clinical Dermatology*, 7th ed. New York, NY: McGraw-Hill; 2013. Figure 8.2.)

Q

A 10-year-old boy is brought to the ED by his parents for a pruritic rash that began 1 week after a camping trip. The rash is most predominant on his legs in a linear pattern, as well as on his both hands. The family dog was present with the family while camping. What is the most likely culprit? Aside from treating the boy's rash, what else should be done to prevent further reaction?

SYMPTOMS/EXAMINATION

- Systemic complaints of pruritus, chills.
- Presence of erythema and scaling involving > 90% of skin surface (Figure 17.4) Skin feels warm, leathery and indurated.

TREATMENT

- Emergent dermatology consultation, hospital admission, correct hypothermia and hypovolemia.
- Identify and treat underlying cause.
- Emollients, low-to-mid potency topical corticosteroids and oral antihistamines are all useful therapies.

COMPLICATIONS

- Disruption of dermis can lead to water loss, excessive heat loss, and high-output congestive heart failure due to widespread vasodilatation.
- Mortality is up to 30%.

See Table 17.3 for additional cutaneous drug eruptions.

A

The rash is most likely a contact dermatitis from a plant exposure while hiking (poison ivy, poison oak, poison sumac). Thoroughly washing the boy's clothes, as well as the family dog, will prevent reexposure to urushiol oils causing the reaction.

TABLE 17.3. Additional Cutaneous Drug Eruptions

Name	Clinical Features	Common Drugs
Phototoxic eruption	Sunburn appearance on sun-exposed skin	NSAIDs Quinolones Tetracycline Phenothiazine Amiodarone
Photoallergic eruption	Eczematous reaction that is intensely pruritic on sun-exposed skin	Phenothiazines Chlorpromazine Sulfa NSAIDs
Fixed drug eruption	Sharply marginated oval or round erythematous plaques that appear and reappear at same site after repeat exposure to same drug	Antibiotics Barbiturates NSAIDs
Hypersensitivity vasculitis	Urticarial papules or palpable purpura with constitutional symptoms; immune-complex mediated	Penicillin Cephalosporin Sulfonamides Phenytoin Allopurinol
Drug rash with eosinophilia and systemic symptoms (DRESS)	Morbilliform rash that may become confluent, fever, malaise and lymphadenopathy; multiorgan involvement may occur; onset. 2-8 wk after drug exposure	Several antiepileptics Sulfonamides Vancomycin

NSAID, nonsteroidal anti-inflammatory drug.

Irritant Contact Dermatitis

An inflammatory reaction of the skin from direct cytotoxic effects (nonallergic) of a chemical, or biological agent. Clothing, jewelry, soaps, plants, and topical medications (such as neomycin) are all causes.

KEY FACT

Rashes with discrete distributions (wrist, ears, neck, belly button, fingers) suggest irritant contact dermatitis.

Symptoms/Examination/Treatment

- Pruritic papules, vesicles, or bullae on an erythematous base in acute reactions.
- Chronic exposure causes the skin to become thickened, hyperkeratotic and fissured.
- Treatment includes avoiding causative agent and using topical steroids and emollients.
- Consider Domeboro or Burow's solution for oozing or vesicular lesions.

Allergic Contact Dermatitis

Most commonly caused by the *Toxicodendron* family of plants (poison ivy/oak/sumac). These weeds are found throughout the United States except Hawaii and Alaska, with poison ivy found east of the Rockies and poison oak to the west.

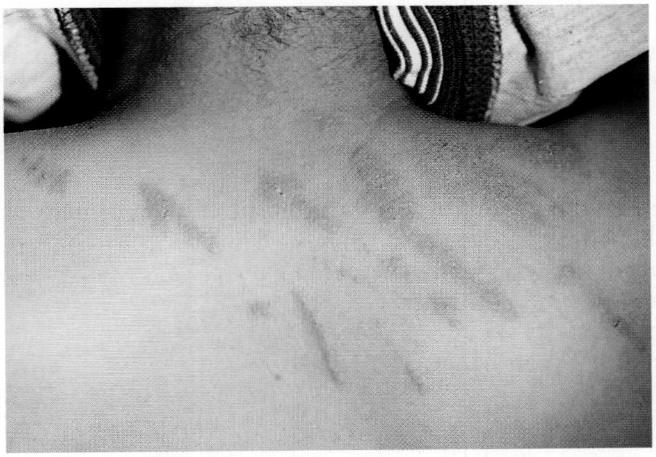

FIGURE 17.5. Allergic contact dermatitis from poison ivy. (Reproduced, with permission, from Knoop KJ, Storrow AB, Stack LB, et al. *The Atlas of Emergency Medicine*. 3rd ed. New York, NY: McGraw-Hill Education; 2010. Figure 16.104. Photographer: Alan B. Storrow, MD.)

The oil **urushiol**, common to all these plants, induces a delayed (type IV) hypersensitivity reaction in approximately 70% of the population. Mango, cashew nut shells, and gingko biloba contain a compound similar to urushiol and may therefore induce a similar reaction.

Symptoms/Examination

- Clinical effects occur 24-48 hours after contact in the sensitized individual (10-14 days with first exposure) and are characterized by linear streaking of papulovesicles with associated pruritus (Figure 17.5). Resolution occurs over 14-21 days in most cases.
- 10%-15% have SEVERE and rapid reactions characterized by early edema and pruritus, followed by extensive vesicles, fevers, malaise. This should be considered a dermatologic emergency.

Treatment

- Wash all contaminated skin and clothing immediately with soap and water to eliminate urushiol.
- Antihistamines and topical therapies (Burow's solution, ultrapotent topical steroids) are often needed.
- Oral steroids are indicated in patients with severe reactions or those involving face, axilla and groin. Taper over **2-3 weeks.**

KEY FACT

"Leaves of three, let them be."

Atopic Dermatitis

Atopic dermatitis is a chronic inflammatory skin disorder due to impaired epidermal barrier function of uncertain etiology. The link between asthma/allergy and atopic dermatitis has been recently called into question. Onset is typically at a young age, most often < 5 years.

Symptoms/Examination

- Inflammatory papular, papulovesicular lesions acutely
- Chronic lichenification (thickening) and hyperpigmentation
- Intense pruritus during flares is a distinguishing hallmark of atopic dermatitis
- May see signs of secondary infections at sites of excoriation.

DIFFERENTIAL

Contact dermatitis, chronic seborrheic dermatitis, scabies, psoriasis, histiocytosis, dermatophytosis, mycosis fungoides

DIAGNOSIS

- Clinical diagnosis
- United Kingdom's Working Party diagnostic criteria of itchy skin PLUS 3 of the following:
  - History of skin crease involvement
  - Current flexural dermatitis
  - Generalized dry skin
  - Onset at < 2 years of age

TREATMENT

- Avoid skin irritants including perfumed soaps and detergents.
- Warm baths followed by emollients
- Topical corticosteroids for flares, consider antihistamines for severe pruritus

Psoriasis

A chronic, immune-mediated skin disorder resulting in epidermal hyperplasia and inflammation. Affects men and women equally. Risk factors include family history, high body mass index, smoking, and alcohol consumption.

SYMPTOMS/EXAMINATION

- Well-defined plaques of salmon-colored erythema with overlying silvery scale (Figure 17.6).

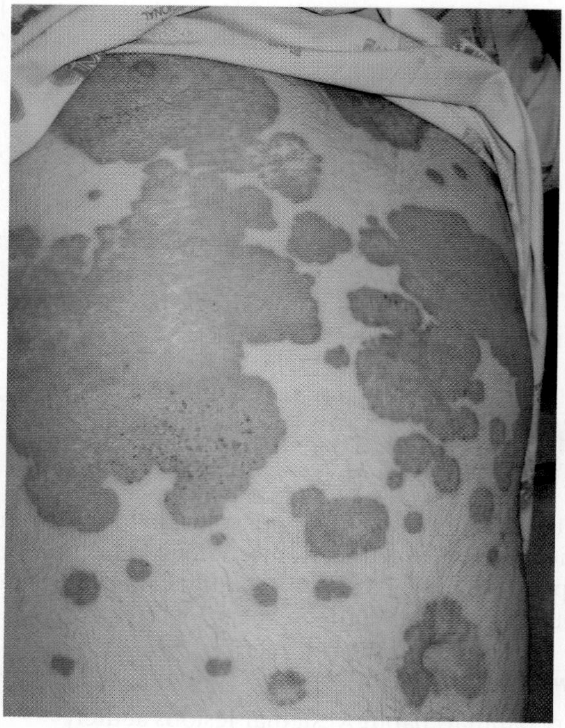

FIGURE 17.6. Psoriasis. (Reproduced, with permission, from Knoop KJ, Storrow AB, Stack LB, et al. *The Atlas of Emergency Medicine*. 3rd ed. New York, NY: McGraw-Hill Education; 2010. Figure 13.22. Photographer: R. Jason Thurman, MD.)

- Commonly seen on scalp, extensor surfaces of extremities, palms, soles, and gluteal cleft.
- Nail abnormalities with pitting, discoloration, and separation from the nail bed are common
- Psoriatic arthritis (rheumatoid factor seronegative) may also be seen.

KEY FACT

Psoriasis is associated with an increased risk of cardiovascular disease.

DIFFERENTIAL DIAGNOSIS

Tinea, seborrheic dermatitis, secondary syphilis, pityriasis rosea, cutaneous lupus erythematosus

TREATMENT

- Topical corticosteroids and emollients are first-line agents for mild to moderate skin disease.
- Systemic treatment (methotrexate, retinoids, cyclosporins, biologics) and ultraviolet therapy may be required for more extensive disease.
- Refer to dermatology for long-term management.

Seborrhea (Seborrheic Dermatitis)

Seborrhea is a superficial inflammatory process in areas with increased activity of sebaceous glands (scalp, ears, eyebrows, central face, upper trunk, intertriginous areas). Most common in infants (cradle cap), adolescents, and the elderly. It is a chronic and relapsing condition with the exception of infant seborrhea where it typically resolves by 1 year of age. The cause is not known, but it may be seen with HIV and Parkinson disease in adults.

SYMPTOMS/EXAMINATION

- Mildest form is dandruff, seen in adolescence and adults; small white powdery scales without erythema.
- More severe forms involve greasy yellow scales with mild underlying erythema (Figure 17.7).

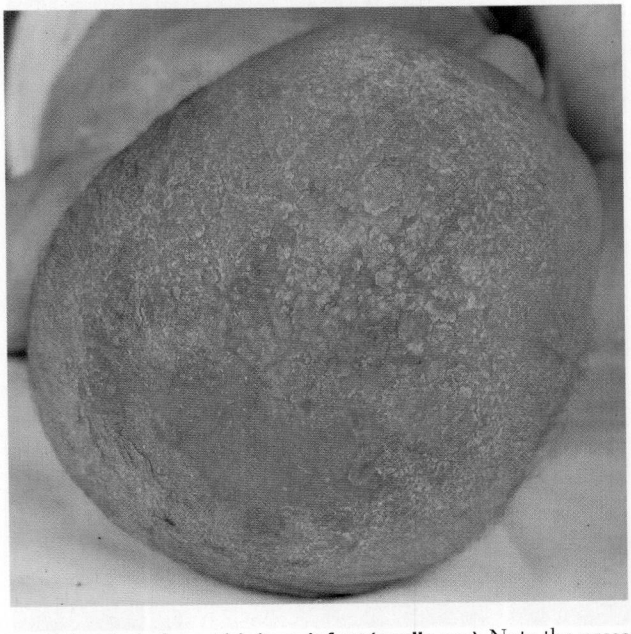

FIGURE 17.7. Seborrheic dermatitis in an infant (cradle cap). Note the presence of greasy yellow scales with mild underlying erythema. (Reproduced with permission from Wolff KL, Johnson R, Suurmond R: *Fitzpatrick's Color Atlas & Synopsis of Clinical Dermatology*, 5th ed. New York: McGraw-Hill Education; 2005.)

DIFFERENTIAL

Tinea, atopic dermatitis, psoriasis

> **KEY FACT**
>
> Low-potency corticosteroids should be used on the face.

TREATMENT

- Cradle cap: Reassurance, emollients, and frequent washing with mild shampoo
- Adolescents and adults: Antifungal shampoo (eg, ketoconazole) or those with coal tar, sulfur, selenium
- Topical corticosteroids can be used for more severe disease.

Impetigo

Superficial bacterial infection of the epidermis commonly around the nose and mouth of children < 6 years with a second peak occurring in the elderly. Very contagious, easily spreading to surrounding skin and other young children. Predisposing factors include poor hygiene, warm weather, overcrowding, and breaks in skin barrier from abrasions or insect bites.

SYMPTOMS/EXAMINATION

Divided into two clinical types:

1. Impetigo contagiosa
   - Caused by *S. aureus* and group A streptococci
   - Superficial vesicles and pustules covered with **honey-colored crusts** (Figure 17.8)

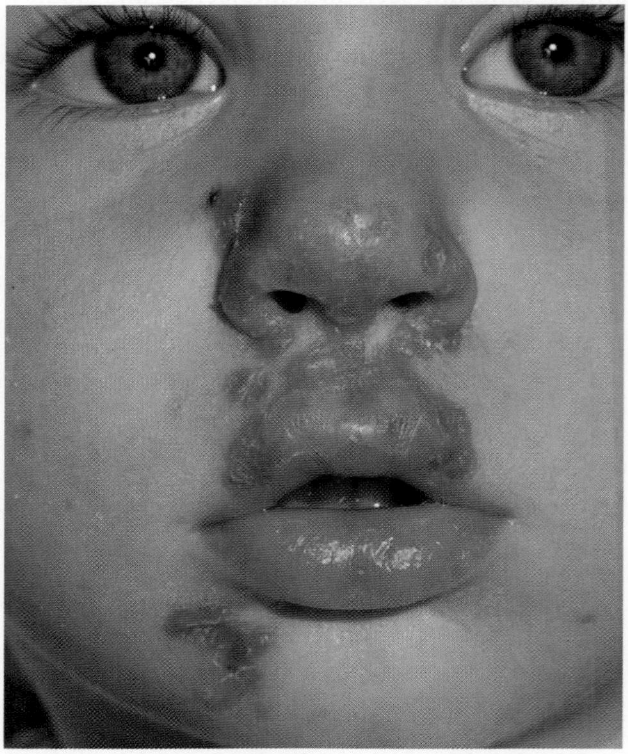

FIGURE 17.8. Impetigo. (Reproduced, with permission, from Wolff K, Johnson RA, Saavedra AP. *Fitzpatrick's Color Atlas and Synopsis of Clinical Dermatology*. 7th ed. New York, NY: McGraw-Hill Education, 2013. Figure 25.8.)

2. Bullous impetigo
   - Caused by epidermolytic, toxin-producing *S. aureus*
   - Flaccid vesicles and bullae up to 3 cm in diameter

TREATMENT

- Limited number of lesions: Topical mupirocin 2% ointment
- Extensive disease: Oral antibiotic, such as dicloxacillin or cephalexin
- Risk for MRSA: Trimethoprim/sulfamethoxazole or clindamycin; doxycycline for those > 8 years
- Meticulous hygiene can prevent spread

COMPLICATIONS

- **Post streptococcal glomerulonephritis** is an uncommon complication that is not prevented by treatment.
- Other complications include cellulitis, sepsis, lymphadenitis, and rarely rheumatic fever.

Erysipelas

A skin infection involving only the **upper dermis and superficial lymphatics**. Typically caused by β-hemolytic streptococcus.

SYMPTOMS/EXAMINATION

- Acute and rapidly progressive illness characterized by raised and intense erythematous plaques with a **sharply demarcated** border (Figure 17.9) and associated fevers/chills.

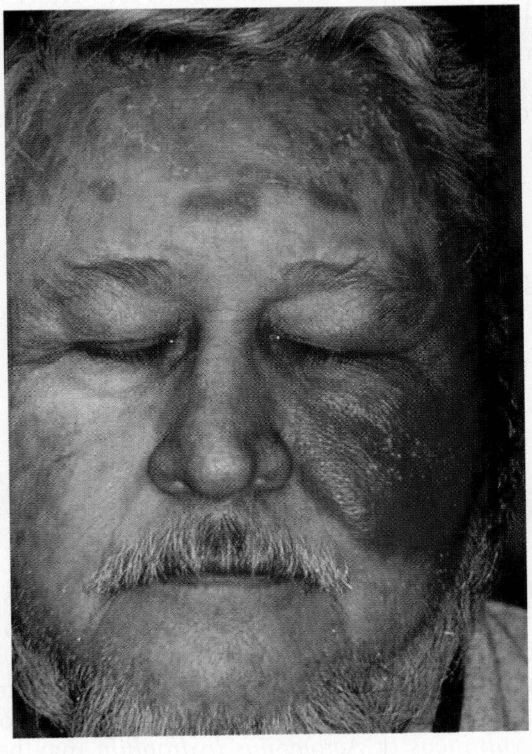

FIGURE 17.9. Erysipelas. (Reproduced with permission from Knoop KJ, Storrow AB, Stack LB, and Thurman RJ. *The Atlas of Emergency Medicine*, 3rd ed. New York, NY: McGraw-Hill; 2010. Figure 13.65. Photographer: The Department of Dermatology, Wilford Hall USAF Medical Center and Brooke Army Medical Center, San Antonio, TX.)

TREATMENT

- Admit patients with systemic manifestations for parenteral therapy with ceftriaxone or cefazolin.
- If no systemic manifestations and otherwise healthy, treat with oral amoxicillin for 5-10 days; second-line therapy includes erythromycin, although macrolides may not be adequate in areas with highly resistant β-hemolytic streptococcus.

Cellulitis

> **KEY FACT**
>
> The most common site of cellulitis and erysipelas is the lower extremity.

Cellulitis is an infection of the deeper dermis and underlying subcutaneous fat. The most common pathogens include *S. aureus* (including MRSA) and *Streptococcus pyogenes* (group A streptococcus). Cellulitis spreads through local trauma, lymphatic, and hematogenous spread. Risk factors include lymphedema (most common), skin break down, immune deficiency, venous stasis, peripheral arterial disease, and obesity.

SYMPTOMS/EXAMINATION

Characterized by erythema, warmth, swelling and tenderness of skin.

> **KEY FACT**
>
> Risk factors for MRSA infection:
> - Recent hospitalization
> - Recent antibiotic use
> - Immunosuppression
> - Resident of long-term care facility
> - Crowded or unsanitary living conditions
> - Men having sex with men
> - Contact sports

TREATMENT

- Consider coverage for staph, strep, and MRSA.
- **Simple nonpurulent cellulitis** (no purulent drainage, abscess, fever, vital sign abnormalities, or mental status changes) may be treated with oral antibiotics, with return to ED if no improvement in 24 hours. Coverage for MRSA is not recommended initially.
- Patients with **purulent cellulitis or risk factors for MRSA** should be covered for MRSA with clindamycin, doxycycline, trimethoprim-sulfamethoxazole.
- If failure of oral antibiotics, consider admission for IV antibiotics.
- Complicated cellulitis (fever, tachycardia, hypotension, immunosuppressed, diabetes), involvement of large body surface area, or failure of oral antibiotics warrants IV antibiotics and admission.

COMPLICATIONS

> **KEY FACT**
>
> Simple abscesses can be treated with incision and drainage, without antibiotics.

- Can progress to bacteremia, sepsis, endocarditis if lymphatic or hematogenous seeding.
- Rapid progression, crepitus, bullae, systemic signs of illness should prompt consideration of necrotizing infection.
- Recurrent cellulitis may suggest a retained foreign body—consider a radiographic study.

Necrotizing Fasciitis

Necrotizing soft tissue infections include necrotizing fasciitis, an uncommon but high-mortality diagnosis. **Type I** necrotizing fasciitis is polymicrobial with an average of 4.6 isolates per specimen and is associated with diabetes and other immunocompromised states. **Type II** is primarily *Streptococcal pyogenes* (previously called "streptococcal gangrene") alone or in combination with *S. aureus*. *Vibrio vulnificus* or *Aeromonas hydrophila* may be seen after salt/fresh water trauma, respectively. Type II can occur in any age group and in patients who do not have complicated medical illnesses.

Symptoms/Examination

- Early in the course, skin may appear relatively normal with **pain out of proportion to examination**.
- Rapidly progressing erythema, warmth, pain, edema.
- Bullae or crepitus are particularly suggestive.
- Systemic toxicity (fever, hypotension, tachycardia) may be out of proportion to clinical examination.

Differential

Cellulitis, erysipelas, abscess, compartment syndrome, myositis, phlegmasia cerulea dolens

Diagnosis

- Necrotizing fasciitis remains a clinical diagnosis, but imaging may be helpful.
  - Plain radiographs and bedside ultrasound may show air in the soft tissues.
  - Computed tomography or magnetic resonance imaging may show air, inflammation, or purulence within the tissue planes.

Treatment

- Emergent surgical consultation when the diagnosis is suspected. Rapid surgical debridement is critical to control spread of infection.
- Broad-spectrum antibiotics to cover staph (including MRSA), strep, Gram negatives, and anaerobes
- Clindamycin is recommended first-line antibiotic for presumed *Streptococcus pyogenes* due to inhibition of toxin formation.
- ICU admission for resuscitation

Complications

High mortality rate, increased with diabetes, older age, and other comorbidities

Tinea (Dermatophyte) Infections

These infections of the outer keratin layer of skin, hair, and nails are caused by fungal species from 1 of 3 genera (*Trichophyton*, *Microsporum*, and *Epidermophyton*). Multiple types of infection are possible and include tinea capitis (scalp), tinea corporis (body), tinea pedis (athlete's foot), and tinea unguium (onychomycosis or nails). Infections are more common in warm, moist environments and are not markedly contagious except for tinea capitis.

Diagnosis

- Usually can be diagnosed clinically
- Tinea corporis: Ringworm-like configuration on the body with sharply marginated, annular lesions, raised or vesicular margins and central clearing
- Tinea capitis: Scaling patch to scalp containing short, broken hairs ("black dots") is most common form of tinea capitis in the United States; much more common in young children so consider alternative diagnosis in healthy adults.
- Kerion: Tinea capitis with secondary immune response to fungus; appears as an indurated, boggy plaque with overlying pustules (Figure 17.10).
- Confirmation by identification of branching hyphae in keratin scrapings after KOH prep

Q

An 85-year-old woman presents to the emergency department with pain, tingling, and a burning sensation along the right side of her face. She also notes a small group of vesicles to the tip of her nose. What examination should be performed in the ED?

KEY FACT

Necrotizing cellulitis (often Clostridial) without involvement of fascia or muscle can occur.

KEY FACT

The definitive diagnosis of necrotizing fasciitis is made surgically.

KEY FACT

The presence of a raised and scaling margin differentiates tinea from EM and erythema migrans.

A

This patient likely has herpes zoster (shingles) with Hutchinson's sign (vesicles to the tip of the nose). This may signify involvement of the ophthalmic branch of cranial nerve V_1, placing this patient at risk for optic involvement. She should receive a slit lamp examination with fluorescein, and an emergent ophthalmology consult if any concerning findings.

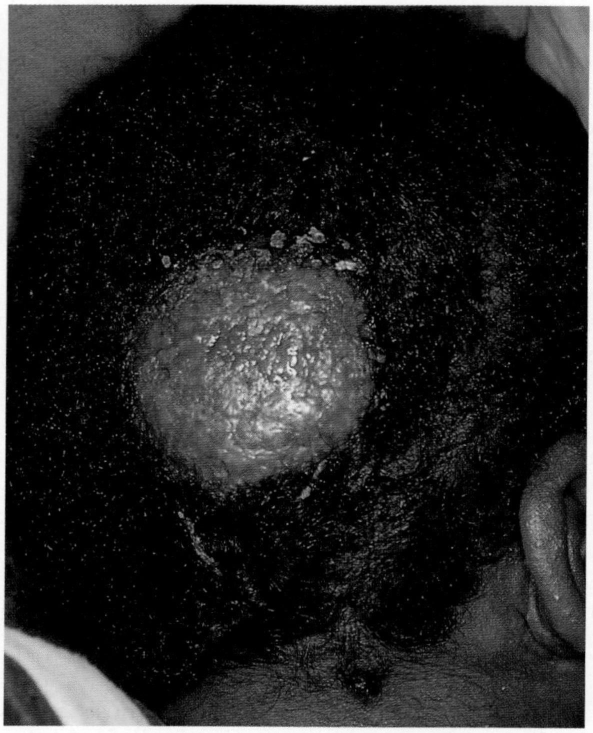

FIGURE 17.10. Kerion with occipital boggy swelling and hair loss. (Reproduced, with permission, from Knoop KJ, Stack LB, Storrow AB. *The Atlas of Emergency Medicine*, 2nd ed. New York, NY: McGraw-Hill, 2002:445. Photographer: Anne W. Lucky, MD.)

Treatment

- Topical antifungal agents are usually effective. Systemic therapy (griseofulvin, itraconazole, or terbinafine) is required for infections of the hair and nails and for recalcitrant disease.
- Kerion is treated the same as tinea capitis (oral antifungals) with the addition of prednisone for 1-2 weeks.

Differential

- **Tinea versicolor:** Superficial fungal infection caused by the yeast *Malassezia* (formerly known as *Pityrosporum*); causes scaling plaques of various colors (pink, tan, white) usually on the chest and trunk; involved areas **fluoresce a yellow to yellow-green under Wood lamp**; definitive diagnosis by KOH prep; treated with topic antifungals (eg, ketoconazole shampoo) or oral itraconazole (extensive disease).
- **Alopecia areata:** Immune-mediated disorder that presents with smooth and circular patches of hair loss; patches also contain short broken hairs, but these hairs narrow near base of shaft (**exclamation point hairs**).
- **Secondary syphilis:** Can present with areas of hair loss that appear patchy (“**moth-eaten**”).

KEY FACT

Findings with hair loss:
"Black dot" hairs = tinea capitis
"Exclamation point" hairs = alopecia areata
"moth-eaten" hair = secondary syphilis

Herpes Simplex

Herpes simplex virus is transmitted through direct contact or infected secretions (saliva or genital). Patients with eczema are at elevated risk for widely disseminated eruptions of HSV. Immunocompromised patients are at risk for systemic dissemination of infection (eg, esophagitis, pneumonia). Neonatal herpes is acquired during delivery.

- **HSV-1** primarily causes oral lesions throughout the mouth; after primary infection a recurrence of lesions usually occur on the lower lip triggered by local trauma, sunburn, or stress.
- **HSV-2** mainly causes genital lesions.

Symptoms/Examination

- Prodrome of local lymphadenopathy, pain, and tingling may occur with lesions appearing within 2 days.
- Small, thin-walled, **grouped vesicles** on an erythematous base.

Diagnosis/Treatment

- A **Tzanck** smear may be used to confirm the diagnosis. Tzanck smears are also positive with varicella/herpes zoster and cannot differentiate between HSV-1 and HSV-2. Viral culture or PCR testing of mucocutaneous lesions may be more effective tests to confirm the diagnosis.
- HSV serum antibody testing may be helpful. Antibodies develop within the first few weeks of initial infection and persist.
- Oral acyclovir, famciclovir, and valacyclovir can shorten duration of symptoms. Topical penciclovir is not effective.
- For sexually transmitted HSV, abstinence is the only method for absolute prevention, condoms are only effective if they cover all lesions; asymptomatic viral shedding still occurs with suppressive drug therapy.

KEY FACT

The Tzanck prep has largely been replaced by culture and PCR testing.

Complications

- **HSV keratitis** (usually due to HSV-1): A leading cause of corneal blindness worldwide. It most commonly presents with a **dendritic** corneal ulcer. Topical or oral antivirals with or without topical steroids are used, depending on location of infection within the cornea. IV antivirals may be necessary in some cases.
- **Eczema herpeticum:** Painful skin and worsening rash in patient with baseline eczema; can be hard to differentiate from severe eczema in appearance.
- **Herpes encephalitis:** Fever, headache, and neurologic symptoms (altered mental status, seizures, deficits); predilection for temporal lobes; most common cause of encephalitis.
- **Herpes esophagitis:** In immunocompromised hosts.

Herpetic Whitlow

Herpetic whitlow is a primary or recurrent HSV-1 or HSV-2 infection of the finger causing painful vesicles on a digit that coalesce and may appear to contain pus, but instead contain necrotic epithelial cells (Figure 17.11).

- It must not be misdiagnosed as a paronychia and incised, which can delay healing and allow secondary infection.
- Treat with local wound care and pain control.

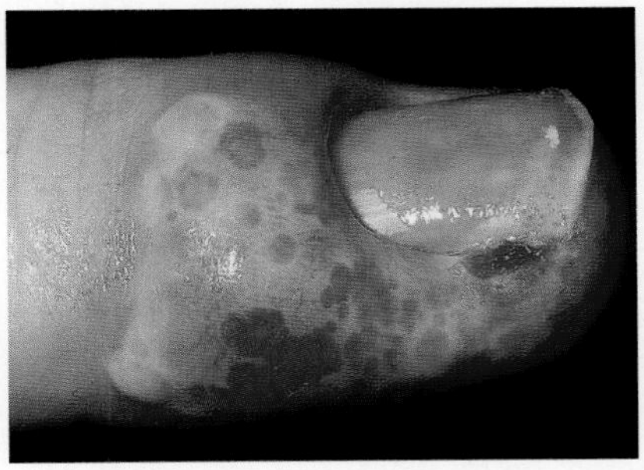

FIGURE 17.11. Herpetic whitlow. (Reproduced, with permission, from Wolff K, Johnson RA, Suurmond D. *Fitzpatrick's Color Atlas and Synopsis of Clinical Dermatology*, 7th ed. New York, NY: McGraw-Hill; 2013. Figure 27.37)

Varicella-Zoster (Shingles)

Shingles results from a reactivation of the latent varicella-zoster virus (VZV) in the dorsal root ganglion. The key risk factor is advanced age, with two-thirds of cases occurring in patients > 50 years. Incidence is also increased in immunocompromised patients.

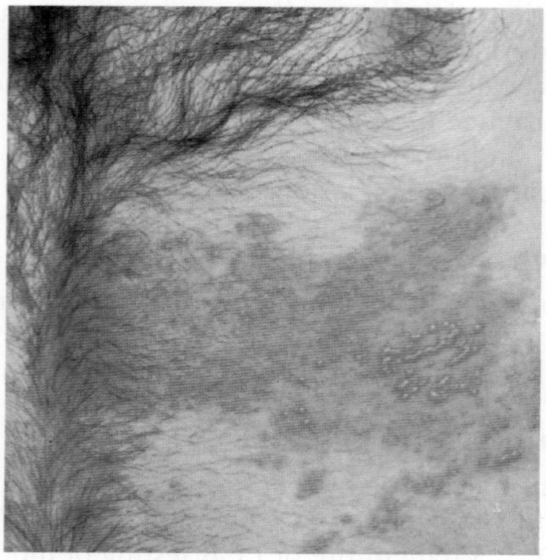

FIGURE 17.12. Herpes zoster (shingles). (Reproduced, with permission, from Goldsmith LA, Katz SI, Gilchrest BA, et al: *Fitzpatrick's Dermatology in General Medicine*, 8th ed. New York, NY: McGraw-Hill, 2012. Figure 194.4A.)

KEY FACT

Hutchinson sign = VZV reactivation of ophthalmic branch of CN V_1, lesion on tip of nose.
Ramsay Hunt syndrome = VZV reactivation of CNs V, IX, and X, lesion in ear canal.

Symptoms/Examination

- Lesions are identical to chickenpox in appearance but have a **unilateral dermatomal** distribution, with thoracic and lumbar areas being most common (see Figure 17.12).
- Lesions appear simultaneously and remain in **congruent stages of healing**, as opposed to smallpox which has variable lesions.
- Infection begins as prodrome of headaches, photophobia, malaise, itching/tingling/pain in the affected area for 1-3 days followed by maculopapular rash → vesicular rash → pustules → ulcers → crusting. The course of the disease is approximately 2 weeks.

Treatment

- Antiviral therapy (acyclovir, famciclovir, valacyclovir) for patients who present within 72 hours of symptoms or if new lesions are still appearing
- Pain control

Complications

- **Herpes zoster ophthalmicus** results from VZV reactivation in the trigeminal nerve first (ophthalmic) division with involvement of its nasociliary branch. Occasionally lesions on the tip of the nose (**Hutchinson's sign**) may be seen before ocular involvement. Staining of the eye typically reveals dendritic lesions or punctate keratitis. This is a vision-threatening condition that requires an ophthalmology consult.
- **Ramsay Hunt syndrome** or herpes zoster oticus results from reactivation of the VZV virus in the geniculate ganglion of the facial nerve with resultant inflammatory changes causing a polycranial neuropathy. It classically presents with ear pain, facial paralysis, and herpetic lesions of the ear canal or auricle. The presentation may mimic Bell's palsy. Vertigo is also common. Ramsay Hunt syndrome is treated with oral acyclovir and steroids.
- **Disseminated disease** with multiple vesicular lesions and end-organ involvement (encephalitis, hepatitis, pneumonia) may be seen in the immunocompromised patient. Treat with IV acyclovir.
- **Postherpetic neuralgia (PHN)**: Severe pain that persists for > 120 days at the site of infection. Incidence is reduced by antiviral treatment at the time of initial illness. The use of corticosteroids to prevent PHN is

KEY FACT

Postherpetic neuralgia is most common in elderly patients.

controversial, though some reliable sources condone their use in high-risk patients without contraindications. Symptoms are treated with tricyclic antidepressants (first-line), gabapentin, opiates, and lidocaine patches.

> **Q**
>
> A Mexican immigrant complains of tender, swollen, red nodules on the lower legs. What rash is suggested by this description? What's the next step?

Infestations

PEDICULOSIS

Pediculosis is infestation by 1 of 3 forms of lice specific to humans, the head louse, the body louse, or the crab (pubic) louse. Adult lice are the size of a sesame seed and live up to 30 days on infested individuals, feeding on blood. Body lice live in clothing and lay eggs (nits) in the seams, while head and crab lice live in infested hair and securely attach their eggs to hair shafts. All can live up to 2 days on inanimate objects. Transmission is through direct contact with infested individuals or their objects such as bedding, clothing, combs, or brushes.

Symptoms/Examination/Diagnosis

- Pruritus is a common feature as an irritant response to lice saliva or excreta.
- Linear excoriations of skin may be present.
- Diagnosis is made by identifying live lice or louse nits. For scalp lice this is best done by combing with a fine-toothed comb. Nits can persistent for months after treatment and fluoresce a pale blue under Wood's lamp.

Treatment

- **Permethrin** 1% rinse or 5% cream is first-line therapy. All close contacts should be treated. Clothing, linens, hairbrushes, carpets, sofas, and similar items should be heat washed or ironed at 65°C (149°F).
- Reevaluate individuals after 9-10 days and retreat if live lice are identified.
- Lindane 1% lotion is second-line therapy. There is concern about **neurotoxicity causing seizures** in children.
- Combing wet hair with a fine-toothed comb every 3-4 days until no lice are identified for 2 weeks is an alternative therapy for head lice.
- Antipruritics may be necessary.

SCABIES

Scabies is a highly contagious, pruritic skin disorder caused by the mite, *Sarcoptes scabiei*. The disease is transmitted through direct contact with an infected individual and less commonly from contact with contaminated objects, which scabies can live on for 2-3 days. Mites live within the epidermis of the skin and make tunnels (burrows) within the skin for laying eggs.

Symptoms/Examination

- **Burrows** are wavy, threadlike, grayish white and 1-10 mm in length, but are not always present.
- Intense pruritus and small erythematous papules with associated excoriations are also common.
- Typical sites of involvement include the **interdigital web spaces** of hands and feet. Penile and scrotal lesions are common in men. Areolae, nipple, and genital areas are commonly affected in women.
- If mite burden becomes high (millions), a form called crusted scabies develops and an immunocompromised state should be suspected.

> **KEY FACT**
>
> Burrows are pathognomonic for scabies.

A

Erythema nodosum. Patient needs further evaluation (start with a review of systems) for causes of erythema nodosum, including *Streptococcus*, tuberculosis, and coccidiomycosis.

MNEMONIC

Causes of Erythema NODOSUM:

NO known cause: Even after a thorough evaluation, the cause of EN remains unknown in 40%-60% of cases
Drugs (OCPs, sulfonamides, PCN, vaccines)
Other (coccidioidomycosis, tuberculosis, Herpes, Epstein–Barr virus, pregnancy)
Strep (most common)/sarcoidosis
Ulcerative colitis/inflammatory bowel disease
Malignancy (leukemia, lymphoma)

Treatment

- **Permethrin**, 5% cream is first line and should be applied from head to toe, excluding scalp. Fingernail areas, web spaces, and the umbilicus should be thoroughly treated. A second treatment should be done 7 days after the first to kill any nymphs that have hatched from eggs.
- **Ivermectin**, an oral antiparasitic, 200 mg/kg given on day 1 and then day 14 is a Centers for Disease Control recommended oral treatment option equivalent to permethrin in nonlactating, nonpregnant adults and in children > 15 kg.
- Lindane was previously recommended, but has fallen out of favor due to its potential for neurotoxicity.
- Crusted scabies requires an aggressive approach using both permethrin and ivermectin.
- All close contacts should be treated and linens washed and dried in a dryer on high heat.
- Pruritus and lesions can persist for 2-4 weeks after successful treatment due to irritant reactions against residuum of dead mites.

Erythema Nodosum

A delayed hypersensitivity reaction to infections (most commonly a recent strep infection), oral contraceptives and a variety of diseases (eg, sarcoidosis, inflammatory bowel disease). Mostly seen in young women, with a female-to-male ratio of 4:1.

Symptoms/Examination

- Numerous, **tender,** erythematous subcutaneous nodules most commonly on the pretibial area of the **lower extremities**; lesions may turn yellow-purple and resemble bruises (Figure 17.13).

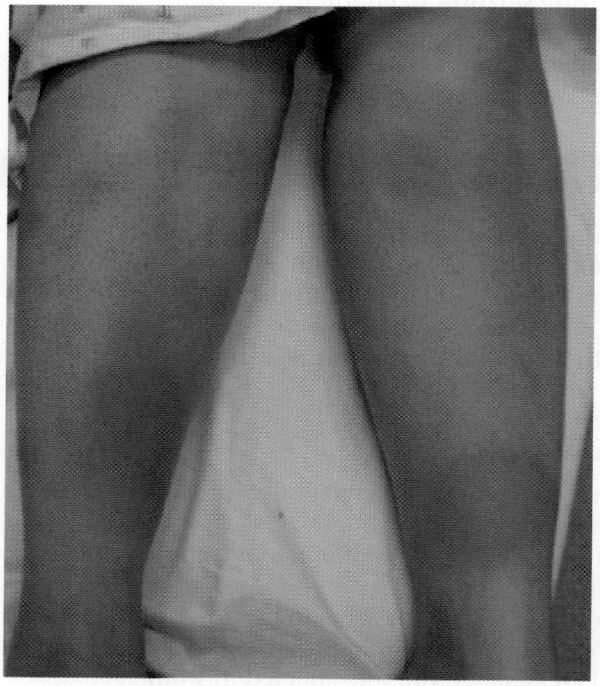

FIGURE 17.13. Erythema nodosum. The nodules are tender, firm, and can resemble bruises. (Reproduced, with permission, from McKean SC, Ross JJ, Dressler DD, et al. *Principles and Practice of Hospital Medicine*. New York, NY: McGraw-Hill Education, 2012. Figure 147.5.)

- Associated symptoms include polyarthralgia, fevers, and malaise.
- Ulceration is not a typical feature and may suggest an alternative diagnosis.

TREATMENT

- Treat underlying cause.
- Symptomatic treatment includes bed rest, leg elevation, and NSAIDs.
- May take 6 weeks to 6 months for full recovery.

> **KEY FACT**
>
> Erythema nodosum is common in patients with inflammatory bowel disease and sarcoidosis.

Pityriasis Rosea

A pruritic, but otherwise benign, self-limited illness of unknown etiology.

SYMPTOMS/EXAMINATION

- Multiple 1- to 2-cm diameter, salmon-colored oval plaques following the ribs in a "Christmas tree" pattern on the trunk (Figure 17.14).
- In half of cases, a larger solitary lesion called a "herald patch" precedes the other lesions by 7 days.
- Lesions may persist for 2-3 months.

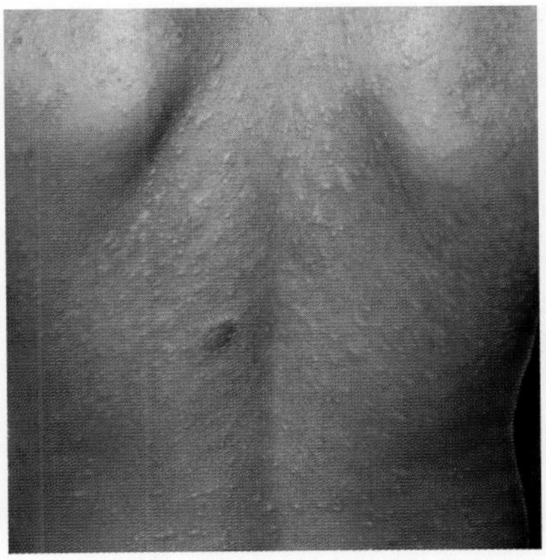

FIGURE 17.14. Pityriasis rosea with visible herald patch. (Reproduced, with permission, from Goldsmith LA, Katz SI, Gilchrest BA, et al: *Fitzpatrick's Dermatology in General Medicine*, 8th ed. New York, NY: McGraw-Hill, 2012. Figure 42.7.)

DIFFERENTIAL

Secondary syphilis, pityriasis rosea-like drug reaction (eg, captopril, barbiturates), guttate psoriasis, nummular eczema, tinea corporis, tinea versicolor

TREATMENT

- Supportive, most do not require therapy.
- May try antipruritics (eg, antihistamines, topical steroids). May be a role for antibiotics, antiviral agents and phototherapy.

> **KEY FACT**
>
> Secondary syphilis can closely resemble pityriasis.

Pemphigus Vulgaris

Pemphigus vulgaris is a life-threatening autoimmune disorder wherein loss of intraepithelial keratinocyte adhesion leads to extensive blistering of skin and mucous membranes and subsequent tissue loss. The disease affects both sexes equally and is most common in 40 to 60 year olds. Use of penicillamine and captopril has been associated with its development.

SYMPTOMS/EXAMINATION

- Symptoms include bullous lesions in the mouth and lips that erode and leave painful ulcers (Figure 17.15).
- Subsequently, small, flaccid bullae form anywhere on the body. They erode easily, forming widespread, **confluent erosions** that are often secondarily infected.
- Nikolsky sign is **positive**. New blisters may be formed by tangential pressure on intact dermis.

> **KEY FACT**
>
> Nikolsky sign is positive in blistering diseases with a very superficial blister, in particular toxic epidermal necrolysis, staphylococcal scalded skin syndrome, and pemphigus vulgaris.

TREATMENT

- Pain control, local wound care, antibiotics for secondary infection, and oral or IV steroids.
- Admission for wound care and IV rehydration may be necessary in widespread disease.

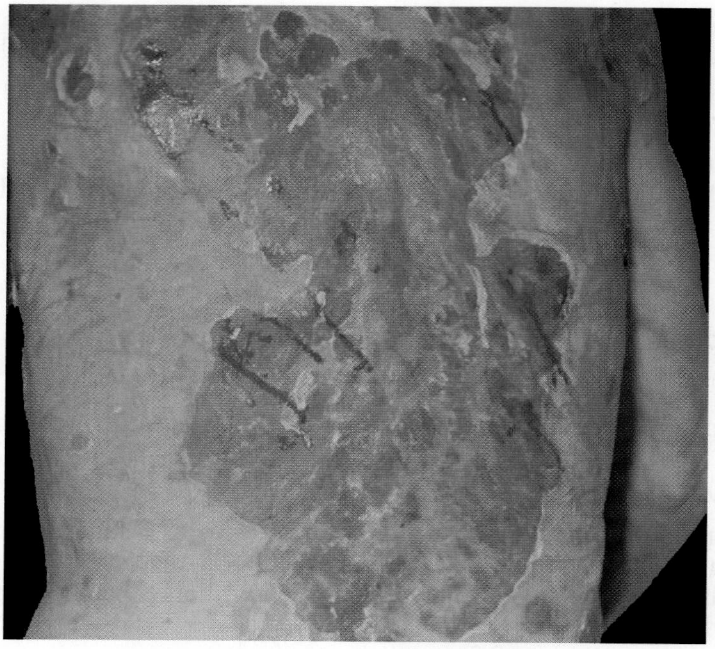

FIGURE 17.15. Pemphigus vulgaris. Typically the blisters are eroded, leaving painful erythematous lesions. (Reproduced, with permission, from Wolff K, Johnson RA, Saavedra AP. *Fitzpatrick's Color Atlas and Synopsis of Clinical Dermatology*. 7th ed. New York, NY: McGraw-Hill Education, 2013. Figure 6.11.)

- Prior to steroid introduction, the mortality rate was 95% due to spread of disease, secondary infection, dehydration, and thromboembolism. The mortality rate is now 10%-15%.

Bullous Pemphigoid

Bullous pemphigoid is a chronic autoimmune blistering disease. Patients are typically older than pemphigus vulgaris patients (> 60 years) and blister formation occurs deeper (subepidermal). Prognosis is better than for pemphigus vulgaris (Table 17.4).

TABLE 17.4. Comparison of Pemphigus Vulgaris with Bullous Pemphigoid

	Patient Population	Lesions	Nikolsky Sign	Treatment and Prognosis
Pemphigus vulgaris	40-60 y old	Small flaccid bullae, erode easily, + oral lesions	Positive	Oral/IV steroids, pain control, wound care Mortality 10%-15%
Bullous pemphigoid	> 60 y old	Large tense bullae, oral lesions rare	Negative	High-potency topical steroids and glucocorticoid sparing agents

IV, intravenous.

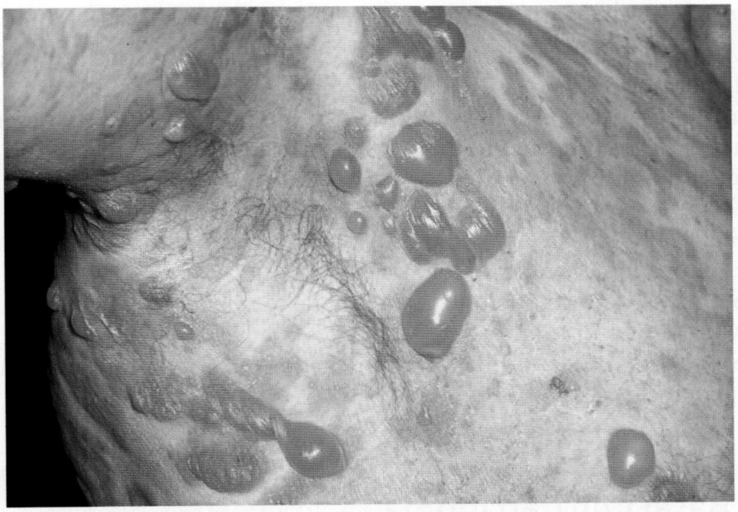

FIGURE 17.16. Bullous pemphigoid with large, tense, fluid-filled bullae that arise from normal or pink skin. (Reproduced with permission from Wolff K, Johnson RA, Saavedra AP: *Fitzpatrick's Color Atlas and Synopsis of Clinical Dermatology*, 7th ed. New York, NY: McGraw-Hill; 2013. Figure 6.15.)

Q

A 45-year-old man, HIV positive with last CD4 count 25 cells/mm^3, no current medications, presents to ED with purple/maroon blotches on his skin, as well as his tongue. What is the most important step in management of this patient?

SYMPTOMS/EXAMINATION

- Large, tense fluid-filled bullae (1-4 cm) arise from normal or pink, urticarial appearing skin (Figure 17.16). Affected skin may be intensely pruritic. Ulceration and tissue loss can follow.
- Axilla and groin are commonly affected sites.
- Oral lesions are rare.
- Due to the depth at which blisters form, Nikolsky sign is **negative** in bullous pemphigoid.

KEY FACT

Blisters are deeper with bullous pemphigoid, so Nikolsky sign is negative.

TREATMENT

- High-potency topical steroids. Oral steroids also work, but are less ideal, due to side effects.
- Glucocorticoid-sparing agents to decrease long-term steroid use: Azathioprine, mycophenolate, methotrexate, dapsone, tetracycline, and nicotinamide

Pressure Ulcers (Decubitus Ulcers)

Pressure ulcers cause significant morbidity in the elderly and the bed bound (eg, obese, neurological impairment, postoperative patients), particularly in nursing homes and in the ICU.

SYMPTOMS/EXAMINATION

- **Stage 1:** Intact skin, local tissue erythema
- **Stage 2:** Penetrate the epidermis or dermis but not the subcutaneous tissue
- **Stage 3:** Extend through the dermis into the subcutaneous tissue
- **Stage 4:** Extend beyond the subcutaneous tissue through to the deep fascia and may involve muscle and bone

DIAGNOSIS

- Clinical diagnosis is based mainly on physical examination.
- Stage 4 ulcers are often underestimated due to fistula formation, eg, a seemingly superficial skin defect may mask extensive deep tissue necrosis. Eschar may also make it difficult to determine depth of wound.

A

This patient has likely Kaposi sarcoma, with typical violaceous lesions. The critical step to managing this process is control of the underlying HIV with antiretroviral therapy.

TREATMENT

- **Prevention:** Ideal positioning of bed-bound patients, position changes at least every 2 hours, pressure reducing devices
- **Treatment:** Fundamentals include proper nutrition, pain management, reducing tissue pressure, maintaining a moist environment, wound debridement, and fighting infection
  - **Stage 1:** More intensive prevention measures
  - **Stage 2:** Occlusive or semipermeable dressing to maintain moist wound environment; avoid wet to dry dressings
  - **Stage 3:** Remove necrotic tissue, manage infections, and maintain moist wound environment
  - **Stage 4:** Undermining and tunneling in consultation with wound specialist (eg, plastic surgeon)

Basal Cell Carcinoma

Basal cell carcinoma (BCC) is the **most common form of skin cancer**. Around 90% occur on sun-exposed skin (especially head and neck), typically in men with age > 50 years. The three main types are nodular, superficial, and morpheaform.

SYMPTOMS/EXAMINATION

- **Nodular:** Pearly papule with visible vessel enlarges over years to nodule with central ulcer (Figure 17.17)
- **Superficial:** Resembles dermatitis, reddish patch with slight scale
- **Morpheaform:** White, waxy papule or plaque

DIAGNOSIS

Requires high index of suspicion followed by, referral to dermatologist for biopsy and pathologic diagnosis.

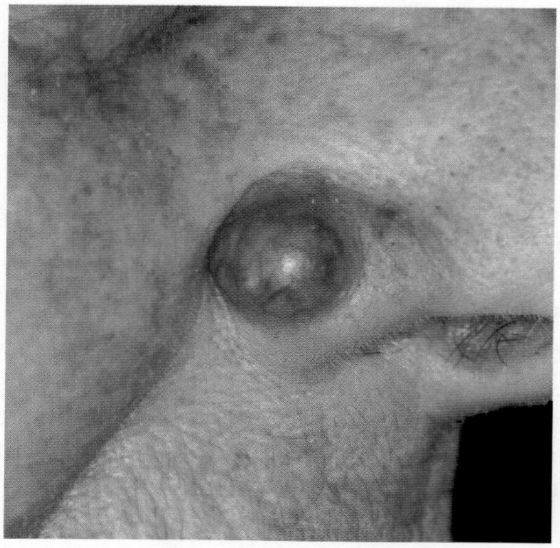

FIGURE 17.17. Basal cell carcinoma: nodular type. Image of a further advanced nodular BCC. A solitary, shiny reddish nodule with large telangiectatic vessels on the ala nasi, arising on skin with dermatoheliosis. (Reproduced, with permission, from Wolff K, Johnson RA, Saavedra AP. Fitzpatrick's Color Atlas and Synopsis of Clinical Dermatology. 7th ed. New York, NY: McGraw-Hill Education, 2013. Figure 11-16B.)

TREATMENT

Depending on stage, may require simple resection (surgical excision or Mohs micrographic surgery) or addition of **chemotherapy.**

Squamous Cell Carcinoma

Squamous cell carcinoma is the second-most common skin cancer after basal cell. Most common in sun-exposed areas (face, scalp, lips, ears, neck, dorsal hands).

SYMPTOMS/EXAMINATION

Quickly growing, erythematous raised lesion with ulcerated center (Figure 17.18)

DIAGNOSIS

Refer to dermatologist for biopsy and pathologic diagnosis.

TREATMENT

Cure rate by resection > 90%. Metastases are more likely when lesion occurs over scarred skin; regional lymphadenopathy is most common manifestation.

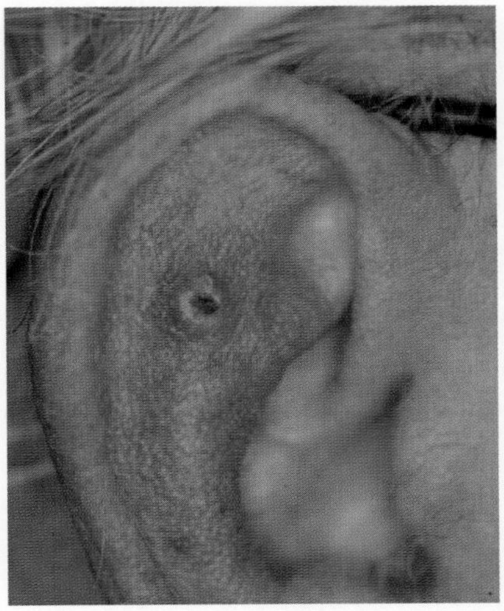

FIGURE 17.18. Squamous cell carcinoma. A rapidly growing, erythematous raised lesion with ulcerated center. (Reproduced with permission from Goldsmith LA, Katz SI, Gilchrest BA, et al: *Fitzpatrick's Dermatology in General Medicine*, 8th ed. New York, NY: McGraw-Hill, 2012. Figure 114.1.)

Kaposi Sarcoma

Kaposi sarcoma manifests as a vascular cutaneous neoplasm, most commonly seen in patients with HIV/AIDS and low CD4 counts. Now relatively uncommon following widespread use of antiretroviral therapy. Related to HHV-8 infection. May also be seen sporadically in African and European populations.

SYMPTOMS/EXAMINATION

- Red or purple papules and plaques (Figure 17.19)
- May involve skin, mucous membranes, GI tract, lungs

DIAGNOSIS

Typically clinical in setting of patient with known HIV; may also require skin biopsy by dermatology.

TREATMENT

- Control of underlying HIV will often control the sarcoma as well.
- Some patients require intralesion or systemic chemotherapy.

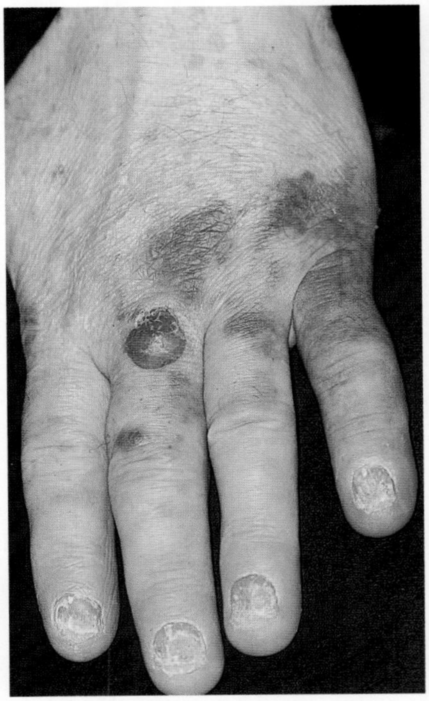

FIGURE 17.19. Kaposi sarcoma. (Reproduced with permission from Wolff K, Johnson RA, Saavedra AP: *Fitzpatrick's Color Atlas and Synopsis of Clinical Dermatology*, 7th ed. New York, NY: McGraw-Hill; 2013. Figure 21.16.)

Melanoma

A pigmented skin cancer, often developing within a prior normal nevus. Makes up only 1% of skin cancer overall, but up to 60% of skin cancer mortalities. Most significant risk factor is a primary relative with melanoma.

SYMPTOMS/EXAMINATION

- May occur in prior nevus.
- New mole in a patient > age 35 years is suspicious.

MNEMONIC

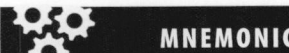

Five cardinal features of melanoma:

ABCDE

Asymmetry
Border irregular
Color mottled
Diameter > 6 mm (size of a pencil eraser)
Enlargement or elevation

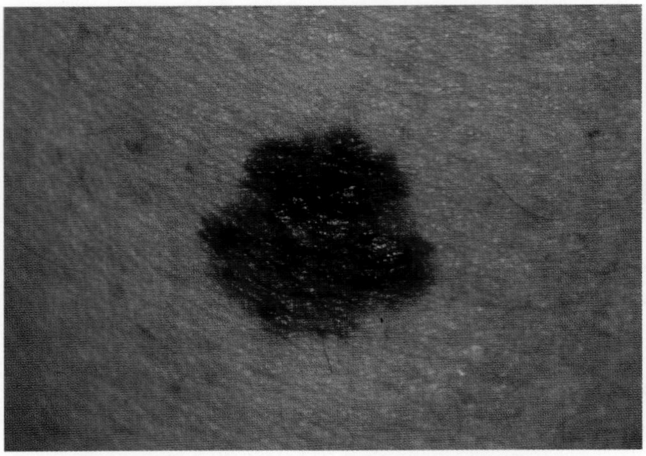

FIGURE 17.20. Melanoma. (Reproduced with permission from Knoop KJ, Storrow AB, Stack LB, and Thurman RJ. *The Atlas of Emergency Medicine*, 3rd ed. New York, NY: McGraw-Hill; 2010. Figure 13.80. Photographer: The Department of Dermatology, Wilford Hall USAF Medical Center and Brooke Army Medical Center, San Antonio, TX.)

- Changing shape, size, color is suspicious (Figure 17.20).
- Friability or ulceration may occur.
- Commonly spreads to lung, liver, brain, and bone.

Diagnosis

Urgent referral Refer urgently to dermatology for biopsy and pathologic diagnosis.

Treatment

Prognosis is determined by the depth of the lesion and presence of metastasis. May be treated with resection alone if early, although chemotherapy and radiation may be required for later disease.

REVIEW QUESTIONS

QUESTIONS

1. A 9-year-old boy presents with several days of progressively worsening rash. He has multiple pruritic, erythematous, raised lesions with central clearing and a scaling margin. Which of the following is the most likely diagnosis?
   A. Erythema marginatum
   B. Erythema migrans
   C. Erythema multiforme
   D. Tinea corporis

2. A 12-week-old infant is brought in to the emergency department with several days of greasy, yellow scales developing on the scalp. Which of the following is the most appropriate treatment?
   A. A short course of antifungal shampoo
   B. Topical corticosteroid cream
   C. Reassurance and washing with a mild shampoo
   D. Daily washing with tar-based shampoo

3. A 62-year-old woman presents with 2 days of painful, vesicular lesions on an erythematous base extending around her right flank. Which of the following is the most appropriate treatment?
   A. Acyclovir
   B. Intramuscular benzathine penicillin G
   C. Oral prednisone
   D. No treatment and reassurance

4. A 28-year-old man presents complaining of a pruritic rash across his back. It initially began as a single, enlarging spot, but now a week later, he notes multiple 1-2 cm salmon-colored plaques on his back. What is the most appropriate treatment?
   A. Acyclovir
   B. Topical corticosteroid cream
   C. Permethrin cream
   D. Topical mupirocin ointment

5. A 19-year-old man, who is a soldier at the local military base, presents complaining of intense pruritus in his groin and between his fingers. Several other soldiers in his barracks have similar symptoms. He has excoriations and small erythematous papules in the affected areas. Which of the following is the most appropriate treatment?
   A. Ivermectin
   B. Lindane
   C. Prednisone cream
   D. Triamcinolone ointment

6. A 59-year-old woman with type 2 diabetes presents with an intensely painful red rash in her right lower extremity. The rash began yesterday around the ankle and now spreads proximally almost to the knee. It is warm to the touch and there is a small bullous lesion over the tibia. Which is the most appropriate first step in treating this patient?
   A. Initiate broad-spectrum antibiotics.
   B. Radiographs to evaluate for subcutaneous gas
   C. Topical corticosteroids
   D. Urgent surgical consultation

7. A 68-year-old farmer presents for evaluation of a 2 cm pearly lesion on his cheek that has been developing over the last 2 years. On examination there is a small area of central ulceration. What is the most likely diagnosis?
   A. Basal cell carcinoma
   B. Kaposi sarcoma
   C. Melanoma
   D. Squamous cell carcinoma

8. A 4-year-old boy is admitted to the ICU with a widespread erythematous rash, blistering, and superficial separation of the skin without mucous membrane involvement. Which of the following is the most appropriate treatment?
   A. Acyclovir
   B. Corticosteroids
   C. Intravenous immunoglobulin
   D. Vancomycin

9. Which of the following is treated with topical mupirocin?
   A. Aphthous ulcer
   B. Atopic dermatitis
   C. Erysipelas
   D. Impetigo

10. A 23-year-old woman presents with multiple tender purple "bumps" over her lower extremities after starting a new antibiotic for a urinary tract infection. Which of the following is true regarding this condition?
   A. It is associated with inflammatory bowel disease.
   B. It involves the mucous membranes.
   C. It is a tick-borne illness.
   D. Ulceration of lesions is common.

ANSWERS

1. **D.** Tinea corporis is the only lesion above that is characterized by a scaling margin. It is a superficial fungal infection that can spread easily. Treatment is with topical antifungals. Erythema marginatum is a migratory annular and polycyclic eruption that is seem in acute rheumatic fever in children. Erythema migrans is an expanding red lesion with central clearing at the site of the tick bite in Lyme disease. Erythema multiforme is an immune-mediated rash most commonly triggered by HSV infection and manifesting as erythematous pupules that evolve to target lesions.

2. **C.** Seborrheic dermatitis of the infant (cradle cap) is a benign condition of infants that typically resolves by age 1. It is treated with emollients and frequent washing with mild shampoo. In contrast, adult seborrhea is a chronic and relapsing condition that is treated with antifungal shampoos or those with coal tar, sulfur or selenium.

3. **A.** Shingles results from reactivation of the latent VZV virus in the dorsal root ganglion. For patients presenting within 72 hours of symptoms or those with new lesions still appearing, treatment with acyclovir is recommended. Prednisone therapy to prevent postthereptic neuralgia is controversial and not universally recommended.

4. **B.** Pityriasis rosea is characterized by multiple 1- to 2-cm-diamter, salmon-colored oval plaques following the ribs in a "Christmas tree" pattern on the trunk. In half of cases a larger solitary "herald patch" is present. Treatment is primarily supportive, but antihistamines and topical steroids may help with itching.

5. **A.** Scabies is a highly contagious, pruritic skin disorder caused by the mite *Sarcoptes scabiei*. Symptoms include intense pruritus of the interdigital web spaces and genital areas. Treatment is with Permethrin, 5% cream applied from head to toe, excluding scalp, repeated on day 7. An alternative is ivermectin, an oral antiparasitic that is given on day 1 and 14. Lindane is not recommended because of its potential for neurotoxicity.

6. **D.** This presentation with pain out of proportion to examination and rapidly progressive erythema and bullae formation is concerning for a necrotizing soft tissue infection. It is primarily a clinical diagnosis, though imaging showing air in soft tissues supports the diagnosis. Immediate surgical consultation should be obtained when the diagnosis is suspected along with broad-spectrum antibiotics.

7. **A.** Basal cell carcinoma is the most common form of skin cancer characterized by a pearly papule with visible vessel that enlarges over years to a nodule with a central ulceration. Kaposi sarcoma is primarily seen in patients with AIDS and is characterized by red or purple papules and plaques. Melanoma is characterized by a change in shape, size or color of a mole is characteristic of melanoma. Squamous cell carcinoma is characterized by a quick growing, erythematous raised lesion with an ulcerated center on sun-exposed surfaces.

8. **D.** This patient likely has staphylococcal scalded skin syndrome cause by an infection (conjunctiva, nasopharynx, umbilicus) with an exotoxin-producing strain of *Staphylococcus aureus*. Treatment is with ICU-level wound care and fluid-resuscitation along with anti-staph antibiotics such as oxacillin or vancomycin.

9. **D.** Impetigo is a superficial epidermal infection caused by *S. aureus* and group A streptococci characterized by superficial vesicles and pustules covered with honey-colored crusts. With limited number of lesions, it can be treated with topical mupirocin alone. Atopic dermatitis is treated with topical steroids, erysepilas with oral/IV antibiotics and aphthous ulcers with topical analgesics and oral rinses.

10. **A.** Erythema nodosum results from a delay-hypersensitivity reaction to infection, oral contraceptives and a number of disease including inflammatory bowel disease. It is treated with bed rest, leg elevation and NSAIDs.

CHAPTER 18

Renal and Genitourinary Emergencies

Jordan Ryan, MD

Proteinuria

Proteinuria can be divided into four basic etiologies: glomerular (increased glomerular permeability), tubular (decreased tubular reabsorption), overflow (excess production exceeding normal kidney capabilities), and postrenal (inflammation in the urinary tract).

SYMPTOMS/EXAMINATION

- Examine patient to gauge severity of protein loss and to look for underlying causes.
- Because most cases are functional, examination is often normal.
- Significant proteinuria leads to edema, ranging from dependent peripheral edema to anasarca (protein wasting in urine → decreased plasma oncotic pressure → increased interstitial fluid).
- Ask about history of recent viral or systemic illness, change in medications, hypertension, diabetes, cardiac, or renal disease, and any signs of systemic illness (weight loss, fatigue, etc).

DIAGNOSIS

- Blood urea nitrogen (BUN)/creatinine (Cr) should be obtained to gauge underlying renal function.
- Proteinuria in combination with other urinalysis findings may be markers of disease:
  - Red blood cell (RBC) casts and hematuria → glomerulonephritis (GN)
  - Fatty casts or oval fat bodies → nephrotic syndrome
  - White blood cells (WBCs), WBC casts without bacteria → interstitial nephritis
  - Hyaline casts → benign causes
- Frequent false-positive proteinuria within 24 hours of iodinated radiocontrast agents, in setting of highly alkaline urine, in presence of gross hematuria, or in presence of specific antiseptics (eg, chlorhexidine, benzalkonium).

TREATMENT

- Patients may be referred for primary care provider follow-up in the absence of edema, azotemia, hypertension, or evidence of systemic illness affecting the kidneys.
- Persistent proteinuria may require referral to a nephrologist, possibly for renal biopsy.

NEPHROTIC SYNDROME

KEY FACT

Nephrotic syndrome: proteinuria, hypoalbuminemia, edema, hyperlipidemia, hypercoagulability.

A form of glomerular proteinuria in which protein losses exceed the liver's capacity to synthesize albumin, resulting in hypoalbuminemia and subsequent systemic effects. It may be caused by a primary glomerular disease process or secondary to diabetes, lupus, etc.

SYMPTOMS/EXAMINATION

- Gradual onset of edema
- Foamy urine, due to high levels of protein

DIAGNOSIS

- Based on characteristic clinical and laboratory findings
  - Peripheral edema and/or ascites.
  - Proteinuria: 3+ or 4+ on dipstick, or 3.5-g protein per 24 hours.

- Fatty casts or oval fat bodies on UA: possibly related to associated hyperlipidemia.
- Hypoproteinemia and hypoalbuminemia.
- BUN and Cr are often normal.

TREATMENT

- Symptomatic: Fluid restriction, intravenous (IV) diuretics, BP control with angiotension-converting enzyme (ACE) inhibitors.
- Corticosteroids may reverse or delay disease progression.

COMPLICATIONS

Increased risk of thrombosis—deep vein thrombosis and renal vein thrombosis (hematuria, flank pain, and worsening renal function)

Q

A 5-year-old boy presents to the emergency department (ED) with 3 days of "brown urine" and facial swelling. One week earlier he had experienced a fever and sore throat. On examination, he is mildly hypertensive and has periorbital edema. His blood urea nitrogen (BUN) and creatinine (Cr) are elevated. What Urinalysis (UA) findings would confirm your suspicion of poststreptococcal glomerulonephritis (GN)?

KEY FACT

Renal vein thrombosis should be considered in all patients with nephrotic syndrome presenting with hematuria, flank pain, and worsening renal function.

Hematuria

Hematuria can be microscopic or gross in nature; it only takes 1 mL of blood in 1 L of urine to turn urine red. While microscopic hematuria is often transient and benign, gross hematuria has a higher incidence of serious underlying pathology. In patients > 60 years, gross hematuria has a positive predictive value for malignancy of 22.1% in men and 8.3% in women.

Pseudohematuria: Red discoloration of urine due to ingestion of foods (beets, berries, rhubarb), medications (rifampin, phenazopyridine, nitrofurantoin), porphyrias (heme precursors enter urine)

Table 18.1 lists the most common etiologies of hematuria by age group.

SYMPTOMS/EXAMINATION

- Some examination findings can give clue to source of bleeding, eg, peripheral edema, atrial fibrillation, abdominal bruit, palpable abdominal mass, flank tenderness, and genitourinary (GU) lesions.
- The character of hematuria may help localize the source.
  - Blood clots indicate a nonglomerular source.
  - Brown-colored urine indicates a renal source.

TABLE 18.1. Common Causes of Hematuria by Age

< 20 years	Glomerulonephritis GU trauma Intense exercise UTI
20-40 years	Stone GU trauma Intense exercise UTI
40+ years	Carcinoma (bladder, kidney) Stone UTI BPH (males)

BPH, benign prostatic hyperplasia; GU, genitourinary; UTI, urinary tract infection.

A

Proteinuria, dysmorphic red blood cells (RBCs), and RBC casts.

TABLE 18.2. Clinical Clues That Suggest a Particular Diagnosis in Patients with Hematuria

CLINICAL FINDINGS	DISEASE
Dysuria, frequency	UTI
Hearing loss	Alport syndrome
Hemoptysis	Goodpasture syndrome, Wegener granulomatosis (patient may also have upper respiratory symptoms such as nosebleeds)
Recent URI	Glomerulonephritis or IgA nephropathy
Proteinuria, RBC casts	Glomerulonephritis
Edema	Glomerulonephritis
Petechiae/purpura, schistocytes on smear	Hemolytic uremic syndrome (children) or TTP (adults)
Nephrotic syndrome, flank pain	Renal vein thrombosis
Developing countries	**Schistosomiasis**

IgA, immunoglobulin A; RBC, red blood cell; TTP, thrombotic thrombocytopenic purpura; URI, upper respiratory infection; UTI, urinary tract infection.

  - Occurring with initiation of voiding or between voids suggests urethral source.
  - Occurring at the end of voiding suggests a source in the bladder neck or prostatic urethra.
  - Occurring throughout the urinary stream suggests a source proximal to the urethra.
- Table 18.2 lists clues from the clinical presentation that suggest a particular diagnosis in patients with hematuria.

KEY FACT

Timing of hematuria with micturition:
Initiation—urethral source
End—bladder neck/prostatic urethral source
Throughout—source proximal to urethra

KEY FACT

If a urine dipstick is positive for heme but no RBCs are seen on microscopic urinalysis, consider rhabdomyolysis.

DIAGNOSIS

- Obtain UA, BUN/Cr, ± complete blood count (CBC).
- Gross hematuria will be dipstick positive for protein.
- Patients with gross hematuria and those with risk factors for serious etiology (age > 35 years, smokers, occupational exposure, abdominal pain, excessive analgesic use) warrant imaging—computed tomography (CT) or ultrasound.
- Other imaging studies—intravenous pyelogram (IVP), angiography, cystoscopy—can be done as an outpatient.
- Presence of anticoagulant use, benign prostatic hyperplasia (BPH), and exercise usually does not directly cause persistent hematuria; evaluate them similarly to other patients.

TREATMENT

- Depends on underlying cause.
- Patients with bladder outlet obstruction from clot formation require 3-way Foley catheter placement and bladder irrigation.
- Belladonna and Opium (B&O) suppositories may alleviate pain from refractory bladder spasms in patients with known bladder cancer and hematuria.

TABLE 18.3. Classification and Causes of Acute Kidney Injury

Prerenal	Intrinsic Renal	Postrenal
Hypovolemia	Glomerulonephritis	Urinary tract obstruction (at any level)
Volume redistribution	AIN	
Decreased effective cardiac output	ATN	
Medications	Vascular causes	

AIN, acute interstitial nephritis; ATN, acute tubular necrosis.

Q

A 65-year-old woman with diabetes mellitus type II (DMII) and hypertension (HTN) presents to the ED with 2 days of nausea vomiting and diarrhea. She appears dry and is mildly hypotensive. She was recently started on an ACE inhibitor. Laboratory work reveals her serum BUN is 45 mg/dL and her serum Cr is now 2 mg/dL, from a baseline of 1.2 mg/dL. In addition to prerenal insults secondary to volume loss, what other etiology for acute kidney injury (AKI) must be considered?

Acute Kidney Injury

Acute kidney injury (AKI) describes a sudden decline in kidney function, marked by the accumulation of nitrogenous waste products, disturbances of fluid balance, and a wide range of other metabolic disturbances. It is classified according to underlying pathophysiology into three groups: **prerenal**, **intrinsic**, and **postrenal** (Tables 18.3 and 18.4).

KEY FACT

The most common cause of community-acquired AKI is hypovolemia.

PRERENAL

Prerenal AKI occurs because of decreased renal perfusion. It is the most common reason for AKI in the nonhospitalized patient.

TABLE 18.4. Urinary Indices in Acute Kidney Injury

	Prerenal	Acute Tubular Necrosis	Intrinsic Renal Acute Glomerulonephritis	Acute Interstitial Nephritis	Postrenal
Serum BUN/Cr ratio	> 20:1	< 20:1	> 20:1	< 20:1	> 20:1
U_{Na} (mEq/L)	< 20	> 20	< 20	Variable	Variable
FENa (%)	< 1	> 2	< 1	Variable	Variable
Urine osmolality	Increased	< 350	Increased	Variable	< 350
Urinalysis	Normal or hyaline casts	Granular (muddy brown) casts, renal tubular casts	Dysmorphic RBCs, RBC casts, proteinuria	WBC, WBC casts, eosinophils	Normal

BUN, blood urea nitrogen; Cr, creatinine; RBC, red blood cell; WBC, white blood cell.

Always suspect bilateral renal artery stenosis in patients with AKI after starting ACE inhibitor therapy.

KEY FACT

Prerenal acute renal failure is associated with a high urine osmolality but a low U_{Na} (< 20 mEq/dL) and a low FENa (< 1%). The kidneys are trying not to lose sodium.

KEY FACT

A low U_{Na} indicates intact urinary concentrating ability and the presence of a stimulus to conserve Na^+.

KEY FACT

Evaluating urinary sodium indices is not helpful in patients with underlying chronic renal failure or diuretic use.

CAUSES

Causes of prerenal AKI include:

- **Hypovolemia**: Hemorrhage, vomiting and diarrhea, diuretic therapy
- **Volume redistribution**: Third-space sequestration, sepsis, hypoalbuminemic states such as cirrhosis
- **Decreased effective cardiac output**: Myocardial infarction (MI), valvular disease, cardiomyopathy, malignant HTN
- **Medications that limit glomerular perfusion**: ACE inhibitors and non-steroidal anti-inflammatory drugs (NSAIDs)

SYMPTOMS/EXAMINATION

Will vary depending on underlying etiology.

DIAGNOSIS

- BUN/Cr ratio > 20:1
- Evidence of **increased renal Na^+ conservation**:
  - Urinary Na^+ (U_{Na}) concentration < 20 mEq/dL.
  - Fractional excretion of sodium (FE_{Na}) < 1%.

$$FENa = \frac{\text{Urine Na} \times \text{Plasma Cr}}{\text{Plasma Na} \times \text{Urine Cr}} \times 100$$

  - Fractional excretion of urea (FE_{Urea}) can be calculated in the setting of diuretic use, with a FE_{Urea} < 35% suggestive of prerenal etiology.
- Urine osmolality increased
- Urinalysis: Normal, may have occasional hyaline casts

TREATMENT

- Treat underlying cause (eg, correct hypovolemia, augment cardiac output).
- Discontinue offending drugs: NSAIDs, ACE inhibitors.
- Correct electrolyte imbalances.
- Dialysis rarely necessary.

INTRINSIC

Intrinsic AKI results from pathology of the glomerulus, interstitium, or renal tubule.

CAUSES

Causes of intrinsic AKI include:

- **GN**
- **Acute interstitial nephritis (AIN)**
- **Acute tubular necrosis**
- **Vascular disease**

Glomerulonephritis

Glomerulonephritis (GN) is a category of renal diseases characterized by inflammation of the glomeruli. It may be a primary process, as in poststreptococcal GN, or secondary to underlying systemic disease, such as lupus, Goodpasture syndrome, and systemic vasculitis.

SYMPTOMS/EXAMINATION

- Patients may be asymptomatic at time of diagnosis.
- Symptoms include dark urine, hematuria, edema, and hypertension.

DIAGNOSIS

- The characteristic findings on urinalysis include hematuria, dysmorphic RBCs, proteinuria, and, most importantly, **RBC casts**.
- Proteinuria may be nephrotic range.
- Renal biopsy is definitive.

> **KEY FACT**
>
> RBC casts are pathognomonic for GN, but may not be picked up by machine urinalysis.

TREATMENT

- Supportive care, control BP.
- Steroids and other immunosuppressives are used to treat underlying systemic disease (when present), but are not indicated in poststreptococcal GN.

Acute Interstitial Nephritis

Acute interstitial nephritis (AIN) results from interstitial inflammation, most commonly in response to medications (penicillins, diuretics, anticoagulants, NSAIDs), but is also associated with infections and autoimmune disease. The mechanism is thought to be immunologic, and there is minimal relationship to medication dosing or duration of therapy.

> **KEY FACT**
>
> NSAIDs can cause AIN, decreased renal perfusion, and nephrotic syndrome.

SYMPTOMS/EXAMINATION

Symptoms variable—fever in 35%, arthralgias in 30%, rash in 20%.

DIAGNOSIS

- Elevated BUN/Cr.
- Presence of eosinophils, WBCs, and WBC casts on UA.
- Renal biopsy is definitive.

TREATMENT

- Supportive care.
- Discontinue offending agent.
- Steroids only needed if no improvement after 3-7 days; no indication in emergency department (ED).

Acute Tubular Necrosis

The most common cause of hospital-acquired AKI. This is (generally) reversible injury to the renal tubule due to:

- **Renal ischemia**: Surgery, trauma, sepsis.
- **Nephrotoxic agents**: Aminoglycosides and radiocontrast agents are most common offenders.
- Risk factors for contrast-induced acute tubular necrosis (ATN) include renal insufficiency, diabetes, intravascular volume depletion, and higher dose of contrast material.
- **Pigments**: Myoglobin (rhabdomyolysis), hemoglobin (hemolysis).

DIAGNOSIS

- Characterized by the **loss of urinary concentrating ability**.
- Urinalysis: Granular (muddy brown) casts and renal tubular casts.
- Suspect rhabdomyolysis if urine is dip positive for heme, but negative for RBCs.

> **KEY FACT**
>
> In ATN, urine osmolality = serum osmolality

TREATMENT

- Treat underlying precipitating cause or discontinue offending agent.
- Use of low-osmolality contrast agents, pretreating with **N-acetylcysteine and/or sodium bicarbonate**, and IV hydration with normal saline may help prevent ATN in high-risk patients (diabetes, preexisting renal insufficiency) receiving radiocontrast agents.
- Renal function typically recovers over days to weeks.

Vascular Disease

Vascular disease of the kidney may be macrovascular (eg, renal artery occlusion, abdominal aortic aneurysm [AAA]) or microvascular (eg, embolus, malignant hypertension, hemolytic uremic syndrome [HUS], thrombotic thrombocytopenic purpura [TTP]).

POSTRENAL

Causes

Results from obstruction at any level of the urinary tract:

- **Bladder outlet obstruction**: BPH, stones, clot, tumor, neurogenic bladder, posterior urethral valve, phimosis, urethral stricture
- **Intrarenal/ureteral obstruction**: Kidney stone, crystalline precipitation (eg, due to tumor lysis, ethylene glycol ingestion), tumor (intrinsic or extrinsic), iatrogenic, papillary necrosis

Symptoms/Examination

Anuria/oliguria, often with systemic symptoms depending on cause

Diagnosis

- Renal and bladder ultrasound to differentiate between upper- and lower-tract obstruction.
- Bedside ultrasound very sensitive for hydronephrosis (Figure 18.1).
- Urinalysis and BUN/Cr ratios are typically **unhelpful**.

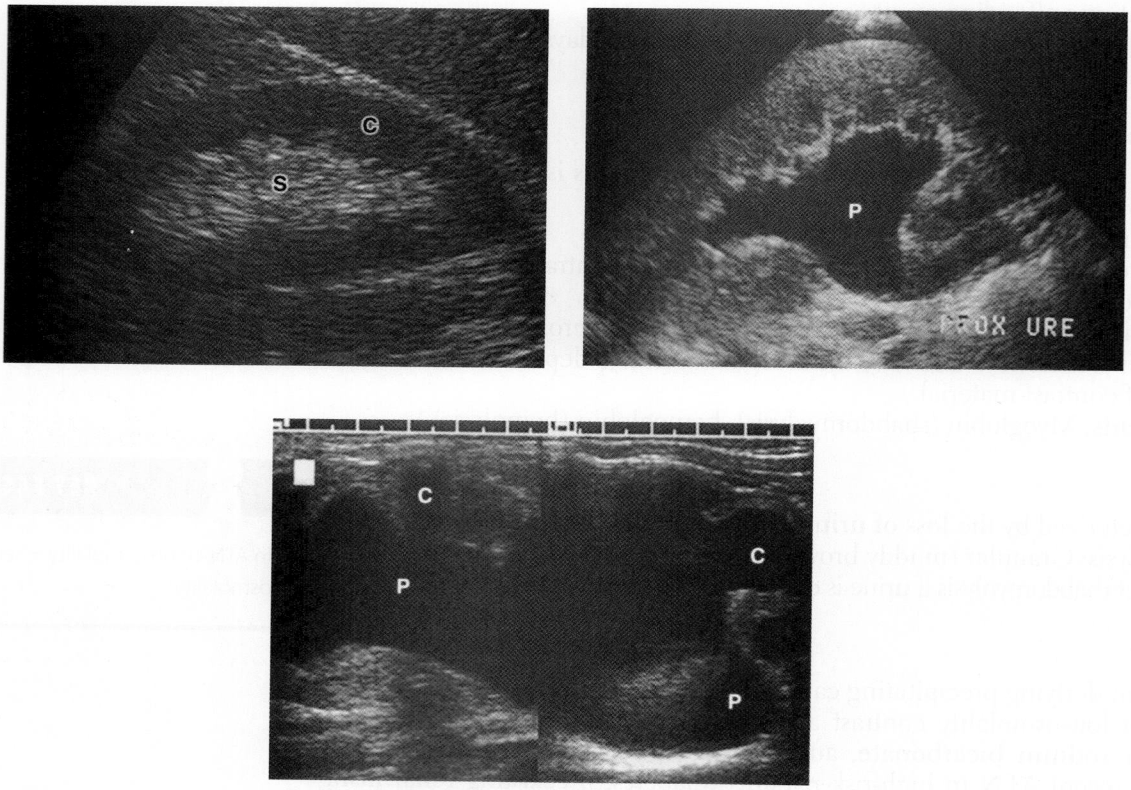

FIGURE 18.1. Normal ultrasound appearance of kidney, then mild-moderate and severe hydronephrosis. (Reproduced, with permission, from McAninch JW, Lue TF. *Smith & Tanagho's General Urology*. 18th ed. New York, NY: McGraw-Hill Education; 2013. Figure 6.21.)

Treatment

- Relieve obstruction (eg, Foley catheter for bladder outlet obstruction).
- Correct electrolyte imbalances.
- Percutaneous nephrostomy tube placement or cystoscopy with retrograde pyelography and stent placement may be necessary; rely on urologist recommendations.
- Start alfuzosin or tamsulosin with initiation of urinary catheter for BPH.

Chronic Kidney Disease

Chronic kidney disease (CKD) is a wide spectrum of disease defined as permanent loss of renal function of > 3 months duration. It is staged based on the estimated glomerular filtration rate (GFR). End-stage renal disease (ESRD, or **kidney failure**) is the final endpoint where GFR is < 10% of normal, and clinical symptoms of uremia will ensue without dialysis or transplant.

Symptoms/Examination

- Uremia:
  - Symptoms of uremia are often nonspecific and include anorexia, nausea, vomiting, and decreased mental function.
  - Uremic frost: Deposition of urea from evaporated sweat; fine white powder on skin.
- Volume overload/pulmonary edema
- Hypertension
- Renal osteodystrophy:
  - Due to loss of vitamin D_3 production and secondary hyperparathyroidism
  - Bone pain, muscle weakness, fractures
- Pericarditis:
  - Consider cardiac tamponade in **any** ill-appearing patient with ESRD.
  - Early tamponade may manifest as hypotension during dialysis.
- Systemic calcification:
  - Deposition of calcium in joints (pseudogout).
  - Deposition in the tunica media of small arteries (calciphylaxis) leading to thrombosis, ischemia, and necrosis of skin and soft tissues. The condition is usually eventually fatal and requires admission.
- Anemia:
  - Normocytic, normochromic
  - Due to decreased erythropoietin production and RBC survival time
- Bleeding:
  - Multifactorial: Decreased platelet function, altered von Willebrand factor (vWF)
  - May include subdural hematomas, gastrointestinal (GI)_ bleeding
- Encephalopathy:
  - May include mental status changes, hiccups, asterixis (hand flapping with dorsiflexion), and myoclonic twitching
- Hyperkalemia (see chapter 14, Head, Eyes, Ear, Nose, and Throat, and Dental Emergencies)
- Immunosuppression
- Peripheral neuropathy

Treatment

- If patient is not ESRD, look for and treat reversible causes of AKI.
- Usual management of HTN, pulmonary edema, hyperkalemia.
- Dialysis.
- Renal transplantation.

KEY FACT

Never give Fleet enema to an ESRD patient due to its high phosphate content.

Violaceous or black skin lesions in a patient with ESRD suggest calciphylaxis.

KEY FACT

Furosemide may have a vasodilating benefit in CKD with pulmonary edema even in patients who cannot produce urine.

- Acute bleeding:
  - **DDAVP**: First line, stimulates release of vWF from endothelial cells
  - **Cryoprecipitate**: Contains factors I (fibrinogen), II (fibronectin), VIII, XIII, and vWF
  - **Conjugated estrogens**: Increases platelet reactivity and decreases nitric oxide generation
  - **Transfusion of packed red blood cells (PRBCs)**: For symptomatic anemia, if Hgb < 7 g/dL

Dialysis-Related Emergencies

Dialysis can be in the form of hemodialysis (HD) where an artificial membrane filters solute and fluids, or peritoneal dialysis (PD) where the peritoneal membrane serves as the dialysis membrane.

INDICATIONS FOR EMERGENT DIALYSIS

Indications for emergent dialysis are listed in Table 18.5.

COMPLICATIONS OF HEMODIALYSIS

Hypotension

Commonly due to fluid shifts and often resolves spontaneously or with a small fluid bolus. Be sure to consider serious causes: tamponade, infection, MI, bleeding, hyperkalemia, air embolism, and anaphylaxis.

Bleeding

Dialysis-related bleeding may be due to underlying platelet dysfunction of ESRD or HD-associated transient thrombocytopenia and anticoagulation.

KEY FACT

Always consider serious causes (eg, tamponade, MI, hyperkalemia) when evaluating the patient presenting with "hypotension during dialysis."

Treatment

- DDAVP, cryoprecipitate, conjugated estrogens, and transfusion as with chronic renal failure (given previously)
- **Protamine**: To reverse heparin, if overanticoagulation is a concern

TABLE 18.5. Indications for Emergent Dialysis

A: Severe acid-base disturbance (metabolic acidosis)
E: Severe electrolyte disturbance (hyperkalemia, hypercalcemia)
I: Certain toxic ingestions (eg, lithium, alcohols, barbiturates, salicylates)
O: Volume overload (pulmonary edema, severe HTN)
U: Symptomatic uremia (pericarditis, twitching, nausea/vomiting, encephalopathy)

HTN, hypertension.

Dialysis Disequilibrium Syndrome

Cerebral edema due to rapid changes in body fluid composition and osmolality. Risk factors include first dialysis session and markedly high BUN prior to dialysis. Symptoms begin during or right after HD.

Symptoms/Examination

- Often includes headache, nausea/vomiting, muscle cramping
- If severe: Altered mental status, seizures, and coma

Treatment

- Symptoms generally resolve over several hours; supportive care.
- Mannitol and hypertonic saline do not improve outcomes.

Fistula-Specific Problems

Fistula-specific problems include:

- **Puncture site bleeding**: The most common complication; treat with pressure (not occlusion), gel foam soaked in thrombin, and/or tissue adhesive.
- **True aneurysms**: Uncommon and rarely rupture.
- **Pseudoaneurysms**: Typically present with swelling, bleeding, or infection.
- **Thrombosis**: Consult a vascular surgeon immediately. Thrombolysis is an option.
- **High-output heart failure**.
  - Branham sign: A drop in HR with temporary compression of HD access site

Vascular Access Infection

Can occur in HD catheters or fistulas (grafts > native vein); typically result from gram-positive skin flora such as *Staphylococcus*, but gram-negative infections are also seen.

Symptoms/Examination

- Fever or history of documented bacteremia.
- Absence of local signs does **not** rule out vascular access infection.

Treatment

- Obtain blood cultures.
- Parenteral antibiotics: IV vancomycin 1-1.5 g to cover gram-positive infection, and gentamycin or third-generation cephalosporin to cover gram-negatives (if suspected). Vancomycin will stay in system for 5-7 days or until next HD.

PERITONITIS

Peritoneal dialysis–related peritonitis is commonly due to gram-positive organisms (*Staphylococcus* and *Streptococcus*), followed by gram-negative bacteria and (rarely) anaerobes and fungi. If the culture shows multiple organisms, suspect bowel perforation.

Symptoms

Fever, abdominal pain, cloudy PD fluid

Q

A 45-year-old woman with ESRD presents to the ED complaining of shortness of breath. Her last dialysis was 1 day prior via a recently placed right arm arteriovenous (AV) fistula. As part of your physical examination, you temporarily occlude her dialysis access site and observe a drop in her heart rate. What diagnosis does this finding support?

KEY FACT

Dialysis disequilibrium is due to transient decrease in blood osmolality and resultant fluid shifts.

KEY FACT

The most common organisms in PD-related peritonitis = *Staphylococcus* and *Streptococcus*

Q

A 50-year-old woman on PD presents to the ED with complaint of fever, abdominal pain, and cloudy PD fluid. On examination, she is well appearing and afebrile, but has a diffusely tender abdomen. The dialysis catheter site is normal. What peritoneal fluid cell counts would confirm your suspicion of peritonitis?

A

The drop in heart rate with occlusion of the dialysis access site is termed Branham sign, which indicates a high-output heart failure from excess flow through the AV fistula. The diagnosis can be confirmed with Doppler ultrasound.

KEY FACT

The differential of acute renal transplant rejection? Renal artery stenosis or occlusion Cyclosporin or tacrolimus toxicity
Obstruction pyelonephritis
Postsurgical lymphocele

KEY FACT

Ureterolithiasis mimics:
Abdominal aortic aneurysm
Acute papillary necrosis
Pyelonephritis
Testicular torsion
Ovarian torsion.

A

Greater than 100 WBC/mm^3 with > 50% neutrophils. A positive Gram stain can also confirm the diagnosis.

Diagnosis

PD fluid with > 100 WBC/mm^3 with > 50% neutrophils **or** a positive Gram stain. This is a lower cutoff than the 250 neutrophils/mm^3 for spontaneous bacterial peritonitis.

Treatment

Intraperitoneal (IP) antibiotics (may give IV if IP not immediately available): Vancomycin or third-generation cephalosporin

Nephrolithiasis

Renal stones most commonly become symptomatic when they obstruct the ureter, causing renal colic (Table 18.6). Complete obstruction may cause irreversible damage after 1-2 weeks.

There are five sites along the GU tract where calculi are likely to cause obstruction: calyx (rare), ureteropelvic junction, pelvic brim, and **ureterovesicular junction (most common)**, and vesical orifice.

Symptoms/Examination

- Abrupt onset of extreme colicky flank pain radiating to the groin.
- Patients frequently are unable to lay still, writhing in their bed.
- Nausea/vomiting, urinary urgency, and frequency may occur.
- Fevers and chills if concomitant infection.

Differential

- The most critical diagnosis in differential is AAA.
- Other considerations include pyelonephritis, testicular torsion in males, and ovarian torsion in females.

TABLE 18.6. Renal Stones

Stone Type	Pathophysiology
Calcium oxalate (most common)	↑ Ca^{2+} production (hyperparathyroidism, neoplasm, sarcoid, RTA) ↑ Oxalate absorption (inflammatory bowel disease)
Struvite	Infection with urea-splitting bacteria (*Pseudomonas, Klebsiella, Staphylococcus, Proteus*) May cause staghorn calculi and alkaline urine
Uric acid	↑ Uric acid excretion in the urine (gout, leukemia, or high-protein diet) Low urine pH supports stone formation
Cystine (rare)	Inborn errors of metabolism

RTA, renal tubular acidosis.

DIAGNOSIS

- Hematuria is common (gross or microscopic), but absent in 10%-20% of CT-proven stones.
- Urinary pH:
  - pH > 7.6 → suspect urea-splitting organisms
  - pH < 5 → suspect uric acid crystalluria
- Bacteriuria suggests infection.
- BUN/Cr—especially if solitary kidney, transplant, chronic renal failure.
- Imaging: Should be performed if the diagnosis is in question, the patient appears toxic, high-grade obstruction is suspected, or it is the patient's first episode of flank pain.
  - **Noncontrast CT**—standard modality; can identify alternative pathology; must weigh benefits versus risks of radiation exposure
  - **Ultrasound**—sensitive for detecting hydronephrosis, less reliable for small stones; can be used in pregnant or pediatric patients
  - **Plain radiographs**—low specificity; only uric acid stones are radiolucent. Use only to track stone progress

> **Q**
>
> A 27-year-old man with no medical history presents with colicky flank pain. He is obviously uncomfortable and fidgety on the stretcher. His urine dipstick reveals 3+ blood. Does this patient need imaging?

> **KEY FACT**
>
> Uric acid stones are radiolucent.
>
> On the boards, suspect AAA in any patient > 50 years presenting with flank pain!

TREATMENT

- Supportive care with IV fluids and analgesia
  - NSAIDs are first line: Shown to decrease both renal capsular pressure (through decreased GFR) and ureterospasm. Should refrain from NSAIDs at least 3 days prior to planned lithotripsy to minimize bleeding risk.
- Opioids are frequently necessary, and the combination of opioids and NSAIDs may be superior to either agent alone
- Stones < 5 mm: 80% pass spontaneously within 4 weeks
- Stones > 8 mm: Only 20% pass spontaneously; often require lithotripsy or surgical intervention
- Ureteral antispasmodic: Tamsulosin (Flomax) may facilitate passage
- Urology follow-up for stones > 10 mm, significant obstruction
- Strain urine
- Admission criteria:
  - Obstruction with concomitant infection (emergent urology consultation)
  - Intractable pain or vomiting
  - Solitary kidney
  - Acute renal insufficiency

Urinary Tract Infection/Pyelonephritis (Adults)

Urinary tract infection (UTI) is an infection of the urinary tract. With the exception of the neonatal period, UTIs are more common in females than males.

DEFINITIONS

- **Cystitis**: Inflammation of the bladder; may be bacterial or nonbacterial
- **Complicated UTI**: UTI associated with factors that may reduce the efficacy of standard antimicrobial therapy (Table 18.7)
- **Pyelonephritis**: Infection of the renal parenchyma and collecting system

> **Q**
>
> A healthy 70-year-old woman presents with 4 days of dysuria and urgency. On clinical examination, there is no evidence for pyelonephritis. UA shows many WBCs and bacteria, + leukocyte esterase, + nitrite, and few RBCs and epithelial cells. Is this patient a candidate for a 3-day course of antibiotic therapy?

A

Yes. Though renal colic is often very apparent clinically, imaging is generally considered appropriate for a first stone, if a patient appears toxic, if there is concern for high-grade obstruction, or if there is diagnostic uncertainty.

TABLE 18.7. Complicated UTIs

Men
Elderly
Pregnant women
Serious medical disease
Immunosuppression
Recent hospitalization
Treatment failure
Structural urinary tract abnormalities
Pyelonephritis
Indwelling catheter
Recent instrumentation

UTI, urinary tract infection.

KEY FACT

The presence of **any** bacteria in an unspun urine sample is significant.

KEY FACT

The presence of nitrite on urine dipstick indicates the presence of gram-negative organisms.

KEY FACT

Urethritis or prostatitis is most likely cause of dysuria or pyuria in sexually active young males, not UTI.

A

No. She needs a 7-day regimen. A 7-day regimen is recommended for pregnant women or those with > 7 days of symptoms, comorbid conditions such as diabetes, previous or recurrent UTI, or > 65 years old.

Etiology

- Organisms causing UTIs usually ascend the urethra from the perineum.
- *Escherichia coli* is the dominant pathogen, followed by *Staphylococcus saprophyticus*. Less common organisms include *Proteus*, *Klebsiella*, and *Enterobacter*.
- Patients at risk for unusual organisms include institutionalized or hospitalized patients and complicated UTIs.

Symptoms/Examination

- Urgency, frequency, dysuria, hematuria
- Flank pain, back pain, suprapubic pain
- Fever, vomiting

Diagnosis

- **Pyuria**: Significant at > 2-5 WBC/hpf
- **Bacteriuria**: Significant for **any bacteria** in an unspun urine sample or > 15/hpf on spun samples
- **Urine dipstick leukocyte esterase**: Indicates presence of WBCs; negative result does not rule out infection
- **Urine dipstick nitrite**: Indicates presence of gram-negative bacteria; negative result does not rule out infection
- **Urine culture**: Definitive test; indicated for all complicated UTIs; positive if > 100 colony-forming unit (CFU)/mL of known uropathogen in males or symptomatic females, > 10^5 CFU/mL in asymptomatic patients

Differential

- Nonbacterial cystitis: Due to inflammation (radiation, interstitial cystitis, medications).
- Urethritis: *Chlamydia* is commonly implicated pathogen. Sexually active males with UTIs should be tested for sexually transmitted infections.
- Prostatitis: consider prostate examination on all males with UTI.
- Vaginitis.

Treatment

- Antibiotic therapy—use local resistance patterns (Table 18.8).
- Criteria for admission:
  - Extremes of age

TABLE 18.8. Antibiotic Therapy in UTI

Condition	Antibiotic (Initial Therapy)	Therapy Duration (Total)
Acute uncomplicated cystitis	Trimethoprim/sulfamethoxazole, nitrofurantoin, second-generation cephalosporin, **or** fluoroquinolone	3-5 d
Acute uncomplicated cystitis with comorbid conditions	Trimethoprim/sulfamethoxazole, nitrofurantoin, **or** fluoroquinolone	7 d
Acute uncomplicated pyelonephritis	Mild to moderately ill: ■ Oral fluoroquinolone or ■ Trimethoprim/sulfamethoxazole Hospitalized: ■ IV fluoroquinolone **or** ampicillin/gentamycin	 7 d 14 d 14 d
Complicated UTI	Mild to moderately ill: ■ Oral fluoroquinolone **or** trimethoprim/sulfamethoxazole Hospitalized: ■ IV ampicillin/gentamycin **or** imipenem/cilastatin **or** fluoroquinolone	 14 d 14 d
Pregnancy	Second-generation cephalosporin **or** nitrofurantoin	7 d
Pregnant with pyelonephritis	Hospitalized: IV ceftriaxone	14 d

IV, intravenous; UTI, urinary tract infection.

  - Systemic toxicity
  - Renal failure
  - Obstruction
  - Intractable vomiting or pain
  - Complicated UTI: Have lower threshold if questionable
- **Pregnancy**: Treat asymptomatic bacteriuria as UTI. Failure to treat can lead to premature labor, perinatal mortality, maternal anemia, and pyelonephritis.
- **Diabetes and sickle cell disease**: Patients are at an increased risk of papillary necrosis, abscess formation, and microvascular complications.
- **Indwelling catheters**: Replacement of the catheter can eliminate bacteria in many patients.

KEY FACT

Asymptomatic bacteriuria in pregnancy should ALWAYS be treated as a UTI.

Complications

- Perinephric abscess: Consider in pyelonephritis patients who do not respond to initial therapy.
- Emphysematous pyelonephritis: High-mortality necrotizing infection of renal parenchyma, primarily in diabetic females. Often necessitates nephrectomy.

Urethritis

Inflammation of the urethra, it is most commonly due to ***Chlamydia trachomatis*** or ***Neisseria gonorrhoeae* (GC)**, but other organisms include *Ureaplasma urealyticum*, *Trichomonas vaginalis*, herpesvirus, or candida.

Symptoms/Examination

- Dysuria, urethral discharge, urinary urgency.
- Many patients are asymptomatic.

Diagnosis

- Nucleic acid amplification test of first-voided urine or urethral swab, **or**
- Culture of urethral secretions

Treatment

- Regimen must be effective at treating both GC and chlamydia: Ceftriaxone **or** cefixime for GC, and doxycycline **or** azithromycin for chlamydia.
- Fluoroquinolones are no longer recommended due to a high prevalence of *N gonorrhoeae* resistance.
- Metronidazole can be considered in patients with persistent symptoms despite treatment for GC and chlamydia, or if otherwise indicated.

Acute Bacterial Prostatitis

Etiology

- **Patients < 35 years**: Sexually transmitted pathogens *C trachomatis* and/or *N gonorrhoeae* predominate.
- **Patients ≥ 35 years:** Most often caused by gram-negative organisms, predominantly *E coli*. Suspect an **acute exacerbation of chronic prostatitis** if there is a history of recurrent UTIs.
- Tuberculosis (TB) should be considered in the presence of renal TB.

Symptoms/Examination

- Fever/chills
- Perineal or low back pain
- Urgency, dysuria, frequency, urinary retention
- Tender swollen prostate (avoid prostatic massage as it may precipitate bacteremia)

Diagnosis

- Clinical examination is key to diagnosis.
- Urinalysis often normal.
- Urine culture may help isolate organism.

Treatment

- Supportive care with analgesia, antipyretics, and hydration.
- Antibiotics:
  - Age < 35 years: Ceftriaxone (IM × 1) or ofloxacin (× 10 days) and doxycycline (× 10 days)
  - Age ≥ 35 years: Fluoroquinolone or trimethoprim/sulfamethoxazole for 2-4 weeks
  - Chronic bacterial: Fluoroquinolone × 4 weeks or trimethoprim/sulfamethoxazole for 1-3 months

KEY FACT

Prostatitis < 35 years: Think sexually transmitted disease (STD). ≥ 35 years: Think ***E coli;*** needs prolonged antibiotic therapy.

TABLE 18.9. Sexually Transmitted Penile Ulcers

Disease	Organism	Clinical	Painful?
Chancroid	*Haemophilus ducreyi*	Sharply demarcated ulcer with undermined edges, often multiple, "kissing lesions," suppurative inguinal nodes	Yes
Herpes	Herpes simplex virus	Grouped vesicles on red base form shallow ulcers	Yes
Syphilis	*Treponema pallidum*	Painless, indurated ulcer; heals spontaneously	No
Lymphogranuloma venereum	*Chlamydia trachomatis*	Transient, painless ulcer; followed by unilateral (mostly) inguinal adenopathy which may suppurate	No
Granuloma inguinale (donovanosis)	*Calymmatobacterium granulomatis*	Subcutaneous nodule(s), becomes beefy red, highly vascular ulcer(s)	No

- **Avoid** urethral catheterization, use suprapubic catheter if urinary retention occurs
- Parenteral antibiotics and admission if patient appears toxic

Penile Ulcers

Sexually transmitted diseases are the likely cause of isolated penile ulcers. Table 18.9 outlines the organisms, diagnosis, and treatment. See Figures 18.2 to 18.4.

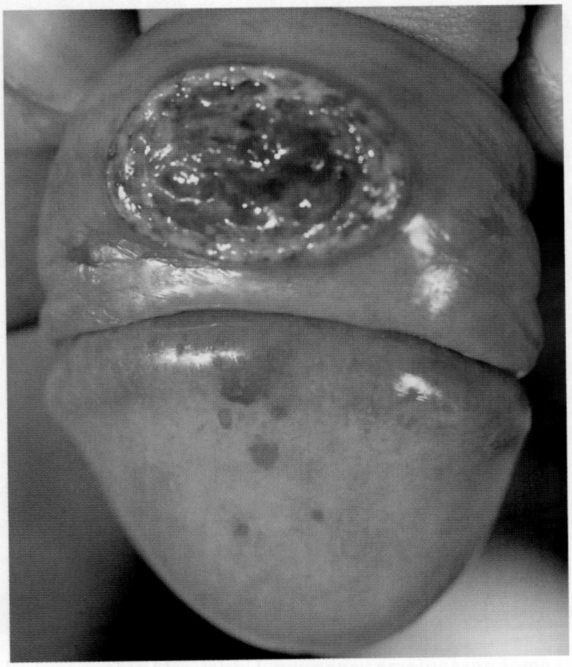

FIGURE 18.2. Chancroid. Painful ulcer with surrounding erythema and edema. (Reproduced, with permission from, A. Wisdom. *Sexually Transmitted Diseases*. London: Mosby-Wolfe; 1992.)

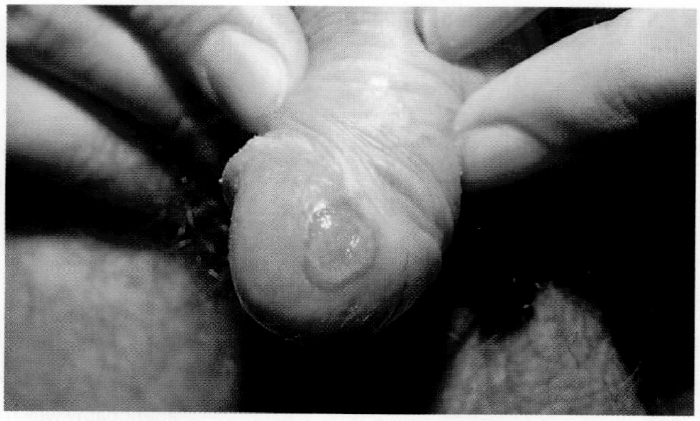

FIGURE 18.3. Syphilis. Painless, indurated chancre. (Reproduced, with permission, from A. Wisdom. *Sexually Transmitted Diseases*. London: Mosby-Wolfe; 1992.)

DIFFERENTIAL

- In the setting of genital ulceration **and** oral ulcerations, consider Behçet disease, Stevens-Johnson syndrome, Reiter syndrome, and pemphigus vulgaris.
- Others causes of isolated genital ulceration include lymphoma, carcinoma, vasculitis, fixed drug eruption, and trauma.

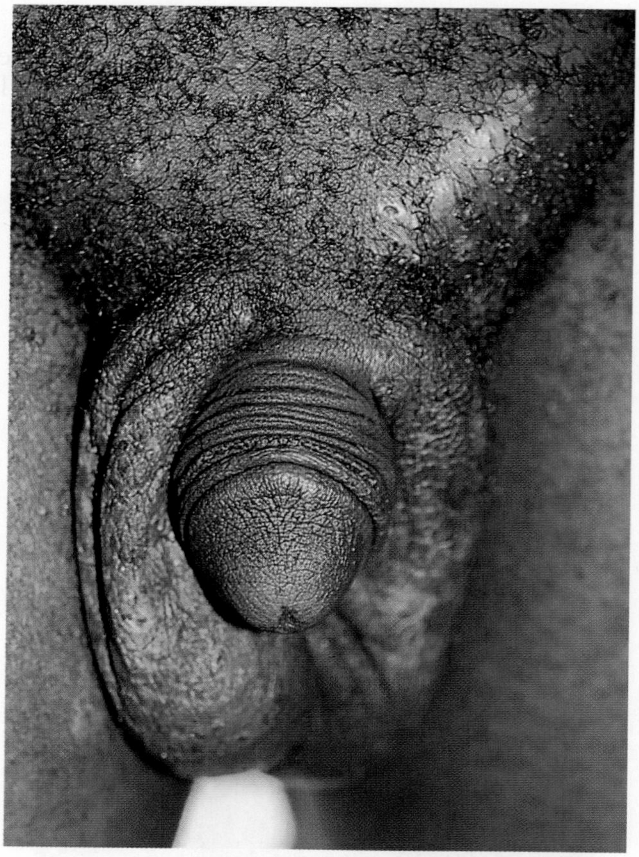

FIGURE 18.4. Lymphogranuloma venereum. Unilateral tender lymphadenopathy. (Reproduced, with permission, from Knoop KJ, Stack LB, Storrow AB, et al. *Atlas of Emergency Medicine*. 3rd ed. New York, NY: McGraw-Hill Education; 2010. Figure 9.21. Photographer: Lawrence B. Stack, MD.)

TABLE 18.10. Treatment of Sexually Transmitted Genital Ulcers

Chancroid	Azithromycin or ceftriaxone or ciprofloxacin
Herpes	Acyclovir
Syphilis	Benzathine penicillin
Lymphogranuloma venereum	Doxycycline
Granuloma inguinale	Doxycycline or trimethoprim/sulfamethoxazole

IM, intramuscular.

Q

A 19-year-old man experiences sudden onset of L flank and testicular pain. He has a history of kidney stones and reports that this pain is as severe as with previous kidney stones. On presentation to the ED, he has minimal costovertebral angle (CVA) tenderness, minimal left lower quadrant tenderness, and a diffusely tender L testicle with loss of cremasteric reflex. What is the next thing you should do?

Diagnosis

- Diagnosis is often clinical.
- Lesions can be swabbed and cultured for bacterial and viral identification.
- Syphilis is diagnosed by a combination of a nontreponemal test (VDRL or rapid plasma reagin [RPR]) followed by confirmatory testing with a treponemal test (TPHA or FTA-Abs).
- Chlamydia can also be diagnosed via nucleic acid amplification testing of swab, lymph node aspirate, and urethral or urine samples.

KEY FACT

SyphiLIS is painLESS
CHANCroid is PAINful
HERPes HURTS

Treatment

Antibiotics: For STD-associated genital ulcers (Table 18.10)

Epididymitis

Epididymitis refers to inflammation **or** infection of the epididymis and may spread to involve the testicle (**epididymo-orchitis**). Inflammation can be due to urinary reflux or obstruction. Common infectious organisms vary with age:

- **Prepubertal boys**: Infection with gram-negative bacteria due to congenital structural urinary tract pathology
- **Men < 35 years**: *Chlamydia* and *N gonorrhoeae*
- **Men ≥ 35 years**: Urinary tract pathogens, predominantly *E coli*

Symptoms

- Gradual onset of pain that may begin in the flank or suprapubic area and progress to scrotal pain
- Fevers/chills
- Dysuria, urgency, frequency

Examination

- Swollen, tender epididymis.
- **Prehn sign**: Relief with elevation of the scrotum.
- Whole testicle may be swollen if associated orchitis.
- Cremasteric reflex is present.

Diagnosis

- Mostly clinical.
- Pyuria in 50%-90%.
- Urethral swab if < 35 years, urine culture if > 35 years.
- Ultrasound can show enlarged epididymis with increased vascularity.

A

The history and examination strongly suggest testicular torsion. The first thing to do is to attempt manual detorsion. If this fails, simultaneous urology consultation and testicular ultrasound with Doppler are appropriate.

KEY FACT

Epididymitis examination findings:
- Swollen tender epididymis
- Relief with elevation of scrotum (Prehn sign)
- Normal cremasteric reflex

TREATMENT

- Supportive care with analgesia, bed rest, elevation of scrotum.
- Antibiotics.
  - **Prepubertal boys**: Augmentin or trimethoprim/sulfamethoxazole
  - **Men < 35 years**: Ceftriaxone and doxycycline
  - **Men ≥ 35 years**: Fluoroquinolone
- Primary care provider (PCP) follow-up with urology referral if symptoms persist.
- Admit patients with systemic signs of toxicity.

Orchitis

Orchitis is an acute infection involving the testis. It most commonly is due to secondary spread of bacterial epididymitis (see previously) but may be viral in nature, most commonly due to mumps in prepubertal boys. Orchitis is unilateral in 70% (even viral).

SYMPTOMS/EXAMINATION

- Testicular pain, swelling, and tenderness.
- Pain may be out of proportion to examination findings.
- Fevers/chills.
- If mumps related, may be preceded by parotitis and other nonspecific viral symptoms.

DIAGNOSIS

As with epididymitis, given previously

TREATMENT

- If viral, supportive therapy only.
- If bacterial, treat as given earlier for epididymitis.

Testicular Torsion

The tunica vaginalis normally surrounds the testicle and attaches to the scrotal wall and epididymis posteriorly, anchoring the testicle in place. In patients at risk for testicular torsion, the tunica vaginalis attaches higher up on the spermatic cord, leaving a redundant spermatic cord and a mobile testicle (**bell-clapper deformity**). Torsion occurs with twisting of the testicle on the spermatic cord resulting in venous, or rarely, arterial occlusion. This results in rapid swelling and edema of the testis.

SYMPTOMS

- May occur at any age, but peaks in the first year of life and at postpubertal boys.
- About half may report prior similar pain that resolved spontaneously.
- Severe onset of unilateral testicular pain that occurs with trauma, hours after strenuous activity, or sometimes during sleep.
- Nausea/vomiting, lower abdominal pain.

KEY FACT

The loss of the cremasteric reflex is the classic sign of testicular torsion, but is not 100% sensitive.

EXAMINATION

- Elevated (or "**high-riding**") testicle with a **transverse lie** (Figure 18.5).
- **Loss of the cremasteric reflex**.

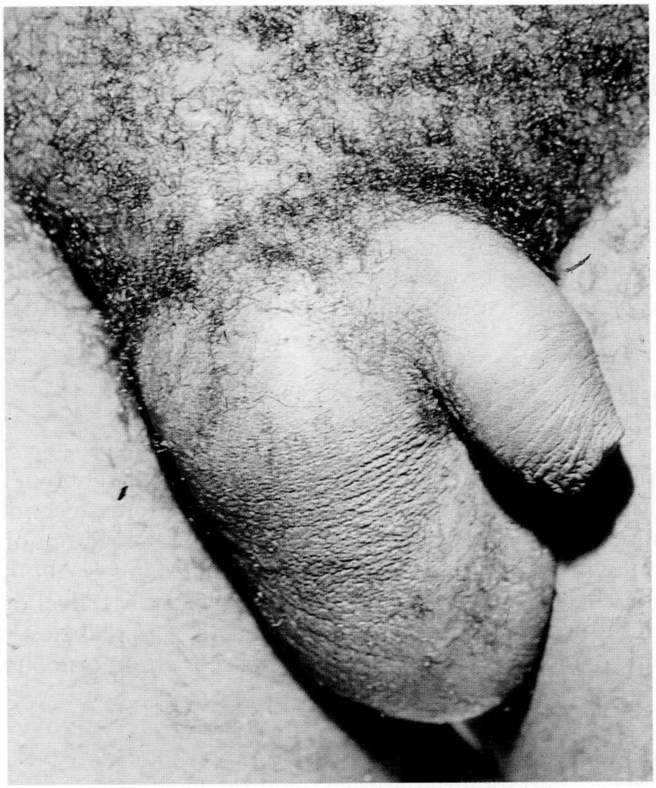

A

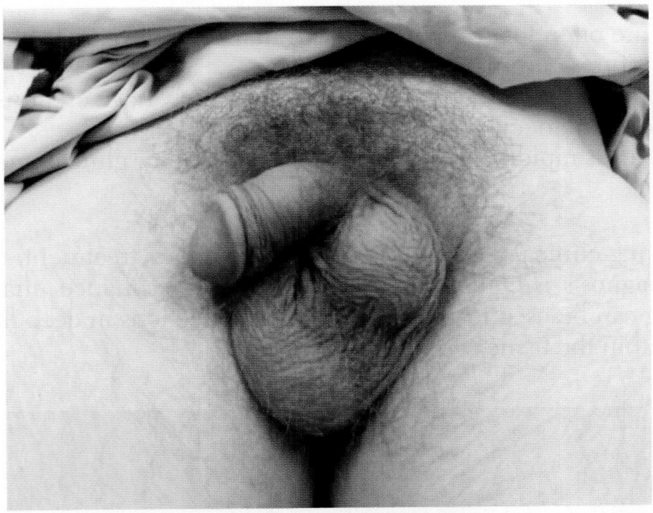

B

FIGURE 18.5. (A&B) Testicular torsion. (Reproduced, with permission, from Knoop KJ, Stack LB, Storrow AB, et al. *Atlas of Emergency Medicine*. 3rd ed. New York, NY: McGraw-Hill Education; 2010. Figure 8.3. Photographer: The Emergency Medicine Department, Naval Medical Center Portsmouth.)

- Tender, firm, swollen testicle.
- Prehn sign (relief of pain with elevation of testicle) is generally **not** present (ie, the testicle still hurts) but is not considered reliable in differentiating torsion from epididymitis.
- Bell-clapper deformity (horizontal lie) of contralateral testicle.

Q

A 60-year-old diabetic man presents to the emergency room (ER) complaining of 2 days of scrotal pain. On examination, the patient has tenderness to palpation of the underside of the scrotum and the perineum, with slight erythema and induration. The patient's pain seems out of proportion to his physical examination findings. What diagnosis should be strongly considered in this patient?

A

Fournier gangrene should be considered, especially in a diabetic man. The patient may complain of scrotal, rectal, or genitalia pain out of proportion to examination findings of warmth, erythema, and edema. Mortality in these patients is about 20%.

KEY FACT

TIME IS TESTIS! Do not let imaging delay detorsion!

Diagnosis

Torsion is a clinical diagnosis, but if this diagnosis is equivocal, Doppler ultrasound can be used to evaluate blood flow to the testicle.

Treatment

- Immediate urology consult for surgical intervention.
- Supportive care with analgesia.
- Attempt manual detorsion (medial to lateral twisting or "open-book" method; if this doesn't work, attempt lateral to medial twisting).
- 96% salvage rate if detorsed before 4 hours, < 10% salvage if > 24 hours.

Fournier Gangrene

Fournier gangrene is a rapidly progressing, necrotizing infection of the scrotum, penis, or perineum, sparing the testicles. It usually occurs secondary to direct spread from infections in the perirectal area, urogenital tract, or skin of the genitalia. Predominant organisms are *Bacteroides fragilis* and *E coli*, but may also include streptococci, staphylococci, and Clostridia (rarely fungal or anaerobic). These infections occur most commonly in patients with diabetes, immunosuppression, obesity, malignancy, chronic steroid use, or chronic alcoholism.

Symptoms

- Scrotal pain or itching is an early symptom.
- Fever, malaise, and intense perineal swelling develop.

Examination

- Patients are often toxic appearing, with marked tachycardia.
- Hypotension is common.
- Involved skin can be tender to palpation and may have crepitus, erythema, edema, or frank necrosis (Figure 18.6).
- Often spreads rapidly up anterior abdominal wall or gluteal muscles.

KEY FACT

Definitive therapy for Fournier gangrene is emergent wide surgical debridement.

Diagnosis

- With strong clinical suspicion, imaging only delays treatment.
- If the diagnosis is equivocal, CT or magnetic resonance imaging (MRI) scanning can be used to demonstrate fluid collections in deep fascial planes or gas within the tissue.

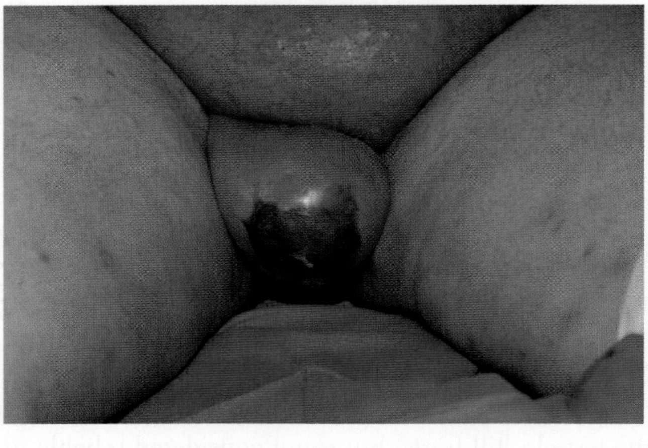

FIGURE 18.6. Fournier gangrene. (Reproduced, with permission, from Knoop KJ, Stack LB, Storrow AB, et al. *Atlas of Emergency Medicine*. 3rd ed. New York, NY: McGraw-Hill Education; 2010. Figure 8.13. Photographer: R. Jason Thurman, MD.)

TREATMENT

- Aggressive supportive care
- Broad-spectrum antibiotics immediately: Imipenem-cilastatin + vancomycin + clindamycin
- Emergent surgical debridement

Balanitis/Balanoposthitis

Results from inflammation of the glans penis (**balanitis**) or the glans and foreskin (**balanoposthitis**). The primary cause is infection, most commonly *Candida*. It is more common in circumcised males, and contributing factors include diabetes, local trauma or irritation, contact dermatitis, and poor hygiene.

SYMPTOMS/EXAMINATION

- Pain, tenderness, and itching are common symptoms.
- The glans may have erythematous, ulcerated, or scaly lesions.
- The foreskin may be adherent or may reveal foul or purulent discharge when retracted.

DIAGNOSIS

- The diagnosis is primarily clinical.
- KOH prep can identify *Candida* sp.
- Finger stick glucose to evaluate for diabetes.

TREATMENT

- Topical antifungal ointment for 1-3 weeks.
- If severe symptoms, also add oral fluconazole 150 mg for 1 dose.
- Antibiotics if presence of cellulitis.
- Treatment of diabetes or underlying immunosuppressive condition.
- If left untreated, may lead to foreskin scarring and phimosis.

Phimosis

Phimosis is a constriction of the foreskin resulting in an inability to retract the prepuce over the glans, from the word phimos meaning "muzzle" in Greek. This is usually physiologic (resolves by age 10) but may occur because of trauma, infections, poor hygiene, or chemical irritation. Phimosis is deemed pathologic when it causes problems, such as difficulty urinating or sexual dysfunction.

SYMPTOMS/EXAMINATION

- Usually asymptomatic; when pathologic may cause pain at the penis, hematuria, abnormal urinary stream, bulging of the foreskin with urination, painful erections.
- Examination classically shows unretractable foreskin with occasional obstruction of the preputial meatus.

DIAGNOSIS

Diagnosis is based on clinical examination.

TREATMENT

- Gentle stretching exercises of the foreskin
- Improved hygiene

Q

A worried mother presents to the ED with her 1-year-old son. The mother is concerned that the child cries uncontrollably when he urinates. She noticed that she is now unable to retract his foreskin, and that when he urinates it swells like a balloon. On examination, you see a well-appearing child with unretractable foreskin. What do you recommend?

KEY FACT

Balanitis = inflammation of the glans penis. Balanoposthitis = inflammation of the glans penis **and** foreskin. Most common cause = Candidal infection.

KEY FACT

In phimosis the foreskin is forward

In paraphimosis you have a pair of problems (swollen foreskin and strangulation).

KEY FACT

Phimosis treatment:

Daily cleaning of foreskin
Topical steroids
Immediate intervention if outlet obstruction or vascular compromise develops

A

The child likely has a pathologic phimosis. Daily cleaning of the foreskin and topical steroids are standard therapy in cases of phimosis. However, with ballooning of the foreskin on voiding, urologic consultation may be required.

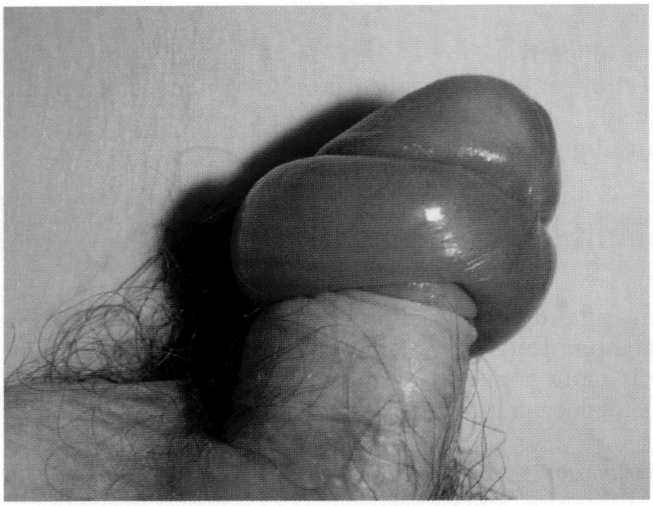

FIGURE 18.7. Paraphimosis. (Reproduced, with permission, from Knoop KJ, Stack LB, Storrow AB, et al. *Atlas of Emergency Medicine*. 3rd ed. New York, NY: McGraw-Hill Education; 2010. Figure 8.15. Photographer: Lawrence B. Stack, MD.)

- Topical steroids for 4-6 weeks (very effective)
- Dilation of the meatus with forceps if signs of urinary outlet obstruction
- Dorsal slit procedure or circumcision in cases of vascular compromise

Paraphimosis

Paraphimosis occurs when the proximal foreskin cannot be reduced distally over the glans penis, resulting in distal vascular congestion and ischemia. This is a true urologic emergency.

Symptoms/Examination

- Patient often reports inability to replace foreskin back over glans.
- Examination reveals a flaccid proximal penis with erythema and engorgement distal to the obstruction (Figure 18.7).

Diagnosis

Diagnosis is largely based on clinical examination.

Treatment

- Supportive care with analgesia—topical anesthetics, local infiltration, dorsal penile nerve block, procedural sedation all appropriate
- Manual reduction with firm circumferential pressure to the glans for 5-10 minutes to reduce edema and slide foreskin distally
- Traction with forceps—constant, steady pressure with forceps at 9- and 3 o'clock
- Invasive reduction by urology if manual reduction is unsuccessful
- Admission for patients unable to void after reduction

KEY FACT

Paraphimosis is a true urologic emergency! Manual reduction with firm pressure for 5-10 minutes is the initial treatment.

Priapism

The penis is composed of two corpora cavernosa and the corpus spongiosa surrounding the urethra. With normal erection the corpora cavernosa fill with well-oxygenated blood (which on blood gas analysis has the appearance of arterial blood).

Priapism is defined as persistent painful erection unrelated to stimulation or desire. Most studies identify priapism as an erection lasting at least 4 hours. Priapism is divided into two types: **ischemic (low-flow) priapism** and **nonischemic (high-flow) priapism**.

ISCHEMIC PRIAPISM

The most common type of priapism, ischemic (low-flow) priapism occurs secondary to venous stasis and blood pooling in the corpora cavernosa with resulting ischemia. This type is a **true emergency because of the risk of permanent erectile dysfunction**.

Predisposing factors for low-flow priapism:

- **Sickle cell disease**
- **Malignancy**: Leukemia, multiple myeloma
- **Substance abuse**: Cocaine, ecstasy
- **Medications**
  - Antihypertensives (hydralazine, CCBs [calcium channel blockers], prazosin), psychiatric medications (trazodone, chlorpromazine, risperidone), erectile dysfunction medications (sildenafil, tadalafil)
- **Penile injection of a vasodilator for erectile dysfunction**
  - Phentolamine, prostaglandin, papaverine

SYMPTOMS/EXAMINATION

The corpora cavernosa are **rigid and tender** with palpation.

DIAGNOSIS

- Primarily based on presence of predisposing factor and clinical examination
- If cause unclear, CBC to screen for hematologic malignancy
- Tests that may confirm diagnosis, if in question:
  - Corpus cavernosum blood gas showing hypercarbia, hypoxia, and acidosis
  - Ultrasound showing diminished cavernous blood flow

TREATMENT

- Supportive care with analgesia and ice packs to perineum; IV hydration.
- Aspiration of the corpus cavernosum: Use butterfly needle to drain 5-mL blood from corpora.
- Injection of 1 mL of dilute phenylephrine (100-500 μg/mL) into the corpus cavernosum with repeated attempts q3-5 minutes until resolution.
- Terbutaline (SQ or PO) and pseudoephedrine (PO) have been used with some success and may be tried while preparing for aspiration/injection.
- Systemic treatment of underlying disorders (eg, exchange transfusion for sickle cell patients).
- Emergent urology consult if unsuccessful.

COMPLICATION

90% of men with ischemic priapism lasting 24 hours suffer permanent erectile dysfunction.

NONISCHEMIC PRIAPISM

High-flow (nonischemic) priapism occurs secondary to unregulated corpora cavernosum arterial inflow. Often the result of a fistula between the cavernosal artery and corpus cavernosum.

Q

A 25-year-old man with history of schizophrenia presents to the ED with priapism. He was recently started on Risperdal and has a history of cocaine use. On examination, the corpora cavernosa are rigid and tender with palpation. What is the most appropriate initial therapy?

KEY FACT

Pharmacologic treatment for ischemic priapism is systemic or local sympathomimetics, which cause vasoconstriction and decreased blood flow into the penis.

KEY FACT

Meds for priapism.

PHENYLephrine (PENILE ephrine)
TerbutaLINE (to make it LEAN)
SUdaFED (patient is SO FED up!)

A

This patient is presenting with low-flow (ischemic) priapism, likely related to risperidone and cocaine use. This is a true urologic emergency. Immediate intervention includes terbutaline (SQ or PO) and pseudoephedrine (PO). If no response, proceed to bilateral corpus cavernosum aspirations and diluted phenylephrine injections.

KEY FACT

With high-flow (nonischemic) priapism the penis is semierect and painless. Observation alone is often effective.

Symptoms/Examination

- Predisposing factor: Straddle or groin injury, spinal cord lesions, penetrating trauma.
- The penis is **semierect and painless**.
- Perineal compression with the thumb (blocking arterial inflow) may cause detumescence (**Piesis sign**).

Diagnosis

Rule out low-flow state, as given earlier.

Treatment

- Urology consultation for evaluation and possible surgical ligation of fistula
- Observation alone may be effective; few long-term consequences and 60% resolve spontaneously

Penile Fracture

Rupture of the tunica albuginea surrounding the corpus cavernosum because of blunt trauma to the erect penis (Figure 18.8).

Symptoms/Examination

- Patient reports a "snapping sound" followed by rapid detumescence.
- The penis appears swollen, deformed, tender, and discolored (Eggplant deformity).

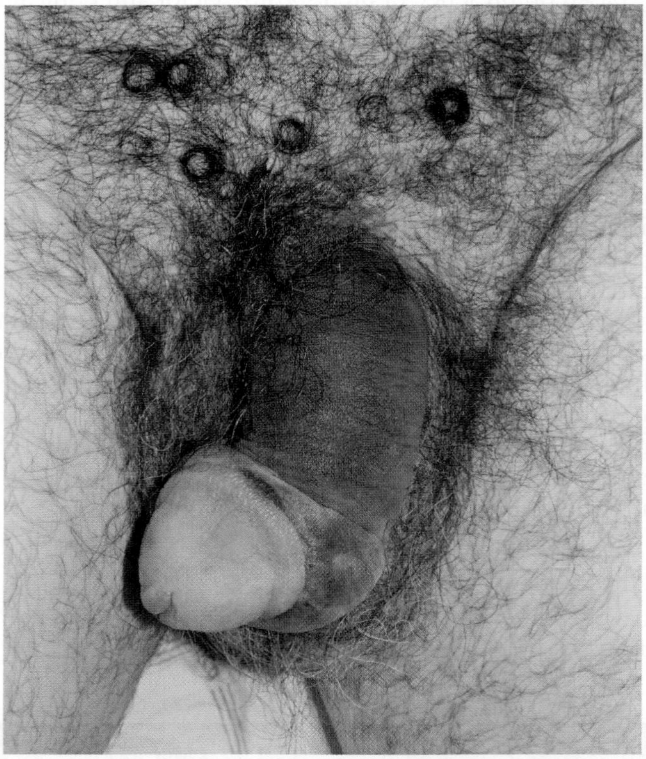

FIGURE 18.8. Penile fracture. (Reproduced, with permission, from Knoop KJ, Stack LB, Storrow AB, et al. *Atlas of Emergency Medicine*. 3rd ed. New York, NY: McGraw-Hill Education; 2010. Figure 8.20. Photographer: Stephen W. Corbett, MD.)

Diagnosis

- Primarily clinical.
- Retrograde urethrogram should be used to evaluate for associated urethral injury (present in 10%-38%).

Treatment

- Supportive care with analgesia
- Suprapubic catheter if urinary drainage needed
- Immediate urologic consult for surgical repair

Q

A 25-year-old man who recently emigrated from Haiti presents to the ED for evaluation of painless scrotal swelling present for several years. Examination reveals unilateral nontender scrotal swelling with homogenous transillumination. What are the diagnosis, likely etiology, and appropriate clinical approach?

Testicular Masses

HYDROCELE

A collection of fluid in the tunica vaginalis. Communicating hydroceles occur when the processus vaginalis fails to obliterate and leaves a potential space between the peritoneum and scrotum. Noncommunicating hydroceles result from an imbalance between the production and absorption of fluid by the tunica vaginalis—can be due to third spacing (congestive heart failure [CHF] exacerbation, nephrotic syndrome) or reactive (testicular neoplasm, epididymitis).

KEY FACT

Hydroceles transilluminate with a homogenous glow.

Symptoms/Examination

- Scrotal fullness, which may be accompanied by pain with palpation.
- Transillumination may illustrate a homogenous glow without presence of shadows (Figure 18.9).

Diagnosis

- Doppler ultrasound can be used to identify and determine the cause of hydrocele.
- Especially warranted if neoplasm or torsion suspected.

Treatment

- Supportive care
- Urology referral for possible surgical intervention

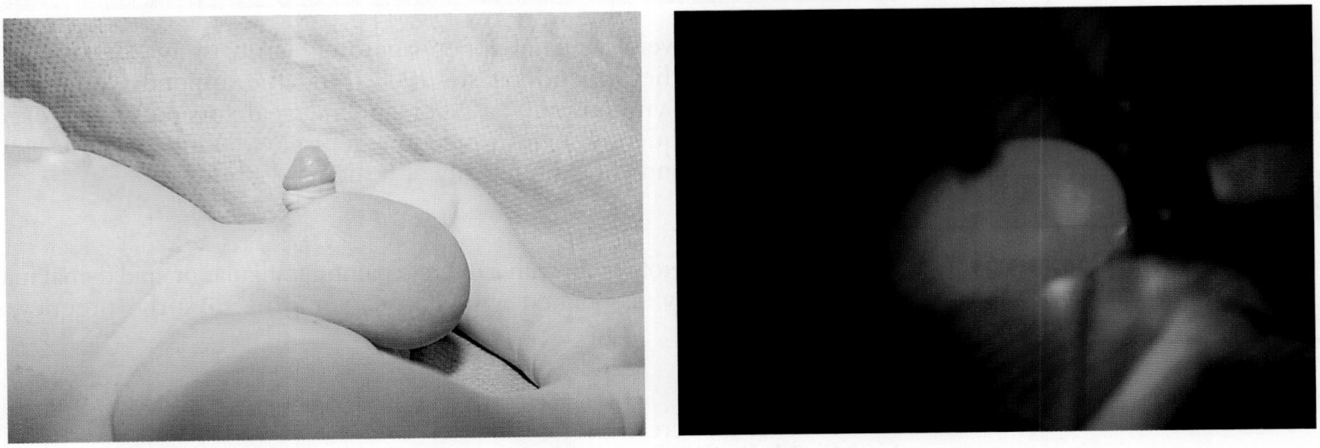

FIGURE 18.9. Hydrocele with transillumination. (Reproduced, with permission, from Knoop KJ, Stack LB, Storrow AB, et al. *Atlas of Emergency Medicine*. 3rd ed. New York, NY: McGraw-Hill Education; 2010. Figure 8.8. Photographer: Michael J. Nowicki, MD.)

A

The patient's physical examination is consistent with hydrocele. The likely etiology with a recent move from an endemic area is lymphatic filariasis. Antihelminthic medical therapy to reduce worm burden and urologic referral would be appropriate next steps, with consideration of ultrasound while in the ED to confirm the diagnosis of hydrocele.

VARICOCELE

Varicocele is a collection of venous varicosities of the spermatic veins due to incomplete drainage of the pampiniform plexus. It is most common in adolescent males. In adults with a new varicocele, suspect inferior vena cava (IVC) compression, thrombosis if R sided, or obstruction of the L renal vein from renal cell carcinoma if L sided.

KEY FACT

On examination, varicoceles feel like a "bag of worms."

Symptoms/Examination

- Scrotal mass or swelling
- Aching scrotal pain worse with standing
- "Bag of worms" with examination and palpation superior and posterior to the testis

Diagnosis

- Clinical examination with abdominal CT if suspected vascular compression.
- Unilateral right varicoceles are rare; think IVC obstruction and consider CT.

Treatment

- Supportive care—scrotal support and NSAIDs.
- Referral for semen analysis; if infertility developing, urology may perform surgical ligation.

TUMORS

KEY FACT

Painless testicular mass = cancer until proven otherwise

Most commonly seminomas, but also may be embryonal cell cancer or teratoma.

Symptoms/Examination

- Hallmark is **asymptomatic** testicular mass, firmness, or induration.
- Examination may show scrotal swelling or a palpable mass.

Diagnosis

Ultrasound can confirm the presence of a mass.

Treatment

Urgent urologic referral; orchiectomy before biopsy is common.

APPENDAGEAL TORSION

The testicle has several vestigial appendages that can twist and become ischemic. Torsion of the **appendix testis** (90%) and the **appendix epididymis** (8%) account for virtually all cases of appendageal torsion. Appendageal torsion is most frequently seen in preadolescent boys. While it causes acute scrotal pain, it has no effect on fertility or testicular viability.

KEY FACT

"Blue-dot sign" with transillumination of scrotal skin = appendageal torsion.

Symptoms

- Acute onset of scrotal pain with a discrete painful testicular or epididymal mass
- Less commonly, associated with nausea/vomiting, dysuria, urgency, or frequency

Examination

- Tender and discrete scrotal "nodule."
- Blue-black dot when present with transillumination of the testicle (blue-dot sign) is pathognomonic (Figure 18.10).

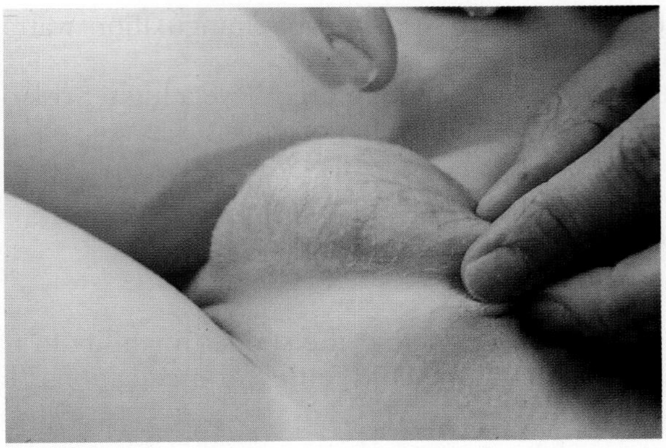

FIGURE 18.10. Blue-dot sign indicating appendageal torsion. (Reproduced, with permission, from Knoop KJ, Stack LB, Storrow AB, et al. *Atlas of Emergency Medicine*. 3rd ed. New York, NY: McGraw-Hill Education; 2010. Figure 8.5. Photographer: Javier A. Gonzalez del Rey, MD.)

Diagnosis

- Primarily clinical.
- Doppler ultrasound illustrates decreased blood flow to the appendage and rules out testicular torsion.

Treatment

- Supportive care only with analgesia, bed rest, scrotal elevation—resolves in 7-10 days
- Surgical excision in cases of severe pain

INGUINAL HERNIA

Inguinal hernias peak in a bimodal distribution, before 1 year of age and then after age 40. A hernia requires surgical consultation in the ED when it becomes incarcerated, strangulated, or causes obstruction.

Anatomy

- Indirect hernia protrudes through the internal ring, **lateral** to the inferior epigastric vessels due to a congenitally patent processus vaginalis.
- Direct hernia protrudes directly through the transversalis fascia and the external inguinal ring **medial** to the inferior epigastric vessels. Are usually **acquired**.
- Clinically, indirect and direct inguinal hernias present identically.

Symptoms/Examination

- Often asymptomatic
- Pain and tenderness if incarceration occurs
- Nausea and vomiting if resultant bowel obstruction
- More toxic appearance with peritonitis or shock if strangulation develops

Diagnosis

- Typically a clinical diagnosis
- Abdominal radiographs or CT if obstruction or perforation is suspected

Treatment

- Incarcerated hernia should be reduced via Trendelenburg position, sedation, and gentle pressure.

- A nonreducible hernia or suspicion of strangulation warrants immediate surgical consultation.
- Inguinal hernias in infants and children have a higher risk of incarceration and should be repaired shortly after diagnosis is made.

Acute Urinary Retention

Acute urinary retention is defined as the sudden inability to pass urine. May be caused by obstruction, neurogenic causes, or medications (Table 18.11).

SYMPTOMS

- Abdominal discomfort and distention (unless neurogenic)
- Hesitancy, decreased force of stream, straining with voiding, sensation of incomplete emptying in patients with obstructive etiology
- Dysuria, urgency, frequency, or discharge with infection

EXAMINATION

- Findings vary with cause of obstruction (eg, enlarged prostate consistent with BPH).
- Abdominal tenderness.
- Palpable bladder (if containing > 150 mL).

DIAGNOSIS

- Bedside ultrasound to estimate bladder volume.
- Greater than 50-100 mL postvoid residual volume is abnormal.

TABLE 18.11. Causes of Acute Urinary Retention

Penile obstruction	Meatal stenosis Paraphimosis Phimosis
Urethral obstruction	Foreign body Hematoma Severe urethritis Stricture Tumor
Prostate obstruction	BPH Cancer Severe prostatitis
Neurogenic causes	Diabetes Multiple sclerosis Cauda equina syndrome
Medications	α-Adrenergic agents Antihistamines Anticholinergics Antispasmodics TCAs

BPH, benign prostatic hyperplasia; TCA, tricycle antidepressant.

- UA to evaluate infection, tumor, calculi.
- BUN and Cr to evaluate renal function.

TREATMENT

- Placement of a Foley catheter.
- Ideal catheter type varies; consider smaller catheter for suspected stricture, and Coudé tip catheter for suspected prostatic obstruction.
- Bladder aspiration if Foley catheter cannot be placed and urology consultant is unavailable.
- Observation of patients with chronic retention and AKI for the development of postobstructive diuresis (4-6 hours).
- Discharge with catheter in place and follow up with urology.
- Antibiotics for infection, as needed.

REVIEW QUESTIONS

QUESTIONS

1. A 24-year-old woman presents to the emergency department (ED) complains of 3 days of dysuria, frequency, and nausea. She a blood pressure of 138/92 mm Hg, a heart rate of 84 bpm, and a temperature of 37°C (98.6°F). On examination, you find her to be well appearing, slightly tender in her suprapubic area, with no unilateral abdominal tenderness, no costovertebral angle (CVA) tenderness, and no extremity or facial edema. Urinalysis demonstrates 31-75 white blood cells (WBCs), 31-75 red blood cells (RBCs), 2+ protein, large leukocyte esterase, negative nitrite, and no casts. What is the appropriate next step in her management?
   A. Obtain BUN/Cr, urine electrolyte studies, and admit to medicine for a renal biopsy.
   B. Discharge home with equipment for a 24-hour urine collection for urine protein measurement.
   C. Discharge home with antibiotics for urinary tract infection (UTI) and steroids for possible nephrotic syndrome.
   D. Discharge home with antibiotics for UTI and primary care provider (PCP) follow-up for a repeat spot urine protein check.
2. A 62-year-old man with history of diabetes and benign prostatic hyperplasia (BPH) presents to the ED with 3 days of progressive lethargy and fever. He has a temperature of 39.4°C, a blood pressure of 86/58 mm Hg, and a heart rate of 118 bpm. Electrocardiogram (ECG) reveals a wide complex, irregular tachycardia with different QRS morphologies. Laboratory findings include a potassium of 6.9, BUN of 72, Cr of 5.4 (baseline of 1.0 mg/dL), and a urinalysis showing > 75 WBCs, large leukocyte esterase, and positive nitrite. After placing two large bore intravenously (IV) and ensuring adequate airway protection, what is the appropriate next step in the management of this patient?
   A. Give IV calcium gluconate, sodium bicarbonate, insulin/D_{50}, and call renal for emergent dialysis.
   B. Begin aggressive fluid resuscitation, give IV calcium gluconate and IV antibiotics, and admit to the ICU.
   C. Shock the patient with 100 J synchronized cardioversion.
   D. Place a central line and initiate pressor therapy and IV antibiotics.
3. Which of the following is **not** an indication for emergency dialysis in a patient with end-stage renal disease?
   A. Magnesium of 2.4 and occasional premature ventricular contractions (PVCs)
   B. BUN of 108 with significant nausea and vomiting
   C. Acute mountain sickness (AMS) with a pH of 6.9
   D. K+ of 7.3 with electrocardiogram (ECG) changes
4. A 38-year-old woman with diabetes presents left flank pain for the past 2 days. She is uncomfortable appearing, vomiting frequently, with a temperature of 38.2°C, blood pressure of 96/60 mm Hg, and a heart rate of 122 bpm. Her urinalysis has 31-75 WBCs and > 75 RBCs with positive nitrite. Computed tomography (CT) of abdomen and pelvis without contrast shows a 3-mm stone at the ureteropelvic junction with moderate hydronephrosis. What is the appropriate next step in the management of this patient?
   A. Begin fluid resuscitation, IV antibiotics, and consult urology for emergent intervention.
   B. Give 2-L normal saline (NS), 1-dose IV antibiotics, and discharge home with 2 weeks of oral antibiotics.
   C. Give PO tamsulosin, oral antibiotics, and observe for 8 hours in the ED.
   D. Obtain CT of abdomen/pelvis with IV contrast to see if the infection has spread to the kidney.
5. In which of these patients with a hydrocele is it most important to get an urgent/emergent testicular ultrasound?
   A. 2-month-old male infant with a fever
   B. 19-year-old healthy man with no other symptoms
   C. 35-year-old man who was hit in the groin by a soccer ball 2 days ago, now pain free
   D. 61-year-old man with known congestive heart failure (CHF) presenting with fluid overload

ANSWERS

1. **D.** The urinalysis has no other findings such as casts to indicate any severe underlying pathology. In addition, the patient does not have severe hypertension, edema, or any signs of severe systemic illness. Therefore, the patient is appropriate for recheck with her PCP.
2. **B.** The patient has severe hyperkalemia, likely related to acute tubular necrosis (ATN) from severe sepsis. The patient emergently needs calcium to stabilize the myocardium. After that, he should be treated like any other patient with severe sepsis—fluids and blood pressure support. While he may ultimately need dialysis depending on how badly his kidneys have been damaged, most likely his renal function will improve and he will lower his own potassium level.
3. **A.** Symptomatic uremia, severe acidosis, and severe hyperkalemia are indications for emergent dialysis, along with severe volume overload and removal of significant toxic ingestions. Hypermagnesemia is not an indication.

4. **A.** An infected obstructive ureteral stone is a urologic emergency, and immediate control of the septic source is mandatory. It should be treated with aggressive fluids and IV antibiotics, with immediate urology consultation for possible intervention, eg, percutaneous nephrostomy tube.

5. **B.** This presentation is most concerning for underlying malignancy. Unless an expedient outpatient testicular ultrasound or urology follow-up can be arranged, strongly consider getting this ultrasound in the ED.

CHAPTER 19

Procedures and Skills

Michael D. Susalla, MD and Sara M. Krzyzaniak, MD

Cardiothoracic Procedures

PERICARDIOCENTESIS

Indications

- Hemopericardium
- Pericardial effusion with tamponade
- Pneumopericardium

Contraindications

- Relative: Coagulopathy, implanted devices and/or valves, ascending aortic dissection, immediately available definitive treatment modalities

Technique

- Use ultrasound guidance when available to identify greatest fluid collection.
- Cardiac monitoring with defibrillator, advanced airway and resuscitation equipment should be readily available.
- Attach a 7.5- to 12.5-cm 18-ga needle or Intracath needle to a syringe. Continuously aspirate syringe while advancing needle.
- **Parasternal approach**:
- Insert needle perpendicular to the skin in the left fifth or sixth intercostal space 1 cm lateral to the sternum.
- Avoid area of internal mammary artery, which lies 3-5 cm from the sternal border.
- **Subxyphoid approach:**
- Insert needle 1 cm inferior to the junction of the xyphoid process and left costal margin at a 30°-45° angle to the skin aiming toward the left shoulder (Figure 19.1).

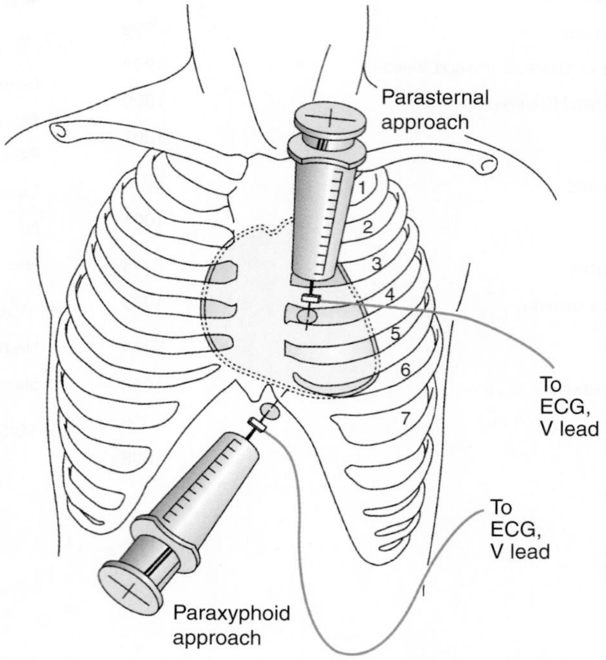

FIGURE 19.1. Pericardiocentesis: Subxyphoid Approach. Insert needle at a 45° angle to the midsagittal plane (A) and at a 45-degree angle to the abdominal wall (B). (Reproduced with permission from Gomella L, Haist S: *Clinician's Pocket Reference*, 11th ed. New York, NY: McGraw-Hill Education; 2006. Figure 13.17.)

- An ECG lead attached to the needle will show a current of injury (wide complex with ST elevation) when the needle touches the ventricular wall. When this occurs, withdraw the needle until the injury pattern is no longer present.
- Needle will penetrate the pericardium about 6-8 cm beneath the skin in adults and < 5 cm in children.
- Post-procedure: Obtain chest x-ray (CXR) to evaluate for pneumothorax or pneumoperitoneum.

COMPLICATIONS

- Failure to yield fluid ("dry tap"), often caused by clotted blood or a skin plug.
- Myocardial injury leading to hemopericardium.
- **Coronary vessel laceration leading to myocardial infarction and/or hemopericardium.**
- Internal mammary artery laceration leading to hemothorax.
- Pneumothorax/pneumoperitoneum.

INTERPRETATION OF RESULTS

- Removal of 30-50 mL may result in marked clinical improvement.
- Except in aortic dissection or ventricular wall rupture, pericardial fluid should have a lower hematocrit than venous blood, otherwise suspect that the needle has entered a cardiac chamber.
- Injection of a small amount of contrast under fluoroscopy can disclose intracardiac placement.

Q

A patient with breast cancer presents with a blood pressure (BP) of 60/30 mm Hg, muffled heart sounds, and distended neck veins. Cardiac monitor shows electrical alternans. Which diagnostic test is indicated? Which therapeutic intervention follows?

KEY FACT

During "blind" pericardiocentesis, the subxyphoid approach is recommended.

THORACOSTOMY

INDICATIONS

- Needle thoracostomy:
  - Emergent decompression for temporary treatment of tension pneumothorax
- Tube thoracostomy:
  - Treatment of large (≥ 3 cm rim of air on CXR) and/or symptomatic pneumothorax
  - Treatment of hemothorax

CONTRAINDICATIONS

- Relative:
  - Anatomic abnormalities: Multiple pleural adhesions, blebs, or pleural scarring
  - Coagulopathy or anticoagulant use

TECHNIQUE

- **Needle decompression**
  - Patient supine, head elevated 30°.
  - Minimum 3 inch, 16-ga needle with angiocatheter
  - Insert needle in second intercostal space, midclavicular line or 4th-5th intercostal space, mid-axillary line.
  - Rush of air will confirm placement. Advance catheter over needle and leave catheter in place.
  - Immediately perform tube thoracostomy after needle decompression, regardless of success.
- **Tube thoracostomy**
  - Place patient on supplemental oxygen and monitor, use sterile technique when possible.
  - Elevate head of bed to 30°-60°.

KEY FACT

The intercostal neurovascular bundle underlies each rib. During thoracentesis or thoracostomy, **enter the chest just above the rib** to avoid the neurovascular bundle.

KEY FACT

A tension pneumothorax is treated with either immediate tube thoracostomy or needle decompression followed by tube thoracostomy.

A

Cardiac ultrasonography to confirm pericardial effusion followed by pericardiocentesis.

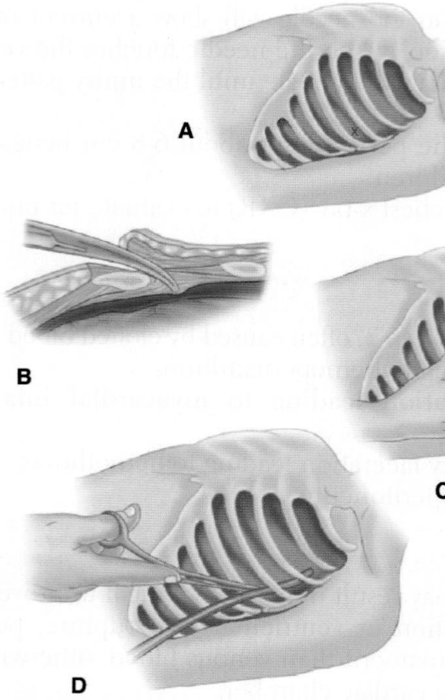

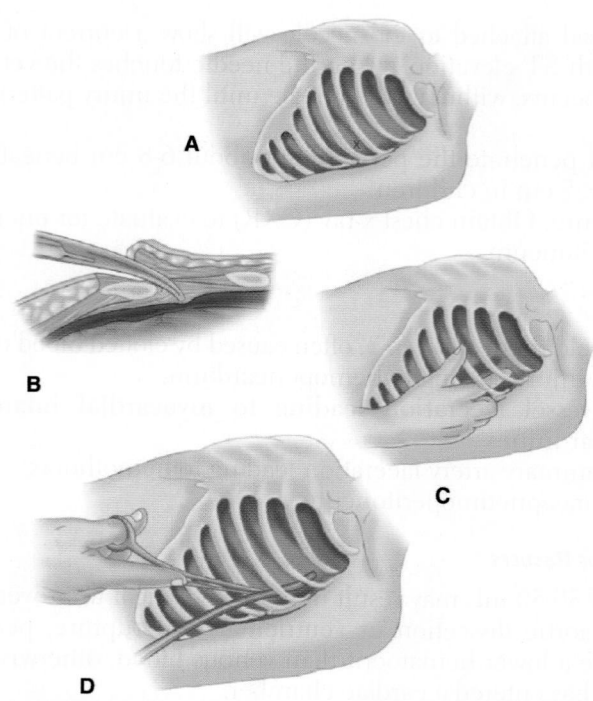

FIGURE 19.2. (A) Site of thoracostomy tube insertion. (B) Blunt dissection with Kelly clamp. (C) Finger confirmation of hole into pleura. (D) Insertion of thoracostomy tube. (Reproduced, with permission, from Brunicardi FC, Andersen DK, Billiar TR, et al. *Schwartz's Principles of Surgery*. 8th ed. New York, NY: McGraw-Hill Education, 2005.)

- Secure arm over patient's head.
- Administer local/regional anesthesia with or without procedural sedation.
- Make an anterior-posterior incision at least 3 cm long at fourth or fifth intercostal space, midaxillary line (Figure 19.2A).
- Perform blunt dissection with long closed Kelly clamp into the pleural space—dissect above rib to avoid nerve/vessel damage (see Figure 19.2B).
- Place finger through hole and feel for lung to confirm entrance into the pleural space—leave finger in pleural space (see Figure 19.2C).
- Use finger to guide tip of Kelly-clamped chest tube into pleural space.
- Insert chest tube posteriorly, medially, and toward lung apex, ensuring all holes are inside pleural space (see Figure 19.2D).
- Connect chest tube to water seal collection device set to wall suction of 10-20 cm H_2O.
- Secure with sutures (0 or 1-0 silk) and occlusive petroleum-impregnated gauze dressing.
- Confirm placement with CXR.

COMPLICATIONS

- Infection
- Injury to diaphragm, spleen, lung, heart, intercostal nerves/vessels, or liver
- Subcutaneous placement of chest tube
- Air leak: Either due to significant air movement from the lung into the pleural space or a leak in the tubing. Temporarily clamp the tube near to the chest—if the leak persists, it is within the tubing system not the patient

INTERPRETATION OF RESULTS

- Rush of air or fluid indicates entrance into pleural space.
- CXR should show improved pneumothorax or hemothorax.
- Immediate drainage of 1000-1500 mL of blood or continued bleeding (ie, > 300-500 mL in first hour or > 200 mL/h for first 3 hours) is indication for surgery.

THORACENTESIS

Indications

- Analysis of pleural effusion
- Treatment of symptomatic pleural effusion

Contraindications

- Use an alternate patient position if overlying cellulitis or zoster.
- Coagulopathy is a relative contraindication.

Technique

- Position patient upright with arms extended on bedside table. The needle insertion site in this position is along the mid-scapular or posterior axillary line. Alternatively, position patient supine with head of bed elevated as much as possible and use a needle insertion site along the mid-axillary or posterior axillary line.
- Localize fluid with ultrasound or percussion.
- Level of needle insertion should be 1-2 intercostal spaces (ICS) below the upper level of effusion but NOT below the eighth intercostal space.
- Using a 25-ga needle with 1% lidocaine, anesthetize the upper edge of the rib below the desired ICS.
- Walk the needle attached to syringe up over rib (to avoid accidental puncture of neurovascular bundle at inferior rib margin) while injecting lidocaine until you enter the pleural space and localize the fluid.
- Insert a needle-catheter into the anesthetized ICS until fluid is withdrawn, then advance catheter into space. Collect fluid via syringe or vacuum bottle.

> **KEY FACT**
>
> Ultrasound guidance has been shown to significantly lower the rate of complications, consider using this modality in patients with coagulopathy or in small effusions.

Interpretation of Results

- First determine if the fluid is exudative or transudative. Send pleural fluid and serum for protein and lactate dehydrogenase (LDH). The fluid is an **exudate** if one of the following is present (Light's criteria).
  - Pleural fluid-serum protein ratio > 0.5.
- Pleural fluid LDH > two-third the upper level of serum reference range.
  - Pleural fluid-serum LDH ratio > 0.6.
- Additional studies for all exudates include complete blood count (CBC) with differential, glucose, cytology, adenosine deaminase. Further studies should be guided by suspicion (eg, pH, Gram stain and culture for suspected infection).
- No further studies are necessary for transudates.

Complications

- Pneumothorax 6%/hemothorax
- Infection
- Puncture of spleen or liver
- Reexpansion pulmonary edema if too much fluid (typically > 1500 mL) is withdrawn

EMERGENCY DEPARTMENT THORACOTOMY

Indications

- **Blunt trauma**
  - Less than 10 minutes of ongoing cardiopulmonary resuscitation (CPR)
    - Unresponsive hypotension (BP < 70 mm Hg) despite resuscitation with echo evidence of cardiac tamponade
    - Rapid exsanguination from a chest tube (>1500 cc output)
- **Penetrating trauma**
  - Prehospital/hospital signs of life with < 15 minutes of ongoing CPR
    - Echo evidence of cardiac activity with cardiac tamponade
    - Unresponsive hypotension (SBP < 70 mm Hg) despite chest decompression and resuscitation with penetrating chest wound

> **KEY FACT**
>
> Signs of life, such as pupillary response, extremity movement, cardiac electrical activity, spontaneous ventilation, or any measurement of blood pressure have been shown to have increased rates of survival in emergency department (ED) thoracotomy.

Contraindications

- Prehospital CPR > 10 minutes (blunt trauma) or > 15 minutes (prehospital/hospital signs of life) without response
- Asystole as presenting rhythm and no echo evidence for cardiac tamponade
- Significant head trauma

Technique

- If possible, analgesia and deep sedation should be provided.
- Patient should be intubated. If necessary, the right lung can be selectively intubated (right mainstem bronchus) to expedite thoracotomy on the left side.
- If possible, a nasogastric tube (NGT) should be placed to help differentiate esophagus from aorta.
- Using #20 blade, make incision into the left chest between fourth and fifth ribs: Just inferior to the nipple in men or along the inframammary fold in women (Figure 19.3A).
- Extend incision from sternum past the posterior axillary line, cutting down through pectoralis and serratus muscles.
- Use blunt nose scissors to divide the intercostal muscles.
- Once the pleural space is entered, stop ventilations temporarily to allow the lung to collapse away from chest wall.
- Place chest wall retractor (rib spreader) to spread ribs. Orient the crank posteriorly, so that the incision can be extended across the sternum into the right chest if necessary.
- If examination suggests any possibility of tamponade, perform pericardiotomy: Lift pericardial sac near diaphragm with forceps, make a small incision with scissors, and extend the incision cephalad along anterior pericardium **parallel to the phrenic nerve** (see Figure 19.3B).
- Retract pericardium to examine heart for injury and repair with staples or sutures. Direct cardiac compressions, internal defibrillation, or intracardiac epinephrine injections can be performed. (see Figure 19.3C/D).
- Aortic cross-clamping if systolic blood pressure (SBP) < 70 mm Hg: Identify aorta which lies anterior to vertebral column and posterior to the esophagus. Place a vascular clamp around the aorta or occlude aorta with digital pressure (Figure 19.4).

KEY FACT

A 20-Fr Foley catheter with 30-mL balloon may be used to temporarily control myocardial wounds. Insert catheter into cardiac chamber, inflate balloon with saline, clamp catheter, and apply gentle traction to tamponade bleeding.

Complications

- Injury to intrathoracic structures (internal mammary artery, phrenic nerve, coronary arteries, aorta, esophagus, lungs)
- Cross-clamping the aorta may cause ischemia of spinal cord, liver, bowel, and kidneys or conversely cerebral hemorrhage or left ventricular failure if pressure elevation is excessive
- Infection

Interpretation of Results

- Patients with SBP > 110 mm Hg within 30 minutes have good survival rates and neurologic outcomes. Those with SBP > 85 mm Hg will likely have brain damage, and those with SBP < 70 mm Hg will likely not survive.

TRANSCUTANEOUS CARDIAC PACING

Indications

- Hemodynamically unstable bradyarrhythmias unresponsive to medication
- Initial stabilization of the patient in the emergency department (ED) while arranging for transvenous pacemaker
- Overdrive pacing for refractory tachyarrythmias

Q

A woman with a family history of sudden cardiac death presents following a syncopal episode. ECG shows intermittent polymorphic ventricular tachycardia and a QT interval of 600 milliseconds. What is the rhythm disturbance? Which treatments are indicated?

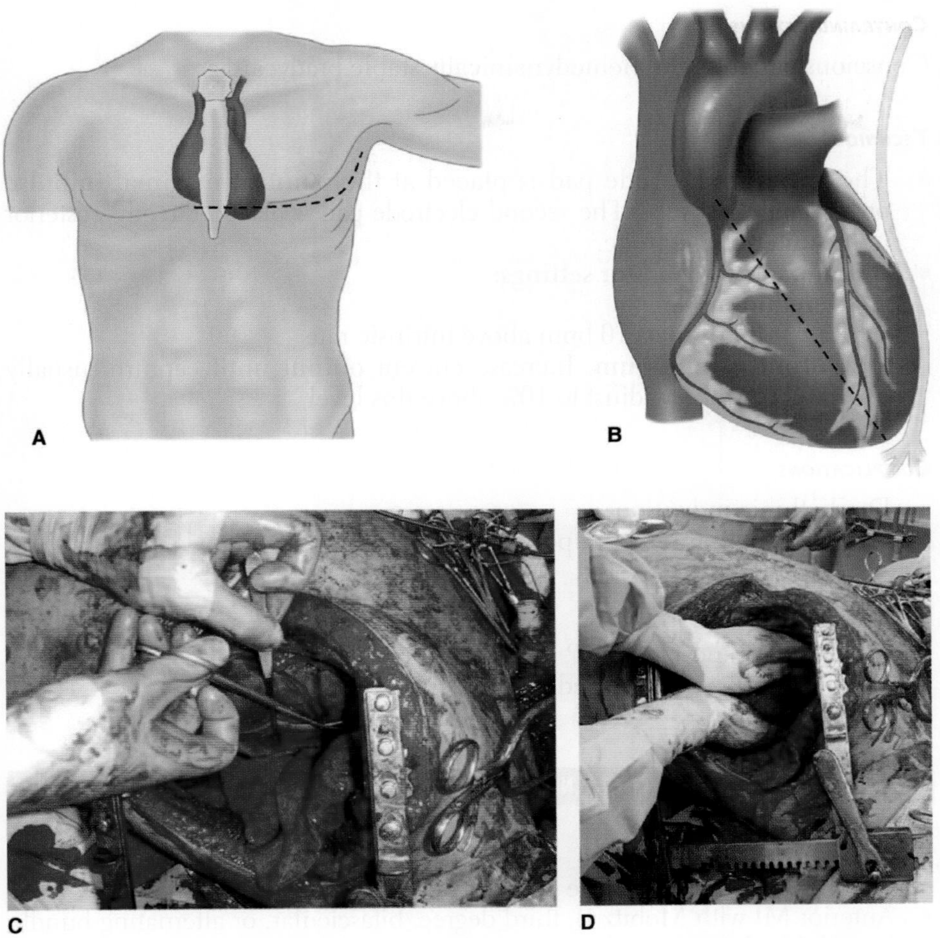

FIGURE 19.3. (A) Site of incision for thoracotomy. (B) Clamping of descending thoracic aorta and site of pericardial window. (C) Visualization of the heart for repairs and (D) open cardiac massage. (Reproduced, with permission, from Brunicardi FC, Andersen DK, Billiar TR, et al. *Schwartz's Principles of Surgery*. 10th ed. New York, NY: McGraw-Hill Education, 2010. Figure 7.12.)

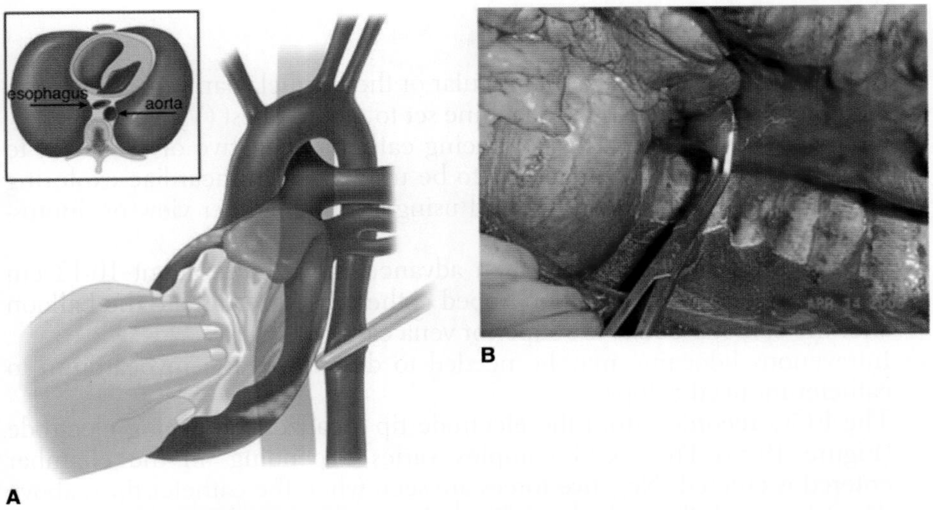

FIGURE 19.4. (A&B) Site of aortic cross-clamp. Puncture through the parietal pleura immediately anterior to the body of the thoracic vertebral body with the tip of a finger to isolate the aorta. (Reproduced, with permission, from Brunicardi FC, Andersen DK, Billiar TR, et al. *Schwartz's Principles of Surgery*, 10th ed. New York, NY: McGraw-Hill, 2010.)

A

Torsade de pointes. Treat with intravenous (IV) magnesium. Consider overdrive pacing.

KEY FACT

Use the asynchronous (or fixed) mode setting rather than demand mode when the pacemaker is unable to sense the intrinsic rhythm.

KEY FACT

With transcutaneous pacing, increase current output until capture, then adjust to 10% above this level.

KEY FACT

When pacing, always confirm electrical capture seen on the monitor by palpating a pulse. Electrical capture without a pulse equals pulseless electrical activity (PEA).

CONTRAINDICATIONS

Conscious patients with hemodynamically stable bradycardias

TECHNIQUE

- The anterior electrode pad is placed at the point of maximal impulse on the left chest wall. The second electrode pad is placed directly posterior to the anterior electrode.
- **Initial pacing generator settings:**
  - **Demand mode**
  - **Rate = 80 bpm** or 10 bpm above intrinsic rate
  - **Output = minimum**. Increase current **output** until capture (usually 40-60 mA) then adjust to 10% above this level

COMPLICATIONS

- Dysrhythmia induction
- Soft tissue discomfort with potential for injury

INTERPRETATION OF RESULTS

Feel for a pulse and check BP to confirm that the electrical capture seen on the monitor results in improved perfusion.

TRANSVENOUS CARDIAC PACING

INDICATIONS

- Hemodynamically unstable bradycardias unresponsive to medication
- Anterior MI with Mobitz II, third degree, bifascicular, or alternating bundle branch block
- Overdrive pacing of certain tachydysrhythmias (most commonly torsades)

CONTRAINDICATIONS

- Severe hypothermia
- Prosthetic tricuspid valve

TECHNIQUE

- Best approach is the R internal jugular or the L subclavian vein.
- Connect patient to an ECG machine set to record chest (V) lead.
- Connect the distal terminal of pacing catheter (negative or "–" lead) to the V lead of the ECG machine to be used as an intracardiac exploring electrode. Alternatively, ultrasound using a four-chamber view or fluoroscopy can be used.
- Insert the introducer sheath, then advance pacing wire about 10-12 cm into selected vein. If a balloon-tipped catheter is used, inflate the balloon after the catheter enters the superior vena cava.
- Intravenous lidocaine may be needed to desensitize the myocardium to catheter-induced ectopy.
- The ECG recorded from the electrode tip localizes the pacing electrode (Figure 19.5). The ECG complex varies depending on the chamber entered is entered: Negative forces are seen when the catheter tip is above the atrium and diminished amplitude is seen if the catheter tip enters the inferior vena cava (IVC) or the pulmonary artery.
- Once ventricular endocardial contact is made, disconnect the pacing catheter from the ECG machine and connect it to the pacing generator.

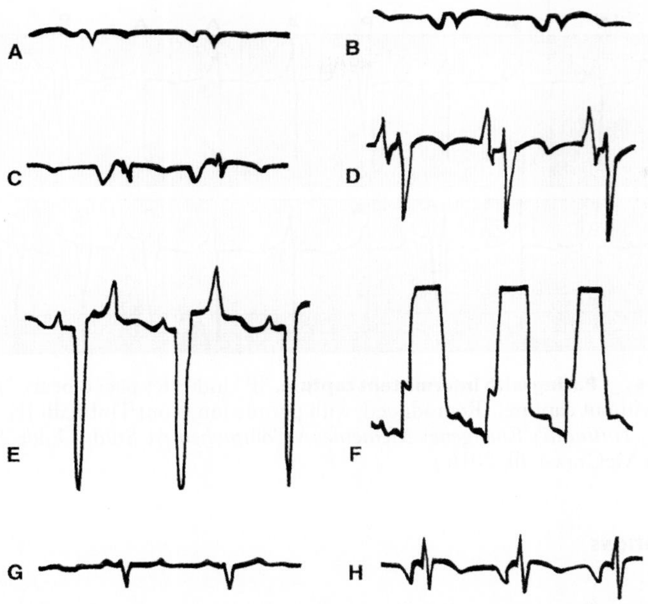

FIGURE 19.5. Typical ECG tracings seen with a transvenous pacing catheter within the different anatomic sites. (**A**) The subclavian or internal jugular vein. (**B**) The superior vena cava. (**C**) The high right atrium. (**D**) The low right atrium. (**E**) Free-floating in the right ventricle. (**F**) Abutting the right ventricular wall. (**G**) The inferior vena cava. (**H**) The pulmonary artery. (Reproduced, with permission, from Reichman EF, Simon RR. *Emergency Medicine Procedures*. New York, NY: McGraw-Hill, 2004.)

- **Initial pacing generator settings:**
  - **Rate = 80 bpm**, or 10 bpm faster than underlying ventricular rhythm above intrinsic rate.
  - **Output = maximum** and reduce until capture is lost, then increase to 2.5 times this threshold (usually between 2 and 3 mA).
  - **Sensitivity = maximum mV** (asynchronous)

COMPLICATIONS

- From introducer sheath: Thrombosis, bleeding, infection, pneumothorax, arterial puncture
- From pacing wire: Dysrhythmias, myocardial wall perforation, hemopericardium/tamponade, mechanical failure, inconsistent pacing

INTERPRETATION OF RESULTS

- Appropriate pacing and CXR indicating proper placement.
- If the catheter is within the right ventricle, a left bundle-branch pattern with left axis deviation should be evident in paced beats (Figure 19.6).

Vascular Access

CENTRAL VENOUS CATHETERIZATION

INDICATIONS

- Central venous pressure (CVP) monitoring
- Rapid volume resuscitation
- Venous access in patients with poor or no peripheral access
- Need to infuse hyperalimentation or other concentrated solutions
- Emergent hemodialysis or plasmapheresis

Q

While you're placing a subclavian line, your patient becomes agitated, hypoxic, tachycardic, and hypotensive. CXR shows Westermark sign (focal oligemia). What's the diagnosis? Treatment?

KEY FACT

Ultrasound can be used to help identify the pacing wire within the right atrium and ventricle.

For transvenous pacing, the initial output is set to maximum and the mode is set to fixed or asynchronous.

A

Air embolism. Clamp the central line. Reposition the tip of the line 2 cm below superior vena cava-right atrium (SVC-RA) junction and aspirate while the patient is in left lateral decubitus position and Trendelenburg. Consider hyperbaric therapy.

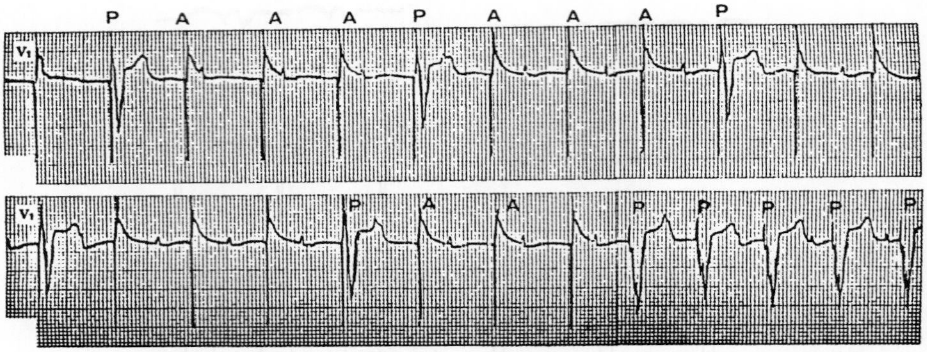

FIGURE 19.6. Pacing with intermittent capture. "P" indicates paced beats; "A" indicates pacer artifact without capture. (Reproduced, with permission, from Tintinalli JE, Kelen GD, Stapczynski JS. *Tintinalli's Emergency Medicine: A Comprehensive Study Guide*, 8th ed. New York, NY: McGraw-Hill, 2016.)

KEY FACT

The use of ultrasound has been shown to increase the rate of successful first puncture and patient satisfaction, while decreasing the number of attempts, time to perform the procedure, and complication rate.

KEY FACT

For IJ and subclavian lines, use Trendelenburg to increase intrathoracic pressure and decrease the risk of an air embolism.

Contraindications

- Absolute:
  - Serious allergy to antibiotic coating an impregnated catheter (eg, tetracycline or rifampin)
- Relative:
  - Distorted local anatomy or landmarks or previous radiation therapy
  - Cellulitis, burns, or abrasions over insertion site
  - Suspected proximal vascular injury
  - Coagulopathy or patient on anticoagulants
  - Current thrombus at site

Technique

- Use strict sterile technique to reduce infectious complications.
- Seldinger (guidewire) technique: Use a thin-walled needle to introduce a guidewire into the vessel lumen. Place the catheter over the guidewire while ensuring you have control over the guidewire at all times and once in place, remove guidewire.
- Use ultrasound guidance for both visualization of landmarks and correct placement of the guidewire at all four central access sites.
- **Infraclavicular subclavian (SC)**
  - Place patient in Trendelenburg position.
  - Vein lies posterior to the medial third of the clavicle. Enter the skin 1 cm inferior and lateral to the curve in the clavicle.
  - Aim needle toward suprasternal notch. Enter vein at a depth of 3-4 cm (Figure 19.7).
- **Supraclavicular subclavian**
  - Place patient in Trendelenburg position.
  - Insert needle 1 cm lateral to the clavicular head of the sternocleidomastoid (SCM) and 1 cm posterior to the clavicle.
  - Aim the needle toward contralateral nipple while maintaining the needle parallel to the bed. Positioning the bevel medially will help prevent the catheter from being blocked by the inferior vessel wall.
- **Internal jugular (IJ)**
  - Place patient in Trendelenburg position with head turned 15°-30° away from puncture site.
  - The vein usually lies anterior and lateral of the carotid artery just deep to the SCM muscle at the level of the thyroid cartilage.
  - Access vein medial to the SCM aiming toward ipsilateral nipple (anterior approach), lateral to the SCM aiming toward sternoclavicular notch (posterior approach), or between the sternal and clavicular heads of the SCM (central approach) (see Figure 19.7).

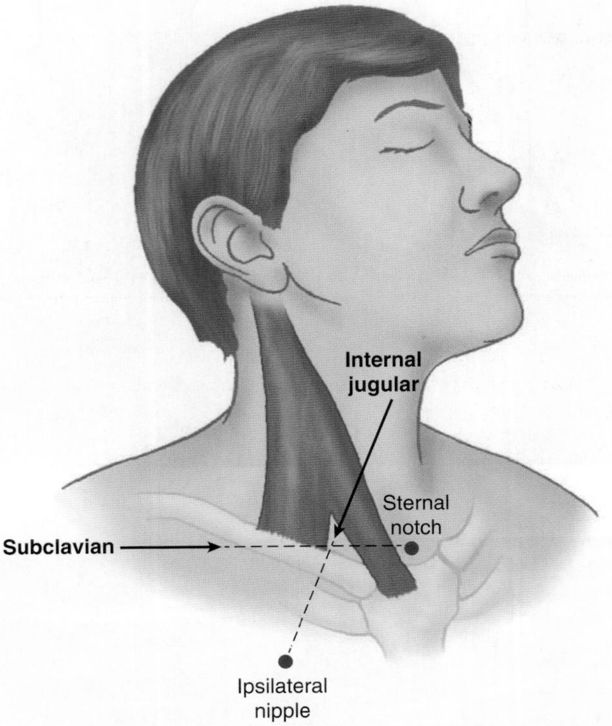

FIGURE 19.7. Access for subclavian and internal jugular central lines. (Modified, with permission, from Wasnick J, Hillel Z, Kramer D, et al. *Cardiac Anesthesia & Transesophageal Echocardiography*. New York, NY: McGraw-Hill Education, 2011. Figure 2.3.)

- Femoral
  - Place patient supine.
  - Vein lies medial to femoral artery below the inguinal ligament.
  - Palpate femoral pulse and place needle just medial to it below inguinal ligament.

Complications

- Air embolism
- Infection
- Pneumothorax, hydrothorax (IJ/SC)
- Vein or artery laceration, bleeding/hematomas (eg, retroperitoneal hematoma with femoral)
- Dysrhythmias from direct irritation of atria or ventricles. Retract guidewire/catheter
- Catheter malposition (eg, subclavian vein catheter ascending IJ)

Interpretation of Results

- Vein has been successfully entered when dark venous blood flows freely into the syringe.
- The return of bright red, pulsatile blood signifies arterial puncture.
- Ultrasound can confirm needle/guidewire in appropriate vessel (Figure 19.8).
- CXR will show appropriate placement of subclavian and internal jugular catheterization.

INTRAOSSEOUS INFUSION

Indications

- Need for emergent, rapid vascular access when venous access is not available.

MNEMONIC

The order of structure in the femoral triangle from lateral to medial:

NAVEL

Nerve
Artery
Vein
Empty canal
Lymphatics

KEY FACT

The femoral vein site has the highest risk for infection after central line placement.

The subclavian vein is not compressible and should not be used in patients with increased risk of bleeding.

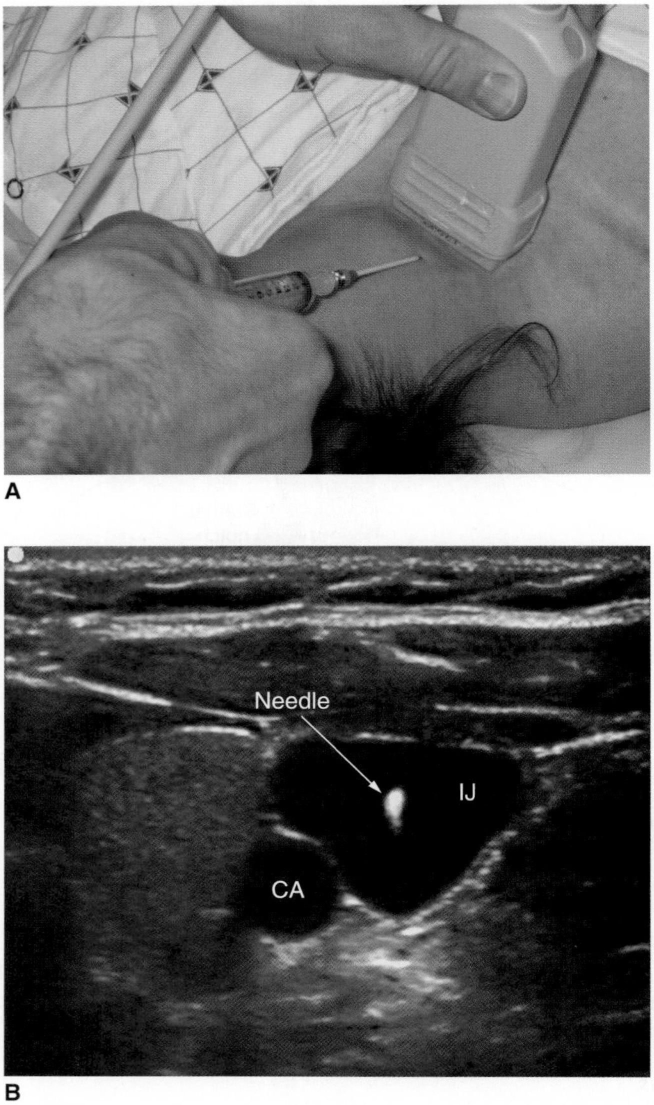

FIGURE 19.8. Ultrasound guided central access. (**A**) Probe in transverse plane. (**B**) Visualization of the needle in the internal jugular (IJ) vein and carotid artery (CA) in view. (Reproduced, with permission, from Knoop K, Stack L, Storrow A, et al. *The Atlas of Emergency Medicine*. 3rd ed. New York, NY: McGraw-Hill Education, 2009. Figure 24.78. Photographer: Paul R. Sierzenski, MD, RDMS.)

- Preferred access over central lines when peripheral access cannot be quickly attained.

KEY FACT

Intraosseous access is a bridge to venous access in critically ill patients.

Once definitive intravenous (IV) access is obtained, the intraosseous line should be removed.

Contraindications

- Avoid in patients with osteogenesis imperfecta and severe osteoporosis (fracture risk) due to fracture risk and in those with R to L intracardiac shunt due to increased risk for cerebral fat/bone marrow embolism.
- Choose alternate site in patients with fracture or prior intraosseous (IO) attempt of selected bone due to risk for extravasation of infused fluid and for those with cellulitis or burns at the insertion site.

Technique

- Can be placed in proximal tibia, distal tibia, distal femur, proximal humerus, and in adults, the sternum. Prox humerus is the preferred site in adults.
- Use sterile technique

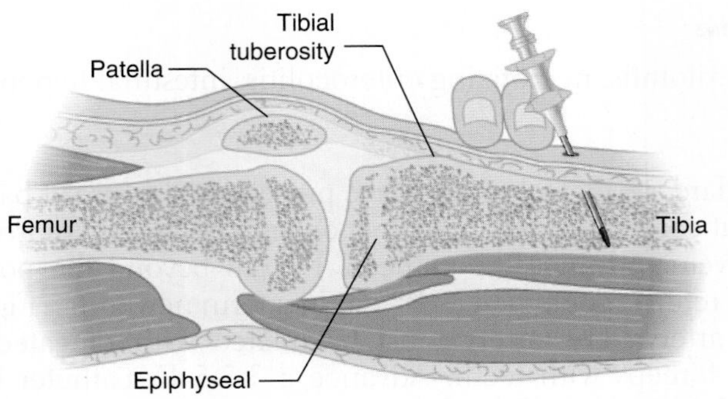

FIGURE 19.9. Insertion of intraosseous needle in the proximal tibia. (Reproduced, with permission, from Tintinalli JE, Kelen GD, Stapczynski JS. *Tintinalli's Emergency Medicine: A Comprehensive Study Guide*. 7th ed. New York, NY: McGraw-Hill Education, 2011. Figure 33.19.)

- When using a manual IO, apply rotatory motion with pressure. With a powered IO, place gentle downward pressure on the drill while actuating the trigger. The distance from the skin through the cortex of the bone is rarely > 1 cm in an infant or child (Figure 19.9)
- Placement site
  - **Proximal tibia:** Anteromedial surface, approximately 1-3 cm (2 finger widths) below the tuberosity on the medial, flat surface of the tibia
  - **Distal tibia:** Medial surface at the junction of the medial malleolus and the shaft of the tibia, posterior to the greater saphenous vein
  - **Distal femur**: 2-3 cm above the external femoral condyles in the anterior midline. May be difficult to palpate bony landmarks
  - **Proximal humerus:** Over greater tubercle with arm in adduction (1 cm above surgical neck)
- Check around the site for extravasation of fluid.

KEY FACT

Damage to the growth plate from IO insertion is feared but has never been reported

Complications

- Cellulitis
- Extravasation of fluid leading to skin sloughing, myonecrosis, or compartment syndrome
- Osteomyelitis, mediastinitis (especially in children)
- Pain with infusion—can be decreased with **slow** infusion of 2-5 mL of 2% lidocaine. Be sure to use IV compatible lidocaine, or "cardiac lidocaine".
- Fracture of the needle within the bone

Interpretation of Results

- Aspiration of blood or marrow contents confirms position.
- The needle's ability to stand **upright without support** and fluids that infuse easily without evidence of swelling or extravasation also confirms position.

UMBILICAL VEIN/ARTERY CATHETERIZATION

The majority of infants are born with a single umbilical vein and paired umbilical arteries. The vein is located at 12 o'clock and is thin walled with a large lumen. The urachus may persist but can be differentiated from the vein by presence of urine. The paired arteries are located at 5 and 7 o'clock and have thick walls with smaller lumens. A single umbilical artery is present in a small percentage of patients.

Indications

- Vein: Need for emergent vascular access in newborns. The umbilical vein remains **patent for 1-2 weeks after birth**.
- Artery: Need for frequent monitoring of arterial blood gases and BP.

CONTRAINDICATIONS

Omphalitis, peritonitis, necrotizing enterocolitis, intestinal hypoperfusion

TECHNIQUE

- Using standard sterile technique place purse-string suture at base of umbilicus then cut cord with a sterile scalpel or iris scissors 1.5 cm from the base.
- Umbilical vein: Advance the catheter 1-2 cm beyond the point at which good blood return is obtained (~4-5 cm in a term newborn) (Figure 19.10).
- Umbilical artery: The artery must be dilated with repeated passes and curved iris forceps with teeth. Advance a 3.5-5 Fr catheter flushed with heparinized saline toward the feet.

COMPLICATIONS

- Vessel or peritoneal perforation, bleeding, infection
- Hepatic ischemia, especially with infusion of vasoconstrictive medications
- Thromboembolism, air embolism, aortic thrombosis, aortic aneurysm

INTERPRETATION OF RESULTS

- Easy aspiration of blood confirms placement in lumen of vessel.
- Findings on x-ray:
  - Umbilical vein catheter travels **cranially** in the umbilical vein to the IVC.
  - Umbilical artery catheter travels **down** toward the pelvis, makes a posterior turn into the common iliac artery **then continues cranially** with the tip ending in the aorta either between T6 and T9 or between L3 and L5 vertebral bodies to avoid the celiac, superior mesenteric, and renal arteries.

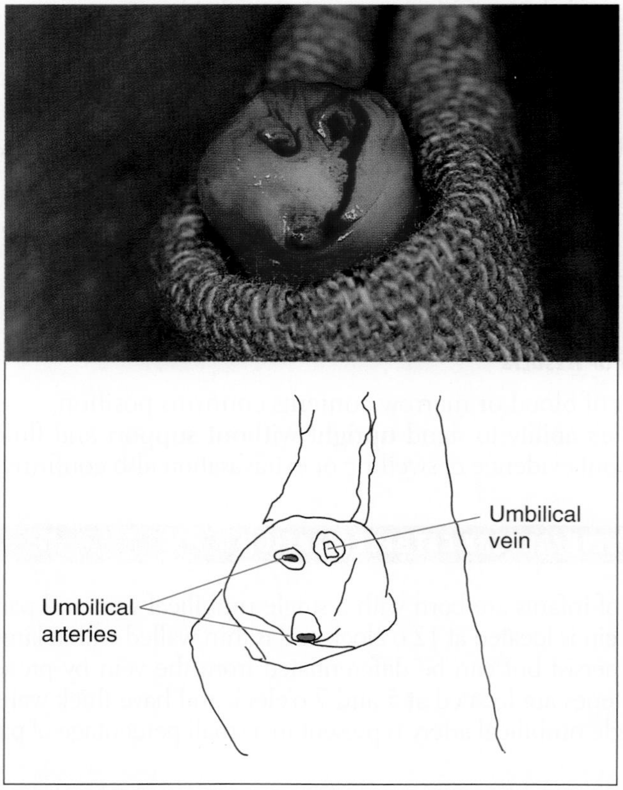

FIGURE 19.10. Cross-section of umbilical cord showing location of vein and arteries. (Reproduced, with permission, from Knoop K, Stack L, Storrow A, et al. *The Atlas of Emergency Medicine*. 3rd ed. New York, NY: McGraw-Hill Education, 2009. Figure 10-40. Photographer: Jennifer Jagoe, MD.)

ARTERIAL CATHETERIZATION

Indications

- Frequent monitoring of arterial blood gases
- Continuous hemodynamic monitoring or inability to use indirect blood pressure monitoring

Contraindications

Use alternate site if there is a traumatic injury proximal to the proposed site, infection or full thickness burn at the site, or evidence of inadequate circulation, Buerger disease or Raynaud in distribution of selected artery.

Technique

- Standard sterile technique should be used and when possible, local anesthesia.
- The radial, brachial, and femoral arteries are usual sites for adult arterial puncture. Pediatric sites include arteries in the foot and the umbilical artery (newborns).
- Perform Allen test prior to radial artery cannulation to ensure collateral flow from ulnar artery.
- Cannulation is usually placed with an over-the-needle catheter with or without a guidewire. When accessing larger vessels, such as the femoral artery, always use needle puncture followed by catheter placement over a guidewire (Seldinger technique) (Figure 19.11).
- Palpate the arterial pulsation with the index and middle fingers and identify the vessel course. Puncture the skin distal to the palpated pulse under the index finger. Advance the needle slowly at a 30° angle with the skin.

Complications

Bleeding, infection, hematoma, pseudoaneurysm, thrombosis → ischemia

Interpretation of Results

- Once in the artery, the syringe should fill on its own due to arterial pressure.
- Once attached to the monitor, the arterial wave form has a distinctive dicrotic notch on the down slope caused by the closure of the aortic valve.

Abdominal and Gastrointestinal Procedures

PARACENTESIS

Indications

- Relieve cardiorespiratory and gastrointestinal (GI) manifestations of tense ascites
- Diagnostic test for patients with new onset ascites or to determine presence of infection in patients with chronic ascites

Contraindications

Cellulitis or engorged veins over site

Technique

- Position patient supine with head of bed slightly elevated or in lateral decubitus position.

Q

You just saw a patient with a history of end-stage liver disease who presents with abdominal pain. What is your concern? What procedure is indicated?

KEY FACT

Ultrasound or handheld Doppler can be used to assist in locating vessel. Evidence shows a 71% improvement in first attempt success.

KEY FACT

Coagulopathy (patients with platelet levels < 50,000/mm^3 and prothrombin times > 20 seconds) is **not** a contraindication and is associated with an acceptably low rate of complications.

A

Spontaneous bacterial peritonitis. This is an indication to perform a diagnostic paracentesis.

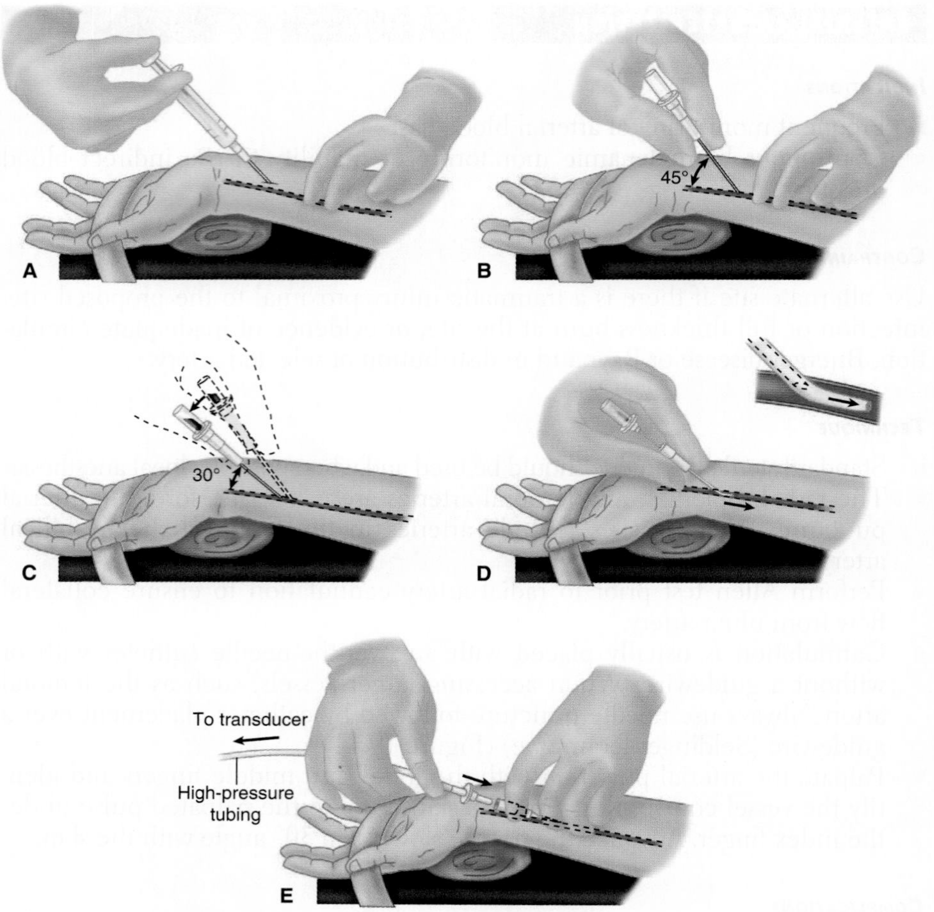

FIGURE 19.11. Radial artery catheterization. (A) Positioning and palpation of the radial artery. (B) Advance catheter at 45° angle. (C) Lower angle of catheter and (D) advance catheter. (E) Connect catheter to transducer and secure. (Reproduced, with permission, from Butterworth J, Mackey D, Wasnick J. *Morgan & Mikhail's Clinical Anesthesiology.* 5th ed. New York, NY: McGraw-Hill Education, 2013. Figure 5.7.)

- Site of entry is 2 cm below the umbilicus in the midline or 4 -5 cm cephalad and medial to the anterior superior iliac spine in the right or left lower quadrant.
- Use sterile technique with local anesthesia. Ultrasound should be used to confirm presence of ascites and avoid bowel injury particularly in patients with previous abdominal surgery, though "blind taps" have a very low complication rate.
- Use the "z-track" method wherein the skin is pulled ~2 cm caudad, then the needle is inserted, and the skin is released when fluid flows from needle into syringe.
- Insert a 1.5-inch needle (with optional catheter) and attached syringe perpendicular to skin. In obese patients a 3.5-inch spinal needle may be used. Advance needle until peritoneal fluid returns. If a catheter is used, advance it over the needle into peritoneal space and tape to the skin.
- Collect fluid via syringe or vacuum bottles. Send fluid for cell count, culture, and Gram stain. Additional studies (depending on clinical suspicion) include protein, glucose, LDH, amylase, albumin, TB culture, cytology, triglycerides, and bilirubin.
- When performing a large-volume paracentesis (≥ 5 L), intravenous albumin may be considered to reduce the likelihood of subsequent hepatorenal syndrome. It is not recommended for removal of volumes < 5 L.

KEY FACT

Avoid surgical scars, visible superficial vessels, and the inferior epigastric artery.

The inferior epigastric artery runs from the midpoint of the inguinal ligament to the umbilicus.

COMPLICATIONS

Persistent leakage of fluid from site (which can be remedied by a single suture), hematoma, hemoperitoneum (rare), perforation of vessels/viscera, peritonitis or abdominal wall abscess

INTERPRETATION OF RESULTS

- Spontaneous Bacterial Peritonitis: > **250 PMN/µL (polymorphonuclear leukocytes)** is considered by many as presumptive evidence of **SBP**. However, other cutoffs have been described, including > 250 WBC/mm^3 (white blood cell) with > 50% PMNs. A positive Gram stain is diagnostic.
- Cirrhosis: < 250 WBC/mm^3, lymphocytes predominant
- Neoplasm: > 1000 WBC/mm^3 with variable cell types
- Serum-ascites albumin gradient (SAAG) > 1.1 g/dL indicates portal hypertension.

KEY FACT

While positive Gram stain is diagnostic for SBP > 250 PMN/µL can make a presumptive diagnosis in the correct clinical scenario.

RECTAL FOREIGN BODY REMOVAL

CONTRAINDICATIONS

- Severe abdominal pain or signs of perforation.
- Nonpalpable rectal foreign bodies (FB) require surgical consultation.

TECHNIQUE

- Use x-ray to confirm the presence of an FB and define its size and position.
- Place patient in knee-chest or lateral decubitus position.
- IV sedation and/or perianal block may be required. Perianal block: Infiltrate anesthetic circumferentially around the anus in the submucosal tissue.
- Perform direct rectal examination to gauge position/orientation of FB.
- Apply suprapubic pressure while patient performs a Valsalva maneuver to deliver FB.
- If unsuccessful, insert an anoscope, vaginal speculum, or retractor into the anus to visualize the FB clearly and use an instrument to secure and remove it.
- A vacuum effect is often present between the FB and mucosa. Release it by passing a Foley catheter or endotracheal tube beyond the FB and then inflate the balloon.
- If there is concern for perforation, either by the process of removal or specific characteristics of FB, observe patient for 12 hours after procedure for complications.

KEY FACT

Use extreme caution to avoid sharps injury when attempting removal of sharp or fragile objects

COMPLICATIONS

- Failure to remove FB.
- Mild mucosal edema and rectal bleeding are common.
- **Perforation or deep mucosal tear** require hospitalization.
- Cracking or shattering of glass FB may require surgical exploration and retrieval.

INTERPRETATION OF RESULTS

Removal of intact FB without abdominal pain or severe bleeding indicates successful removal.

NASOGASTRIC TUBE PLACEMENT

INDICATIONS

- Decompression of stomach/small bowel with obstruction, ileus, perforation, or postintubation

- GI bleed (differentiate upper from lower source and quantify bleed)
- Administration of food or medication

CONTRAINDICATIONS

- Absolute: Facial or basilar skull fractures
- Relative:
  - Varices (multiple studies suggest it's safe to place nasogastric (NG) tube in presence of varices)
  - Severe coagulopathy
  - Esophageal strictures, gastric bypass or lap band
  - Patient with elevated intracranial pressure
  - Recent oropharyngeal surgery

> **KEY FACT**
>
> In a patient with facial fractures or severe coagulopathy, consider placing an orogastric tube through mouth rather than nose.

TECHNIQUE

- Conscious patients should be sitting upright in bed.
- Measure NG tube by placing tip at xiphoid then to earlobe and tip of nose; add 15 cm.
- Spray topical vasoconstrictor (eg, phenylephrine or oxymetazoline) into both nares 5 minutes before procedure. Combinations of tetracaine, benzocaine, and lidocaine gel (2%) may be used.
- Antiemetics such as ondansetron and metoclopramide may be helpful.
- Insert the tube into naris along floor of nose, under inferior turbinate.
- Ask the patient to sip water from a straw and swallow as the tube is advanced from oropharynx into esophagus. Flexing the patient's neck will help direct the NG tube into esophagus rather than trachea.
- Once NG tube is in esophagus, advance rapidly to predetermined depth.
- Secure with tape attached to both tube and nose.

COMPLICATIONS

- Coiling of NG tube in oropharynx
- Placement into trachea or lungs; suspect if choking, laryngospasm, coughing, change in voice, or condensation in tube occurs.

INTERPRETATION OF RESULTS

Successful placement can be determined by auscultation (insufflate air into NG tube and assess rush of air over stomach), aspiration of stomach contents, or x-ray.

GASTRIC TUBE REPLACEMENT

INDICATIONS

- Accidental removal/dislodgement of gastric tube (G-tube)
- Dysfunctional tube secondary to clogs, leakage, or breakage

CONTRAINDICATIONS

- Immediate postoperative period (< 1-3 weeks depending on rate of healing)
- Signs of complication (eg, infection, ileus, intestinal obstruction)
- Use caution if tube has been dislodged for > 2-3 hours, as the stoma may have already closed

TECHNIQUE

- Use cotton applicator to determine patency and direction of tract.
- Insert fresh G-tube into stoma.
- If no G-tube is available, a Foley catheter may be substituted as a temporizing measure.

- The end of a cotton applicator may be inserted through "eye" of Foley or a silicone Foley catheter can be placed in ice water to add rigidity.
- Inflate balloon with saline unless there is question whether the tube terminates in the jejunum, where inflation of the balloon could lead to intestinal obstruction.
- Create a bolster using a cut 3-cm segment of the proximal end of Foley
- Once tube is placed and secure, order a contrast "G-tube study" (abdominal radiograph using water-soluble contrast through tube) to confirm gastric position and exclude gastric perforation.

Q

A patient with known esophageal varices presents with hematemesis and hypotension. After blood, antibiotics, octreotide, and proton pump inhibitor, the patient continues to bleed. Upper endoscopy is not available. What other interventions should be considered?

Complications

- Creation of false tract with placement into the peritoneum
- GI obstruction or perforation

Interpretation of Results

- Insufflation and auscultation of air over stomach and/or aspiration of intestinal contents
- Contrast radiography to verify position (use water-soluble contrast such as Gastrografin)

BALLOON TAMPONADE OF GASTROESOPHAGEAL VARICES

Indications

Patient with known or suspected portal hypertension or varices with substantial ongoing upper GI bleeding despite optimal medical therapy and for whom endoscopy is unavailable.

Contraindications

Endoscopy readily available

Technique

- Strongly consider endotracheal intubation prior to placement of gastroesophageal balloon tamponade (GEBT) tube in order to prevent aspiration.
- If not intubated, use topical anesthetic to posterior pharynx and nostrils during procedure.
- Elevate head of bed to 45° if possible or place patient in left lateral decubitus position.
- Evacuate stomach with gastric lavage and remove NG tube.
- There are two types of GEBT tubes commonly used in the U.S.:
  - The 3-lumen Sengstaken-Blakemore (SB) tube (gastric balloon, esophageal balloon, and gastric aspiration port) (Figure 19.12).
  - The 4-lumen Minnesota tube (which adds an esophageal aspiration port).
  - For SB tube, secure a standard NG tube to the SB tube using silk suture to create a esophageal aspiration port.
- Collapse all balloons and clamp the balloon ports. Pass tube through mouth/nose into stomach. Apply suction to gastric and esophageal aspiration lumens and confirm position by x-ray.
- Introduce increments of 100 mL of air through the gastric balloon inflation lumen until the recommended total volume (usually 250-300 mL for SB tube, 500 mL for Minnesota tube) fills the gastric balloon. Once the gastric balloon is inflated, pull back the tube until the resistance of the diaphragm is firmly felt and secure the proximal end using a traction device.
- If blood is still detected with gastric or esophageal aspiration, inflate the esophageal balloon to the pressure recommended in the accompanying instructions (generally 30-45 mm Hg).

KEY FACT

Chilling the GEBT tube in an ice water bath while prepping the patient facilitates placement by making the tube temporarily more rigid.

A

Balloon tamponade of gastroesophageal varices may serve as a bridge to upper endoscopy in patients with massive upper GI bleeds. Surgical consultation should also be obtained for possible operative intervention and because of the substantial risk of esophageal perforation.

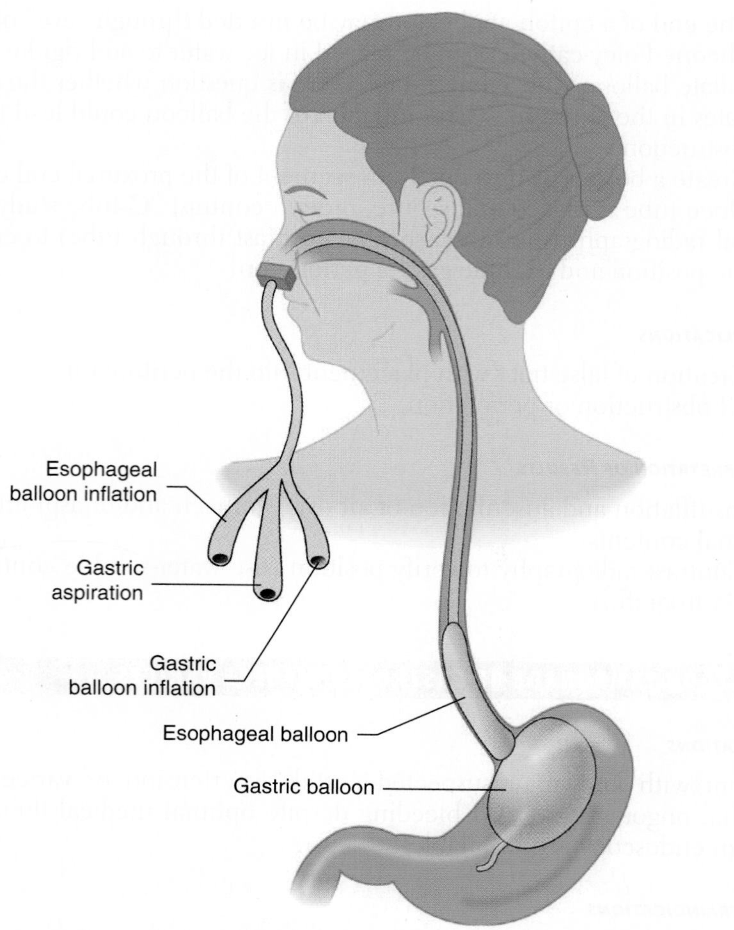

FIGURE 19.12. Placement of Sengstaken-Blakemore tube. (Reproduced, with permission, from Tintinalli JE, Kelen GD, Stapczynski JS. *Tintinalli's Emergency Medicine: A Comprehensive Study Guide*, 8th ed. New York, NY: McGraw-Hill, 2016. Figure 75.1.)

KEY FACT

Monitor the intragastric balloon pressure. If high, the balloon is likely in the esophagus and should be deflated and replaced into stomach.

- After bleeding has been controlled by tamponade, reduce the pressure in the esophageal balloon by 5 mm Hg every 3 hours until an intraesophageal balloon pressure of 25 mm Hg is achieved without ongoing bleeding.

Complications

Ulceration of mucosal surfaces, mucosal ischemia → esophageal necrosis/perforation, aspiration pneumonia, airway obstruction

Interpretation of Results

Pressure should be maintained at the lowest level that will stop bleeding from each of the aspiration suction ports.

EXCISION OF THROMBOSED HEMORRHOIDS

Indications

Patient presenting within 48 hours of onset of pain

Contraindications

Relative: > 48 hours of symptoms, bleeding disorder, serious systemic illness

Technique

- Place patient in prone or lateral decubitus position with buttocks taped apart to aid in visualization.

- Infiltrate local anesthesia over dome of hemorrhoid.
- Using forceps to grasp skin overlying thrombosis, excise an elliptical-shaped piece of skin overlying the clot. Incision should be directed radially from anal orifice. Remove the clot.
- Pack the wound loosely to prevent premature closure of skin edges. Some consider packing wounds optional.
- Advise patient to avoid prolonged standing or straining for the next few days.
- The patient should avoid using toilet paper for several days, instead washing in the shower or bath with mild soap. Frequent sitz-baths are recommended.
- After packing has fallen out (~24 hours), patient may use a soothing cream (eg, Preparation H, Anusol HC, witch hazel) for several days.

Complications

Uncontrolled bleeding, infection, premature closure of skin edges, reaccumulation of clot

Interpretation of Results

Clots should be manually removed with forceps or digital pressure; there may be > 1 clot present.

ANOSCOPY

Indications

Suspicion of internal hemorrhoids, rectal mucosal tears, foreign bodies, anorectal masses

Contraindications

- Absolute: Imperforate anus
- Relative: Patient tolerance of procedure

Technique

- Place patient in prone or lateral decubitus position with knees and hips flexed.
- First perform digital rectal examination to localize sources for pain or masses.
- Apply lubricant to anoscope and gently insert scope into anus with obturator in place.
- Once anoscope is fully inserted, remove obturator and use light source for direct visualization of mucosa.
- Gradually withdraw anoscope while inspecting for pathology.

KEY FACT

To help reduce patient discomfort during and after anoscopy, viscous lidocaine may be used as a lubricant.

Complications

Patient discomfort, local irritation with bleeding

Interpretation of Results

Direct visualization of bleeding or cause of patient's pain during.

Neurologic Procedures

LUMBAR PUNCTURE

Indications

- Evaluation for meningoencephalitis, subarachnoid hemorrhage, inflammatory/demyelinating CNS process, or carcinomatous/metastatic disease
- Diagnosis and therapy for pseudotumor cerebri (idiopathic intracranial hypertension)

Q

A 34-year-old woman presents with 3 days of headaches and intermittent blurry vision. She is neurologically intact and you find papilledema on your retinal examination. Brain computed tomography (CT) is normal. What is your suspected diagnosis? How do you confirm diagnosis?

KEY FACT

Obtain CT scan before lumbar puncture in patients with immune compromise, focal neurologic signs, papilledema, recent seizure, or AMS.

KEY FACT

Seated patients will usually have higher than normal opening pressures that do not reflect the true ICP.

KEY FACT

In newborns, topical EMLA can be used in place of local anesthetic.

A

Idiopathic intracranial hypertension. Perform a lumbar puncture and check opening pressure.

CONTRAINDICATIONS

- Absolute:
  - Infection near the puncture site (eg, cellulitis or epidural abscess)
  - Extra-axial intracranial mass lesion causing midline shift on brain CT
- Relative:
  - **Increased intracranial pressure** due to space occupying lesion
  - Lateralizing signs (eg, hemiparesis) or evidence of uncal herniation (eg, unilateral third nerve palsy with altered mental status)
  - Coagulopathy

TECHNIQUE

- Position patient in lateral decubitus or seated position.
- Provide parenteral anxiolysis or analgesia as needed.
- Use sterile technique and administer local anesthesia.
- Needle placement:
  - L2-L3 to L5-S1 interspaces in adults (cord ends at L2 in adults)
  - L4-L5 or L5-S1 in infants (cord ends at L3 level at birth)
  - The L4 spinous process is at the level of the iliac crests
- Insert the needle at midline, aiming toward the umbilicus and with the bevel facing the flanks. Keep the stylet in place while advancing, and remove stylet to see if the subarachnoid space has been reached.
- If the needle tip hits bone, partially withdraw the needle and redirect. Redirect either caudally or in a grid-like pattern until successful penetration of subarachnoid space.
  - If the patient complains of pain radiating down their side or leg, it indicates impact of needle on a spinal root and the needle should be directed slightly away from that side or leg.
- Once the needle is in proper position, measure opening pressure and collect cerebrospinal fluid (CSF) for analysis. After this is complete, replace stylet and remove needle.

COMPLICATIONS

- Postlumbar puncture headache from CSF leak
- Bleeding with resultant spinal epidural or subdural hematoma
- Brain herniation, infection/abscess, backache
- Late onset of epidermoid tumors of the thecal sac

INTERPRETATION OF RESULTS (TABLE 19.1)

- Opening pressure (OP)
- Normal = **7-20 cm H_2O in adults,** 1-10 cm H_2O in children < 8 years old
  - Low OP = CSF leak, dehydration
  - High OP = pseudotumor, infection, bleeding, tumor, falsely elevated with sitting position/valsalva/crying
- Color
  - Normal = clear
  - Xanthochromia (yellow) = seen in subarachnoid hemorrhage (byproduct of red blood cell [RBC] breakdown)
- Cells
  - Normal WBC = < 5 cells/mm^3 in adults with < 3 PMN/mm^3, < 20 cells/mm^3 in neonates with < 1 PMN/mm^3
  - Elevated WBC = infection, leukemia, vasculitis, traumatic tap. PMN predominance = bacterial infection
  - Normal RBC = < 10 cells/mm^3
  - Elevated RBC = subarachnoid hemorrhage, herpes simplex virus encephalitis, traumatic tap

TABLE 19.1. Interpretation of CSF Results

	Normal	Bacterial Meningitis	Viral Meningitis	SAH
Color	Clear	Purulent	Clear or purulent	Bloody or xanthochromia
Opening pressure, cm H_2O	7-18	> 20 cm H_2O	Normal/high	High
WBC/mm^3	0-5	25-10,000+	10-500	Slightly high
Diff	Lymphocytes	PMNs	Lymphocytes	WBC/RBC same as blood
RBC/mm^3	0-5	Normal	Normal	> 500
Glucose, mg/100 mL	45-80	< 20	Normal/low	Normal
Protein, mg/100 mL	15-50	50-10,000	50-200	60-150

PMN, polymorphonuclear leukocytes; RBC, red blood cell; SAH, subarachnoid hemorrhage; WBC, white blood cell.

- Glucose
  - Normal = 50-80 mg/dL
  - Decreased in bacterial/tuberculous meningitis or central nervous system tumors
- Protein
  - Normal = < 45 mg/dL in adults, < 20 mg/dL in children
  - Increased in bacterial/tuberculous meningitis, presence of blood (subarachnoid hemorrhage or traumatic tap), multiple sclerosis, and Guillain-Barré syndrome
- Miscellaneous
  - India ink or cryptococcal antigen = *Cryptococcus*
  - VDRL/RPR = neurosyphilis
  - Polymerase chain reaction for HSV or cytomegalovirus infections

KEY FACT

In a traumatic tap, elevated WBC can be corrected for by using peripheral blood WBC:RBC ratio, ie, typically 1:1000.

Obstetrical Procedures

PERIMORTEM CESAREAN DELIVERY

Indications

- Cesarean delivery must be considered in any woman who suffers a cardiac arrest **after 24 weeks' gestation** and is unresponsive to brief resuscitation.
  - If age of gestation is not known, estimate based on fundal height (height of fundus from symphysis pubis in centimeters = gestational age).
- C-section performed **within 5 minutes of mother's death** usually results in an excellent neonatal outcome; 5-10 minutes, good; 10-15 minutes, fair; and 15-20 minutes, poor.

KEY FACT

In pregnant women with cardiac arrest and unknown gestational age, if the fundus of the uterus is palpated above the umbilicus, assume that the fetus is viable.

Contraindications

- **Relative**:
  - Performance before the point of fetal viability (~24 weeks)
  - Absence of immediate obstetric/neonatal backup—**the procedure should not be delayed regardless of availability**

Technique

- Maternal CPR should begin the time of maternal cardiac arrest and resuscitative efforts should be continued after delivery of the infant.

- A midline vertical incision is made through the abdominal wall extending from the symphysis pubis to the umbilicus and carried through all abdominal layers to the peritoneal cavity (Figure 19.13A/B). Retract the bladder inferiorly.

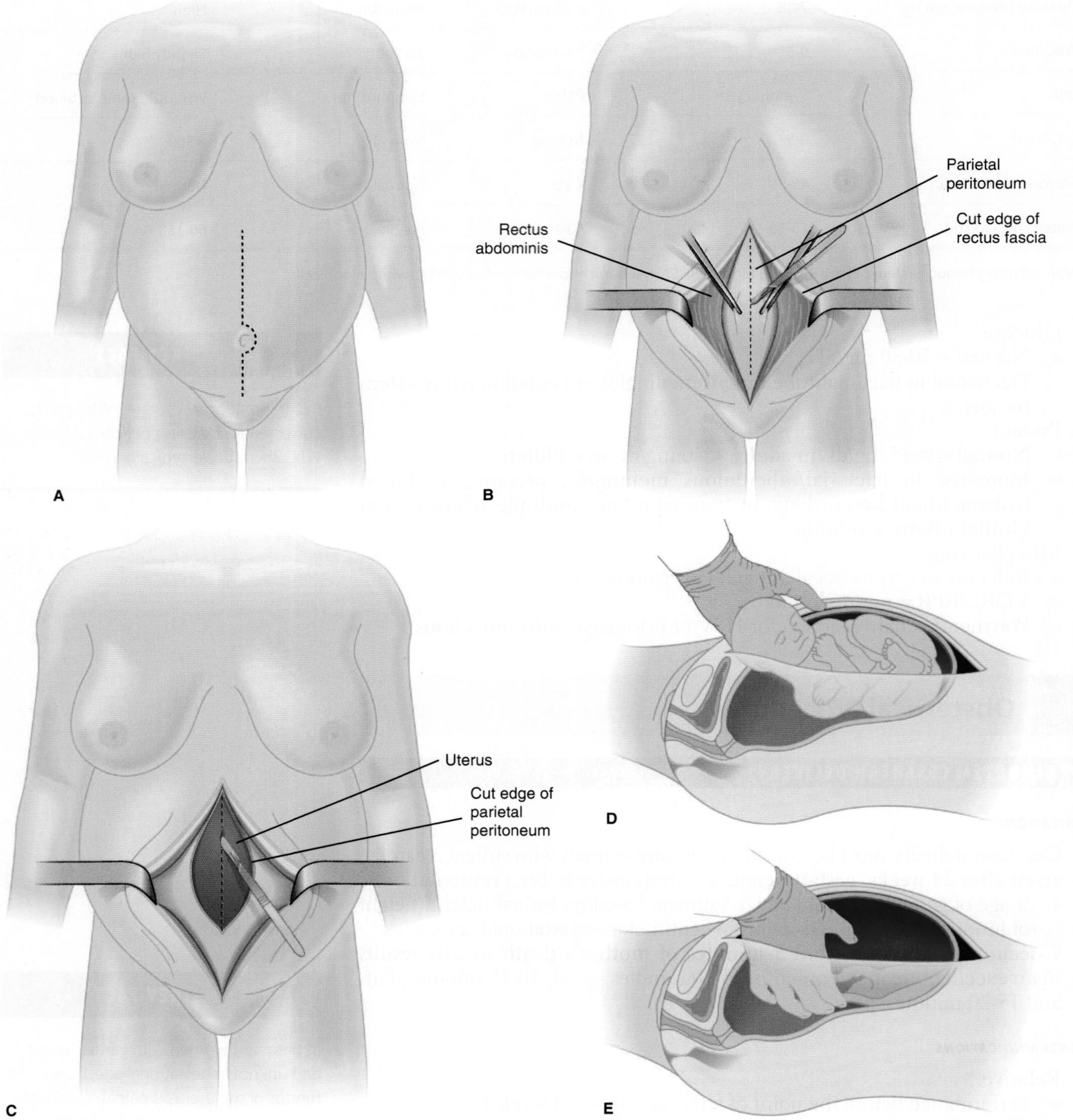

FIGURE 19.13. Delivery of neonate with perimortem cesarean section. (A) Abdominal incision. (B) Extend into fascia and muscles. (C) Vertical uterine incision. (D) Delivery of fetus. (E) Removal of placenta and membranes. (Reproduced, with permission, from Pearlman MD, Tintinalli JE, Dyne PL. *Obstetric & Gynecologic Emergencies: Diagnosis and Management*. New York, NY: McGraw-Hill Education, 2004. Figure 11.4.)

TABLE 19.2. Apgar Scoring System

	0	1	2
Appearance (color)	Blue/pale	Pink body, blue extremities	Completely pink
Pulse	Absent	< 100 bpm	> 100 bpm
Grimace (reflex irritability)	No response	Grimace	Cough or sneeze
Activity (muscle tone)	Limp	Some flexion	Active movement
Respirations	Absent	Slow, irregular	Good, crying

(Reproduced, with permission, from Gomella LG, Haist SA, eds. *Clinician's Pocket Reference: The Scut Monkey*, 11th ed. New York: McGraw-Hill, 2006.)

- A small (~5 cm) vertical incision is made through the lower uterine segment until amniotic fluid is obtained or until the uterine cavity is clearly entered (see Figure 19.13C). Extend this incision with blunt scissors to the uterine fundus.
- The infant is then gently delivered, the mouth and nose suctioned, and the cord clamped and cut. Deliver placenta and membranes (see Figure 19.13D/E). The infant may require active resuscitation measures, including bag-valve mask, intubation, CPR, and/or administration of medications including epinephrine, naloxone, dextrose 10%, intravenous fluid, or bicarbonate depending on the situation.

KEY FACT

There is no evidence that perimortem C-section worsens maternal outcome, and there is evidence suggesting it may improve it.

Complications

- Maternal death or poor neurologic outcome
- Neonatal death or poor neurologic outcome

Interpretation of Results

Traditionally, Apgar scores (Table 19.2) are used in the standard newborn evaluation. Apgar scores are recorded at 1 minute and 5 minutes after delivery. A score of 7-10 is considered normal, while 4-7 might require some resuscitative measures, and a baby with Apgar of 3 and below requires immediate resuscitation.

Anesthesia

ACUTE PAIN MANAGEMENT

Indications

Provide adequate analgesia in the ED for painful conditions and procedures

Contraindications

Allergic reactions/anaphylaxis, renal or liver failure (depending on specific drug clearance), patient respiratory and cardiovascular status (can potentiate respiratory depression and/or hypotension)

KEY FACT

Equipotent doses of IV opiates:
Morphine 10 mg
Hydromorphone 1.5 mg
Fentanyl 100 mcg

KEY FACT

Naloxone is available in IV, intramuscular, subcutaneous, and nebulized preparations. Duration of action is 45 minutes. Titrate 0.2-mg IV doses with smallest dose possible to reverse respiratory depression.

KEY FACT

Am**i**de local anesthetics include: L**i**docaine, bup**i**vacaine, rop**i**vacaine

Ester local anesthetics include: Procaine, benzocaine, tetracaine, novocaine, cocaine.

Technique

- PO: Provides mild-moderate analgesia
  - Acetaminophen: 650-1000 mg (10-15 mg/kg in peds) q 4-6 hours, max 75 mg/kg or 4 g per day
  - Ibuprofen: 400 mg for analgesic dose q 4-6 hours (40 mg/kg/day in divided doses q 6-8 h for peds)
  - Oxycodone: 0.15 mg/kg, duration 3-4 hours
  - Hydrocodone: 5-15 mg, duration 3-4 hours (not available for peds)
- IV: Provides moderate-significant analgesia
  - Morphine: 0.1 mg/kg, duration 3-4 hours
  - Hydromorphone: 0.015 mg/kg, duration 2-4 hours
  - Fentanyl: 1.5 mcg/kg, duration 0.5-1.5 hours
  - Ketorolac: 30 mg (0.5 mg/kg in peds), duration 4-6 hours

Complications

- Nausea and vomiting, pruritus (mast cell-mediated histamine release)
- Sedation and respiratory depression with opioid analgesia: Reversal with naloxone
- Hypotension with IV opioid administration
- Constipation

Interpretation of Results

Appropriate analgesia is achieved when the patient's pain or discomfort is alleviated or satisfactorily decreased.

LOCAL ANESTHESIA

Indications

Used for the majority of minor surgical procedures such as excision of skin lesions, abscess incision and drainage, and wound repair

Contraindications

- Local infiltration distorts the tissues that will be incised or repaired, making it undesirable in areas requiring precise anatomic alignment (eg, lip repairs).
- Epinephrine can theoretically cause ischemia thus should be avoided in digital blocks, penis, tip of nose, or earlobe.

Technique

- **Pain from local anesthesia can be diminished by:**
  - Using a fine needle (27 ga)
  - Slow infiltration
  - Buffering the local anesthetic with bicarbonate (exception is bupivacaine because the combination will crystallize)
  - Warming the local anesthetic to body temperature
  - Injecting into the wound margins (instead of intact epidermis)
- **Lidocaine** (0.5%-2%).
  - Onset: 2-5 minutes, duration: 1-2 hours
  - **Maximum dose = 3-5 mg/kg without epinephrine, 7 mg/kg with epinephrine**
    - 1% solution = 1 g lidocaine/100 mL or 10 mg/mL
    - 2% solution = 2 g lidocaine/100 mL or 20 mg/mL
- Procaine is useful for patients who are allergic to amide anesthetics. Diphenhydramine can also be used.

- Bupivacaine (Marcaine) has a longer duration and may be preferred for prolonged procedures.
  - Onset: 2-5 minutes, duration: 4-6 hours
  - Maximum dose (0.25%) = 1.5 mg/kg without epinephrine, 3 mg/kg with epinephrine
- Anesthetic **plus** epinephrine
  - Prolongs anesthesia duration
  - Provides excellent wound hemostasis
  - Slows systemic absorption of anesthetic
- **Phentolamine** can be used to reverse epinephrine-induced tissue ischemia by providing postsynaptic α-adrenergic blockade).
- Pretreatment with topical anesthetic.
  - Intact skin: EMLA (eutectic mixture of local anesthetics)
  - Mucosal surfaces: Cocaine (excellent vasoconstriction, used in epistaxis), lidocaine (used in nasal procedures, Foley placement), tetracaine (ocular anesthesia), benzocaine spray (oropharyngeal procedures, caution with methemoglobinemia)
  - Open skin: LET (lidocaine, epinephrine, tetracaine)—20-minute onset

Complications

- Allergic reaction
  - True allergic reactions account for only 1%-2% of all adverse reactions.
  - Ester solutions (eg, procaine, tetracaine), which produce the metabolite **para-**aminobenzoic acid (PABA), account for the great majority of these reactions.
  - Amide solutions (eg, lidocaine, bupivacaine) are rarely involved. Allergic reactions are usually caused by the preservative methylparaben, which is structurally similar to PABA.
- **Dose-related CNS toxicity**: Early paresthesias, tinnitus, vertigo, restlessness → slurred speech, muscle fasciculations → seizures
- **Dose-related cardiac toxicity:** Conduction delays, ventricular dysrhythmias, depressed myocardial contractility
- Drugs that are more lipophilic are generally more toxic (eg, bupivacaine).
- Epinephrine can cause headache, hypertension, palpitations, tremors, tachycardia, diaphoresis, and cardiac arrest.

> **KEY FACT**
>
> For CNS/cardiac toxicity, administer 20% IV lipid emulsion 1.5 mL/kg as bolus, may repeat 1-3 times and then start 0.25 mL/kg/min infusion.

Interpretation of Results

Local anesthesia is achieved when the patient no longer feels the tip of the needle in area requiring suturing/procedure. Typically pressure sensation will remain intact.

HEMATOMA BLOCK

Indications

Anesthesia for reduction of fractures, particularly of distal forearm and hand

Contraindications

- Overlying cellulitis
- Grossly contaminated wound

Technique

- Clean skin overlying fracture site with antiseptic solution.
- Anesthetize skin with wheal of 1% lidocaine.
- Insert 18-ga needle into fracture site, aspirating blood to confirm entrance into hematoma.
- Slowly inject 5-15 mL 1% lidocaine, infiltrating fracture cavity, and periosteum.
- Wait 5-10 minutes, then perform reduction.

Complications

- Worsened pain
- Infection

Interpretation of Results

- Adequate anesthesia of affected area

REGIONAL NERVE BLOCKS

Indications

- Anesthetize areas where swelling caused by local infiltration is undesirable, eg, lips, forehead, and midface. They are also useful for providing anesthesia to the hands and feet.
- Control dental pain (Figure 19.14).

Contraindications

Infection overlying site of injection

Technique

See Table 19.3

Complications

- Placement of the needle or injection of anesthetic into the nerve or a foramen can produce pain and neurovascular damage.
- Posterior-superior alveolar nerve block: Puncture of the pterygoid plexus and hematoma formation if the syringe is not aspirated before injection. Also, if the needle is advanced too far posteriorly, a division II block of cranial nerve V will result.

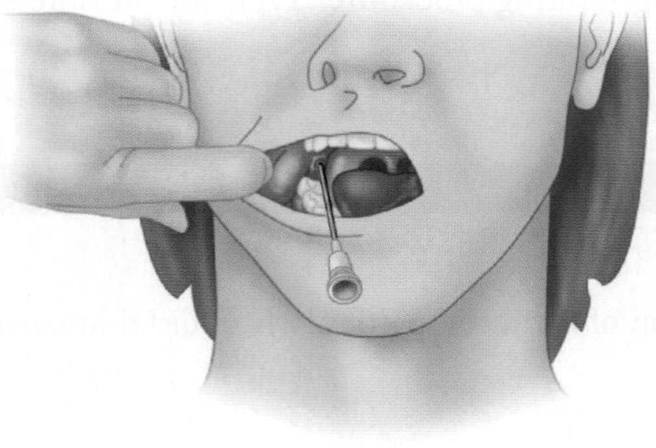

FIGURE 19.14. Insertion site for needle during inferior alveolar nerve block. (Reproduced, with permission, from Butterworth J, Mackey D, Wasnick J. *Morgan & Mikhail's Clinical Anesthesiology*. 5th ed. New York, NY: McGraw-Hill Education, 2013. Fig 47.8F.)

TABLE 19.3. Regional Nerve Blocks

TECHNIQUE	INJECTION LOCATION/ANATOMY	TISSUES AND/OR TEETH AFFECTED	COMMENTS
Supraperiosteal injection (local infiltration)	1-2 mL anesthetic to apex of affected tooth—anesthetic will diffuse across the bone to reach the nerve root of the involved tooth	One selected tooth	Straightforward, highly successful; ideal for relief of a toothache
Mental nerve block	1-2 mL anesthetic to foramen below the second mandibular premolar (just medial to pupil in sagittal plane when looking straight ahead)	Buccal soft tissues from midline to second mandibular premolar; lower lip and chin	Technically simple, highly successful; ideal for repairing lower-lip lacerations
Infraorbital (anterior superior alveolar) nerve block	2-3 mL anesthetic, insert needle in mucosa adjacent to upper second bicuspid and direct toward foramen on inferior border of infraorbital ridge (a depth of approximately 2.5 cm)	Maxillary teeth and buccal soft tissues, midline to premolar, upper lip, lateral aspect of nose, and lower eyelid	Highly safe and successful; ideal for repairing lacerations to upper lip
Posterior superior alveolar nerve block	Distal to the distal buccal root of the upper second molar toward maxillary tuberosity at depth of 2-2.5 cm	Second and third maxillary molars; sometimes also first maxillary molar	Highly effective but carries significant risk of hematoma, so frequent aspiration during injection is crucial
Inferior alveolar nerve block (see Figure 19.14)	1-2 mL anesthetic, in the pterygomandibular triangle, at a point that is 1 cm above the occlusal surface of the molars	All mandibular teeth to midline; anterior 2/3 of tongue and floor of oral cavity; distribution of mental nerve	Failure rate 15%-20% even in experienced hands; extremely useful and, when successful, extremely effective
Ophthalmic (V1) nerve block	1-3 mL anesthetic, aim near the supraorbital notch, above a midline pupil, along the superior orbital rim	The forehead and the scalp back to the lambdoid suture	Suturing or debridement of the forehead, scalp, or delicate upper eyelid
Median nerve block	3-5 mL anesthetic, on the radial border of the palmaris longus tendon just proximal to the proximal wrist crease	The radial aspect of palm and, the anterior thumb, index finger, and middle finger	Suturing or debridement of the hand and/or palm
Ulnar nerve block	5-15 mL anesthetic, on the ulnar aspect of the wrist at the proximal palmar crease, directed horizontally under the *flexor carpi ulnaris*	The ulnar aspect of hand along with ring and little fingers, both dorsal and palmar surfaces	Suturing or debridement of the fourth and fifth digits
Radial nerve block	10 mL anesthetic infiltrated subcutaneously starting on dorsal surface of wrist just proximal and medial to radial styloid and extending laterally in a field block	The radial aspect of dorsal hand along with dorsal thumb	Suturing or debridement of the dorsal hand or thumb
Digital nerve blocks	1-2 mL anesthetic, can be administered in the webspace just distal to the metacarpal-phalangeal joint on both sides of digit.	Any digit	Epinephrine should not be used since it vasoconstricts digital blood supply

- Inferior alveolar block: Injection of anesthetic posteriorly in the region of the parotid gland will anesthetize the facial nerves and cause temporary facial paralysis → inability to close the eyelid. Should this occur, the eye must be protected until the local anesthetic has worn off (~2-3 hours or up to 10-18 hours if Marcaine is used).

INTERPRETATION OF RESULTS

Anesthesia of intended area signifies successful nerve block.

PROCEDURAL SEDATION

INDICATIONS

- Relieve the pain and anxiety associated with diagnostic and therapeutic procedures performed in various settings
- Allow the provider to perform procedures in uncooperative patients
- Facilitate fracture and dislocation reductions by providing muscle relaxation

KEY FACT

Ketamine should not be used in patients with schizophrenia or age < 3 months. Globe rupture is a relative contraindication.

CONTRAINDICATIONS

- Lack of support staff or monitoring equipment
- Comorbidities (ie, cardiac, hemodynamic, or respiratory compromise)
- Patient refusal (providing they are competent)

KEY FACT

"Ketofol," half-dose ketamine (0.5 mg/kg) and half-dose propofol (0.5-1 mg/kg) has been proposed as a procedural sedation agent that is thought to mitigate side-effects from both drugs.

TECHNIQUE

- Assess airway and cardiopulmonary status.
- Have necessary equipment in the room and ready for use: O_2, nonrebreather mask, bag-valve mask, suction, oral airway, intubation materials, including laryngoscope and endotracheal tubes, and cardiac resuscitation equipment and medications.
- Monitoring is essential for procedural sedation: Oxygenation (via pulse oximetry), ventilation (via capnography), and hemodynamic status (including BP and cardiac rhythm) should all be monitored.
- Obtain and document informed consent.
- Identify desired level of sedation (Table 19.4).
- Select appropriate medication and dose accordingly (Table 19.5).
- Discharge criteria: Patients should be alert and oriented (or returned to age-appropriate baseline), vital signs should be stable and patient should be escorted by a reliable adult who will observe them after discharge. Except for lower extremity injuries, patients who walk in should walk out.

KEY FACT

Ketamine provides both amnesia and analgesia.

TABLE 19.4. Continuum of Sedation and Analgesia (Levels of Procedural Sedation)

Level	Patient Response	Ventilatory Response	Cardiovascular Response
Minimal	Anxiolysis	Maintained	Maintained
Moderate (formerly "conscious sedation")	Depression of consciousness Responds purposefully to commands	Maintained	Maintained
Deep	Not easily aroused Responds purposefully to repeated stimuli	May be impaired	Maintained
General anesthesia	Cannot be aroused even by painful stimuli	Impaired	May be impaired
Dissociative sedation	Analgesia/amnesia by ketamine	Maintained	Maintained

TABLE 19.5. Drug Characteristics Used in Procedural Sedation

Drug	Onset Time	Duration	Adverse Effects	Notes
Midazolam Children: 0.05-0.1 mg/kg IV, 0.2 mg/kg intranasal Adults: 0.03-0.1 mg/kg IV	3 min IV	30 min IV	Paradoxical hyperexcitability (children) Apnea Hypotension (rare)	reverse with flumazenil No analgesia
Propofol 0.5-1 mg/kg bolus followed by 0.5 mg/kg every 2-3 min PRN	30-45 s IV	5-10 min IV	Apnea Hypotension	No analgesia
Etomidate 0.1-0.2 mg/kg IV followed by 0.05 mg/kg IV every 3-5 min PRN	30-60 s IV	3-5 min IV	Transient myoclonus Respiratory depression	Can cause myoclonus or laryngospasm No analgesia
Ketamine Children: 1-2 mg/kg IV; 4-5 mg/kg IM Adults: 1 mg/kg IV followed by 0.5-1 mg/kg every 5-15 min PRN	1 min IV 5 min IM	10-20 min IV 15-45 min IM	Laryngospasm Emergence reaction Transiently increased ICP/IOP (not significant) Hypersalivation Hypertension and tachycardia	Consider benzodiazepines to prevent emergence reaction **Analgesia** + amnesia
Fentanyl 1-1.5 μg/kg IV	3 min IV	30 min IV	Apnea Myoclonus Chest wall rigidity (>5 μg/kg dose)	Reverse with naloxone or nalmefene Minimal sedation
Adjunct medications				
Atropine Children: 0.01-0.02 mg/kg IM or IV Min 0.1 mg Max 0.5 mg	30-60 s IV 5 min IM	2 h	Tachycardia Anticholinergic symptoms	Use in children < 5 y old to counteract vagal effects of ketamine
Glycopyrrolate 4 μg/kg IV/IM	1 min IV 15-30 min IM	2-7 h	Tachycardia Anticholinergic symptoms	Use in children < 5 y old to counteract vagal effects of ketamine
Flumazenil Children: 0.01 mg/kg IV Adults: 0.2 mg IV	< 30 s IV	30-60 min IV	Unmasking of seizures Status epilepticus in patients on chronic benzodiazepines	
Naloxone Children < 5 yr: 0.1 mg/kg IV (max 2 mg) Adults: 0.4-2 mg IV/IM; 4 mg IN	1-2 min IV 2-5 min IM 8-13 mg IN	30-120 min	May precipitate withdrawal reactions May make pain difficult to control	May require repeat dosing due to short duration

ICP, intracranial pressure; IM, intramuscular; IOP, intraocular pressure; IV, intravenous; IN, intranasal.

COMPLICATIONS

- Delayed awakening from prolonged drug action; also consider hypoxemia or hypercarbia
- Agitation due to pain or paradoxical/emergence reactions
- Nausea/vomiting from sedative agents, premature administration of oral fluids after procedure
- Tachycardia from pain, hypovolemia, or impaired ventilation
- Bradycardia due to vagal stimulation, opioids, or hypoxia
- Hypoxia from laryngospasm, airway obstruction, or oversedation

Head, Eyes, Ears, Nose and Throat Procedures

INTRAOCULAR PRESSURE MEASUREMENT

INDICATIONS

- Confirm the diagnosis of glaucoma
- Determine the ocular pressure after blunt ocular injury, or in patients with uveitis, chemical burn (after appropriate irrigation), or topical/oral steroid use

CONTRAINDICATIONS

- Suspected open globe injury is the only absolute contraindication.
- Relative:
  - Examination of infected eyes unless a sterilized cover can be used
  - The presence of corneal defects that may be further injured with tonometry

> **KEY FACT**
>
> Manual retraction of the eyelids can create false elevations in IOP. In patients with periorbital swelling, paperclips can be used to retract the eyelids for accurate IOP measurement.

TECHNIQUE

- Topical ocular anesthesia (proparacaine) must be instilled prior to procedure.
- Methods of measuring intraocular pressure (IOP):
  - Applanation tonometry: Measures the pressure required to create a flat surface on the globe as determined by visual inspection of globe; used by the Goldmann tonometer.
  - Electronic indentation tonometry: Used by the Tono-Pen.
  - Impression tonometry: Measures depth of deflection of cornea created by a known weight; Used by the Schiotz tonometer.
  - Pneumotonometry (air puff tonometry): Measures deflection of the cornea in response to a puff of air.

COMPLICATIONS

- Corneal abrasion
- Transmission of infection
- Extrusion of ocular contents with penetrating injuries

INTERPRETATION OF RESULTS

- Normal IOP is 10-20 mm Hg.
- Tono-Pen: After a set number of valid readings (4-10 depending on model), a mean IOP is displayed and a single bar measures standard deviation. If this is > 20%, the measurement is unreliable and should be repeated.

LATERAL CANTHOTOMY AND CANTHOLYSIS

Indications

- Retrobulbar hemorrhage with afferent pupillary defect, ophthalmoplegia, cherry-red macula, optic nerve head pallor, or severe pain in affected eye. Irreversible vision loss can occur if retina ischemia time is > 90-120 minutes.
- Retrobulbar hemorrhage with IOP > 40 mm Hg (normal IOP is 10-21 mm Hg).

Contraindications

Suspected globe rupture (hyphema, irregular pupil, exposed uveal tissue, Siedel sign)

Technique

- Use local anesthesia with epinephrine on the lateral canthus and conscious sedation as needed so that patient doesn't move during procedure.
- Quickly clear debris with normal saline.
- Crush skin at the lateral corner of patient's eye with hemostat for 1-2 minutes to minimize bleeding.
- Use iris or Stevens scissors to make a 1- to 2-cm incision from lateral corner of the eye extending laterally, to gain exposure (Figure 19.15).
- Visualize infero-lateral canthus tendon by pulling down on inferior lid.
- With scissors pointing away from the globe, dissect the inferior crux of lateral canthus tendon and cut it.
- If IOP remains elevated (> 40 mm Hg), cut the superior crux of the lateral canthus tendon.

Complications

Iatrogenic globe injury, bleeding, infection

Interpretation of Results

A successful procedure is marked by improved visual acuity, resolution of a previously detected afferent pupillary defect, and decrease in IOP to below 40 mm Hg.

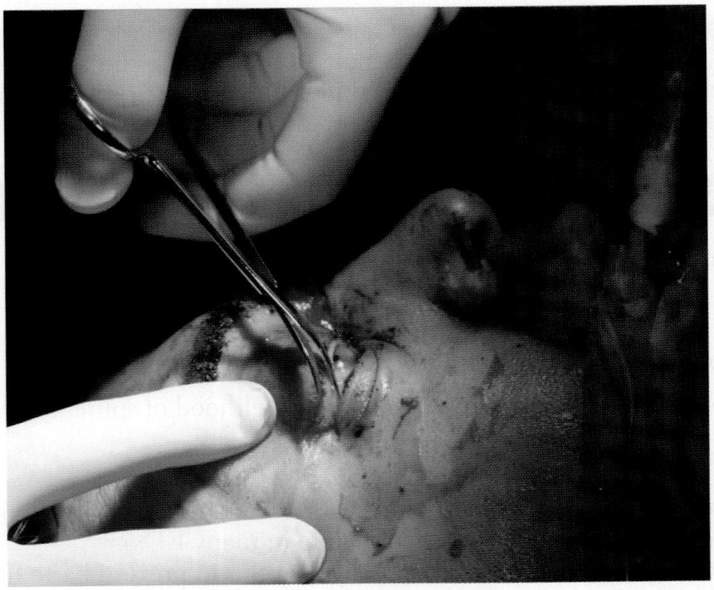

FIGURE 19.15. Lateral canthotomy. (Reproduced, with permission, from Knoop K, Stack L, Storrow A, et al. *The Atlas of Emergency Medicine*. 3rd ed, New York, NY: McGraw-Hill Education, 2009. Figure 1.44. Photographer: Kevin J. Knoop, MD, MS.)

Q

A young woman presents with a laceration of the upper right lip after being bitten by her dog. How would you anesthetize this wound prior to examination, irrigation, and possible closure?

KEY FACT

It is often helpful to protect the globe by inserting the handle of a capped scalpel, the handle of forceps or a cotton applicator between the globe and the lateral canthus.

A

Infraorbital nerve block.

SLIT LAMP EXAMINATION

Indications

- Diagnose corneal abrasions, FBs, and iritis
- Aid in foreign body removal

Contraindications

Patients who cannot sit in an upright position (in absence of a portable slit lamp).

Technique

- A slit lamp has three basic components: A light source, an apparatus to immobilize the head, and a binocular microscope. The adjustment knobs and dials are arranged differently on each slit lamp according to manufacturer.
- Turn the slit lamp on and have the patient positioned so that the forehead is pressed against the head rest and the eyes are in line with the eye mark by adjusting the chin rest.
- Screen the anterior portion of the eye:
  - Set the slit beam to maximum height and minimum width and place light at 45° angle, slowly inspecting all parts of the cornea.
  - Examine and evert eyelids to expose pathology or foreign bodies.
- Examine for iritis or microscopic hyphema:
  - Adjust the beam to 3-4 mm in height and direct the beam to the center of the cornea. Adjust the focus halfway between the cornea and the lens to identify cells floating on the black background of the pupil.
- Fluorescein examination:
  - After applying anesthetic, place fluorescein stain in each eye.
  - Repeat the anterior examination with a blue light and widen the beam. Identify corneal defects.

Complications

Patient discomfort

KEY FACT

In a patient with multiple vertical corneal abrasions, consider the possibility of a retained foreign body within the eyelids.

Interpretation of Results

- Iritis appears as "cell-and-flare": Cells floating in the anterior chamber and small proteins that light up when focused on with the slit lamp beam.
- Corneal abrasions will stain green under fluorescein and the mark will not disappear with blinking of the eyes.

TOOTH STABILIZATION

Indications

Avulsed or luxated teeth

Contraindications

Lack of proper equipment leading to higher likelihood of splint failure

Technique

- Prepare periodontal paste by mixing catalyst and base together (brands such as Coe-Pak are commonly available in many EDs).
- Lubricate gloves with lubricating jelly or water to prevent paste from sticking. Dry gingiva and enamel completely before application.
- Press the paste around the groove of injured tooth and adjacent teeth. Splinting works best with application on the facial and buccal surface,

however, paste to only the (facial surface) is acceptable. Allow splinting material to completely harden.

COMPLICATIONS

Aspiration of tooth and splinting material from splint failure

INTERPRETATION OF RESULTS

In the emergency setting, teeth do not need to be perfectly aligned. Adequate splinting and prompt follow-up should be the priority.

EPISTAXIS CONTROL

INDICATIONS

- Management of anterior epistaxis: Typically from Kiesselbach's plexus
- Temporization of posterior epistaxis: Typically from the sphenopalatine artery

CONTRAINDICATIONS

Massive facial trauma with possibility of basilar skull fracture

TECHNIQUE

- Place patient in sitting position and have patient blow nose to evacuate all clotted blood.
- Apply topical vasoconstrictor (eg, lidocaine with epinephrine, phenylephrine, oxymetazoline, cocaine).
- Have patient hold direct pressure by pinching nasal alae against septum for 10-15 minutes.
- Anterior epistaxis:
  - If bleeding is ongoing and a source is identified, attempt cautery with silver nitrate.
  - If this is unsuccessful, proceed to anterior packing. Multiple methods and products exist, including gauze, nasal tampon (eg, Merocel), and the Rapid Rhino kit. Gauze has largely been replaced by packing products.
- Posterior epistaxis:
  - Suspect when no anterior source is visualized and there is profuse bleeding in the oropharynx.
  - Balloon packing: Use either a 12-Fr Foley catheter or dual-balloon tamponading system. Anesthetize the naris and advance tube parallel to floor to the posterior part of the nasopharynx. Partially inflate Foley or posterior balloon and slowly pull it into place behind the middle turbinate. Once in the correct place, fully inflate the balloon. With a Foley, use bilateral anterior packing to avoid deviation of the septum. With the dual-balloon, gently inflate the anterior portion.
  - Most, if not all, patients should be admitted for cardiac monitoring and observation. Consider ENT consult if unsuccessful with posterior packing.

COMPLICATIONS

- Anterior packing: Sinusitis, nasal mucosal pressure and necrosis, aspiration of packing, ethmoid plate fracture.
- Posterior packing: Tissue necrosis, infection, dysphagia, aspiration of packing materials. Rare reports of hypoxia, hypercapnia and bradycardia.

INTERPRETATION OF RESULTS

Achieving control of epistaxis

Q

You are performing a FAST examination on a patient in a car accident with abdominal pain but the image appears white. What do you do?

KEY FACT

Keep anterior packing in for 2-5 days. Oral antibiotics may be given; however, no data exists to show efficacy of antibiotics to prevent infectious complications.

A

Decrease the gain. Consider also the possibility of subcutaneous air from a pneumothorax.

DRAINAGE OF PERITONSILLAR ABSCESS

Contraindications

Severe trismus, coagulopathy, lack of patient cooperation

Technique

- Provide local anesthesia via spray (eg, Cetacaine) as well as parenteral analgesia.
- The carotid artery is located posterior and lateral to the tonsil.
- Identify landmarks (including carotid artery) and abscess cavity via endocavitary ultrasound probe if available.
- Needle aspiration is recommended over scalpel I&D. Use a long 18- to 20-ga needle and 10-mL syringe. The end of the plastic needle cover can be cut 1 cm to act as a guard to prevent going too deep.
- Aspirate over the superior pole first and advance to the middle and then inferior pole of the abscess if unsuccessful at each location.
- Do not direct needle laterally to avoid carotid artery injury.

Complications

- 10% failure rate → need for subsequent repeat drainage
- Hemorrhage from mistaken pseudoaneurysm of carotid artery

Interpretation of Results

- Improvement of swelling and pain
- Infections are often polymicrobial, provide antibiotics (cephalexin or clindamycin) to all patients afterward.

Ultrasound

Indications

Numerous diagnostic and therapeutic indications.

Contraindications

Lack of sonographic training and experience

Technique

- Lower-frequency probes (3-7 MHz) are used for viewing deeper structures but produce lower resolution images.
- Higher-frequency probes (7-20 MHz) are used for viewing superficial structures and provide higher resolution images.
- The "gain" controls the amplification of the returning signal. High gain will cause the image to appear white, low gain will produce dark images.
- The depth gain control is a set of slide bars that allow you to set individual gains (brightness) at different depths.
- The "magnify" function causes the field to be magnified with the skin surface remaining in the image.
- The "zoom" function causes the boxed area of interest to be magnified. Other portions of the image are cut.

KEY FACT

Use a low frequency probe to see deep structures. For example, a 3.5-MHz probe is appropriate for a FAST examination.

Complications

Ultrasound is generally considered safe because it does not produce cancer-causing ionizing radiation. However, prolonged ultrasound causes increased inflammatory response and heats soft tissue.

Interpretation of Results

- Catheters, wires, and needles appear as brightly reflective structures within fluid-filled anechoic spaces.
- Arteries and veins appear as anechoic circular structures when viewed in the transverse plane. Veins are easily compressed, arteries are less easily compressed, and veins filled with clot are noncompressible. Color flow option may also be used to delineate if a structure is a blood vessel.

Orthopedic Procedures

EXTENSOR TENDON LACERATION REPAIR

Management of upper extremity extensor tendon injuries is determined by anatomic zones of injury.

Indications

- Most common indication is an isolated extensor tendon laceration in **zone 6** (dorsum of hand from wrist to metacarpophalangeal joint).
- Zones 3 (proximal interphalangeal joint) and 4 (proximal phalanx) lacerations require consultation with a hand surgeon for repair in the ED.
- Most tendon lacerations can be repaired up to 10 days after initial injury.

Contraindications

- Absolute:
  - Lacerations involving joints, tissue loss, gross contamination, or flexor tendons.
  - **Zone 5** (over metacarpophalangeal joint) should be presumed to be from a human bite and repaired by a hand surgeon after 7-10 days of antibiotics.
  - **Zones 7 and 8** (dorsal wrist and forearm) injuries are not repaired in the ED due to risk of adhesions and possible retraction of tendons past retinaculum, making repair more difficult.

Technique

- Assess neurovascular status of injured hand and fingers. After sensory examination using 2 point discrimination use, regional or digital block to reduce pain from swollen/injured joints to fully assess motor strength.
- Obtain x-ray to evaluate for associated fractures/dislocations and foreign bodies.
- Visualize location of tendon injury and locate both ends to be repaired.
- Laceration of extensor tendon at zones 1 (distal interphalangeal joint) or 2 (middle phalanx) should be repaired via sutures that simultaneously approximate both the skin and tendon.
- Larger tendons may allow sutures to pass through the core of the tendon (eg, horizontal mattress or figure-of-eight) but smaller tendons require a modified Kessler or Bunnell core suture technique with 4-0 **nonabsorbable** suture.
- The affected joint should be splinted after repair.

Complications

- Infection
- Tendon rupture
- Restriction of PIP and MCP joint flexion due to tendon shortening or adhesions

Interpretation of Results

Return of tendon function demonstrates adequate repair. However, all patients will need reevaluation and most require assistance with improving range of motion.

KEY FACT

Extensor tendon zones of injury for the hand and wrist:

Zone 1: Distal interphalangeal joint
Zone 2: Middle phalanx
Zone 3: Proximal interphalangeal joint
Zone 4: Proximal phalanx
Zone 5: Metacarpophalangeal joint
Zone 6: Dorsum of hand
Zone 7: Wrist
Zone 8: Proximal forearm

Q

An 8-year-old boy falls backward off a swing. He is diagnosed with a supracondylar fracture, splinted, and sent home with next-day orthopedic follow-up. The child returns to the ED the same evening complaining of arm pain. What limb-threatening diagnosis must be considered?

ARTHROCENTESIS

Indications

- Evaluate a "red, hot joint" to determine the etiology of joint effusion
- Determine if a laceration communicates with the joint space
- Relieve pain from hemarthrosis by removing blood from joint space

Contraindications

- Absolute: Infection in the tissues overlying the puncture site
- Relative: Known bacteremia may lead to hematogenous spread of bacteria into the joint.

Technique

- Always use sterile technique to prevent infection.
- Apply local anesthesia from the skin down to the area of the joint capsule.
- Ultrasonography may be used to assess for the presence and location of synovial fluid.
- **Elbow:** The elbow is flexed to 90° with forearm pronated and palm flat on a table. A 22-ga needle is inserted in depression in center of triangle formed by radial head, lateral epicondyle and olecranon and directed medially.
- **Shoulder:** The patient should sit upright with arm at side and hand in lap. A 20-ga needle is inserted at a point inferior and lateral to the coracoid process and directed posteriorly toward the glenoid rim.
- **Knee:** The knee can either be fully extended or flexed to 15°-20° by placing a towel under the knee to open up the joint space. An 18-ga needle is inserted at the midpoint or superior portion of the patella and directed between the posterior surface of the patella and the intercondylar femoral notch.
- **Ankle:** The patient is positioned supine with the foot plantar flexed. A 20- to 22-ga needle is inserted at a point just medial to the anterior tibial tendon and directed inward at the anterior edge of the medial malleolus. The needle must be inserted 2-4 cm to penetrate the joint space.
- Order cell count with differential, crystal analysis, Gram stain, bacterial culture, and sensitivity analysis. Consider rheumatoid factor analysis, fungal and acid-fast stains, Lyme titer, fungal and TB culture, and complement analysis.

Complications

Infection, bleeding, allergic reaction to local anesthesia

Interpretation of Results

	Normal	Noninflammatory	Inflammatory	Septic
Clarity	Transparent	Transparent	Cloudy	Cloudy
WBC/mm^3	< 200	< 2000	2000-50,000	> 50,000
PMNs (%)	< 25	< 25	> 50	> 75
Crystals	None	None	Multiple or none	None
Associated conditions		Osteoarthritis, trauma, rheumatic fever	Gout, pseudogout, rheumatoid arthritis, Lyme disease, SLE	Nongonococcal or gonococcal septic arthritis

KEY FACT

If you suspect septic arthritis, perform an arthrocentesis. No other test allows you to exclude the diagnosis with confidence.

KEY FACT

Pseudogout is caused by calcium pyrophosphate crystals that are positively birefringent.

KEY FACT

Gonococcal arthritis can have neutrophil predominant cell counts at less than 50,000 WBC/mm^3 and diagnosis requires plating the synovial fluid on standard chocolate agar NOT Thayer Martin media.

A

Compartment syndrome.

- A typical presentation of septic joint is suggested by synovial fluid WBC > 50,000/mm³ with high percentage of neutrophils.
- Synovial fluid WBC > 50,000/mm³ may also be seen with gout. The presence of both intracellular and extracellular crystals in the absence of bacteria on Gram stain and culture confirms the diagnosis.
  - Gout = monosodium urate crystals, negatively birefringent
  - Pseudogout = calcium pyrophosphate crystals, positively birefringent
- Presence of fat globules in joint fluid indicates presence of a fracture extending into the joint.

KEY FACT

Septic arthritis can occur in patients with gout.

COMPARTMENT PRESSURE MEASUREMENT

Indications

- Suspected compartment syndrome based on: Tight muscle compartment in patients with extremity trauma or bleeding, pain out of proportion to exam, pain on passive muscle stretch, or otherwise unexplained limb ischemia.
- Limb may be salvageable for up to 10-12 hours, but with very high pressures, the time period may be as little as 4 hours.

KEY FACT

The most common cause and location of compartment syndrome is in the lower leg following mid-shaft tibial fractures. It is wise to observe all mid-shaft tibial fractures for compartment syndrome.

Contraindications

Infection overlying site of needle insertion, coagulopathy

Technique

- Use sterile technique and local anesthesia.
- The compartment to be measured should be at the same level as the heart.
- For the **lower extremity**, needle placement is at the junction of the proximal and middle thirds of the lower leg, perpendicular to the skin (unless noted) with the following needle entry points (Figure 19.16):
  - Anterior compartment: 1 cm **lateral** to the anterior border of the tibia to a depth of 1-3 cm
  - Deep posterior compartment: Just posterior to the medial border of the tibia to a depth of 2-4 cm.

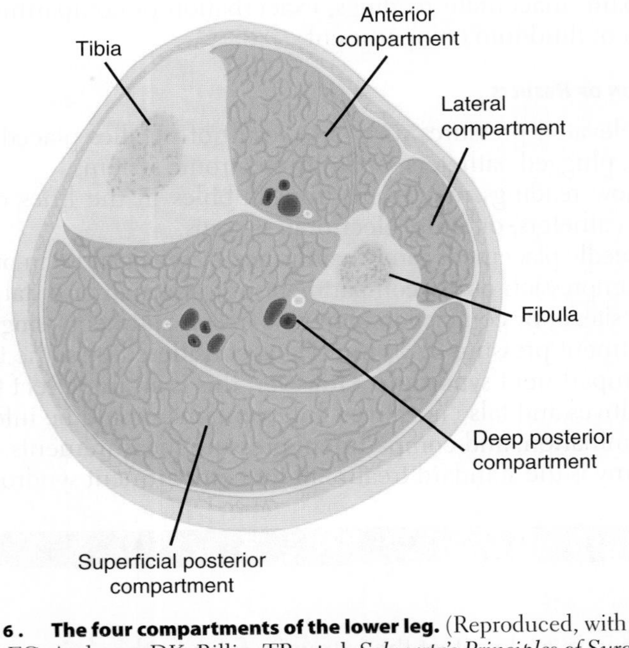

FIGURE 19.16. The four compartments of the lower leg. (Reproduced, with permission, from Brunicardi FC, Andersen DK, Billiar TR, et al. *Schwartz's Principles of Surgery*. 10th ed. New York, NY: McGraw-Hill Education, 2010. Figure 23.62.)

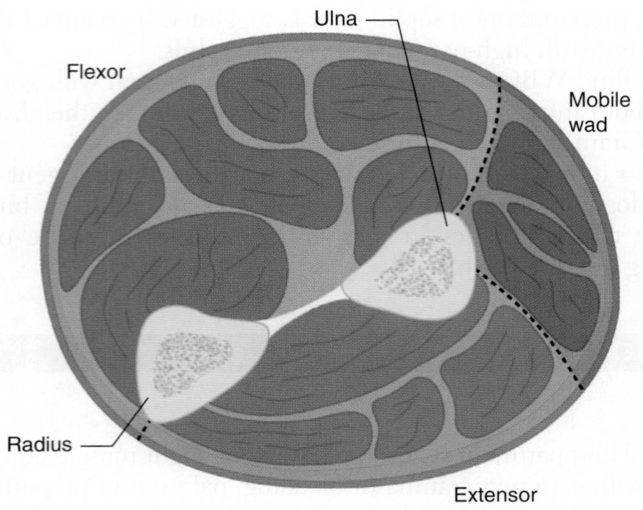

FIGURE 19.17. Forearm compartments. (Reproduced, with permission, from Tintinalli JE, Kelen GD, Stapczynski JS. *Tintinalli's Emergency Medicine: A Comprehensive Study Guide*, 8th ed. New York, NY: McGraw-Hill, 2016.)

  - Lateral compartment: Just anterior to the posterior border of the fibula to a depth of 1-1.5 cm. Direct needle toward the fibula.
  - Superficial posterior compartment: 3-5 cm on either side of a vertical line drawn down the middle of the calf to a depth of 2-4 cm.
- For the **forearm** the needle insertion site is at the junction of the proximal and middle thirds of the forearm, perpendicular to the skin, with the following needle entry points (Figure 19.17):
  - Volar compartment: Just medial to the **palmaris longus** to a depth of 1-2 cm
  - Dorsal compartment: 1-2 cm lateral to the posterior aspect of the ulna to a depth of 1-2 cm
- Pressures can be measured either with an arterial line pressure measurement system or with a Stryker intracompartmental pressure monitor system.

Complications

Infection, pain, inaccurate readings, exacerbation of compartment syndrome by injection of fluid into compartment

Interpretation of Results

- Falsely elevated pressures may be a result of needles placed into tendons or fascia, plugged catheters, or faulty electronic systems.
- Falsely low readings may result from bubbles in the lines or transducer, plugged catheters, or faulty electronic systems.
- Proper needle placement can be confirmed by seeing a rise in pressure during digital compression of the compartment just proximal or distal to the needle insertion site, or by contraction of muscle in compartment being measured.
- Compartment pressure of 30 mm Hg is considered by some to be diagnostic of compartment syndrome. However, this is an imperfect test with both false positives and false negatives. Interventions should be informed by history, examination, and compartment pressure measurements.
- Fasciotomy is the standard treatment for compartment syndrome.

SPLINTING

Indications

- Decrease pain and protect the extremity from further injury
- Facilitate the healing process in certain types of injury

Contraindications

Patient tolerance and cooperation

Technique

- Equipment required: Padding and/or stockinette, splinting material (plaster of Paris or prefabricated splint rolls), elastic bandage or outer wrapping, water, tape.
- Use hematoma block, IV analgesia, or conscious sedation to provide adequate patient comfort.
- Measure appropriate length of splint on contralateral extremity. Ensure there are enough layers of splinting material to provide adequate immobilization. Prepare affected extremity by applying stockinette or padding.
- Soak splinting material in cool water and wring out excess water. Place splint on affected extremity and mold splint to desired position, making sure to avoid any bumps or pressure points. Use the palms of the hands for molding.
- Wrap splint in bandage or elastic material and keep the extremity immobilized until the splint has completely hardened. Ensure that the distal portion of the extremity has good circulation and all exposed skin is adequately protected by padding.
- See Tables 19.6 and 19.7 for types of splints and indications.

Complications

- **Overheated splinting material** leading to burns
- **Compartment syndrome** resulting in ischemic injury and contracture
- Also pressure sores, skin infection, or dermatitis

Interpretation of Results

- Confirm proper reduction and splinting by postprocedure radiographs.
- Ensure extremity has intact neurovascular function postsplinting.

> **KEY FACT**
>
> Layers of plaster required:
>
> 8-10 layers for upper extremity splints
>
> 10-15 layers for lower extremity splints

> **KEY FACT**
>
> Prefabricated splint rolls will typically require less water and have faster drying times than plaster of Paris.

SPINE IMMOBILIZATION

Indications

Traumatic injuries with a concerning mechanism, tenderness, focal neurologic deficit, unreliable examination/AMS, or distracting injury

Contraindications

Harm to the patient, logistically impossible

Technique

- Keep patient flat on a bed or solid surface.
- Maintain in-line stabilization while placing cervical collar.
- Perform logroll maneuver for any transport between bed locations or off a prehospital stretcher or backboard. Ensure there is a dedicated provider for the head/neck region during any patient positioning.

Complications

Improper size or position of collar → movement and injury, risk of aspiration with emesis

Interpretation of Results

- Clearance of the spine can be performed after the indications above have been addressed/resolved.
- Radiographs and/or clinical criteria can be used to aid in cervical spine clearance.

TABLE 19.6. Upper Extremity Splints

Type of Splint	Indications/Uses	Application	Comments
Posterior long arm	Elbow or proximal forearm injuries	Extend splint from proximal part of arm along the ulnar aspect of the forearm to the MCP joint. Keep elbow flexed at 90°.	Does not fully limit supination and pronation—unstable fractures may require a more advanced splint.
Volar splint	Soft tissue hand/wrist injuries, triquetral fractures, lunate/perilunate dislocations, second to fifth metacarpal head fractures	From the metacarpal heads over the volar surface, extending to proximal forearm	Can add dorsal splint for increased stabilization. Does not fully limit supination and pronation.
Sugar tong	Distal radius or ulna fractures	From the metacarpal heads on the dorsal surface of the hand, wrapping around the elbow and extending to the palmar MCP joints.	Compared to volar splint, eliminates pronation and supination as well as elbow movement.
Double sugar-tong splint	Elbow or proximal forearm injuries	Construct 2 splints: (1) From the metacarpal heads on the dorsal surface of the hand, wrapping around the elbow and extending to the palmar MCP joints. (2) Proximal arm, wrapping around the elbow.	Fully limits supination and pronation. Keeps elbow flexed at 90°.
Thumb spica	Scaphoid, lunate, first metacarpal and thumb fractures	**Positioning:** Forearm: Neutral Wrist: 25° extension Thumb: Wineglass position Extend splint from thumb IP joint to mid-forearm. Wrap splint circumferentially around thumb and along radial side of forearm.	Make a small incision in the splint over the first MCP joint to aid in molding around the thumb. (See Figure 19.18)
Ulnar gutter	Fractures/soft tissue injuries of fourth and fifth digits and metacarpals	**Positioning:** Forearm: Neutral, wrist: 10-20° extension MCP: 50° flexion PIP/DIP: 10-15° flexion Extend splint from beyond DIP to mid-forearm	When splinting a Boxer's fracture, immobilize MCP to 90° flexion. Add additional padding between fourth and fifth digits.
Radial gutter	Fractures/soft tissue injuries of second and third digits and metacarpals	**Positioning:** Forearm: Neutral, wrist: 10°-20° extension MCP: 50° flexion PIP/DIP: 5°-10° flexion Extend splint from beyond DIP to mid-forearm.	When splinting a metacarpal neck fracture, immobilize MCP to 90° flexion and fingers extended.

DIP, distal interphalangeal; IP, interphalangeal; MCP, metacarpophalangeal; PIP, proximal interphalangeal.

TABLE 19.7. Lower Extremity Splints

Type of Splint	Indications/Uses	Application	Comments
Knee immobilizer	Mild to moderate ligamentous and soft tissue knee injuries	Choose appropriate size and place splint under affected knee. Secure straps.	Advantage of being removable, able to place over clothes.
Posterior knee splint	Ligamentous and soft tissue knee injuries, treatment of angulated knee fractures, temporary immobilization before surgery	Extend splint from below the buttocks crease to mid-leg. Alternative: Medial and lateral slabs across knee	Can also be used in patients that are too large to fit into knee immobilizer.
Posterior ankle splint	Severe ankle sprains, distal fibula/tibia fractures, reduced ankle dislocations	Extend splint from plantar surface of great toe to level of fibular head. Keep ankle flexed at 90°.	A U-splint (similar to sugar tong) can be used along the medial and lateral surfaces to increase immobilization in unstable fractures or dislocations.
Walking boot	Moderate to severe soft tissue ankle injuries, nondisplaced lateral malleolar fractures	Choose appropriate size. Remind patients of non- and partial-weight bearing as indicated by injury.	Allows easy transition to full weight bearing. Ensure proper specialist follow-up.
Hard shoe	Reduces pain in weight-bearing fractures and soft-tissue injuries of the foot	Buddy tape the toes to aid in immobilization prior to hard shoe application.	Removable. Can aid in ambulation with painful toe fractures.

Soft Tissue Procedures

ESCHAROTOMY

Indications

- Clinical evidence of elevated compartment pressures indicative of compartment syndrome in burned extremities. This procedure is typically performed in circumferential burns.
- Circumferential burns of the torso or neck resulting in impaired ventilation or tracheal obstruction.

Contraindications

There are no absolute contraindications to emergent escharotomy.

Technique

- Full thickness burns are insensate. Deep partial thickness burns and crush injuries will require analgesia and/or sedation.
- Extend incision through the entire thickness of skin and expose fat and subcutaneous tissue. Use a scalpel or electrocautery.
- **Limbs:** Incise over the medial and lateral aspects of the affected area. Extend incision 1 cm proximal to the burn and 1 cm distal to the area of injury. Take care to avoid vasculature and vital nerves (Figure 19.19).
- **Chest:** Patients should be intubated and ventilated. Incise from the clavicle to the costal margin on the anterior axillary line bilaterally. This may be joined by transverse incisions over the subcostal margin (Figure 19.20).

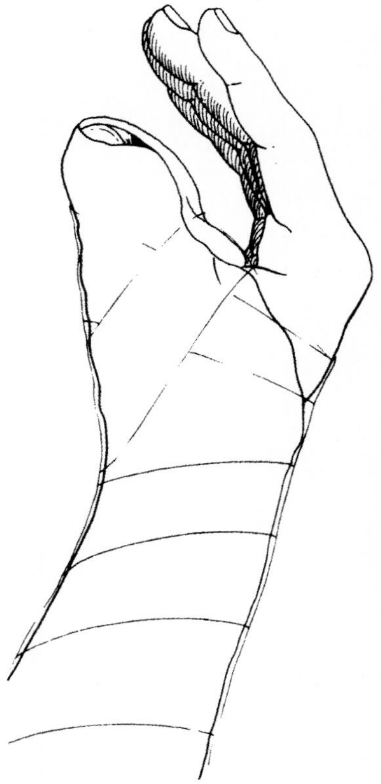

FIGURE 19.18. Thumb spica splint. (Figure 28.8 Current Dx and Treatment, EM) (Reproduced, with permission, from Stone C, Humphries R. *Current Diagnosis & Treatment, Emergency Medicine*. 7th ed. New York, NY: McGraw-Hill, 2011.)

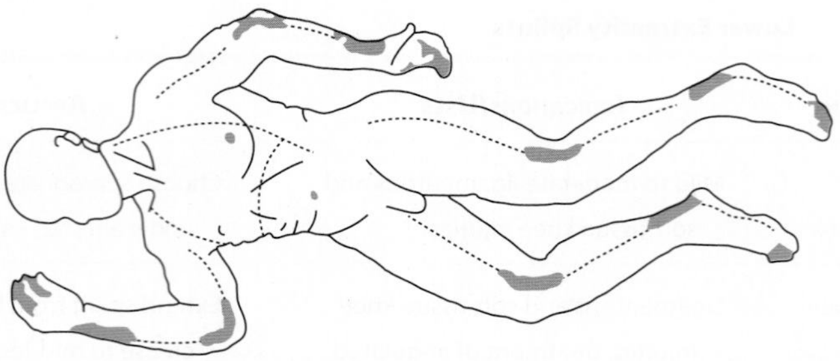

FIGURE 19.19. Escharotomy incision sites. (Reproduced with permission from *Emergency War Surgery*, 3rd rev. The Department of Defense United States of America, 2004.)

- **Neck:** Incise laterally and posteriorly to avoid jugular veins and carotid arteries.
- **Penis:** Incise laterally to avoid dorsal vein.

Complications

- Bleeding, infection, damage to underlying structures
- Inadequate decompression can lead to the effects of compartment syndrome.

Interpretation of Results

Improved distal perfusion, softening of compartment, return of sensation and improved Doppler flow signal strength are all indications of successful compartment pressure release.

ABSCESS INCISION AND DRAINAGE

Indications

Definitive treatment of a soft tissue abscess (antibiotics alone are ineffective)

Contraindications

Incision prior to localization of pus (size, proximity to tendon, nerve, vascular structures)

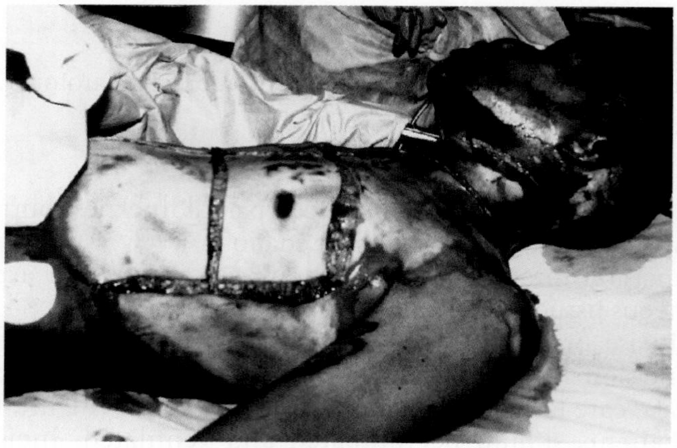

FIGURE 19.20. Chest escharotomy. (Reproduced, with permission, from Tintinalli JE, Kelen GD, Stapczynski JS. *Tintinalli's Emergency Medicine: A Comprehensive Study Guide*, 8th ed. New York, NY: McGraw-Hill, 2016. Figure 216.9.)

TECHNIQUE

- Ultrasound may be used to guide drainage.
- Regional blocks are preferred to local anesthesia as local anesthetic agents function poorly in the low pH of infected tissue and local injection is painful. Parenteral analgesia and/or conscious sedation may be appropriate.
- Patients at risk for endocarditis should receive IV antibiotics prior to I&D.
- Incise abscess along total length of the cavity for noncosmetic areas. For cosmetic areas, a stab incision or simple aspiration may be attempted.
- Probe abscess to break open loculations with a hemostat or hemostat wrapped in gauze.
- Gently pack cavity with gauze.
- Prescribe packing change periodically and follow up in 1-3 days.
- The use of antibiotics following I&D is a clinical decision that depends on host factors (immunocompromised status, diabetes) and wound characteristics (associated cellulitis).

COMPLICATIONS

- Bleeding
- Extension of infection
- Recurrence

INTERPRETATION OF RESULTS

- Drainage of pus indicates correct localization but follow-up must be provided to ensure progression of adequate drainage.
- Principles of Wound Management and Closure.

INDICATIONS

- Restore function of injured tissue
- Achieve optimal cosmetic appearance
- Reduce risk of infection

CONTRAINDICATIONS

Relative: Increased risk for wound infection

TECHNIQUE

- Perform complete history and physical examination of affected area:
  - Assess host risk factors for infection.
  - Achieve bloodless field and adequate anesthesia.
  - Perform distal neurovascular evaluation.
  - Examine active and passive range of motion.
  - Extend wound as needed for exploration.
- Evaluate presence of foreign body (ultrasound, radiographs, CT scan).
- Debride wound of foreign material and devitalized tissue.
- Irrigate with water/saline under high pressure.
- Determine type of closure to be used: Primary, delayed primary, secondary intention.

COMPLICATIONS

- Missed foreign body, neurovascular, tendon injury
- Wound infection
- Poor cosmesis

INTERPRETATION OF RESULTS

- Approximation of tissue
- Acceptable healing and scar formation

KEY FACT

In draining abscesses of IV drug users, use caution on avoid FBs (needles). Radiographs can be ordered to aid in localization of needle fragments.

KEY FACT

A wound should be assessed for infectious risk. A clean linear laceration on face may be closed up to 24 hours after injury, while a contaminated crush injury to the leg should never be closed primarily.

Risk factors for wound infection

- Injury > 8-12 hours old
- Crush mechanism
- High risk location: leg/thigh > arms > feet > chest > back > face > scalp
- Deep wound
- Elderly
- Significant peripheral vascular disease
- Immunocompromised
- High velocity impact
- Contamination (eg, saliva, feces, soil)

KEY FACT

High pressure irrigation is the most effective means of infection control. You can achieve the recommended force of 7psi by attaching an 18-ga needle to a 30-mL syringe.

KEY FACT

Delayed primary closure technique:

- Debride and irrigate
- Pack wound to prevent closure
- Splint and dress if on an extremity
- Wound check 24 hours
- Close 96-120 hours after injury

LACERATION REPAIR

Indications

Lacerations or wounds with separation of skin, subcutaneous tissue, and/or fascia

Contraindications

- Relative:
  - Risk for infection based on mechanism of injury and contamination
  - Cooperation of patient

Technique

- Anesthetize the wound with local anesthetic. In certain cases, nerve blocks may be more suitable (see sections on local anesthesia and regional blocks). In extremities perform a full neurovascular examination prior to anesthesia.
- Explore the wound for FBs and injuries to deep structures, including joints, tendon and muscle belly, nerves, or blood vessels.
- Determine mechanism for closure based on site, size, shape and depth of laceration (Table 19.8).
- Suture material characteristics include:
- **Absorbable (Vicryl, PDS, catgut) vs nonabsorbable (silk, nylon, polypropylene) material.**
  - Absorbable material will lose tensile strength within 60 days (range 5-60 days)
  - Silk has the lowest tensile strength of the nonabsorbable sutures
  - Chromic catgut—used for lacerations in oral mucosa
  - Fast absorbing catgut—used for facial lacerations when follow-up/removal is concern
  - Vicryl, PDS—used for subcutaneous sutures
- **Monofilament vs multifilament** (eg, braided) material. Multifilament material is easier to tie but has a **higher infection rate**.
- **Tensile strength** is graded by number of zeros (0 to 6-0 for ED use) with more zeros = small size and lower tensile strength.

Complications

- Too loose → poor wound closure, too tight → local ischemia
- Infection, retained foreign body, missed neurovascular, muscle/tendon, or joint injury

Interpretation of Results

- Successful approximation of wound edges
- Local hemostasis

NAIL TREPHINATION

Indications

Subungual hematoma, usually >50% of the nail bed.

Contraindications

- Relative:
  - Greater than 24-36 hours after injury, as blood has coagulated and will be more difficult to remove
  - Artificial nails (if hot cautery is used)

TABLE 19.8. Laceration Repair

Type of Repair	Indications/Uses	Technique	Comments
Tissue glue	Superficial wounds with minimal edge separation and tension	Place manual pressure to keep the wound edges together and apply glue 5-10 mm past each edge of the wound. Hold for 1 min while glue dries.	Caution with wounds in close proximity to the eye to prevent seepage of glue onto the eyelid. There is increased risk of dehiscence with glue compared to sutures.
Staples	Linear lacerations with straight, sharp edges. Avoid in deep lacerations, or those on face, hands, feet, or neck	A second provider ideally should evert wound edges. Squeeze trigger/handle to release staple. Repeat until desired closure is achieved.	Pressing too hard can cause local ischemia within the staple loop. Staples do not provide the same hemostasis as sutures.
Deep sutures	Closure of fascial and subcutaneous layers in wounds deep layer involvement	Place suture starting at the bottom of the wound, exiting subcutaneous tissue in a more superficial location. Re-insert needle at same dermal level on opposite side and tie off. The knot should be in the deepest part of the wound.	Use absorbable suture material for deep sutures.
Simple interrupted	Mainstay for suturing. Used in all shapes, sizes and locations of wounds	Insert needle perpendicular to epidermis and into wound. Reposition needle and insert at same level of dermis on opposite side of wound. Use instrument tie to secure.	Can use simple interrupted between mattress sutures on large, high-tension wounds. Achieve better wound closure by bisecting open areas of the laceration with each new suture.
Running/continuous	Long, linear lacerations with little-no tension on immobile skin surfaces	Start with a simple interrupted stitch at the edge of the wound. Instead of cutting the thread continue to make successive stitches over the length of the wound and tie at the end.	A variation is the continuous locking stitch. Loop the needle behind the thread to lock each stitch down without tying off.
Vertical mattress	Used to evert skin edges. Combines deep and epidermal suture	Start with a simple interrupted stitch. In same plane re-insert needle at a deeper level, ending the stitch on the same side as initial needle insertion. Instrument tie.	Combines a deep suture and simple interrupted on deep wounds to save time. See Figure 19.21.
Horizontal mattress	Wounds with high tension and little subcutaneous tissue available	Start with simple interrupted stitch. Reinsert needle 5mm from exit point and drive suture back to initial edge of wound. Instrument tie.	See Figure 19.22. A variation of this is a half-buried mattress suture—combining a horizontal mattress with a subcutaneous stitch. This is ideal for corners.

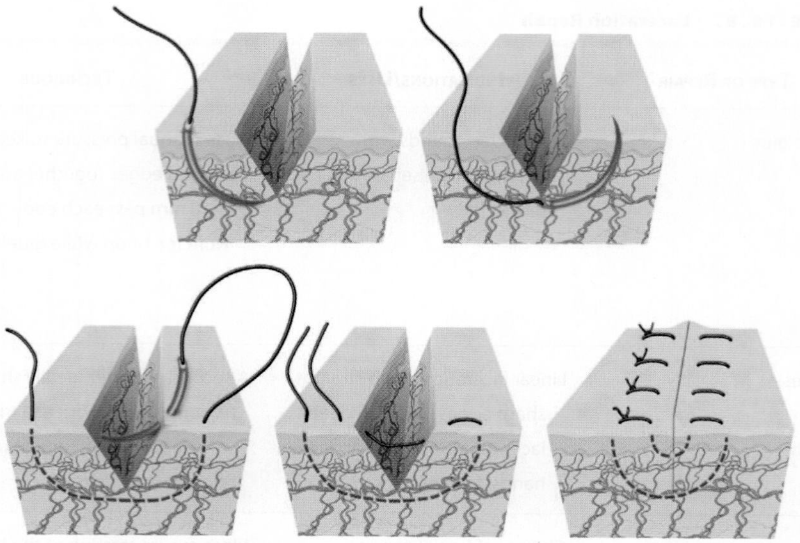

FIGURE 19.21. Vertical mattress suture. (Reproduced with permission from Goldsmith L, Katz S, Gilchrest B, et al: *Fitzpatrick's Dermatology in General Medicine*, 8th ed. New York, NY: McGraw-Hill Education; 2012. Figure 242.9.)

TECHNIQUE

- Perform full neurovascular examination of affected digit.
- Perform digital block, if needed.
- Hot cautery (heated straightened paperclip or commercial cautery tool) is applied to the nail until resistance is no longer felt and there is a return of blood. An alternative is a No. 11 scalpel blade or 18- or 21-ga needle.
- After drainage, apply antibiotic ointment and dressing and instruct patient to keep the nail dry for 24 hours.

COMPLICATIONS

Damage to nail bed

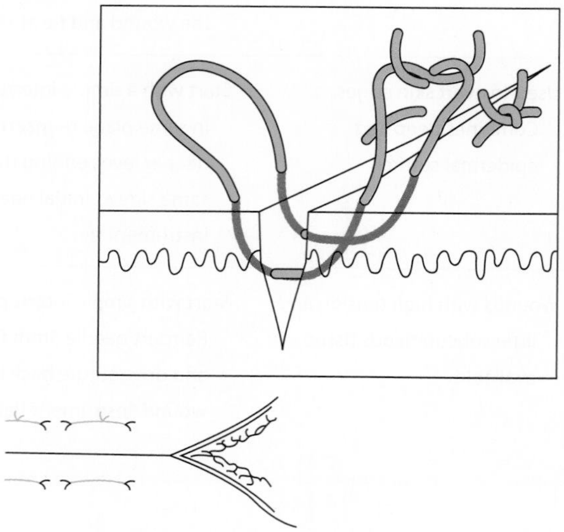

FIGURE 19.22. Horizontal mattress suture. (Reproduced, with permission, from Gomella L, Haist S. *Clinician's Pocket Reference.* 11th ed. New York, NY: McGraw-Hill Education, 2006. Figure 17.5.)

INTERPRETATION OF RESULTS

- Return of blood, indicating evacuation of hematoma
- Immediate improvement of patient discomfort and appearance of nail

NAIL REMOVAL

INDICATIONS

- Unstable or avulsed nail
- Need for nail bed repair

CONTRAINDICATIONS

Patient tolerance

TECHNIQUE

- Perform digital block and use a tourniquet for a painless, bloodless field.
- Hold iris scissors parallel to nail bed and spread blades to loosen nail working proximally.
- Upon reaching the base of the nail, hold tip of nail with hemostats and pull the nail from the base.
- Repair any nail bed lacerations with **absorbable** sutures or tissue adhesive.
- Make sure nail is clean and replace nail into eponychial fold. Suture nail in place with nonabsorbable sutures or use tissue adhesive to glue nail in place.

COMPLICATIONS

- Damage to nail bed
- Poor cosmesis and improper regrowth of nail

INTERPRETATION OF RESULTS

- Successful replacement of nail postprocedure
- Proper growth of new nail (6 months until nail growth to fingertip)

Genitourinary Procedures

URETHRAL CATHETERIZATION

INDICATIONS

- Acute urinary retention
- Bladder irrigation to relieve clots
- Need for close monitoring of urinary output in critically ill patient (eg, rhabdomyolysis)
- Collection of sterile urine sample for diagnostic purposes
- Prolonged immobilization (eg, pelvic or hip fractures)
- Improve comfort for end of life care
- Facilitate healing of sacral/perineal wounds in incontinent patients

CONTRAINDICATIONS

- Suspected traumatic urethral injury (rule out with urethrogram prior to placement of catheter).
- Consider urologic consultation for history of difficult catheterization or false-passage.

Q

A patient presents with right thumb pain after crushing his finger in a car door prior to arrival. On examination, you see a large hematoma under the nail. Besides pain medication, how would you relieve the patient's discomfort?

KEY FACT

If the nail is too damaged or lost for removal/replacement, a nonadherent piece of gauze or foil can be used to maintain the germinal matrix and ensure proper nail regeneration.

KEY FACT

Strict adherence to indwelling catheter guidelines is critical. Hospitals may be penalized for inappropriate use of urinary catheters, and Medicare no longer reimburses hospitals for catheter-associated urinary tract infections (UTIs).

A

Nail trephination.

Technique

- Use aseptic technique and sterile equipment that is the appropriate size for patient's age.
  - 10 Fr is adequate for small children
  - 14-16 Fr is a common starting size in adults
- Use antiseptic solution to cleanse urethral meatus and surrounding tissue. The foreskin (males, if present) should be fully retracted prior to establishing sterile field (be sure to return foreskin to normal position after the procedure). 2% viscous lidocaine can be injected into urethra for topical anesthesia (males).
- Slowly and gently pass the lubricated catheter into the urethra and toward the bladder. To minimize mechanical obstruction in males due to long urethra or prostate, hold the penis taught and upright.
- Stop if you encounter resistance or the patient complains of pain.
- When catheter has been inserted, inflate the balloon with 10 mL of air or tap water. In males the catheter must be fully inserted prior to balloon inflation. This is not true for females due to the short length of the female urethra (4 cm).
- Gently withdraw catheter until you reach resistance of balloon against bladder neck and secure to thigh or abdomen. Attach catheter to collection system of choice (eg, leg bag).

Complications

- If initial passage of a standard catheter is unsuccessful (eg, history of prostatic hypertrophy), try either a **larger** catheter or a coudé catheter (Figure 19.23).
- Iatrogenic injury may occur if the balloon is inflated prematurely, insertion is forced against an obstruction (creation of false passage), or catheter is not secured properly (traumatic removal).
- Failure to use aseptic technique may lead to catheter-associated infection.
- Inability to obtain urine sample may be due to several factors, including clogged catheter, improper placement (eg, false passage, not advance far enough), lack of urine in bladder (eg, recent voiding, anuria).

Interpretation of Results

- Return of urine through the catheter indicates successful placement.
- Urine specimen may be sent for diagnostic testing.
- Bladder irrigation may be performed as indicated until there is no sign of hematuria.

SUPRAPUBIC BLADDER ASPIRATION

Indications

- Collection of sterile urine sample in children < 2 years
- Inability to obtain urethral sample in adults (eg, phimosis, urethral stricture)
- Determine presence of true pathogens rather than contaminants

Contraindications

Inability to palpate bladder or visualize with ultrasound

Technique

- Locate bladder by palpation, percussion, or ultrasound.
- Point of entry is 2-4 cm above the pubic symphysis, in the midline of abdomen.
- Prepare skin of infraumbilical abdomen and drape area around point of entry.

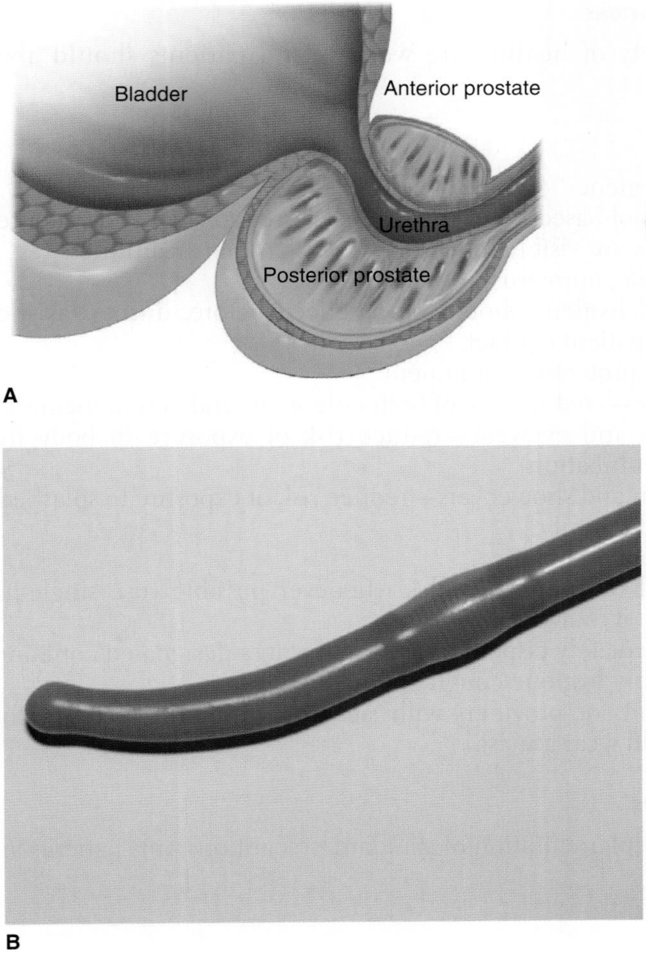

FIGURE 19.23. Insertion of coudé catheter. (Reproduced, with permission, from Brunicardi FC, Andersen DK, Billiar TR, et al. *Schwartz's Principles of Surgery*. 10th ed. New York, NY: McGraw-Hill Education, 2010. Figure 40.8.)

- Infiltrate skin and subcutaneous tissue with local anesthetic.
- For adult patients, use a 22-ga, 3.75- to 8.75-cm needle.
- Direct needle toward bladder (cephalad direction in children and caudad in adults), aspirating as you advance.

COMPLICATIONS

Microscopic hematuria, but not gross hematuria, is expected following this procedure.

INTERPRETATION OF RESULTS

- Return of urine through by aspiration indicates successful entry to bladder.
- Urine specimen may be sent for diagnostic testing as indicated.

Universal Precautions

INDICATIONS

- Protect and prevent health care workers from transmission of infection among patients.
- Use appropriate precautions whenever there is any possibility of contact with body fluids.

Q

An elderly gentleman who is on Coumadin for atrial fibrillation presents with hematuria. He has been passing clots all day, but now has been unable to urinate for over 6 hours. He complains of pelvic pain and nausea. He is tachycardic and hypertensive. A bedside ultrasound reveals > 600 mL of urine in his bladder. What is the most appropriate next step?

KEY FACT

The ED population has a high prevalence of communicable diseases such as HIV and hepatitis.

A

Place a Foley catheter to relieve his obstruction and begin bladder irrigation.

KEY FACT

Reference: http://www.cdc.gov/HAI/pdfs/guidelines/Outpatient-Care-Guide-withChecklist.pdf

CONTRAINDICATIONS

None: Safety of health care workers and patients should always be first priority.

TECHNIQUE

- Hand hygiene:
  - Alcohol-based hand rubs are preferred to soap and water, except when hands are visibly soiled or patient has diarrheal illness (eg, *Clostridium difficile*, norovirus).
  - Hand hygiene should be practiced before, during (as indicated) and after patient contact.
- Personal protective equipment:
  - Gloves—reduce risk of both cutaneous and percutaneous exposure
  - Mask and eyewear—reduce risk of exposure to body fluid aerosols (eg, intubation)
  - Gown and shoe covers—reduce risk of exposure to splashed body fluids (eg, chest tube)
- Safe injection practice:
  - Avoid recapping needles whenever possible (use single-handed technique if unavoidable).
  - Immediately dispose of used sharps in a designated container.
- Respiratory hygiene/cough etiquette:
  - Patients or providers with signs or symptoms of respiratory infection should wear a mask.

COMPLICATIONS

Improper implementation of standard precautions puts patients and providers at risk.

REVIEW QUESTIONS

QUESTIONS

1. A 25-year-old woman presents with fever, headache, and nuchal rigidity. You perform a lumbar puncture to evaluate for meningitis. Which of the following results is most suggestive of bacterial meningitis?
   A. Xanthochromia
   B. Neutrophil predominance
   C. > 500 RBC/mm^3
   D. 0-5 WBC/mm^3
2. Ketamine is associated with which of the following adverse effects?
   A. Myoclonus
   B. Hypotension
   C. Apnea
   D. Laryngospasm
3. A 30-year-old man is struck in the face with a baseball during a game. He presents with tense swelling around his right eye. Which of the following is an indication for emergent lateral canthotomy and cantholysis?
   A. Intraocular pressure > 40 mm Hg
   B. Irregular pupil
   C. Large hyphema
   D. Exposed uveal tissue
4. An ED thoracotomy would be indicated in which of the following scenarios?
   A. 58-year-old man found unresponsive at the bottom of his stairs with agonal respirations and sinus bradycardia.
   B. 34-year-old woman with a stab wound to the left chest, breathing during EMS transport, in PEA on arrival to ED.
   C. 22-year-old unrestrained passenger in a roll-over MVC who has received 15 minutes of prehospital CPR.
   D. 42-year-old man with gunshot wound to left chest, no signs of life at scene, who arrives to ED apneic and in asystole.
5. A 47-year-old man with alcoholic-induced liver failure presents with diffuse abdominal pain. On examination he is noted to have ascites and generalized pain without rebound or guarding. You perform a diagnostic paracentesis. The results show 270 PMN/μL with pending Gram stain/culture. The next appropriate step is:
   A. Admit and initiate antibiotic therapy for spontaneous bacterial peritonitis
   B. Perform a CT scan to evaluate for bowel perforation
   C. Consult GI for liver biopsy
   D. Consult social work for alcohol cessation therapy
6. Which regional nerve block is indicated for pain relief of lower molar pain?
   A. Infraorbital nerve block
   B. Mental nerve block
   C. Inferior alveolar nerve block
   D. Posterior superior alveolar nerve block
7. You perform procedural sedation on a 32-year-old man to reduce a shoulder dislocation. After administration of propofol, the patient is not easily aroused and does not response purposefully to commands. What level of sedation have you achieved?
   A. Minimal
   B. Moderate
   C. Deep
   D. General anesthesia

ANSWERS

1. **B.** The yellow color of xanthochromia is due to bilirubin and indicates the presence of old RBCs, most commonly seen in SAH. A CSF RBC count > 10 cells/mm^3 is seen in SAH, HSV encephalitis or a traumatic tap, but not usually bacterial meningitis. A normal CSF WBC count is < 5 cell/mm^3 in adults (< 20 cells/mm^3 in neonates). Findings of bacterial meningitis include an elevated CSF WBC count with neutrophil predominance. The Gram stain may also be positive.
2. **D.** Ketamine is a dissociative anesthetic that provides both amnesia and analgesia. It is associated with laryngospasm, emergency reaction, transient increased ICP/OPD (not significant), and hypersalivation. Myoclonus occurs after administration of fentanyl. Although most sedative/hypnotics in high enough doses can cause respiratory depression, propofol is known for causing both hypotension and apnea.
3. **A.** Indications for lateral canthotomy and cantholysis include patients with suspected or confirmed retrobulbar hemorrhage and an elevated IOP > 40 mm Hg, or the presence of an afferent pupillary defect, ophthalmoplegia, cherry-red macula, optic nerve head pallor, or severe eye pain.
4. **B.** Indications for ED thoracotomy in penetrating trauma include prehospital signs of life, echo evidence of cardiac activity with cardiac tamponade, and unresponsive hypotension (BP < 70 mm Hg) despite resuscitation in the presence of a penetrating chest wound. Indications for ED thoracotomy in the setting of blunt trauma include < 10 minutes of ongoing

CPR, unresponsive hypotension (BP < 70 mm Hg) despite resuscitation with echo evidence of cardiac tamponade, and rapid exsanguination from a chest tube (> 1500 mL output).

5. **A.** A peritoneal fluid PMN cell count > 250 PMN/μL is presumptive evidence of SBP and warrants admission and empiric antibiotic coverage. A positive Gram stain or culture is also diagnostic.

6. **C.** The inferior alveolar nerve block anesthetizes all the mandibular teeth, the anterior two-third of the tongue and floor of oral cavity as well as the distribution of the mental nerve (see the following text). The infraorbital nerve block anesthetizes the maxillary teeth and buccal soft tissues from midline to premolars as well as the upper lip, lateral aspect of nose and lower eyelid. The mental nerve block anesthetizes the buccal soft tissues from midline to the second mandibular premolar as well as the lower lip and chin soft tissue. The posterior superior alveolar nerve block anesthetizes the second and third (sometimes also the first) maxillary molars.

7. **C.** Minimal sedation is characterized by anxiolysis alone; moderate sedation by depression of consciousness with quick purposeful response to commands; deep sedation by depression of consciousness with purposeful response only to repeated commands and general anesthesia by no response to any stimuli along with impaired ventilation.

CHAPTER 20

EMS and Disaster Medicine

Elena D. Garcia, MD and Justin McLean, MD

Origins of Emergency Medical Services

Modern emergency medical service (EMS) systems began to evolve in the 1960s and 1970s to deliver emergency care in the prehospital environment rather than simply as a means of transport to the hospital. Several important steps in the development of modern EMS in the United States resulted in improved training, regulation, and quality of prehospital care.

- Highway Safety Act (1966)
  - Authorized the U.S. Department of Transportation (DOT) to develop prehospital services
  - Established the National Highway Traffic Safety Administration (NHTSA)
- Emergency Medical Services System Act (1973)
  - Provided government funding and training to encourage development of regional, county, and local EMS systems
  - Identified essential components of an EMS system
- Development of communication and ambulance standards (1973-1974)
  - 911 system
  - Dedicated radio frequencies for EMS
  - Federal specifications for ambulances
- Emergency Medical Treatment and Active Labor Act (EMTALA) 1985
  - Part of the Consolidated Omnibus Budget Reconciliation Act (COBRA)
  - A condition of Medicare funding that requires a medical screening examination and stabilization of any emergent medical condition (including active labor) for any patient who presents to a hospital with an emergency department
- Trauma Care Systems Planning and Development Act (1990)
  - Authorized government funds to states for development of trauma systems

KEY FACT

The Highway Safety Act of 1966 established the initial government funding for prehospital services.

EMS System Designs

Multiple EMS system designs exist and depend on the type of community served. In general, there should be 1 ambulance per 7000-10,000 people.

- **Volunteer model:** Used primarily in rural areas where there are no funds to pay personnel.
- **Public utility model:** Allows a local government to contract calls for service to a **private** company that provides basic life support (BLS) and/or advanced life support (ALS); the government oversees and regulates performance.
- **Third service model:** A separate department of local government owns, operates, and staffs ambulances.
- **Fire department-based model:** The fire department provides all EMS services as well as fire suppression services.
- **Combined public/private model: Parts of the EMS response come from different organizations,** eg, the fire department provides first response while transportation to the hospital is provided by a private ambulance service or government "third service."
- **Hospital-based EMS model:** Not as common as in the past; EMS services are provided by the local hospital.

All models rely on lesser-trained medical (or "first") responders, but the subsequent level of care of an EMS system varies:

- **Single-tier system:** Provides **only** BLS or **only** ALS (including EMT-Intermediate and/or EMT-Paramedic) response.
- **Multitiered system:** Provides a mixed BLS/ALS response (becoming less common). In a multitiered system, the level of response (BLS or ALS) depends on the nature of the call.

Components of an EMS System

EDUCATION

Multiple levels of EMS training and credentialing exist. The old nomenclature recognizes first responders, EMT-Basic, EMT-Intermediate, and EMT-Paramedic. The National Registry of Emergency Medical Technicians recently changed its classification system to comply with the National Scope of Practice Model which recognizes four levels of EMS licensure: EMR, EMT, AEMT (Advanced EMT), and Paramedic. In addition, some states recognize Critical Care Paramedics. Each level represents a unique role, skill set, and knowledge base.

- **Emergency medical responders (EMRs)**
  - Often the first to arrive on scene (eg, firefighters, police officers, community EMS responders)
  - Trained in cardiopulmonary resuscitation (CPR) and automated external defibrillator (AED) use, BLS, and basic trauma care, the primary focus of the EMR is to provide lifesaving interventions while awaiting additional EMS response
- **Emergency medical technician (EMT)**
  - Possess the basic knowledge and skills necessary to provide patient care and transportation
  - Perform BLS and basic trauma care, including CPR and AED use, basic assessments, administer some medications, and assist ALS personnel
- **Advanced EMT**
  - EMT skills plus intravenous (IV)/intraosseous (IO) access, placement of supraglottic airway devices, manual defibrillation, and an expanded scope of practice for drug administration
- **Paramedic**
  - The most advanced EMT level
  - Can perform advanced airway procedures including endotracheal (ET) intubation and cricothyrotomy and administer bilevel positive airway pressure (BiPAP)/continuous positive airway pressure (CPAP), perform needle decompression of chest, electrocardiogram (ECG) interpretation, external pacing, and advanced drug therapy

COMMUNICATION

After activating the system via 911, the goal is to get the right resources to the right location in an appropriate amount of time depending on the nature of the call. An **enhanced 911** system displays the caller's telephone number and address.

The emergency medical dispatcher must:

- Take and triage the call and categorize the nature of the emergency.
- Locate the address of the call.
- Alert the appropriate unit(s).
- Assist victim until arrival by providing medical care instructions to the caller.

Communication must also be available between hospital and field or dispatch center via designated radio frequencies.

KEY FACT

The Emergency Medical Service Act of 1973 identified 15 essential components of an EMS system.

In a single-tier EMS system, only one level of response (eg, BLS) is provided for every call.

KEY FACT

EMT and AEMT providers can assist in medication administration and provide BLS, AED, and basic care.

KEY FACT

Paramedic can perform advanced drug therapy, ECG interpretation, external pacing, surgical airway, and needle decompression of chest.

FACILITIES

There are three ways to conceptualize relationships between categories of hospital facilities, which are the usual destinations for EMS transports.

- **Vertical**
  - Describes a level of care provided at the hospital
  - Not standardized (eg, a Level 1 trauma center is the most sophisticated, with all specialty services immediately available 24 hours a day, whereas a Level 3 nursery has the most sophisticated NICU services)
- **Horizontal**
  - Describes the specialty care provided at the hospital (eg, neurosurgery, burn, cardiac care, and trauma)
- **Circular**
  - Transfer agreements among hospitals of different vertical and horizontal levels so they can get to most appropriate care (eg, regionalization of trauma centers).

TRANSPORTATION

Ground Transportation

- Ground transportation is used for the majority of acutely ill or injured patients.
- Ambulances staffed by two persons of varying training levels.
- There are various types of ambulances used by EMS which can transport patients, which vary from a pickup truck or van-style design to a commercial-style chassis with modular patient care compartment.

Rotary-Wing Air Transportation

Indications for helicopter transport: Benefit by the personnel and equipment must outweigh the risks of transport. Air transport is most beneficial over moderate to long distances, rough terrain, and in heavy ground traffic conditions. Helicopter transport is most effective between 15 and 100 miles. The 4 S's can help determine the benefit of helicopter transport: speed, special skills, smoothness, and access. Helicopter transport is reliant on favorable weather conditions to safely perform transport.

Fixed-Wing Air Transportation

For distances > 100 miles, when rapid transport is essential. Limited by weather, lack of runways, and refueling. Possible altitude problems for the patient due to barometric pressure, including worsening of a pneumothorax, increases in ET cuff and balloon catheter volumes. Always consider securing a concerning airway prior to transport.

PATIENT TRANSFER

- Refusal of care: Lawsuits number approximately 1 per 24,000 calls. However, ambulance crashes result in the main litigation against EMS.
  - An impaired patient cannot refuse (definition varies, and may include dementia, intoxication, head injury, or other state causing altered mentation).
  - Patient with capacity may sign waiver form, perhaps with online (over the phone) medical physician consultation.
- On-scene physician: A physician bystander may be able to assist with EMS protocols after identity check, depending on local protocols and practice.

KEY FACT

An impaired patient cannot refuse prehospital care.

- If an on-scene physician assumes full medicolegal responsibility for patient care, then she/he may treat the patient, depending on local regulations, but she/he must accompany the patient to hospital and their instruction does not supersede provider scope of practice or protocols.

REVIEW AND EVALUATION

The EMS medical director is a physician who provides administrative and medical oversight for an EMS system.

Means of medical control and evaluation:

- **Direct medical control and evaluation**
  - Infield observation
  - Real-time "online" discussion with prehospital providers, includes providing medical orders, usually as per protocol
- **Indirect medical control and evaluation**
  - **Prospective** via development of standing orders, medical care protocols, and education
  - **Retrospective** via review of EMS patient care, quality assurance through EMS education

Disaster and Mass Gathering Medicine

In medical terms, a disaster is defined as any event where the needs exceed the available resources. It is not defined by the type of event (chemical, nuclear, biological attack, terrorist incident, natural catastrophe), but rather is dependent on the response capabilities of a community. A "mass casualty incident" (MCI) is often a "disaster" event because it leads to multiple patients whose needs may quickly exceed the available health care resources. Conversely, not all disasters are MCIs, because the needs may not be related to casualties (eg, may only have infrastructure damage after a flood and no patient victims). Disasters may be natural (floods, tornadoes, earthquakes, etc), manmade (plane and train crashes, industrial explosions, fires, radiation leaks, chemical spills), and even terrorist related (biological, chemical, nuclear events). Within a hospital, disasters may be further categorized as **internal** (within the hospital) and **external** (outside the hospital grounds).

A "mass gathering" is an event of over 1000 people gathered at a specific location for a specific amount of time (eg, sporting event, music festival). Mass gathering medicine may be thought of as planning and responding to an "expected" MCI.

Disaster: Needs > Resources

Classically, disasters have been categorized into levels denoted in Table 20.1. However, newer nomenclature replaces the term "disaster" with an acronym

TABLE 20.1. Disaster Classification

Level	Projected Need	Response Time
I	Local resources only	Hours
II	Regional mutual aid	Up to 1 d
III	Statewide or federal assistance required	Up to 3 d

Q

A patient presents to your ED with 30 minutes of chest pain and found to have a ST-elevation myocardial infarction (STEMI). You work in a single provider mountain town ED without an airport, 50 miles from the nearest cardiac cath laboratory. What are some of the considerations when deciding on type of transport?

KEY FACT

Direct medical control = Providing direction to EMTs during actual patient care.

KEY FACT

Indirect medical control = Off-line direction and training for EMTs including development of protocols and quality assurance reviews.

KEY FACT

Classic disaster terminology: Three levels, based on projected need for resources.

KEY FACT

PICE classification: Four stages, 0-III, based on potential for further victims, state of local resources, and extent of geographic involvement.

Q

A metropolitan EMS system receives a call that there has been an explosion at a sports stadium with an unknown number of injured victims. Source of the explosion is unclear. They are the single EMS agency in the city. What would define this event as a medical disaster?

A

In this case there are four options: helicopter transport, critical care ground transport, ALS transport, or no transport. General considerations include the patient's medical injury or illness, optimal interhospital transport time or scene time, distance, special skills of the transport team, weather, and cost.

TABLE 20.2. Potential Injury-Creating Event Classification

	A	B	C
PICE Stage	Potential for Further Victims?	State of Local Resources?	Extent of Geographic Involvement
0	No = static	Controlled (**ok**)	Local
I	Yes = dynamic	Disrupted	Regional
II		Paralytic (overwhelmed)	National
III			International

for "**potential injury-creating event**" **(PICE)**. There are further categories assigned based on need for mutual aid, potential for casualties, and the nature of the event (static or dynamic). Because these things may change in the course of an event, the assigned PICE stage may also change accordingly (Table 20.2).

KEY FACT

JCAHO phases of disaster preparedness: Mitigation, preparedness, response, implementation.

KEY FACT

Communication is the most important component of any disaster response!

DISASTER PREPAREDNESS

The Joint Commission on Accreditation of Health Care Organizations (JCAHO) requires all hospitals to have a written plan for both internal and external disasters and to perform practice drills twice yearly. There are four phases of disaster preparedness: mitigation, preparedness, response (activation, implementation), and recovery (Table 20.3).

TABLE 20.3. Phases of Disaster Preparedness

Phase	
Mitigation	Activities to lessen impact of a **potential** disaster Occurs before and after emergencies
Preparedness	Plans and preparations to help with response and rescue operations in a disaster
Response	
Activation	Notification for response Organization of incident command post
Implementation	Assessment of event Scene: Search and rescue, triage and transport, definitive management ED: Coordinating treatment
Recovery	Scene withdrawal Debriefing Return to normal operations

ED, emergency department.

A

This event would be defined as a disaster if the local health care system is unable to meet the needs of the event.

THE INCIDENT COMMAND SYSTEM

The incident command system is the standard incident management system for a single scene disaster. It can be expanded or contracted to match the needs of the incident. The National Incident Management System (NIMS) standardizes the structure used by EMS agencies, law enforcement, fire departments, hospitals, local governments, and other stakeholders to enhance response coordination for all levels and all types of incidents. Common components include:

- **Incident command**: The **incident commander** has overall management responsibility for the incident. The incident commander relies on several "sections" of the system:
  - **Planning** (determines what is needed to manage the incident)
  - **Logistics** (supplies what is needed to manage the incident)
  - **Operations** (uses what is needed to manage the incident)
  - **Finance** (manages money and tallies budgets)

In the hospital, additional considerations may be given to establishing treatment areas (which may be usual patient care areas or "surge" spaces employed in an emergency), ensuring documentation for and identification of patients, providing security, and managing potentially hazardous waste.

Table 20.4 summarizes the federal response resources that are available in the event of a disaster.

KEY FACT

The standard prehospital management system for a single scene disaster = Incident Command System.

DISASTER AND MASS CASUALTY TRIAGE

The need for patient triage arises when available resources require prioritizing the treatment of one patient over another in order to deliver the greatest good to the greatest number of people (ie, a community-minded "altered standard of care"). Many triage systems provide a means of assigning priority for the ill or injured. This is a dynamic process of sorting that may change as a victim's disease

TABLE 20.4. Disaster Response Organizations

Organization	Example of Resource Provided
Department of Homeland Security	FEMA state and local assistance
NDMS	Federally coordinated system of government and private institutions which uses DMATs
Centers for Disease Control	Public health emergency preparedness and response
Department of Veterans Affairs	Highly trained disaster medical personnel
Urban search and rescue	Highly trained medical, fire, and rescue personnel
Metropolitan Medical Response Systems	Personnel and equipment to enhance local planning and disaster response
The military	Response personnel

DMAT, Disaster Medical Assistance Team; FEMA, Federal Emergency Management Agency; NDMS, National Disaster Medical System.

Q

You are in the ambulance that is first to arrive on scene after the explosion at the sports complex. You see panicked sports fans running out of the stadium and see many casualties on the ground. Some are moaning and moving, and others appear unconscious and lifeless. How would you prioritize patients for treatment and transport?

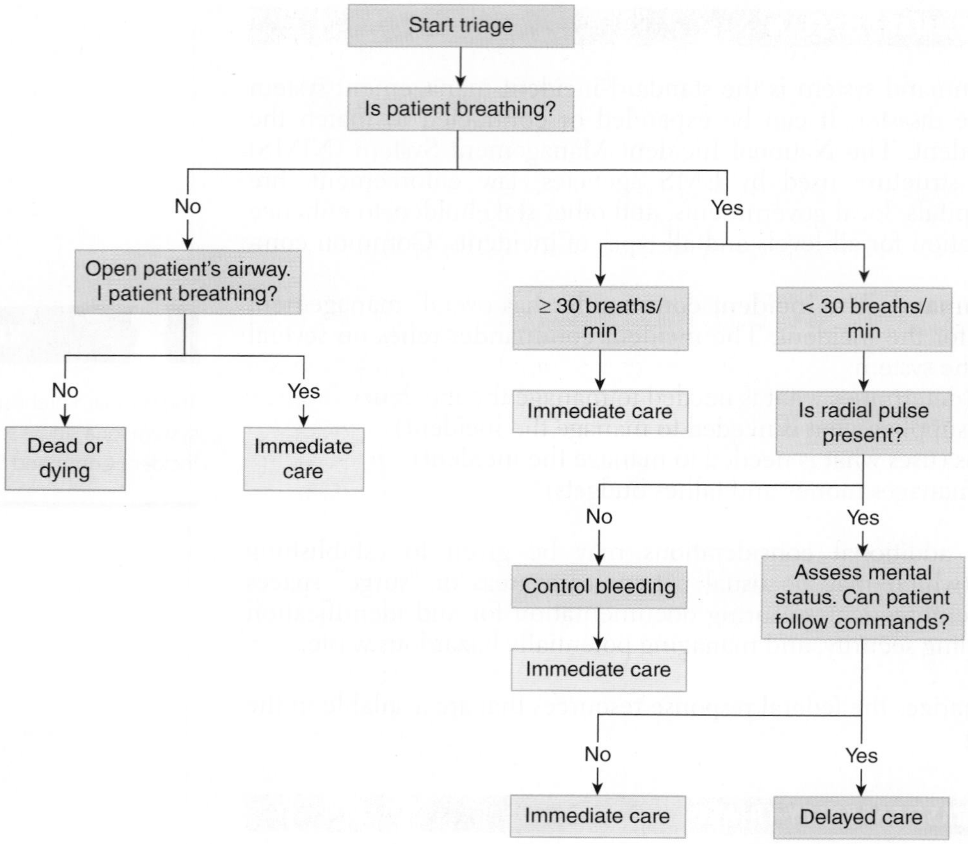

FIGURE 20.1. START triage. (Reproduced with permission from Benson M, Koenig KL, Schultz CH: Disaster triage: START, then SAVE—a new method of dynamic triage for victims of a catastrophic earthquake. *Prehosp Disaster Med.* 1996;11:117.)

state progresses, which creates a "double funnel" of triage and retriage. Simple Triage and Rapid Treatment (START) is probably the most widely used form of triage, although multiple other systems have been developed to take into consideration special populations (such as the pediatric version termed Jump-START), or the role that limited resources play in a disaster response (eg, the Grey designation in SALT triage for those patients who would survive if sufficient resources were available) (Figure 20.1).

KEY FACT

A disaster triage category "red" patient requires immediate care.

"RPM: 30 to 2, can do" mnemonic for START triage: Respiration rate < 30 breaths/min, perfusion < 2 seconds, and mental status (can do).

A

A triage system such as START can provide a way to rapidly assess victims from a disaster to ensure resources are utilized with maximal effectiveness to provide aid to the greatest number of people.

SIMPLE TRIAGE AND RAPID TREATMENT

The national triage system of the United States adopted by health care agencies worldwide. Simple Triage and Rapid Treatment (START) has four color designations:

- **Red** ***(immediate)***: Critical or immediate life-threatening illness or injury (eg, tension pneumothorax, hypovolemic shock)
- **Yellow** ***(delayed)***: Serious but not immediately life-threatening illness or injury (eg, most long bone fractures)
- **Green** ***(minor)***: The walking wounded (eg, anxiety attack after witnessing event, minor burns)
- **Black** ***(dead/dying, or expectant)***: Dead or resource-intensive victims (eg, 100% TBSA burn)

Red patients are prioritized for initial stabilization (such as inserting an oropharyngeal airway to assist with breathing or performing a needle decompression for a tension pneumothorax) as well as transport, followed by yellow patients. Green patients may not need an in-hospital evaluation (may be cleared on scene), or may be transported en masse (eg, a school bus). Black patients may have palliative interventions (such as morphine for pain control) if resources permit.

Q

A secretary for a government official shows up in a Washington, DC emergency department complaining of an itchy red sore on his right index finger that he thought was an insect bite but now is becoming swollen and blistered. The patient also complains of swollen lymph nodes in the same arm pit and a low-grade fever. What diagnosis should be considered?

Biological Weapons of Mass Destruction

Throughout history, terrorists have attempted to use biological agents as weapons to produce widespread disease and therefore disable or kill an enemy. Some agents are more able to cause rapid, widespread disease (ie, an "epidemic") than others. The spectrum of disease spread includes "**endemic**" (the chronic low-level presence of disease in a community), "**epidemic**" (a rapid increase or outbreak and spread of disease in a specific area), and "**pandemic**" (an epidemic that becomes very widespread, affecting continents or the world).

The "ideal" characteristics of an agent for bioterrorism are easy to disseminate (eg, able to be aerosolized), transmissible from person to person, high mortality rate, and potential for inciting panic and social disruption. Biological weapons of mass destruction are typically divided into three groups: bacteria, viruses, and toxins. All share the ability for aerosol dispersal.

The agents considered to have the most severe potential (Class A agents) include:

- *Bacillus anthracis* (anthrax)
- *Yersinia pestis* (plague)
- Variola major (smallpox)
- *Francisella tularensis* (tularemia)
- *Clostridium botulinum* (botulism): See Botulism in Chapter 8, Infectious Disease
- Filoviruses and arenaviruses (viral hemorrhagic fevers)

ANTHRAX

Organism: *B anthracis*, a gram-positive spore-forming bacterium.
Appears as long chains, resembling bamboo or boxcars (Figure 20.2)

Anthrax is found worldwide in grass-eating mammals that ingest or inhale the spores while feeding. In normal circumstances, humans may become infected by eating infected animals or through contact (skin or inhalation) with spores on the fur or hide of animals (thus the term Woolsorters disease).

Forms of disease:

- **Inhalational anthrax:** Most deadly (90% mortality rate)
- **Cutaneous anthrax:** Most common, rarely fatal if treated (20% mortality without treatment, 1% with treatment)
- **Oropharyngeal or gastrointestinal anthrax:** Less common, 50% mortality rate

Pathophysiology

Exposure to spore via dermal contact, ingestion, or inhalation → spores germinate into bacilli inside cell macrophages → transported to **regional lymph nodes** → **release toxins** → symptoms

A

Cutaneous anthrax. Anthrax is caused by the bacterium *B anthracis* and was spread as a white powder through the US Postal Service in 2001 as a weapon of bioterrorism. Diagnosis can be made via history of exposure and clinical findings, and confirmed with culture. Ciprofloxacin has been the antibiotic of choice, though most strains are sensitive to a broad range of antibiotics including penicillin and doxycycline.

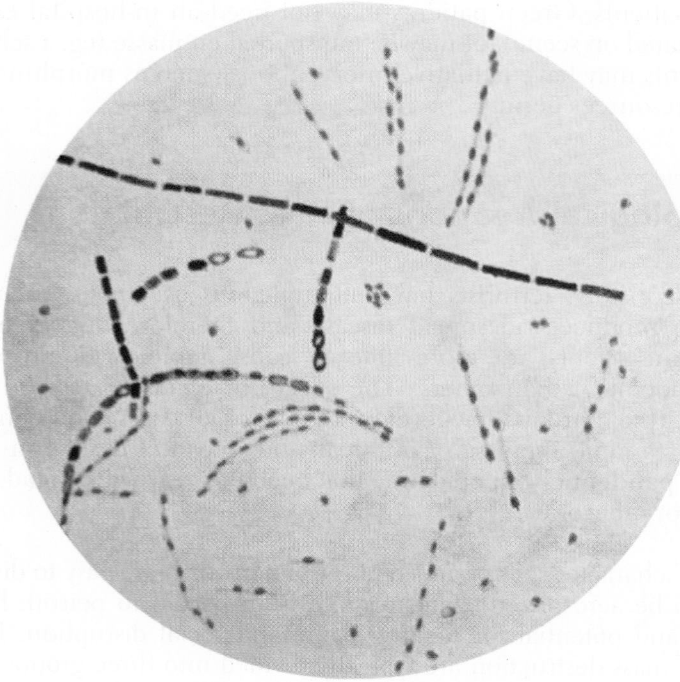

FIGURE 20.2. Bacillus anthracis. (Reproduced with permission from Centers for Disease Control and Prevention Public Health Image Library.)

SYMPTOMS/EXAMINATION

Inhalational Anthrax

- Flulike prodrome (2-10 days) followed by rapid progression (24-48 hours) of hemorrhagic mediastinitis, dyspnea, stridor, sepsis, and shock

Cutaneous Anthrax

- Incubation period of 5 days followed by painless papules that become itchy and vesicular with significant edema and regional lymphadenitis.
- Progresses to ulcerated black eschar (*anthrax* is Greek for "coal") after 1 week. Within 2-3 weeks, the eschar either sloughs off and illness resolves or the infection disseminates, leading to sepsis and possible death.

Oropharyngeal and Gastrointestinal Anthrax

- Incubation period of 2-5 days followed by pharyngitis, lymphadenitis, (cervical, submandibular, or mesenteric); gastrointestinal (GI) bleeding and acute abdomen may also develop.

KEY FACT

Cutaneous anthrax is the most common form of anthrax. Inhalational anthrax is the most deadly form of anthrax.

DIAGNOSIS

- Primarily a clinical diagnosis
- Chest x-ray (CXR) (inhalational disease)—may be normal, otherwise may show mediastinal lymphadenopathy, pleural effusions, or consolidations. Computed tomography (CT) more sensitive than CXR
- Gram stain and culture of skin lesions
- Tissue or pleural fluid evaluation (caution as risk for transmission to health care personnel)

TREATMENT

- Supportive care.
- Simple cutaneous anthrax (nontoxic): Ciprofloxacin, doxycycline, or amoxicillin.

KEY FACT

Anthrax treatment requires prolonged (60 days) antibiotic therapy.

- Toxic patients or inhalational disease: Requires triple antibiotic therapy with ciprofloxacin or doxycycline **plus** 2 additional antibiotics (eg, rifampin, clindamycin, aminoglycoside, imipenem).
- Antibiotic therapy must continue for 60 days. Vaccination is also additionally given as 3 doses (on days 0, 14, and 28).
- Prophylaxis: An FDA-approved vaccine is available (given to military personnel). Postexposure prophylaxis with ciprofloxacin or doxycycline: 30 days (with vaccination) or 60 days (no vaccination).

PLAGUE

Organism: *Y pestis*, a gram-negative bacillus.

Plague is normally a disease of rodents transmitted to humans via inhalation of infected flea feces or cutaneous inoculation by flea bite.

Forms of disease:

- **Bubonic** (skin):
  - Bacilli migrate to regional lymph nodes → bubo
- **Pneumonic** (inhalational): Highly fatal (near 100% mortality)
  - Most common, may be transmitted person-to-person
- **Septicemic** (from secondary dissemination)

SYMPTOMS/EXAMINATION

Bubonic Plague

- Approximately 2-3 days incubation followed by:
  - Regional **painful** lymph node inflammation and necrosis (bubo, Figure 20.3).
  - Associated with fevers, chills, malaise; infection may disseminate in 50% of patients and lead to secondary pneumonic plague or septicemic plague.

Pneumonic Plague

- Approximately 2-3 days incubation followed by fevers, chills, and flu-like illness

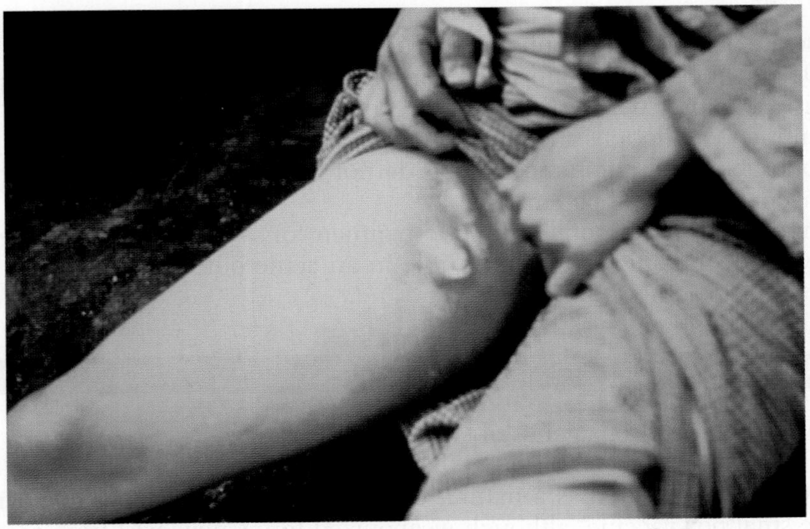

FIGURE 20.3. Plague: An inguinal bubo. (Reproduced from Centers for Disease Control and Prevention.)

Q

A 50-year-old woman presents to the emergency department in southwestern Colorado with complaint of shortness of breath. She notes that she had been feeling feverish with malaise and mild cough the past several days. Over the course of her visit, she begins coughing up blood, her oxygen saturation drops to 70%, and she requires intubation. Her blood pressure plummets to 76/50 mm Hg despite 3 L of normal saline and vasopressors are started. Her CXR shows florid pulmonary edema. She is admitted to the ICU in critical condition. Her family provides additional history that she was cleaning out an old barn that had "piles of mouse poop." What diagnosis should be considered?

KEY FACT

Pneumonic plague is due to inhalation of *Y pestis* (gram-negative bacillus), normally found in flea feces and can be transmitted person-to-person.

KEY FACT

Half of untreated patients with bubonic plague will develop septicemia from bacterial dissemination.

A

This patient may have pneumonic plague, which is associated with high mortality despite aggressive treatment. Family members should be closely monitored for symptoms.

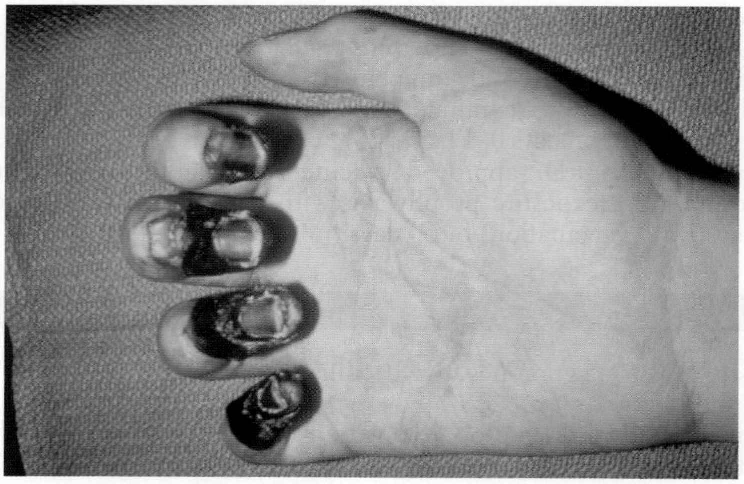

FIGURE 20.4. Plague: Acral gangrene. (Reproduced from Centers for Disease Control and Prevention.)

- Fulminant pneumonia develops within 24 hours, leading to cardiopulmonary collapse.
- Patients may develop meningitis, liver injury, coagulopathy, and acral gangrene (black death) (Figure 20.4).

Septicemic Plague

- Characterized by endotoxemia, shock, disseminated intravascular coagulation (DIC), and coma

Diagnosis

- Suspect in any healthy individual who develops overwhelming gram-negative sepsis and painful lymphadenitis (bubonic) or pneumonia with hemoptysis (pneumonic).
- CXR may show lobar pneumonia, acute respiratory distress syndrome (ARDS), or other pattern.
- Diagnosis can be confirmed by Gram stain and culture of body fluids (caution for secondary transmission).

Treatment

- Isolate patients. Mild bubonic plague may be treated at home.
- Do **not** incise and drain fluctuant lymph nodes because this may spread disease to providers (aspiration is acceptable).
- Antibiotics: Options include streptomycin, gentamycin, doxycycline, ciprofloxacin, and chloramphenicol (do not use chloramphenicol or streptomycin in pregnant patients).
- Prophylaxis: Same oral antibiotic regimen for 7-day course. Vaccine also exists for bubonic form but no role in an acute outbreak because it takes months to achieve immunity.

SMALLPOX

Organism: *Variola* sp, a genus of large DNA viruses.

Successfully eradicated as a natural disease in 1980 with global deployment of the smallpox vaccine, although weaponized forms now exist from research repositories in Russia and the United States. Highly infectious via aerosol and can survive 24-48 hours in the environment.

There are several clinical forms of disease:

- **Variola major:** The classic form of disease (30% mortality)
- **Variola minor:** Milder form (1% mortality)
- **Hemorrhagic smallpox:** Petechiae and hemorrhages (> 90% mortality)
- **Malignant smallpox:** Soft, flat lesions (> 90% mortality)

Symptoms/Examination

Incubation period of 2 weeks after infection via aerosolized exposure. The virus replicates in the lymph nodes and travels to lymphoid tissue (spleen, bone marrow) and liver. Viremia follows and is associated with fever, headache, and malaise. Rash begins as maculopapular and spreads distally from the face to include palms and soles. All lesions are **in the same stage** and change from vesicular to pustular over 1-2 weeks, eventually leaving scars (Figure 20.5).

Diagnosis

The CDC developed an algorithm to assist with clinical diagnosis, which is based on major and minor criteria. Major criteria are febrile prodrome, classic smallpox lesions, and lesions in same stage of development. Minor criteria are centrifugal distribution of pustules, toxic appearance, first lesions in mouth, face, or forearms, slow evolution of lesions, and pustules on the palms and soles. A patient with all 3 major criteria should be isolated immediately, and authorities

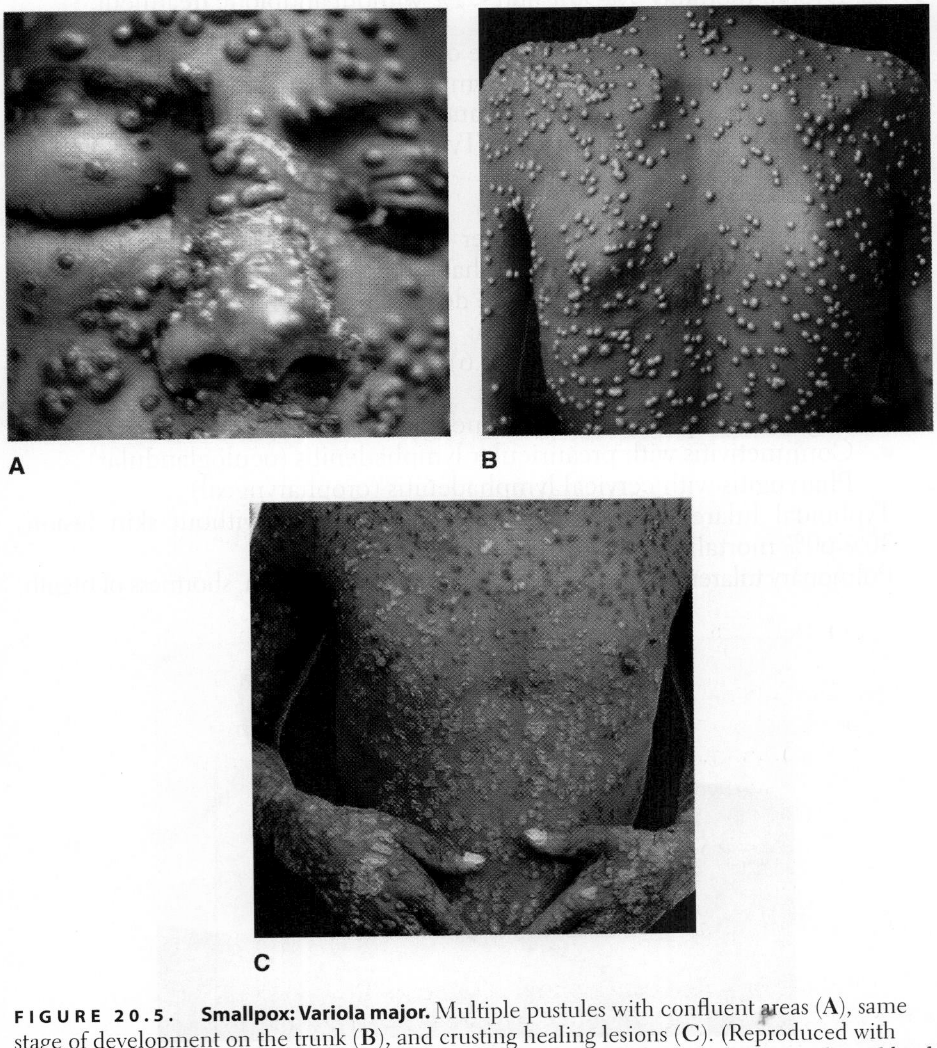

FIGURE 20.5. Smallpox: Variola major. Multiple pustules with confluent areas (**A**), same stage of development on the trunk (**B**), and crusting healing lesions (**C**). (Reproduced with permission from K Wolff, RA Johnson: *Color Atlas and Synopsis of Clinical Dermatology*, 6th ed. New York, NY: McGraw-Hill; 2009.)

Q

A patient presents to the emergency department with a rash. He notes the rash began on the face and forearms and now has spread to his entire body. On examination, you see pustules that have coalesced in areas and are in the same stage of development. What is an important step in treatment of this patient?

KEY FACT

Classic smallpox lesions change from maculopapules → vesicles → pustules with ALL LESIONS IN THE SAME STAGE OF DEVELOPMENT.

KEY FACT

Smallpox starts in the face and forearms and spreads inward (centrifugal), whereas chickenpox starts in the trunk and spreads outward (centripetal).

A

This patient likely has smallpox, and thus airborne isolation is crucial to prevent spread of the disease (the patient is contagious until his rash forms scabs and the scabs fall off).

KEY FACT

Vaccinia immunoglobulin is given to limit the complications of smallpox vaccination (not disease).

KEY FACT

The most common form of tularemia = Ulceroglandular.

should be notified. Those with fever and 4 minor criteria or 1 other major criterion are at moderate risk and warrant confirmatory testing (ie, varicella polymerase chain reaction [PCR]). Those with fever and no major criteria and fewer than 4 minor criteria are at low risk and can be expectantly managed.

Treatment

- Airborne isolation, supportive care (no definitive treatment). Patients are contagious until all scabs fall off.
- Exposed persons → vaccinate within 3 days to prevent or attenuate disease.
- Vaccinia immunoglobulin is given simultaneously with vaccine and redosed as needed to limit complications of vaccination.
- Antivirals (such as ribavirin) are being investigated as treatment.

TULAREMIA

Organism: *F tularensis*, a gram-negative coccobacillus.

Tularemia (commonly called "rabbit fever") is transmitted primarily by ticks, lagomorphs, and rodent hosts (also isolated in prairie dogs and domestic cats) or via direct contact or ingestion of infected water, soil, or fomites. An aerosolized form was developed as a biologic warfare agent in the United States in the 1950s. Overall mortality 5%-30% and < 1% without antibiotic treatment.

Several forms exist depending on route of contact:

- **Localized disease** with regional lymph node involvement: Ulceroglandular (80% cases), glandular, oculoglandular, oropharyngeal
- **Invasive and generalized disease**: Typhoidal, pulmonary

Symptoms/Examination

- Incubation period of 2-6 days after exposure to organism (possibly from tick feces) via skin, ingestion, inhalation, or conjunctival transmission. Multiple presentations are possible depending on which form is present.
- Localized disease may present with:
  - Slow-healing ulcer (Figure 20.6) with associated regional lymphadenopathy (ulceroglandular form)
  - Regional lymphadenopathy alone (glandular)
  - Conjunctivitis with preauricular lymphadenitis (oculoglandular)
  - Pharyngitis with cervical lymphadenitis (oropharyngeal)
- Typhoidal tularemia: Fevers, chills, GI symptoms without skin lesions. 30%-60% mortality rate.
- Pulmonary tularemia: Fevers, chills, nonproductive cough, shortness of breath.

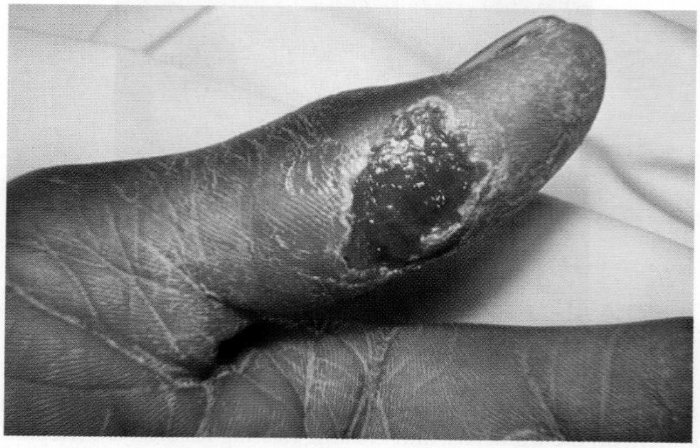

FIGURE 20.6. Tularemia: Ulcerated skin lesion. (Reproduced from Centers for Disease Control and Prevention/Emory Univ.; Dr. Sellers.)

May also manifest as pericarditis, endocarditis, meningitis, peritonitis, appendicitis, osteomyelitis, and Guillain-Barré syndrome.

Diagnosis

- Based on clinical findings
- Antibody titers, rapid PCR

Treatment

- Isolation is **not** required.
- Antibiotic: Streptomycin is drug of choice. Gentamycin also effective.
- Prophylaxis = doxycycline (14-day course). Vaccine in experimental stages.

VIRAL HEMORRHAGIC FEVER

Organisms: Filoviruses (eg, Marburg and Ebola); Arenaviruses (eg, Lassa fever).

Possible reservoir in nature (such as monkeys for Ebola, rats for Lassa fever). Transmission via body fluids. Mortality rate may exceed 90%.

Symptoms/Examination

Incubation period from 4 to 21 days, followed by fevers, myalgias, and prostration, leading to diffuse coagulopathy (hemorrhage, DIC) and eventual multisystem organ dysfunction and cardiovascular collapse.

Diagnosis

Enzyme-linked immunosorbent assay (ELISA) or PCR

Treatment

- Supportive care
- Possible role for antivirals, immunoglobulins (experimental). Ribavirin highly effective for Lassa fever

See Figure 20.7 of recent decontamination efforts in the Democratic Republic of Congo.

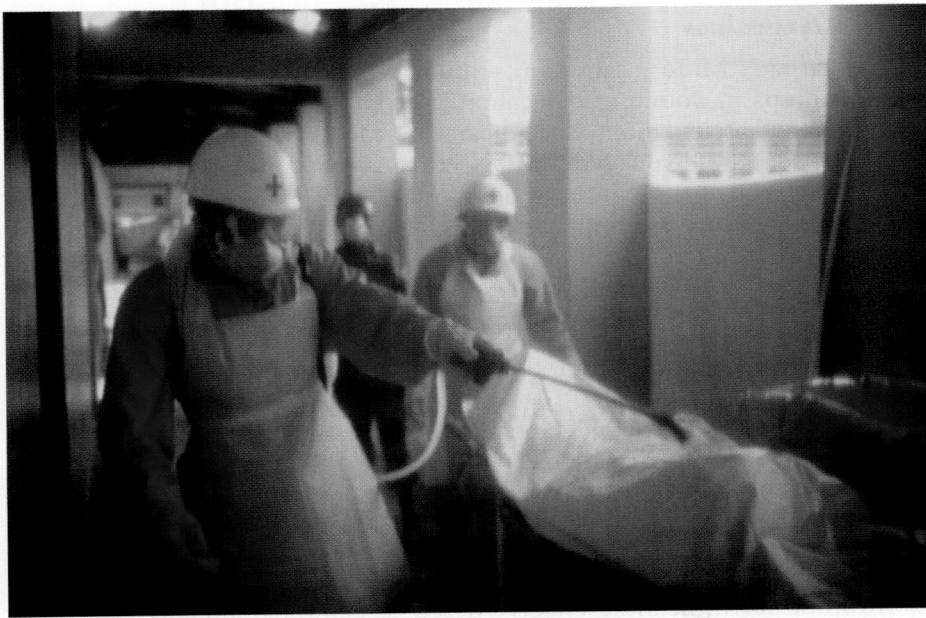

FIGURE 20.7. Disinfection of body bag of a patient who died of Ebola virus disease in the Democratic Republic of Congo. (Reproduced from Centers for Disease Control and Prevention/Ethleen Lloyd.)

Q

A pet store owner presents with an ulcer on his hand and a painful lymph node. He reports that he just got a new shipment of rabbits to his store. What is the treatment of choice for this patient?

Q

A health care worker returns from a medical trip to Liberia, where she was working with a relief organization to manage the Ebola epidemic there. She reports that she was adherent to strict precautions and wore personal protective equipment (PPE) the entire time she was there. Over what period of time may she develop symptoms?

A

He likely has ulceroglandular tularemia. The treatment of choice is streptomycin.

TOXINS

There are weaponized forms of botulism, ricin, T2 mycotoxins (yellow rain), and staphylococcal enterotoxin B that have been developed for use as bioterrorism agents.

Chemical Weapons of Mass Destruction

Agents include nerve agents, vesicants (blistering), pulmonary (choking), and blood agents (see Chapter 6, Toxicology for further and broader descriptions of toxidromes). Because nerve agents and vesicants are thought to have the highest potential for use as bioterrorism agents, they will be the focus of this review. Regarding disaster preparedness, important considerations for chemical weapons are decontamination protocols as well as access to antidotes, and staff should protect themselves from exposure with the use of personal protective equipment (PPE).

NERVE AGENTS

Nerve agents are organophosphates and therefore cause classic symptoms of cholinergic poisoning. Agents include sarin, tabun, soman, and VX. Sarin was used in a 1995 terrorist attack in the Tokyo subway system, resulting in 12 deaths VX is a thick liquid with low volatility and is highly lethal after skin exposure and can cause death in < 30 minutes (LD^{50} for VX is 10 mg, a droplet the size of a pinhead). Effects from nerve agents are immediate (seconds to minutes). Asymptomatic patients after sarin exposure can be discharged after 1 hour of observation, while those exposed to VX should be observed for 18 hours to ensure no delayed symptoms develop.

Pathophysiology

Inhibit acetylcholinesterase → accumulation of acetylcholine at muscarinic and nicotinic receptors → cholinergic toxidrome

KEY FACT

Nerve agents inhibit acetylcholinesterase, producing a cholinergic toxidrome.

Symptoms/Examination

- Muscarinic: Miosis, salivation, rhinorrhea, lacrimation, bronchorrhea, bronchospasm, vomiting, defecation (SLUDGE and killer BBBs).
- Nicotinic: Fasciculations, flaccid paralysis, tachycardia, hypertension.
- Direct central nervous system (CNS) toxicity: Seizures, coma, apnea, and psychological changes in survivors.
- Unlike other organophosphates, nerve agents typically do NOT cause bradycardia or urination.

KEY FACT

Antidotes for nerve agent poisoning = Atropine and pralidoxime, available in Mark 1 autoinjector kit.

Diagnosis

- Based on history of exposure and clinical presentation (muscle fasciculations, miosis).
- Laboratory testing for red blood cell cholinesterase levels may confirm diagnosis, but should not delay management.

A

Ebola viral disease (EVD) has an incubation period of 4-21 days, so she may not be symptomatic until 3 weeks after exposure.

Treatment

- Supportive care.
- **Atropine** for muscarinic effects—dosed to control respiratory secretions, may not reverse miosis or tachycardia in nerve agent poisoning. Dosed as 2-4 mg every 5-10 minutes.

- **Pralidoxime** chloride (**2-PAM**) for nicotinic effects (reverses paralysis) removes the organophosphate from acetylcholinesterase, reactivating it. Most effective if used within 4-6 hours of exposure. May cause hypertension with administration, which can be controlled with phentolamine.
- **Benzodiazepines** (such as diazepam) for seizures.
- All medications may need to be redosed at frequent intervals.

VESICANTS

Agents that induce blistering via cellular damage, including sulfur and nitrogen mustards, named because they smell like mustard. Cell injury occurs within minutes, although symptoms may not develop for 4-8 hours.

Symptoms/Examination

- Local skin effects: Severe pain, vesicle formation, and inflammation to site of contact (Figure 20.8)
- Inhalation effects: Pharyngeal edema and pulmonary necrosis → varying degrees of respiratory distress
- Systemic effects: Bone marrow suppression—leads to decreased white blood cell (WBC) counts, which correlate with mortality (survival rare with levels < 200)

Treatment

- Supportive care, skin and mucous membrane decontamination with irrigation, topical care for burns and eye injuries (do not require aggressive fluid resuscitation as not a typical burn), intubation for severe respiratory exposures
- Experimental—topical iodine preparations

PULMONARY AGENTS (PHOSGENE, CHLORINE)

Cause inflammatory reaction in airways via direct contact with upper airway and eyes; may be fatal if inhaled. Treatment is decontamination and supportive care.

BLOOD AGENTS (CYANIDE)

Bind to cytochromes in mitochondria and inhibit cellular oxygen use, leading to tachypnea, headache, dizziness, vomiting, anxiety, and can progress

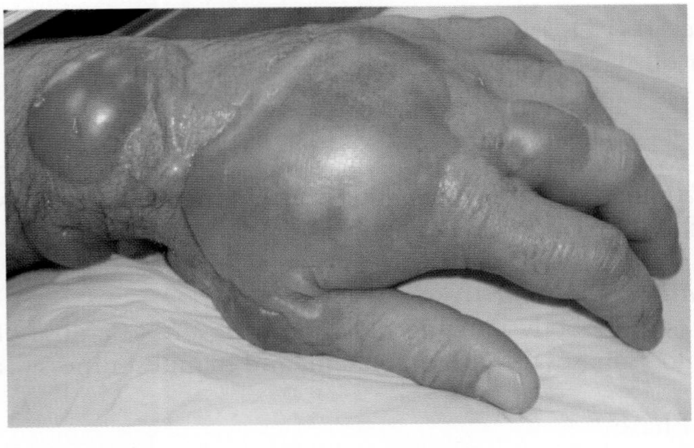

FIGURE 20.8. Blistering from mustard gas exposure. (Reproduced with permission from Kasper DK, Fauci AS, Hauser SL, et al: *Harrison's Principles of Internal Medicine*, 19th ed. New York, NY: McGraw-Hill; 2015.)

Q

A patient presents to the emergency department drooling excessively and having difficulty speaking. He is wearing a jersey and baseball cap of the local sports team. Physical examination reveals miosis and muscle fasciculations. Minutes later, 3 more patients arrive with similar symptoms, also dressed in fan gear. What diagnosis are you considering, and what are your priorities for management?

KEY FACT

The hallmark of mustard injury is skin blistering that resembles second-degree burns.

to seizures, respiratory arrest, and asystole. Treatment includes decontamination as well as antidote (Cyanokit, hydroxocobalamin).

A

This patient has symptoms of nerve agent exposure, and with multiple patients with similar symptoms, a terrorist attack should be considered. Priorities include decontamination with removal of clothing, staff should wear PPE to minimize their exposure, and symptomatic patients should be given a Mark 1 kit (atropine and pralidoxime).

Radiation Injuries

Most radiation exposures occur accidentally in an industrial setting, with hands as the most common overall site of injury. Dose expressed as gray (Gy, where 1 Gy = 1 joule of radiation absorbed per kilogram of tissue) and radiation absorbed dose (rad, where 1 rad = 0.01 Gy). Also expressed as roentgen equivalent man (rem), which is equal to 1 rad of x-radation (1 rad = 1 rem). Exposure can be reduced by time, distance, and shielding. Management involves decontamination (most industrial and laboratory facilities will have protocols); contaminated items are radioactive.

Types of exposure:

- **Contamination:** Either external via skin or internal via inhalation or ingestion
  - These patients are "radioactive." For example, the 2006 intentional poisoning of a former Russian agent with Polonium-210.
- **Irradiation:** Occurs when a radioactive substance passes through an object/person
  - Patients pose no risk to other people (eg, cancer patient postradiation therapy).

Pathophysiology

KEY FACT

Higher radiation exposure is associated with earlier prodrome phase and shorter latent phase.

- **Ionizing radiation** has short wavelength, high frequency, and high energy.
  - **α Particles**: Dissipate quickly, travel only few centimeters (do not go through paper), harmful if ingested/internalized
  - **β Particles**: Tissue penetration of 8 mm to exposed skin, can degrade to gamma emission
  - **Gamma rays**: Travel quickly and penetrate deeply, primary cause of acute radiation syndrome
  - **Neutrons**: Source of radioactive fallout, can also cause gamma radiation
- High-level exposure → direct cell death.
- Low-level exposure → formation of free radicals → breakage of DNA and RNA strands → cell injury and/or death.
- Rapidly dividing cells (bone marrow, GI, and reproductive) are most sensitive.

Lethal dose 50 (LD_{50}) is the dose that will kill 50% of the exposed population within 60 days = approximately 450 radiation-absorbed dose (rad) or 4.5 gray (Gy).

Local Skin Exposure

Results in cutaneous changes ranging from erythema to overt skin necrosis and ulceration, depending on dose.

Acute Radiation Syndrome (ARS)

Occurs after whole body ionizing radiation exposure to a dose of > 2 Gy. It is divided into 3 phases: prodromal, latent, and manifest illness (Table 20.5).

Prodromal Phase

Autonomic nervous system response to radiation, leading to primarily GI symptoms. Higher exposure = earlier, longer, more severe symptoms, including bloody diarrhea

Latent Phase

Symptom-free interval prior to onset of bone marrow suppression; generally lasts 2-4 weeks. Higher exposure = shorter latent period

Manifest Illness Phase

Consists of following "syndromes" that correlate with increasing radiation dose (see Table 20.5)

DIAGNOSIS

- Exposure history.
- A Geiger-Mueller counter can detect contaminating ionizing radiation.
- The actual exposure dose is often not known, but can be estimated by clinical or laboratory findings ("biologic dosimetry"):
  - The timing of onset of prodromal symptoms
    - No vomiting by 4 hours → nonlethal dose
    - Vomiting in < 2 hours → serious/lethal dose (correlates to dose > 3.5 Gy)
  - Timing of onset of lymphocyte depletion
    - Rapid decline (over hours) = serious/lethal dose

TREATMENT

- Immediate decontamination.
  - Remove clothing (rids approximately 90% of radiation), wash skin.
  - Enhance elimination of ingested particles (cathartics, lavage etc).
  - Blocking agents, eg, potassium iodine for radioiodine exposure.
  - Chelating agents, eg, calcium disodium edetate and penicillamine for radioactive lead exposure.
  - Ferric hexacyanoferrate (Prussian blue) for Cesium-137 and thallium exposure.
  - Ca- and Zn-diethylenetriamine pentaacetate (DTPA) for plutonium, americium, curium exposure.
- Supportive care, bone marrow stimulating factors, treatment of fever and neutropenia with antibiotics.

TABLE 20.5. Acute Radiation Syndrome

Approximate Dose	Onset of Prodrome	Duration of Latent Phase	Manifest Illness
> 2 Gy (200 rad)	Within 2 d	1-3 wk	Hematopoietic syndrome with pancytopenia, infection, and hemorrhage; survival possible
> 6 Gy (600 rad)	Within hours	< 1 wk	GI syndrome with dehydration, electrolyte abnormalities, GI bleeding, and fulminant enterocolitis; uniformly fatal
> 30 Gy (3000 rad)	Within minutes	None	Cardiovascular/CNS (neurovascular) syndrome with refractory hypotension and circulatory collapse; fatal within 24-72 h

CNS, central nervous system; GI, gastrointestinal.

(Reproduced, with permission, from Tintinalli JE, Kelen GD, Stapczynski JS. *Emergency Medicine: A Comprehensive Study Guide*. 6th ed. New York, NY: McGraw-Hill; 2004:56.)

Q

A nuclear physicist presents to the ED shortly after total-body radiation exposure of uncertain dose. On arrival he appears acutely ill with nausea, vomiting, and disorientation. What can you predict regarding his likely clinical course?

KEY FACT

Estimating exposure dose after whole body radiation: Timing of onset of prodromal symptoms (earlier = higher dose) and/or onset of lymphocyte depletion (earlier/rapid = higher dose).

KEY FACT

Exposure to > 10 Gy should be considered "expectant" or black in triage setting.

Q

A young scuba diver is brought into the ED after her tank exploded during a refill. On arrival, she is complaining of shortness of breath and appears in acute distress. What is the most common cause of primary blast injury death?

A

The rapid onset of prodromal GI and CNS symptoms indicates an extremely high-exposure dose. This patient will likely develop refractory hypotension, circulatory collapse, and death in 24-72 hours despite aggressive intensive care.

TABLE 20.6. Predicting Survival After Radiation Injury

Prognosis	Absolute Lymphocytes (at 48 h)
Excellent	Normal range (1400-30,000/mm^3)
Good	1000-1400/mm^3
Fair	500-999/mm^3
Poor	100-499/mm^3
Death	< 100/mm^3

- Absolute lymphocyte count at 48 hours can be used to predict survival (Table 20.6).

KEY FACT

The absolute lymphocyte count is both the earliest indicator of significant radiation exposure and the best predictor of survival.

Complications

- Malignancy in survivors (leukemia can occur in as little as 2 years)
- Mutagenesis in offspring

Blast Injuries

KEY FACT

Primary blast injury = Blast pressure wave. Secondary blast injury = Projectiles from the explosion. Tertiary blast injury = Blunt trauma resulting from victim being thrown by blast wind.

PRIMARY BLAST INJURY

- Barotrauma resulting from the blast pressure wave.
- Air-containing structures are most commonly affected (eg, ears, lungs, intestines, sinuses).

SECONDARY BLAST INJURY

Results from solid projectiles from the explosive itself or the surrounding structures

KEY FACT

Most common blast injury = TM rupture at the pars tensa

TERTIARY BLAST INJURY

- Seen when victim is thrown against a solid structure or caught in a structural collapse
- Most lethal injury

QUATERNARY BLAST INJURY

Exposure to contaminants in bomb (eg chemical or biological "dirty" bombs)

A

Blast lung is the most common cause of death from primary blast injuries. Tympanic membrane (TM) ruptures are also common but are a poor predictor for more serious injuries.

QUINARY BLAST INJURY

Induced medical effects from blast (eg asthma exacerbation, acute MI)

SYMPTOMS/EXAMINATION

Depends on organs involved and presence of secondary or tertiary injuries

Primary Blast Injury

- Ear involvement: Hearing loss, vertigo, nystagmus, and TM rupture
- Pulmonary
  - Barotrauma (pneumothorax, air embolism, pneumomediastinum)
  - Pulmonary hemorrhage: Increasing respiratory distress and poor air exchange
- Intestinal
  - Less common than ear or lung injury
- Intestinal wall hemorrhage and edema → abdominal pain, nausea/vomiting

Secondary and Tertiary Blast Injury

- Findings of penetrating injuries, fractures/dislocations, closed head injuries
- If suicide bomber, possible human foreign material embedded

DIAGNOSIS

- Standard trauma evaluation
- Careful evaluation to rule out primary blast injury:
  - CXR in all cases
  - Chest CT if significant pulmonary symptoms
  - Abdominal CT if any GI symptoms

TREATMENT

- Supportive care.
- Treat associated injuries.
- Risk of pneumothorax and air embolism is particularly high in blast lung injury.
  - Minimize peak airway pressures and allow permissive hypercapnia in ventilated patient.
  - Immediate hyperbarics if suspected air embolism.
- Consider hepatitis B vaccine and immunoglobulin G (IgG) if suicide bomber.

KEY FACT

TM rupture does not predict other significant injury.

KEY FACT

Following blast injury, obtain abdominal CT if any GI symptoms are present.

REVIEW QUESTIONS

QUESTIONS

1. Which of the following is true regarding rotary wing transport?
   A. Used when transport time to hospital is < 30 minutes.
   B. Medical equipment such as endotracheal or chest tubes are not affected by altitude.
   C. Appropriate for distances between 15 and 100 miles.
   D. Weather is not a consideration.
2. What is the definition of a disaster?
   A. An event when the needs exceed available resources
   B. A natural calamity that causes structural damage to a community
   C. An event identified by the federal government as requiring national assistance
   D. An incident leading to numerous victims
3. Which are the correctly paired triage designations and colors?
   A. Yellow = expectant, red = delayed, green = immediate, black = minor
   B. Green = immediate, black = delayed, red = expectant, yellow = minor
   C. Black = expectant, red = delayed, yellow = minor, green = immediate
   D. Red = immediate, yellow = delayed, green = minor, black = expectant
4. Which is the most lethal form of anthrax?
   A. Oropharyngeal
   B. Gastrointestinal
   C. Cutaneous
   D. Inhalational
5. What distinguishes smallpox (variola) from chickenpox (varicella)?
   A. Chickenpox lesions are all in the same stage of development, whereas smallpox lesions are not.
   B. Smallpox has centrifugal distribution, whereas chickenpox has centripetal distribution.
   C. There is a prodrome of febrile illness with chickenpox, but not with smallpox.
   D. A patient who has had smallpox can get it again.
6. Which of the following is true regarding nerve agents?
   A. They produce an anticholinergic syndrome.
   B. The antidote includes sodium nitrite.
   C. Treatment is dosed at frequent intervals.
   D. They typically smell like mustard.
7. In acute radiation syndrome with gastrointestinal (GI) symptoms, electrolyte abnormalities, GI bleeding, and fulminant enterocolitis, when is the onset of prodrome expected?
   A. Within minutes
   B. Within hours
   C. Within days
   D. Within months
8. What is the name of the emergency medical service (EMS) system model that allows a local government to contract calls for service to a private company that provides basic life support (BLS) and/or advanced life support (ALS)?
   A. Third service model
   B. Volunteer model
   C. Public utility model
   D. Hospital-based model

ANSWERS

1. **C.** Helicopter transport is most effective between 15 and 100 miles. Longer distances may require fixed-wing transport, and shorter distances may be better served by an ambulance. Weather is always a consideration and altitude can cause problems both for the patient and the medical equipment because of changes in barometric pressure.
2. **A.** A medical disaster varies from institution to institution and system to system depending on the capability of that institution or system. When the needs for any given disaster exceed the available resources for a hospital or EMS system, then there is a disaster or mass casualty incident. Numerous victims do not necessarily define a disaster, because the system may have sufficient resources to handle them.
3. **D.** In a mass casualty situation, patients are designated a color based on the severity of their injury. The walking wounded are generally labeled green. Patients with serious but not immediately life-threatening injuries or illness are labeled yellow. Red patients require immediate attention for a life-threatening illness such as tension pneumothorax or hypovolemic shock. Dead or resource intensive victims such as 100% total body surface area (TBSA) burns are categorized as black according to the START triage algorithm.

4. **D.** Bacillus *anthracis*, a gram-positive spore forming bacterium, has many forms of disease. Inhalational anthrax is the most deadly with a mortality rate of 90%. Cutaneous anthrax is the most common form and is rarely fatal if treated. Oropharyngeal and GI anthrax are less common, and each has a 50% mortality rate.

5. **B.** Smallpox, considered a potential Class A biologic agent, can be seen in several clinical forms: variola major, variola minor, hemorrhagic smallpox, and malignant smallpox. The smallpox rash begins as maculopapular and spreads from the face downward to include the palms and soles with all lesions being in the same stage. The lesions classically have a centrifugal distribution and change from papules to vesicles to pustules. This differs from chickenpox, in which lesions are in various stages and progress centripetally. Both begin with a febrile prodrome. Chickenpox can recur in the form of varicella zoster (shingles), while smallpox is not known to recur.

6. **C.** Nerve agents produce a cholinergic toxidrome by inhibiting acetylcholinesterase. Treatment includes supportive care and benzodiazepines for seizures. Atropine is used for muscarinic effects, dosed to control respiratory secretions every 5-10 minutes. Pralidoxime chloride (2-PAM) is used to reverse nicotinic effects such as paralysis. All medications may require redosing at frequent intervals.

7. **B.** Higher radiation exposure is associated with earlier prodrome phase and a shorter latent phase. In the prodrome phase, higher radiation exposure means earlier, longer, and more severe symptoms including bloody diarrhea. Vomiting that occurs within 2 hours of exposure corresponds to a serious/lethal dose (dose > 3.5 Gy).

8. **C.** The public utility model of an EMS systems design allows a local government to contract calls for service to a private company. The third service model is when a separate department of local government owns, operates, and staffs ambulances. In a single-tier system only BLS crews or only ALS crews respond. In a multitiered system, a mix of BLS and ALS may respond. Volunteer model, as the name suggests, are staffed by volunteers (eg, a rural fire department), and a hospital-based model, also as the name suggests, is staffed by emergency medical technicians (EMTs) and paramedics who are employees of the hospital.

CHAPTER 21

Ethical/Legal Issues

Graydon Goodman, MD and
Abhi Mehrotra, MD, MBA, FACEP

Accreditation, Licensure, and Credentialing

LICENSURE

To become a licensed physician in the United States, you must:

- Successfully complete a required course of education in a school that is licensed and accredited.
- Pass a standardized examination (USMLE for MD or DO, COMPLEX for DO).
- Obtain at least one state's permission to practice.

To become a board-certified emergency physician (EP), you must also:

- Complete a required course of training in an accredited postgraduate emergency medicine residency program approved by the Accreditation Council for Graduate Medical Education (ACGME).
- Pass a qualifying examination and an oral certification examination as specified by the American Board of Emergency Medicine (ABEM) or American Osteopathic Board of Emergency Medicine (AOBEM).

KEY FACT

Medical licenses are granted and regulated by **states**.

KEY FACT

Licensure is general, but hospital privileges are specific.

State medical practice statutes vest authority in state medical boards to control access to licensure and regulate the profession. Courts usually cannot be persuaded to intervene unless the physician has exhausted administrative remedies. Unlike in the podiatric, chiropractic, dental, or other professions, medical licenses are **unrestricted**. Any licensed physician can perform neurosurgery or practice emergency medicine—if they can convince a hospital to allow it.

Grounds for denial of license and basis for revocation, sanction, and discipline of established license holders include:

- Fraudulent application statements
- Conviction of a felony
- Suspension or reduction of hospital privileges
- Unprofessional or immoral conduct

State boards of medicine discipline 2%-3% of physicians.

CREDENTIALING

Hospital credentialing is specific to each institution. A committee of physicians and administrators grants an approved list of activities and procedures based on education, training, and experience. Hospitals may accept ABEM certification as a sufficient indicator of competence, but that may not always be the case. State boards, insurers, regulatory agencies, and others organizations may use denial and revocation of credentials as a basis for adverse action on payment, participation, and licensing.

Compliance and Confidentiality

In health law, compliance refers to conformity with rules, especially federal medical billing rules and patient confidentiality laws.

BILLING

Billing for services requires both the CPT® (Current Procedural Terminology) and International Classification of Diseases (ICD) codes. One way to look at the two is that the CPT is what you did and the ICD is why you did it.

Current Procedural Terminology

- Forms the basis of Evaluation and Management (E&M) codes
- Consists of five levels of E&M codes plus the critical care code
- Owned and published by the American Medical Association
- Mandated by insurers for all billing submissions
- Enforced by Medicare

Intentional billing for services not performed is fraud. Inaccurate or unsupported coding of charges often results from the use of billing agencies or the hospital's system. Error can subject the physician, not the billing company, to investigation by insurers, principally Medicare or Medicaid.

CONFIDENTIALITY AND HEALTH INSURANCE PORTABILITY AND ACCOUNTABILITY ACT

The Health Insurance Portability and Accountability Act (HIPAA) of 1996 was intended to:

- Improve portability and continuity of health insurance coverage.
- Protect confidential protected health information (PHI).
- Standardize health information transfers.
- Require identification numbers for providers, health plans, and employers.

The law penalizes disclosures of confidential health information that are not authorized in writing by the patient. PHI includes (but is not limited to) name, postal address, telephone numbers, e-mail addresses, social security numbers, medical record numbers, health plan beneficiary numbers, vehicle identifiers, driver's licenses, and biometric identifiers such as facial photographs and fingerprints.

The Secretary of Health and Human Services imposes civil monetary penalties for violation of any HIPAA requirement, up to $50,000 per violation.

Important Points About HIPAA and Confidentiality

- Most releases of PHI to another health provider (eg, getting information from another hospital) must be accompanied by a signed release from the patient.
- Mandatory reporting requirements to an agency (eg, a local health authority) must include a written note of such disclosure in the patient's medical record.
- Law enforcement does **not** have automatic access to a patient's medical record.
- Disclosures for the purposes of treatment are permitted, except for **psychotherapy notes**, which have a special status. Disclosures for billing are allowed, but may be limited by "minimum necessary" rules.

Q

A newly hired EP is scheduled to work tonight, but the state has not yet issued his license. Can he work his shift?

KEY FACT

CPT is what you did and the ICD is why you did it.

KEY FACT

A medical bill submitted in your name can subject you to penalties and fines based on lack of compliance.

KEY FACT

Disclosures of confidential health information must comply with the privacy rules of HIPAA.

Q

An emergency department (ED) patient in police custody is being discharged and the officer wants a copy of the medical record. Can you give it to him?

A

No. In addition to likely violating the group's contract with the hospital and medical staff rules regarding privileges, it would violate state law that prohibits practicing medicine without a license.

Ethical Principles/Values

Ethical dilemmas occur when there is conflict between core ethical principles/values or when understanding or application of a core value is not clear in a specific situation.

- **Autonomy**: Recognizing a person's right to make health care decisions
- **Beneficence**: Acting for the good of the patient
- **Confidentiality**: The presumption that information disclosed to the physician will not be revealed to any other person or institution without the patient's permission
- **Nonmaleficence (*primum non nocere*)**: "First, do no harm." Acting to prevent harm and not cause harm
- **Personal integrity**: Acting according to one's own values and moral standards
- **Justice**: Acting to provide medical care fairly regarding resources, patient rights, and legal restrictions
- **Honesty**: Disclosing the truth to the patient

Common dilemmas might include knowing whether to honor the autonomy of a patient who refuses a needed intervention and the physician's desire to do what he/she thinks is best medically (beneficence); keeping a patient's human immunodeficiency virus (HIV) status confidential or disclosing to his or her partner (nonmaleficence); or deciding on how to allocate ventilators in a disaster (justice).

The resolution of ethical dilemmas will vary with practitioners and the details of the clinical situation. Some can be resolved or become clearer by using the following process:

1. Identify the ethical issues causing conflict.
2. Clarify your own and patient/family values and goals.
3. Analyze barriers and influencing factors.
4. Identify resolutions that are ethically acceptable.
5. Consult your institution's ethics board if the situation remains unresolved.
6. Choose a plan to go forward with patient care.

Consent and Refusal of Care

Consent refers to the process by which a physician informs and communicates with a patient and the patient authorizes a medical intervention. The goal of obtaining informed consent is to encourage patient autonomy, and the written forms serve to document the conversation. Without proper consent, the EP can be liable for negligence or battery.

KEY FACT

Battery = Unpermitted touching.

Consent can be **expressed** in written or verbal form by the patient, or, if the patient lacks decisional capacity, by a surrogate. In an emergency, when the patient is incapacitated and no surrogate or directives for care are available, EPs should act to save and stabilize the patient under the principle of **implied consent**.

INFORMED CONSENT

A

Only if the patient/arrestee consents.

Obtaining informed consent should be considered in any of the following:

- When the procedure is not routine

- When the procedure carries significant risks
- When it is the community standard
- Where hospital rules require it

In general, the patient or a surrogate decision maker should know:
- The **current state** of the patient and **likely course** of the medical problem
- The **nature of the intervention** being proposed
- The **expected outcome** of the intervention and likelihood of success
- The **risks** and **problems** associated with the proposed interventions
- What **alternative** management options exist, including the option of doing nothing
- A **recommendation from the physician** based on clinical judgment

The law contains two standards that address what information must be disclosed to the patient:
- **The reasonable physician standard** is required in most states. In this standard the physician must disclose information that a reasonable physician would tell a patient.
- **The reasonable patient standard.** Under this standard, the physician must disclose information that a reasonable patient would want to know before undergoing the procedure.

The signed form or the chart note is not informed consent. It is a representation of what information was communicated. The documentation should include the essential elements of an informed consent.

In obtaining informed consent, include all risks of high severity (eg, death, permanent limb and organ impairment) and high frequency. Precise means of injury and causation do not need to be disclosed in detail.

Most forms require the **signature of a witness**. If you want the witness to be able to testify as to what was said in the informed consent session, that person has to be present throughout the conversation. More commonly, the witness is only confirming that the patient signed the document and has to be present only for the signing.

The Emergency Exception Doctrine

Emergency physicians may treat the patient without consent **only if all of the three** following conditions are met:
1. The patient is unable to express his or her wishes.
2. The patient has a condition that demands **immediate** attention.
3. No family or other substitute decision maker is immediately available to consent.

The physician must document the reasons why obtaining consent was not possible.

Harry says, "I don't want to know. Just do it." If you use this exception, you should document witnessed offers to inform **and** the patient's mental ability to make this choice.

Waiver of Consent

Patients sometimes respond, "Whatever you say, doctor. I trust you." Both case law and statute recognize that a patient's rejection of attempts to give information is a defense to a suit. Witnessed notes in the chart and signed statements from the patient can help prove the patient insisted on not knowing.

Q

Tom is more intoxicated than usual, or is he? His head computed tomography (CT) shows an epidural hematoma. Does the neurosurgeon need consent before she drills?

KEY FACT

A signed form can be a manifestation of, but not a substitute for, actual consent.

KEY FACT

The emergency exception is **not** a blanket covering all ED patients. Do not presume this exception applies unless the patient or surrogate cannot consent and the treatment must take place **immediately**.

Q

The nurse objects to getting Harvey's consent for the procedure. "He'll freak out and try to leave." Can you skip informing Harvey for his own good?

A

No, unless his family is readily available.

KEY FACT

The capacity to make a decision requires that the patient have the ability to understand the relevant information, appreciate consequences of the situation, communicate a choice, and reason about treatment choices.

CAPACITY TO CONSENT

Decision-making capacity (DMC) refers to the patient's ability to adequately appreciate his or her condition and proposed treatment. The capacity to consent requires the patient be able to:

- Take in what the physicians are saying.
- Appreciate his or her medical condition and its consequences.
- Communicate a choice.
- Reason about treatment choices (eg, give a reason for choices).

Capacity is contextual. EPs have to assess—and document—a patient's capacity. Capacity can wax and wane with time or medical condition. A physician must attempt to maximize capacity and recruit a surrogate decision maker if capacity is in question.

Infants and children are considered incompetent under the law; medical care is judged by a "best interest" standard. Parents are authorized to make medical decisions for their children. When parental preferences go counter to medical recommendations, physicians have legal recourse to override parental decisions, acting according to the child's "best interests." In addition, as children grow older, their voice in assenting, particularly to complex and difficult treatments, needs to be considered.

States can make exceptions to the requirement to obtain parental consent. Such exceptions vary by state, but can include:

- Emancipated minors:
  - Minors who are legally married or have dependent children
  - Minors living independently and supporting themselves
  - Those with court-approved independence from their parents or guardians
  - Minors serving the US Armed Forces
- Minors seeking medical attention for:
  - Reproductive issues (including pregnancy and contraceptives)
  - Communicable diseases
  - Drug abuse

KEY FACT

Patients can refuse treatment, even life-saving treatment.

SUBSTITUTED CONSENT

If a court decides that the patient is under the guardianship of another individual for medical decisions, or if a patient, prior to their infirmity, has signed advance directives that authorize a health care agent (eg, medical durable power of attorney), then the proxy decision maker for consent is clear.

Without a formal guardian or an advance directive, physicians sometimes look to the "next-of-kin." Many states have statutes prescribing which relative and in what order a proxy decision maker should be derived.

REFUSAL TO CONSENT

If a patient has DMC, they have the right to refuse treatment. Different philosophical or religious beliefs do not necessarily mean that the patient lacks capacity. However, a choice which the patient cannot explain or one that is clearly inconsistent with a patient's lifelong value system does raise questions about capacity.

A

No, but it can be limited in detail.

Refusal, like consent, has to be "informed." Therefore, try to **make the discussion into an informed refusal**, to the extent the patient will allow. Patients who are willing to listen should be warned of the risks they are taking by refusing care or choosing a nonrecommended option. The physician may need to make a judgment about whether the patient lacks DMC and should be detained to continue treatment and assess him further, or whether a "poor" decision is one which the patient has capacity to make, by the criteria cited previously. The patient's reasons and the physician's assessment process should be documented in the chart. Patients who refuse to engage in such a discussion need to have their rejection of the discussion documented.

Arrestees and incarcerated prisoners have not automatically lost the right to refuse medical care.

Patients who refuse treatment or leave against medical advice should have the following documented in the medical record:

- Decisional capacity to refuse treatment
- Understanding of the risks of refusing treatment and explanation of alternative treatment, if any
- Discharge instructions
- Follow-up care options

Advance Directives/Do Not Attempt Resuscitation (DNAR)

- **Advance directives**: Indicate a **patient's** wishes regarding medical treatments when the patient is unable to direct his or her own care.
- **DNAR: Physician's orders** alerting other medical professionals not to initiate cardiopulmonary resuscitation (CPR). Such orders are hospitalization specific.
- **CPR directives**: State-authorized forms alerting emergency medical service (EMS) personnel and physicians to withhold CPR in the event of a cardiac arrest.
- Physician's Orders for Life-Sustaining Treatment (**POLST**)-**type documents**: More recent physician or provider-initiated orders to be honored in all situations and by all medical personnel which reflect patient preferences regarding a wide range of life-sustaining care. They include orders regarding CPR, antibiotics, and artificially administered nutrition and other medical interventions.

Emergency Medical Treatment and Active Labor Act

The Emergency Medical Treatment and Active Labor Act (EMTALA) mandates that unstable patients cannot be discharged or transferred except for medical necessity.

The EMTALA:

- Encourages **"equal"** treatment for patients
- Discourages poor and high-risk patients from being transferred from one emergency department (ED) to another for financial advantage
- Mandates that hospitals keep **on-call records** of specialty physicians

EMTALA Basics:

- Any patient coming to the ED has the right to a timely **medical screening examination (MSE)** to determine if an emergency medical condition (EMC) exists without regarding the patient's ability or willingness to pay for any services rendered.
- If an EMC exists, the hospital must, given its resources (including staff and facilities), **stabilize the condition**. The term "stabilize" means to ensure that no material deterioration of the condition is likely to result from or occur during a transfer, which includes mother and unborn child.

Q

Tonight, Fred is obviously intoxicated, but he has a fever and seems more impaired than his blood alcohol level indicates. Can he consent to a lumbar puncture?

KEY FACT

Treat refusal of recommended care like informed consent. Make it an "informed refusal."

People in another's custody, be it police, family, or nursing home may still retain the right to refuse treatment.

KEY FACT

Advance Directives: Patient INSTRUCTIONS

DNAR, CPR, POLST: Physician ORDERS (which should reflect patient preferences).

KEY FACT

Any individual patient must have medical screening and stabilization before discharge from the ED.

A

No, he lacks the decisional capacity.

- If the hospital cannot stabilize the condition, the staff are further obligated to **transfer the patient** to a facility that can.
- Normal registration processes may be followed as long as screening and stabilizing treatment are NOT delayed.
- As of this writing, a hospital's EMTALA obligation ends with hospital admission.

What Is "Coming to the Emergency Department"?

- Presenting with a request for emergency treatment or appearing to need emergency treatment according to a prudent layperson, to either:
  - A "**dedicated emergency department**" including those licensed by the state as an ED and facilities where medical services are provided on an urgent basis without needing an appointment
  - Within 250 yd of the main hospital buildings, excluding nonmedical facilities, physician's offices, and medical buildings that have a separate Medicare identity

An EMC Is One in Which:

- A delay in treatment would cause loss of body functions or impairment to organs or limbs.
- A pregnant woman is contracting and there isn't time to transfer her before she delivers, or the transfer may pose a threat to mother or child. In reality, if a woman is in active labor in the ED, she should deliver in that hospital.
- **Nonemergent conditions** in patients who have a received an MSE do not invoke an EMTALA obligation. For example, patients coming for suture removal, without any other concerning findings, are exempt from EMTALA.

An MSE:

- **Is not triage!** MSE can require a workup, including ancillary tests and consultations, as necessary to determine if an EMC exists.
- Can be performed by anyone the hospital designates as its standard of practice; in practice, this is usually the physician, but the task can be delegated, eg, to a nurse, physician assistant, etc. For example, a nurse on labor and delivery can be delegated this responsibility.

Transfers, When the EMC Is not Yet Stabilized, Cannot Take Place Unless:

- The patient or representative requests it, knowing the risks and the hospital's EMTALA obligations.
- The transferring physician certifies the benefits outweigh the risks.
- The transfer is medically appropriate.

An "Appropriate" Transfer Includes the Following Elements:

- The transferring hospital must do all it can to **minimize the risks of transfer**.
- The receiving hospital has **available space and personnel** (capability and capacity) and has agreed to take the case.
- The transferring hospital sends **copies of records**, including the name and address of any on-call physician who has refused or failed to appear within a reasonable time to help stabilize the patient.
- The transfer must use qualified personnel and equipment.
- Medical records must be maintained by the hospital for a period of 5 years from the date of transfer.

If a receiving hospital, such as burn or shock-trauma unit, has capacity it cannot refuse "appropriate transfers." This leaves open the possibility of rejecting inappropriate transfers, but many authorities point to the difficulty of proof and suggest a "Just Say Yes" policy.

KEY FACT

Referral center hospitals, eg, burn centers, with capacity cannot refuse transfers.

EMTALA VIOLATIONS

Enforcement of EMTALA is complaint driven. To that end, the law requires hospitals receiving transfers to report violations within 72 hours. EMTALA is enforced by the Office of the Inspector General. Civil penalties include:

- A hospital that negligently violates an EMTALA requirement may have to pay up to $50,000 per violation.
- The responsible EP and the on-call physician who negligently violate may also have to pay up to $50,000 per violation. **Civil monetary penalties such as EMTALA are not covered by malpractice insurance.**
- Violation may result in loss of Medicare/Medicaid billing privileges for the hospital.

KEY FACT

Civil monetary penalties are not covered by malpractice insurance.

External Quality Measures

External quality measures are implemented primarily by insurance companies and more specifically the Centers for Medicare and Medicaid Services (CMS) as they transition from a pay for service system to pay for performance system. The goal is to provide better care to a larger population of patients and it is incentivized by reimbursement. Multiple different measures spanning diagnostic, therapeutic, and organizational aspects are included. These measures are decided upon by various national committees and are routinely reevaluated.

The CMS has three main programs that affect EM physicians:

- Physician Quality Reporting System (PQRS): A reporting program that will both positively and negatively adjust payments based on reporting of quality information. Examples of PQRS measures:
  - Percentage of patients > 40 with nontraumatic chest pain who received an ECG
  - Percentage of Rh-negative pregnant patients with possible blood exposure who received RhoGam
- Hospital Outpatient Quality Reporting (OQR) Program: Quality of care reporting for outpatient hospitals. Examples of OQR measures:
  - OP-4: Administration of aspirin to patients with acute myocardial infarction (MI) or probable cardiac chest pain.
  - OP-21: ED median time to pain management for long bone fractures.
- Hospital Inpatient Quality Reporting (IQR) Program: Quality of care reporting for acute inpatient stays. Examples of IQR measures:
  - ED-1: Median time from ED arrival to ED departure for admitted ED patients
  - AMI-8: Median time to primary percutaneous intervention

How each hospital performs on the measures they report is publicly reported and can be viewed online by the general public to compare performance. Hospitals' payments are tied to their performance. Physician payments will soon be tied to performance on these types of measures (currently only tied to reporting on the measures). These systems are evolving, with new measures and systems being approved almost annually.

Liability and Malpractice

A "statute of limitations" is the time period in which a person can file a claim for malpractice. They vary from state to state but are usually within 2 or 3 years from the date of the injury or when the discovery of negligence is made.

These statutes carry exceptions for disability, legal minority or mental illness, but even these extensions are not open ended.

Most potential malpractice cases are rejected by at least 1 lawyer. Of those filed, some are settled, some dismissed by judges, and some—estimates suggest only approximately 10%—go to trial. Of malpractice trials, physician defendants win more than half. Statistics also suggest that most EPs will be sued at least once in their professional lifetimes.

THE LEGAL PROCESS

Required Elements of a Malpractice Lawsuit

KEY FACT

Negligence forms the basis of most malpractice cases.

The four main elements of a malpractice:

1. Duty
2. Breach of duty
3. Damages
4. Causation

To go to trial, the plaintiff must offer proof that four things occurred:

1. The defendant had a **duty** to the plaintiff. Anyone who comes or is brought to the emergency room (ER) has a physician–patient relationship with the physician who sees him or her, attaching that duty via EMTALA.
2. There was a **breach** of duty. This is the "negligence" in a medical negligence case.
3. There were **damages**. What would the plaintiff's condition have been if the duty had been fulfilled? If the outcome would have been the same, there are no damages.
4. There was **causation**. The breach in duty led to the damages.

The Standard of Care and Expert Witnesses

In a malpractice suit, the standard against which a defendant physician is judged:

"How would a reasonable emergency physician have performed in the same or similar circumstances?"

This community/state standard does not demand the highest skill level, although physicians have set themselves up against that threshold by advertising the highest or best practices. The standard depends on what is actually done, not a theoretical ideal.

Internal guidelines and policies for quality assurance procedures and peer review are often protected by statute, but any information accessible to plaintiffs may potentially be used in litigation.

Admission of **expert testimony** remains at the discretion of the judge. At least one state requires EP experts in malpractice cases against EPs. Medical malpractice involves a professional standard. The expert answers the previous question about standard of care. The expert is also usually asked about the causation element—did the claimed negligence cause the harm?

Standard of Proof

KEY FACT

The standard for a malpractice case is the "preponderance of evidence."

Judges instruct juries that, to find for the plaintiff, they must conclude that there was duty, breach of duty, damages, and causation through preponderance of the evidence or "likely based on the evidence." This is a significantly **lower** threshold than the criminal standard of "beyond a reasonable doubt."

Compensation

Juries award the plaintiff damages, which are the amount of the verdict. The amount of damages is intended to make the victim of malpractice "whole."

- Economic damages: Lost income and medical bills
- Noneconomic damages: Pain and suffering compensation

Lawyers estimate potential verdict amounts based on all involved factors, but sometimes use a rule of thumb that applies a multiplier to the more easily demonstrated real damages.

In addition to the two types of damages listed previously, a plaintiff may be entitled to **punitive damages,** which can be awarded if the jury feels that the conduct of the defendant was particularly loathsome and unprofessional.

KEY FACT

Tort reform efforts seek caps on the possible amount of noneconomic damages.

Commonly, however, the verdict should be restorative for the plaintiff. The plaintiff should never come out ahead of where she would have been had the malpractice not occurred. Tort reform efforts often seek caps on the possible amount of noneconomic damages.

INSURANCE

There are two types of medical malpractice insurance policies:

- **Occurrence**: Coverage for events which occur during the life of the policy, no matter when the allegation is eventually initiated
- **Claims made**: Coverage only if there is a claim made (or, sometimes, a report of an incident) during the coverage period of that policy or renewal of that policy

Claims-made insurance policies are cheaper and more common. If an EP leaves a group, they should make sure that renewals will include them, or that the group will buy a "**tail**" covering later filed suits. Effectively, the tail converts a "claims made" policy into an occurrence policy.

Right to approve settlement: A defendant can ask that the insurer offer policy limits to any plaintiff, but most policies today do **not** provide for any control by the physician or group policyholders. Insurers want to be able to make economic choices about the terms and conditions of a settlement, free of the visceral and professional concerns driving physician defendants.

Security of coverage: Domestic insurers are inspected and regulated by state insurance commissioners. Offshore companies can be less secure. Some hospitals insist that staff and contract physicians and physician groups carry US insurance and usually at required minimum amounts.

Reporting: Responsibilities to the Whole of Society

KEY FACT

Claims-made malpractice—insurance should be renewed or have tail coverage—purchased if an EM physician leaves a practice setting.

The list of conditions that must be reported varies from state to state.

When a medical illness exists that may harm others, it is the physician's duty to protect society by reporting that condition. This duty can be in direct conflict with the patient's right to confidentiality and privacy and may impede the patient's desire to seek help. Thus, reporting has required legislation to help protect the physician–patient relationship and instill patient's confidence that only "required" conditions will be reported. The law takes away any decision making once the diagnosis is made; even if the patient demands otherwise, the doctor has an obligation to report. Many hospitals identify laboratory personnel as reporting officers for infectious diseases and inpatient caregivers often handle admitted patients' reports. EPs still retain shared responsibility for compliance with the laws. Reportable conditions infrequently carry criminal penalties for the failure to report, but they are nonetheless a legal requirement.

COMMUNICABLE AND INFECTIOUS DISEASE

Typical state reporting lists include:

- Sexually transmitted infections, including HIV
- Community outbreaks, eg, food poisoning
- Illnesses related to foreign travel, eg, malaria
- Suspected biological terrorist threats, eg, anthrax

RESULTS OF CRIMINAL ACTIVITIES

Assault

Not all injuries that are or could be the result of assault must, or even can, be reported. At present, five states do not have reporting requirements for assault-related injuries. Forty-two states have reporting requirements for injuries from weapons, usually guns only, but knives and even martial arts weapons have been included.

Domestic Violence

Intimate partner violence often causes a dilemma for EPs. Many of the victims do not want reports made. Some states have mandatory reporting rules for injuries resulting from domestic violence. In those states, a decision not to report should include clear documentation of the risk of harm to the particular patient and of your reasoning. In some states, if the patient does not want a report made, you cannot call the police, even if you feel future danger exists.

Child Abuse

Child abuse is another form of assault, but it deserves its own category because the reporting rules are clearer and more consistent. **All states have laws protecting children and require mandatory reporting of child abuse.** Some even include express immunity from suit for reporting health professionals.

Emergency physicians are responsible for learning the variations of the law in the state where they practice.

- Definition of "child" may vary with statutory language or by reference to other concepts, such as emancipated minors.
- What constitutes abuse may vary. Generally, abuse is any nonaccidental, serious physical injury inflicted by any adult responsible for the child. Some states include neglect as a form of abuse.
- Mechanisms of reporting vary. Many states require a verbal report followed by a written one.

Child abuse is 1 of only 2 situations where patients may be held in the ED against their and their parents' wishes. Sometimes the only way ED staff can assure protection for the child is to arrange admission. Hospitals have been successfully sued for failing to report abuse in children who are subsequently reinjured. Criminal penalties for failing to report appear in many state laws.

Elder Abuse

Neglect and abuse can also present as apparent self-care deficit. Many states now have adult protection laws, some for all adults, some only above a stated age. These reporting rules usually call for initial contact with a social service agency, like adult protective services, in the case of suspected elder abuse. To qualify as elder abuse, the abuser must be in a "trust relationship" with the patient, meaning that the patient relies on the abuser for services.

REVIEW QUESTIONS

QUESTIONS

1. Involving the patient in decision making and respecting the wishes of the patient displays what form of ethical principle?
   A. Beneficence
   B. Justice
   C. Autonomy
   D. Nonmaleficence

2. The rules governing emancipated minors may vary between states however one may be considered an emancipated minor for the following reasons EXCEPT:
   A. Minors who are legally married or have dependent children
   B. Minors who both live and are financially independent
   C. Minors serving the US Armed Forces
   D. Minors who state they do not want parents involved

3. The name of the law which dictates that any patient who presents to the emergency department has the right to a timely medical screening examination to determine if an emergency medical condition exists is:
   A. Emergency Medical Treatment and Labor Act (EMTALA)
   B. Health Insurance Portability and Accountability Act (HIPAA)
   C. Physician Quality Reporting System (PQRS)
   D. Do Not Attempt Resuscitation (DNAR)

4. When initiating a transfer of a patient to another hospital it is important to insure that all of the following are met except:
   A. The receiving hospital has the capability and capacity to accept the patient.
   B. You have discussed the patient with the receiving hospital and they have accepted the transfer.
   C. The benefits of transfer outweigh the risks.
   D. You have arranged transport back for the patient when/if the patient is discharged from the receiving hospital.

ANSWERS

1. **C.** Autonomy is the principle that people have the right to make their own health care decisions. Beneficence is acting for the good of the patient. Justice is the idea that everyone must be cared for fairly regarding resources, patient rights, and legal restrictions. Nonmaleficence is the concept of do no harm.

2. **D.** Minors who state they do not want parents involved. Minors may be emancipated if they have been given court-approved independence; however, simply stating they do not want parental involvement does not grant them emancipation. Certain exceptions regarding parental consent may be obtained in situations dealing with reproductive issues, communicable diseases, and drug abuse.

3. **A.** The EMTALA established medical screening guidelines for patients without regarding capacity to pay. The HIPAA helped establish guidelines regarding protection of confidential health information and improving continuity of health insurance coverage. The PQRS is a reporting program that adjusts hospital payments based on reporting of quality information. A DNAR form is a physician's order alerting other medical professionals not to initiate cardiopulmonary resuscitation (CPR).

4. **D.** You have arranged transport back for the patient when/if the patient is discharged from the receiving hospital. This is not required and should not delay appropriate transfers of patients. Transfers of patients prior to complete stabilization may take place only under certain circumstances which include if the patient or representatives request it and they acknowledge the risks and the hospital's EMTALA obligations, the benefits outweigh the risks, if the transfer is medically appropriate, if the risks of transfer are minimized (including transport with an appropriate level of care), if the receiving hospital has capability and capacity, and if the medical records are sent with the patient.

Index

Page numbers followed by *f* or *t* indicate figures or tables, respectively.